Modern Trends in Infertility and Conception Control

Volume 4

Under the auspices of
The American Fertility Society

Modern Trends in Infertility and Conception Control

Volume 4

Edited by

Edward E. Wallach, M.D.
Professor and Chairman
Department of Gynecology and Obstetrics
The Johns Hopkins University School of Medicine
Baltimore, Maryland

Roger D. Kempers, M.D.
Professor of Obstetrics and Gynecology
Mayo Medical School
Consultant, Department of Obstetrics and Gynecology
Mayo Clinic
Rochester, Minnesota

Year Book Medical Publishers, Inc.
Chicago • London • Boca Raton

1 2 3 4 5 6 7 8 9 0 CC 92 91 90 89 88

Library of Congress Cataloging-in-Publication Data
(Revised for v. 4)
Modern trends in infertility and conception control.
Vol. 2- published by Harper & Row, Philadelphia.
Vols. 3-4 published by Year Book Medical Publishers, Chicago.
Includes bibliographical references and indexes.
1. Infertility, Female. 2. Endocrine gynecology.
3. Contraception. 4. Infertility, Male. I. Wallach,
Edward E., 1933- . II. Kempers, Roger D.
III. American Fertility Society. [DNLM: 1. Contraception—collected works. 2. Sterility—collected works.
WP570 M689]
RG201.M62 618.1'78 78-27202
ISBN 0-683-08706-1 (v. 1)
ISBN 0-06-142605-9 (Harper & Row : v. 2)
ISBN 0-8151-9092-1 (v. 4)

Sponsoring Editor: Nancy E. Chorpenning
Assistant Director, Manuscript Services: Frances M. Perveiler
Production Project Manager: Nancy C. Baker
Proofroom Supervisor: Shirley E. Taylor

Contributors

Nancy J. Alexander, Ph.D.
Professor, Obstetrics and Gynecology
Director, Applied Fundamental Research, CONRAD
Section of Reproductive Immunology
Department of Obstetrics and Gynecology
Eastern Virginia Medical School
Norfolk, Virginia

Nancy C. Allen, M.D.
Resident, Obstetrics and Gynecology
University of Tennessee
Memphis, Tennessee

Deborah J. Anderson, Ph.D.
Fearing Research Laboratory
Department of Obstetrics and Gynecology
Harvard Medical School
Boston, Massachusetts

Ricardo H. Asch, M.D.
Professor, Obstetrics and Gynecology
University of California, Irvine
Irvine, California

Bruce G. Bateman, M.D.
Associate Professor, Obstetrics and Gynecology
University of Virginia School of Medicine
Charlottesville, Virginia

Alan E. Beer, M.D.
Professor of Obstetrics and Gynecology and Microbiology and Immunology
University of Michigan Medical Center
Ann Arbor, Michigan

Richard E. Blackwell, Ph.D., M.D.
Professor, Obstetrics and Gynecology, Physiology and Biophysics
Director of the Division of Reproductive Biology and Endocrinology
Department of Obstetrics and Gynecology
University of Alabama at Birmingham Medical Center
Birmingham, Alabama

Beverly L. Brodie, M.D., F.R.C.S.C.
Fellow, Center for Fertility and Reproductive Research
Department of Obstetrics and Gynecology
Vanderbilt University Medical Center
Nashville, Tennessee

Robert G. Castadot, M.D., M.P.H.
Population and Public Health Specialist
World Bank
Washington, D.C.

Elizabeth B. Connell, M.D.
Professor, Department of Gynecology and Obstetrics
Department of Gynecology and Obstetrics
Emory University School of Medicine
Atlanta, Georgia

Marian D. Damewood, M.D.
Assistant Professor, Gynecology and Obstetrics
Director, IVF Program
Department of Gynecology and Obstetrics
The Johns Hopkins Hospital
Baltimore, Maryland

James F. Daniell, M.D.
Clinical Associate Professor, Obstetrics and Gynecology
Vanderbilt University
Private Practitioner
The Woman's Health Group
Nashville, Tennessee

Alan H. DeCherney, M.D.
John Slade Ely Professor of Obstetrics and Gynecology
Department of Obstetrics and Gynecology
Yale University School of Medicine
New Haven, Connecticut

Michael P. Diamond, M.D.
Assistant Professor, Obstetrics and Gynecology
Mellon Fellow, Reproductive Sciences
Department of Obstetrics and Gynecology
Yale University School of Medicine
New Haven, Connecticut

Paul R. Gindoff, M.D.
Assistant Professor, Department of Reproductive Endocrinology
Department of Obstetrics and Gynecology
Division of Reproductive Endocrinology
George Washington University
Washington, D.C.

Ruth M. Greenblatt, M.D.
Robert Wood Johnson Clinical Scholar
Assistant Clinical Professor, Medicine
Department of Medicine
Division of Infectious Diseases
University of California
San Francisco, California

Louise B. Grochow, M.D.
Assistant Professor, Oncology and Medicine
Department of Medicine
Division of Oncology
The Johns Hopkins University School of Medicine
Baltimore, Maryland

Gilbert G. Haas, Jr., M.D.
Associate Professor and Chief
Section of Reproductive Endocrinology and Infertility
Department of Obstetrics and Gynecology
University of Oklahoma Health Sciences Center
Oklahoma City, Oklahoma

Jouko Halme, M.D., Ph.D.
Associate Professor
Department of Obstetrics and Gynecology
UCLA School of Medicine
Los Angeles, California

H. Hunter Handsfield, M.D.
Associate Professor of Medicine
Department of Medicine
Division of Infectious Diseases
Harborview Medical Center
University of Washington
Seattle, Washington

Carl M. Herbert III, M.D.
Assistant Professor
Center for Fertility and Reproductive Research (C-FARR)
Division of Reproductive Endocrinology
Department of Obstetrics and Gynecology
Vanderbilt University School of Medicine
Nashville, Tennessee

King K. Holmes, M.D., Ph.D.
Professor and Vice-Chairman
Department of Medicine
University of Washington
Seattle-King County Department of Public Health
Seattle, Washington

George R. Huggins, M.D.
Associate Professor and Chairman, Department of Obstetrics and Gynecology
Francis Scott Key Medical Center
The Johns Hopkins School of Medicine
Baltimore, Maryland

Jaroslav Hulka, M.D.
Professor, Department of Obstetrics and Gynecology
The University of North Carolina
Chapel Hill, North Carolina

Raphael Jewelewicz, M.D.
Associate Professor and Director
Division of Reproductive Endocrinology
Department of Obstetrics and Gynecology
College of Physicians and Surgeons
Columbia University
New York, New York

Elton Kessel, M.D., M.P.H.
Consultant, International Federation for Family Health
Chapel Hill, North Carolina

James D. Kitchin III, M.D.
Professor, Obstetrics and Gynecology
University of Virginia School of Medicine
Charlottesville, Virginia

Gad Lavy, M.D.
Assistant Professor
Department of Obstetrics and Gynecology
Division of Reproductive Endocrinology
Yale University School of Medicine
New Haven, Connecticut

Patricia P. Mahlstedt, Ed.D.
Clinical Instructor
Department of Obstetrics and Gynecology
Baylor College of Medicine
Houston, Texas

Wayne S. Maxson, M.D.
Assistant Professor
Center for Fertility and Reproductive Research (C-FARR)
Division of Reproductive Endocrinology
Department of Obstetrics and Gynecology
Vanderbilt University
Nashville, Tennessee

Stephen D. Mumford, Dr.P.H., M.P.H.
President, Center for Research on Population and Security
Research Triangle Park, North Carolina

Ana Alvarez Murphy, M.D.
Assistant Professor
Department of Reproductive Medicine
University of California
San Diego UCSD Medical Center
San Diego, California

Wallace C. Nunley, Jr., M.D.
Department of Obstetrics and Gynecology
University of Virginia Hospital
Charlottesville, Virginia

David L. Olive, M.D.
Assistant Professor
Department of Obstetrics and Gynecology
The University of Texas Health Science Center at San Antonio
San Antonio, Texas

Alik Peretz, M.D.
Clinical Assistant Professor
Department of Obstetrics and Gynecology
Rambam Medical Center
Haifa, Bat-Galim, Israel

William G. M. Ritchie, M.D.
Clinical Associate Professor
Department of Radiology
University of Pennsylvania School of Medicine
Pennsylvania Hospital
Philadelphia, Pennsylvania

John A. Robertson
Baker and Botts Professor of Law
School of Law
The University of Texas at Austin
Austin, Texas

John A. Rock, M.D.
Director of Reproductive Endocrinology
Division of Reproductive Endocrinology and Infertility
The Johns Hopkins Hospital
Baltimore, Maryland

B. Jane Rogers, Ph.D.
Associate Professor
Center for Fertility and Reproductive Research (C-FARR)
Director, Semenology Laboratory
Division of Reproductive Endocrinology
Department of Obstetrics and Gynecology
Vanderbilt University School of Medicine
Nashville, Tennessee

Allen W. Root, M.D.
Professor of Pediatrics and Biochemistry
Department of Pediatrics
University of South Florida College of Medicine
Tampa, Florida
All Children's Hospital St. Petersburg
St. Petersburg, Florida

Michael J. Rosenberg, M.D., M.P.H.
Director, Reproductive Epidemiology Division
Reproductive Epidemiology
Family Health International
Research Triangle Park, North Carolina

Zev Rosenwaks, M.D.
Director, Jones Institute for Reproductive Medicine
Professor, Department of Obstetrics and Gynecology
Eastern Virginia Medical School
Norfolk, Virginia

Benjamin P. Sachs, M.D., D.P.H.
Director, Maternal and Fetal Medicine
Division of Maternal and Fetal Medicine
Department of Obstetrics and Gynecology
Harvard Medical School
Beth Israel Hospital
Boston, Massachusetts

Merlin H. Sayers, M.D., Ph.D.
Assistant Professor, Medicine
University of Washington
Puget Sound Blood Center
Seattle, Washington

William D. Schlaff, M.D.
Assistant Professor
Gynecology and Obstetrics
The Johns Hopkins University School of Medicine
Baltimore, Maryland

Cecilia L. Schmidt, M.D.
Director, Reproductive Endocrinology/Infertility
Department of Obstetrics and Gynecology
University of Medicine and Dentistry of New Jersey
New Jersey Medical School
Newark, New Jersey

Anthony R. Scialli, M.D.
Director, Reproductive Toxicology Center
Assistant Professor
Department of Obstetrics and Gynecology
Georgetown University School of Medicine
Reproductive Toxicology Center
Columbia Hospital for Women Medical Center
Washington, D.C.

Sander S. Shapiro, M.D.
Associate Professor
Department of Obstetrics and Gynecology
Division of Reproductive Endocrinology
University of Wisconsin
University Hospital
Madison, Wisconsin

Dorothy I. Shulman, M.D.
Assistant Professor of Pediatrics
Department of Pediatrics
University of South Florida College of Medicine
Tampa, Florida
All Children's Hospital
St. Petersburg, Florida

Alvin M. Siegler, M.D., D.Sc.
Clinical Professor
State University of New York Health Sciences Center
Brooklyn, New York

Joe Leigh Simpson, M.D.
Professor and Chairman
Department of Obstetrics and Gynecology
University of Tennessee
Memphis, Tennessee

Carol Grace Smith, Ph.D.
Associate Professor
Department of Obstetrics and Gynecology
University of Texas Health Science Center at San Antonio
San Antonio, Texas

Robert J. Stillman, M.D.
Associate Professor
Director of the Division of Reproductive Endocrinology and Fertility
Department of Obstetrics and Gynecology
George Washington University School of Medicine
Washington, D.C.

Marianne Styler, M.D.
Assistant Professor
Department of Obstetrics and Gynecology
Academic Health Science Center
New Brunswick, New Jersey

Craig H. Syrop, M.D.
Assistant Professor
Obstetrics and Gynecology
Division of Reproductive Endocrinology and Fertility
University of Iowa Hospitals and Clinics
Iowa City, Iowa

Howard J. Tatum, M.D., Ph.D.
Professor, Department of Gynecology and Obstetrics
Emory University School of Medicine
Atlanta, Georgia

Alan Trounson, Ph.D.
Centre for Early Human Development
Monash University
Queen Victoria Medical Center
Melbourne, Australia

Anne Colston Wentz, M.D.
Professor, Obstetrics and Gynecology
Director, Division of Reproductive Endocrinology
Center for Fertility and Reproductive Research (C-FARR)
Department of Obstetrics and Gynecology
Vanderbilt University School of Medicine
Nashville, Tennessee

Howard A. Zacur, M.D., Ph.D.
Associate Professor
Department of Gynecology and Obstetrics
The Johns Hopkins University School of Medicine
Baltimore, Maryland

Luciano Zamboni, M.D.
Professor and Chairman, Department of Pathology
University of California
Los Angeles County Harbor-UCLA Medical Center
Torrance, California

Jaime Zipper, M.D.
Hospital Sotero del Rio
Puente Alto, Chile

Peter K. Zucker, M.D.
Assistant Professor
Obstetrics and Gynecology
Department of Gynecology and Obstetrics
The Johns Hopkins School of Medicine
Baltimore, Maryland

Preface

When the *Modern Trends* section of *Fertility & Sterility* was first established in December 1975, the purpose was to provide monthly reviews of contemporary subject matter provided by recognized authorities. The approach was immediately successful. The section was widely read from the outset and the material was often cited as reference sources. When the suggestion was initially made to amalgamate the first 36 contributions into a book, the idea was considered with skepticism. Yet, once the book was published, the response was once again strongly positive. The attraction of the book was that it served as a composite compendium containing up-to-date material of practical value arranged into sections and indexed. This arrangement of material appeals to the requirements of the practicing physician needing a ready reference to meet clinical situations with expert advice from the authoritative sources. This type of text appeals also to house officers and fellows during their ongoing process of acquainting themselves with the literature. At the same time, the comprehensive format has provided a solid resource for the academician in preparing teaching materials.

From the editor's standpoint the mission has been enjoyable. Over a 12-year period, we have reviewed a large number of manuscripts of the highest quality and have become acquainted with many outstanding leaders in the field of reproduction. That the original text was successful enough to re-enact the publication process three times in 12 years represents an achievement in itself, and provides a sense of permanence to the concept of the *Modern Trends* text.

This text is comprised of the 36 *Modern Trends* selections from *Fertility & Sterility* appearing between 1984 and 1987. The text can be viewed as representing 3 years of progress and achievement in diagnostic procedures and in therapeutic measures. The rapid growth of in vitro fertilization and related technology makes this volume contrast vividly with the first volume of *Modern Trends* published in 1979, in which in vitro fertilization had only just been clinically proved, sonography was in its infancy, and lasers had not yet been applied to infertility surgery. In addition, environmental aspects of reproduction are now highlighted as never before. We've come a long way since *Modern Trends* was established. Scanning the contents of each of the four volumes of *Modern Trends* serially creates a feeling of humility as one advance in our field eclipses the last. Volume 4 readily falls into seven sections: General Aspects of Reproduction; Reproductive Endocrinology; Developmental Abnormalities and Reproductive Potential; Female Reproductive Tract Surgery; In Vitro Fertilization; Male Infertility; and Contraception and Sterilization. Each section is preceded by an introduction that synthesizes the material encompassed by that section.

No textbook can be developed without significant input from various sources. All of the authors need to be acknowledged once again not only for their contributions, but also for meeting deadlines and being flexible enough to make requested revisions. My co-editor, Roger Kempers, continues to reflect the finest qualities of journal editorship. Herbert Thomas, Executive Director of The American Fertility Society, needs to be acknowledged for having given the original impetus for a text. The understanding and support of Marcia Kempers and Joanne Wallach, as their husbands toiled away, contributed significantly to this project.

Carol Olson, Maria Esquela, and Lorraine Tamberino spurred on the editorial process with their secretarial and administrative talents. Nancy Chorpenning and the staff at Year Book Medical Publishers, Inc., were always there with their technical assistance. Finally, Volume 4 of *Modern Trends* is dedicated to our readers, who have encouraged us and provided the incentive for us to continue to prepare the monthly article for the *Fertility & Sterility* section and this book at 3-year intervals. The editors salute all of the above for their roles in making this text possible.

Edward E. Wallach, M.D.

Contents

SECTION I

General Aspects of Reproduction

In 1986 a record 125.8 million Americans, approximately 69% of the working age population, held full-time or part-time jobs. Of particular significance is the statistic that 57 million women were included in this work force. The trends indicate that this number will continue to rise. Many of yesterday's housewives are today's doctors, lawyers, teachers, secretaries, executives, computer programmers, reporters, and editors. Between 1960 and 1987, the percentage of women in the work place rose from 35.7% to 55.8%. In today's society with an increasing number of delayed marriages, employment-related stress, high divorce rate, and serious consideration of single parenthood, the implications for reproductive performance among American women are changing rapidly.

Oral contraceptives and intrauterine devices (IUD) were introduced in the United States during the early 1960s. Along with these new technologies developed specifically for prevention of fertility, we've experienced an increase in sexual freedom, deferment of both marriage and childbearing to an older age, and a prominent role for women in the work force. These sociologic changes in today's society, among others, have had a profound influence on the demographic pattern of reproduction. Entrance of the "baby boom" segment of our population (1942 to 1961) into the reproductive age together with their postponement of childbearing has changed the first-birth rate of women 30 to 35 years of age. In this group of women with at least 4 years of college education, the first-birth rate will have increased from 19.11/1000 in 1970 to 39.6/1000 by the end of this decade. In 1985 the number of births in the United States increased to almost 3.75 million with fewer deliveries of women in the 20 to 25 age range and more deliveries among women aged 30 to 35 years.[1] The implications of these figures are significant and they raise the issue of fecundity as an age-related phenomenon.

Changes in sexual mores affect patterns and incidence of sexually transmitted disease. The increase in number of women in careers has expanded and prolonged possibilities for their exposure to environmental hazards and to stress phenomena in the work place. Deferment of childbearing also prolongs the interval of risk for acquiring a variety of medical disorders prior to exercising their options for reproduction. Placing these considerations in practical terms, for a woman delaying pregnancy to beyond age 30 is associated with decreased fecundity. Among women seeking infertility evaluation, those older than 35 have cumulative pregnancy rates one half that of younger women.[1] The fact that this figure applies to women over 35 undergoing artificial insemination with husband's semen suggests factors attributable to age and not to decreased coital frequency. Exposure to multiple partners as well as a prolonged time interval during which sexual exposure may occur increases the risk of acquiring pelvic inflammatory disease. The presence of endometriosis also correlates with voluntary delays in childbearing.

The genetics of maternal aging clearly indicate a strong correlation of fetal chromosomal abnormalities with advancing age. In patients 40 to 44 years of age, 6% of conceptuses demonstrate a chromosomal defect as compared to 1.6% between ages 35 and 39.[2] Although 95% to 99% of anomalous conceptuses are lost prior to viability, the risk of a trisomic birth continues to represent a significant problem for older women contemplating pregnancy. It is obvious that the pathogenesis of such genetic mishaps remains to be determined, but as Gindoff and Jewelewicz indicate in their chapter on age and reproduction, the "production line theory" may shed light on the problem. This theory suggests that oocytes ovulate in the order in which they were formed during fetal life, a proportion of the oocyte population suffering chromosomal damage during early prophase of the first meiotic division. Evidence suggests that endocrine abnormalities may alter the intrafollicular as well as the intrauterine environment, resulting in abnormal offspring or spontaneous abortion. An anti-estrogen preparation has been shown to reduce blastocyst formation when the oocyte has been exposed to this influence while still contained within the follicle prior to ovulation and fertilization.[3] Biologic aging may influence not only patterns of sexual behavior and the physiology of ovary and uterus, but also hypothalamic-pituitary function, resulting in defects in the corpus luteum, alterations in the duration of the follicular phase, and diminished ovarian estrogen synthesis.

When considering the influence of environment on reproductive performance, substance abuse must be among the prominent environmental hazards. An increasing percentage of women and teenagers now smoke. The high prevalence of smoking and its hazards to health, specifically the respiratory tract and cardiovascular system, are well known. Also appreciated during the past 25 years is the strong association between low birth weight infants and maternal smoking. We know less, however, about the influence of nicotine and other components of tobacco on early reproduction. That nicotine can act as an aromatase inhibitor raises speculation about its potential influence on the oocyte which may be dependent upon intrafollicular estrogen levels for normal function.[4] Stillman and his coauthors reveal the negative effect which smoking exerts on the many sites of action necessary for normal procreation. The chapter concludes with the hope that this knowledge may stimulate further investigation of the potential reproductive toxins associated with cigarette smoke and may help to persuade individuals to cease smoking. This is an optimistic, if not attainable, objective. Substance abuse and its effects on reproduction also form the theme for the Smith and Asch chapter. Unfortunately, the use of marijuana, cocaine, and other preparations has permeated our society such that an estimated 5% to 10% of women in the childbearing years use these illicit substances regularly.

Alcohol abuse is also prevalent among a significant number of women of reproductive age. The short-term effects of alcohol abuse during pregnancy on the fetus are well recognized as the "fetal alcohol syndrome." The normal function of the hypothalamic-pituitary gonadal system is extremely complex, involving not only hormonal interactions among several endocrine organs, but also metabolic pathways and cellular function. It is not surprising, therefore, that agents which have multiple sites of action, including central nervous system, liver, and cellular function in general, may exert diverse and profound effects on reproduction. Marijuana, one of the more widely used agents, for example, acts as an antigonadotropin and may inhibit ovulation in the female; in the male testis marijuana inhibits protein and nucleic acid synthesis in the testis, impairing spermatogenesis. That a significant number of adolescents are being exposed to these agents also raises the concern over future impairment of their physiologic development and reproductive potential.

As an aftermath of the thalidomide tragedy in the early 1960s a conservative approach has been established with regard to drug use during pregnancy. The effects of any agent on the outcome of pregnancy and immediate condition of the fetus are frequently vividly apparent. However, the most subtle effects on reproductive performance and on the fetal germ cells are not so clear cut. Cigarette smoking is the most common addiction among women in the reproductive age group. Legal and moderately socially acceptable, cigarette smoking jeopardizes reproductive performance and the chances for a normal healthy life for the offspring if pregnancy is established. It is important to appreciate the likelihood of reproductive impairment by other agents even more dangerous, illicit, and socially unacceptable than tobacco.

Nicotine and anabasine, low molecular weight components of cigarette smoke, inhibit granulosa cell aromatase in a dose dependent manner.[5] Nicotine has also been shown to delay ovum cleavage in the rat.[5] Inhibition of aromatase activity and estradiol production by granulosa cells has important implications regarding drug-induced and environmental effects on estrogen dependent processes.[4] Cannabinoids may affect gonadal function, but their effects on fertilizability of ova and embryonic development have not been studied. The intrafollicular preovulatory environment is important for nuclear and cytoplasmic maturation of the oocyte and may affect its fertilizability and govern its potential for full and normal development. This concept has significant implications with respect to a relationship between environmental influences on the intrafollicular oocyte and subsequent fertility.

Responsiveness of many malignancies to chemotherapy and to radiation has led to sustained remissions or cure. Specifically success with treatment of Hodgkin's disease, leukemias, and certain cancers of childhood has yielded a sizeable number of adolescents and young adults who contemplate marriage and pregnancy. To this group of patients the potential injury to the reproductive system by the therapy which has spared their lives is a real concern. To those physicians who treat malignancies in the young, the realization that long-term cures are likely necessitates awareness of the effects of treatment on reproductive function. In contrast to pharmacologic agents used electively for benign conditions and to abused substances, the use of potent drugs and radiation therapy in cancer treatment is critical and not usually optional. The prospects for fertility after such treatment require the reproductive endocrinologist to possess a fine appreciation of the chances for conception, pregnancy outcome, and generational genetics of the offspring of those exposed to chemotherapy and radiation. The chapter prepared by Damewood and Grochow represents a cooperative effort of reproductive endocrinologist and oncologist to provide a resource for our counselling. They review the effects of chemotherapy and radiation on gonadal function in both men and women. Alkylating agents such as cyclophosphamide and chlorambucil produce azoospermia and premature ovarian failure in a dose-dependent manner. Isolated cases of reversible amenorrhea and restoration of spermatogenesis have been reported. Since the prepubertal gonad seems to have more resistance than that after puberty, the age at which therapy is provided may be an important variable. Interval since cessation of therapy also appears to be a factor in gonadal recovery. Sex differences in response to radiation therapy have been described. As Damewood and Grochow point out, knowledge of the pharmacology of agents used, awareness of the reproductive aspirations of patients under therapy, and counselling about potential sexual and emotional problems following treatment are important issues for the physician. Cryopreservation of gametes offers prospects for fertility for patients who are at risk for gonadal failure following therapy for malignant disease. The contemporary procedure of ovum donation and in vitro fertilization provide new hope for such patients.

Agents used socially or for therapeutic purposes may have subtle and unanticipated influences on reproductive performance. Clearly, therefore, preparations used for their specific effects on the reproductive tract may exert "toxicity" which runs counter to the underlying purposes for employing them. Scialli, of the Reproductive Toxicology Center in Washington, directs his attention to three agents widely used for ovulation induction: clomiphene citrate, human menopausal gonadotropins, and bromocriptine. The discrepancy between ovulation rate and pregnancy rate with clomiphene therapy suggests that clomiphene may exert simultaneous proconceptional effects as well as antagonistic effects. Luteal phase defect may represent one possible explanation for the discrepancy, but Scialli provides reassuring data regarding pregnancy outcomes. Once pregnancy is achieved after clomiphene, the only complication reproducibly related to therapy is an increased incidence of multiple pregnancy. This complication is considerably more prevalent with gonadotropin therapy; the majority of adverse outcomes are associated with prematurity which usually accompanies multiple gestation. The question of whether to discontinue bromocriptine during pregnancy also receives a critical review. That the rates of congenital malformation associated with bromocriptine treatment do not differ from statistics for patients in general is also reassuring.

An understanding of the soundness of an experiment is a key in evaluation of its results and conclusions. Olive's chapter on the validity of studies regarding reproductive performance needs to be read and re-read by any physician, scientist, or counsellor bombarded with data, claims, and decision-making dilemmas. Indeed, it should be required reading before approaching the rest of this text. First, understand the study design. Is the study prospective or retrospective? Is there a source of comparison, i.e., control group? When no control group is used, we tend to attribute all pregnancies to success of the therapeutic intervention, a distinct pitfall. Do randomized controls always indicate equal allocation? Do we analyze data by pregnancy rates, or life table analysis? The intent of this chapter is to emphasize the possible shortcomings of study design, analysis, and conclusions. The tools for designing a sound study are clearly represented in Olive's chapter, helping us to understand biases, flaws, distortions, and limitations of clinical investigation. That the conduct of sound clinical investigation is more difficult than experiments performed in the more controllable confines of the laboratory is apparent.

Stress is an unavoidable component of an infertility problem. Environmental pressures can participate in reducing fertility. This phenomenon has been experimentally described in colonies of mice and rats in which population density and supply of food and water could be regulated. Despite ample food supply, increased crowding of cages has been shown to lead to combative behavior, infertility, smaller litter size, and increased infant mortality. Supplement the basic underlying cause of infertility in a given couple with the frustrations of being infertile, the stress of a demanding evaluation and treatment, and the depression, anger, and guilt associated with being unable to conceive, and the original problem is markedly compounded. Awareness of these pressures is a vital part of the management. Mahlstedt views these phenomena through the eyes of a psychologist and underscores the importance of insight and communication in the successful physician-couple relationship.

Since the relationship between T-mycoplasma colonization of the reproductive tract and infertility was first postulated, the organism has been more commonly referred to as *Ureaplasma urealyticum* and *Mycoplasma hominis*. Now Styler and Shapiro refer to the taxonomic class in which these organisms are classified, Mollicutes. These are small self-replicating prokaryotes, possessing a trilaminar cell membrane but no cell wall. Virtually millions of dollars have been spent clinically, once an association had been suggested of these organisms to infertility, both for cultures and antibiotic therapy. But are all the facts regarding this association conclusive? Styler and Shapiro summarize for us, in their chapter, what is known to date about these organisms and their possible role in infertility, concluding that the role of genital Mollicutes organisms in induction of infertility can only be generalized. If such a relationship is ultimately established, *U. urealyticum* and *M. hominis* will probably be the organisms of note. The chapter leaves us hanging, not because of any lack of diligence on the part of the authors, but because of inadequacy of the existing evidence. On the contrary, they provide us with a thorough rendition of the current status of this organism. The reader should review the data carefully and make a choice as to whether or not to culture, if so when to culture, and if positive what antibiotic to use, whom to treat, and how to confirm a cure.

Edward E. Wallach, M.D.

REFERENCES

1. Azziz R, Wallach E: The change in human female reproductive capacity with age fecundability and fertility. Postgrad Obstet Gynecol 7:1, 1987
2. Tsuji K, Nakano R: Chromosome studies of embryos from induced abortions in pregnant women age 35 and over. Obstet Gynecol 52:542, 1978
3. Yoshimura Y, Hosoi Y, Atlas SJ, Wallach EE: Effect of clomiphene citrate on in vitro ovulated ova. Fertil Steril 45:800, 1986
4. Barbieri RL, McShane PM, Ryan KJ: Constituents of cigarette smoke inhibit human granulosa cell aromatase. Fertil Steril 46:232, 1986
5. Yoshinaga K, Rice C, Krenn J, Pilot R: Effects of nicotine on early pregnancy in the rat. Biol Reprod 20:294, 1979

Chapter 1

Reproductive potential in the older woman

Paul R. Gindoff, M.D.
Raphael Jewelewicz, M.D.

Division of Reproductive Endocrinology, Department of Obstetrics and Gynecology, College of Physicians & Surgeons, Columbia University, New York, New York

"Then Abraham fell upon his face and laughed, and said in his heart, shall a child be born unto him that is an hundred years old? And shall Sarah that is ninety years old bear?"

The Bible, *Genesis, 17:17*

"For Sarah conceived, and bore Abraham a son."

The Bible, *Genesis, 21:2*

Fecundity, defined as reproductive potential, and its relation to age has become an important issue for many women. In the United States, we are witnessing a marked change in the patterns of childbearing that has developed over the past decade. The U.S. fertility rate rose slightly, from 67 births per 1000 women 18 to 44 years old in 1976 to 71/1000 in 1980, according to the Current Population Surveys for those years. Yet the most notable increases occurred among women who were 30 years and older. Almost one-half of births to college graduates were first births, indicative of delayed childbearing among this group of women.[1]

The post-World War II cohorts (the "baby boom" generation), comprising individuals currently in their 30s and early 40s, have been the source of this change. Those individuals were the first group to be able to exercise control over fertility almost completely, with available contraception and abortion services. Many women deferred marriage until their late 20s and early 30s.[2, 3] Thus rates of childlessness remained high at ages 30 and 35 years, and at the same time rates of first births at ages 30 to 34 years rose.[4] Thus far, the post-baby boom generation, though fewer in number, seems to be following the example of the baby boom generation by deferring age at marriage and first birth.

Historical data suggest that in a natural population, when women marry in their late 30s or early 40s, perhaps one-third to one-half of couples will remain involuntarily childless.[5] Henry[6] estimated that a couple becomes infertile when the median age of the woman is around 40 years. The decrease in the fecundity of women who have passed a certain age is generally acknowledged. In an analysis of data from several large studies, Leridon[5] suggested that fecundity is decreased in women older than 30 years of age (Fig. 1).[7] A decline in fecundability with age would provide an explanation for the relationship of maternal age with the incidence of overdue conceptions[8] and the length of their delay. That fecundability

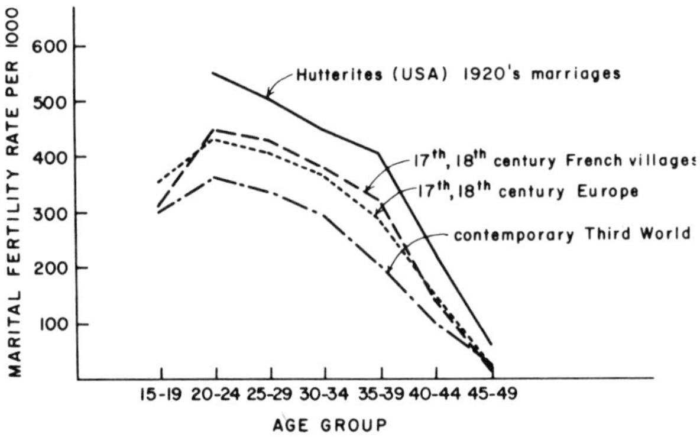

Figure 1
Age-specific fertility in selected noncontracepting populations. Based on data from Leridon,[5] reproduced from Stein.[7]

does decline with age is generally accepted, but the starting point and rate of decline, as well as its causes, are very much in dispute. Infectious, occupational, and environmental factors have a longer time to exert their cumulative effect on infertility. The inherent age-related biologic factors further reduce the ability to conceive. The fact remains that a larger proportion of women become infertile as they get older. Biologic reasons include hypothalamic aging, progressive luteal defects, and increased rates of early pregnancy wastage. Thus, because women are delaying childbearing in their early years, they are faced with reduced chances of becoming pregnant in their later reproductive years.

James[9] argues that fecundability declines more or less linearly from age 20 through age 40, due almost entirely to the progressive decline in the frequency of coitus. In a study by The Fédération des Centres d'Etude et de Conservation du Sperme Humain (CECOS), the effects of coital behavior were separated from the biologic capacity to conceive by studying 2193 women who were receiving artificial donor insemination and whose husbands were azoospermic.[10] The study demonstrated that the decrease in fecundability (conception rate per cycle) as a function of a woman's age is slight but significant after 30 years of age and marked after 35 years. The probability of success of artificial donor insemination for 12 cycles, which was 73% and 74% for two groups of women younger than 31 years of age, dropped to 61% for those 31 to 35 and to 54% for those older than 35 years.

The relative share of infertility-related visits increased from 95.6/100,000 visits to private physicians' offices for all causes in 1976 to 101.9/100,000 in 1980.[11] This increasing concern with infertility services seems to be concentrated in a unique cohort of the American population—the "baby boom" generation. As they have aged, their reproductive health concerns have evolved from preventing unintentional fertility to treating unintended infertility. The tendency to delay childbearing into the later reproductive years has increased the number of infertile couples. Because a larger proportion of American couples have delayed childbearing until their later reproductive years, they have condensed the interval of desired fertility into a shorter time span than have previous generations. This reduced period of intended childbearing has influenced the demand for infertility services. Individual couples would feel greater pressure to conceive within a shorter period of time, and thus might have a lower threshold for seeking infertility services if they were unsuccessful. Simultaneously, the avoidance of early childbearing has enhanced the age-related biologic risks of infertility. In addition to a rise in the number of these couples who are infertile, an increased proportion are seeking health care to evaluate their condition.

Before the menopause, most women will experience a phase of infertility lasting a decade or less. Yet during this phase, menstrual cycles will usually continue, often in a regular fashion and with ovulation. Experimental data from animal studies have implicated an aging process in the hypothalamic-pituitary-ovarian axis.[12] The influence of this aging process on the intactness and functioning of ova and their genetic material, as well as the pattern of oocyte depletion and atresia, seem to determine the reproductive potential in older women. Biologic, and not simply chronologic, age is the main determinant.

PHYSIOLOGY OF THE TRANSITION TO MENOPAUSE—ENDOCRINOLOGY OF THE OLDER WOMAN

To advise the older woman about her reproductive capacity and potential, the physician must first be aware of the natural endocrinologic history of menstrual physiology during these years, which coincide in many cases with the preperimenopause or the perimenopause. This prodromal period of failing ovarian function may cover 5 to 10 years before the complete cessation of menses at menopause.

Table 1. *Changes in Menstrual Cycle Length During Reproductive Life*[a]

Age	No.	Total cycle length	Follicular phase	Luteal phase
yrs				
18–30	10	30.0 ± 3.6	16.9 ± 1.8	12.9 ± 1.8
40–45	7	25.4 ± 2.3	10.4 ± 2.9	15.0 ± 0.9
46–56	8	23.2 ± 2.9	8.2 ± 2.8	15.9 ± 1.3

[a]Based on data and reproduced from Sherman et al.[20]

The initial findings are an elevated follicle-stimulating hormone (FSH) during the early follicular phase at a time of the nadir of serum estradiol (E_2). In their editorial, Jones and Jones[13] reported that in older women, following an ovulation induction protocol for in vitro fertilization, if the patient has an elevated E_2 on day 3 of the cycle, her FSH and luteinizing hormone (LH) may well be in the normal range, whereas if in another cycle she had a low E_2 her FSH may be above the normal range. The findings[14-18] of a shorter follicle phase and a normal luteal phase associated with an increased FSH with a normal LH during the early follicular phase can be identified sometimes many years before the actual menopause. This is associated with chronologic age but seems to be more of a function of biologic age, because it interfaces with medical decision making concerning the statistical success of achieving a pregnancy in the older woman, either spontaneous or through various technologic interventions.

Prospective studies of menstrual cycle length have shown that during the years just before menopause there is a marked increase in the variability of intermenstrual intervals.[19] The decade preceding menopause is characterized by generally regular menses and a slow, steady decrease in cycle length, which is due to a shortened follicular phase of the cycle. This was confirmed in a small group of women by measurement of serum FSH, LH, E_2, and progesterone (P) throughout the menstrual cycle.[15] When studies were carried out in women who were 40 and 41 years of age and with regular menses, the patterns of FSH, LH, E_2, and P concentrations did not differ from those observed in women 18 to 30 years of age. Hormonal changes reflecting altered function were detected in regular menstruating women who were older than 45 years of age. These older women had a significantly shorter follicular phase (Table 1). In these perimenopausal women, E_2 levels during active follicular maturation, at the midcycle peak, and during the luteal phase were lower than in women 18 to 30 years of age. Concentrations of FSH in the early follicular phase were strikingly elevated when compared with those of younger women and fell as E_2 increased during follicular maturation. LH concentrations during these cycles were indistinguishable from those observed in younger women.[14-16, 21]

Other studies have demonstrated that an elevation of FSH could predict the absence of ovarian follicles in patients with primary or secondary amenorrhea before surgery.[22] Although there are several possible interpretations, the elevated concentration of serum FSH observed in perimenopausal women may be indicative of the reduced number of functional residual ovarian follicles. Yet ovulation has been documented in cycles occurring during this phase.[15-17] One can see how the potential for conception could exist even during this transitional phase of reproductive life.

Because E_2 concentrations remained substantial, an explanation other than that of estrogen feedback inhibition is required for the discordant regulation of FSH and LH. Evidence that FSH is more sensitive than LH to the suppressive effects of exogenous E_2[23] argues against an increase in FSH due only to a decreased estrogen concentration. Moreover, during menopause FSH and LH appear to change proportionally when estrogen is given. However, these findings are consistent with the possibility that a decrease in estrogens may sometimes result in a greater response of FSH than LH because of differential regulation of LH and FSH secretion at the hypothalamic or pituitary level. Altered sensitivity of the aging hypothalamus-pituitary to sex steroids may manifest itself in the perimenopause by differential regulation of the gonadotropins. Alternatively, there may be another ovarian hormone that regulates FSH secretion. Such a factor, inhibin,[24] would be reduced with age consequent to a reduced number of follicles. A loss of inhibin would explain the elevated FSH in older women with relatively normal E_2 and LH and the marked fluctuations in concentrations of FSH observed in the presence of very modest changes in E_2.[15, 16]

Women who have menopause at an early age have a relatively short duration of cycle variability before amenorrhea ensues.[19] By contrast, later menopause is accompanied by unusually long and short intermenstrual intervals and an overall increased mean cycle length and variance. It has been claimed that there is an inverse relationship between age and ovulatory frequency in women older than 40 years.[25] Metcalf[26] reported that the onset of oligomenorrhea, and not age, per se, is associated with a decline in the incidence of ovulation in older women. More than 89% of the women who were older than 50 years of age reported recent changes in menstrual cycle length, compared with only 23.5% of women 40 to 44 years of age. The difference was reflected in the lower frequency of ovulatory cycles in the older group. When women with oligomenorrhea were excluded, however, the age effect disappeared, and almost all of the women with an unchanging record of 21- to 35-day menstrual cycles ovulated in every cycle during the study, irrespective of age.

These observations are in accord with reports[15-17] that there may be gross disturbances in gonadotropin levels (particularly FSH) in pre-perimenopausal and perimenopausal women, but with no significant difference in luteal P. This confirms that there are primordial follicles with apparently normal oocytes in the ovaries of older women.[27] In women who are 40 years of age and older, the incidence of ovulation can be deduced if reliable information about menstrual periodicity is available. Metcalf and Livesey[17] identified an age-related rise in urinary FSH that occurred before the break in regular menstrual cyclicity in women who were older than 40 years of age, compared with younger women. The difference was greatest at the time of the perimenstrual phase and occurred in women with regular menstrual cyclicity. These cycles were almost all ovulatory. More dramatic increases in urinary FSH and a statistically significant rise in urinary LH was observed in older women (older than 40 years of age) with irregular cyclicity. Again, the majority of these cycles were ovulatory. The marked variations in FSH and LH excreted during a typical ovulatory menstrual cycle mean not only that no simple estimate of the effect of age can be made, but also that early ovarian failure may be difficult to recognize.

Regardless of the mechanism by which it is brought about, any age-related change that involves the functional relationship between the hypothalamus-pituitary and the ovary must result in a qualitative (bioactivity) and/or quantitative (immunoactivity) change in the gonadotropins that are released or a change in the ability of the ovary to respond to these hormones. Because increased levels of gonadotropins occur in the setting of ovulatory cycles, qualitative changes or the ovarian response to gonadotropins may be more important in characterizing ovarian senescence and perimenopause.

AGING OF THE FEMALE REPRODUCTIVE SYSTEM

It is common knowledge that the human menstrual cycle tends to be irregular in length during the last few years of reproductive life. It has not been firmly established whether these irregularities are initiated in the ovary or centrally (hypothalamus-pituitary). Even after menopause, there is some evidence of cyclic changes in the ovary. In humans, the period of reproductive potential cannot extend much beyond the menopause because of progressive atresia and exhaustion of all oocytes. But in an indefinite percentage of women, reproduction ceases up to several years before this time, either naturally or prematurely, which may result from age-related changes in the hypothalamic-pituitary axis. An ovary-dependent, neuroendocrine aging syndrome of laboratory rats and mice was described by Finch et al.[28] This syndrome can be attenuated during aging by longstanding ovariectomy and can be prematurely induced in young rodents by sustained exposure to E_2. The limited follicular stock in the ovary is proposed to be a major pacemaker of aging in this neuroendocrine syndrome; ovarian aging may interact with neuroendocrine aging. Ovary-independent neuroendocrine changes occur as well.

Aged rats show an increased incidence of irregular estrous cycles and a decline in fertility with advancing age.[12] The hypothalamus, pituitary, ovary, and uterus each has been implicated as the primary site responsible for this age-related decline in reproduction.[29-31] Krohn[32] suggested that the age of the ovary played a major role in maintenance of estrous cycles, because transplants of young ovaries into acyclic old colored black agouti mice restored estrous cycles, whereas acyclic old ovaries transplanted into young mice resulted in irregular cycles or failure to cycle. With the use of young ovaries transplanted into acyclic old rats, Aschheim[33] and Peng and Huang[34] reported that the hypothalamus-pituitary was the primary site of aging that led to the termination of cyclic activity. Aschheim's original observations[33] on a limited number of rats suggested that persistent estrus rats aged 2 years did not regain cycles with young grafts unless the old hosts were ovariectomized when young and allowed to age in the absence of ovaries. Because old ovaries could support some cycles when grafted to young hosts, this study set two fundamental principles for the neuroendocrinology of aging by providing a basis for the hypotheses: (1) that an age-related change occurs in the hypothalamic sensitivity to ovarian steroids, which impairs its capacity to drive ovarian cycles; and (2) that in the absence of the ovary, hypothalamic aging is attenuated.

Sopelak and Butcher[35] investigated the influence of age of the ovary (to be transplanted) and age of the recipient on cyclicity. Among all rats with ovarian transplants, more recipients with young and prepuberal ovaries cycled (35%) than recipients with old ovaries (6%), indicating that old ovaries are not as capable of maintaining cyclicity as younger ovaries. In the rats with ovarian transplants that became acyclic, the distribution of constant estrus and anestrus was different. More old than young recipients became constantly estrous (56% versus 15%), and more young than old recipients became anestrous (85% versus 44%). These results provide evidence for age-related differences in both the ovary and the hypothalamic-pituitary axis. The age of the ovary and the age of the hypothalamus-pituitary both contributed to the termination of reproductive cyclicity in that study. A decrease in number of oocytes, and therefore number of follicles, appears to be the ovarian aging factor, because a reduction in number of oocytes following ovary transplant is associated with an age-like reduction in estrous cyclicity.

The finding that young rats with old transplanted ovaries failed to maintain regular cycles agrees with work in colored black agouti mice by Krohn[32] but appears to conflict with the reports of Aschheim,[33] who often used acyclic rats as donors and recipients. From the Sopelak and Butcher study,[35] it was concluded that old rats with regular estrous cycles before receiving an ovarian transplant were capable of continuing cyclicity, provided that transplants of young ovaries were used. However, once the number of oocytes and follicles fell below the minimum number required for maintenance of estrous cycles, age-related hypothalamic-pituitary differences became evident. This tendency for aged rats to become constantly estrous and young rats to become anestrous when both have a similar number of transplanted oocytes probably is due to a change in the sensitivity of the hypothalamic-pituitary axis to ovarian steroid feedback and could be caused by the duration of exposure to steroids such as E_2.[28, 36]

It appears that as the population of oocytes decreases, there is an associated decrease in cyclic activity and an increase in concentration of gonadotropins. This increase in gonadotropins cannot be explained by changes in steroids alone, because a significant decline in ovarian steroids was not found at this particular sampling time.[35] Likewise, it appears that a reduced number of follicles or responsive ovarian tissue plays a major role in the decline in reproductive function. However, because young rats respond to decreases in the amount of ovarian tissue (after unilateral oophorectomy or ovarian transplant) by becoming anestrous, whereas old rats become constantly estrous, a central factor (i.e., hypothalamic-pituitary) is responsible. Further evidence for ovarian-dependent central aging was reported by Lu et al.[37] Their study demonstrates that the stimulatory feedback actions of E_2 and P on LH secretion, which are present in acutely ovariectomized old pseudopregnant rats, are absent in old constant estrous females immediately following ovariectomy. Because pituitary LH responses to LH-releasing hormone administration in this study are intact in both constant estrous and pseudopregnant rats, it would appear that the functional defect involved in the lack of stimulatory feedback of ovarian steroids on LH secretion in the constant estrous animal lies in the central nervous system.

Altered neurotransmitter dynamics may occur in aging rats,[38] as may an age-dependent decrease in the kinetics of hypothalamic-pituitary axis estrogen receptors in the brain of mice.[39] Positive and negative feedback actions of steroid occur mainly within the central nervous system (i.e., hypothalamus). Steroid feedback actions within the hypothalamus are accomplished by affecting monoamine dynamics and/or affecting the synthesis, storage, and release of LH-releasing hormone. It is possible that aging may not involve primary spontaneous defects in neuronal function or in gonadal steroid secretion, but instead influence steroid feedback to the brain. Several studies[37, 40-42] suggest that aging affects both negative and positive feedback of E_2. Changes in concentrations of estrogen and or P receptors in the brain account for the diminished ability of the brain to respond. Changes in steroid receptor number may be important in attenuated steroid responsiveness during the middle-aged transition to acyclicity. Attenuated E_2-induced LH surges have been correlated with decreased E_2 nuclear receptors in the preoptic area and with decreased P cytosol receptors in the preoptic area and medial basal hypothalamus of middle-aged ovariectomized steroid-treated rats.[43] Aging of the reproductive system may involve a cumulative impact of ovarian steroids on the hypothalamus and pituitary.[44]

Age-related changes at the level of the ovary in humans are well recognized. Exhaustion of follicles has been a popular hypothesis as the primary trigger for the menopausal transition. The majority of follicles have either been ovulated or undergone atresia by the time a women is acyclic; nevertheless, Costoff and Mahesh[27] found normal primary oocytes in all postmenopausal ovaries examined. Although differentiating follicles were found, all of them were in various stages of atresia. These data suggest that follicular exhaustion is not the only cause of the menopausal transition. E_2 production by the postmenopausal ovary is greatly diminished, but estrone and androgen production are not as affected.[45] Measurement of ovarian and peripheral venous estrogens and androgens demonstrated that substantial concentrations of androstenedione and testosterone and very little estrogen are secreted by the postmenopausal ovary.[46] Thus the majority of circulating estrogen concentrations are the result of peripheral conversion of androgens.[47] This is supported by the fact that E_2 concentrations did not change after gonadectomy in postmenopausal women.[48] Ovarian changes are not due to decreased hypothalamic-pituitary input, because pituitary responsiveness to LH-releasing hormone is comparable to premenopausal and postmenopausal women.[49]

Whether age-related changes in the ovary occur prior to hypothalamic and/or pituitary age-related changes in women is not clear. Reyes et al.[14] found that estrogen concentrations remain normal until at least 1 year after the postmenopausal state is reached, again discounting the importance of estrogen concentrations as the trigger for transition to menopause. It is intriguing that changes occur in middle-aged women that indicate increasing neurotransmitter imbalance at this critical age,[43] which is manifested as vasomotor instability,[50] for example. Several subtle changes have been observed in middle-aged animals and women that may be important triggers culminating in ovarian senescence and age-related acyclicity. Continuously changing interactions among the aging hypothalamus, pituitary, and ovary may be important in humans as well as in experimental animal models.

FACTORS AFFECTING THE AGE AT MENOPAUSE

The potential for ovulation during the perimenopausal period, although reduced, is present. No basis is known, other than clinical experience, for judging whether a given interval without menses is likely to represent permanent amenorrhea. The probability that natural menopause was associated with various intervals without menses was calculated by Treloar et al.[19] for women aged 45 to 49 years, 50 to 52 years, and 53 years of age and older. For each age group an increasing duration of amenorrhea was associated with an increased likelihood that menopause had occurred. Also, for any given interval of amenorrhea the older women were more likely to have reached menopause. The results indicated that 6 months of amenorrhea was predictive of menopause in only 52% of women aged 45 to 49 years and 70% of women aged 53 years of age or older.

The median age at menopause was 51.7 years, as reported by Van Keep et al.[51] from data obtained by postal questionnaire in The Netherlands. The influence of marital status on the age at menopause has been investigated, and it was found that single women had an earlier menopause. Older age at the time of last pregnancy was associated with later menopause. Menarche and the age at menopause were correlated in this survey,[51] in that a late menarche was associated with an early menopause and vice versa. There was not a significant association between age at menopause and parity. However, there was a weak trend to a later median age at menopause with an increase in parity. Although the study did not show an effect of former oral contraceptive use on the median age at menopause, there was a tendency toward a later median age with duration of pill use.

Gray[52] reported the median age of menopause in the United States to be 49.8 years. Essentially, the median age of menopause in industrialized population lies within this narrow range.[51, 52] However, in developing countries the median age at menopause may be < 44 years, and other studies indicate that women of lower socioeconomic class may reach menopause at a younger age than women of higher class.[53] There is associated evidence that inadequate nutrition can lead to delayed menarche and anovulation, and thus premature menopause.

PATTERNS OF FERTILITY IN THE OLDER WOMAN—EPIDEMIOLOGY OF LATE FERTILITY

LEVELS AND TRENDS OF LATE FERTILITY

The decline of fertility, as evidenced during demographic transition, has been much greater for late fertility than for overall fertility. Data from southeastern France demonstrated this trend, comparing age-specific fertility rates among women who were married at 20 to 24 years of age during four different time intervals: 1690 to 1739, 1770 to 1789, 1790 to 1819, and 1935 to 1937. The fertility rate for the women aged 20 to 24 years remained stable over the first three time intervals. However, by 1790 to 1819, the fertility rate for women 40 to 44 years of age was only 50% of the 1690 to 1739 rate. For the years 1935 to 1937, the fertility rate for women 20 to 24 years of age was only 60% of that for the 20- to 24-year-old women during the 1690 to 1739 time interval, whereas in women who were 40 to 44 years of age fertility had decreased to 11% of the level observed from 1690 to 1739.[54] In the United States from 1964 to 1974, age-specific fertility rates (births per 1000 women) for mothers aged 35 years or more has steadily dropped. That is, the older the woman, the lower the overall fertility rate. This trend is repeatedly found in all western industrialized nations.

CHARACTERS OF BIRTH ORDER

In England and Wales, the mean order of births to mothers aged 35 years and older in 1975 was 3.3. The proportion of births of order 1 among these births to women aged 35 years and older increased from 10% in 1965 to 15% in 1975.[55] The same trend was evidenced for the proportion of births of order 2 and 3 as well, essentially because the absolute number of higher-order births is compared with all first births, regardless of age.[54] Essentially, if a woman has a child after the age of 35 years, there is an increased likelihood that it will be her first, though at the same time, the overall age-specific fertility rate declines with advancing age.

Recent trends[4] show an increase in the age at first birth and postponement of the first birth after marriage. In England and Wales[54] and in other developed nations, the most significant trend has been the increasing delay between marriage and first birth.

Recently Bloom[55] analyzed the cross cohort trends in the age pattern of women at first birth in the United States, reaching much the same conclusions as the earlier study. The results indicate that the proportion of women who will never have a first birth is increasing across cohorts and can be expected to be as high as 0.25 and 0.20 for recent white and nonwhite cohorts, respectively. The mean age at first birth and the proportion of first births occurring between 25 and 35 years of age is increasing across cohorts of white women but is stable across cohorts of nonwhite women. At the same time, a relatively high proportion of births to older women in the Northeast were first births (21%), demonstrating a greater tendency to delay childbearing in the Northeast than in the rest of the United States.[1]

Decline in fecundity with advancing age was demonstrated in the Fédération CECOS study[10] and in a recent study by Hendershot,[56] who reconfirmed increased conception delays in women older than 30 years of age. However, the effect of age on fertility decisions also has a sociobiologic component that is not related to fecundity. Rather, it deals with the concern that with increasing age, the partners may not have sufficient time and energy to cope with a child.[3] Essentially, taking epidemiology, fecundity, and sociobiologic factors into account, voluntary delay in childbearing may be expected ultimately to result in a reduction in the level of voluntary fertility desired.

BIOLOGIC AND SOCIAL INTERACTIONS IN THE DETERMINATION OF FERTILITY IN THE OLDER WOMAN

Demographic studies have shown that there is a consistent decline in fecundity with advancing age after 30 to 35 years. In many societies this fall in birth rate is due to deliberate fertility control by the use of contraception, abortion, or decreased frequency of sexual intercourse. Such factors can mask any interactions between biologic factors of the aging female reproductive system and other social factors that might otherwise determine fertility during the later reproductive years. To assess the effects of these latter factors, it is necessary to examine reproductive patterns in selected societies that do not practice deliberate fertility regulation.[52] As shown in Figure 1, regardless of the level of fertility during the reproductive years, there is, in all populations, a marked decrease in fertility during the fourth and fifth decades of life, and the shape of the fertility distributions at older ages follows a remarkably similar pattern in different populations. These data are obtained from societies with "natural fertility," as defined by Henry,[6] which is reproduction in the absence of deliberate fertility control. In particular, fertility in the 40- to 44-year age group is between 40% and 50% lower than in the 35- to 39-year age group.

The mean age at last childbirth in a number of historical European populations experiencing "natural fertility" is estimated to be approximately 40 years, and it is remarkable how consistently this observation has been reported.[6] There are few data available from 20th century populations, but it is noteworthy that among the Hutterites of North America, who have one of the highest levels of fertility ever recorded, the mean age of last confinement is 40.9 years.[57]

A comparison of the age-specific curves of the proportions of the population sterile and postmenopausal show that in developing countries, the median age of sterility antedates the age at menopause by an average of 10 years.[58] Similar differences exist between the age at menopause and the mean age of the mother at the birth of her last child, which is generally around 40 years. From these data, it is clear that fertility declines substantially before the menopause and that the median or mean age of terminal reproduction antedates the median age at menopause by up to a decade.[52]

The biologic and social factors that might explain the decline of fertility during this decade before menopause can be divided into those factors that influence the probability of conception and those that influence the probability that a conception will result in a live birth.

FACTORS AFFECTING PROBABILITY OF CONCEPTION

This decade of the preperimenopausal and perimenopausal period is characterized by an increase in menstrual irregularity, which indicates a decreased incidence of ovulation. However, in the 40- to 44-year age group, only 16% to 30% of cycles can be considered abnormal, whereas 40 years represents the median age of terminal reproduction, and the birth rate declines by 50% between the age groups 35 to 39 years and 40 to 44 years. From these data, it would appear that anovulation or failure of corpus luteum function can explain only a relatively small proportion of the decline in fertility before the menopause.

The observed decline in birth rates could be due in part to a reduction in male fertility. Although Anderson[59] analyzed Irish census data to show a decline of fertility among men older than the age of 57.5 years, regardless of the age of the wife or duration of the marriage, this reduction in male fertility is relatively small and, given the usual age difference between spouses, would occur too late substantially to affect female fertility rates before menopause.

The use of oral contraceptives has been associated with increased conception delays. A cross-sectional study by Linn et al.[60] indicated a longer interval from cessation of pill use to conception, relative to a corresponding interval for previous users of other methods of contraception. The longer conception delay was not confined to primigravida women. It was considerable and statistically significant, even for women who had proven fertility. Harlop and Baras[61] found a highly significant interaction between pill use and age, older women having a greater temporary reduction in conceptions shortly after stopping pill use. There was also an interaction involving age and duration of use. In women who used the pill for a short time, there was little age effect, and in younger women there was little age effect with the duration of use. Older women who had used the pill for several years, however, had a marked temporary reduction in fertility on stopping it.

FACTORS AFFECTING THE FREQUENCY OF SPONTANEOUS ABORTION

The incidence of spontaneous abortions rises markedly with age, and this age-related increase is independent of prior obstetric history.[62, 63] The majority of these spontaneous abortions occur during the first trimester of pregnancy. Cytogenetic studies have shown that in 40% to 60% of all first-trimester abortions, there is evidence of chromosomal abnormalities, and the majority of these anomalies are autosomal trisomic defects in

Table 2. *Risk of Spontaneous Abortion Related to Maternal Age (Presbyterian Hospital Data)*[a]

Maternal age	Spontaneous abortion
yrs	%
15–19	9.9
20–24	9.5
25–29	10.0
30–34	11.7
35–39	17.7
40–44	33.8
≥ 45	53.2

[a]Based on data and reproduced from Warburton et al.[66]

which an extra chromosome is present.[64, 65] The majority of autosomal trisomies and all autosomal monosomic anomalies lead to early spontaneous fetal wastage, and only a small minority of trisomies involving chromosomes 13, 18, and 21 survive to full-term delivery and give rise to conditions such as Down's syndrome.[63, 65] The frequency of trisomy among spontaneous abortions increases with maternal age.[64] The incidence of a live-born child with Down's syndrome increases with age, in parallel to the increasing age-specific incidence of spontaneous abortion after age 34.[52]

Confirmatory data were collected by Warburton and colleagues[66] at Columbia-Presbyterian Medical Center (Tables 2 and 3). As maternal age increases, the risk of spontaneous abortion rises. This association is quite dramatic after 40 years of age. In addition, the risk for a trisomic abortus actually decreases in younger women with repeated miscarriage, but the risk remains constant and higher for women older than 35 years of age.[67]

GENETICS AND MATERNAL AGING

The risk of a trisomic birth remains the single most outstanding problem for the older woman who does conceive successfully. Nondisjunction during meioses is facilitated when the chiasmata joining pairs of chromosomes are fewer. Smaller chromosomes have fewer chiasmata, and perhaps these are further depleted over the decades of the reproductive years in ova awaiting their turn to ovulate, from the time when the woman was herself a fetus.[7] It has been shown[68] that advancing maternal age is associated with trisomy of the small chromosomes. According to the "production line" hypothesis,[69] trisomy is predetermined by the order of formation of oocytes during fetal development, the last formed oocytes with fewer chiasmata and more univalent pairs being the last to be ovulated, late in life. Others have proposed that it is some factor in the adult maternal environment and dependent on physiologic aging of the reproductive system that is important. Thus delayed ovulation might lead to a higher incidence of spindle defects in overripe eggs[70] or to asynchrony between chiasma terminalization and chromosome alignment on the spindle.[71] The hormonal imbalance and irregular cyclicity associated with the perimenopausal period[72] could be critical. This is an obvious contrast between the hypothesis that the risk of aneuploidy is determined before birth and may be influenced by environmental factors and the latter hypothesis that the occurrence of chromosomal anomalies is linked to the physiologic age of the female reproductive system. Brook et al.[73] investigated this question by advancing the process of aging, by performing unilateral ovariectomy early in adulthood in colored black agouti mice. An earlier onset of irregular cyclicity and an earlier rise in aneuploidy was noted. The clinical implications are that the probability of conceiving a Down's fetus will be determined by the time from approaching menopause (i.e., biologic age) rather than the absolute or chronologic age of the woman. Further support for the concept that maternal endocrine irregularity is responsible for the occurrence of chromosomal anomalies is the observation that there is an increased frequency of severe chromosomal abnormalities in abortuses from women who had recently ceased to use oral contraceptives.[74] In addition, Ford[75] pointed out that when pH of cultures of actively dividing human fetal fibroblasts is raised for 15 to 30 minutes, numerical chromosomal errors are induced in up to 60% of the cells, and the effect is greatest if the cells are treated at the time of deoxyribonucleic acid replication. The female reproductive tract is not subject to such sensitively buffered

Table 3. *Estimates of the Probability of Spontaneous Abortion for Recognized Conceptions with Trisomy 21, by Maternal Age*[a]

Maternal age	Trisomy 21 among abortions	Trisomy in live births	Abortion of trisomy 21
yrs	%	%	%
15–19	0.79	0.059	0.54
20–24	0.84	0.074	0.55
25–29	0.90	0.088	0.53
30–34	2.06	0.145	0.65
35–39	1.90	0.374	0.52
40–44	9.26	1.496	0.76
≥ 45	28.57	6.210	0.84

[a]Based on data and reproduced from Warburton et al.[66]

conditions as most other tissues of the body, and a slight decrease in estrogen concentration leads to an increased pH.[76] Estrogen levels are diminished at the end of reproductive life, therefore chromosomal errors may reflect changes in pH due to the changed endocrine milieu. Documentation of the influence of a changing endocrine milieu on the aging of the female reproductive system has been shown by differences in the surface ultrastructure of the aged uterus as a function of age-related changes in hormone levels.[77]

OBSTETRIC IMPLICATIONS OF THE OLDER GRAVID WOMAN

The older primigravid woman has historically been labelled "high risk." Despite modern perinatal and neonatal care, several series continued to show a high fetal wastage from a variety of causes. Morrison,[78] in a 5-year review of 127 primigravid women (aged 35 years or older) defined a risk to the fetus in terms of perinatal death and neonatal morbidity. With the equivalent of a perinatal mortality rate of 94/1000, an 11% incidence of small-for-date infants, and a neonatal morbidity rate of 18%, there still appeared to be a need for increased awareness of the fetal risks in this group and an increased emphasis on their prevention by prenatal care and more liberal abdominal delivery. A recent study[79] again looked at these issues and did not show an increase in the stillbirth or neonatal death rate for neonates of older women. For nulliparous mothers, there was no age-related difference in preterm labor or neonatal intensive care unit admissions of neonates. Apgar scores, congenital anomalies, and birth weight categories showed some age-related differences. There was an increased incidence of low 1-minute Apgar scores and congenital anomalies in the infants of the older healthy pregnant women. Despite the lower 1-minute Apgar scores, there was no increase in meconium or cesarean births for fetal distress in this group. There was an increase in macrosomic babies for the older women, independent of the incidence of glucose intolerance. The overwhelming majority of studies in the obstetric literature report a higher rate of cesarean births in older women.[78-80]

TREATMENT OF THE OLDER INFERTILE WOMAN

Clearly, the older woman can ovulate, conceive, and have a normal child. The probability of these events occurring, though, are compromised as the chronologic age of the individual approaches the age of her menopause. Certain endocrinologic parameters can be checked to identify, as best as possible, where on the reproductive continuum she lies. In addition to the basal body temperature chart, endometrial biopsy study, and luteal P, gonadotropin levels should be studied, because, to date, FSH is the most sensitive marker readily available to delineate the perimenopausal state and, together with LH, the menopausal state. The older woman should be counselled on her increased risks of spontaneous abortion and chromosomal anomaly, which can be detected efficiently with the use of either chorionic villus biopsy study or amniocentesis.

Because of the intrinsic decreased fertility rates and increased conception delays in the older woman, she should be considered in the category of idiopathic or unexplained infertility, at least until the biologic and endocrinologic effects of aging can be determined. Essentially, we recommend empiric ovulation induction, which would be expected statistically to enhance her fecundity by superovulation. At the same time, this should not exaggerate her already higher risk for a chromosomally anomalous conceptus. We could not identify any difference in response to human menopausal gonadotropin/human chorionic gonadotropin based simply on chronologic age.[81] More aggressive intervention may be necessary and applied after a shorter trial of ovulation induction or other therapies needed for the older woman who is racing a biologic time clock, especially if other confounding variables (i.e., male factor, peritoneal factors) are identified. As long as the endocrine profile of the woman is within the normal range for younger women, ovulation induction is indicated, and she should be allowed entry into an in vitro fertilization or gamete intrafallopian tube transfer program, despite an age $>$ 40 years.

Although success in the older woman should be less on a statistical basis, therapeutic decisions are not easily reached and will require high motivation by the patient with a full understanding of the odds. Tuboplasty, per se, should not be routinely recommended in the woman who is older than 40 years of age with a structural/mechanical factor, because she will suffer a statistical defeat due to the advancing aging of the reproductive system. In vitro fertilization would be the recommended alternative as long as her gonadotropins are normal. Elevated gonadotropins would preclude intervention, because all available data indicate that there may be chromosomal effects due to the changing endocrine milieu. In essence, the older woman with a conception delay deserves an expedited full workup and aggressive therapy.

SUMMARY

There is a definite increase in the number of women bearing children in the 30- and 40-year-old age groups. The total number of women who are 35 to 40 years of age in the United States is projected to increase 42% and the percent births to this age group is projected to increase 37%. This is apparently because of a trend to postpone childbearing and first birth due to women's career priorities, advanced education, control over fertility, financial concerns, late and second marriages, and infertility. Associated with this is an increase in visits to the infertility specialist for older women who have an intrinsic decrease in fecundity with advancing age.

Although, on the average, a woman will not experience menopause until about 50 years of age, her effective childbearing period may stop almost a decade earlier. A woman in her late 30s and, especially, early 40s is at some disadvantage in terms of conception delay, ability to carry a chromosomally normal fetus until term, and risk of trisomic conception.

Certain endocrinologic parameters have been identified for the woman entering the transition to menopause. Biologic aging of the hypothalamic-pituitary-ovarian axis is intertwined with changes in the endocrine milieu of the perimenopause and preperimenopause. Despite a clear association of decreased fecundity in older women due to multiple biologic and social influences, so long as the individual has regular cycles and essentially normal endocrine parameters, she should be a candidate for an expedited infertility workup and ovulation induction, if not more aggressive treatment. Her obstetric profile is much improved, except for an increase in congenital anomalies and chromosomal defects. Chorionic villus biopsy study or amniocentesis is advised in all cases, regardless of therapy.

Acknowledgment. We thank Ms. Bambi Aharon for her special efforts in typing the manuscript.

REFERENCES

1. O'Connell M, Rogers C: Differential fertility in the United States: 1976-1980. Fam Plann Perspect 14:281, 1982
2. Gibson C: The U.S. fertility decline, 1961-1975: the contribution of changes in marital status and marital fertility. Fam Plann Perspect 8:249, 1976
3. Rindfuss R, Bumpass L: How old is too old? Age and the sociology of fertility. Fam Plann Perspect 8:226, 1976
4. Ventura S: Trends in first births to older mothers, 1970-1979. Washington, DC, National Center for Health Statistics, Series 31, No. 2, Suppl. 1, 1982 (Department of Health and Human Services Publication no. Public Health Service 82-1120)
5. Leridon H: Human Fertility: The Basic Components. Chicago, University of Chicago Press, 1977, p 107
6. Henry L: Some data on natural fertility. Eugenics Quart 8:81, 1961
7. Stein Z: Review and commentary—a woman's age: childbearing and child rearing. Am J Epidemiol 121:327, 1985
8. Hendershot G: Maternal age and overdue conceptions. Am J Public Health 74:35, 1984
9. James W: The causes of the decline in fecundability with age. Soc Biol 26:330, 1979
10. Fédération CECOS, Schwartz D, Mayaux MJ: Female fecundity as a function of age: results of artificial insemination in 2193 nulliparous women with azoospermic husbands. N Engl J Med 306:404, 1982
11. Aral S, Cates W: The increasing concern with fertility: why now? JAMA 250:2327, 1983
12. Talbert G: Effect of maternal age on reproductive capacity. Am J Obstet Gynecol 102:451, 1968
13. Metcalf M, Livesey J: Gonadotropin excretion in fertile women: effect of age and the onset of the menopausal transition. Editorial Review by HW Jones Jr, GS Jones. Obstet Gynecol Surv 41:101, 1986
14. Reyes F, Winter J, Faiman C: Pituitary-ovarian relationships preceding the menopause. Am J Obstet Gynecol 129:557, 1977
15. Sherman B, Korenman S: Hormonal characteristics of the human menstrual cycle throughout reproductive life. J Clin Invest 55:699, 1975
16. Sherman B, West J, Korenman S: The menopausal transition: analysis of LH, FSH, estradiol and progesterone concentrations during menstrual cycles of older women. J Clin Endocrinol Metab 42:629, 1976
17. Metcalf M, Livesey J: Gonadotropin excretion in fertile women: effect of age and the onset of the menopausal transition. J Endocrinol 105:357, 1985
18. Korenman S, Sherman B, Korenman J: Reproductive hormone function: the peri-menopausal period and beyond. Clin Endocrinol Metab 7:625, 1978
19. Treloar A, Boynton R, Benn B, Brown B: Variation of the human menstrual cycle through reproductive life. Int J Fertil 12:77, 1967
20. Sherman B, Wallace R, Treloar A: The menopausal transition: endocrinologic and epidemiological considerations. J Biosoc Sci [Suppl] 6:19, 1979
21. Van Look P, Lothran H, Hunter W, Michie E, Baird D: Hypothalamic-pituitary-ovarian function in perimenopausal women. J Clin Endocrinol 7:13, 1977
22. Goldenberg R, Grodin J, Rodbard D, Ross G: Gonadotropins in women with amenorrhea: use of plasma follicle stimulating hormone to differentiate women with and

without ovarian follicles. Am J Obstet Gynecol 116:1003, 1973

23. Vaitukaitis J, Bernudez J, Cargille C, Lipsett M, Ross G: New evidence of an anti-estrogenic action of clomiphene citrate in women. J Clin Endocrinol Metab 32:503, 1971
24. Marrs R, Lobo R, Campeau J, Nakamura R, Brown J, Uzita E, DiZerega G: Correlation of human follicular fluid inhibin activity with spontaneous and induced follicle maturation. J Clin Endocrinol Metab 58:704, 1984
25. Doung G: The incidence of anovular cycles in women. J Reprod Fertil [Suppl] 6:77, 1969
26. Metcalf M: Incidence of ovulatory cycles in women approaching the menopause. J Biosoc Sci 11:39, 1979
27. Costoff A, Mahesh U: Primordial follicles with normal oocytes in the ovaries of postmenopausal women. J Am Geriatr Soc 23:5, 1975
28. Finch C, Felicio L, Mobbs C, Nelson J: Ovarian and steroid influences on neuroendocrine aging processes in female rodents. Endocr Rev 5:467, 1984
29. Adams C: Aging and reproduction in the female mammal with particular reference to the rabbit. J Reprod Fertil [Suppl] 12:1, 1970
30. Finch C: Reproductive senescence in rodents: factors in the decline of fertility and loss of regular estrous cycles. In The Aging Reproductive System, Vol 4, Edited by EL Schneider. New York, Raven Press, 1978, p 193
31. Talbert G: Effect of aging of the ovaries and female gametes on reproductive capacity. In The Aging Reproductive System, Vol 4, Edited by EL Schneider. New York, Raven Press, 1978, p 59
32. Krohn P: Review lectures on senescence. II. Heterochronic transplantation in the study of aging. Proc R Soc Lond (Biol) 157:128, 1962
33. Aschheim P: Resultats fournis par la greffe heterochrone des ovaries dans l'étude de la regulation hypothalamo-hypophyso-ovarienne de la ratte sénile. Gerontologia 10:65, 1965
34. Peng M-T, Huang H-H: Aging of hypothalamic-pituitary-ovarian function in the rat. Fertil Steril 23:535, 1972
35. Sopelak V, Butcher R: Contribution of the ovary versus hypothalamic-pituitary to termination of estrous cycles in aging rats using ovarian transplants. Biol Reprod 27:29, 1982
36. Brawer J, Schipper H, Naftolin F: Ovary-dependent degeneration in the hypothalamic arcuate nucleus. Endocrinology 107:274, 1980
37. Lu J, Damassa D, Gilman D, Judd H, Sawyer C: Differential patterns of gonadotropin responses to ovarian steroids and to LH-releasing hormone between constant-estrous and pseudopregnant states in aging rats. Biol Reprod 23:345, 1980
38. Cooper R, McNamara C, Linnoila M: Catecholaminergic-serotonergic balance in the CNS and reproductive cycling in aging rats. Neurobiol Aging 7:9, 1986
39. Belisle S, Bellabarba D, Lehoux J-G: Age-dependent, ovary-independent decrease in the nuclear binding kinetics of estrogen receptors in the brain of the C57BL/6J mouse. Am J Obstet Gynecol 153:394, 1985
40. Huang S, Steger R, Sonntag W, Meites J: Positive feedback by ovarian hormones on prolactin and LH in old versus young female rats. Neurobiol Aging 1:141, 1980
41. Hunag H, Marshall S, Meites J: Capacity of old versus young female rats to secrete LH, FSH and prolactin. Biol Reprod 14:528, 1976
42. Everett J, Tyrey L: Comparison of luteinizing hormone surge responses to ovarian steroids in cyclic and spontaneously persistent estrous rats of middle age. Biol Reprod 26:663, 1982
43. Wise P: Aging of the female reproductive system. Rev Biol Res Aging 1:195, 1983
44. Finch C, Felicio L, Flurkey K, Gee D, Mobb C, Nelson J, Osterberg H: Studies on ovarian-hypothalamic-pituitary interactions during reproductive aging in C57BL/6J mice. Peptides 1:163, 1980
45. Vermeulen A: The hormonal activity of the postmenopausal ovary. J Clin Endocrinol Metab 42:247, 1976
46. Judd H, Judd G, Lucas W, Yen SSC: Endocrine function of the postmenopausal ovary: concentration of androgens and estrogens in ovarian and peripheral vein blood. J Clin Endocrinol Metab 39:1020, 1974
47. Poortman J, Thijssen J, Schwarz F: Androgen production and conversion to estrogens in normal postmenopausal women and in selected breast cancer patients. J Clin Endocrinol Metab 37:101, 1974
48. Judd H, Lucas W, Yen SSC: Serum 17β-estradiol and estrone levels in postmenopausal women with and without endometrial cancer. J Clin Endocrinol Metab 42:272, 1976
49. Hashimoto T, Miyai K, Izumi K, Kumahara Y: Gonadotropin response to synthetic LH-RH in normal subjects: Correlation between LH and FSH. J Clin Endocrinol Metab 37:910, 1973
50. Meldrum D, Tataryn I, Fruman A, Erlik Y, Lu K, Judd H: Gonadotropins, estrogens, and adrenal steroids during the menopausal hot flush. J Clin Endocrinol Metab 50:685, 1980
51. Van Keep P, Brand P, Lehert P: Factors affecting the age at menopause. J Biosoc Sci [Suppl] 6:37, 1979
52. Gray R: Biological and social interactions in the determinations of late fertility. J Biosoc Sci [Suppl] 6:97, 1979
53. Gray R: The menopause: epidemiological and demographic considerations. In The Menopause, Edited by RJ Beard. Lancaster, MTP Press, 1976, p 25
54. Leridon H: Patterns of fertility at later ages of reproduction. J Biosoc Sci [Suppl] 6:59, 1979
55. Bloom D: What's happening to the age at first birth in the United States? A study of recent cohorts. Demography 19:351, 1982
56. Hendershot G: Maternal age and overdue conceptions. Am J Public Health 74:35, 1984
57. Tietze C: Reproductive span and rate of reproduction among Hutterite women. Fertil Steril 8:89, 1957
58. Pittenger D: An exponential model of female sterility. Demography 10:113, 1973
59. Anderson B: Male age and fertility: results from Ireland prior to 1911. Popul Ind 41:561, 1975
60. Linn S, Schoenbaum S, Monson R, Rosner B, Ryan K: Delay in conception for former pill users. JAMA 247:629, 1982
61. Harlap S, Baras M: Conception waits in fertile women after stopping oral contraceptives. Int J Fertil 29:73, 1984
62. Leridon H: Biostatistics of human reproduction. In Measuring the Effects of Family Planning Programs on Fertility, Edited by B Chandrasekaran, A Hermalen. Belgium, Ordina Editions, 1975, p 93
63. Warburton D, Fraser F: Spontaneous abortion risks in man: data from reproductive histories collected in a medical genetics unit. Hum Genet 16:1, 1964

64. Wright E: Chromosomes and human fetal development. In The Biology of Human Fetal Growth, Edited by D Roberts, A Thomson. London, Taylor and Francis, Publishers, 1976, p 237
65. Creasy M, Crolla J, Alberman E: A cytogenetic study of human spontaneous abortion using banding technique. Hum Genet 31:177, 1976
66. Warburton D, Kline J, Stein Z, Strobino B: Cytogenetic abnormalities in spontaneous abortions of recognized conceptions. In Perinatal Genetics: Diagnosis and Treatment, Edited by IH Porter, A Willey. New York, Academic Press, 1986, p 133
67. Warburton D: Unpublished data
68. Hassold T, Jacobs P, Kline J: Effect of maternal age on autosomal trisomies. Ann Hum Genet 44:29, 1980
69. Henderson S, Edwards R: Chiasma frequency and maternal age in mammals. Nature 218:22, 1968
70. Sugawara S, Mikamo K: An experimental approach to the analysis of mechanisms of meiotic dysjunction and anaphase lagging in primary oocytes. Cytogenet Cell Genet 20:251, 1980
71. Crowley P, Guleh D, Hayden T, Lopez P, Dyer R: A chiasma-hormonal hypothesis relating Down's syndrome and maternal age. Nature 280:417, 1979
72. Read S: The distribution of Down's syndrome. J Ment Defic Res 26:215, 1982
73. Brook D, Gosden R, Chandley A: Maternal aging and aneuploid embryos-evidence from the mouse that biological and not chronological age is the important influence. Hum Genet 66:41, 1984
74. Alberman E, Creasy M: Factors affecting chromosome abnormalities in human conceptions. In Chromosome Variations in Human Evolution, Edited by A Boyce. London, Taylor & Frances, 1976, p 83
75. Ford J: Induction of chromosomal errors. Lancet 1:54, 1973
76. Simpson J: Disorders of Sexual Differentiation. New York, Academic Press, 1976
77. Craig, Jollee W: The response of the uterine surface to ovarian hormones in the aged rat. Anat Embryol [Berl] 169:205, 1984
78. Morrison I: The elderly primigravida. Am J Obstet Gynecol 121:465, 1975
79. Kirz D, Dorchester W, Freeman R: Advanced maternal age: the mature gravida. Am J Obstet Gynecol 152:7, 1985
80. Blum M: Is the elderly primipara really at high risk? J Perinat Med 7:108, 1979
81. Gindoff P, Jewelewicz R: Use of gonadotropins in ovulation induction: analysis of treatment protocols and pregnancy outcome. NY State J Med 85:580, 1985

Chapter 2

Smoking and reproduction

Robert J. Stillman, M.D.
Michael J. Rosenberg, M.D., M.P.H.
Benjamin P. Sachs, M.D., D.P.H.

The George Washington School of Medicine, Washington, District of Columbia; Reproductive Epidemiology, Family Health International, Research Triangle Park, North Carolina; and Beth Israel Hospital, Harvard Medical School, Boston, Massachusetts

Approximately 30% of women and 36% of men of reproductive age in the United States smoke, as do an increasing percentage of adolescents and teenage girls.[1] In addition to those who voluntarily expose themselves to the recognized hazards of smoking, nonsmokers are also affected by inhaling "sidestream" smoke from burning cigarettes and from exhaled "passive smoking". The high prevalence of smoking and its variety of deleterious health effects has led the Surgeon General of the United States to label smoking "the chief single avoidable cause of death in our society, and the most important public health issue of our time."[1]

Cigarette smoke contains several hundred substances, including nicotine, carbon monoxide, and recognized carcinogens and mutagens, such as radioactive polonium, benzo(a)pyrine, dimethylbenz(a)anthracene, dimethylnitrosamine, napthalene, and methylnapthalene.[2] Many constituents, however, have not been evaluated for their toxicity. The full ingredients of cigarettes remain unknown; they are not required to be revealed. Inhalation of cigarette smoke, whether through active or passive smoking, leads to absorption of these substances through the pulmonary vasculature and bloodborne circulation throughout the body.

In August 1985, a two-part article by Fielding, "Smoking: Health Effects and Control," appeared in the Medical Progress section of the *New England Journal of Medicine*.[3] It is at once a sobering and an enlightening review of the magnitude of the public health risks attributed to cigarette smoking:

> The estimated annual excess mortality from cigarette smoking in the United States exceeds 350,000. . . . It has been estimated that an average of 5½ minutes of life is lost for each cigarette smoked, on the basis of an average reduction in life expectancy for cigarette smokers of five to eight years. . . . One recent analysis of mortality suggests that differences in the rates of cigarette smoking between men and women over the age of 30 are the overwhelming cause of male–female longevity differences, and that increases in the difference in life expectancy between the sexes since 1930 are largely attributable to cigarette smoking.

Except for a short section on in utero effects of maternal smoking, the effect of smoking on reproductive health is not addressed in Fielding's review.[3] Thus, given the importance of the subject matter to reproductive biologists, clinicians, and their patients, a review of the currently available epidemiologic and experimental data on this subject is warranted. We address the evidence for and possible causes of a perturbation of physiologic characteristics in three major areas of reproduction: female fertility, male fertility, and the effect of smoking in pregnancy. Numerous other important aspects of smoking and women's health care, including effects on genital tract and breast cancers, osteoporosis, contraceptives, public policy, and smoking prevention, were addressed in the recent International Conference on Smoking and Reproductive Health in San Francisco. These subjects will be dealt with in the forthcoming publication of the symposium proceedings[4] and are beyond the scope of this review.

EFFECT OF SMOKING ON FEMALE FERTILITY

A number of epidemiologic studies address the effects of cigarette smoking on fecundity (ability to conceive during a given menstrual cycle).[5–17] Methodologic issues, such as patient selection, choice of controls, and treatment of potentially confounding variables, may be raised against most of these studies when addressed individually, but viewed as a whole this literature clearly demonstrates a reduction in the fecundity of women who smoke. In support of these studies, there exist experimental data that address the biologic plausibility and the proposed mechanisms by which cigarette smoking may affect the ability of these women to conceive.

EPIDEMIOLOGIC DATA

Thirteen studies that touch upon this subject (Table 1) warrant discussion.

1. Tokuhata[5] retrospectively evaluated reproductive history in a cohort of 2016 deceased, married women. Data, including infertility (defined as never being pregnant) and smoking history, were obtained by interview or questionnaire of surviving family members. Sixteen percent of the cohort (314 women) were never pregnant. "Habitual" cigarette smokers had significantly increased frequency of infertility (21%), compared with both nonsmokers (14%) and users of tobacco, snuff, or chew (12%) (Table 2). Potential confounding risk factors were evaluated, including the cause, age, and year of death, education, race, occupation, and the husband's tobacco use, education, and occupation. The adjusted odds ratios (OR) averaged 1.46,* suggesting that there were 46% more cases of infertility among smokers than among nonsmokers. The observed differences were not accounted for by any of the nine attributes considered within the analysis. Some methodologic issues should be mentioned. The use of the death registry for patient acquisition to the study limits the randomness of selection and the ability to generalize the results of the study, but it does allow use of an older population whose reproductive history is completed. Information obtained from family members may not be accurate, but actually it may be biased against including infertile women, who may not have had family members to contact, and therefore would have been excluded from the study. Defining infertility as those women who were never pregnant does not allow exclusion of male factor infertility or voluntary childlessness. However, this latter group may represent a small percentage of never-pregnant women but not a higher percentage of smoking than nonsmoking women.

2. Howe et al.[6] reported results from the Oxford Family Planning Association contraceptive study, which followed 17,032 white married women of childbearing age for an average of 11.5 years. Of these women, 4104 stopped birth control methods to plan a pregnancy on a total of 6199 occasions. The influence of various factors, including smoking, on fertility of this cohort of women was assessed by measuring the time taken to give birth to a child and the time to conceive.

A consistent and highly significant trend of decreasing fertility with increasing number of cigarettes smoked per day was seen, especially in women smoking $\geq$ 16 cigarettes/day. Exsmokers did not show any decrease in fertility relative to non (never)–smokers. The inverse dose–response between smoking and decreased fertility suggested a causal relationship (Table 3). The large number of women with long follow–up periods improves the power of this study to detect even small differences that may have existed. The differences appear minimal for women smoking $<$ 16 cigarettes/day but are striking thereafter. One criticism of this study is the potential misclassification of smokers. Smoking habits were classified when patients first entered the contraceptive study and may have changed by the time the women started to try to conceive. Women who quit smoking cigarettes after entry would be misclassified as nonsmokers, and vice versa. However, because this study revealed a decreased fecundity among smokers but not among exsmok-

---

*The odds ratio (OR) is a calculated estimate of risk in a case–control study design, comparable to a relative risk or risk ratio in a cohort study. It represents the proportion of smokers with an adverse result, compared with the proportion of nonsmokers with the same result. An odds ratio $>$ 1.0 suggests an increased risk and $<$ 1.0 a protective effect. When the 95% confidence interval for the odds ratio excludes 1.0, the risk is significant, designated, for example, OR 2.1; 1.3 to 2.5 95% confidence interval (CI).

Table 1. *Summary of the Epidemiologic Studies Evaluating the Effect of Smoking on Fecundity*[a]

Author, year	Study design	Sample size	Adjusted OR (95% CI if available)[b]	Potential confounders controlled
Tokuhata, 1968[5]	Retrospective cohort	2016	1.5	Cause, age, and year of death, education, occupation, tobacco use, education and occupation of husband
Howe et al., 1985[6]	Retrospective cohort	6199	1.3 (1.1–1.4)	Contraception, age, social class, age at marriage, parity
Friedman, 1977[7]	Cohort	227	1.0	None
Olsen et al., 1982[8]	Case-control	1069 infertile 4305 matched control	2.1 (1.7–2.5)	Alcohol, contraception, age, residence, education, parity, male factor
	Retrospective cohort[c]	4305[c]	1.8 (1.3–2.5)	
Linn et al., 1982[9]	Retrospective cohort	3214	1.0 (0.9–1.2)	Contraception, age, parity, menarche, body mass, education, history of spontaneous abortion, induced abortion, ectopics, pelvic inflammatory disease, DES exposure, race, religion
Daling et al., 1985[10]	Case-control	159 primary tubal infertility 159 matched controls	3.3 (1.9–5.6)	Race, residence, age
Daling, 1986[11]	Case-control	170 primary tubal infertility 170 matched controls[d]	2.7 (1.4–5.3)[e]	IUD use, no. of sexual partners, age, race, payment status, income, husband smoking, herpes, gonorrhea, pelvic surgery, education, religion
Cramer et al., 1983[12]	Case-control	388 tubal infertility 1380 infertility 4023 matched controls	1.6 (1.3–2.0) 1.1 (1.0–1.2)	Age, race, payment status, education, no. of sexual partners
Phipps et al., 1986[13]	Case-control	225 primary tubal infertility 901 primary infertility 1264 matched controls[f]	1.6	Age, religion, education, no. of sexual partners, contraceptive use
Harlap and Barras, 1982[14]	Retrospective cohort	5880	1.0	None
Mai et al., 1977[15]	Case-control	50 fertile 50 infertile	> 1.0	None
Baird and Wilcox, 1984[16]	Retrospective cohort	678	1.4 (1.1–1.7)	Age, parity, infertility, intercourse frequency, oral contraception, recent pregnancy, alcohol, body mass
de Mouzon, 1985[17]	Prospective	1576	1.1 (0.8–1.7)	Contraception, parity, occupation, reference year

[a]Modified from Spira.
[b]OR, odds ratio.
[c]Separate analyses among the control patients assessing time to conceive by smoking habits.
[d]From same cohort as Daling.[10]
[e]Further increased risk noted with increased pack years, earlier age at start of smoking, coincident IUD use and/or increasing number of sex partners.
[f]From same cohort as Cramer.[12]

ers, both of these misclassifications actually would minimize the magnitude of risk attributed to smoking.

3. Friedman[7] studied the pregnancy rate of 227 women entering a donor insemination program. He mentioned that no influence of cigarette smoking was found. No method of analysis or evaluation is discussed. Other confounding factors that influence pregnancy rate are not accounted for, such as additional female infertility factors. Ma-

Table 2. *Percentage of Women Never Pregnant Compared By Race and Cigarette Use*[a]

Race	% Women never pregnant			
	No. of women	All	Non-smokers	Smokers
All	2016	15.6	14.2	21.3
White	1297	13.9	12.4	18.6
Nonwhite	719	18.6	18.8	28.1

[a]Modified from Tokuhata.[5]

jor methodologic deficiencies and the small sample size unfortunately limit the usefulness of this study's conclusions.

4. Olsen and colleagues[8] recruited 927 women evaluated for infertility at a university hospital and 3728 contemporaneous delivery controls from the same hospital in a case control study. Analysis was by logistic regression, adjusting for age and parity, residence, education, and alcohol consumption. Smoking history is defined simply as "yes" or "no." Cigarette smoking increased the odds ratio (OR) of infertility to 2.1 (1.7 to 2.5, 95% CI), compared with delivery controls. The increased risk of infertility in smokers was found to persist after separating primary infertility (no prior liveborn) (OR = 1.6; 1.1 to 2.2, 95% CI) or secondary infertility (OR = 2.1; 1.3 to 3.6, 95% CI) and after infertility due to male factor was excluded (OR = 2.3; 1.8 to 2.9, 95% CI). Selection bias may have been introduced because only those couples seeking infertility care were included. Infertility couples seeking care are not necessarily representative of all infertile couples and may not be representative regarding smoking habits. Another potential bias includes the delivery control group. This group may be biased against smoking, because their smoking habits were ascertained in the year of delivery, which coincides with their pregnancy—a time when some of these individuals may have stopped smoking and therefore may be classified as nonsmokers. These two potential weaknesses are adequately managed by a separate evaluation and analysis done among the delivery control patients themselves: an evaluation of the relative time to conception among delivery patients in relation to their smoking history. Delivery control patients who smoked had a significantly increased risk of a conception delay greater than 1 year, compared with those who did not. This relationship held whether conception delay before a past pregnancy (OR = 1.6), before the current pregnancy (OR = 1.5), or before both a past and the current pregnancy (OR = 2.0) was assessed. The results of both types of analyses in this study provide consistent evidence for an association between smoking and infertility/conception delay. This study was also the first to report a significant association between smoking and tubal cause of infertility ($P < 0.05$) compared with other causes in smokers. This theme is expanded upon below.

5. Linn et al.[9] evaluated conception delays after stopping various contraceptives in 3214 fertile married women interviewed after delivery. As part of their analysis, they compared women who smoked during pregnancy, with those who had never smoked or who had stopped smoking before the pregancy. No differences in the time to conception (OR = 1.0; 0.9 to 1.2, 95% CI) were found between these two groups. Logistic regression analysis adjusted for confounding factors, including age, previous reproductive history, and type of contraception that was stopped to conceive. Unfortunately, smokers and nonsmokers may have been misclassified, dampening any effect of smoking that might be present, because women who smoked during pregnancy (classified here as smokers) may not have smoked during any of the time they attempted to conceive, and women who smoked throughout their attempts at conceiving but who stopped just before becoming pregnant would have been classified as nonsmokers. Further evaluation and appropriate classification would be needed to measure the effect of smoking on delayed conception in this study.

6. In a paper addressing tubal infertility and the intrauterine device (IUD), Daling et al.[10] reported evaluating the smoking habits in 159 pa-

Table 3. *Dose-Response Effect of Cigarette Smoking on the Time to Conception in Women After Stopping Contraception*[a]

Smoking status (number/day)	No. of episodes attempting pregnancy	No. of months follow-up	Fertility	
			Relative rate[c]	95% CI
Never smoked	3672	134	1.0	
Former smoker	843	111	0.99	(0.92–1.07)
1–5	389	54	0.99	(0.9–1.11)
6–10	485	94	0.97	(0.88–1.07)
11–15	374	105	0.93	(0.84–1.04)
16–20	334	93	0.79	(0.7–0.89)
≥ 21	97	29	0.78	(0.62–0.97)

[a]Modified from Howe and colleagues.[6]

[b]Some women followed through attempting more than one pregnancy.

[c]P (trend) < 0.0001 time to conception, adjusted for type of contraception stopped.

Table 4. *Relation of Cigarette Smoking to the Risk of Primary Tubal Infertility*[a]

Smoking status	IUD Use	Cases	Controls	Relative risk[b]	95% confidence interval
		No.	*No.*		
Never smoked	Never	52	98	1.0	
Current smoked	Never	48	25	2.6	1.2–5.6
Never smoked	Ever	27	17	2.3	1.0–5.3
Current smoker	Ever	19	2	6.7	1.4–32.2

[a]From Daling.[11]

[b]Risk relative to that of women who never smoked and never used an IUD, adjusted for income and number of sexual partners.

tients who had a diagnosis of primary tubal infertility, compared with 159 matched controls who delivered. They found that 38% of patients who had primary tubal infertility were current cigarette smokers, compared with 16% of the controls (OR = 3.3; 1.9 to 5.6, 95% CI), the greatest risk to fertility attributed to smoking in any study to date. There were no analyses of other confounding factors in this part of their study.

7. In a follow–up study of the above IUD paper, Daling[11] more closely evaluated the smoking habits of 170 patients with primary infertility due to tubal factor and again compared them with matched controls. IUD use, number of sexual partners, and income were controlled in this study in the logistic regression analysis. After control of these confounding factors, the significant risk of smoking to tubal infertility remained, with 39% of patients smoking at the time they started trying to conceive, compared with only 16% of controls (OR = 2.7). The smoking habits of husbands did not affect ability to conceive, nor did former (not current) smoking habits. Heavy smoking (smoking ≥ 5 pack–years) increased the OR for tubal infertility to 4.2, compared with smokers smoking < 5 pack–years. The size of the smoking/infertility association also increased markedly with earlier age of starting smoking and the usual number of cigarettes smoked per day. For smokers who also wore an IUD, there was a multiplicative effect of risk of tubal infertility (OR = 6.7) compared with either the risk of smoking and tubal infertility without IUD use (OR = 2.7) or IUD use and tubal infertility without smoking (OR = 2.6) (Table 4). The same multiplicative risk is observed when evaluating patients with tubal infertility for smoking habits and number of sexual partners, compared with nonsmokers. Current smokers with a history of one to four sexual partners had an OR = 2.7 of having tubal infertility; this increased to 5.7 for current smokers with ≥ 5 sexual partners (Table 5).

8. Cramer and colleagues[12] studied smoking as one of the risk factors in a multicollaborative study of prior IUD use and subsequent tubal infertility. Their profile of 1880 patients seeking infertility care revealed 47.9% who had ever smoked, similar to 45.6% smokers among 4023 matched delivery control patients (OR = 1.1; 1.0 to 1.2, 95% CI). However, among the 1880 infertility patients were 388 with tubal infertility, 56.7% of whom smoked—a significant increase in the OR to 1.6. In general, the profile patients with tubal disease were older, more likely to be smokers, less educated, and had had more sexual partners than women in general. These variables, including smoking, were controlled for in a multivariate regression analysis as each having had independent effect in the risk of tubal infertility, independent of the IUD. This observation is consistent with the findings of Daling[11] and Olsen et al.[8] that at least part of smoking's apparent association to infertility is its relationship to tubal disease. A potential bias in the study[12] is enrolling only women who attended pregnancy classes as controls, the women who by the author's definition had not miscarried nor had unplanned pregnancies, thereby excluding a group who may smoke more. In addition, prior pelvic inflammatory disease (PID), ectopic pregnancy, and spontaneous abortions were not controlled for in the analysis.

Table 5. *Relation of Cigarette Smoking to the Risk of Primary Tubal Infertility According to Lifetime Number of Sexual Partners*[a]

Smoking status	No. of sexual partners	Cases	Controls	Relative risk[b]	95% confidence interval
		No.	*No.*		
Never smoked	1–4	57	96	1.0	
Current smoker	1–4	28	18	2.7	1.2–6.2
Never smoked	≥ 5	22	19	1.6	0.7–3.6
Current smoker	≥ 5	39	9	5.2	2.1–12.5

[a]From Daling.[11]

[b]Risk relative to women who never smoked and who had one to four sexual partners, adjusted for income and IUD use.

9. To answer some of the above concerns, Phipps and colleagues[13] further evaluated the Boston collaborative cohort just described, comparing in more detail the smoking history of 901 women with primary infertility of various causes with 1264 matched delivery controls. Controlling for a variety of potentially confounding factors, including contraception, number of sexual partners, age, and education, there was a significant ($P < 0.01$) risk association with smoking among the 225 patients with tubal infertility (OR = 1.6). A dose–response relationship of increasing risk of tubal infertility with greater amount of smoking was also found. Ninety-six patients with cervical factor infertility had a slightly increased risk association with smoking, and for 191 patients with endometriosis and 389 patients with ovulatory factor infertility no association with smoking was detectable. The conclusion that cigarette smoking is associated significantly with infertility, and primarily with tubal infertility, is strongly supported.

10. To study the effect of contraception on subsequent time to conception, Harlap and Barras[14] did postpartum interviews on 5880 women who had stopped using contraceptives to conceive. Although the data are not shown or discussed, it was stated that neither education, social class, nor smoking had an effect on fertility. Methodologic concerns (e.g., interviewing only patients who delivered, thereby eliminating patients who miscarried) and other issues that may affect the validity of these negative conclusions are difficult to assess, not having been included in the methods or discussion.

11. Mai and colleagues[15] compared psychiatric interviews between 50 consecutive infertile couples and 50 fertile women. The infertile women were found to have significantly more variability in the number of cigarettes smoked per day (standard deviation 6.27 versus 4.85; $P < 0.05$) and a somewhat higher average number of cigarettes per day (7.8 versus 7.0). These differences are, however, due to a few of the infertile women who smoked excessively. A variety of methodologic problems, including sample size, method of interview, and choice of controls, limit any conclusions from this study.

12. Baird and Wilcox[16] conducted a retrospective cohort study specifically designed to test the hypothesis that women who smoke have reduced fecundity. This study, like the studies of Howe et al.,[6] Linn et al.,[9] and Harlap and Barras,[14] compared delay in conception after stopping contraception in smoking versus nonsmoking women. Of 678 women, 35% of nonsmokers and only 28% of smokers conceived in the first cycle off contraception. The overall mean pregnancy rate per cycle for smokers was 22%, significantly lower than the 32% per cycle for nonsmokers. Even after adjusting for age, body mass, husband's smoking habits, parity, previous infertility, frequency of intercourse, oral contraceptive as the last contraception used, recent pregnancy or nursing, and alcohol consumption, smokers still had a conception rate per cycle of only 72% of that of nonsmokers (OR = 1.4; 1.1 to 1.7, 95% CI). A trend toward a dose–response effect of heavier smoking on fecundity was observed: the fertility of light smokers ($\leq$ 20 cigarettes/day) was 75% that of nonsmokers and the fertility of heavy smokers ($>$ 20 cigarettes/day) fell to 57% that of nonsmokers. Smokers were 3.4 times more likely to have taken more than 1 year longer than nonsmokers to conceive.

13. In his review, Spira[17] mentioned (as a personal communication) a prospective study of 1576 French couples desiring to conceive were recruited as volunteers from newspaper announcements. The authors, de Mouzon and colleagues, were reported to find a highly significant decrease in fecundity among smokers. However, after controlling for various factors, including contraception, parity, occupation, and reference year, this significance was lost (risk ratio 1.1; 0.8 to 1.7, 95% CI). These data, including the patient population enlisted, methods of recruitment, and analyses, should be critically evaluated, if the text is published.

Of the epidemiologic studies that can be evaluated for the influence of smoking on fecundity, most reveal a decreased rate of conception or fertility associated with smoking, versus control, patients. Spira[17] appropriately emphasized the difference between an association and causation. In evaluating causation, one must look at the strength of the association, at dose–response effect, and at the specificity of the association, its consistency, and its biologic plausibility. The strength of association of smoking and decreased fecundity, although significant, is not overwhelming in most studies. There is the suggestion of a dose–response effect in those studies, but this phenomenon needs more evaluation. The specificity of the association is not great, but the consistency of the findings is good, although not completely uniform. In studies such as those of Howe et al.,[6] Olsen et al.,[8] Daling et al.,[10] Daling,[11] Cramer et al.,[12] Phipps et al.,[13] and, especially, Baird and Wilcox,[16] the association of smoking to decreased fecundity is well supported, especially in relationship to primary tubal infertility. The possibility that this association is related to the different life styles of smokers, such as increased number of sexual partners, increased risk and frequency of pelvic inflammatory disease,[18] and a direct effect of smoking on the likelihood of acquiring pelvic inflammatory disease, remains an important unresolved issue. However, these potentially confounding factors have been controlled in the analyses of a number of these studies, supporting the significance of this epidemiologic association and helping in part to satisfy the stringent medical definition of causation. Biologic plausibility of an effect of smoking on fecundity would further help the "causation" argument. Thus evidence for such biologic plausibility and mechanisms of action need to be evaluated.

BIOLOGIC PLAUSIBILITY AND MECHANISM OF ACTION OF SMOKING AND DIMINISHED FECUNDITY

Effects on Tubal Function and Embryo Transport

Support for a mechanism of action explaining the effect of smoking on tubal infertility comes from both human and animal data. Neri and Eckerling[19] evaluated the influence of smoking and epinephrine on uterotubal insufflation. They evaluated 50 women in each of four groups: (1) intramuscular epinephrine; (2) smoking one cigarette; (3) intramuscular saline (placebo); and (4) no treatment (placebo). They performed a Rubin's test before and 5 minutes after the therapy (or after no therapy). Significant increases in uterotubal wave amplitude and tonus were seen after both epinephrine and cigarette smoking, in marked contrast to patients given placebo or no therapy, who usually demonstrated decreases in these parameters during the second test. In a later study, Neri and Marcus[20] injected nicotine into rhesus monkeys and recorded in vivo measurements of tubal function through an indwelling tubal catheter. Follicular-phase responses were biphasic, with first a higher tone and amplitude, followed by a marked inhibition of tubal activity. Luteal-phase injections resulted in little alteration of baseline function. Similar stimulatory responses on the rabbit oviduct were demonstrated by Ruckebusch,[21] after exposure of the rabbits to either cigarette smoke or adrenergic drugs. The smoking/nicotine-induced effects generally are believed to be mediated via epinephrine and/or vasopressin release, shown to increase in blood and urine studies after smoking.[22] Although many gaps exist in our information, these animal and human effects of cigarettes/nicotine may translate into altered uterine tubal function. A clinical manifestation of alterations in gamete transport might be decreased fecundity. On one hand, potential delay in embryo transport might decrease embryo viability or increase the frequency of ectopic tubal gestation from retained embryos. On the other hand, impairment of implantation/nidation from accelerated embryo transport and early entrance into the uterus also might affect fertility .

Ectopic tubal gestation, although not technically a decrease in fecundity, affects fertility and is often a manifestation of tubal dysfunction. An important piece of evidence linking smoking and ectopic gestation in humans comes from Campbell and Gray,[23] who reported the results of a multinational case control study from the World Health Organization in which 1108 women with confirmed ectopic tubal gestation were matched to both a pregnant woman who delivered and a nonpregnant control. The data were adjusted for confounding variables, such as history of PID, gonorrhea, prior ectopic gestation, contraceptives, tubal ligation, and induced abortion. Significantly more women with ectopic gestation were smokers, compared with controls (OR = 2.2 to 4.0, depending upon whether pregnant or nonpregnant controls were matched and whether the case came originally from a developed or developing country). Matsunaga and Shiota[24] supported these data in describing an excess of smokers among women with ectopic pregnancy, compared with women having induced abortions, as a finding in their cross-sectional study on teratogenicity. Unfortunately, no adjustment for confounding variables, such as sexual history or PID, were included. Levin et al.,[25] in evaluating ectopic gestation risk from prior induced abortion, also noted that smoking tended to increase the risk for tubal ectopic gestation.

In numerous studies, cigarette smoking has been demonstrated to affect adversely both the humoral and cellular immune systems.[26] Such alterations might affect tubal epithelial response to inflammation and, it is speculated, result in an increased frequency of tubal infection and subsequent infertility. Thus, overall, some human studies and animal work support the possibility of altered tubal physiologic features, with altered tubal transport, possible early or delayed entry of blastocyst into the uterus, and alterations in the immune system that can account for the epidemiologic association between smoking and decreased fecundity from tubal causes.[19–26]

Effects of Preimplantation Embryo and Implantation

Alterations in tubal physiologic features may not be the sole factor in the effect of smoking on fecundity. The effect of smoking on human endometrial response to estrogen and progesterone or the ability of the conceptuses to implant are unknown. The increased frequency of spontaneous abortions of chromosomally normal conceptuses observed in women who smoke[27] (discussed below) suggests possible interference with placentation or implantation. Card and Mitchell[28] demonstrated that nicotine treatment impaired decidualization in the pseudopregnant rat, possibly through an effect of decreasing progesterone. Yoshinaga and colleagues[29] demonstrated a nicotine-induced delay in conceptus cleavage from two- to four-cell stage, delayed conceptus entry into the uterus, delayed blastocyst formation, delayed shedding of the zona pellucida, and delayed implantation in response to pharmacologic doses of nicotine. Nicotine treatment also altered the spacing of implantation sites, producing considerable crowding at the tubal end of the uterus, perhaps due to altered uterotubal motility. These observations confirmed and extended previous observations indicating that nicotine prolonged gestation and delayed implantation in the rat. Because Yoshinaga and colleagues[29] also demonstrated lower progesterone levels, an indirect effect caused by nicotine's effect on corpus luteal function cannot be excluded. However, these delays in conceptus cleavage, blastocyst formation, and zona shedding may be due to nicotine's presence in the fallopian tube and/or uterus. In elegant studies, McLachlan and colleagues[30] demonstrated that nicotine concentrated in uterine and oviductal fluid of six-day-pregnant rabbits. The uterine fluid concentrations were ten times that in the plasma. Nicotine was also concentrated directly in preimplantation blastocysts, giving evidence for direct interaction of the drug on the developing zygote while still in the tube and uterus.

Effects on Gametes

Effects of smoking on gamete maturation and function also can affect male or female fertility. Effects on spermatogenesis and sperm function are discussed later. Direct effects on oocyte viability or maturation or an acceleration of the rate of oocyte atresia may affect female fecundity. A large body of experimental evidence in animals supports the hypothesis that smoke, or its toxic components, such as nicotine or polycyclic aromatic hydrocarbons, results in oocyte/follicle destruction and leads to accelerated loss of reproductive function.[27] Oocyte destruction in rats and mice has been shown to encompass not only primordial follicles, but growing preovulatory follicles and even oocyte meiosis. These experiments demonstrate deleterious dose-response effects on oocyte/follicle destruction and function in histologic-sectioned ovaries. Also noted is a dose-response effect of these compounds on fertility of rats bred after exposure to smoke or its selected components. The oocyte or the process of fertilization also may be altered: nicotine has been shown to prevent cortical granule formation, inhibiting the block to polyspermy.[31] A polyspermic embryo might fail to develop (seen clinically as decreased fecundity) or later abort. Species differences in oocyte sensitivity to these compounds, dose effects of injected nicotine or polycyclic aromatic hydrocarbons are, of course, among other concerns that limit extrapolation of these animal data to humans. However, the weight of experimental evidence and the similarity of effects to those seen after known hazards (e.g., ionizing radiation and alkylating agents) make for a reasonable and biologically plausible hypothesis.[27]

Epidemiologic evidence in humans to support the animal data of the adverse effects of smoking on oocyte viability would add to the reasonableness of the hypothesis. The only such data come from a number of human studies that associate cigarette smoking with the decreasing age of menopause.[27] Jick et al.[32] demonstrated a clear inverse dose-response relationship between smoking and age at menopause: increasing cigarette consumption results in decreasing age of spontaneous menopause. Mattison[27] summarized the data from six other studies, all confirming the same association. His review of this (and of smoking's effect on the reproductive process) is especially worthwhile. Some of these studies also eliminated potentially confounding factors, such as the body weight of smokers, that could affect the age at menopause. Thus based on animal models and human effects on age at menopause comes a hypothesis that cigarette smoking depletes oocyte viability and/or number. This depletion in humans may result in an earlier age of the loss of reproductive function: menopause. This earlier menopause may be the endpoint of a process taking place throughout a smoker's reproductive life, namely the effect of smoking on oocyte meiosis, follicular maturation, and oocyte viability. A decrease in fecundity might result.

Effects of smoking on the ovulatory mechanism and granulosa cell function are more speculative and may be difficult to separate from smoking's effects on the central hormonal control of the menstrual cycle.[22]

Effects on Menstrual Cyclicity

Some anecdotal clinical support for the effect of cigarette smoking on menstrual function in women exists, although no detailed study with appropriate experimental design has been organized to evaluate this important issue.[22] Pettersson and colleagues observed a higher frequency of secondary amenorrhea among smokers, compared with nonsmokers.[33] In 1961, Hammond[34] studied physical complaints of more than 24,000 women. He found an increase in abnormal vaginal bleeding in smokers, with heavy smokers (> 1 pack/day) demonstrating a 67% increase (OR = 1.7), significantly greater than nonsmokers. He also found current smokers, and especially heavy smokers, more likely to have had irregular menses in the fourth and fifth decades of life than nonsmokers. More smokers than nonsmokers between the ages of 30 and 39 years had had hysterectomy, and fewer had had pregnancies. These effects also were exaggerated with heavier smoking. Bernhardt[35] also suggested that menstrual disorders (and infertility) were more common among smokers. MacMahon and colleagues[36] reported that smokers have significantly lower concentrations of urinary estriol, estradiol, and estrone during the luteal phase of ovulatory cycles, compared with former smokers. Follicular-phase estrogens were diminished, but not significantly so. These data are supported by reports of decreased frequency of breast cancer,[37] endometrial cancer,[38] and endometriosis[39] and an increase in the risk of osteoporosis[40] (unrelated to weight) among smokers. Because these are estrogen-dependent phenomena, diminished estrogen secretion or altered metabolism associated with cigarette smoking has been suggested.

Numerous animal studies demonstrate that nicotine or cigarette smoke can, in a dose-dependent fashion, alter mechanisms controlling the release of gonadotropins and cyclicity. Most studies performed have evaluated the female rat hypothalamus and pituitary. Nicotine is suggested as the primary constituent in smoke that produces these effects, although other constituents in cigarette smoke may or may not modify the nicotine-induced changes. Nicotine itself may act directly or may work through its well-described enhancement of vasopressin, which can diminish luteinizing hormone (LH).[27] Blake et al.[41] demonstrated that nicotine itself diminished LH in a dose-dependent fashion by delaying, blunting, or completely abolishing the LH surge in preoestrus rats. Similar, but less demonstrable, effects were seen on prolactin secretion. No abnormality in the pituitary response to luteinizing hormone-releasing hormone (LHRH) was noted, suggesting that the effect of nicotine was not at the pituitary level. Similar findings were made by McLean and colleagues,[42] who also found that there was a decrease in the percentage of rats ovulating after exposure to nicotine. Catecholaminergic and adrenergic adrenal responses (increasing cortisol) and an increase in growth hormone have been demonstrated in a number of studies, including human studies, although these human studies have been generally restricted to men. Little work is available on women.[22, 27] Taken together, these clinical reports in human and animal studies emphasize the effect of nicotine/smoke on the central hormonal homeostasis of women, which may affect ovulatory cyclicity and hence fecundity.

In summary from the evidence available today, a strong association exists between smoking and decreased female fecundity and fertility, including dose-response effects. Continued assurance is needed that potential confounding variables, already controlled for in many studies, do not cloud the association. The argument supporting causation is growing but needs further study. The association between smoking and fecundity seems most clear for patients with tubal factor infertility. Biologic plausibility and experimental evidence exists to support altered tubal function, transport, immune surveillance, and even increased ectopic gestations, further implicating a tubal mechanism of action as one means of decreasing fecundity in smokers. Other possible mechanisms with experimental support suggest that cigarette smoke and its constituents may have adverse effects along a continuum of preimplantational and implantation reproductive processes in women, including gamete production and function, ovulation and cyclicity, fertilization, early embryonic cleavage, embryo transport, and implantation. Most encouraging are the epidemiologic data suggesting that for former smokers, the risk to fecundity is minimized. Thus stopping smoking may diminish the risks inherent with its continuation. This path, therefore, seems most prudent for all women wishing to conceive, especially for those experiencing difficulty.

EFFECT OF SMOKING ON MALE FERTILITY

Recent interest in the effects of smoking on male reproduction has come about for two reasons. First, smoking is probably the most prevalent voluntary action that modifies susceptibility to a diverse variety of diseases in a generally deleterious fashion. Twenty eight million men, or 36% of the adult population, individually smoke an average of 20 cigarettes per day. Second is the growing realization that male reproduction can be impared by a small but increasing number of environmental and occupational exposures.[43] Reproductive problems such as fetal loss traditionally have been associated with women, and reproductive research, including that dealing with the effects of tobacco, has centered on women. The growing realization of a paternal component of reproductive impairment suggests that studying men is also appropriate.

Smoking's influence on men's ability to reproduce may be studied by two methods. The most direct method is to examine a reproductive outcome, such as ability to achieve pregnancy, among smokers and nonsmokers, while controlling for maternal smoking and other factors that might influence this relationship. The number of such studies are few, perhaps because of the relatively recent interest in reproductive aspects of smoking. The second method is to hypothesize a mechanism whereby smoking might impair reproduction and to investigate how smoking affects that mechanism. Postulating that smoking adversely affects reproduction by impairing sperm, however, involves two links: first, that smoking can adversely affect sperm numbers, motility, or morphologic features; and second, that this impairment results in difficulty conceiving or carrying a pregnancy to term and producing a healthy baby. The first of these links is the subject of a number of studies, but the second is methodologically challenging and the subject of a limited amount of data. Although the data suggest that impaired sperm are associated with decreased ability to conceive (most clearly in the case of instances of reduced sperm count), increased rates of spontaneous fetal loss, and possibly increased rates of congenital malformations, data also exist to the contrary, and are not sufficient to draw firm conclusions.

EPIDEMIOLOGIC DATA

Only two studies have been done to examine the relationship between paternal smoking and reproduction by using the first method, examining a reproductive outcome. The first, by Tokuhata,[5] investigated the role of smoking on infertility and fetal loss among 1608 couples. The effects on female fecundity were discussed earlier. Among the group in which none of the women smoked, the risk of infertility among couples in which the man smoked, compared with couples in which the man did not, was 0.7, and for fetal loss, 1.1. For couples in which the women smoked, the risk of infertility among those in which the man smoked (compared with those in which the man did not), was the same. This part of the study, however, is subject to methodologic limitations that may limit its credibility. For example, information on men's smoking was described as "less complete" than for the women. Also, the risk estimates were not adjusted for age or other potentially influencing factors. The recent study designed to investigate the influence of smoking on conception, by Baird and Wilcox,[16] revealed that, after considering a woman's smoking history, paternal smoking did not influence the probability of conception. This study, limited to women who had become pregnant, was analyzed by means of a logistic model that considered maternal smoking, age, frequency of intercourse, and seven other factors potentially related. Neither this nor the previously mentioned study, however, was designed to address the issue of men's smoking, and the presence of selection and other forms of bias probably limits their ability to detect a subtle effect of men's smoking.

Twelve investigators have studied how smoking affects spermatozoa.[43–54] These represent a variety of populations studied, methodologies employed, parameters evaluated, means of controlling confounding, and statistical evaluations. Methodologic details and how each affects the interpretation are discussed elsewhere[4] but should also be considered by the critical reader in evaluating these studies. In this format, we discuss this literature as a whole and attempt to facilitate comparisons of these diverse studies. Therefore, we present the mean values for sperm density, percentage of motile sperm, the proportion of normally shaped sperm, and the *P* values that result from the comparison of these means. Because *P* values reflect the number of subjects as well as the magnitude of the difference in values, we also calculated the odds ratio of an abnormal result (Table 6).

Sperm density is reduced in smokers in 11 of the 12[43-54] evaluations in which mean values for smokers and nonsmokers were reported and approximately equal in the remaining study.[49] For all studies, density averaged 22% lower in smokers than in nonsmokers, with the greatest reduction being 57%. Additional information comes from examining dose-response relationships of sperm density with differing levels of smoking. In the two studies that included this type of evaluation, a strong relationship existed, which indicated that higher levels of smoking are associated with lower levels of sperm density. Persons smoking zero, < 20, and ≥ 20 cigarettes per day had sperm concentrations of 55.5, 54.4, and 51.8 $\times 10^6$/ml, respectively.[49] The remaining study showed an equivocal relationship.[43] A third study followed sperm counts of men who stopped smoking.[44] While smoking, these men had a mean sperm density of 5.2 $\times 10^6$/ml; 6 months after stopping smoking, the mean density had risen more than nine times to a mean of 47.3 $\times 10^6$/ml.

Twelve studies include evaluations of sperm motility.[43-54] Of these, a lower proportion of motile sperm was found among smokers, compared with nonsmokers, in eight,[43, 45, 46, 50–53] a higher proportion in two,[49] and approximately equal proportions in two.[44, 45] The last study includes only the report of a nonsignificant difference between the two groups. For the first eight studies in which impairment was reported, the level of impairment averages 20% lower motility in smokers. Three studies include further information regarding the changes in sperm motility. Increased cigarette smoking was significantly associated with successively lower proportion of motile sperm in one study.[43] Among three men studied as they stopped smoking, the average number of sperm with "very good" motility improved from 27% to 45%.[44] The motility of former smokers did not differ from that of smokers or nonsmokers in another study,[54] and did not differ between nonsmokers, men smoking < 20 cigarettes/day, and men smoking > 20 cigarettes/day.[49]

Eleven studies include evaluations of the proportion of sperm with normal morphologic features. Five showed a lower proportion of such sperm among smokers,[43, 47, 48, 50, 51] one an increased proportion in smokers,[49] and four approximately equal proportions.[49, 52-54] The magnitude of the decrease averaged 17%, compared with the single study that showed an increase of 5%. Of the four evaluations of the relationship of morphologic features with differing levels of smokers, two showed increasing levels of smoking associated with increasing levels of abnormally shaped sperm[43, 47] and two showed no such association.[43, 54]

Any study may have weaknesses, but some of those included in this summary are important enough to affect the assessment of this body of literature. Perhaps the most important limitation of some of these studies is the relatively small number of subjects. When differences between groups are judged with a continuous sample test, such as the *t*-test, small numbers can limit the ability to detect a difference even if one actually exists. Although individual studies can fail to reflect significant differences in means, the body of literature as a whole is rather consistent in reflecting impairment of all three parameters of sperm function in smokers compared with nonsmokers.

A second consideration is the populations from which comparisons are made about the effects of smoking. Most studies are drawn from volunteers of infertility clinics. Bias that may be induced by using volunteers is difficult to quantitate, but generally, volunteers can be expected to be in better health than nonvolunteers. If nonsmoking volunteers are healthier as a group than smoking

Table 6. *Summary of Epidemiologic Studies Evaluating the Effect of Smoking on Semen Parameters*

Author, year	Study group	No. of subjects	Sample source	Sperm density			Motility			Morphology		
				Mean	Relative risk[a]	P-value[b,c]	Mean	Relative risk[a]	P-value[b,c]	Mean	Relative risk[a]	P-value[b,c]
				10^6/ml			%			% normal		
Viczian, 1969[43]	Smokers	120	Volunteers	61			53			73		
	Nonsmokers	50	Volunteers of proven fertility	74			69			81		
Schirren & Gey, 1968[44]	Smokers	1377			1.2			1.0				
	Nonsmokers	580										
Campbell & Harrison, 1979[45]	Smokers	134	Infertility clinic		1.6			1.3				
	Nonsmokers	119			(1.2–2.1)			(1.0–1.9)				
Vogel et al., 1979[46]	Smokers	17	Not specified		2.1		65.4		0.2			NS
	Nonsmokers	39			(1.4–3.3)		75.0					
Evans et al., 1981[47]	Smokers	43	Infertility clinic						> 0.5	52.9	1.4	
	Nonsmokers	43								57.7	(1.1–1.7)	
Godfrey, 1981[48]	Smokers	75	Infertility clinic			> 0.05			> 0.5	61.6		0.05
	Nonsmokers	74								65.4		
Rodriguez-Rigau et al., 1982[49]	Smokers	58	Infertility clinic excludes men with varicocele	55.5	0.9		58.5		> 0.05	44.8		< 0.05
	Nonsmokers	101		52.4	(0.6–1.5)		58.4			44.7		
	Smokers	38	Infertility clinic men with varicocele	52.3	0.9		60.3		> 0.05	44.0		> 0.05
	Nonsmokers	59		53.2	(0.6–1.4)		52.6			42.1		
Shaarawy, 1982[50]	Smokers	25	Healthy volunteers of unproven fertility	74.8		> 0.5	52.0		< 0.0005	52.0		< 0.0005
	Nonsmokers	20		80.8			78.0			75.0		
Spira, 1981[51]	Smokers	122	Vasectomy candidates	83.8		< 0.01	52.4		< 0.05	48.2		NS
	Nonsmokers	173		112.1			56.2			51.2		
	Smokers	292	Infertility clinic	67.0		NS	48.8		NS	40.2		< 0.02
	Nonsmokers	228		78.3			50.3			44.1		
Handlesman, et al., 1984[52]	Smokers	71	Healthy sperm donors	64.1		NS	67.0		0.001	73.4		NS
	Nonsmokers	23		95.5			72.0			74.8		
Kulikauskas et al., 1985[53]	Smokers	103	Infertility clinic and premarital exam	55.5		< 0.001	49.3		< 0.001	73.0		0.09
	Nonsmokers	135		27.3			63.2			74.3		
Vogt et al., 1986[54]	Smokers	150	Healthy volunteers	59.0		0.07	73.0		NS	68.8		
	Nonsmokers	52		72.9			74.0			68.0		

[a]Risk of abnormal result in smokers as compared to nonsmokers.
[b]Difference between means.
[c]NS, nonsignificant.

volunteers, this bias may extend to and explain some of the apparently better sperm parameters among nonsmokers. Only one of the studies summarized here includes evaluations of smokers and nonsmokers from groups of fertile men and men with fertility problems; both groups showed impairment of sperm density, motility, and morphologic features among smokers.[53] Sperm parameters of fertile men differed from those of the infertile men, pointing out the difficulty of generalizing results from many of these studies to the larger population.

There is a clear indication that smoking results in fewer sperm, less motile sperm, and a lower proportion of normally shaped sperm. The perspective afforded by the literature as a whole varies with the conclusions of individual investigators,[43-54] even those whose results support the existence of an effect. The pitfall of drawing faulty conclusions based on small numbers of subjects needs careful attention in future studies of sperm and in critically appraising such work.

BIOLOGIC PLAUSIBILITY AND MECHANISM OF ACTION OF THE EFFECT OF SMOKING ON MALE FERTILITY

Evidence suggests that tissues that turn over rapidly, including sperm produced by the testes, may be particularly sensitive to the mutagenic and carcinogenic materials found in cigarette smoke.[55] Smokers have increased numbers of sister chromatid exchange in peripheral lymphocytes[56] and increased numbers of covalent desoxyribonucleic acid (DNA) adducts in placentas,[57] compared with nonsmokers.

As reviewed and summarized by Mattison,[27] a solid body of experimental evidence suggests that exposure to nicotine, cigarette smoke, and/or polycyclic aromatic hydrocarbons is able to produce testicular atrophy, block spermatogenesis, and alter sperm morphologic features in experimental animals. These effects may be seen in a time-dependent and dose-dependent fashion. Cigarette smoke condensates have been demonstrated to possess compounds that are able to produce DNA mutations, either directly or after metabolism by enzyme systems similar to those found in rodent and human gonads. There are also ample experimental data to support the acute and chronic adverse effects of smoking (especially nicotine exposure) on the hypothalamic/pituitary/testicular axis, showing effects on LH, testosterone, adrenal corticotropic hormone (ACTH), growth hormone, thyroid stimulating hormone (TSH), and prolactin concentrations. These animal experimental data support the epidemiologic observation of male smokers' alterations in sperm morphologic features, concentration, and motility and give plausibility to the suggestion that cigarette smoke is directly or indirectly toxic to spermatogenesis.

Whether such impairment in spermatogenesis translates into clinical impairment of fertility remains unclear. One might argue that because each ejaculate results in several million sperm, impairment of even a substantial proportion might not be of clinical importance. Animal and human data to support effects on fertility in exposed males but unexposed females are needed. Controlled studies done using the hamster zona free sperm penetration assay and data from human in vivo fertilization may provide some of this information and are suggested. In the meantime, the clear consequences of smoking on sperm and spermatogenesis suggest that the most prudent course for couples experiencing difficulty in having a child, especially in men in whom semen characteristics are marginal and in couples in whom no factors can be implicated as a cause of their problems, is to stop smoking.

EFFECT OF SMOKING ON EARLY PREGNANCY OUTCOME

Along the continuum of the pathophysiologic effects of smoking on reproduction already reviewed, early pregnancy outcome also may need to be included. Cigarette smoke toxins that affect gamete viability, fertilization, early embryonic cleavage, embryo transport, and implantational events may, at one or more stages, predestine an adverse pregnancy outcome.[27] Decreased fecundity may be the result of failure of the steps leading to fertilization or may be the clinical view of what actually is an occult "preclinical" abortion. Somewhat later miscarriages will be detected as a clinical spontaneous abortion. Here we review what data exist on the effect of smoking on clinical spontaneous abortion.

An association of maternal smoking to spontaneous abortion was suggested as early as the 1940s.[58] These data and animal data reviewed by Abel[58] supported these early reports, as did a limited series of reports from 1963 to 1973. These reports, as reviewed by Harlap,[59] were seriously flawed epidemiologically, having small, limited groups of patients, limited or no control groups, and little or no understanding of characteristics of smokers that might predispose them to spontaneous abortion independent of smoking itself. Harlap[59] described the difficulties inherent in this research, an example of which is the exclusion from evaluation of an unknown percentage of women who abort, by including only those women who come to medical care. Not all women who abort seek medical help or are hospitalized. There are also many confounding variables that must be accounted for, some of which include prior obstetric history, age, social class, education, drug use, alcohol intake, body fat, and even legal statutes. Kullander and Källen,[60] in their report from Scandinavia, found that before there were laws legalizing induced abortion, many patients were falsely registered as having spontaneous abortion. The rate of spontaneous abortion associated with cigarette smoking also varied based on the patient's interest in keeping the pregnancy. Patients who smoked who had an unwanted pregnancy (and not undergoing induced abortion) had a higher rate of spontaneous abortion than patients wanting their pregnancy, emphasizing confounding variables in the smoking and spontaneous abortion studies. Thus crude comparison of abortion rates in smokers versus nonsmokers is obviously not satisfactory.

More recent studies[59-65] have been attempts to address these epidemiologic concerns with a variety of multivariate regression analyses. As a whole, they have demonstrated a significant increase in the risk of spontaneously aborting a chromosomally normal fetus in association with cigarette smoking.[27, 59] Although not of complete uniformity, these studies suggest a significant increase in the odds ratio, ranging from 1.2 to 1.8.[60-64] Based on these figures, Harlap[59] estimated that smokers have a 2.5% to 10% increase in miscarriages per 100 pregnancies, compared with nonsmokers. In addition, a dose-response effect of heavier smoking to greater frequency of spontaneous abortion has been suggested.[63]

Some of the studies addressing spontaneous abortion detail late first-trimester and second-trimester losses, opposed to earlier abortion.[58, 60, 65] This may suggest that some of the effects of smoking on spontaneous abortion are not the end of the continuum of effects on fertilization and preimplantation events, but rather more closely tied by cause to the beginning of a new continuum of adverse effects of smoking on fetal growth and well-being.

EFFECT OF SMOKING ON LATE PREGNANCY OUTCOME: BIRTHWEIGHT

In 1957, Simpson[66] reported the effect of smoking on pregnancy, showing that in a population of 7499 women in San Bernardino County there was a near doubling of the prematurity rate among smokers. The rate of premature births correlated with the number of cigarettes smoked. Since this report, many others on this same subject have appeared, but not all support her findings. We evaluate the epidemiologic evidence for smoking being associated with or causative to low birthweight (LBW) and whether this LBW is due to intrauterine growth retardation and/or to prematurity. Also, we discuss the biologic plausibility and the mechanism for the observed outcomes.

EPIDEMIOLOGIC DATA

Many researchers have considered the effect of smoking on LBW.[67-72] Some studies show an increased incidence of small for gestational age infants (SGA)[67, 68, 71] and decreased birth length[68, 69] and others show a higher incidence of premature infants appropriate for gestational age (AGA).[67, 68]

Yerushalmy,[69, 70] in 1971, argued that the cause of lower-birthweight infants was due to attributes of the smoker and not to smoking. The effect of birthweight was seen in mothers who had not yet smoked when the infant was born but who acquired the habit later. In essence, he was pointing out the problem of inferring causation from observed associations. It is clear that many potential confounding variables could have an impact on birthweight, including maternal age, race, sex, and maternal weight gain. Yerushalmy[69, 70] and Hickey et al.[71] argued that the poor maternal weight gain in pregnancy commonly seen among smokers accounts for the lower birthweight. In a 1978 report supported by the Council for Tobacco Research,[71] this argument was taken further without substantiating evidence. Further, this paper claimed the possibility that nicotine could induce a physiologic response "serving to alleviate bioenergetic deficiency in some individuals." In this view, both smoking and low birthweight are "symptoms of deficient maternal bioenergetic systems." The authors, in fact, claimed that for some patients, nicotine from cigarette smoke may be beneficial for the mother and the fetus. This point of view is difficult to substantiate.

These reports are in the minority in discrediting a link between cigarette smoking and low birthweight. At the very least, the data demonstrate a strong association, if not actual causation[67, 68] (Table 7). The 1983 report of the Surgeon General[67] on the consequences of smoking in women reviewed five studies with respect to the issue of low birthweight. These studies comprise nearly 113,000 births in the United States,

Table 7. *Association Between Cigarette Smoking and Birthweight*[a]

	No. of cigarettes			
	0	1–10	11–20	> 20
Birthweight (gm) (white)	3399	3272	3185	3128
Birthweight (gm) (black)	3128	2977	2957	2945
% LBW (< 2500 gm) (white)	4.8	8.0	9.0	13.4
% LBW (< 2500 gm) (black)	8.3	13.6	17.7	22.7

[a]From Abel.[58]

Canada, and Wales. It was found that 21% to 39% of the incidence of low birthweight could be attributed to maternal cigarette smoking.

An important study addressing this issue was conducted by Naeye[73] on 8000 pregnancies. The effect on birthweight was found to be independent of dietary intake or nutritional status, and the effect was present regardless of prepregnancy weight or weight gain. Further, a dose-response relationship was seen: the more cigarettes smoked, the lower the birthweight. Genetic factors were ruled out by studying information obtained from two successive pregnancies in which the mother smoked in only one. In these cases, a clear link was found between smoking and low birthweight. Further, the analysis showed that the effect on birthweight was independent of socioeconomic class, maternal age, or birth order.

Two arguments counter the belief that smoking mothers eat less and therefore have smaller babies. First, one would expect poor maternal weight gain if the fetus is growth-retarded, because 30% to 45% of the weight in the last trimester is due to fetal growth. Second, there is no clear connection between poor maternal nutrition and the incidence of SGA infants.[74] Even in studies conducted in a situation as extreme as World War II, the mother had to be severely malnourished for there to be any effect on birthweight. Further, these results were confounded by poor prenatal care at that time.[75, 76]

A recent clinical trial, by Sexton and Hebel,[77] supported a relationship between smoking and low birthweight. These authors randomly assigned 935 pregnant mothers to a treatment or a control group. The treatment group achieved a 43% reduction in smoking and the control group a 20% reduction. Salivary thiocyanate levels were measured between the two groups to quantify cigarette exposure. The authors reported that even though 57% of the treatment group continued to smoke, they had a mean birthweight for singleton live births 92 gm heavier and a birth length 0.6 cm longer than the control group infants, independent of the gestational age. The only similar experimental study was that of Donovan,[78] which failed to demonstrate an adverse effect of smoking on birthweight. He was, however, unable to quantify the amount of smoking, viz., the salivary thiocyanate levels. Cnattingius et al.[79] recently demonstrated, in a prospective clinical study, that smoking was the most important and highly significant risk factor for intrauterine growth retardation among 636 patients matched to 536 controls. The risk was magnified in heavier smokers, as well as in older smokers, although advancing maternal age alone did not influence the standardized birthweights evaluated. The effect of smoking cessation in pregnancy requires further research. Does this alteration in habit reverse the adverse effects of smoking and, if so, how quickly? Is this situation analogous to the opiate addict, in whom withdrawal of the drug can adversely affect the fetus? If former smokers experience pregnancies as do nonsmokers and the fetus is not affected by withdrawal, how do we influence or predict changes in smoking habits in pregnancy?[80]

Some studies have shown an increase in the incidence of premature deliveries in women smokers[67, 68, 81, 82] and attributed LBW to this prematurity. However, many of these studies were based on birth record data, which are notoriously poor in the assessment of gestational age. The birthweight differential between smokers and nonsmokers is between 150 gm and 300 gm.[67] Vital Records data are not sensitive enough to detect these changes in gestational age. Overall, the magnitude of the effect of smoking on the incidence of prematurity is unknown. There is a strong association between cigarette smoking (especially nicotine) and abruptio placentae[67-71] and premature rupture of membranes,[67-71] two clinical conditions that can lead to premature birth. However, a number of studies done to assess decreased fetal weight showed an association with smoking even when adjusting for gestational age.[67-71]

BIOLOGIC PLAUSIBILITY AND MECHANISM OF ACTION OF THE EFFECT OF SMOKING ON BIRTHWEIGHT

An understanding of the physiologic adaptation of the fetus to life in utero is a prerequisite to appreciating the effects of smoking in pregnancy. The fetus is in a state of "physiologic hypoxia."[83] The low oxygen tension maintains the patency of the ductus arteriosus and the constriction of the pulmonary vasculature in utero. The fetus adapts to this state of physiologic hypoxia through a number of mechanisms: fetal hemoglobin (HbF), which has a greater oxygen affinity than adult hemoglobin (HbA); higher hematocrit; and higher fetal cardiac output from a more rapid heart rate and higher stroke volume. All of these physiologic adaptations allow the fetus to survive at low PO_2—adaptations that also make the fetus susceptible to alterations in that physiology, as may occur from cigarette smoke.

In response to acute or chronic hypoxia, there is an elevation in 2,3 diphosphoglycerate (2,3-DPG) and a decrease in Hb-O_2 affinity.[84, 85] These changes maintain the end capillary PO_2 at a level that exhibits minimum demand on cardiac output. Carbon monoxide from cigarette smoke can not only cause fetal hypoxia, but also prevents an adequate physiologic response to this insult. Carbon monoxide has 200 times the affinity for hemoglobin than does oxygen.[86] Further, HbF has a higher affinity for carbon monoxide than does HbA. When HbF combines with carbon monoxide, there is a left shift in the O_2 dissociation curve. These changes lead to a decrease in oxygen-carrying capacity of the blood and a decrease in offloading of oxygen at the tissue level, resulting in a functional anemia. After 5 to 6 hours, carbon monoxide levels in the fetus are in equilibrium with maternal levels,[86] but carbon monoxide will last longer in the fetus, which is less able than the mother to metabolize it.[87] Only two packs of cigarettes per day result in a 10% concentration of carboxyhemoglobin, which is equivalent to a 60% reduction in the blood flow.[87] Because the fetus normally exists in a low-oxygen environment, there is little margin for safety with respect to tissue oxygenation. Further, the fetus is unable to compensate by increasing the cardiac output, because it is already at or near peak levels.[87] Thus the fetus is unable to compensate adequately for carbon monoxide from cigarette smoke.[87, 88]

These findings were also observed in a major study of the effect of smoking on 100 maternal-infant pairs equally divided between smoking and nonsmoking mothers.[89] For the smokers, there was no significant change in the levels of 2,3-DPG values, but there was a small but significant increase in their hematocrit. For the newborns, however, there was a significant difference for the exposed infants in their HbF but no change in the 2,3-DPG levels. These changes reflect an inefficient compensatory mechanism and emphasize the sensitivity of the fetus to an increased concentration of carbon monoxide from cigarettes. The fetus can be compared with the canary that used to be taken underground by miners to detect carbon monoxide.

Burning of the tobacco leaf results in gases and tiny droplets of tar. Two principal gaseous ingredients, besides carbon monoxide, are nicotine and cyanide, and there are numerous cancer-producing substances.[90] Besides the effects on the fetus from carbon monoxide, one puff of a cigarette is equivalent to an intravenous injection of 0.1 mg of nicotine or 2 mg of nicotine per cigarette.[81, 89] Nicotine acts on the adrenal glands in pregnancy and causes an increase in norepinephrine, epinephrine, and acetylcholine.[91, 92] It leads to decreased uteroplacental perfusion and crosses the placenta to affect the fetal cardiovascular system.[91, 92] Nicotine has been shown to cause a rise in the blood pressure and respiratory rate of the fetus and affects the gastrointestinal, genitourinary, and central nervous systems.[91, 92] Nicotine is the principle in tobacco that causes addictive or habituating behavior.[81, 89, 93]

Placental changes reflect smoking's adverse affect on oxygenation and circulation. Van der Veen and Fox[94] examined placentas from 72 smokers and 28 nonsmokers. They found changes consistent with chronic ischemia and chronic hypoxia in placentas of smokers, including a relative placental hypertrophy. These morphologic changes in the placenta and vasculature[95, 96] are consistent with our understanding of the effects of carbon monoxide and nicotine on the fetus.

Smoking has been shown to cause a decrease in term infant birthweight of between 150 and 300 gm.[67] This figure is equivalent to approximately 50 mg of fetal weight lost for each cigarette smoked by a woman smoking one pack per day through pregnancy. The majority of studies have shown that this reduction in weight is an effect of smoking and not of the smoker, and may be related to hypoxia, vascular, and direct fetal effects of smoking constituents. For LBW infants (< 2500 gm) in the United States, Canada, and Wales, 21% to 39% of the cases could be attributed to maternal smoking.[67] An increased incidence of prematurity also has been associated with cigarette smoking. The relative risk of a preterm birth reported is 36% to 47% higher in women who smoke, and the attributable risk for all preterm births is 11% to 14%. For some studies, it is unclear whether the effect of smoking is on fetal growth or prematurity. However, there is a clear dose-response effect on birthweight, with light smokers having 54% and heavy smokers 130% increase in the frequency of infants weighing less than 2500 gm at birth.[73]

EFFECT OF SMOKING ON LATE PREGNANCY OUTCOME: OTHER

PERINATAL MORTALITY

It has been estimated that maternal smoking is strongly associated with 4600 infant deaths in the United States per year.[67] A number of studies have shown an increase in the incidence of stillbirths, neonatal, and postneonatal deaths.[67, 72, 82, 97, 98] Some of these reports indicate that the increase in perinatal mortality was independent of decreased birthweight.[67, 68, 72] However, a few studies[99-101] have shown no increase in the incidence in perinatal mortality. Some of the controversy may be explained by the fact that the sample size required to examine the effect of smoking on perinatal mortality would have to exceed 10,000 women. Further, the effect on perinatal mortality rate is likely to be very small, especially for those babies weighing > 3000 gm. The randomized clinical study by Sexton and Hebel[77] revealed no difference in the incidence of perinatal mortality, although this study was not designed specifically to show such a difference and had too few subjects. Of interest, though, is a study by Meyer and Tonascia[72] analyzing data from the Ontario Perinatal Mortality Study, which showed a 20% increased risk of a perinatal demise for women who smoked less than one pack of cigarettes per day and a 35% increase for those who smoked more than one pack of cigarettes per day. The deaths were associated with a high incidence of bleeding during pregnancy due to abruptio placentae, placenta previa, and premature rupture of the membranes.

LOW APGAR SCORES

Garn and colleagues,[102] using data from the Collaborative Perinatal Project on the 1- and 5-minute Apgar scores of 43,492 infants, showed that there was a four times increased incidence of low Apgar scores if the mother smoked more than two packs of cigarettes per day. These findings were independent of race or gestational age of the baby. Further, the babies exposed to cigarette smoke had higher hematocrits and cord carbon monoxide levels.

ABRUPTIO PLACENTAE AND OTHER ANTEPARTUM HEMORRHAGE

A number of studies[67, 68, 72] have shown an increased incidence of abruptio placentae among smoking mothers. Others have reported an increase in the incidence of placenta previa.[67, 72] The cause-and-effect relationship between cigarette smoking and abnormal localization of the placenta is difficult to explain, although hypoxia and vasoconstriction might favor the placenta's seeking a larger or richer internal vascular bed. In addition, many of these studies were conducted before placental localization by ultrasound was used, which may have limited diagnostic accuracy.

PREMATURE RUPTURE OF MEMBRANES

A few studies have associated smoking with an increased incidence of premature rupture of membranes.[67, 72, 103] The mechanism is unknown, but confounding factors of vaginal flora and infection that may be different in smokers versus nonsmokers must be considered before postulating immune compromise due to cigarette smoke.[26]

RESPIRATORY DISTRESS SYNDROME

The Collaborative Group on Antenatal Steroid Therapy in their study on the efficacy of steroids for prevention of respiratory distress syndrome (RDS) found that there was a lower incidence of RDS in babies exposed to cigarette smoke in utero.[104] The findings were significant after adjustment for treatment and risk factors. This relationship is not surprising, because it is known that the incidence of RDS is lower in "stressed" or SGA infants.[105]

BIRTH DEFECTS

In a study on 67,609 singleton pregnancies in Cardiff, Wales[106] between 1965 and 1976, the overall incidence of congenital anomalies was 2.8% for both smokers and nonsmokers. There was no dose-response effect for malformations except for neural tube defects. There was an increased incidence of neural tube defects for heavy smokers. However, the potential confounding variable in this study was socioeconomic status, which appeared to be a stronger correlate than smoking per se. In a case-control study from Sweden[107] that examined 66 infants with cleft lip and/or cleft palate, 66 with closure defects and 261 controls, significantly more women having infants with cleft lip or cleft palate smoked, compared with controls. The findings were independent of other drug use. Hemminki and colleagues[63] studied 3300 affected children between 1967 and 1977 in the Finnish Register of Congenital Malformations. They carried out a multivariate analysis of this retrospective data set and found that, when controlling for 13 possible confounding variables, smoking was not a teratogen. Most of the large controlled studies have not shown a teratogenic effect of cigarette smoking.

LONG-TERM MORBIDITY

There appears to be a long-term effect of cigarette smoking on surviving children,[67, 108-112] but it is unclear whether the effect on child development can be separated completely from such potential confounding variables as socioeconomic status, education, and passive smoking. In a study of more than 5000 children in the British National Child Development Study using a multifactorial analysis, Davie and colleagues[111] and Goldstein[112] showed reduced reading attainment at 7 years of age among children exposed to cigarette smoke. When the same children were examined at 11 years of age,[109] if the mother had smoked more than ten cigarettes per day, there was a 3-month retardation in general ability, 4 months in reading skills, and 5 months in mathematics. However, none of these findings was statistically significant.

LONG-TERM RISK OF CANCER FOLLOWING IN UTERO EXPOSURE TO CIGARETTES

Everson[113] hypothesized that there is an association between cigarette smoking and long-term risk of cancer to the infant. His argument was based on clinical observations and animal experimentation. More than 30 agents have been identified as active transplacental carcinogens. The best known of these is diethylstilbestrol (DES), which has been associated with vaginal clear cell adenocarcinoma after in utero exposure.[114] Further, hydantoin, used to treat epilepsy, has been associated with neuroblastomas and a malignant mesenchymoma.[115] A number of agents found in cigarettes are potent transplacental carcinogens in animals. These include benzopyrene, urethane, anthracenes, nitrosamines, and hydrazines.[27] However, at present, there is only indirect evidence for their ability to cross the placenta in humans. The fetus undergoes rapid growth in utero, which is thought to make it more susceptible to transplacental carcinogens. This hypothesis is supported by experimental evidence in animals.[27] In addition, the carcinogens may increase the sensitivity of that individual to later exposure to carcinogens.[116] Epidemiologic studies in humans have not been conclusive. Neutal and Buck,[117] for a cohort of 89,302 infants in 1971, reported an OR of 1.3; (0.8 to 2.2, 95% CI) for cancer among offspring of women who smoke during pregnancy. Most of the other studies examining this issue contained too few subjects to study what is probably a problem of low incidence.

FETAL TOBACCO SYNDROME

It has been recommended that the findings discussed above be described as fetal tobacco syndrome.[118] With the introduction of the term "fetal alcohol syndrome," it was clear that the consciousness level of the public and the medical profession was increased as to the hazards of drinking in pregnancy. The introduction of the term fetal tobacco syndrome has a number of potential benefits: (1) uniform diagnostic criteria, (2) heightened awareness on behalf of the public and medical profession, (3) more precise epidemiologic assessment of populations at risk, and (4) more careful evaluation of smoking intervention programs. The criteria that the Centers for Disease Control proposed are (1) the mother should have smoked five or more cigarettes per day throughout the pregnancy; (2) the mother had no evidence of hypertension during pregnancy, specifically (a) no preeclampsia and (b) documentation of normal blood pressure at least once after the first trimester; (3) the newborn has symmetric growth retardation ($>$ 37 weeks), defined as (a) birthweight $<$ 2500 gm and (b) a ponderal index [weight gm/length $(cm)^3$] $>$ 2.32; (4) there is no other obvious cause of intrauterine growth retardation (e.g., congenital infection or anomaly).

It may be stated simply that to avoid the fetal tobacco syndrome any expectant mother should stop smoking, especially if she has a history of prior miscarriage or adverse late pregnancy outcome. Programs aimed at altering pregnant women's smoking habits must be strengthened, especially because it has been estimated that even among women with planned pregnancies entering early prenatal care, less than 18% have stopped smoking.[4, 80]

CONCLUSION

Smoking presents a challenging dilemma for the health care provider. He or she must convince patients who may be single-mindedly entrenched in pursuing a habit with well-defined, direct, varied, and significant adverse health effects to give up that habit. Indeed, the health care provider may him or herself be entrenched, through either true addiction or persuasion of massive advertising, and thus be unconvincing in altering their patients' behavior. This behavior can be defined only as physically self-destructive. Promotion of nonsmokers' rights and support of economic disincentives for smoking may help to alter some patients' habits; our best professional resource, however, is health promotion. Anyone who smokes should be advised to stop. Joseph Califano, former Secretary of Health, Education, and Welfare, summarized the health problem in women smokers by saying bluntly, "Women who smoke like men, die like men."[119] Yet the changes in sex ratios for lung cancer and cardiovascular mortality that correlate with changes in sex ratios of people who smoke have not done enough to convince women to give up their cigarettes. We review increasing epidemiologic evidence that smoking adversely affects female fertility, male fertility, early pregnancy, and late pregnancy outcomes. We have also presented the biologic plausibility and mechanisms of action of cigarette smoke and its components on these reproductive processes. The argument against smoking holds true for anyone wishing to conceive, but it is particularly imperative for individuals having difficulty in conceiving or having prior miscarriages. Of those women smokers who are fortunate enough to conceive, all must be counseled to stop smoking, or otherwise risk exposing their fetus to the effects of the fetal tobacco syndrome.

Perhaps illuminating these adverse effects that smoking imparts on their reproductive health will persuade individuals to stop. It is our hope to aid in the process of illumination and to stimulate further research into this health problem, not out of a sense of militancy but out of a sense of urgency and responsibility any of us should feel when one of our patients ingests a known toxin.

Two recent publications are noteworthy, suggesting a direct effect of cigarette smoke constituents on granulosa-cell function in vitro[120] and the separate significant effects of both active maternal and passive paternal smoking on infant birthweight.[121]

Acknowledgments. We thank Ms. Katherine O'Mahoney, Ms. Angela Sylvestre, Ms. Carol Williamson, and Ms. Martha Lonzana for their expertise in the preparation of the manuscript and Susan Harlap, M.B.B.S., Oona Campbell, Sc.M., Janet Daling, Ph.D., and Alfred Spira, M.D., Ph.D., for allowing us to review preprints of their articles still in press.[4]

REFERENCES

1. U.S. Department of Health and Human Services: The health consequences of smoking. a report of the Surgeon General. Washington, D.C., U.S. Government Printing Office, 1984
2. Stedman RL: The chemical composition of tobacco and tobacco smoke. Chem Rev 68:153, 1968
3. Fielding JE: Smoking: health effects and control. N Engl J Med 313:491, 1985
4. Rosenberg MJ, ed: Smoking and Reproductive Health. Littleton, MA, P.S.G. Publishers, 1986
5. Tokuhata GM: Smoking in relation to infertility and fetal loss. Arch Environ Health 17:353, 1968
6. Howe G, Westhoff C, Vessey M, Yeates D: Effects of age, cigarette smoking, and other factors on fertility: findings in a large prospective study. Br Med J 290:1697, 1985
7. Friedman S: Artificial donor insemination with frozen human semen. Fertil Steril 28:1230, 1977
8. Olsen J, Rachootin P, Schiodt AV, Damsbo N: Tobacco use, alcohol consumption and infertility. Int J Epidemiol 12:179, 1982
9. Linn S, Schoenbaum SC, Monson RR, Rosner B, Ryan KJ: Delay in conception for former "pill" users. JAMA 247:629, 1982
10. Daling JR, Weiss NS, Metch BJ, Chow WH, Soderstrom RM, Moore DE, Spadoni LR, Stadel BS: Primary tubal infertility in relation to the use of an intrauterine device. N Engl J Med 312:937, 1985
11. Daling JR: Cigarette smoking and primary tubal infertility. In Smoking and Reproductive Health, Edited by MJ Rosenberg. Littleton, MA, P.S.G. Publishers, 1986
12. Cramer DW, Schiff I, Schoenbaum SC, Gibson M, Belisle S, Albrecht B, Stillman RJ, Berger MJ, Wilson E, Stadel B, Seibel M: Tubal infertility and the intrauterine device. N Engl J Med 312:941, 1985
13. Phipps WR, Cramer DW, Schiff I, Belisle S, Gibson M, Wilson E, Albrecht BH, Stillman RJ, Berger MJ: Cigarette smoking and primary female infertility (Abstr 337P). Published by the Society for Gynecologic Investigation, 33rd Annual Meeting, March 19, 1986, Toronto, Canada

14. Harlap S, Barras M: Conception-waits in fertile women after stopping oral contraceptives. Int J Fertil 29:73, 1984
15. Mai FM, Munday RN, Rump EE: Psychiatric interview comparisons between infertile and fertile couples. Psychosom Med 34:431, 1972
16. Baird DD, Wilcox AJ: Cigarette smoking associated with delayed conception. JAMA 253:2979, 1985
17. Spira A: Smoking and fecundity. In Smoking and Reproductive Health, Edited by MJ Rosenberg. Littleton, MA, P.S.G. Publishers, 1986
18. Malcolm S, Shephard RJ: Personality and sexual behavior of the adolescent smoker. Am J Drug Alcohol Abuse 5:87, 1978
19. Neri A, Eckerling B: Influence of smoking and adrenaline (epinephrine) on the uterotubal insufflation test (Rubin test). Fertil Steril 20:818, 1969
20. Neri A, Marcus SL: Effect of nicotine on the motility of the oviducts in the rhesus monkey: a preliminary report. J Reprod Fertil 31:91, 1972
21. Ruckebusch Y: Relationship between the electrical activity of the oviduct and the uterus of the rabbit in vivo. J Reprod Fertil 45:73, 1975
22. Weathersbee PS: Nicotine and its influence on the female reproductive system. J Reprod Med 25:243, 1980
23. Campbell OM, Gray RH: Smoking and ectopic pregnancy: a multinational case-control study. In Smoking and Reproductive Health, Edited by MJ Rosenberg. Littleton MA, P.S.G. Publishers, 1986
24. Matsunaga E, Shiota K: Ectopic pregnancy and myoma uteri: teratogenic effects and maternal characteristics. Teratology 21:61, 1980
25. Levin AA, Schoenbaun SC, Stubblefield PG, Zimicki S, Monson RR, Ryan KJ: Ectopic pregnancy and prior induced abortion. Am J Public Health 72:253, 1982
26. Burton RC: Smoking, immunity and cancer. Med J Aust 5:411, 1983
27. Mattison DR: The effects of smoking on fertility from gametogenesis to implantation. Environ Res 28:410, 1982
28. Card JP, Mitchell JA: The effects of nicotine administration on deciduoma induction in the rat. Biol Reprod 19: 326, 1978
29. Yoshinaga K, Rice C, Krenn J, Pilot RL: Effects of nicotine on early pregnancy in the rat. Biol Reprod 20:294, 1979
30. McLachlan JA, Dames NM, Sieber SM, Fabro S: Accumulation of nicotine in the uterine fluid of the six-day pregnant rabbit. Fertil Steril 27:1204, 1976
31. Longo FJ, Anderson E: The effects of nicotine on fertilization in the sea urchin, Arbacia punctulata. J Cell Biol 46:308, 1970
32. Jick H, Porter J, Morrison AS: Relation between smoking and age of natural menopause. Lancet 1:1354, 1977
33. Pettersson F, Fries H, Nillius SJ: Epidemiology of secondary amenorrhea. 1. Incidence and prevalence rates. Am J Obstet Gynecol 117:80, 1973
34. Hammond EC: Smoking in relation to physical complaints. Arch Environ Health 3:28, 1961
35. Bernhardt P: Dir Wirkung des Ranchens auf Frau und Mutter. Munch Med Wochenschr 104:1826, 1962
36. MacMahon B, Trichopoulous D, Cole P, Brown J: Cigarette smoking and urinary estrogens. N Engl J Med 307:1062, 1982
37. Vessey M, Baron J, Doll R: Oral contraceptives and breast cancer, final report of an epidemiological study. Br J Cancer 47:455, 1983
38. Baron JA: Smoking and estrogen-related disease. Am J Epidemiol 119:9, 1984
39. Cramer DW, Wilson E, Stillman RJ, Berger MJ, Belisle S, Schiff I, Albrecht B, Gibson M, Stadel BV, Schoenbaum SC: The relation of endometriosis to menstrual characteristics, smoking, and exercise. JAMA 255:1904, 1986
40. Daniell HW: Osteoporosis of the slender smoker. Arch Intern Med 136:298, 1976
41. Blake CA, Norman RL, Scaramuzzi RJ, Sawyer CA: Inhibition of the proestrous surge of prolactin in the rat by nicotine. Endocrinol 92:1334, 1973
42. McLean BK, Rubel A, Nikitovitch–Winer MB: The differential effects of exposure to tobacco smoke on the secretion of luteinizing hormone and prolactin in the proestrous rat. Endocrinol 100:1566, 1977
43. Viczian M: Ergelovisse von Spermauntersuchungen bei Zigarettenranchern. Z Haut Geschlechtskr 44:183, 1969
44. Schirren C, Gey G: Der Einfluss des Ranchens and die Fortplanzungsfahighert bei Mann and Frau. Z Haut Geschlechtskr 44:175, 1969
45. Campbell JM, Harrison KL: Smoking and infertility. Med J Aust 1:342, 1979
46. Vogel W, Broverman DM, Klaiber EL: Gonadal, behavioral, and electroencephalographic correlates of smoking. In Electrophysiological Effects of Nicotine, Edited by A Remond, C Izard. Amsterdam, Elsevier Biomedical Press, 1979, p 201
47. Evans HJ, Fletcher J, Torrance M, Hargreave TB: Sperm abnormalities and cigarette smoking. Lancet 1: 627, 1981
48. Godfrey B: Sperm morphology in smokers. Lancet 1:948, 1981
49. Rodriguez–Rigau LJ, Smith KD, Steinberger E: Cigarette smoking and semen quality. Fertil Steril 38:115, 1982
50. Shaarawy M, Mahmoud KZ: Endocrine profile and semen characteristics in male smokers. Fertil Steril 38: 255, 1982
51. Spira A: Consummation de tabac et caracteristique du sperme. In Human Fertility Factors, with Emphasis on the Male, Edited by P Jouannet, A Spira. Paris, Institut National de la Santé et de la Recherche Médicale, 1981, p 363
52. Handelsman DJ, Conway AJ, Boylan LM, Turtle JR: Testicular function in potential sperm donors: normal ranges and the effects of smoking and varicocele. Int J Androl 7:369, 1984
53. Kulikauskas V, Blaustein D, Ablin RJ: Cigarette smoking and its possible effects on sperm. Fertil Steril 44:526, 1985
54. Vogt HJ, Heller WD, Borelli S: Sperm quality of healthy smokers, ex-smokers, and never-smokers. Fertil Steril 45:106, 1986
55. Ravenholt RT: Circulating mutagens from smoking. N Engl J Med 307:312, 1982
56. Lambert B, Lindblad A, Nordenskjold M, Werelius B: Increased frequency of sister chromatid exchanges in cigarette smokers. Hereditas 88:147, 1988
57. Everson RB, Randerath E, Santella RM, Cefalo RC, Avitts TA, Randerath K: Detection of smoking-related

covalent DNA adducts in human placenta. Science 231: 54, 1986
58. Abel EL: Smoking during pregnancy: a review of effects on growth and development of offspring. Hum Biol 52: 593, 1980
59. Harlap S: Smoking and spontaneous abortion. In Smoking and Reproductive Health, Edited by MJ Rosenberg. Littleton, MA, P.S.G. Publishers, 1986
60. Kullender S, Källen B: A prospective study of smoking and pregnancy. Acta Obstet Gynecol Scand 50:83, 1971
61. Klinc J, Stein ZA, Susser M, Warburton D: Smoking: a risk factor for spontaneous abortion. N Engl J Med 297: 793, 1977
62. Himmelberger DU, Brown BW Jr, Cohen EN: Cigarette smoking during pregnancy and the occurrence of spontaneous abortion and congenital abnormality. Am J Epidemiol 108:470, 1978
63. Hemminki K, Mutanen P, Saloniemi I: Smoking and the occurrence of malformations and spontaneous abortions: multivariate analysis. Am J Obstet Gynecol 145:61, 1983
64. Harlap S, Shiono PH: Alcohol, smoking and incidence of spontaneous abortions in the first and second trimester. Lancet 2:173, 1980
65. Alberman E, Elliott M, Creasy M, Dhadial R: Previous reproductive history in mothers presenting with spontaneous abortions. Br J Obstet Gynaecol 82:366, 1975
66. Simpson WJ: A preliminary report on cigarette smoking and the incidence of prematurity. Am J Obstet Gynecol 73:808, 1957
67. U.S. Department of Health and Human Services: The Health Consequences of Smoking for Women: A report of the Surgeon General. Washington, D.C., U.S. Government Printing Office, 1983
68. United States Department of Health, Education and Welfare: Pregnancy and Infant Health. In Smoking and Health. Washington, D.C., U.S. Government Printing Office, 1979
69. Yerushalmy J: The relationship of parents' cigarette smoking to outcome of pregnancy: implications as to the problem of inferring causation from observed associations. Am J Epidemiol 93:443, 1971
70. Yerushalmy J: Infants with low birth weight born before their mothers started to smoke cigarettes. Am J Obstet Gynecol 112:277, 1972
71. Hickey RJ, Clelland RC, Bowers EJ: Maternal smoking, birth weight, infant death, and the self-selection problem. Am J Obstet Gynecol 131:805, 1978
72. Meyer NB, Tonascia JA: Maternal smoking, pregnancy complications and perinatal mortality. Am J Obstet Gynecol 128:494, 1977
73. Naeye RL: Influence of maternal cigarette smoking during pregnancy on fetal and childhood growth. Obstet Gynecol 57:18, 1981
74. Stein Z, Susser M, Rush D: Prenatal nutrition and birthweight: experiments and quasi experiments in the past decade. J Reprod Med 21:287, 1978
75. Antonov AW: Children born during the siege of Leningrad in 1942. J Pediatr 30:250, 1947
76. Smith CA: Effects of maternal undernutrition upon the newborn infant in Holland. J Pediatr 30:299, 1947
77. Sexton M, Hebel JR: A clinical trial of change in maternal smoking and its effect on birthweight. JAMA 251: 911, 1984
78. Donovan JW: Randomized controlled trial of anti-smoking advice in pregnancy. Br J Prevent Soc Med 31:6, 1977
79. Cnattingius S, Axelsson O, Eklund G, Lindamark G: Smoking, maternal age and fetal growth. Obstet Gynecol 66:449, 1985
80. Kruse J, LeFevre M, Zweig S: Changes in smoking and alcohol consumption during pregnancy: a population-based study in a rural area. Obstet Gynecol 67:627, 1986
81. United States Department of Health, Education and Welfare: Harmful Constituents. In The Health Consequences of Smoking: A report of the Surgeon General. Washington, D.C., U.S. Government Printing Office, 1972
82. Frazier TM, Davis GH, Goldstein H, Goldberg ID: Cigarette smoking and prematurity: a prospective study. Am J Obstet Gynecol 81:988, 1961
83. Meschia G: Placental respiratory gas exchange and fetal oxygenation: In Maternal and Fetal Medicine Principles and Practice, Edited by R Creasy, R Resnick. Philadelphia, WB Saunders Co., 1984, p 274
84. Oski FA, Gottlieb AJ, Delivoria–Papadopoulos M, Altman A: Red cell, 2,3-diphosphoglycerate levels in subjects with chronic hypoxemia. N Engl J Med 280:1165, 1967
85. Lenfant C, Warp P, Aucutt C: Effect of chronic hypoxia on the O_2-Hb dissociation curve and respiratory gas transport in man. Respir Physiol 7:7, 1969
86. Longo LD: Carbon monoxide effects on oxygenization of the fetus in utero. Science 194:523, 1976
87. Longo LD: The biological effects of carbon monoxide on the pregnant woman, fetus and newborn infant. Am J Obstet Gynecol 129:69, 1977
88. Bureau MA, Shapcott D, Berthiaume Y: Maternal cigarette smoking and fetal oxygen transport; a study of P50, 2,3-diphosphoglycerate, total hemoglobin, hematocrit, and type F hemoglobin in fetal blood. Pediatrics 72:22, 1983
89. Royal College of Physicians of London: The Chemistry and Pharmacology of Tobacco Smoke. In Smoking and Health Now. London, Pitman Medical, 1971
90. Fried PA, Oxorn H: Smoking For Two: Cigarettes and Pregnancy. Ontario, Canada, The Free Press, 1980
91. Monheit AG, van Vunakis H, Key TC, Resnik R: Maternal and fetal cardiovascular effects of nicotine infusion in pregnant sheep. Am J Obstet Gynecol 145:290, 1983
92. Resnik R, Brink GW, Wilkes M: Catecholamine-mediated reduction in uterine blood flow after nicotine infusion in the pregnant ewe. J Clin Invest 63:1133, 1979
93. Royal College of Physicians of London: Smoking or Health. The Third Report of the Royal College of Physicians of London. London, Pitman Medical, 1977, p 128
94. Van der Veen F, Fox H: The effects of cigarette smoking on the human placenta: a light and electron microscopic study. Placenta 3:243, 1982
95. Lehtovirta P, Forss M: The acute effect of smoking on intervillous blood flow of the placenta. Br J Obstet Gynaecol 85:729, 1978
96. Verma RC, Chansoriya M, Kaul KK: Effect of tobacco chewing by mothers on fetal outcome. Indian Pediat 20: 105, 1983
97. Butler NR, Bonham DG: Perinatal Mortality: The First Report of the 1958 British Perinatal Mortality Survey, Edinburg, E & S Livingstone, Ltd., 1963

98. Ravenholt RT, Levinski MJ, Nellist DJ, Takenaga M: Effects of smoking upon reproduction. Am J Obstet Gynecol 96:267, 1966
99. Peterson WF, Morese KN, Kaltreider DF: Smoking and prematurity: a preliminary report based on study of 7740 caucasians. Obstet Gynecol 26:775, 1965
100. Underwood PB, Kesler KF, O'Lane JM, Callagan DA: Parental smoking empirically related to pregnancy outcome. Obstet Gynecol 29:1, 1967
101. Yerushalmy J: Mother's cigarette smoking and survival of infant. Am J Obstet Gynecol 88:505, 1964
102. Garn SM, Johnston M, Ridella SA, Petgold AS: The effect of maternal cigarette smoking on Apgar scores. Am J Dis Child 135:503, 1981
103. Rush D, Kass EH: Maternal smoking: a reassessment of the association with perinatal mortality. Am J Epidemiol 96:183, 1972
104. Curet LB, Vyayario A, Zachman RD, Mornson J, Burkett G, Poole WK: Maternal smoking and respiratory distress syndrome. Am J Obstet Gynecol 147:446, 1983
105. Russell CS, Taylor R, Law CE: Smoking in pregnancy, maternal blood pressure, pregnancy outcome, baby weight and growth, and other related factors: a prospective study. Br J Prev Soc Med 22:119, 1968
106. Evans DR, Newcombe RG, Campbell H: Maternal smoking habits and congenital malformations: population study. Br Med J 2:171, 1979
107. Ericson A, Kallen B, Westerholm P: Cigarette smoking and etiologic factors in cleft lip and palate. Am J Obstet Gynecol 61:539, 1983
108. Dunn HG, McBurney AK, Ingram S, Hunter CM: Maternal cigarette smoking during pregnancy and the child's subsequent development: I. Physical growth to age 6½ years. Can J Public Health 67:499, 1976
109. Butler NR, Goldstein H: Smoking in pregnancy and subsequent child development. Br Med J 4:573, 1973
110. Naeye RL, Peters EC: Mental development of children whose mothers smoked during pregnancy. Obstet Gynecol 64:60, 1984
111. Davie R, Butler NR, Goldstein H: From Birth to Seven: The Second Report of the National Child Development Study. London, Longmans, 1972, p 198
112. Goldstein H: Factors influencing the weight of seven year old children: results from the National Child Development Study. Hum Biol 43:92, 1972
113. Everson BE: Individuals transplacentally exposed to maternal smoking may be at increased cancer risk in adult life. Lancet 2:123, 1980
114. Stillman RJ: In utero exposure to diethylstilbestrol: adverse effects on the reproductive tract and reproductive performance in male and female offspring. Am J Obstet Gynecol 142:905, 1982
115. Seeler RA, Israel JN, Royal JE, Kaye CI, Rao S, Abulaban M: Ganglioneuroblastoma and fetal hydantoin–alcohol syndrones. Pediatrics 63:524, 1979
116. Vesselinovitch SD: Comparative studies on perinatal carcinogenesis. In Transplacental Carcinogenesis, No. 4, Edited by L Tomatis, U Mohr. Lyon, I.A.R.C Science Publications, 1973, p 14
117. Neutel CI, Buck C: Effect of smoking during pregnancy on the risk of cancer in children. J Natl Cancer Inst 47:59, 1971
118. Division of Nutrition, Center for Health Promotion and Education. Centers for Disease Control, Atlanta: the fetal tobacco syndrome. JAMA 253:2998, 1985
119. Okie S: Smoking now a threat to women's health. Washington Post, November 11, 1985, p A1
120. Barbieri RL, McShane PM, Ryan KJ: Constituents of cigarette smoke inhibit human granulosa cell aromatase. Fertil Steril 46:232, 1986
121. Rubin DH, Krasilnikoss PA, Leventhal JM, Weile B, Berget A: The effect of passive smoking on birthweight. Lancet 2:415, 1986

Chapter 3

Drug abuse and reproduction

Carol Grace Smith, Ph.D.
Ricardo H. Asch, M.D.

The University of Texas Health Science Center at San Antonio, San Antonio, Texas, and University of California Irvine Medical Center, Orange, California

Drug abuse has so permeated our society that the use of marijuana, alcohol, cocaine, and other mood-altering substances has become commonplace among young adults (Table 1).[1] Today, an estimated 5% to 10% of women of childbearing years (more in some sociodemographic groups) use illicit drugs on a regular basis, and 5% are classified as "heavy" drinkers of alcoholic beverages (two or more drinks per day).[2] Although the research on the reproductive effects of drug abuse is relatively new, it shows potentially serious risks to reproduction and fertility.

REPRODUCTIVE RISKS OF DRUG ABUSE

The degree of reproductive risks from drug abuse depends on many factors. A major factor is extent of drug use, i.e., the amount of a drug that is taken, its frequency of use, and the amount of active ingredients (and contaminants) in the street drugs. A single episode of drug intoxication carries much less risk to reproductive hormones than does daily use. Another factor is the age of the user and the length of time the drug is used. Frequent drug use in adolescence or any drug use during pregnancy is potentially more hazardous. Additionally, individuals with hypogonadal syndromes may be at increased risk to the damaging effects of these drugs.

The reproductive system is unusual among the bodily systems in the complexity of the mechanisms that control it and that must operate in order for it to function. Many classes of drugs can disrupt aspects of these controlling mechanisms and thereby alter reproductive function. Drugs that disrupt nervous system function (either voluntary or autonomic) can inhibit reproduction. The hypothalamic nervous pathways that control the secretion of gonadotropins are inhibited by such central nervous system (CNS) drugs as marijuana, the narcotics, barbiturates, and tranquilizers, making these pathways a major mechanism for the effects of drugs on reproductive hormones. Other classes of drugs include those that inhibit protein or nucleic acid synthesis or cell division; agents that inhibit endocrine or exocrine secretion mechanisms; and agents that alter the biotransformation of hormones by the liver. Few other bodily systems require the intricate interaction of so many components for efficient operation. However, disruption of reproduction is a subtle process that may only be detected when fertility is desired. For this reason, drug effects on reproduction in a population may not be detected for many years.

LIMITATIONS ON REPRODUCTIVE RESEARCH WITH DRUGS OF ABUSE

Almost all drug abuse research has been fraught with contradictions and controversies. Research on the reproductive effects of drugs has had numerous methodologic and interpretive problems, and several important questions remain unanswered. Because ethical considerations prohibit controlled human experiments in this area, clinical research has been limited to epidemiologic and retrospective studies, case reports, and small studies of volunteers. Controlled human studies seldom have been done. Regulations prohibit administration of drugs of abuse to women who might become pregnant or to anyone who has not previously used the drug. The life-styles of regular drug abusers frequently involve conditions that may be hazardous to gen-

Table 1 Current Drug Use by Age Group[a]

Drug	Age group	1979	1982	1985
	yrs	%	%	%
Alcohol	12–17	37.2	26.9	31.5
	18–25	75.9	67.9	71.5
	26+	61.3	56.7	60.7
Marijuana	12–17	16.7	11.5	12.3
	18–25	35.4	27.4	21.9
	26+	6.0	6.5	6.2
Stimulants	12–17	1.2	2.6	1.8
	18–25	3.5	4.7	4.0
	26+	0.5	0.6	0.7
Cocaine	12–17	1.4	1.6	1.8
	18–25	9.3	6.8	7.7
	26+	0.9	1.2	2.1
Hallucinogens	12–17	2.2	1.4	1.1
	18–25	4.4	1.7	1.6
	26+	<0.5	<0.5	<0.5

[a] Percent of the overall household population reporting drug use within the past month at the time of the survey (highlights of the 1985 National Household Survey of Drug Abuse, National Institute on Drug Abuse[1]).

eral health and reproductive health, such as poor nutrition, inadequate medical care, use of contaminated drug paraphernalia, and multiple drug use. These investigations also entail problems of adequacy of the endocrine data collected, validity of self-reports of drug use, and possible bias in participant interviews. Such confounding variables have made it difficult to detect disruptive effects on reproductive function and to document associations with drug abuse practices.

Many of the studies of drug effects on reproduction have been done using laboratory animals. In our opinion, the best animal model for the study of drug abuse effects on reproduction has been the nonhuman primate. Most of the reported drug-effects animal studies have been confirmed by clinical observations, although there have been examples wherein the magnitude of the drug effect has not been that predicted in animal studies. Some of the early studies in laboratory animals used drug dosages far in excess of those used by humans and reported devastating disruption of reproductive function. Recent developments in assay technologies have provided the means to measure blood concentrations of the various drugs, so that the drug dosages used in laboratory studies can actually reflect the usual pattern of drug use by people. Recent advances in our knowledge of hypothalamic-pituitary-gonadal function also have provided important new insights into how the drugs produce their effects. These new developments have resulted in more accurate and reliable data and greater collaboration among laboratory and clinical studies.

NEUROACTIVE DRUGS AND HYPOTHALAMIC-PITUITARY-GONADAL FUNCTION

The evidence now strongly indicates that the major pathways involved in the hypothalamic control of gonadotropins are adrenergic and dopaminergic. A multitude of pharmacologic agents can modify neurotransmitter levels by altering synthesis, release, receptor activation, and reuptake. The best known drugs that produce actions of this type are the neuropharmacologic agents that either inhibit CNS activities—the anesthetics, analgesics, sedatives, and tranquilizers; or stimulate CNS activities—the antidepressants, stimulants, and hallucinogens (Table 2). These drugs can modify the hypothalamic-pituitary control of the gonadotropins and prolactin (PRL) because of their action on CNS pathways. The changes in luteinizing hormone (LH), follicle-stimulating hormone (FSH), and PRL concentrations can result in adverse side effects on the reproductive system, including

Table 2 Pharmacologic Classes of Drugs of Abuse

CNS stimulants
- Amphetamines
- Caffeine
- Cocaine
- Nicotine
- Phenmetrazine (Preludin[a])

CNS depressants
- Anesthetics
- Barbiturates
- Benzodiazepine tranquilizers (Valium[b]; Librium[b]; Dalmane[b]; Serax[c])
- Ethanol
- Inhalants (volatile solvents)
- Marijuana

Psychiatric drugs
- Antipsychotics
  - Phenothiazines (Thorazine[d]; Mellaril[e])
  - Butyrophenones (haloperidol)
  - Thioxanthenes (Taractan[b]; Navane[f])
- Antidepressants
  - Tricyclics
  - MAO inhibitors

Hallucinogens
- Lysergic acid diethylamide (LSD)
- Dimethyltryptamine (DMT)
- Mescaline
- Psylocibin
- Dimethoxyamphetamine (DOM; STP)
- Phencyclidine (PCP)
- Cannabinoids (THC, high doses)

Opiate drugs
- Heroin
- Morphine
- Codeine, oxycodone (Percodan[g])
- Dihydromorphone (Dilaudid[h])
- Meperidine (Demerol[i])
- Propoxyphene (Darvon[j])
- Pentazozine (Talwin[i])
- Paregoric
- Methadone (Dolophine[j])
- L-alpha-acetyl methadol (LAAM)
- Illicit synthetic narcotics ("designer drugs")

[a] Boehringer Ingelheim, Ridgefield, CT; [b]Roche Products, Manati, PR; [c]Wyeth Laboratories, Philadelphia, PA; [d]Smith, Kline and French Laboratories, Philadelphia, PA; [e]Sandoz, Inc., East Hanover, NJ; [f]Roerig, New York, NY; [g]DuPont Pharmaceuticals, Wilmington, DE; [h]Knoll Pharmaceutical Co., Whippany, NJ; [i]Winthrop-Breon Laboratories, New York, NY; [j]Eli Lilly and Company, Indianapolis, IN.

changes in libido, sexual dysfunction, and disruption of fertility.

Marijuana

During the past several years, new concerns have arisen over the possibility of adverse effects on the reproductive system from marijuana use. Several studies show changes in reproductive hormone levels that are consistent with the development of infertility and sexual dysfunction. In response to these concerns, new emphasis has been given to the study of marijuana's effects on reproduction, and several significant findings, both in laboratory animals and clinical studies with human subjects, have contributed to our understanding. Although most of these studies show clear changes in reproductive function, there are also conflicting reports and apparent inconsistencies in the findings.

Studies with laboratory animals clearly show that marijuana and Δ^9-tetrahydrocannabinol (THC), the principal psychoactive ingredient, inhibit secretion of the pituitary hormones, LH and FSH, as well as PRL. These changes in pituitary hormone levels produce decreases in sex steroid hormones. Because of its potent antigonadotropic activity, THC inhibits ovulation. However, ovulation can be induced by exogenous gonadotropins or gonadotropin-releasing hormone (GnRH), even in the presence of high concentrations of THC, suggesting that the antiovulatory effect of THC does not occur at the gonadal or pituitary level, but rather at the hypothalamic level.

Most of the reported findings on the effect of marijuana and its main constituents on primate pituitary hormones have been obtained in the rhesus monkey. Acute administration of THC results in marked reductions (50% to 80%) of serum FSH and LH that last up to 24 hours, depending on the dose administered. As in nonprimate animals, the inhibition of gonadotropin levels by THC appears to take place at the level of the hypothalamus, as both LH and FSH are released from the pituitary gland in response to GnRH in monkeys treated with THC, and THC does not interfere with the estrogen-induced LH surge in castrate female monkeys.[3] Acute administration of THC produces marked suppression of PRL levels.[4] The maximal effect is observed between 30 and 90 minutes after drug treatment. It is likely that the psychoactive properties of THC are related to these effects on reproductive hormones, as nonpsychoactive components of marijuana have no effect on these hormones.

Several studies have examined the effects of marijuana and/or THC on the menstrual cycle. At dose levels that elicit blood concentrations of THC similar to those found in regular human marijuana users, THC disrupted the menstrual cycle in the rhesus monkey. When THC was given during the follicular phase, ovulation was inhibited and hormones remained at basal levels throughout the treatment cycle,[5] and when THC was given during the luteal phase, only slight changes were observed in the hormones of the treatment cycle,[6] but in both cases there was a continued disruption following cessation of the drug treatment. Normal ovulation and hormonal concentrations were restored several months after the cessation of THC administration. Simultaneous administration of exogenous gonadotropins during chronic treatment with THC inhibits the drug effect. Ovulation was restored and normal hormone concentrations were observed. These studies further demonstrate that the antiovulatory effect of THC in the nonhuman primate does not occur primarily at the ovarian level.[7] The mechanism for the prolonged disruption of the menstrual cycle after discontinuation of short-term THC treatment is not known. PRL levels, which were markedly elevated during this post-treatment period, may be involved.

Further studies in monkeys examined the effect of continuous THC treatment on the menstrual cycle and the development of tolerance to the drug effects.[8] All monkeys exhibited normal hormone concentrations and ovulation during the control and vehicle treatment cycles, and menstrual cycle lengths were within normal limits of the colony. The monkeys were given THC (2.5 mg/kg or 1.25 mg/kg) three times per week. After the drug injections began, none of the monkeys ovulated or showed normal hormone levels. The duration of the drug effect (days until next normal menstruation) was 135, 110, and 103 days for the monkeys treated with the 2.5 mg/kg dose of THC and 120 and 70 days for the monkeys treated with the 1.25 mg/kg dose. After tolerance to the drug effects developed, normal cycles were re-established. Ovulation was again detected by laparoscopy and normal concentrations of gonadotropins and steroids were observed. Comparisons were made of PRL concentrations during control cycles, during the period of disruption, and after menstrual cycles were restored. There were no significant differences in PRL concentrations. The previously observed elevations in PRL levels following discontinuation of short-term drug treatment were not observed with chronic drug treatment. Since both gonadotropins and sex steroids were at basal levels during the period of disruption, it is likely that THC inhibited the hypothalamic control of pituitary activity; however, with chronic drug treatment, tolerance develops to this inhibitory effect of THC and normal cycles are re-established. Pharmacokinetic data from this study showed no increase in drug metabolism or clearance that could have produced tolerance. Thus, it is likely that the tolerance that develops to the reproductive effects of THC is due to adaptation of neural mechanisms in the hypothalamus.

These studies in rhesus monkeys are consistent with the clinical studies of young women who regularly use marijuana. Twenty-six women who reported using marijuana at least four times per week were compared with 16 age-matched controls who stated that they had never used marijuana. Marijuana users had shorter menstrual cycles and shorter luteal phases.[9] A recent double-blind study demonstrated the acute suppression of LH concentrations when women smoked marijuana during the luteal phase of the menstrual cycle.[10] These women smoked a single 1-gm marijuana cigarette containing 1.8% THC, and LH concentrations were decreased by 30%. Placebo cigarettes caused no change in LH concentrations. Additional studies indicate the development of tolerance and return to apparently normal hormone concentrations in young women who regularly used marijuana.[11] It is clear now that development of tolerance must be considered as a variable in reproductive studies in young men and women who use marijuana and may help to explain some of the conflicting data in human and laboratory animal studies.

In male laboratory animals, acute or chronic administration of THC results in lower serum concentrations of testosterone (T).[12] In the male rhesus monkey, a single dose of THC causes a significant decrease in blood levels of T as early as 60 minutes after administration; this decrease lasts as long as 24 hours. The decrease in T can be reversed by administration of human chorionic gonadotropin (hCG) (indicating that THC does not directly inhibit testicular synthesis of T) and by GnRH (suggesting a lack of effect at the pituitary gland).[13] Studies with chronically exposed male monkeys show that tolerance develops to the hormonal effects of THC. After tolerance develops, testosterone levels are still decreased by THC treatment, but for shorter periods of time.

Conflicting reports exist on the effects of marijuana on T concentrations in men. Kolodny et al.[14] reported a lowering of plasma T in heavy marijuana users as compared with age-matched controls who had never used marijuana. A later, well-controlled prospective study failed to confirm earlier findings.[15] Studies of hormone levels in marijuana users are hard to interpret. The actual amount of drug that reaches the circulation can be evaluated only by careful measurement of THC levels in the blood. Concentrations of T vary considerably even in normal men, so it is difficult to evaluate the biologic significance of drug-induced changes when they do occur. Other questions remain to be answered, including what role tolerance plays in the effects of THC on hormone levels in men and what are the possible effects of even moderate changes in sex hormones on fertility and sexual function in men.

The effects of marijuana and THC on spermatogenesis has been studied in humans and laboratory animals. Studies in laboratory rodents[16,17] and in dogs[18] have shown that chronic treatment with marijuana or THC can cause decreased testicular size, degenerative changes in spermatogenesis, and abnormal sperm morphology. In vitro studies have shown that cannabinoids inhibit protein and nucleic acid synthesis and glucose metabolism in the rat testes. Inhibition is greatest in the seminiferous tubule cells.[19,20] Inhibition of these processes could account for the decreased sperm production associated with marijuana exposure in animals. Several studies have examined sperm counts and sperm morphology in men who are chronic marijuana users. Kolodny et al.[14] first reported that 6 out of 17 chronic marijuana smokers had sperm counts below 30×10^6/ml. Hembree et al.[21] studied chronic marijuana smokers in a hospital setting. Subjects smoked up to a minimum of ten cigarettes per day (each containing 20 mg of THC) for a 4-week period. Sperm counts were significantly lowered after the treatment period. In a later study, Hembree et al.[22] conducted a similar study in men with an initial sperm count of >100 million and normal sperm motility. As in the previous study, sperm concentrations were significantly lower during the 2 weeks after the 4-week smoking period (motility not studied) and had returned to normal by 3 to 4 weeks after marijuana smoking ceased. In summary, studies in which animals were treated with marijuana or THC are consistent with studies in humans who use marijuana. Both show decreased sperm production following chronic marijuana use. The significance of these observations is unclear, since there are no clinical studies evaluating the effects of marijuana on infertility in men. It is clear from the current evidence that marijuana use should be considered as a factor that may contribute to unexplained infertility in men.

Cocaine

Cocaine is a CNS stimulant, acting mainly on the catecholamine neurotransmitters. Cocaine acts peripherally to inhibit nerve conduction (local anesthetic) and to prevent norepinephrine uptake at nerve terminals. Increased concentrations of norepinephrine at the nerve terminals causes vasoconstriction and tachycardia with an abrupt rise in blood pressure. Some reports indicate that cocaine may actually heighten sexual powers and sexual arousal temporarily. Cocaine has been applied topically to male and female genitalia to increase sexual performance in human males, probably due to its effect as a local anesthetic, thereby prolonging erection and delaying ejaculation. In addition, many claims that cocaine is an aphrodisiac may be attributed to the fact that, like other CNS drugs, it suppresses inhibitions. The acute effect of cocaine at low to moderate dosages is an increase in LH, whereas at higher doses, cocaine appears to inhibit LH release.[23,24] Therefore, at low to moderate dosages, an increase in T should be expected, and at higher dosages, T levels should be inhibited. Studies in female ovariectomized rats show that moderate doses (10 to 20 mg/kg of cocaine) increase and high doses (40 mg/kg cocaine) decrease serum LH. FSH was unaffected at any dosage, whereas serum PRL levels were decreased by cocaine at either dosage level.[25] The effects of cocaine on LH and PRL appear to be due, in part, to their effect on the neurotransmitters, norepinephrine and dopamine. Cocaine prevents reuptake of released norepinephrine at nerve endings, leading to increased levels of neurotransmitter in the nerve terminals and enhanced effect. Cocaine also has been shown to block the reuptake of dopamine. Inhibition of PRL and stimulation of LH release by cocaine may be due to these actions on neurotransmitters. It is not known whether pharmacologic stimulation of gonadotropin release and inhibition of PRL release can cause disruption of reproductive function in humans. It is likely that chronic cocaine use would result in temporary depletion of hypothalamic neurotransmitters and inhibition of gonadotropins and elevated PRL concentrations; however, no studies on the effects of cocaine on reproductive hormones in humans have been published. This may be because the other life-threatening toxicities of cocaine on other bodily systems and the clear risk of cocaine dependency overshadow the concern about effects on reproductive hormones.

Narcotics

The effects of narcotic drugs on reproductive function have been observed in heroin addicts. Clinical manifestations, such as decreased sexual desire and performance, menstrual irregularities, and infertility among narcotics users are attributed, in part, to altered gonadal functions.[26–28]

Acute doses of morphine have been found to prevent ovulation in laboratory animals,[29] and chronic doses of morphine or heroin totally disrupt the estrous cycle in rodents and the menstrual cycle in women.[26,30] It is clear that the narcotics produce these disruptions in female reproductive function by altering reproductive hormone levels. Significant reductions in both serum LH and FSH have been observed in narcotic-treated female rodents and humans.

Heroin addicts have decreased fertility and atrophy of male accessory sex organs. Similar findings were observed in laboratory animals, with marked decreases in seminal vesicle and prostate weights in narcotic-treated rats. This disruption of male fertility by narcotics appears to be produced by alteration of reproductive endocrine function; however, serum concentrations of FSH and LH in male addicts have been reported as unchanged,[31] significantly decreased,[32] or slightly increased.[33] In rodents, significant decreases in LH levels were observed after administration of morphine.[34]

Studies in the male rhesus monkey described the effect of acute morphine administration on plasma LH and T levels.[35] In these studies, morphine sulfate (0.25 to 1.0 mg/kg) or saline vehicle was given to adult monkeys by an intravenous injection through an indwelling jugular catheter. Significant decreases in LH levels were observed 40 to 100 minutes after drug treatment. LH levels remained below pretreatment levels for at least 140 minutes. Significant depressions in plasma T levels occurred by 80 minutes after morphine administration, and T remained significantly depressed for at least 100 minutes. The decrease in LH levels preceded the depression of circulating T by approximately 40 minutes. This difference in time of drug effect on the hormones corresponds with the typical physiologic lag period between LH changes and subsequent T changes.

The majority of current evidence concerning the opioid-induced decrease in plasma T levels suggests a CNS-mediated action. A lack of a direct testicular effect is supported by studies in monkeys pretreated with hCG to remove the effects of endogenous LH on T production.[35] Morphine administration subsequent to hCG had no direct effect on T levels. Numerous studies indicate that narcotics act via the hypothalamus and not through a direct pituitary effect. GnRH, administered to monkeys after the administration of morphine, produces a LH response that is indistinguishable in magnitude, duration, and time of onset from that observed in monkeys pretreated with vehicle.[36] The absence of a direct pituitary effect of narcotics has been demonstrated further by in vitro studies in which addition of morphine sulfate to an incubation system containing rat anterior pituitary tissue had no effect on gonadotropin release stimulated by GnRH.[37] Thus, it appears that the effects of narcotics on gonadotropin levels are elicited at a level above the pituitary, probably involving modulation of the endogenous opioid peptides (EOP). Studies have been done using the EOP and opioid drugs to evaluate the interaction of EOP with reproductive endocrine function. Administration of the Leu-enkephalin analog D-Ala^2,D-Leu^5-enkephalin to male monkeys decreased both T and LH levels.[36] This decrease in LH concentration is consistent with decreases observed in normal human males administered a Met-enkephalin analog.[38] In contrast, no statistically significant alterations in plasma LH levels were observed in male monkeys administered a 10.0-mg/kg dose of beta-endorphin; however, studies in human male volunteers administered a 40 mg/kg dose of beta-endorphin showed a decrease in serum LH.[39] When compared on a relative basis, the pharmacologic effects of morphine and various EOP may be used to infer differential actions on these various narcotic receptor subtypes. Morphine has been shown to have greatest selectivity for mu receptors; D-Ala,^{2} D-Leu^5-enkephalin is delta-selective; and beta-endorphin has about equal actions upon mu and delta receptors. When compared on a molar basis, these findings suggest that the receptor subtypes responsible for opioid-induced inhibition of plasma LH are delta. Further studies have been done using the opiate receptor antagonist, naloxone. Naloxone administration produces increases in plasma LH levels, presumably by blocking the tonic inhibitory effects of the EOP. This effect has been demonstrated with naloxone administration in humans,[40,41] monkeys,[36] and rats.[42] When administered to monkeys after pretreatment with opioids, naloxone completely reversed the opioid effects and produced increases in plasma LH levels that did not differ significantly from those seen with naloxone alone. These results indicate that naloxone can reverse the tonic inhibitory effect of the EOP on gonadotropin secretion and that this effect is mediated through opiate receptors. The precise mechanism by which opioids modulate neuroendocrine function is unknown. The most likely mechanism would appear to involve one of the various putative synaptic transmitters that regulate hypothalamic endocrine neurons.[43–45]

Alcohol

Alcohol is another example of a commonly abused drug that affects the reproductive system. Its effects on reproduction have been studied primarily in male subjects. In a study of 16 normal men, LH and T levels were determined during a period of acute alcohol intoxication.[46] Careful monitoring of both T and LH levels demonstrated that the primary effect of alcohol is on the testicular synthesis and secretion of T. Both ethanol and its major metabolite, acetaldehyde, inhibit the testicular enzymes involved in T synthesis.[47] This testicular effect of alcohol is worsened by the increased metabolic clearance rate of T by the liver, which also is caused by acute alcohol consumption.[48] As expected, male alcoholics and animals treated chronically with alcohol produce less T and have lower serum T levels.[49,50] Multiple endocrine abnormalities are seen in men with alcoholic cirrhosis. Hypogonadism and gynecomastia are common manifestations of alcoholic cirrhosis in men. These manifestations emphasize how important normal liver function is to the maintenance of reproductive function. With destructive liver disease, the pattern of circulating sex steroids changes. Increased levels of estrogenic steroids are observed in these men. These estrogenic steroids secondarily suppress gonadotropins and T production and inhibit the functioning of accessory sex glands.[49]

Thus, the primary toxic effect of alcohol appears to be testicular.[51] Reduction in circulating T concentrations and decreased responsiveness to exogenous hCG are consistent with Leydig cell damage. This does not preclude inhibition of hypothalamic-pituitary function as being involved in alcohol-related effects. LH concentrations tend to be normal in alcoholics instead of being elevated as might be expected, and there is good evidence of a dual effect on gonadal and hypothalamic-pituitary function in men with alcoholic liver disease.[52]

Alcohol can directly inhibit penile tumescence and ejaculatory capability through a direct action on spinal reflex centers.[53,54] In alcoholic and nonalcoholic men, a blood alcohol level of 40 to 50 mg/dl inhibits penile tumescence, and with a blood alcohol level of above 100 mg/dl, penile tumescence is almost completely inhibited. Chronic alcoholism may result in permanent impotence in men, even after years of sobriety.[55]

Both acute and chronic alcohol exposure can cause abnormal spermatozoa. After acute alcohol consumption (0.4 to 0.8 gm/kg), sperm samples from a group of men revealed spermatozoa with heads broken off, tails curled, and distended midsections.[56] Sperm specimens from alcoholic men able to produce an ejaculate were grossly abnormal with fewer total cells and many abnormal cells.[50]

A few studies have examined the effects of alcohol on reproductive hormones in the female. Alcohol does appear to inhibit gonadal activities in female rodents.[57,58] These effects may not be as pronounced in women and laboratory primates. In clinical studies, there was no significant effect of acute alcohol ingestion on either sex steroids or gonadotropins.[59] A similar lack of effect was observed in female rhesus monkeys when alcohol was administered at various phases of the menstrual cycle.[60] These results demonstrate that women and female nonhuman primates may be less sensitive to the acute gonadal effects of alcohol, although females may not be less vulnerable to the toxic effects of chronic alcohol use on reproductive endocrinology. Chronic use of alcohol and alcoholism have been related to infertility[61,62] and menstrual disorders in women,[63,64] and disruption of reproductive function has been shown with alcohol self-administration in female monkeys.[65]

Other Central Nervous System Drugs

The barbiturates are classified pharmacologically as sedative-hypnotic agents. They are general depressant drugs, and the CNS has a particular sensitivity to this effect. Although the exact mechanism of action is not known, barbiturates are known to depress neural activity in various brain regions. Their potent depressant effects have made them popular as drugs of abuse, both for their sedative effects and for the effect they produce in combination with other drugs of abuse. Barbiturates have been used as anesthetic agents in reproductive studies in laboratory animals for many years. These studies provided the description of the inhibitory effects of these drugs on reproductive hormones, observations that resulted in the use of these drugs as important tools in the study of reproductive function. Most of these investigations concerned the neuroendocrine control of female reproductive cycles, but some information is available on the effects of barbiturates in male animals.

The general effect of barbiturates is an inhibition of both LH and FSH, with subsequent depression of steroid hormone secretion. Barbiturate anesthesia blocked both spontaneous and steroid-induced LH release in rats[66] and hamsters.[67] In these animals, the spontaneous release of LH is controlled by the light-dark cycle and occurs at a specific hour and day of the estrous cycle. Prolonged barbiturate anesthesia did not block the steroid-induced LH surge in rhesus monkeys.[68] This suggests that barbiturates act on neural elements—in the medial preoptic area—that generate the circadian stimulus mediating LH release and not at the medial basal hypothalamus, where steroid hormones have their action. The effect of barbiturate anesthesia in male animals is similar to the effect in females. Phenobarbital inhibits gonadotropin secretion and blocks the rise in serum gonadotropin levels that normally follows castration.[69] Both of these effects can be reversed by the administration of GnRH. LH secretion and ovulation can be restored in barbiturate-treated animals by infusion of GnRH, indicating a hypothalamic site of action for the barbiturates.[70] Studies in both male and female animals showed that barbiturate pretreatment can even potentiate the effect of GnRH on LH release.[69,71]

The effect of barbiturates on PRL concentrations is less well established. Nonspecific stresses, such as anesthesia and blood drawing, increase PRL release. Studies employing these techniques in the evaluation of PRL concentrations are difficult to interpret. Acute administration of barbiturates in relatively small doses appears to cause the release of PRL.[72,73] However, barbiturate anesthesia blocks the release of PRL caused by ether or estrogen administration.[74]

An additionally well-recognized effect of the barbiturates is stimulation of hepatic mixed-function oxidases. The same enzyme systems are involved in the metabolism of the steroid hormones. Thus, the barbiturates have the potential for disrupting reproductive hormones by several mechanisms. Such effects have not, however, been demonstrated in clinical studies.

Phencyclidine hydrochloride (PCP) was one of a group of related drugs developed as anesthetic agents and animal tranquilizers. PCP is now a frequently abused drug commonly referred to as "angel dust." It has been classified as a schedule I controlled substance, and legal manufacture and sale of the drug was discontinued in 1978.

Many areas of the brain are affected by PCP. It has been shown to alter the catabolism, steady state levels and turnover rates of a number of neurotransmitters in the CNS, and current evidence indicates that the effects of PCP are caused by alterations in the function of several neurotransmitters. There have been several investigations of the effect of PCP and ketamine (a PCP analog) on reproductive hormones. Ferin et al.[75] showed that release of LH, growth hormone, and PRL persisted under prolonged sedation with PCP, but the secretion of PRL in response to the administration of thyrotropin-releasing hormone (TRH) was increased in animals under sedation. Zaidi et al.[76] reported that serum T levels and production rates were not significantly different in conscious or ketamine-anesthetized male rhesus monkeys. Numerous endocrine studies in laboratory primates have used PCP or ketamine as an anesthetic agent for minor surgical and blood-drawing procedures because these agents have less effect on reproductive hormones than do other anesthetic agents.

Another study examined the acute and chronic effects of PCP on reproductive hormone levels in male rats. Acute administration of PCP at recreational dosage levels produced only a slight depression of serum T and LH levels. However, both hormones were strongly reduced after nine daily treatments, and after discontinuation of drug treatment, both hormones were significantly elevated above control levels and returned to normal value by 60 days. A similar period of elevated serum T and LH was found in adult male rats that received nine daily injections of PCP during sexual maturation. The magnitude of the increased hormone levels in the PCP-treated juvenile rats was several times that of the rats that received the drug as adults, and the period of elevation persisted for 80 days.[77] It is not known whether PCP inhibits reproductive hormones in humans.

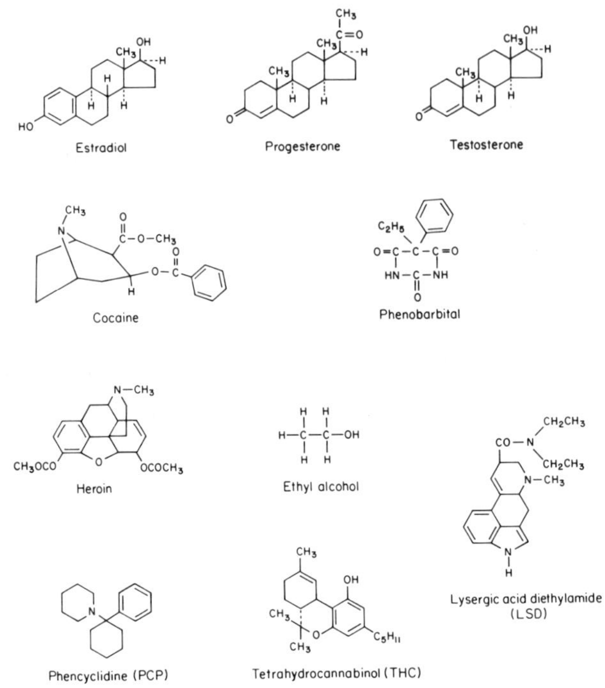

Figure 1 Representative chemical structures of the drugs of abuse and steroid reproductive hormones.

Summary

It is clear that a number of CNS agents, including drugs of abuse, can inhibit reproductive function. Figure 1 shows the chemical diversity of some of the drug groups that affect reproductive hormones. Their structural dissimilarity to the steroid hormones is also readily apparent in the figure. These chemically diverse drugs share an important pharmacologic property: they are highly potent neuroactive drugs, and they can disrupt hypothalamic-pituitary function. Although it is frequently difficult to distinguish between direct drug actions on the hypothalamic-pituitary axis and subsequent effects on gonadal hormones and sex accessory gland function, the distinction is an important one. Most neuroactive drugs produce only transient effects on the central nervous pathways necessary for normal gonadotropin secretion. The disruptive effects of these drugs are likely to be transient and completely reversible, and tolerance to the inhibitory drug effects may occur even with continued drug use. Under these circumstances, normal adults may experience only subtle changes in sexual function. However, individuals with compromised reproductive function may exhibit major problems. It is also likely that adolescents may be at substantial risk for reproductive damage from these neuroactive drugs since the endocrine events associated with puberty are dependent on the normal development of the hypothalamic-pituitary axis.

DRUG ABUSE EFFECTS ON PREGNANCY AND FETAL/PERINATAL DEVELOPMENT

It is well recognized that drugs taken during pregnancy can produce devastating effects on fetal development. Dysmorphic teratology is considered to be the major risk associated with drug use in pregnancy, but additional concern is behavioral teratology. Behavioral effects are less obvious and, therefore, not as easily recognized as dysmorphic effects. Although most drugs of abuse do not produce obvious congenital malformations, there is increasing evidence of neurologic and behavioral effects that can impair a child's development. Recent developments in the methods used to evaluate neonatal behavior and neurologic development are providing a better understanding of behavioral teratology.

The maternal-placental-fetal unit is a complex pharmacologic model. Each component is an independent and dependent contributor to the overall picture of drug disposition and toxicity. Additionally, the pharmacologic and physicochemical properties of the drug(s) or its metabolites can play an important role in the development of teratologic effects. Drug abuse frequently represents an optimal combination of the factors favoring adverse effects on pregnancy (Table 3). The drugs produce potent and reinforcing CNS effects on the pregnant mother. She is likely to use them frequently and throughout pregnancy. The highly potent CNS drugs that readily cross the blood–brain barrier (lipid-soluble; low molecular weight) also readily cross the placenta. The preferred routes of administration (intravenous or inhalation) produce high serum concentrations that may not undergo first-pass metabolism and may cross the placenta in large quantities. The illicit drugs of abuse are readily available, but they are expensive and frequently contain toxic contaminants. Most drugs of abuse have pharmacologic actions that are undesirable in pregnancy, apart from their direct fetotoxic actions. Both stimulants and depressant drugs can decrease appetite and result in inadequate nutrition during pregnancy, and the cardiovascular effects of the drugs can hinder placental circulation and placental metabolic function. At birth, the drugs can persist in fetal circulation and interfere with neonatal adaptation. Most of the drugs of abuse have no specific antagonist for neonatal resuscitation and certain drugs cause a newborn abstinence syndrome. Maternal drug abuse that continues after the pregnancy can result in continued drug exposure of the infant during nursing and disruption of infant care.

Table 3 Teratogenic Potential of Drug Abuse

Maternal factors
Amount and duration of drug use
Poly-drug abuse
Routes of administration of drugs
Altered pharmacokinetics in pregnancy
Prenatal medical care
Parenting abilities
Placental factors
Placental transfer of drugs
Placental metabolism of drugs
Direct placental toxicity of drugs (e.g., effects on placental growth and development and effects on placental circulation)
Fetal factors
Genetic susceptibility to drug toxicity
Stage of embryonic/fetal development
Immaturity of drug biotransformation activities
Drug factors
Pharmacologic actions
Potency
Contaminants in illicit drugs

Since drug abuse has such a potential for harmful effects on pregnancy, it is perhaps surprising that the associations are not well documented in the clinical literature. There are several reasons why this is not the case. Drug and alcohol dependency in pregnancy has been described as one of the most frequently missed diagnoses in obstetrics. This situation could be significantly improved with routine urine toxicology during prenatal visits. Excellent guidelines recently have been published for the recognition, management, and/or referral to treatment facilities for drug dependence in pregnancy.[78] Even the research on drug abuse in pregnancy reflects a somewhat ambivalent approach to the problem. Many of the studies are retrospective, based on the recall of the pregnant woman during or after the pregnancy. Prospective studies are complicated by the intervention strategies that attempt to persuade women to discontinue or modify their drug use to minimize the risk to the pregnancy and unborn child. Statistical interpretation of all of the studies is overwhelmed by the presence in the subjects and controls of other serious risk factors, so we may never learn the independent risk of drug abuse in pregnancy. The studies are further complicated by the inability to perform the types of research on the fetus that might yield data on drug effects on human development. Despite the limitations of such studies, there are some useful observations that show the risks of drug abuse during pregnancy.

Effects on Pregnancy Hormones and Length of Gestation

There is convincing evidence that the neuroactive drugs of abuse can inhibit both gonadotropins and sex steroids during the menstrual cycle. It is reasonable to presume that similar inhibitory effects on chorionic gonadotropins and sex steroids may occur if these drugs are used during pregnancy. Inhibition of pregnancy hormones could result in a range of toxicities from insufficient placental growth and function to pregnancy termination. In order to determine whether such toxicities are produced through a disruption of the endocrine function of the placenta, careful endocrine studies must be done throughout the course of the pregnancy and in close proximity to the episodes of drug use. Such studies are difficult to accomplish, particularly with the illicit drugs. There are, however, several studies that indicate that disruption of pregnancy hormones may be partly responsible for some of the problems when marijuana is used during pregnancy.

The extent of marijuana use by pregnant women is thought to be comparable to the estimated 14% of women (ages 18 to 25) who use marijuana in the general population. This is sufficient to represent a serious health hazard if marijuana is found to have a deleterious effect on pregnancy or fetal growth and development. Several studies have presented evidence linking certain maternal and fetal risk factors with marijuana use during pregnancy. A prospective study examined women who reported use of marijuana before and/or during pregnancy.[79] Infants born to heavy users showed significantly more symptoms of CNS immaturity (inability to self-quiet, heightening of tremors and startles, failure to react to visual stimuli). A recent study examined the effect of marijuana use during pregnancy on length of gestation and infant birth weight.[80] Compared to nonuse, an average use of marijuana six or more times per week during pregnancy was associated with a significant reduction in the length of gestation after consideration of the effects of nicotine, alcohol, parity, prepregnancy weight, and sex of the infant. Among heavy marijuana users, the effect on gestation length was dose-dependent.

An examination of labor and delivery of mothers who had used marijuana during pregnancy demonstrated an increased incidence of meconium in the amniotic fluid in the newborn infants. Need for neonatal resuscitation was also greater, particularly when the mother had used marijuana close to delivery.[81] When Hingson and associates examined the effects of using marijuana, alcohol, or both during pregnancy, they found a relationship between maternal marijuana smoking and poor fetal development.[82] Women who used marijuana during pregnancy delivered infants with significantly decreased birth weight, body length, and head circumference, and these infants were five times more likely to have dysmorphic features usually associated with fetal alcohol syndrome.

The effect of THC, the principal psychoactive component in marijuana, has been studied in pregnant rhesus monkeys.[83] The THC or vehicle was administered during different periods of gestation and effects on pregnancy outcome and hormone concentrations during pregnancy were studied. The most obvious effects were observed when THC was administered from early in the pregnancy. Three of the five pregnancies were aborted within days after the drug injections began; one pregnancy resulted in stillbirth at term; and one pregnancy resulted in the birth of an infant of normal size and appearance. The three abortions were associated with a premature decrease in chorionic gonadotropin and progesterone (P) concentrations. Estradiol (E_2) concentrations were significantly higher than in vehicle control pregnancies in the two pregnancies that continued until term. Daily THC administration during the middle or third portions of gestation resulted in less pregnancy loss (one premature birth and four live births at term with THC treatment during the middle portion; two premature births and three live births at term with THC treatment during the third portion of gestation). All of the premature infants died within 2 weeks of birth of the complications of prematurity. The weights of the infants at birth and weaning were not significantly different for the full-term infants of vehicle control pregnancies and full-term infants that were exposed to THC during gestation. Since no effects on intrauterine growth and development were detected (by ultrasound) in the drug-treated pregnancies, the most likely cause of the early pregnancy loss was disruption of placental endocrine function.

There is evidence that a LH-releasing hormone-like hormone of placental origin controls the secretion of chorionic gonadotropin in human and nonhuman primates.[84] It is reasonable to postulate that the inhibitory effects of THC on placental function early in pregnancy are due to an effect on the placental LH-releasing hormone-like substance in a manner similar to its effect on hypothalamic LH-releasing hormone. If, in the monkey studies, the THC administration began after the physiologic decline in macaque chorionic gonadotropin (mCG), no effect on P concentrations was observed, and no effect on mCG or P concentrations was observed during the remainder of the pregnancy. The implication is that there is a critical interval for the inhibition of mCG by THC administration. This fact may explain why Braunstein et al.[85] observed no significant differences in hCG concentrations or outcomes of pregnancy in women who used marijuana during pregnancy and those who did not.

Effects on Fetal Growth, Development, and Malformations: The Fetal Alcohol Syndrome

Fetal alcohol syndrome (FAS) was first recognized as a syndrome in 1973.[86,87] Unlike other problems associated with drug abuse in pregnancy, FAS is a clinically observable entity with specific parameters for diagnosis. Three parameters make up the primary presentation of FAS: (1) prenatal growth deficiency in length and weight; (2) microcephaly; and (3) short palpebral fissures. Infants with FAS are small for their gestational age and, unlike other small infants, they remain small for their age through childhood.

A prospective study of over 800 women examined the effect of maternal drinking during pregnancy using regression analysis, which adjusted for such factors as smoking, maternal height, maternal age and parity, gestational age, and sex of the child. This study found that, for each ounce of alcohol consumed per day during late pregnancy, there was a resultant depression in birth weight of 160 gm.[88] Numerous studies have confirmed alcohol use during pregnancy as a risk factor for intrauterine growth retardation.[2,89,90] There also is the possibility that drinking prior to pregnancy may have residual effects on subsequent prenatal growth. Little et al.[91] found that birth weights of children born to alcoholic women who abstained during pregnancy were about 260 gm below those infants of nonalcoholic women, and the average birth weights for infants of alcoholic women who drank during pregnancy was about 490 gm below normal. Other risk factors related to alcohol use during pregnancy may contribute to the decreased birth weight. In one study, maternal smoking was found to have an additive effect to that of alcohol.[2] Alcohol abuse alone resulted in a 2.4-fold increase in intrauterine growth retardation, smoking had a 1.8-fold increase, and the combination of alcohol abuse and smoking was associated with a 3.9-fold increase. Since chronic alcoholics tend to be undernourished, it is possible that growth deficiency in FAS may be due, in part, to alcohol-related nutritional deficiencies.[92] Alcohol impairs absorption and metabolism of nutrients, vitamins, and minerals.[93] Although animal studies that use "pair-feeding" techniques minimize the importance of altered nutrition in the production of FAS,[94] alcohol-related inhibition of transport across membranes may be important in the nutritional contribution to FAS.[95] Thus, altered nutrition cannot be ruled out as an indirect factor in FAS. Other alcohol-related illnesses, socioeconomic conditions, and related stresses also may contribute to the toxic effects of alcohol abuse. However, unlike infants of the women in many of the drug-abuse studies, infants of alcoholic women who come from mostly Caucasian, middle socioeconomic backgrounds clearly demonstrate the manifestations of FAS.[88]

It was the similarity of the facial features associated with FAS that first drew clinical attention to the syndrome. Clarren and Smith[96] noted that the key facial features are short palpebral fissures, hypoplastic upper lip with thinned vermilion, a diminished-to-absent philthrum, and, frequently, midfacial and mandibular growth deficiency. The facial features of FAS are thought to result from midfacial hypoplasia. Studies in an animal model have shown that facial features similar to FAS can be produced in mice when exposure occurs during the gastrulation stage of embryogenesis.[97] Other anomalies include cardiac septal defects,[98] skeletal defects,[99] urogenital defects,[100] and structural and developmental anomalies of the brain and spinal cord.[101] Behavioral teratology is another remarkable feature of the FAS. There is good evidence that children born to alcoholics are at risk for various behavioral problems, the most serious of which is mental retardation. Studies in laboratory animals demonstrate deficits in learning/memory function with prenatal exposure to alcohol.[102,103]

FAS represents a spectrum of anomalies that are manifest to a different extent in different individuals. The full FAS is seen only in some of the infants of chronic alcoholic women. Other infants of alcoholic mothers have few or none of the fetal alcohol affects. A recent study discovered one difference in alcoholic women whose infants had FAS and those who did not. Women who gave birth to infants with FAS had lower E_2 and estriol concentrations throughout pregnancy and tended to have lower P concentrations than those alcoholic women whose infants did not have FAS. PRL levels were elevated in all alcoholic women, and hCG concentrations were not different in alcoholic women and abstinent women.[104]

The actual mechanisms by which alcohol produces the effects of fetal alcohol exposure are unknown. The mechanism by which alcohol produces the growth-retarding effect may be different from the mechanism that produces congenital abnormalities. Since there are no clear relationships between quantity of alcohol used during pregnancy and the severity of the FAS, it is reasonable to presume that factors such as maximum blood alcohol concentrations, stage of gestational development, adequacy of nutrition before and during pregnancy, smoking, and other drug use in pregnancy contribute to the severity of FAS. Attempts have been made to establish a safe level of alcohol use in pregnancy, but with so many uncertainties, such information is speculative. In 1981, the Surgeon General of the United States recommended that women abstain from alcohol throughout pregnancy.

Complications of Pregnancy and Labor/Delivery

Heroin addiction was once the only major drug abuse concern in the treatment of pregnant patients. At the present time, cocaine addiction (either alone or in combination with alcohol and/or tranquilizers) is a major drug abuse problem. An estimated 10 million Americans have used cocaine at least once and 5 million use it on a regular basis.[105] The factors that have contributed to this are thought to be the ready availability of cocaine, the ease of administration of cocaine, and the drug's popularity among prominent individuals. Cocaine is recognized as a particularly attractive drug to women as their first drug of abuse.

Significant complications in pregnancy and adverse effects on infants have been reported in women who use cocaine during pregnancy. The use of cocaine during the first trimester of pregnancy was associated with an increased rate of spontaneous abortion and third trimester cocaine use increased the risk of abruptio placentae within 30 minutes of use.[106] It is likely that the increased rate of spontaneous abortion caused by cocaine in early pregnancy is due to decreased blood flow to the fetus as a result of placental vasoconstriction and an increase in uterine contractility caused by increased norepinephrine concentrations. Women who used cocaine in the third trimester reported feeling contractions and increased fetal activity within minutes of cocaine use. The hypertension and placental vasoconstriction in these women caused by cocaine is thought to increase their risk of abruptio placentae. Maternal cocaine use also may cause fetal tachycardia and hypertension. One recent report of perinatal cerebral infarction was thought to be caused by use of a large amount of cocaine by the mother before delivery.[107] Another study of eight newborns who were positive on urine toxicology screening for cocaine demonstrated no potentially life-threatening symptoms at birth.[108]

Impairment of newborn interactive behavior and poor organizational response to environmental stimuli has been demonstrated in infants of women who use cocaine during pregnancy.[107] Similar neurobehavioral impairments have been shown to result from prenatal drug exposure to opiate drugs[109] and to PCP.[110] A recent study demonstrated abnormal sleeping ventilatory patterns in infants of mothers who abused cocaine and PCP during pregnancy.[111] These abnormalities have been implicated as a risk factor for sudden infant death syndrome (SIDS). Infants born to mothers who abuse opiates during pregnancy have a 5- to 10-fold increased risk of dying from SIDS,[112] so the abnormal sleep ventilatory patterns in infants exposed in utero to cocaine and PCP mean that these infants may carry an increased risk of SIDS.

Neonatal Complications

The narcotic abstinence syndrome in newborns is the best-documented neonatal complication of drug abuse in pregnancy. The syndrome consists of a wide variety of features that mimic aspects of the adult narcotic abstinence syndrome. Most significant for the neonate are tremors, high-pitched cry, sweating, exoriation of the extremities, and gastrointestinal upset.[113] Most of the infants of heroin- or methadone-addicted mothers will undergo some degree of withdrawal within hours to days after birth. The incidence of withdrawal may be related to the degree of maternal addiction but not to the severity of the withdrawal symptoms.[114] The severity of the withdrawal symptoms appears to be more related to the degree of poly-drug abuse by the mother and the maternal dosage of methadone.[115]

Infants delivered to mothers who abuse heroin have a higher incidence of perinatal morbidity and mortality than do infants in the general population. It has been well established that infants born to heroin-addicted mothers have low birth weights (half below 2500 gm) and are small for gestational age.[116–118] There is evidence that this is due to both prematurity and intrauterine growth retardation. Narcotic drug exposure during pregnancy produces growth delays that are not related to inadequate maternal nutrition or prenatal care[119] and that result from a subnormal number of cells in all organs of the developing fetus.[120] Infants born to mothers on methadone maintenance weigh more at birth than the infants of mothers using heroin, so the usual procedure is to initiate methadone replacement early in the pregnancy.[113,121] Methadone maintenance during pregnancy is, at best, a tradeoff. Although the intrauterine stress of narcotics abstinence syndrome is avoided, the newborns suffer a greater postnatal weight loss[122,123] and have a higher incidence of withdrawal and more severe withdrawal symptoms than do the newborns of heroin-addicted mothers.[113] There is evidence that heroin may accelerate lung and liver maturation,[124] which would be helpful in premature birth.

Other perinatal complications of narcotic addiction that have been reported include a higher incidence of meconium staining and perinatal asphyxia and neonatal death following narcotic withdrawal in the last trimester of pregnancy.[120,125] Some studies have found a high incidence of respiratory distress in the neonates,[115,126] and there are reports of an increased incidence of SIDS among infants of women addicted to the narcotic drugs.[111]

Behavioral symptoms that continue through infancy in these drug-exposed infants include irritability, hyperactivity, and feeding and sleep disturbances. Psychological and educational problems may continue throughout early and middle childhood, but the available studies are insufficient to permit definitive conclusions.[127]

Polydrug Abuse in Pregnancy

A significant problem in drug abuse research in pregnancy is lack of control over polydrug use. The prevalence of polydrug abuse among pregnant women who use drugs makes it complex, if not impossible, to determine the effect of abuse of a single drug. The concurrent use of alcohol, stimulants, tranquilizers, PCP, and combinations including sedative/stimulant and pentazocine/tripelennamine (so-called Ts and blues), is common in women who use drugs during pregnancy. In one program, the Perinatal Services Project of Northwestern University, specialized prenatal care for these women results in successful drug abstinence throughout the remainder of the pregnancy of only about 20%. However, with close supervision of nutritional intake in women enrolled in this special program, there was no significant reduction in fetal growth parameters. Intrauterine exposure to the nonopiate drugs and combinations did not reduce birth weight, length, and head circumference as compared with non-drug-exposed infants.[128] The newborn infants exposed to drugs, however, showed significant impairment of their interactive abilities, motor maturity, and organizational responses to environmental stimuli. They were more tremulous and irritable than the control infants and showed significant and unpredictable emotional responses. These studies demonstrated the beginning of the cycle of poor infant responsiveness and maternal rejection: a behavioral pattern that must be interrupted if the mother/infant relationship is to be established. Among the polydrug abuse problems, the use of PCP is of particular concern. PCP has been shown to cross the placenta in both animals and humans.[129,130] The use of PCP during pregnancy has adverse effects on the newborn. A withdrawal syndrome in two infants exposed prenatally to PCP has been reported.[131] PCP-exposed infants were particularly labile and showed marked deficits in their responses to mothering attempts by caretakers.[132]

A 2-year follow-up of the drug-exposed and control infants demonstrated a downward trend in developmental scores, but all of the infants were from a low socioeconomic population, a factor known to adversely affect developmental scores. There has been no long-term follow-up of children who have been exposed to multiple-drug abuse before birth, so their prognosis for emotional and educational development remains unknown. Infants and children of women who use drugs during pregnancy remain at increased risk for various problems, including SIDS,[110] increased rate of infections, including acquired immunodeficiency syndrome (AIDS),[133] and a high rate of child abuse.[134]

DRUG ABUSE AND ADOLESCENT REPRODUCTIVE DEVELOPMENT

Surveys indicate that young Americans have been gradually moderating their use of illicit drugs in recent years; however, adolescent drug abuse is still acknowledged as a national problem. The age of first use of virtually all drugs has steadily declined; and, while the strength of many street drugs has increased, their cost has sharply decreased, increasing their availability to younger buyers. The 1985 National Household Survey found that 1 in 5 (22%) of 12- to 17-year-olds has used marijuana. About half of those who have ever used marijuana have continued to use it (i.e., had used it in the month preceding the survey).[1] Typically, persons who have a degree of experience with marijuana (used it more than ten times) will become involved in the use of another illicit drug and those who use illicit drugs other than marijuana are likely to continue using at least three substances concurrently.[135] By the time they are high school seniors, the majority of adolescents have tried alcohol, tobacco, and marijuana, and 1 in 20 uses alcohol or marijuana daily.[136]

Since adolescence is a critical developmental period of life, heavy drug use and involvement in a drug lifestyle have a greater negative impact than they do in adults. Research shows that adolescents use drugs because they are readily available; they provide a quick, easy, cheap way to feel good; they offer a means of gaining peer acceptance. They may also help modify unpleasant feelings, reduce disturbing emotions, alleviate depression, reduce tension, and help cope with life pressures.[137] Some adolescents (as many as 5% of teens aged 14 to 18 years) have serious drug-related problems and need treatment. These youngsters are generally compulsive, dedicated users with serious personal problems who rely on drugs as self-medication to cope with their problems.[138,139]

The physiologic events associated with normal adolescent development rely on the maturation of the hypothalamic centers that control the release of GnRH. The earliest indication that this process is beginning is an increase in episodic secretion of GnRH and gonadotropins; throughout the course of adolescent development, the secretion of GnRH is of paramount importance. There is evidence that most of the drugs of abuse can interfere with the secretion of GnRH. Inhibition of GnRH during adolescent development is physiologically more significant than inhibition of GnRH in an adult. Thus, drug abuse by adolescents may result in delayed or arrested reproductive development. It is difficult to predict the magnitude of such disruption, but it is reasonable to presume that the developing system is particularly sensitive to pharmacologic inhibition of GnRH. It would also be difficult to identify drug-related disruption of adolescent development without careful evaluation because there is considerable age variation and irregular progress in the normal developmental process. In addition to the risks of long-term disruption of reproductive function, the emotional trauma of arrested sexual development may contribute to the drug-seeking behavior.

The effect of THC or marijuana administration on aspects of pubertal development has been studied in laboratory rodents.[140–142] Treatment with THC lowers plasma LH and T concentrations in male mice and inhibits prostate growth. Interference with testicular development was shown in rats treated daily during puberty with THC,[143] and chronic administration of cannabis extract has been shown to suppress spermatogenesis in rodents.[144,145] Alterations in sexual behavior also has been observed in rats treated early in life or in adulthood with various cannabis derivatives.[146] In prepubertal, female rats, daily THC administration caused a 5-day delay in sexual maturation.[147] These studies indicate that THC and other cannabis derivatives have effects on sexual development in nonprimate species. No clinical studies or studies of drug effects in primates have been done. Concerns have been expressed in the pediatric literature over cases of arrested pubertal development associated with marijuana use,[148] but there are no definitive answers.

Age-dependent effects of the opiate drugs on gonadotropin secretion in rodents have led to the speculation that changes in the activity of the endogenous opioid system might be part of the physiologic mechanism for the initiation of increased GnRH secretion and onset of pubertal development.[149] Since T and LH concentrations have been shown to be significantly depressed in current heroin users, it is reasonable to predict that heroin use might cause a disruption in pubertal development. The one study that has examined hormone concentrations and psychosocial development in young men after chronic heroin use found no significant impairment of reproductive development.[150] It is likely that tolerance develops to the inhibitory effect of the opiate drugs on neuroendocrine function in both adolescence and adulthood.

The impact of drug abuse on adolescent reproductive development has not been researched adequately. In 1981, the Institute of Medicine's report on Marijuana and Health recognized the lack of information on drug abuse effects on adolescent development as an area of particular concern and emphasized the need for new information about the possible adverse effects of marijuana use on the developing reproductive system.[151] Five years after the publication of the Institute of Medicine's report, this critical issue remains largely uninvestigated.

CONCLUSION

It is clear that drug abuse has the potential for disrupting reproductive function. This is especially true since young men and women of reproductive age are the segment of the population most heavily involved in drug abuse. There is convincing evidence that the drugs of abuse can disrupt neuroendocrine and gonadal function with sufficient magnitude to cause infertility and sexual dysfunction. There is some documentation of such effects in the clinical literature. As a result, most protocols for the evaluation of unexplained infertility now include investigation of drug abuse history as a possible cause of hormonal problems,[152] drug abuse is now recognized as a possible cause of delayed or arrested pubertal development,[153] and the problems of drug abuse and dependency in pregnancy are being recognized and programs are being developed to minimize the risks to mother and baby.[71,121]

There are still many unanswered questions. To what extent does drug abuse contribute to unexplained infertility? Are the effects always reversible if drug use is discontinued? Does disruption of reproductive development (real or perceived) contribute to the drug-seeking behavior of adolescents? What are the medical-legal issues of drug abuse in pregnancy? The research on the reproductive consequences of drug abuse must be given a high priority by the funding agencies if these questions are to be answered. Since it appears unlikely that our drug abuse problems will be solved in the immediate future, the issue of the risks to reproductive function cannot be ignored.

REFERENCES

1. 1985 National Household Survey on Drug Abuse, National Institution on Drug Abuse, Washington, D.C., Government Printing Office, 1987
2. Sokol RJ, Miller SI, Reed G: Alcohol abuse during pregnancy: an epidemiological study. Alcoholism (NY) 4:134, 1980
3. Smith CG, Besch NF, Smith RG, Besch PK: Effect of tetrahydrocannabinol on the hypothalamic-pituitary axis in the ovariectomized rhesus monkey. Fertil Steril 31:335, 1979
4. Asch RH, Smith CG, Siler-Khodr TM, Pauerstein CJ: Acute decreases in serum prolactin concentrations caused by Δ^9-tetrahydrocannabinol in nonhuman primates. Fertil Steril 32:571, 1979
5. Asch RH, Smith CG, Siler-Khodr TM, Pauerstein CJ: Effects of Δ^9-tetrahydrocannabinol during the follicular phase of rhesus monkeys. J Clin Endocrinol Metab 52:50, 1981
6. Asch RH, Smith CG, Siler-Khodr TM, Pauerstein CJ: Effects of Δ^9-tetrahydrocannabinol administration on gonadal steroidogenic activity in vivo. Fertil Steril 32:576, 1979
7. Almirez RG, Smith CG, Asch RH: The effects of marijuana extract and Δ^9-tetrahydrocannabinol on luteal function in the rhesus monkey. Fertil Steril 39:212, 1983
8. Smith CG, Almirez RG, Berenberg J, Asch RH: Tolerance develops to the disruptive effects of Δ^9-tetrahydrocannabinol on the primate menstrual cycle. Science 219:1453, 1983
9. Bauman JE: Marijuana and the female reproductive system. In Health Consequences of Marijuana Use. Washington, D.C., U.S. Government Printing Office, 1980
10. Mendelson JH, Mello NK, Ellingboe J, Skupny AST, Lex BW, Griffin M: Marihuana smoking suppresses luteinizing hormone in women. J Pharmacol Exp Ther 237:862, 1986
11. Mendelson JH, Mello NK: Effects of marijuana on neuroendocrine hormones in human males and females. In Marijuana Effects on the Endocrine and Reproductive Systems. NIDA Research Monograph Washington, D.C., Government Printing Office, 1984
12. Harclerode J: Endocrine effects of marijuana in the male: preclinical studies. In Marijuana Effects on the Endocrine and Reproductive Systems. NIDA Research Monograph. Washington, D.C., Government Printing Office, 1984
13. Smith CG, Besch NF, Asch RH: Effects of marihuana on the reproductive system. In Advances in Sex Hormone Research, Edited by JA Thomas, R Singhal. Baltimore-Munich, Urban and Schwartzenberg, 1980, p 273
14. Kolodny RC, Masters WH, Kolodner AB, Toro G: Depression of plasma testosterone levels after chronic intensive marihuana use. N Engl J Med 290:872, 1974
15. Mendelson JH, Kuenhle JC, Ellingboe J, Babor TF: Plasma testosterone levels before, during and after chronic marihuana smoking. N Engl J Med 291:1051, 1974
16. Zimmerman AM, Zimmerman S, Raj AY: Effects of cannabinoids on sperm morphology. Pharmacology 18:143, 1979
17. Huang HFS, Nahas GG, Hembree WC: Effects of marijuana inhalation on spermatogenesis of the rat. In Marihuana: Biological Effects, Edited by GG Nahas, WDM Paton. Oxford, Pergamon Press, 1980, p 419
18. Dixit VP, Gupta CL, Agrawal M: Testicular degeneration and necrosis induced by chronic administration of cannabis extract in dogs. Endokrinologie 69:299, 1977
19. Jakubovic A, McGeer EG, McGeer PL: Effects of cannabinoids on testosterone and protein synthesis in rat testis Leydig cells in vitro. Mol Cell Endocrinol 15:41, 1979
20. Husain S, Lame M, DeBoer B: Rat testicular tissue glucose metabolism in the presence of delta-9-tetrahydrocannabinol. Proc West Pharmacol Soc 22:355, 1979
21. Hembree WC, Zeidenberg P, Nahas GG: Marihuana's effect on human gonadal function. In Marijuana, Chemistry, Biochemistry and Cellular Effects, Edited by GG Nahas. New York, Springer-Verlag, 1976, p 521
22. Hembree WC, Nahas GG, Zeidenberg P, Huang HFS: Changes in human spermatozoa associated with high-dose marijuana smoking. In Marihuana: Biological Effects,

Edited by GG Nahas, WDM Paton. Oxford, Pergamon Press, 1980, p 429

23. Scher PM, Almirez RG, Smith CG: The effects of cocaine on reproductive hormones in the primate. Pharmacologist 24:185, 1982
24. Gordon LA, Mostofsky DI, Gordon GG: Changes in testosterone levels in the rat following intraperitoneal cocaine HCl. Int J Neurosci 11:139, 1980
25. Steger RW, Silverman AY, Johns A, Asch RH: Interactions of cocaine and Δ^9-tetrahydrocannabinol with the hypothalamic-hypophyseal axis of the female rat. Fertil Steril 35:567, 1981
26. Gaulden EC, Littlefield DC, Putoff OE, Sievert AL: Menstrual abnormalities associated with heroin addiction. Am J Obstet Gynecol 90:155, 1964
27. Mintz JH, O'Hare K, O'Brien CR, Goldschmidt J: Sexual problems of heroin addicts. Arch Gen Psychiatry 31:700, 1974
28. Hollister LE: Human pharmacology of drugs of abuse with emphasis on neuroendocrine effects. Prog Brain Res 39:373, 1973
29. Barraclough CA, Sawyer CH: Inhibition of the release of pituitary ovulatory hormones in the rat by morphine. Endocrinology 57:329, 1955
30. Stoffer SS: A gynecologic study of drug addicts. Am J Obstet Gynecol 101:779, 1986
31. Wang C, Chan V, Yeung RTT: The effect of heroin addiction on pituitary testicular function. Clin Endocrinol 9:455, 1978
32. Brambilla F, Resele L, DeMaio D, Nobile P: Gonadotropin response to synthetic gonadotropin hormone releasing hormone (GnRH) in heroin addicts. Am J Psychiatry 136:314, 1979
33. Kley HK, Oellerick M, Wiegelmann W, Herrmann J, Rudorff KH, Nieschlag E, Kruskemper HL: The effect of methadone on hypophyseal and peripheral glandular hormones during withdrawal. Horm Metab Res 9:484, 1977
34. Bruni JF, Van Vugt D, Marshall S, Meites J: Effects of naloxone, morphine and met-enkephalin on serum prolactin, luteinizing hormone, follicle stimulating hormone, thyroxine stimulating hormone and growth hormone. Life Sci 21:461, 1977
35. Gilbeau PM, Almirez RG, Holaday JW, Smith CG: The role of endogenous opioid peptides in the control of androgen levels in the male non-human primate. J Androl 5:339, 1983
36. Gilbeau PM, Almirez RG, Holaday JW, Smith CG: Opioid effects on blood concentrations of luteinizing hormone and prolactin in the adult male rhesus monkey. J Clin Endocrinol Metab 60:299, 1985
37. Cicero TJ, Badger TM, Wilcox CE, Bell RD, Meyer ER: Morphine decreases luteinizing hormone by an action on the hypothalamic-pituitary axis. J Pharmacol Exp Ther 203:548, 1977
38. Stubbs WA, Jones A, Edwards CRW, Delitala G, Jeffcoate WJ, Ratter SJ, Besser GM, Bloom SR, Albert KG: Hormonal and metabolic responses to an enkephalin analogue in normal men. Lancet 2:1223, 1978
39. Reid RL, Hoff JD, Yen SSC, Li CH: Effects of exogenous β-endorphin on pituitary hormone secretion and its disappearance rate in normal human subjects. J Clin Endocrinol Metab 52:1179, 1981
40. Lightman SL, Jacobs HS, Maguire AK, McGarrick G, Jeffcoat SL: Constancy of opioid control of LH on different pathophysiological states. J Clin Endocrinol Metab 52:1260, 1981
41. Ropert JF, Quigley ME, Yen SSC: Endogenous opiates modulate pulsatile LH release in humans. J Clin Endocrinol Metab 52:583, 1981
42. Cicero TJ, Wilcox CE, Bell RD, Meyer ER: Naloxone-induced increases in serum LH in the male: mechanisms of action. J Pharmacol Exp Ther 212:573, 1980
43. Alper RH, Demarest KT, Moore KE: Morphine differentially alters synthesis and turnover of dopamine in central neuronal systems. J Neural Transm 48:157, 1980
44. Van Vugt DA, Bruni JF, Sylvester PW, Chen HT, Iliri T, Meites J: Interaction between opiates and hypothalamic dopamine on prolactin release. Life Sci 24:2361, 1979
45. Yarbrough GG, Buxbaum DM, Sanders-Bush E: Biogenic amines and narcotic effects. II. Serotonin turnover in the rat after acute and chronic morphine administration. J Pharmacol Exp Ther 185:328, 1979
46. Mendelson JH, Mello NK, Ellingboe J: Effects of acute alcohol intake on pituitary-gonadal hormones in normal human males. J Pharmacol Exp Ther 202:676, 1977
47. Johnston DE, Chiao Y, Gavaler JS, Van Wiel DH: Inhibition of testosterone synthesis by ethanol and acetaldehyde. Biochem Pharmacol 30:1827, 1981
48. Gordon GG, Altman K, Southern AL, Rubin E, Lieber CS: Effect of alcohol (ethanol) administration on sex hormone metabolism in normal men. N Engl J Med 295:793, 1976
49. Gordon GG, Southern AL, Lieber CS: The effects of alcoholic liver disease and alcohol ingestion on sex hormone levels. Alcoholism (NY) 2:259, 1978
50. Lester R, Van Thiel DH: Gonadal function in chronic alcoholism. Adv Exp Med Biol 85A:399, 1977
51. Van Thiel DW, Gavaler JS, Lester R, Goodman MD: Alcohol-induced testicular atrophy: an experimental model for hypogonadism occurring in chronic alcoholic men. Gastroenterology 69:326, 1975
52. Van Thiel DH, Lester R, Sherins RJ: Hypogonadism in alcoholic liver disease: evidence for a double effect. Gastroenterology 67:1188, 1974
53. Farkas M, Rosen RC: Effect of alcohol on elicited male sexual response. J Stud Alcohol 37:265, 1976
54. Hart BL: Effects of alcohol on sexual reflexes and mating behavior in the male dog. J Stud Alcohol 29:839, 1968
55. Lemere F, Smith JW: Alcohol-induced sexual impotence. Am J Psychiatry 130:212, 1973
56. Dixit VP, Agarwal M, Lohiya NK: Effects of a single ethanol injection into the vas deferens on the testicular function of rats. Endokrinologie 67:8, 1976
57. Van Thiel DH, Gavaler JS, Lester R: Ethanol: a gonadal toxin in the female. Drug Alcohol Depend 2:327, 1977
58. Van Thiel DH, Gavaler JS, Lester R, Sherins RJ: Alcohol-induced ovarian failure in the rat. J Clin Invest 61:624, 1978
59. Mendelson JH, Mello NK, Ellingboe J: Effects of acute alcohol intake on pituitary-gonadal hormones in normal human females. J Pharmacol Exp Ther 218:23, 1981
60. Mello NK, Ellingboe J, Bree MP, Harvey KL, Mendelson JH: Alcohol effects on estradiol in female macaque monkey. In Problems of Drug Dependence 1981, NIDA Research Monograph Series, Washington, D.C., Government Printing Office, 1981, p 210
61. Kinsey BA: Psychological factors in alcoholic women from a state hospital sample. Am J Psychiatry 124:1463, 1968

62. Wilsnack SC: Sex role identity in female alcoholism. J Abnorm Psychol 82:253, 1973
63. Belfer M, Shader RI, Carrol M, Harnatz JS: Alcoholism in women. Arch Gen Psychiatry 25:540, 1971
64. Podolsky E: The woman alcoholic and premenstrual tension. J Am Med Wom Assoc 18:816, 1963
65. Mello WK, Bree MP, Mendelson JH, Ellingboe J, King NW, Sehgal P: Alcohol self-administration disrupts reproductive function in female macaque monkeys. Science 221:677, 1983
66. Everett JW, Sawyer CH: A 24-hour periodicity in the "LH-releasing apparatus" of female rats, disclosure by barbiturate sedation. Endocrinology 47:198, 1950
67. Siegel HI, Bast JD, Greenwald GS: The effects of phenobarbital and gonadal steroids on periovulatory serum levels of luteinizing hormone and follicle stimulating hormone in the hamster. Endocrinology 98:48, 1976
68. Knobil E: On the control of gonadotropin secretion in the rhesus monkey. Recent Prog Horm Res 30:1, 1974
69. Nansel DD, Aiyer MS, Meinzer H, Bogdanove EM: Rapid direct effects of castration and androgen treatment on luteinizing hormone-releasing hormone-induced luteinizing hormone release in the phenobarbital-treated male rat: examination of the roles direct and indirect androgen feedback mechanisms might play in the physiological control of luteinizing hormone release. Endocrinology 104:524, 1979
70. Arimura A, Schally AV, Satio T, Miller E, Bowers CY: Induction of ovulation in rats by highly purified pig LH-releasing factor (LRF). Endocrinology 80:515, 1967
71. Wedig JH, Gay VL: Potentiation of luteinizing hormone-releasing factor activities following pentobarbital anesthesia in the steroid-blocked castrated rat. Proc Soc Exp Biol Med 144:993, 1973
72. Azika D, Krulick L, McCann S: On the effect of pentobarbital (Nembutal) on prolactin release in the rat. Proc Soc Exp Biol Med 141:203, 1972
73. Wuttke W, Meites J: Effects of ether and pentobarbital on serum prolactin on LH levels in proestrous rats. Proc Soc Exp Biol Med 135:648, 1970
74. Azika K, Kalra SP, Krulick L, Fawcett CP, McCann SM: The effect of stress and Nembutal on plasma levels of gonadotropins and prolactin in ovariectomized rats. Endocrinology 90:707, 1972
75. Ferin M, Carmel PW, Warren MP, Himsworth RL, Frantz AG: Phencyclidine sedation as a technique for handling rhesus monkeys: effects on LH, GH, and prolactin secretion. Proc Soc Exp Biol Med 151:428, 1976
76. Zaidi P, Wickings EJ, Nieschlag E: Effects of ketamine hydrochloride and barbiturate anesthesia on the metabolic clearance and production rates of testosterone in the male rhesus monkey *Macaca mulatta*. J Steroid Biochem 16:436, 1982
77. Harclerode J, Bird L, Sawyer H, Berger V, Mooney R, Smith R: Sex hormone levels in adult rats injected with Δ^9-tetrahydrocannabinol and phencyclidine hydrochloride. In The Cannabinoids: Chemical, Pharmacologic and Therapeutic Aspects, Edited by S Augurell, WL Dewey, RE Willette. Orlando, Academic Press, 1984, p 471
78. Chisum GM: Recognition and initial management of the pregnant substance-abusing woman. In Drug Use in Pregnancy—Mother and Child, Edited by IJ Chasnoff. Norwell, Mass., MTP Press, 1986, p 17
79. Fried PA, Watkinson B, Grant A, Knights RM: Changing patterns of soft drug use prior to and during pregnancy. Drug Alcohol Depend 6:323, 1980
80. Fried PA, Watkinson B, Willan A: Marijuana use during pregnancy and decreased length of gestation. Am J Obstet Gynecol 150:23, 1984
81. Greenland S, Staisch KJ, Brown N, Gross SJ: The effects of marijuana use during pregnancy. I. A preliminary epidemiologic study. Am J Obstet Gynecol 143:408, 1982
82. Hingson R, Alpert JJ, Day N, Dooling E, Kayne H, Morelock S, Openheimer E, Zuckerman B: Effects of maternal drinking and marijuana use on fetal growth and development. Pediatrics 70:539, 1982
83. Asch RH, Smith CG: Effects of delta-9-tetrahydrocannabinol, the principal psychoactive component of marijuana on pregnancy and lactation in the rhesus monkey. J Reprod Med 31:1071, 1987
84. Khodr GS, Siler-Khodr TM: Placental LRF and its synthesis. Science 207:315, 1980
85. Braunstein GD, Buster JE, Soares JR, Gross SJ: Pregnancy hormone concentrations in marijuana users. Life Sci 33:195, 1983
86. Jones KL, Smith DW, Ulleland CN, Streissguth AP: Pattern of malformations in offspring of chronic alcoholic mothers. Lancet 1:1267, 1973
87. Jones KL, Smith DW: Recognition of the fetal alcohol syndrome in early infancy. Lancet 2:999, 1973
88. Little RE: Moderate alcohol use during pregnancy and decreased infant birth weight. Am J Public Health 67:1154, 1977
89. Ouellette EM, Rosett HL, Rosman NP, Weiner L: Adverse effects on offspring of maternal alcohol abuse during pregnancy. N Engl J Med 297:528, 1977
90. Russell M: Intrauterine growth in infants born to women with alcohol-related psychiatric diagnoses. Alcoholism (NY) 1:225, 1977
91. Little RE, Streissguth AP, Barr HM, Herman CS: Decreased birth weight in infants of alcoholic women who abstained during pregnancy. J Pediatr 96:974, 1980
92. Neville JN, Eagles JA, Samson G, Olson RE: Nutritional status of alcoholics. Am J Clin Nutr 21:1329, 1968
93. Olson RE: Nutrition and alcoholism. In Modern Nutrition in Health and Disease, Edited by RS Goodhart, ME Shils. Philadelphia, Lea & Febiger, 1973, p 1037
94. Abel EL, Dintcheff BA: Effects of prenatal alcohol exposure on growth and development in rats. J Pharmacol Exp Ther 207:916, 1978
95. Henderson GI, Hoyumpa A, Patwardhan R, Schenker S: Effect of acute and chronic ethanol exposure on placental uptake of amino acids. Alcoholism (NY) 5:183, 1981
96. Clarren SK, Smith DW: The fetal alcohol syndrome. N Engl J Med 298:1063, 1978
97. Sulik KK, Jonston MC, Webb MA: Fetal alcohol syndrome: embryogenesis in a mouse model. Science 214:936, 1981
98. Steeg CN, Woolf P: Cardiovascular malformations in the fetal alcohol syndrome. Am Heart J 98:635, 1979
99. Randall CL, Taylor WJ: Prenatal ethanol exposure in mice: teratogenic effects. Teratology 19:305, 1979
100. Boggan WO, Randall CL, DeBeukelaer M: Renal abnormalities in mice prenatally exposed to ethanol. Res Commun Chem Pathol Pharmacol 23:127, 1979
101. Clarren SK, Alvoid EC, Sumi SM, Streissguth AP: Brain malformations related to prenatal exposure to ethanol. J Pediatr 92:64, 1978

102. Lee MH, Haddad R, Rabe A: Developmental impairments in the progeny of rats consuming ethanol during pregnancy. Neurobehav Toxicol Teratol 2:189, 1980
103. Abel EL: Prenatal effects of alcohol on adult learning in rats. Pharmacol Biochem Behav 10:239, 1979
104. Halmesmäki E, Acutti I, Granström M-L, Stenman U-H, Ylikorkala O: Estradiol, estriol, progesterone, prolactin, and human chorionic gonadotorpin in pregnant women with alcohol abuse. J Clin Endocrinol Metab 64:153, 1987
105. Fishburne PM: National survey on drug abuse: main findings, 1979. National Institute on Drug Abuse, 1980 (DHHS publication no. ADM 80976), Rockville, MD, 1980
106. Chasnoff IJ, Burns WJ, Schnoll SH, Burns KA: Cocaine use in pregnancy. N Engl J Med 313:666, 1985
107. Chasnoff IJ, Bussey ME, Savich R, Stack CM: Perinatal cerebral infarction and maternal cocaine use. J Pediatr 108:456, 1986
108. Madden JD, Payne TF, Miller S: Maternal cocaine abuse and effect on the newborn. Pediatrics 77:209, 1986
109. Chasnoff IJ, Hatcher R, Burns WJ: Polydrug and methadone-addicted newborns: a continuum of impairment? Pediatrics 70:210, 1982
110. Chasnoff IJ, Burns WJ, Hatcher RP, Burns KA: Phencyclidine: effects on the fetus and neonate. Dev Pharmacol Ther 6:404, 1983
111. Davidson Ward SL, Scheutz S, Krishna V, Bean X, Wingert W, Wachsman L, Keens TG: Abnormal sleeping ventilatory pattern in infants of substance-abusing mothers. Am J Dis Child 140:1015, 1986
112. Chavez CJ, Ostrea EM Jr, Stryker JC, Smialek Z: Sudden infant death syndrome among infants of drug-dependent mothers. J Pediatr 95:407, 1979
113. Zelson C, JaLee S, Casalino M: Neonatal narcotic addiction: comparative effects of maternal intake of heroin and methodone. N Engl J Med 289:1216, 1973
114. Kron RE, Kaplan SL, Phoenix MD, Finnegan LP: Behavior of infants born to drug-dependent mothers: effects of prenatal and postnatal drugs. In Drug Abuse in Pregnancy and Neonatal Effects, Edited by JL Rementeria. St. Louis, CV Mosby, 1977, p 129
115. Ramer CM, Lodge A: Neonatal addiction: a two-year study. I. Clinical and developmental characteristics of infants of mothers methodone maintained. Addict Dis Int J 2:227, 1975
116. Fricker HS, Segal S: Narcotic addiction, pregnancy and the newborn. Am J Dis Child 132:360, 1978
117. Reddy AM, Harper RG, Stern G: Observations on heroin and methadone withdrawal in the newborn. Pediatrics 48:353, 1971
118. Zelson C, Rubio E, Wasserman E: Neonatal narcotic addiction: ten-year observation. Pediatrics 48:178, 1971
119. Rosen T, Pippenger C: Pharmacologic observations on the neonate withdrawal syndrome. J Pediatr 88:1044, 1976
120. Naeye KL, Blanc W, Leblanc W, Khatamee MA: Fetal complications of maternal heroin addiction: abnormal growth, infections, and episodes of stress. J Pediatr 83:1055, 1973
121. Kandall SR, Album S, Dreyer E, Comstock M, Lowinson J: Differential effects of heroin and methadone on birth weights. Addict Dis Int J 2:347, 1975
122. Ostrea EM, Chavez CJ, Strauss ME: A study of factors that influence the severity of neonatal narcotic withdrawal. Addict Dis Int J 2:187, 1975
123. Strauss ME, Andresko M, Stryker JC, Wardell JN, Dunkel LD: Methadone maintenance during pregnancy: pregnancy, birth, and neonatal characteristics. Am J Obstet Gynecol 120:895, 1974
124. Gluck L, Kulovich MV: Lecithin/sphingomyelin ratio in amniotic fluid in normal and abnormal pregnancy. Am J Obstet Gynecol 115:539, 1973
125. Desmond MM, Wilson GS: Neonatal abstinence syndrome: recognition and diagnosis. Addict Dis Int J 2:113, 1975
126. Zelson C: Neonatal narcotic addiction. In The Neonate: Clinical Biochemistry, Physiology and Pathology, Edited by JM Hicks. New York, John Wiley & Sons, 1976, p 113
127. Householder J, Hatcher R, Burns W, Chasnoff I: Infants born to narcotic-addicted mothers. Psychol Bull 92:453, 1982
128. Chasnoff I: Perinatal addiction: consequences of intrauterine exposure to opiate and nonopiate drugs. In Drug Use in Pregnancy: Mother and Child, Edited by I Chasnoff, MA Norwell. MTP Press, 1986, p 52
129. Cummings AJ, Jones HMR, Cooper JE: Transplacental disposition of phencyclidine in the pig. Xenobiotica 9:447, 1979
130. Nicholas TM, Lipshitz G, Schreiber EC: Phencyclidine: its transfer across the placenta as well as into breast milk. Am J Obstet Gynecol 143:143, 1982
131. Golden NL, Kuhnert BR, Sokol RJ, Martier S, Bagby BS: Phencylidine use during pregnancy. Am J Obstet Gynecol 148:254, 1984
132. Strauss AA, Modanlou HD, Bosu SK: Neonatal manifestations of maternal phencyclidine (PCP) abuse. Pediatrics 68:550, 1981
133. Oleske J, Minnefor RT, Cooper R, Thomas K, de la Cruz A, Adieh H, Guerrero I, Joski VV, Desposito F: Immune deficiency syndrome in children. JAMA 249:2345, 1983
134. Wiet MJ: Legal issues in perinatal addiction. In Drug Use in Pregnancy: Mother and Child, Edited by I Chasnoff, MA Norwell. MTP Press, 1986, p 147
135. Miller JD, Cisin I: Highlights from the National Survey on Drug Abuse: 1982 DHHS pub. no. (ADM) 83-1277 Rockville, MD, National Institute on Drug Abuse, 1983
136. Johnston LD, O'Malley PM, Bachman JG: Highlights from Drugs and American High School Students: 1975–1983 DHHS pub. no. (ADM) 84-1317, Rockville, MD, National Institute on Drug Abuse, 1984
137. Beschner GM, Friedman AS: Youth Drug Abuse: Problems, Issues, and Treatment. Lexington, MA, Lexington Books, 1979, p 169
138. Kandel D: Epidemiological and psychosocial perspectives on adolescent drug abuse. J Am Acad Child Psychiatry 21:328, 1982
139. Wesson DR, Carlin AS, Adams KM, Beschner GM: Polydrug Abuse. New York, Academic Press, 1977
140. Symons AM, Teale JD, Marks V: Effect of Δ^9-tetrahydrocannabinol on the hypothalamic-pituitary-gonadal system in the maturing male rat. J Endocrinol 68:43, 1976
141. Collie R: Endocrine effects of chronic intraventricular administration of Δ^9-tetrahydrocannabinol to prepubertal and adult male rats. Life Sci 18:223, 1976
142. Collie R, Letarte J, Leboeuf G, Ducharme JR: Endocrine effects of chronic administration of psychoactive drugs to prepubertal male rats. I. Δ^9-tetrahydrocannabinol. Life Sci 16:533, 1974

143. Harmon JW, Locke D, Aliapoulious MA, MacIndoe J: Interference with testicular development by Δ^9-tetrahydrocannabinol. Surg Forum 27:350, 1976
144. Zimmerman AM, Bruce WR, Zimmerman S: Effects of cannabinoids on sperm morphology. Pharmacology 18:143, 1979
145. Block E, Thipen B, Morrill GA, Gardner E, Fujimoto G: Effects of cannabinoids on reproduction and development. Vitam Horm 36:203, 1978
146. Dalterio S, Bartke A: Perinatal exposure to cannabinoids alters male reproductive function in mice. Science 205:1420, 1979
147. Field E, Tyrey L: Delayed sexual maturation in the female rat during chronic exposure to delta-9-tetrahydrocannabinol. Life Sci 35:1725, 1984
148. Copeland KC, Underwood LF, Van Wyk JJ: Marijuana smoking and pubertal arrest. J Pediatr 96:1079, 1980
149. Wilkinson M, Bhanol R: Puberty-related attenuation of opiate peptide-induced inhibition of LH secretion. Endocrinology 110:1046, 1982
150. Mendelson JH, Mellow NK: Plasma testosterone levels during chronic heroin use and protracted abstinence: a study of Hong Kong addicts. Clin Pharmacol Ther 17:529, 1975
151. Institute of Medicine of the National Academy of Sciences: Marijuana and Health. Washington, D.C., National Academy Press, 1982
152. Conrad MJ, Ross LS: Evaluation and treatment of the infertile man. Primary Care 12:687, 1985
153. Styne DM, Grumbach MM: Puberty in the male and female: its physiology and disorders. In Reproductive Endocrinology, Physiology, Pathophysiology and Clinical Management, Edited by SSC Yen, RB Jaffe. Philadelphia, WB Saunders, 1986, p 313

Chapter 4

Prospects for fertility after chemotherapy or radiation for neoplastic disease

Marian D. Damewood, M.D.
Louise B. Grochow, M.D.

The Johns Hopkins University School of Medicine, Baltimore, Maryland

In recent years, chemotherapy and radiation of patients with cancer has become increasingly successful, and sustained remissions have been achieved. In addition, more effective therapy of childhood cancers and leukemias has led to an emergence of a generation of patients who approach adolescence and adulthood. The acute toxicity of anticancer treatment regimens is well recognized, with effects including nausea, neutropenia, mucosal lesions, and delayed effects of pulmonary fibrosis, myocardiopathy, and peripheral neuropathy.[1] However, the chronic side effect of potential injury to the reproductive system in long-term survivors is of particular concern. Drug- and radiation-induced azoospermia and amenorrhea are associated with depletion of testicular and ovarian germ cells and sterility after therapy with these therapeutic modalities for cancer in adults.[2] Treatment of adolescents and children with these modes of therapy as well has raised questions regarding the ability of these individuals to progress through puberty and achieve normal reproductive function.[3]

Certain neoplastic disease states have lent themselves to close scrutiny regarding gonadal function after therapy. In particular, Hodgkin's disease primarily affects young patients. Present treatment may now produce long-term remissions in > 50% of patients, irrespective of initial extent of disease.[4] Therefore, it is important to establish the effects of therapy on female and male fertility. Other diseases of young women, such as breast cancer and carcinoma of the cervix, lead to further questions regarding reproductive potential in these individuals.

The prospects for fertility after chemotherapy and radiation for neoplastic disease are multifaceted. The issues of pregnancy, pregnancy out come, and the generational genetics of the offspring of those exposed to chemotherapy and radiation may stimulate exploration of avenues such as sperm or oocyte banking to prevent complete loss of germ cell productivity. Treatment of the gonadal damage may alleviate some of the emotional consequences of cancer therapy for those patients afflicted not only with a malignant disease but possible impairment of their reproductive potential.[2]

HISTORICAL BACKGROUND

Gonadal destruction by cytotoxic agents was first described in 1948.[5] Absent spermatogenesis at autopsy in 27 of 30 men treated with nitrogen mustard, the first antineoplastic agent, was noted, as were menstrual irregularity and amenorrhea with intravenous administration of the same agent.[6] Since 1948, the gonadal effects of chemotherapy and radiation have expanded with the introduction of new drugs and protocols. In 1963, procarbazine was noted to affect spermatogenesis[7] adversely, and in 1971 cyclophosphamide and chlorambucil were described as toxic to the human testis,[8, 9] with an unpredictable reversibility.[10] In 1978, Chapman et al.[11] reported evidence of widespread sexual dysfunction and decreased fertility in male patients with Hodgkin's disease. In 1981, these authors showed that only one or two cycles of nitrogen mustard, vinblastine, procarbazine, and prednisolone (MVPP) were necessary to produce azoospermia in most men.[12] Since the first report of amenorrhea following nitrogen mustard therapy,[6] the same effect was noted in women receiving busulfan as adjunctive therapy for breast cancer.[13] In 1971, a loss of ova was demonstrated on examination of an ovarian biopsy specimen after cytotoxic therapy with cyclophosphamide,[14] a possibly reversible depletion.[15] In 1973, ovarian failure at a mean age of 29.6 years was reported after one cycle of cyclophosphamide therapy. In this case, ovarian failure has been progressive, rather than occurring as an "all-or-none" phenomenon.[16] In 1971, ovarian failure was reported in women treated for Hodgkin's disease,[17] and in 1979 MVPP was described as producing premature ovarian failure that was *age*- and *dose*-related.[4] On examination of an ovarian biopsy specimen, a loss of primordial follicles was confirmed, particularly in older patients.

World War II directed attention to the effects of radiation on germ cells and on the reproductive potential of offspring of survivors exposed to the atomic bomb. Before the atomic age, shortly after the discovery of x-rays[18] and radioactivity,[19] the profound effect of radiation on normal cells and tumor cells was appreciated. The marked germ cell damage within a short time of exposure led to consideration of the gonadal effects of therapeutic radiation.[20] In 1939, Jacox[21] reported that 500 rads to the ovaries produced permanent castration in most patients. With the introduction of infradiaphragmatic radiation therapy for use in Hodgkin's disease, a high dose of radiation was given incidentally to the ovaries. Subsequently, surgical oophoropexy with uterine shielding in women of reproductive age was devised.[22] In the late 1970s, inverted Y radiation therapy for Hodgkin's disease in men was found to produce at least 70% azoospermia.[23] Full-dose versus fractionated irradiation and testicular shielding were then investigated.

CHEMOTHERAPY AND GONADAL FUNCTION

The marked cytotoxicity of most anticancer drugs, in particular the alkylating agents, imparts an expectation of adverse affects on reproductive potential.[2, 24] Cytotoxic agents produce azoospermia, compromised Leydig cell function, and perifollicular agenesis, progressing to premature ovarian failure. The severity of gonadal dysfunction is a function of total dose in both sexes and of patient age in women at the time of therapy.[2] Gonadal damage is attributed to single agents, such as cyclophosphamide,[10, 25-28] chlorambucil,[29, 30] and methotrexate,[31] combination regimens for Hodgkin's disease,[4, 12, 17, 23, 32, 33] and multiple therapies for breast cancer. The disease state of malignancy or neoplasm, which initially requires the use of chemotherapy, may have an early adverse effect on gonadal function as well.[34]

PHARMACOLOGY OF CHEMOTHERAPY AGENTS

For a more detailed discussion of the mechanisms of action, clinical pharmacology, and conventional use of antineoplastic agents, exhaustive reviews are available.[35, 36] This section is a review of the general mechanisms of action of classes of antineoplastics as they may relate to impaired fertility and a discussion of specific characteristics of important drugs and combinations and their conventional use in the treatment of malignant diseases.

The alkylating agents, whose cytotoxic activity is thought to be mediated through covalent bonding of saturated carbon atoms to critical biologic molecules, are most commonly associated with persistent infertility, in addition to a host of other toxicities, including teratogenesis, mutagenesis, and carcinogenesis. Inhibition of deoxyribonucleic acid (DNA) synthesis is one of the effects of alkylating drugs at conventional cytotoxic concentrations. Specific DNA bases are preferentially alkylated by different drugs; bifunctional alkylating agents (mechlorethamine, cyclophosphamide) produce DNA-DNA cross-links, and nonfunctional alkylators result in single strand breaks. Inactivation of the DNA template is thought to result in single strand breaks and eventual cell death. Because this damage can occur in resting cells as well as in cells that are actively dividing, these drugs are described as cell cycle-nonspecific. However, misreading of the DNA code may inhibit ribonucleic acid (RNA) and protein synthesis and cause more damage to rapidly dividing tissues. The relative specificity of these drugs in eliminating malignant cells is far from completely understood; relative susceptibility and resistance may be based on several factors, including transport into the cell, enzymatic inactivation, protection from alkylation by increased intracellular thiols, and DNA repair mechanisms. In addition, the relative size of the stem pool for replacement of lost cells and its selective recruitment after tissue damage provide some vital organs (e.g., gut and bone marrow) with the critical resilience needed for a favorable therapeutic index. The concept of first-order cell kill, which presumably applies to normal as well as malignant cells, may explain in part the increased infertility observed at equivalent drug exposures in older women, whose ova are more depleted, than in younger patients.

The combination of several of these agents, with the addition of antitumor antimetabolites, has been dramatically useful in achieving long-term remission and cure in patients with malignancies, including leukemias, lymphomas, Hodgkin's disease, testicular and ovarian cancer, and breast cancer. The rational design of these combinations has taken advantage of nonoverlapping acute toxicities, but little attention was paid at the time these programs were initiated to toxicities that would affect the new long-term survivors. In particular, the combinations of mechlorethamine, vincristine, and procarbazine in the MOPP (mechlorethamine, vincristine, procarbazine, and prednisone) regimen for Hodgkin's disease could retrospectively have been expected to affect reproductive potential adversely in at least an additive fashion.

Nitrogen mustard, or mechlorethamine, was originally derived from an agent used for chemical warfare. It is highly reactive in solution and must be rapidly administered intravenously. It can cause severe local injury if extravasated into the skin, and it causes acute nausea and vomiting, which are only partially suppressed with currently used antimetics. It was included in the first combination chemotherapy regimen that cured patients with advanced Hodgkin's disease and continues to be used primarily in that setting. A dose of 6 mg/M^2 is given intravenously once weekly for 2 of 4 weeks over six complete cycles, resulting in a total dose of 72 mg/M^2 in a traditional regimen.

Other drugs with the bis-chloroethylamine structure, including melphalan (1-phenylalanine mustard), chlorambucil, and cyclophosphamide, have better therapeutic indices and are simpler to use. Cyclophosphamide, now the most commonly used alkylating drug, must be metabolized, primarily by hepatic microsomes, to an active alkylating species. It is well absorbed orally, and nausea is well controlled with high-dose steroids. It is not a vesicant and can be given orally or intravenously. It causes more myelosuppression than thrombocytopenia and also can cause alopecia, hemorrhagic cystitis, and inappropriate antidiuretic hormone (ADH) secretion. Doses range from 100 mg/M^2 orally for 14 days monthly for 6 to 24 months in combination with methotrexate and 5-fluorouracil (5-FU) for adjuvant treatment of stage II breast cancer, to 600 mg/M^2 intravenously days 1 and 8 out of each 21 days in combination for lymphomas, to 2000 mg/M^2 delivered over 1 to 4 days in bone marrow transplantation and other intensive regimens producing severe aplasia.

Melphalan, which is used extensively for ovarian carcinoma and for breast cancer, lymphomas, and myeloma, also enters cells by active transport. Its absorption after oral administration is variable, and doses are generally adjusted for marrow suppression. It is commonly used at a dose of 8 mg/M^2 daily for 5 days. Chlorambucil, a close congener of melphalan, is available only for oral use, most commonly for breast cancer and lymphoma, and is used in low doses daily or in higher doses every 2 to 3 weeks.

The nitrosoureas were originally found to have modest antitumor activity in animal models, leading to extensive structure function studies demonstrating that chloroethyl derivatives possess greater antitumor activity. In addition to producing DNA-DNA and DNA-protein cross-links, it produces isocyanate, which inhibits DNA polymerase, repair of strand breaks, and RNA synthesis and protein production, which may play a significant role in the toxicity of these drugs. These very reactive compounds disappear rapidly from the blood after administration. A delayed and protracted granulocytopenia and thrombocytopenia commonly occur after carmustine (BCNU) or lomustine (CCNU) administration. With repeated doses, progressive marrow damage occurs, in addition to pulmonary fibrosis and renal damage. BCNU is commonly used at 100 to 225 mg/M^2 at 6-week intervals.

Cis (II) platinum diaminedichloride (cis-DDP, cis-platin) is the first in a series of heavy metal compounds that can interact with nucleophilic sites on DNA, RNA, or proteins to form bifunctional covalent links analogous to alkylation reactions, changing DNA conformation and preventing DNA transcription and synthesis. The dose-limiting toxicities are nephrotoxicity and ototoxicity, severe nausea and vomiting, and moderate myelosuppression. Cis-DDP is also mutagenic, teratogenic, and carcinogenic. In combination with other drugs, doses of 100 mg/M^2 are given every 4 weeks, usually divided into intravenous doses for 5 days. For testicular germ cell neoplasms, three to four 3-week cycles of 300 to 400 mg/M^2 are usually in curative regimens.

Busulfan, the important alkylating agent in the class of alkylalkane sulfonate compounds, forms carbonium ions after oral administration, leading to DNA alkylation. Although this drug has traditionally been used orally in low doses for chronic granulocytic leukemia, it is used in very high doses for preparation for bone marrow transplantation (16 mg/kg in divided doses over 4 days). It can cause irreversible bone marrow stem cell depletion when used chronically.

The podophyllotoxins, extracts of the mandrake, bind to tubulin and inhibit microtubular assembly. However, VP-16 (etopside) and VM-26 are synthetic glycosidic derivatives whose mechanism of action is uncertain. Cells are arrested in G2 rather than in mitosis, and DNA strand breaks are involved in cytotoxicity. They are now widely used for the treatment of lymphoma, small cell lung cancer, testicular cancer, and head and neck cancer, which may be seen in increasing frequency in young men as the prevalence of snuff use increases. Typical doses are 80 mg/M^2 two or three times weekly, followed by a 3-week break to recover normal marrow function.

Doxorubicin and daunomycin are anthracyclines derived from *Streptomyces* sp. These antitumor antibiotics are widely used for many different malignancies. These drugs and several new analogs intercalate between strands of the DNA helix, in addition to chelating divalentations and engaging in oxidation-reduction reactions and reacting directly with cell membranes. The anthracyclines are also mutagenic, carcinogenic, and teratogenic, causing single-stranded DNA breaks and impairing DNA repair. Other serious side effects include bone marrow suppression, mucositis, alopecia, severe extravasation injuries, and a cumulative cardiotoxicity. In the treatment of breast cancer and Hodgkin's disease and other lymphomas, doxorubicin is commonly used at doses of 30 to 60 mg/M^2 every 3 to 4 weeks. In the adriamycin, bleomycin, vinblastine, and decarbazine (ABVD) regimen for Hodgkin's disease, a total dose of 300 mg/M^2 would be administered over 6 months.

Bleomycin, another important antitumor antibiotic, is a mixture of small peptides isolated from *Streptomyces*. It produces single- and double-strand breaks in DNA. It penetrates into cells slowly and can be inactivated by an enzyme that has been detected in normal tissue and in resistant tumor line. It is minimally myelosuppressive but can cause life-threatening pulmonary toxicity and unusual cutaneous toxicity. It is an important component of combination chemotherapy for testicular cancer, for which it is usually given as 30 U intravenously weekly for 9 to 12 weeks.

Procarbazine, a substituted hydrazine, and decarbazine (DTIC), a triazine derivative, are nonclassical alkylating agents that show no cell cycle specificity or schedule dependency. Both cause myelosuppression and nausea and vomiting. Procarbazine is also a neurotoxin, especially if given parenterally, and can cause an anabuse-like reaction if combined with alcoholic beverages. Although DTIC is only modestly mutagenic in the Ames assay, it is highly carcinogenic in animals and produces fetal malformations. Procarbazine is highly mutagenic and has also been demonstrated to ablate spermatogenesis, playing a significant role in the infertility seen in men treated with MOPP. Procarbazine is used orally at 100 mg/M^2 for 14 days monthly in the MOPP regimen; DTIC is used intravenously at 375 mg/M^2 every other week in the ABVD regimen for Hodgkin's disease.

The vinca alkaloids, vincristine, vinblastine, and vindesine, cause cytotoxicity by binding to tubulin, inhibiting the mitotic spindle, and arresting cells in metaphase. They enter the cell by active transport. Vincristine dose is limited by neurotoxicity and vinblastine dose by myelotoxicity and mucositis. Both are used in combination for the treatment of leukemia, lymphoma, testicular cancer, and breast cancer.

The other major group of anticancer drugs, the antimetabolites, primarily cause cytotoxicity in rapidly dividing tissues. These agents generally pass as fraudulent substrates for critical biosynthetic pathways and are generally rationally designed for structural similarity with their physiologic counterpart. Thus, although these drugs may acutely interrupt fertility, in general they are not thought to have long-term effects.

Methotrexate is an antifolate and depletes cells of reduced folates, inhibiting synthesis of purine nucleotides and thymidylate by binding to dihydrofolate reductase. Methotrexate enters the cell by a carrier-mediated active transport system unless it is given in massive doses. Its effect on rapidly dividing tissues causes myelosuppression and mucositis. Toxicities manifested by nondividing tissues are less predictable in their incidence; they include hepatotoxicity and neurotoxicity, possibly mediated by the persistence of polyglutamylated methotrexate in some tissues. Methotrexate is used in doses ranging from 50 to 5000 mg/M^2 for a wide variety of malignancies, including lymphomas and breast cancer.

The fluorophymidines, of which 5-FU is the most commonly used, are converted to fluoronucleotides, which can both be incorporated into RNA, inhibiting its synthetic function and be bound to thymidylate synthetase, inhibiting DNA synthesis. Toxicity to rapidly dividing mucosal lining cells and the bone marrow are dose-limiting but vary with the schedule of drug administration. Acute neurotoxicity caused by a neurotoxic metabolite is also seen. 5-FU is widely used in combination chemotherapy for breast and ovarian cancer and in gastrointestinal malignancies and as a radiosensitizer with external beam radiation therapy. Doses range from 500 mg/M^2 intravenously weekly to 1200 mg/M^2/24 hours by continuous infusion.

Cytosine arabinoside (Ara-C) is an analog of 2′-deoxycytidine, which is activated to Ara-CTP to inhibit DNA polymerase in competition with deoxycytidine triphosphate and to damage newly synthesized DNA by direct incorporation. Cells are selectively killed during S phase. The timing and duration of exposure are important to cytotoxicity, with increased damage occurring during rapid DNA synthesis, for instance in the recovery period after another cytotoxic exposure. Side effects include gastrointestinal toxicity and myelosuppression and mild hepatotoxicity. Conventional doses for the treatment of leukemia range from 100 mg/M^2/day to 2000 or more mg/M^2 for up to 6 days in intensive antileukemic regimens.

The purine analogs, 6 mercaptopurine and 6 thioguanine (6-MP and 6-TG), are used extensively for pediatric leukemic therapy. After activation to nucleotides, these drugs inhibit de novo purine biosynthesis and are incorporated into DNA. As with the other antimetabolites, their primary toxicity is evidenced in tissues with a rapid turnover, but the marrow and liver are particularly susceptible to these drugs. These drugs and azathioprine, which releases 6-MP after hepatic metabolism, are also used in organ transplantation and to treat autoimmune processes. For immunosuppression, doses of 50 mg/M^2 daily are used; twice that dose is commonly used in antileukemic therapy.

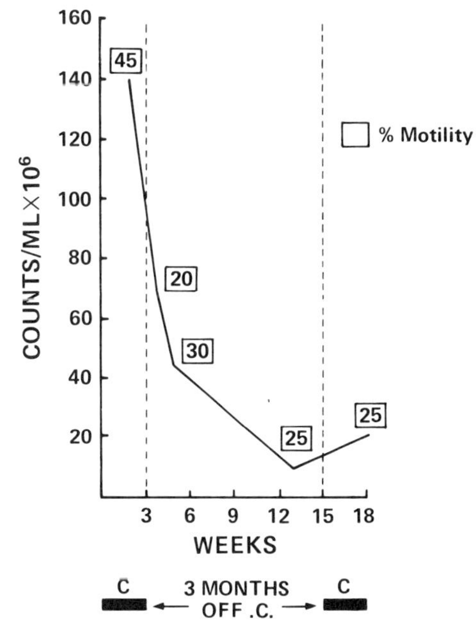

Figure 1
Rate of fall of absolute sperm count and motility during treatment with cyclophosphamide. (From Fairley et al.[28] Reproduced with the permission of the publisher, The Lancet, London, England.)

CYTOTOXIC-INDUCED GONADAL DYSFUNCTION IN MEN

The most extensively studied chemotherapeutic drugs, with respect to male fertility, are the alkylating agents. Here the predominant lesion is localized to the germinal epithelium of the testis.[24] Light-microscopic studies of testicular biopsy specimens obtained from patients treated with cyclophosphamide show germinal aplasia, absent spermatogonia, and spermatozoa with normal-appearing Leydig cells.[25, 28] Single-agent daily therapy with cyclophosphamide results in a rapidly progressive decrease in sperm count to azoospermia in approximately 90 to 120 days[9, 28] (Fig. 1). Further duration of therapy potentiates continued azoospermia with progression to testicular atrophy.[15] In patients who demonstrate azoospermia and oligospermia plasma levels of follicle-stimulating hormone (FSH) and luteinizing hormone (LH) are elevated with normal levels of plasma testosterone.[25] The onset of testicular compromise is dose- and possibly duration-dependent.[24] With doses of cyclophosphamide ranging from 2 to 4.6 mg/kg/day (mean, 3.5

mg/kg/day) for periods of 2 months or less, gonadal function and semen parameters remain essentially normal.[25] However, with a dose of 3.5 to 3.7 mg/kg/day for 3 months or longer, azoospermia and oligospermia occur. Men treated with > 18 gm total, regardless of length of treatment, develop definitive azoospermia. When cyclophosphamide therapy is discontinued, a return of spermatogenesis may be anticipated and has been documented within a period of 15 to 49 months (mean, 31 months)[27] after discontinuation. However, full recovery to the baseline count occurs in only a few situations,[15] with isolated reports of paternity in patients after stopping therapy with substerilizing doses.[26]

The same pattern of response is seen with chlorambucil and other alkylating agents. The germinal cell line disappears with only Sertoli cells, remaining along with moderate peritubular fibrosis. Within 2 to 3 months of therapy, a decrease in sperm count to azoospermia is seen, in addition to an increase in seminal fluid fructose, a deleterious effect.[29] In an evaluation of chlorambucil effect on spermatogenesis in the human with malignant lymphoma, urinary FSH and LH excretion remained normal, despite the arrest of spermatogenesis,[8] suggesting uninjured Leydig cells. The degree of compromise is dose-dependent, with a minimal total dose of 400 mg of chlorambucil for development of azoospermia.[8] Recovery occurs only if the drug is suspended before this threshold dose is given. After withdrawal of treatment, some remission of the germinal lesion is observed in up to 66% of patients, with paternity reported in a small number of cases.[30]

Thus a germinal lesion of the testis and a decline in semen analysis parameters occur within 2 to 4 months of initiation of therapy with alkylating agents. The effect is dose- and duration-related, with recovery of spermatogenesis in a small number of cases of patients who have received less than the threshold dose.

Other agents, such as the folic acid antagonist methotrexate, adversely affect tissues with high mitotic activity, such as the rapidly dividing spermatogonia and spermatocytes. A rapid decrease in sperm count within 2 to 3 weeks of the onset of chemotherapy is thus due to inhibition of the early steps of spermatogenesis, with progressive increase of early and late spermatids with continued use of the drug.[37] Alkaloids, such as vinblastine, are associated with mitotic arrest of spermatogenesis and binding to microtubular proteins, altering the flagella of mature sperm.[38] Corticosteroids cause oligospermia and low sperm motility after 30 mg/day for 15 days,[39] with testicular biopsy specimens showing spermatogenic arrest, sloughing of germinal cells, and a decrease in spermatogonia numbers.

CYTOTOXIC-INDUCED TESTICULAR DAMAGE IN PREPUBERTAL AND POSTPUBERTAL BOYS

Impairment of testicular function is observed following the use of cyclophosphamide before or during puberty.[40] The pubertal germinal epithelium is susceptible to cytotoxic-induced damage, with aplasia, high serum FSH levels, and abnormal testicular histologic features observed in patients who received cyclophosphamide and chlorambucil during prepubertal life.[41-43] Those treated at puberty sustain moderately severe damage to the tubular system of the testis unassociated with Leydig cell impairment.[24] The dose of cyclophosphamide or chlorambucil necessary to cause oligo- or azoospermia in prepubertal or pubertal boys is > 365 mg/kg. Boys that receive ≤ 200 mg/kg have minimal alteration of spermatogenesis. With doses between 200 and 365 mg/kg, spermatogenesis diminishes, but persistent azoospermia does not occur.[40] Resumption of normal testicular function occurs in those treated with < 12 gm, but those treated with > 14 gm experience long-term impairment of spermatogenesis.[44] Follow-up studies of adolescents will adequately assess the cytotoxicity to the germinal epithelium as a factor in adult fertility. A safe regimen is thus not established for either the immature or the mature gonad in boys.

CYTOTOXIC-INDUCED OVARIAN FAILURE IN WOMEN

The alkylating agents, such as cyclophosphamide, impart significant effects on reproductive function in women. Uldall et al.[45] reported amenorrhea developing within 7 months in 18 of 34 menstruating women treated with the maximum of 40 to 120 mg of cyclophosphamide daily. Twelve developed amenorrhea within 1 month of starting treatment. Urinary estrogens were low and FSH and LH were elevated, suggesting that the amenorrhea was due to cyclophosphamide-induced compromise at the ovarian level. Menses returned in < 10% of patients who had discontinued the drug 12 months earlier. Warne et al.[16] reviewed ovarian biopsy specimens in the patients who received cyclophosphamide; they

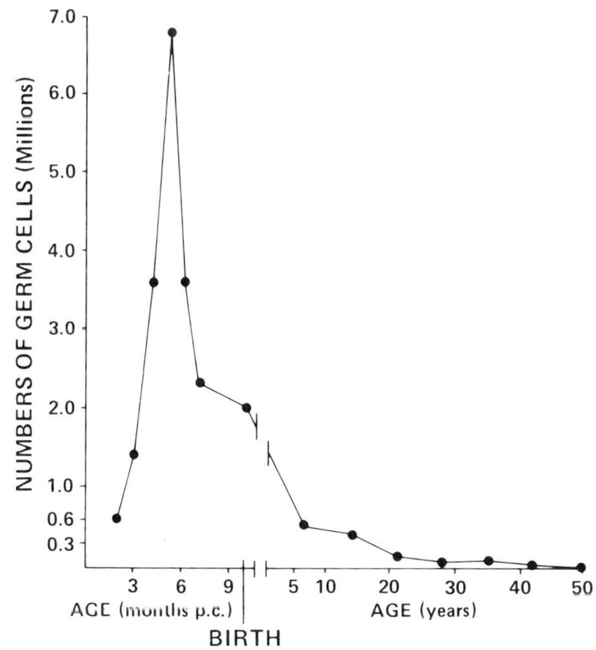

Figure 2
Changes in the total number of germ cells in the human ovary from the prenatal to the postmenopausal period. (From Baker.[20] Reproduced with the permission of the publisher, The C.V. Mosby Company, St. Louis, MO.)

found an absence of thecal cells and ova, suggesting a direct action of the drug on the oocyte. There was no evidence of follicular maturation or primordial follicle development. The time of maximum ovarian effect may thus be before meiosis and separation of the first polar body, with the follicular and oocyte depletion appearing to be progressive, not an abrupt process. Similar histologic changes have been observed in ovaries of women who received chlorambucil therapy. Other agents, such as vinblastine and busulfan, produce ovarian atrophy.[46] Ovarian function is not compromised with corticosteroid therapy.[44]

The dose of cytotoxic agent is an important determinant of its gonadal effect, with an additional variable in women of age-related susceptibility. The total dose of cyclophosphamide received before the onset of amenorrhea in patients 40 years of age or older is 5.2 gm. However, in patients 30 to 39 years of age, a dose of 9.3 gm results in amenorrhea and in women 20 to 29 years of age, 20.4 gm is necessary to induce absence of menses.[24] Women who were older than 40 years had ovarian failure much sooner and at a smaller dose.[46] From 2 million follicles at birth, 200,000 remain at puberty, and approximately 400 at menopause (Fig. 2). The number of oocytes decreases steadily with age, thus ovarian function in older women is more easily compromised. Recovery of ovarian function after cessation of cyclophosphamide is rare,[45, 46] although there are isolated reports of reversible amenorrhea. Less than 10% of patients have a return of menses if there is associated hormonal evidence of ovarian hypofunction, absent oocytes, or poor follicular maturation.[46] Younger women treated for less than 9 months with cyclophosphamide may have potentially reversible amenorrhea.[15]

CYTOTOXIC-INDUCED GONADAL DAMAGE IN PREPUBERTAL AND POSTPUBERTAL GIRLS

Although the prepubertal gonad may be more resistant than the postpubertal gonad to damage by alkylating agents, primary ovarian failure is reported in patients with cyclophosphamide therapy before puberty.[24, 47] High FSH levels are noted, along with morphologic changes consistent with impaired follicular maturation and a reduction in the number of small nongrowing follicles. Antral follicle size is reduced in young leukemic girls treated for more than 2 months with cyclophosphamide. This concept is controversial, however, because other studies show abnormal ovarian function in $<$ 10% of exposed prepubertal girls,[3] with only one third temporarily amenorrheic. In girls treated at prepubertal and pubertal ages, cyclophosphamide in doses of 525 mg/kg or less did not prevent ovulation, as detected by basal temperatures in the majority (90%). A factor in resistance may be the larger number of primordial follicles in prepubertal adolescents, compared with older patients.

CHEMOTHERAPY FOR HODGKIN'S DISEASE: GONADAL EFFECTS

Since the introduction of combination chemotherapy for Hodgkin's disease, up to 80% of patients may achieve complete remission, with 66% remaining in remission after 10 years.[48] The presence of many survivors of a disease primarily affecting young patients arouses interest in the effects of these regimens on reproductive potential.[49]

SPERMATOGENESIS

Primary gonadal dysfunction may exist at the time of diagnosis of Hodgkin's disease. In a study

Hodgkin's disease patients before treatment, 33% of men had inadequate sperm counts with decreased motility. One sixth had raised blood FSH levels, and at least 40% had impairment of the testosterone-LH axis, suggesting compromised Leydig cell function,[12] with degeneration of seminiferous tubules on examination of testicular biopsy specimens. Testicular dysfunction before therapy contrasts with that of women, in whom gonadal function appears to be unaffected by the presence of active Hodgkin's disease.[4] Possibly, a nonspecific depression of spermatogenesis results from a metabolic disturbance imparted by the disease or by mechanisms unique to the individual's geneteic component.[12]

The effect of single-agent chemotherapeutic regimens on testicular function has been reviewed, but Hodgkin's disease therapy invariably involves combination regimens, such as MVPP or MOPP. A prospective study of men receiving cyclic chemotherapy with MVPP showed elevated serum FSH and LH levels after therapy.[2] Testicular biopsy specimens demonstrated complete hyalinization and collapse of almost all seminiferous tubules, with no germinal epithelium or Sertoli cells, and Leydig cell atrophy. After one or two cycles of chemotherapy, > 90% of the men were persistently azoospermic, which is not unexpected considering the effect of the individual MVPP agents on the testis. Mechlorethamine kills mature germ cells.[5] Alkylating agents produce azoospermia and destruction of germinal epithelium. Vinblastine arrests primitive germ cells in mitosis and prevents replacement of killed spermatogonia between cycles of therapy and may effect mature sperm by depressing motility.[50] This occurs within *12 weeks* from onset of therapy. Thus extensive germ cell damage may occur after only one cycle of combination chemotherapy.

The outlook for recovery of spermatogenesis from combination therapy such as MVPP or MOPP is poor, with azoospermia common up to 4 years after therapy. Isolated case reports exist of paternity after chemotherapy-induced sterility in Hodgkin's disease,[33] but the low frequency and unpredictability of spermatogenesis dictates a need for sperm banking in young patients with prolonged survival who wish to be fertile.

Germinal aplasia, high serum FSH levels, and normal LH levels are also found in boys who received MOPP therapy for Hodgkin's disease when pubertal or prepubertal. The Leydig cell thus seems to be spared in the prepubertal adult. However, a study of gonadal function in 19 adolescent boys with Hodgkin's disease who survived for at least 2 years after the onset of combination chemotherapy reported the development of gynecomastia, suggesting a clinical sign of Leydig cell dysfunction.[51] Testes of these boys in early or middle puberty are also sensitive to the germinal-depleting effects of combination chemotherapy, as shown by continued postpubertal azoospermia. Follow-up studies of young patients throughout pubertal maturation are necessary to determine whether the testicular injury persists at a later age.

OVARIAN FUNCTION

Hodgkin's disease per se does not impair ovarian function, in contrast to the testicular impairment in men. The ovarian dysfunction is associated with the chemotherapeutic regimens. The mechanism of action of alkylating agents, cytotoxicity in a direct, dose-dependent manner independent of the cell cycle, in contrast to antimetabolites, which are dependent on active DNA synthesis, could explain the effect on the resting oocyte. Toxicity may also be directed at the supporting pregranulosa cells of the follicle and their metabolic activity.[49] Sobrinho et al.[17] studied young women with Hodgkin's disease who developed amenorrhea or oligomenorrhea shortly after regimens including at least one alkylating agent. In 50% of the women, high levels of FSH and LH were obtained in association with amenorrhea. Only 20% of the patients experienced a return of menses after 14 months of therapy. Histologic examination of the ovaries showed destruction of resting oocytes and absent primordial follicles. Thus arrest of follicular maturation and a decrease in estrogen secretion occur. A large study[2] of reproductive function of 41 women with advanced Hodgkin's disease addressed MVPP chemotherapy. Patients 21 to 51 years of age (median, 30 years) having discontinued chemotherapy for 10 to 78 months (median, 36 months) were observed for 16 months. At the end of the observation period, 12% of the patients had regular ovulatory menstrual cycles, 26% had oligomenorrhea, and 62% had complete amenorrhea with gonadotropic evidence of premature ovarian failure (Table 1). Ovarian biopsy specimens showed a reduction in primordial follicles and clinical dete-

Table 1. *Forty-One Women Treated with MVPP Hodgkin's Disease*

	Age (years)		Cycles of Chemotherapy	
	<29	≥30	6	≥7
No. of patients	(16)	(25)	(21)	(20)
Functioning (%)	5 (31%)	1 (4%)	5 (24%)	1 (5%)
Failing (%)	6 (38%)	3 (12%)	3 (14%)	6 (30%)
Failed (%)	5 (31%)	21 (84%)	13 (62%)	13 (65%)
	0.01<p<0.025		0.05<p<0.10	

Relation of ovarian function to age and number of cycles of chemotherapy with MVPP. (From Chapman et al.[4] Reproduced with the permission of the publisher, The Journal of the American Medical Association, Chicago, IL.)

rioration of ovarian function after the discontinuation of chemotherapy.

Prospects for fertility after treatment of Hodgkin's disease (i.e., the probability of maintaining ovarian function, becoming pregnant, and delivering a normal child) are important to young women anticipating successful therapy.[32]

Horning et al.[32] showed the probability of regular menses after combined modality therapy for five or more cycles to decline after 30 years of age (Fig. 3), with an increased probability of regular menses after chemotherapy significant only in patients younger than 30 years of age. In a study of patients wishing to become pregnant, women with regular menses and no menopausal symptoms had a 59% conception rate. Those with amenorrhea or menopausal symptoms had a low conception rate. A marked decline in pregnancy rate also occurred in the normal and abnormal menses group after 30 years of age (Fig. 4). Therefore, age of initiation of therapy and ovarian function after therapy by menstrual and gonadotropin parameters are predictable as to fertility potential after chemotherapy for Hodgkin's disease. This principle also applies to the prepubertal girls, in that prolonged treatment for 1 to 2 years may cause a reduction in the number of resting follicles.[24]

BREAST CANCER CHEMOTHERAPY

Breast cancer is another major female malignancy with an associated abnormality of reproductive function after chemotherapy. Administration of 10 gm or more of cyclophosphamide produces permanent amenorrhea, invariably in women in their 40s with breast cancer.[52] It is interesting that the prolonged disease-free interval observed in breast cancer patients given adjuvant therapy might be attributed to a treatment-induced endocrine ablation. Fisher et al.[53] studied the relationship between disease-free interval and depression of ovarian function in premenopausal patients with primary breast cancer who received adjuvant chemotherapy. Those in the less-than-40-years age group showed a greater improvement in disease-free survival at 4 years relative to those in the older age group. Although ovarian function was most affected in the older age group, suppression of ovarian function accounts for some adjuvant chemotherapeutic effects in the premenopausal woman, and in this situation may be a beneficial side effect.

CHILDHOOD LEUKEMIAS

Long-term survival in children with acute lymphocytic leukemia is increasing in frequency.[54] Unfortunately, the child with leukemia brings to the process the twofold problem of coexistent systemic disease and exposure to various chemotherapeutic agents.[3] Children prepubertal at diagnosis have normal reproductive function, whereas 30% of those who were pubertal when leukemia developed have abnormal function. Thus the disease state itself has a deleterious effect on reproductive function. The fertility potential of boys with acute lymphoblastic leukemia appears to carry a worse prognosis than that of girls,[55] pos-

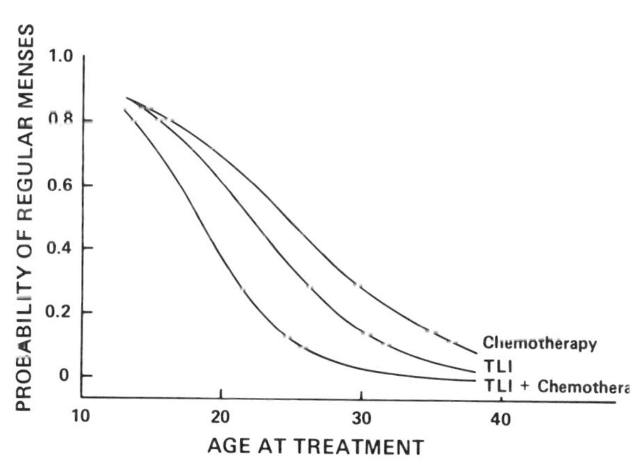

Figure 3
Probability of regular menses after chemotherapy, total lymphoid irradiation (TLI), or combined modality therapy, according to age at time of therapy. (From Horning et al.[32] Reproduced with the permission of the publisher, The New England Journal of Medicine, Boston, MA.)

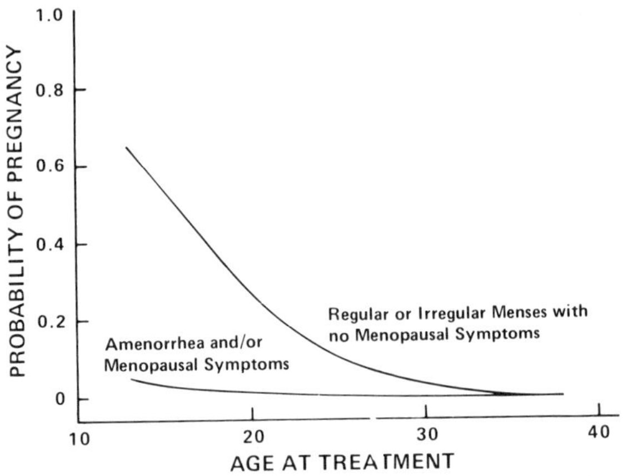

Figure 4
Probability of pregnancy after chemotherapy or combined modality therapy, according to menstrual states, menopausal symptoms, and age at treatment. (From Horning et al.[32] Reproduced with the permission of the publisher, The New England Journal of Medicine, Boston, MA.)

sibly because the testis acts as a sanctuary for residual disease after chemotherapy.[56] Female fertility following *all* treatment, however, is not as impaired. Siris et al.[3] showed that 80% of girls had normal pubertal progression during a median of 74 months after a diagnosis of leukemia and after 49 months of chemotherapy that did include alkylating agents. The degree of pubertal development present at the time of initial diagnosis of leukemia was a variable in the preservation of a normally functioning hypothalamic-pituitary-ovarian axis. Treatment of leukemia before puberty has a less adverse effect on the hypothalamic-pituitary axis that treatment of disease with onset after puberty or menarche.[3]

RADIATION THERAPY

Radiation therapy has achieved long-term control of cancer such as Hodgkin's disease, lymphosarcoma, and testicular tumors. Because many of these patients become ill before or during the childbearing age, the quality of prolonged life, including reproduction, is a major clinical management concern. In some situations there is no other alternative but to irradiate the pelvis, and subsequently the germinal epithelium of the gonad may be seriously impaired.[57] Obviously, controlled radiation experiments cannot be performed on humans. Data on the response of human ovary and testis to radiation are based mainly on middle-aged cancer patients who have been subjected to radiotherapy or on the examination of survivors of the nuclear explosion at Nagasaki and Hiroshima.[20, 58, 59] Ionizing radiation has adverse effects on gonadal function at all ages, with the percent of damage and the ability to recover dependent on the total dose.

Susceptibility to radiation-induced cell death depends on the developmental stage of the germ cell at the time of the exposure.[20, 60] Cells next to each other in development and spatial placement in the seminiferous tubule, interestingly, have different radioresistances. The type B spermatogonium is the most radiosensitive cell, but cells arising from the B spermatogonium, such as the preleptotene spermatocyte, require 10 times the amount of radiation than the type B cell to be damaged similarly. Spermatids are 40 times as resistant to radiation damage as spermatogonia.[61] Regarding oocytes, as is well known, a prolonged resting phase is entered shortly after birth. Arrest in the prophase of the first meiotic division persists throughout follicular growth before ovulation. If the ovary is irradiated in the prenatal period, sensitivity is high in oogonia that are undergoing mitosis, with some cells undergoing immediate death at interphase. As the human oocyte passes through the leptotene, zygotene, and pachytene stages of meiotic prophase, the resistance to radiation increases.[20] Microscopic studies of the human oocyte after irradiation show rapid onset of pyknosis,[62] condensation of the chromosomes, interruption of the nuclear envelope, and cytoplasmic vacuolization. Affected oocytes undergo either repair or elimination from the ovary by phagocytosis. The time at which the degenerative change occurs is independent of the dose administered to the cell. Dosage, however, affects the proportion of oocytes destroyed.[63] In animal studies, doses sufficient to destroy most small primordial follicles have not affected oocytes in Graafian follicles.[60] The radiation insult in large follicles occurs first in the granulosa cells, which become pyknotic within a few hours of exposure.[20]

IRRADIATION OF THE HUMAN TESTIS

Radiation effects on spermatogenesis depend on total dose received and stage of spermatogenesis exposed. For discussion purposes, 1 rad represents the energy transfer of 100 ergs/gm to any absorbing tissue. In an experiment in which the testes of normal men were exposed to known in-

Table 2. *Effects of Ionizing Radiation on Testicular Function*

Testicular Dose (RAD)	Results
10-30	Temporary oligospermia
30-50	100% Temporary aspermia from 4-12 months post-irradiation Full recovery by 48 months
50-100	100% Temporary aspermia from 3-17 months Full recovery *beginning* at 8-38 months
100-200	100% temporary aspermia at 2-15 months Recovery beginning at 1-20 months
200-300	100% aspermia at 2 months No recovery observed up to 40 months

Effects of radiation on testicular function. (Modified from Ash.[63] Reproduced with the permission of the publisher, The British Journal of Radiology, London, England.)

crements of radiation, the sperm count was assessed before and after irradiation. At doses of 200 to 300 rads, spermatocytes were unable to complete maturational divisions, resulting in decreased spermatid numbers. At 400 to 600 rads, spermatocytes were overtly damaged, and at doses > 400 to 600 rads, the numbers of spermatozoa and spermatids were significantly decreased. No changes in FSH and LH were noted at 8 rads of exposure, a slight increase at 20 rads, and a very significant rise at 175 to 600 rads.[61]

After 100 rads, a 67-day interval exists for the development of azoospermia. After 200 to 300 rads, the decrease in count begins at 46 days after irradiation, because it takes approximately 46 days for the preleptotene spermatocytes to develop into spermatozoa. Following irradiation with 400 to 600 rads, the drop in count occurs within the first 46 days, because the more mature spermatids and spermatocytes have been damaged.[61, 63] Temporary oligospermia is seen in those patients receiving < 30 rads. Overall recovery occurs in about one fourth of men treated with 30 to 100 rads within 1 year, but the majority of patients exposed to 200 to 300 rads continue to produce no sperm 40 months later. In another study, recovery of oligo- or azoospermia by return to preirradiation sperm concentrations occurred within 9 to 18 months for doses of ≤ 100 rads, 30 months for doses of 200 and 300 rads, and 5 or more years if at all for doses of 400 to 600 rads[63] (Table 2). Thus at doses > 200 rads, testicular function is associated with permanent or long-term azoospermia. Fertility in isolated cases leading to conception of normal offspring has been documented at 3 to 68 months after treatment.[64] If both tests are included in a single-dose field with 600 to 800 rads, permanent sterility occurs in almost all cases and prolonged azoospermia of > 5 years in the remainder.[1, 65, 66]

IRRADIATION OF THE HUMAN OVARY

The ovary is sensitive to radiation at higher doses than the testis, because of the constant cell division in the seminiferous tubule, in contrast to the meiotic activity of only a few cells in each ovarian cycle. Gonadal impairment is related to age at the time of radiotherapy, or, more pre-

Table 3. *Effects of Ionizing Radiation on Ovarian Function*

Ovarian dose	Results
60	No deleterious effect
150	No deleterious effect in young women; some risk for sterilization in women older than 40
250-500	In women aged 15-40, 60% permanently sterilized; remainder may suffer temporary amenorrhea. In women older than 40, 100% permanently sterilized
500-800	In women aged 15-40, 60%-70% permanently sterilized; remainder may experience temporary amenorrhea. No data available for women over 40.
>800	100% permanently sterilized

Effects of radiation on ovarian function. (Modified from Ash[63] and Kay and Mattison.[44] Reproduced with the permission of the publishers, The British Journal of Radiology, London, England, and The Medical Economics Company [Contemporary Obstetrics and Gynecology], Oradell, NJ, respectively.)

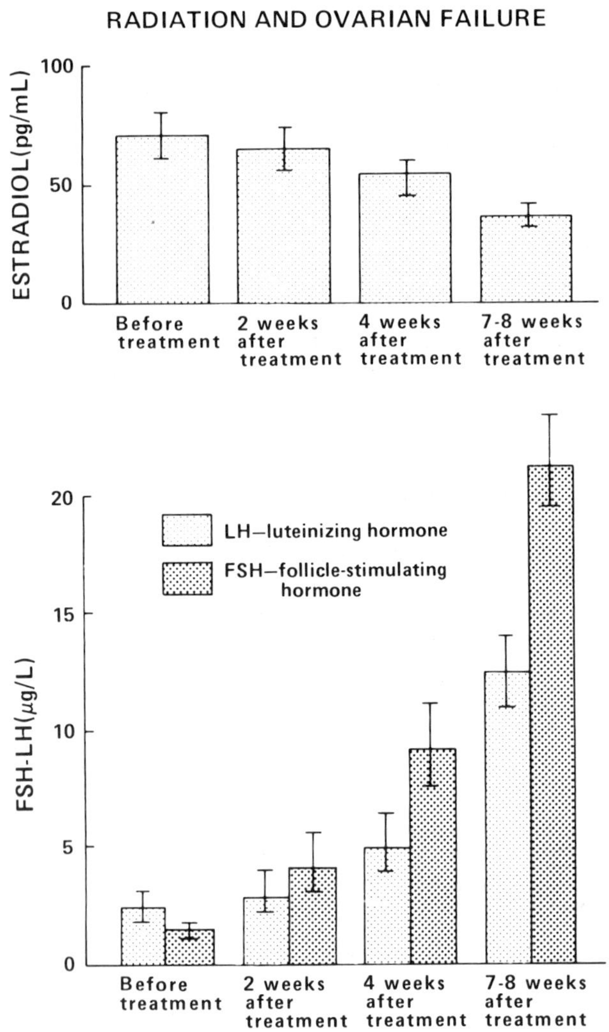

Figure 5
Estradiol, FSH, and LH levels before and after radiation therapy for cervical cancer. (Modified from Janson et al.[67] and Kay and Mattison.[44] Reproduced with the permission of the publisher, The Medical Economics Company [Contemporary Obstetrics and Gynecology], Oradell, NJ.)

cisely, to the number of oocytes that remain.[63] In women 40 years of age or older, 600 rads is associated with menopause. Women in their 30s and 20s may have up to 2000 rads over 5 to 6 weeks with a lesser chance of permanent sterility.[65, 66] A dose of 60 rads or less has no deleterious effect in most age groups. Doses of 150 rads do not appear to affect young women in their 30s and 20s, but women older than 40 years are at risk for sterilization. Women in all age groups exposed to 250 to 500 rads experience menstrual problems. Subsequently, 60% of these patients become permanently sterile, as do all women older than 40 years. In the range of 500 to 800 rads, 70% of all women are permanently sterilized. With doses > 800 rads, 100% of all women are permanently sterilized[63] (Table 3). Concurrently, FSH and LH levels are shown to rise and indicate progressive ovarian failure within 4 to 8 weeks after treatment, along with a decline in estradiol during the same time frame[65] (Fig. 5).[67]

RADIATION THERAPY FOR HODGKIN'S DISEASE

Patients with Hodgkin's disease are often treated with external irradiation, with the inverted Y, modified inverted Y, mantle, and inguinal fields[23] as common radiation approaches when radiation below the diaphragm is required (Fig. 6). The testis receives a total dose of 140 to 300 rads, with an average daily dose of 12.0 rads with inverted Y therapy.[23] Within 6 weeks of irradiation, a significant decrease in sperm viability, motility, and concentration develops (Fig. 7). Internal scatter from the thighs, however, can be prevented by shielding the testes or elongating the areas of the Y field, which can be incorporated into the therapy of men who wish to be fertile.[68] However, despite these precautions, inverted Y irradiation seems to produce 70% to 100% azoospermia.[2]

In Hodgkin's disease therapy, any of the fields mentioned will include the ovaries, which is the case with the standard inverted Y radiation tech-

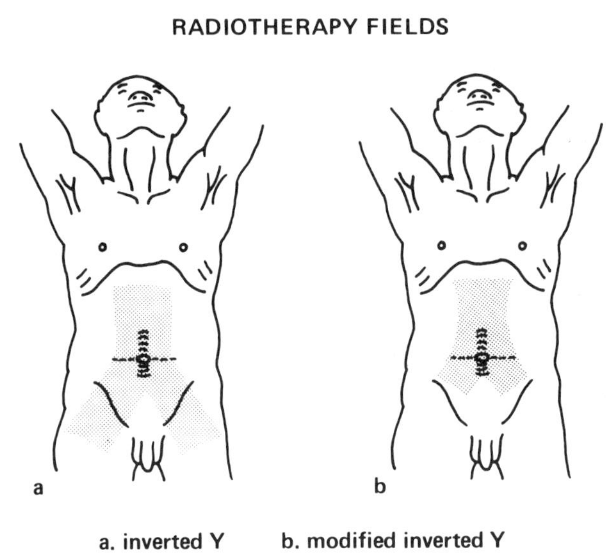

Figure 6
Radiation fields for Hodgkin's disease that can include the gonads. (From Maguire.[1] Reproduced with the permission of the publisher, McGraw-Hill Book Company [Postgraduate Medicine], Minneapolis, MN.)

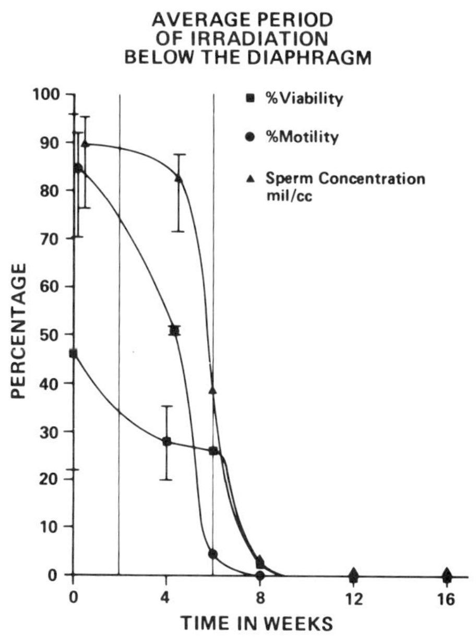

Figure 7
Development of aspermia in relation to testicular irradiation. (Adapted from Speiser et al.[23] Reproduced with the permission of the publisher, J.B. Lippincott Company [Cancer], Philadelphia, PA.)

nique. Minimizing the dose of radiation received by the ovaries without jeopardizing the chances of eradicating tumor in adjacent lymph nodes is important. An operative procedure, oophoropexy, was thus devised to move the ovaries medially or laterally from the treatment field at the time of staging laparotomy (Fig. 8).[10, 22, 69] Dosage received with medial displacement is 600 to 3500 rads, and the majority of these patients become amenorrheic. With lateral displacement in the area of the superior iliac crest, the ovaries are exposed to only 9% of the total dose.[1] However, the alteration of tubo-ovarian anatomic relationships with oophoropexy may compromise fertility by interfering with ovum transport. Reduction of the dose of radiation to the transposed ovary may also be achieved with shaped lead blocks prepared for the individual ovary to ensure maximum shielding.[68] Pelvic shielding or ovarian transposition is thus only partially successful at preserving fertility.[69] In Hodgkin's disease patients not requiring radiation below the diaphragm, 66% achieved pregnancy. Those receiving inverted periaortic radiation of 150 rads to each ovary had minimal impairment of menstrual function. However, inverted Y irradiation with ovarian shielding resulted in 75% of patients having persistent permanent amenorrhea,[32] a bleak outlook in general.

GENERATIONAL GENETICS AND PREGNANCY OUTCOME

The possibility of cytotoxic therapy and radiation of germ cells inducing mutations that result in congenital abnormalities in the progeny of those treated patients who can reproduce is a major consideration for prospects of future fertility. With radiation therapy, the incidence of mutation in germ cells increases linearly with dose; in addition, radiation may cause breakage of chromosomes. Studies on human populations exposed to large amounts of radiation and nuclear hazards, in particular the atomic bomb,[58, 59] have indicated a higher rate of abortion, stillbirth, and complications of pregnancy. The risk of serious hereditary ill health within the first two generations after irradiation of either parent is 100 cases per million per rad of exposure.[63] The additional damage to later generations is of the same magnitude. When considering numbers, a woman 35 years of age may have a population of 80,000 oocytes. If 10% of these oocytes were affected and carried recessive mutations, they would not necessarily be detected, because at most only ten pregnancies could occur. What is unclear is the incidence of recessive mutations

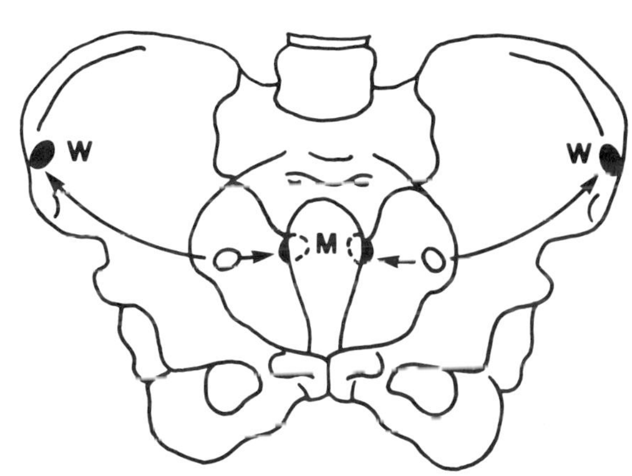

Figure 8
Oophoropexy sites. M, medial displacement; W, wide lateral displacement. (Adapted from Maguire.[1] Reproduced with the permission of the publisher, McGraw-Hill Book Company [Postgraduate Medicine], Minneapolis, MN.)

that are unlikely to show their effects for several generations, thus sequelae of any cancer therapy may be only partially expressed in the progeny of treated individuals, or the F1 generation.

Recent clinical studies,[70-73] however, have shown no increase in chromosomal abnormalities or congenital abnormalities in offspring of individuals exposed to either radiation or chemotherapy. The rate of spontaneous abortion is not any higher than that of the general population.[2, 70] The incidence of fetal abnormality was the same as the normal population in 93 conceptions in 29 women and the spouses of 19 men treated for Hodgkin's disease.[71] There were no abnormal findings in 268 pregnancies in 146 patients (72 of whom had cytotoxic chemotherapy) for a variety of cancers[72] and for 107 pregnancies in 17 men and 29 women who had been treated for cancer in childhood.[73]

THERAPEUTIC CONSIDERATIONS FOR GONADAL DYSFUNCTION

Implications for chemotherapy- or radiation-induced gonadal dysfunction go far beyond the diagnosis of azoospermia, amenorrhea, or altered gonadotropin parameters. The impact of these changes on sexuality and the quality of life for the patient is also a consideration. Premature menopause exacts a heavy toll on women, especially in those younger than 30 years of age. In addition to loss of libido, women with complete ovarian failure also manifest hot flashes, insomnia, and irritability. Disruption of stable partnerships and families has occurred after chemotherapy- and/or radiation-induced castration. Counseling should be available to such patients, along with cyclic estrogen replacement therapy and calcium supplements, which should be instituted early in patients with erratic ovarian function and in women symptomatic from premature ovarian failure.[4] In men with Hodgkin's disease, loss of libido has resulted from the physical damage caused by the chronic illness, anxiety over the uncertainty of prognosis, and the associated gonadal dysfunction. In one study,[12] approximately one half of the men experienced alteration of libido with onset of illness, with 80% noting that libido was greatly suppressed by the end of three cycles of therapy.

The therapies briefly mentioned are palliative, useful only after gonadal insult has occurred. The question arises: Is there a possibility of protection against induced gonadal damage? In an animal model, pretreatment with a synthetic analog of gonadotropin-releasing hormone (GnRH) produced "protection" from histologically detectable chemotherapeutic-induced damage from cyclophosphamide. D-leu GnRH was shown to protect spermatogenesis, possibly by down-regulation of GnRH receptors, and diminished pituitary responsiveness. Temporary interruption of the pituitary-gonadal axis may thus ameliorate the gonadal toxicity of systemic chemotherapy.[74] The GnRH analog may also affect the sensitivity of the seminiferous tubule to cyclophosphamide.[75] Another avenue of therapy for patients with neoplastic disease requiring chemotherapy or radiation is the option for storage of gametes. Sperm banking can be performed in men with acceptable sperm counts before initiation of cancer therapy, providing a possibility for pregnancy at a later date after therapy has been completed and remission achieved. The advent of in vitro fertilization programs has allowed potential expansion of techniques for the cancer patient with possible induction of multiple follicles with subsequent cryopreservation of the retrieved oocytes prior to therapy.

CONCLUSION

The major group of drugs responsible for cytotoxic-induced gonadal damage are the alkylating agents, such as cyclophosphamide and chlorambucil. Agents such as vinblastine have also been incriminated.

Gonadal insult in men and women depends on the total dose of the drug received, but it is unclear whether the duration of therapy is an important variable.

Age at time of therapeutic intervention is an important variable in the chemotherapeutic- and radiation-induced gonadal impairment in women but not in men.

Chemotherapeutic drugs compromise the testis by affecting the germinal epithelium. Leydig cell function may be impaired, but these cells appear in general to be resistant.

The duration of time after cessation of single-agent chemotherapy is an important determinant of gonadal recovery. The outlook for Hodgkin's disease patients treated with combination chemotherapy, such as MVPP or MOPP, appears poor, regardless of time of discontinuation.

The disease state itself, particularly Hodgkin's disease in men, may impair testicular function even before chemotherapy and radiation. This should be considered in prescreening evaluations for Hodgkin's disease therapy. This is in contrast to women, whose gonadal function seems to be unaffected by the presence of active disease.

The dose of radiation received appears to be the major prognostic indicator for gonadal function after therapy. Greater than 800 rads in women of any age and 700 rads in men produces permanent sterility. The difference in sensitivity to radiation may be due to the spermatozoon's constant state of mitotic division. No deleterious effects on reproductive function appear with 60 rads in women and 30 rads in men by ovulation parameters or semen analysis, respectively.

There is no documented increase in congenital anomalies, spontaneous abortions, or pregnancy complications in patients who reproduce after chemotherapy and radiation. The risk to the gene pool of subsequent generations has not been assessed adequately.

Sexual and emotional problems and loss of libido may ensue as a result of the stress of the disease process and the chemotherapy and radiation. Proper counseling, when indicated, and hormonal replacement therapy may improve the quality of life even for short-term survivors.

Banking of gametes, such as sperm banking, ovulation induction, oocyte retrieval, and cryopreservation offer some prospects for fertility for patients who will have permanent gonadal failure after chemotherapy or radiation for neoplastic disease.

REFERENCES

1. Maguire L: Fertility and cancer therapy. Postgrad Med 65(5):293, 1979
2. Chapman RM: Effect of cytotoxic therapy on sexuality and gonadal function. Semin Oncol 9:84, 1982
3. Siris ES, Leventhal BG, Vaitukaitis JL: Effects of childhood leukemia and chemotherapy on puberty and reproductive function in girls. N Engl J Med 294:1143, 1976
4. Chapman RM, Sutcliffe SB, Malpas JS: Cytotoxic-induced ovarian failure in women with Hodgkin's disease. JAMA 242:1877, 1979
5. Spitz S: The histological effects of nitrogen mustards on human tumors and tissues. Cancer 1:383, 1948
6. Gilman A: The initial clinical trial of nitrogen mustard. Am J Surg 105:574, 1963
7. Bollag W, Theiss E: Methylhydrazine derivatives. In Proceedings of the International Symposium on Chemotherapy of Cancer, Edited by PA Plattner. New York, Elsevier Publishing, 1964, p 311
8. Richter P, Calamera JC, Morgenfeld MC, Kierszenbaum AL, Lavieri JC, Mancini RE: Effect of chlorambucil on spermatogenesis in the human with malignant lymphoma. Cancer 23:1026, 1970
9. Miller DG: Alkylating agents and human spermatogenesis. JAMA 217:1662, 1971
10. Qureshi MSA, Pennington JH, Goldsmith HJ, Cox PE: Cyclophosphamide therapy and sterility. Lancet 2:1290, 1972
11. Chapman RM, Sutcliffe SB, Rees L: Gonadal dysfunction in patients with Hodgkin's disease (Abstr). J R Soc Med 71:96, 1978
12. Chapman RM, Sutcliffe SB, Malpas JS: Male gonadal dysfunction in Hodgkin's disease: a prospective study. JAMA 245:1323, 1981
13. Rose DP, Davis TE: Ovarian function in patients receiving adjuvant chemotherapy for breast cancer. Lancet 1:1174, 1977
14. Miller JJ, Williams GF, Leissring JC: Multiple late complications of therapy with cyclophosphamide, including ovarian destruction. Am J Med 50:530, 1971
15. Kumar R, Biggart JD, McEvoy J: Cyclophosphamide and reproductive function. Lancet 1:1212, 1972
16. Warne GL, Fairley KF, Hobbs JB, Martin FIR: Cyclophosphamide-induced ovarian failure. N Engl J Med 289:1159, 1973
17. Sobrinho LG, Levine RA, DeConti RC: Amenorrhea in patients with Hodgkin's disease treated with antineoplastic agents. Am J Obstet Gynecol 109:135, 1971
18. Roentgen WC: Radiation Biology (1895): Cited by Patt HM, Brues AM, Part 2, Vol 1, Edited by A Hallaender. New York, McGraw-Hill Book Company, 1954, p 959
19. Bequerel H: Sur les radiations invisibles emises par les corps phosphorescents. C R Acad Sci (Paris) 122:501, 1896
20. Baker TG: Radiosensitivity of mammalian oocytes with particular reference to the human female. Am J Obstet Gynecol 110:746, 1971
21. Jacox HW: Recovery following human ovarian irradiation. Radiology 32:538, 1939
22. Ray GR, Trueblood HW, Enright LP, Kaplan HS, Nelson TS: Oophoropexy: a means of preserving ovarian function following pelvic megavoltage radiotherapy for Hodgkin's disease. Radiology 96:175, 1970
23. Speiser B, Rubin P, Casarett G: Aspermia following lower truncal irradiation in Hodgkin's disease. Cancer 32:692, 1973
24. Shalet SM: Effects of cancer chemotherapy on gonadal function of patients. Cancer Treat Rev 7:141, 1980
25. Etteldorf JN, West CD, Pitcock JA, Williams DL: Gonadal function, testicular histology, and meiosis following cyclophosphamide therapy in patients with nephrotic syndrome. J Pediatr 88:206, 1976
26. Blake DA, Heller RH, Hsu SH, Schacter BZ: Return of fertility in a patient with cyclophosphamide-induced azoospermia. Johns Hopkins Med J 139:20, 1976
27. Buchanan JD, Fairley KF, Barrie JU: Return of spermatogenesis after stopping cyclophosphamide therapy. Lancet 2:156, 1975
28. Fairley KF, Barrie JU, Johnson W: Sterility and testicular atrophy related to cyclophosphamide therapy. Lancet 1:568, 1972
29. Calamera JC, Morgenfeld MC, Mancini RE, Vilar O: Biochemical changes of the human semen produced by chlorambucil, testosterone propionate and human chorionic gonadotropin administration. Andrologia 11:43, 1979

30. Cheviakoff S, Calamera JC, Morgenfeld M, Mancini RE: Recovery of spermatogenesis in patients with lymphoma after treatment with chlorambucil. J Reprod Fertil 33:155, 1973
31. El-Beheiry A, El-Mansy E, Kamel N, Salama N: Methotrexate and fertility in men. Arch Androl 3:177, 1979
32. Horning SJ, Hoppe RT, Kaplan HS, Rosenberg SA: Female reproductive potential after treatment for Hodgkin's disease. N Engl J Med 304:1376, 1981
33. Stricker S, Crosby K, Carey RW: Paternity after chemotherapy-induced sterility in Hodgkin's disease. N Engl J Med 304:1175, 1981
34. Pahdke A, MacKinnon KJ, Dossetor JB: Male fertility in uremia: restoration by renal allografts. Can Med Assoc J 102:607, 1970
35. Devita VT Jr, Hellman S, Rosenberg SA: Cancer: Principles and Practice of Oncology, Second edition. Philadelphia, J. B. Lippincott Co., 1985
36. Chabner B: Pharmacologic Principles of Cancer Treatment. Philadelphia, W. B. Saunders Co., 1982
37. Sussman A, Leonard J: Psoriasis, methotrexate, and oligospermia. Arch Dermatol 116:215, 1980
38. Greenwald ES: Cancer Chemotherapy. New York, Medical Examination Publishing Co., 1979, p 28
39. Mancini RE, Lavieri JC, Muller F, Andrada JA, Saraceni DJ: Effect of prednisolone upon normal and pathologic human spermatogenesis. Fertil Steril 17:500, 1966
40. Lentz RD, Bergstein J, Steffes MW, Brown DR, Prem K, Michael AF, Vernier RL: Postpubertal evaluation of gonadal function following cyclophosphamide therapy before and during puberty. J Pediatr 91:385, 1977
41. Guesry P, Lenoir G, Broyer M: Gonadal effects of chlorambucil given to prepubertal and pubertal boys for nephrotic syndrome. J Pediatr 92:299, 1978
42. Lendon M, Hann IM, Palmer MK, Shalet SM, Morris Jones PH: Testicular histology after combination chemotherapy in childhood for acute lymphoblastic leukemia. Lancet 2:439, 1978
43. Matus-Ridley M, Nicosia SV, Meadows AT: Gonadal effects of cancer therapy in boys. Cancer 55:2353, 1985
44. Kay H, Mattison D: How radiation and chemotherapy affect gonadal function. Contemp Obstet Gynecol 109:106, 1985
45. Uldall PR, Kerr DNS, Tacchi D: Amenorrhea and sterility. Lancet 1:693, 1972
46. Belohorsky B, Siracky J, Sandor L, Klauber E: Comments on the development of amenorrhea caused by Myleran in cases of chronic myelosis. Neoplasma 4:397, 1960
47. Nicosia SV, Matus-Ridley M, Meadows AT: Gonadal effects of cancer therapy in girls. Cancer 55:2364, 1985
48. Rostom AY, White WF: Hodgkin's disease, chemotherapy and fertility (Letter to the Editor). Lancet 1:555, 1979
49. Viviani S, Sanroro A, Ragni G, Bonfante V, Bestetti O, Bonadonna G: Gonadal toxicity after combination chemotherapy for Hodgkin's disease: comparative results of MOPP vs ABVD. Eur J Cancer Clin Oncol 21:601, 1985
50. Cutts JH: The effect of vincaleukoblastine on dividing cells in vivo. Cancer Res 21:168, 1961
51. Sherins RJ, Olweny CLM, Ziegler JL: Gynecomastia and gonadal dysfunction in adolescent boys treated with combination chemotherapy for Hodgkin's disease. N Engl J Med 299:12, 1978
52. Koyama H, Wada T, Nishizawa Y, Iwanaga T, Aoki Y, Terasawa T, Kosaki G, Yamamoto T, Wada A: Cyclophosphamide-induced ovarian failure and its therapeutic significance in patients with breast cancer. Cancer 39:1403, 1977
53. Fisher B, Sherman BM, Rockette H, Redmond C, Margolese R, Fisher ER: L-Phenylalanine mustard (L-PAM) in the management of premenopausal patients with primary breast cancer: lack of association of disease-free survival with depression of ovarian function. National Surgical Adjuvant Project for Breast and Bowel Cancers. Cancer 44:847, 1979
54. Hinkes E, Plotkin D: Reversible drug-induced sterility in a patient with acute leukemia. JAMA 223:1490, 1973
55. Lilleyman JS: Male fertility after successful chemotherapy for lymphoblastic leukemia (Letter to the Editor). Lancet 2:1125, 1979
56. Evenson DP, Arlin Z, Welt S, Claps ML, Malamed MR: Male reproductive capacity may recover following drug treatment with L-10 protocol for acute lymphocytic leukemia. Cancer 53:30, 1984
57. Hahn EW, Feingold SM, Nisce L: Aspermia and recovery of spermatogenesis in cancer patients following incidental gonadal irradiation during treatment: a progress report. Radiology 119:223, 1976
58. Blot WJ, Shimizu Y, Kato H, Miller RW: Frequency of marriage and live birth among survivors prenatally exposed to the atomic bomb. Am J Epidemiol 102:128, 1975
59. Seigel DG: Frequency of live births among survivors of Hiroshima and Nagasaki atomic bombings. Radiat Res 28:278, 1966
60. Mandl AM: The radiosensitivity of germ cells. Biol Rev 39:288, 1964
61. Rowley MJ, Leach DR, Warner GA, Heller CG: Effect of graded doses of ionizing radiation on the human testis. Radiat Res 59:665, 1974
62. Mandl AM: A quantitative study of the sensitivity of oocytes to X-irradiation. Proc R Soc Biol 150:53, 1959
63. Ash P: The influence of radiation on fertility in man. Br J Radiol 53:271, 1980
64. Sandeman TF: The effects of X irradiation on male human fertility. Br J Radiol 39:901, 1966
65. Lushbaugh CC, Casarett GW: The effects of gonadal irradiation in clinical radiation therapy: a review. Cancer 37:1111, 1976
66. Shapiro E, Kinsella TJ, Makuch RW, Fraass BA, Glatstein E, Rosenberg SA, Sherins RJ: Effects of fractionated irradiation on endocrine aspects of testicular function. J Clin Oncol 3:1232, 1985
67. Janson PO, Jansson I, Skryten A, Dambler J, Lindstedt G: Ovarian endocrine function in young women undergoing radiotherapy for carcinoma of the cervix. Gynecol Oncol 11:218, 1981
68. Jackson HL, Hass AC, Sooby D, Marschke CH: The gonadal exposure of boys and young men treated with inverted "Y" fields: its reduction and genetic significance. Radiology 96:181, 1970
69. Thomas PRM, Winstantly D, Peckham MJ, Austin DE, Murray MAF, Jacobs HS: Reproductive and endocrine function in patients with Hodgkin's disease: effects of oophoropexy and irradiation. Br J Cancer 33:226, 1976
70. Ross GT: Congenital anomalies among children born of mothers receiving chemotherapy for gestational trophoblastic neoplasms. Cancer 37:1043, 1976
71. Holmes GF, Holmes FF: Pregnancy outcome of patients treated for Hodgkin's disease. Cancer 41:1317, 1978

72. Li FP, Fine W, Jaffe N, Holmes G, Holmes F: Offspring of patients treated for cancer in childhood. JNCI 62:1193, 1979
73. Li FP, Jaffe N: Progeny of childhood cancer survivors. Lancet 2:707, 1974
74. Glode LM, Robinson J, Gould SF: Protection from cyclophosphamide-induced testicular damage with an analogue of gonadotropin-releasing hormone. Lancet 1:1132, 1981
75. Johnson DH, Linde R, Hainsworth JD, Vale W, Rivier J, Stein R, Flexner J, Van Welch R, Greco FA: Effect of a luteinizing hormone releasing hormone agonist given during combination chemotherapy on posttherapy fertility in male patients with lymphoma: preliminary observations. Blood 165:832, 1985

Chapter 5

The reproductive toxicity of ovulation induction

Anthony R. Scialli, M.D.

Reproductive Toxicology Center, Columbia Hospital for Women Medical Center, Washington, D.C.

Disorders of ovulation resulting in impaired fertility constitute one of the most common causes of involuntary childlessness. Medications to cause or at least facilitate ovulation have been in clinical use for two decades. An increasing number of pregnancies are being conceived during or shortly after therapy with these agents. It is relevant, then, to determine whether the use of ovulation induction places a pregnant woman at greater risk of an abnormal outcome, such as spontaneous abortion, fetal malformation, or intrauterine growth disturbance.

In any consideration of the reproductive toxicity of a group of agents, it is important to bear in mind that abnormal pregnancy outcomes are relatively common events and that some abnormal outcomes, such as spontaneous abortion, are found more readily if they are sought. For example, a supervised woman on basal body temperature charts who has an early measurement of serum human chorionic gonadotropin (hCG) will have a pregnancy identified earlier than would an unsupervised woman. An early spontaneous abortion in a supervised infertility patient will be recognized promptly, whereas the unsupervised woman may pass off the same episode of bleeding as a late menstrual period. This may lead to the impression that infertility patients have a higher rate of spontaneous abortion than do women with normal fertility. Although this higher rate of abortion may be due to the lack of a suitable control population of closely supervised "normal" women, it may also be due to some feature of the fertility patients themselves or to the drugs given to these patients, which is the subject of this discussion.

A number of chemical agents have been used clinically or experimentally to induce ovulation or to improve the quality of the follicle and/or the corpus luteum around the time of ovulation. I will consider the three medications most commonly used in clinical practice, clomiphene citrate (CC), human menopausal gonadotropins (hMG), and bromocriptine.

CLOMIPHENE CITRATE

The triphenylethylenes include a number of compounds with the ability to bind estrogen receptor. Some, such as chlorotrianisene (TACE; Merrell Dow Pharmaceuticals, Inc., Cincinnati, OH), appear to activate the receptor and exert estrogenic activity, and others, such as tamoxifen, apparently block the activity of endogenous hormone and therefore act as antiestrogens. CC appears to possess both agonist and antagonist activities. Although it is widely believed that CC acts by displacing endogenous estrogens from hypothalamic receptors (thereby augmenting the release of gonadotropin-releasing hormone), a case may be made for a direct estrogenic effect of CC on the pituitary and/or the ovary.[1] The potential of CC to block estrogen receptor has, however, raised the concern that the normal estrogen-dependent events surrounding ovulation may be altered by this compound, resulting in impaired functioning of the preovulatory follicle, the early corpus luteum, and/or the endometrium/decidua. It is often noted, in fact, that with CC therapy the ovulation rate (70% to 90%) is much higher than the pregnancy rate (30% to 40%).[2] This suggests that the female genital system exposed to CC may have a decreased ability to transport or sustain the ovum, spermatozoan, or early embryo.

LUTEAL PHASE DEFICIENCY

Inadequate luteal phase progesterone (P) levels and/or endometrial histologic response, seen both in infertile and normal women, has been referred to as luteal phase deficiency (LPD). The association between CC therapy and LPD has been considered a major cause of impaired reproductive capability in women taking CC. Although CC has been used to treat LPD, such treatment may be less effective than supplemental P and may induce LPD in normally cycling women.[3] Garcia and co-workers,[4] in addition, found 10 of 34 endometrial biopsies in the luteal phase of CC-induced pregnancy cycles to be out of phase with the date of ovulation. Human corpus luteum slices incubated with CC show a reduced ability to incorporate radiolabeled acetate into P. Although high culture levels of CC (20 μg/ml) are necessary to reduce acetate incorporation by as much as 95%, some effect is seen with CC concentrations as low as 0.02 μg/ml; this is comparable to clinically achievable drug levels.[5] It is interesting that the addition of hCG to the medium counteracts the inhibitory effect of CC.

More recent investigations into the mechanism of CC-induced LPD suggests that abnormalities of preovulatory follicular steroidogenesis may be responsible for the luteal phase problem. Rat preovulatory follicles in culture show an inhibition of steroid accumulation after exposure to high concentrations of CC. Concentrations of CC of 1.2 mg/ml are associated with a 90% reduction in estradiol (E_2) accumulation, a 97% reduction in P accumulation, and a 65% reduction in testosterone accumulation. The inhibitory effects of CC are seen both in basal and luteinizing hormone (LH)-stimulated steroid accumulation and are not reversed by the addition of pregnenolone or a brominated cyclic adenosine monophosphate (cAMP) to the medium, suggesting a block in follicular steroidogenesis distal to the cAMP-mediated stimulatory activity of LH.[6] This study has been criticized because of culture medium concentrations of CC much higher than those encountered in clinical practice; however, results permitting a similar interpretation were reported by Marut and Hodgen[7] in the monkey. Doses of CC of 25 mg/day given to normal ovulatory animals for 5-day intervals at various times in the follicular phase are accompanied by an elevation in serum gonadotropins but a decrease in serum E_2 during therapy. Ovulation is delayed, with the effects of CC greatest when the drug is given during cycle days 9 to 13, after the dominant follicle has already been selected. The luteal phase is shortened and serum P levels are decreased in treated cycles. These abnormalities are consistent with inhibition of E_2-mediated gonadotropin receptor formation in the follicle.

Work in human in vitro fertilization programs has confirmed that CC therapy decreases intrafollicular E_2. Dlugi et al.[8] compared eight women in whom oocyte maturation had been stimulated by CC with a similar number of women prepared with hMG. Serum and follicular fluid E_2 were higher in the hMG group. By contrast, diZerega and co-workers[9] noted that women prepared with either CC or hMG had reduced intrafollicular E_2, compared with untreated controls. Follicular E_2 levels were not less after CC than after hMG in this study.

It is possible that CC exerts an antiestrogenic effect in the follicle and may inhibit the induction of gonadotropin receptors. This may lead to LPD with failure of pregnancy to be achieved or supported. It is difficult, however, to determine whether or how often CC gives rise to clinical LPD, because it is not clear how often and with what significance evidence of LPD may be found in normally ovulating women. In addition, women given CC have ovulatory dysfunction from the outset. It is possible that LPD in these patients represents an incomplete correction of the ovulatory problem, and not a drug effect at all.

SPONTANEOUS ABORTION

A related issue is whether CC-induced pregnancies are more likely to abort than pregnancies after spontaneous ovulation. A number of authors have reported miscarriage rates after CC that are much higher than rates in the general population; however, the special surveillance accorded a woman on fertility drugs may predispose to a bias in favor of identifying their early pregnancy losses. Several authors have attempted to select control groups to eliminate this and other sources of bias. For example, a comparison of 93 pregnancies conceived after CC therapy with 270 pregnancies conceived after other (unspecified) therapies for infertility resulted in a 23.6% abortion rate in the CC group and an 8.9% rate in the controls ($P < 0.005$).[10] There was a particular dependence in the CC group of abortion on the cycle of conception, with nearly one half of the miscarriages occurring in women who had been on CC for more than 6 months. Another report was that 25.3% of pregnancies conceived in cycles on CC miscarried and only 11% of pregnancies conceived in cycles after CC had been discontinued ended in abortion.[4] By contrast, a nonconcurrent retrospective comparison of abortion rates in pregnancies conceived after ovarian wedge resection and after CC therapy showed 21.6% miscarriages after wedge resection and 26.5% miscarriages after CC, rates that are not statistically different.[11] This comparison is of particular interest because in the reporting institution, CC therapy replaced wedge resection over time for treatment of the same disorder (oligo/anovulation), suggesting that women comprising the two groups had similar characteristics and a similar innate potential for reproductive success. Finally, a prospective 5-year study in nine Japanese university hospitals compared adverse pregnancy outcomes in 1034 pregnancies conceived after CC, 186 pregnancies conceived after hMG/hCG, and 29,900 pregnancies conceived after spontaneous ovulation. Early pregnancy wastage was not different among the groups (14.8% after CC, 19.4% after hMG/hCG, and 13.9% after spontaneous ovulation).[12]

Although an increase in the abortion rate after CC has been identified by some authors as due to LPD,[4] other investigators believe the quality of the ovum/conceptus to be deficient after ovulation induction. High doses of CC in vitro may cause degenerative changes in rat oocytes.[6] In mice exposed to CC before ovulation, the number of ovulated ova is reduced and the potential of the ovum to fertilize diminished.[13] Those ova that do fertilize, however, appear able to develop normally in vitro to the blastocyst stage. In human beings, preparation of in vitro fertilization patients with CC does not appear to impair oocyte quality or to reduce the number of embryos that will implant after embryo transfer.[8]

The classic studies of Boué and co-workers[14, 15] have raised the possibility that ovulation induction increases the incidence of chromosomal abnormalities in the conceptus. Abortus tissue was carefully collected and karyotyped as soon as possible after pregnancy loss. If ovulation induction (with either CC, hMG, hCG, or any combination of these) had been used in the cycle of conception or the cycle immediately preceding the cycle of conception, chromosomal abnormalities were present in more than 80% of abortuses. If ovulation induction was used two or more cycles before the cycle of conception or if no ovulation induction had been used, chromosomal abnormalities were seen in only 60% of abortuses. These data have been interpreted as demonstrating an adverse effect of ovulation induction on the maintenance of a normal karyotype during oocyte maturation and early embryogenesis. Another explanation, however, is tenable. If ovulation induction improves the hormonal and/or decidual support of the conceptus, fewer chromosomally normal embryos would abort, because abortion of a normal embryo is likely to be related to abnormality of the environment provided by the mother.[16] There would, therefore, be an overrepresentation of abnormal karyotypes among abortuses in these women.

COMPLICATION IN CONTINUING PREGNANCIES

Multiple gestations occur in 8% to 13% of pregnancies conceived after ovulation induction with CC.[11, 17-20] Twins comprise nearly all of the multiple pregnancies with higher-order pregnancies occurring infrequently. The complications that occur more commonly in twin than in singleton pregnancy, such as prematurity, toxemia, and gestational diabetes mellitus, probably occur at the same rate in CC-induced twin pregnancies as in spontaneous twin pregnancies, although this has not been systematically studied. There have been reports of bilateral tubal pregnancies and coexisting tubal and intrauterine pregnancies after ovulation induction,[21, 22] but these phenomena are attributable to fraternal twinning without the need to invoke a separate CC-mediated mechanism of heterotopic pregnancy.

Isolated studies have reported an increased incidence of various pregnancy abnormalities other than multiple gestation. Hack and co-workers[19] found toxemia to occur in 16.7% of 96 CC pregnancies that reached 20 gestational weeks or more. The cases of toxemia occurred exclusively in singleton pregnancies. Although there was no control group in this study, this rate appeared higher than the 7% toxemia incidence in the general population. The details of the report, however, do not permit a conclusion as to whether the women conceiving on CC differed in important ways (e.g., age, parity, and nutritional status) from the general population. In addition, 14 of the 16 toxemic patients were classified as having "mild" disease, raising the possibility that the criteria for toxemia may have included women with borderline presentations. In other surveys, such women might have been considered normal.

An older report from the Shelton Clinic in Los Angeles[20] found that 50 of 140 CC pregnancies with known outcome were "complicated." Many of these complications, however, would not currently be listed as adverse pregnancy outcomes for purposes of reproductive toxicity evaluation. Among the 50 complications were 16 cesarean sections (for various indications), 4 breech presentations, 12 twin gestations, and 1 chronic hypertensive pregnancy. Of interest was the finding that 6 of 140 pregnancies demonstrated "placental insufficiency." The lack of definition of this condition in the study makes it difficult to evaluate the intriguing possibility that CC treatment interferes with normal placentation. Twelve patients were reported to have cervical incompetence, but it is unclear how this condition was diagnosed and whether the diagnosis was established before or after CC therapy. Nine of the 12 patients with cervical incompetence are reported to have had abnormal uterine contours on hysterography. If this was the basis of the diagnosis, it would not be expected that such a high incidence of this disorder would be seen with current diagnostic criteria.

Perinatal mortality in CC pregnancies has been reported as 1.8% to 3.1% for singletons[17, 19]; however, these figures are from studies published in 1968 and 1972 and must be interpreted with caution. The lack of mortality statistics from a suitable control population further detracts from the usefulness of these numbers. Encouraging results were reported in the comparison of pregnancy after CC with pregnancy after wedge resection; it was shown that the chance of pregnancy resulting in delivery of a living child was not reduced by CC therapy.[11]

Fetal/neonatal growth does not appear to be affected by ovulation induction with CC. Birth weights are not different when infants born after CC are compared with controls born after ovarian wedge resection[11] or with controls matched for sex, length of gestation, maternal parity, and maternal smoking.[23] Six- and 12-month follow-up of infants born after CC therapy show normal length and weight by general population standards.[19]

BIRTH DEFECTS

Case reports from the early 1970s called attention to the occurrence of neural tube defects in women conceiving after therapy with CC.[24-27] There has also been a report of an infant with multiple musculoskeletal anomalies conceived one to two cycles after CC was stopped (the mother also took dimenhydrinate during the first trimester).[28] Although such reports have been taken as evidence of a link between CC ingestion and teratogenicity, it is not possible to consider such a connection without information on how often birth defects occur in an entire population of CC-exposed infants. Uncontrolled studies have reported congenital anomaly rates of 2% to 9%, which did not differ from background anomaly rates in the authors' communities.[17-20, 23, 29] In a controlled prospective study, major and minor malformations occurred in 1.0% and 1.3%, respectively, of CC-induced pregnancies and in 1.1% and 0.6% of spontaneously conceived pregnancies, an insignificant difference.[12]

EVALUATION

Ovulation induction with CC may cause LPD with consequent failure of implantation or early pregnancy loss. This may be due to the antiestrogenic action of this medication within the preovulatory follicle or on the endometrium. There are few adequately controlled studies on the possible adverse pregnancy effects of CC. It appears, however, that once pregnancy is established, the only complication reproducibly related to CC therapy is an increase in twinning. Miscarriage (not due to LPD) and other adverse pregnancy outcomes have not been shown to be increased in pregnancies conceived after therapy with CC. Fetal growth and development appear to be normal in these pregnancies.

HUMAN MENOPAUSAL GONADOTROPINS

It should be recognized that studies on the effects of hMG do not deal with a discrete exposure given in a standard manner. Ovulation induction with hMG involves a number of agents. Commercially available hMG is a mixture of follicle-stimulating hormone and LH. In some patients, estrogens or CC are also used with hMG therapy. After obtaining evidence of sufficient follicular maturation, it is customary to give hCG as a surrogate for the LH surge. In addition, monitoring of follicle size may incorporate the use of serial ultrasound examinations,[30] although it is doubtful that diagnostic ultrasound is a reproductive toxin.[31] The administration of hMG may be monitored with clinical estimates of estrogen effect, serum or urinary estrogen measurements, and/or ultrasound evaluation of follicular development, and differences in monitoring techniques may give rise to differences in dosing and in effects. Finally, the older literature includes the use of gonadotropins of pituitary origin instead of the more standard menopausal urine extracts.

LUTEAL PHASE DEFICIENCY

Abnormalities of the luteal phase have been reported to occur after hMG induction of ovulation. Olson and co-workers[32] studied 126 hMG cycles in 24 women. Ninety-eight cycles were presumed ovulatory, with 20 resulting in pregnancy. A luteal phase less than 11 days long was found in 18 cycles (14% of presumed ovulatory cycles). When cycles with short luteal phases were compared with cycles resulting in pregnancy, it was found that the abnormal cycles had either very low (< 200 pg/ml) or very high (> 2000 pg/ml) preovulatory serum E_2 levels, suggesting a dysfunction of the follicular phase. Dlugi et al.[33] reported similar findings in a study of in vitro fertilization patients prepared with hMG. A comparison of conception and nonconception cycles showed successful outcome to be associated with a higher serum P in the midluteal and late luteal phases and with higher serum E_2 before laparoscopy and in the midluteal phase. As appears to be the case with respect to CC, hMG treatment may lead to a reduction in intrafollicular E_2 in some cases.[9]

It is not known how often hMG-induced ovulation is followed by clinically significant LPD, but many current regimens include a repeat dose of hCG 4 to 8 days after ovulation to help maintain the corpus luteum.[30]

SPONTANEOUS ABORTION

Determination of the miscarriage rate after hMG is subject to the same problems as those discussed above for CC. Abortion rates between 11.5% and 57% have been reported.[12, 32, 34-40] In a prospective study of 186 hMG pregnancies and 29,900 spontaneous pregnancies, early pregnancy loss occurred in 19.4% of induced and 13.9% of control gestations, an insignificant difference.[12] Ben-Rafael et al.[34] studied 34 women with hMG-induced pregnancies followed by spontaneously conceived pregnancies. Miscarriages occurred in 29% of the hMG pregnancies (24.1% if twins were excluded) and only 8.8% of second pregnancies. The study was extended to include 203 women with hMG pregnancies, of whom 116 conceived subsequently. Second pregnancies included 32 spontaneously conceived and 84 conceived again after hMG. The abortion rate in the 203 initial hMG pregnancies was 28.5%, with second pregnancy abortion rates of 9.3% and 11.9% in spontaneous and hMG pregnancies, respectively.[35] The authors interpreted the higher pregnancy loss rates in first hMG pregnancies as suggesting uterine hypoplasia; however, they and others[38] have noted an association between ovarian hyperstimulation and abortion. It is possible that nonconcurrent comparisons favoring the later treatment groups reflect more careful monitoring of estrogen levels in the later cycles. This interpretation is supported by the finding of the highest rates of miscarriage in older reports, in which estrogen effect was estimated clinically or not at all.

Gemzell and co-workers[41] called attention to another possible effect of ovarian hyperstimulation on early pregnancy loss. They identified 10 tubal pregnancies in 379 gestations conceived after hMG. Of these, four were combined with an intrauterine pregnancy. Although a control population was not used, the extrauterine pregnancy rate of 2.6% appears higher than generally quoted rates (1.2% to 1.8%). The authors postulated that abnormally elevated estrogens in stimulated cycles might predispose to ectopic pregnancy by altering tubal motility.

The possibility that hMG treatment causes a higher incidence of chromosomal abnormalities was suggested by Boué and co-workers.[14, 15] Their data, discussed above with respect to CC, pertained to abortuses from pregnancies conceived after therapy with CC, hMG, hCG, or any combination. Although chromosomally abnormal abortuses were found more often immediately after ovulation induction than remote from ovulation induction, no estimate of the total spontaneous abortion rate was included. It is not known, then, whether ovulation induction induces chromosomal abnormalities or serves better to maintain chromosomally normal conceptuses at risk for abortion from other factors.

MULTIPLE GESTATION

Twin and higher-order pregnancies have been reported to occur in 11% to 42% of hMG-induced gestations.[18, 36-40] The multiple pregnancy rate appears to depend on the care with which estrogen levels are monitored, and it would appear that a multiple pregnancy rate of 10% is achievable.[30] Most multiple gestations after hMG are twins; however, higher-order pregnancies are much more common after hMG than after spontaneous ovulation or CC. Triplet rates with hMG therapy are as high as 5% to 6%.[36, 38, 39]

The occurrence of multiple pregnancy is responsible for the majority of perinatal deaths in hMG-induced gestations. In 78 pregnancies reported by Hack et al.,[39] the perinatal mortality rates for singletons and twins were 6.8% and 21.7%, respectively. All neonatal deaths in this population were among infants weighing < 2000 gm. In the report of Caspi and co-workers,[36] there were five neonatal deaths among 62 pregnancies. Four of the five deaths occurred among twins or triplets, with three of these deaths attributed to prematurity.

BIRTH DEFECTS

The congenital anomaly rate after hMG induction of ovulation has been reported to be no higher than expected for the general population.[18, 39, 40] A controlled prospective study[12] showed major and minor malformations to occur in 1.4% and 0.5% of pregnancies after hMG and in 1.1% and 0.6% of spontaneous pregnancies. These differences were not significant. Growth and development at 6 and 12 months of age are normal in infants born after hMG therapy.[39] Evaluation of physical, psychomotor, and mental development in adolescent girls who were born after hMG therapy does not show any deviation of this group from population norms, and puberty does not appear to be altered in these children.[42]

EVALUATION

Although hMG may be responsible for LPD in some patients, there is no evidence that this therapy increases spontaneous abortion or abnormalities in growth and development of the conceptus. The multiple gestation rate is increased to at least 10%, and the majority of adverse pregnancy outcomes are related to prematurity accompanying these multiple gestations.

BROMOCRIPTINE

Hyperprolactinemia may be the cause of childlessness in as many as one third of infertile women (reviewed by Molitch[43]). Elevated prolactin (PRL) decreases hypothalamic gonadotropin-releasing hormone, decreases the positive feedback of estrogens on gonadotropin release, and may inhibit P production by granulosa cells. PRL secretion is inhibited by dopamine. Bromocriptine, an ergot derivative, is a dopamine receptor agonist that acts directly on the pituitary, and possibly on the hypothalamus as well.

Many practitioners administer bromocriptine to hyperprolactinemic women until the diagnosis of pregnancy is made and then discontinue the drug to avoid any potential effects of the medication on the conceptus. Some, in fact, have advocated discontinuing bromocriptine as soon as ovulation is suggested to minimize any exposure of the conceptus to the drug.[44] There are, however, many cases in which bromocriptine has been used during much of the pregnancy (and occasionally until term), either for the treatment of macroadenomas, for the prevention and/or treatment of neurologic symptoms from adenomas of any size, or for acromegaly.[45-57] In addition, treatment of acromegaly generally involves doses much higher than those used for hyperprolactinemic women. These cases permit an evaluation of the pregnancy effects of bromocriptine therapy.

BIOCHEMICAL ALTERATIONS

Maternal serum PRL levels increase during normal pregnancy. There is also a rise in fetal and amniotic fluid PRL during gestation. When bromocriptine is given for ovulation induction and withheld after a diagnosis of pregnancy is made, maternal serum PRL increases as expected during pregnancy.[47, 52] Continuation of bromocriptine during pregnancy causes a suppression of maternal serum PRL to low levels.[46, 47, 50, 52, 58] PRL levels in cord and neonatal blood are also low, but amniotic fluid PRL levels are normal, suggesting that decidual PRL production is not inhibited.[46, 50]

Other maternal hormones have generally been found to be unaffected by bromocriptine. Canales et al.[52] studied eight patients who conceived on bromocriptine. Four discontinued the drug early in pregnancy and four continued it throughout pregnancy and the puerperium. There was no difference between the groups in maternal serum values of human placental lactogen, growth hormone, or estriol. Other workers[46, 50, 58] also found no deviation from normal values for serum E_2, estriol, P, human placental lactogen, testosterone, and alkaline phosphatase in pregnant women on bromocriptine. An exception was noted by Yuen,[53] who found E_2 to be lower and estriol to be higher than normal in pregnant women on bromocriptine.

SPONTANEOUS ABORTION AND MULTIPLE GESTATION

The miscarriage rate associated with bromocriptine treatment is not greater than that in the general population, although published reports have not included concurrently monitored control groups. Data collected by a manufacturer of the drug showed early pregnancy loss to occur in 14% of 1410 bromocriptine-related pregnancies.[48, 59] These 197 losses included 157 spontaneous abortions, 25 induced abortions, 12 ectopic gestations, and 3 molar pregnancies. Similar rates of spontaneous abortion, ectopic gestation, and molar pregnancy were found in a review of the literature encompassing 1858 pregnancies.[47]

The incidence of multiple gestation (almost all twins) associated with bromocriptine use is 1.2% to 1.8%.[47, 48, 59] Higher rates of multiple gestation may be associated with concurrent use of CC or hMG.[48]

OTHER COMPLICATIONS OF PREGNANCY

Although there have been reports of premature delivery associated with bromocriptine exposure during pregnancy,[57, 60] most patients deliver at term.[46, 49, 50, 52, 53, 56] The prematurity rate associated with bromocriptine therapy early in pregnancy is similar to that in the general population.[47, 59] Similarly, intrauterine growth retardation has been reported in bromocriptine-exposed pregnancies,[45] but the majority of publications document normal newborn weights and early childhood development after such pregnancies.[46, 49, 52, 54-56, 60]

Congenital malformations have been reported to occur in 0.9% to 3.5% of large series.[47, 48, 59] Although controlled studies are not available, these rates compare favorably with general population statistics.

NURSING

Suppression of PRL levels might be expected to interfere with lactation; however, there is a report of a woman who successfully nursed her infant while continuing bromocriptine therapy.[52] Nursing does not appear to be contraindicated by bromocriptine therapy.[43, 47]

EVALUATION

Bromocriptine therapy may successfully induce ovulation in hyperprolactinemic women. Published experience does not identify a risk of adverse pregnancy outcome attributable to the medication. Although it has been said that bromocriptine should be stopped as soon as possible after a diagnosis of pregnancy is made, a number of cases in which high-dose bromocriptine is continued through much of pregnancy have not identified a hazard of this medication for the fetus. Although these case reports are encouraging, it should be remembered that there are no controlled studies establishing the safety of this medication during pregnancy.

REFERENCES

1. Adashi EY: Clomiphene citrate: mechanism(s) and site(s) of action—a hypothesis revisited. Fertil Steril 42:331, 1984
2. Wu CH: A rational and practical approach to clomiphene therapy. Clin Obstet Gynecol 27:953, 1984
3. Cook CL, Schroeder JA, Yussman MA, Sanfilippo JS: Induction of luteal phase defect with clomiphene citrate. Am J Obstet Gynecol 149:613, 1984
4. Garcia J, Jones GS, Wentz AC: The use of clomiphene citrate. Fertil Steril 28:707, 1977
5. Hammerstein J: Mode of action of clomiphene. I. Inhibitory effect of clomiphene citrate on the formation of progesterone from acetate-1-^{14}C by human corpus luteum slices in vitro. Acta Endocrinol (Copenh) 60:635, 1969
6. Laufer N, Reich R, Braw R, Shenker JG, Tsafriri A: Effect of clomiphene citrate on preovulatory rat follicles in culture. Biol Reprod 27:463, 1982
7. Marut EL, Hodgen GD: Antiestrogenic action of high-dose clomiphene in primates: pituitary augmentation but with ovarian attenuation. Fertil Steril 38:100, 1982
8. Dlugi AM, Laufer N, Botero-Ruiz W, DeCherney AH, Polan ML, Haseltine FP, Mezer HC, Behrman HR: Altered follicular development in clomiphene citrate versus human menopausal gonadotropin-stimulated cycles for in vitro fertilization. Fertil Steril 43:40, 1985
9. diZerega GS, Campeau JD, Nakamura RN, Ujita EL, Lobo R, Marrs RP: Activity of human follicular protein(s) in spontaneous and induced ovarian cycles. J Clin Endocrinol Metab 57:838, 1983

10. Toshinobu T, Seiichiro F, Noriaki S, Kihyoe I: Correlation between dosage or duration of Clomid therapy and abortion rate. Int J Fertil 24:193, 1979
11. Adashi EY, Rock JA, Sapp KC, Martin EJ, Wentz AC, Jones GS: Gestational outcome of clomiphene-related conceptions. Fertil Steril 31:620, 1979
12. Kurachi K, Aono T, Minagawa J, Miyake A: Congenital malformations of newborn infants after clomiphene-induced ovulation. Fertil Steril 40:187, 1983
13. Laufer N, Pratt BM, DeCherney AH, Naftolin F, Merino M, Markert CL: The in vivo and in vitro effects of clomiphene citrate on ovulation, fertilization, and development of cultured mouse oocytes. Am J Obstet Gynecol 147:633, 1983
14. Boué JG, Boué A: Increased frequency of chromosomal anomalies in abortions after induced ovulation. Lancet 1:679, 1973
15. Boué J, Boué A, Lazar P: Retrospective and prospective epidemiological studies of 1500 karyotyped spontaneous human abortions. Teratology 12:11, 1975
16. Fabro S, Scialli AR: The perinatal environment. In Pediatric Pathophysiology, Edited by AR Colón, M Ziai. Boston, Little, Brown & Co., 1985, p 129
17. Macgregor AH, Johnson JE, Bunde CA: Further clinical experience with clomiphene citrate. Fertil Steril 19:616, 1968
18. Harlap S: Ovulation induction and congenital malformation. Lancet 2:961, 1976
19. Hack M, Brish M, Serr DM, Insler V, Salomy M, Lunenfeld B: Outcome of pregnancy after induced ovulation. Follow-up of pregnancies and children born after clomiphene therapy. JAMA 220:1329, 1972
20. Karow WG, Payne SA: Pregnancy after clomiphene citrate treatment. Fertil Steril 19:351, 1968
21. Falk RJ, Lackritz RM: Bilateral simultaneous tubal pregnancies after ovulation induction with clomiphene-menotropin combination. Fertil Steril 28:32, 1977
22. Koroly MV, Belsky DH: Heterotopic pregnancy as a result of induced ovulation. A report of two cases. J Reprod Med 27:476, 1982
23. Lee F, Nelson N, Faiman C, Choi N, Reyes FI: Low-dose corticoid therapy for anovulation: effect upon fetal weight. Obstet Gynecol 60:314, 1982
24. Dyson JL, Kohler HG: Anencephaly and ovulation stimulation (Letter). Lancet 1:1256, 1973
25. Sandler B: Anencephaly and ovulation stimulation (Letter). Lancet 2:379, 1973
26. Barrett C, Hakim C: Anencephaly, ovulation stimulation, subfertility, and illegitimacy. Lancet 2:916, 1973
27. Field B, Kerr C: Ovulation stimulation and defects of neural tube closure. Lancet 2:1511, 1974
28. Berman P: Congenital anomalies associated with maternal clomiphene ingestion. Lancet 2:878, 1975
29. Ahlgren M, Källén B, Rannevik G: Outcome of pregnancy after clomiphene therapy. Acta Obstet Gynecol Scand 55:371, 1976
30. March CM: The use of Pergonal for the induction of ovulation. Clin Obstet Gynecol 27:966, 1984
31. Fabro S, Brown NA, Scialli AR: Ultrasound in industry and medicine. Reprod Toxicol Med Lett 3:17, 1984
32. Olson JL, Rebar RW, Schreiber JR, Vaitukaitis JL: Shortened luteal phase after ovulation induction with human menopausal gonadotropin and human chorionic gonadotropin. Fertil Steril 39:284, 1983
33. Dlugi AM, Laufer N, DeCherney AH, MacLusky NJ, Haseltine FP, Polan ML, Mezer HC, Tarlatzis B, Naftolin F: The periovulatory and luteal phase of conception cycles following in vitro fertilization and embryo transfer. Fertil Steril 41:530, 1984
34. Ben-Rafael Z, Mashiach S, Oelsner G, Farine D, Lunenfeld B, Serr DM: Spontaneous pregnancy and its outcome after human menopausal gonadotropin/human chorionic gonadotropin-induced pregnancy. Fertil Steril 36:560, 1981
35. Ben-Rafael Z, Dor J, Mashiach S, Blankstein J, Lunenfeld B, Serr DM: Abortion rate in pregnancies following ovulation induced by human menopausal gonadotropin/human chorionic gonadotropin. Fertil Steril 39:157, 1983
36. Caspi E, Levin S, Bukovsky I, Weinraub Z: Induction of pregnancy with human gonadotropins after clomiphene failure in menstruating ovulatory infertility patients. Isr J Med Sci 10:249, 1974
37. Marshall JR, Wider JA: Results of human menopausal gonadotropins (HMG) therapy for anovulatory infertility using a nonvariable treatment schedule: comparison with previous reports. Fertil Steril 22:19, 1971
38. Schwartz M, Jewelewicz R, Dyrenfurth I, Tropper P, Vande Wiele RL: The use of human menopausal and chorionic gonadotropins for induction of ovulation. Sixteen years' experience at the Sloane Hospital for Women. Am J Obstet Gynecol 138:801, 1980
39. Hack M, Brish M, Serr D, Insler V, Lunenfeld B: Outcome of pregnancy after induced ovulation. Follow-up of pregnancies and children born after gonadotropin therapy. JAMA 211:791, 1970
40. Spadoni LR, Cox DW, Smith DC: The use of menopausal gonadotropin for the induction of ovulation. Am J Obstet Gynecol 120:988, 1974
41. Gemzell C, Guillome J, Wang CF: Ectopic pregnancy following treatment with human gonadotropins. Am J Obstet Gynecol 143:761, 1982
42. Ben-Rafael Z, Blankstein J, Sack J, Lunenfeld B, Oelsner G, Serr DM, Mashiach S: Menarche and puberty in daughters of amenorrheic women. JAMA 250:3202, 1983
43. Molitch ME: Pregnancy and the hyperprolactinemic woman. N Engl J Med 312:1364, 1985
44. Coelingh Bennink HJT: Intermittent bromocriptine treatment for the induction of ovulation in hyperprolactinemic patients. Fertil Steril 31:267, 1979
45. Cundy T, Grundy EN, Melville H, Sheldon J: Bromocriptine treatment of acromegaly following spontaneous conception. Fertil Steril 42:134, 1984
46. Bigazzi M, Ronga R, Lancranjan I, Ferraro S, Branconi F, Buzzoni P, Martorana G, Scarselli GF, del Pozo E: A pregnancy in an acromegalic woman during bromocriptine treatment: effects on growth hormone and prolactin in the maternal, fetal, and amniotic compartments. J Clin Endocrinol Metab 48:9, 1979
47. Ruiz-Velasco V, Tolis G: Pregnancy in hyperprolactinemic women. Fertil Steril 41:793, 1984
48. Turkalj I, Braun P, Krupp P: Surveillance of bromocriptine in pregnancy. JAMA 247:1589, 1982
49. Yuen BH, Cannon W, Sy L, Booth J, Burch P: Regression of pituitary microadenoma during and following bromo-

criptine therapy: persistent defect in prolactin regulation before and throughout pregnancy. Am J Obstet Gynecol 142:634, 1982

50. Miyakawa I, Taniyama K, Koike H, Mori N, Nagaminc M, Kurıbayashi T, Araki S: Successful pregnancy in an acromegalic patient during 2-Br-α-ergocryptine (CB-154) therapy. Acta Endocrinol (Copenh) 101:333, 1982
51. Maeda T, Ushiroyama T, Okuda K, Fujimoto A, Ueki M, Sugimoto O: Effective bromocriptine treatment of a pituitary macroadenoma during pregnancy. Obstet Gynecol 61:117, 1983
52. Canales ES, García IC, Ruíz JE, Zárate A: Bromocriptine as a prophylactic therapy in prolactinoma during pregnancy. Fertil Steril 36:524, 1981
53. Yuen BH: Bromocriptine, pituitary tumors, and pregnancy. Lancet 2:1314, 1978
54. Luboshitzky R, Dickstein G, Barzilai D: Bromocriptine-induced pregnancy in an acromegalic patient. JAMA 244:584, 1980
55. Modena G, Portioli I: Delivery after bromocriptine therapy. Lancet 2:558, 1977
56. Konopka P, Raymond JP, Merceron RE, Seneze J: Continuous administration of bromocriptine in the prevention of neurological complications in pregnant women with prolactinomas. Am J Obstet Gynecol 146:935, 1983
57. Espersen T, Ditzel J: Pregnancy and delivery under bromocriptine therapy. Lancet 2:985, 1977
58. Ylikorkala O, Kivinen S, Rönnberg L: Bromocriptine treatment during early human pregnancy: effects on the levels of prolactin, sex steroids and placental lactogen. Acta Endocrinol (Copenh) 95:412, 1980
59. Molitch ME, Reichlin S: Hyperprolactinemic disorders. DM 28:1, 1982
60. Randall S, Laing I, Chapman AJ, Shalet SM, Beardwell CG, Kelly WF, Davies D: Pregnancies in women with hyperprolactinaemia: obstetric and endocrinological management of 50 pregnancies in 37 women. Br J Obstet Gynaecol 89:20, 1982

Chapter 6

Analysis of clinical fertility trials: a methodologic review

David L. Olive, M.D.

Division of Reproductive Endocrinology, Department of Obstetrics and Gynecology, University of Arkansas for Medical Sciences, Little Rock, Arkansas

The process of clinical investigation is a unique hybrid that requires a firm foundation in clinical medicine, statistics, and scientific method. To shed some light on a designated question, a proper design must first be formulated. This design would be expected to produce data that should provide clues regarding the point in question. Data analysis must then be performed in a manner to yield the maximal amount of information. Finally, this analysis must be extrapolated in an attempt to achieve the initial purpose: helping to answer a general clinical query.

In recent years, the variety of study designs and analytic methods for clinical experimentation has increased sharply, producing a growing need on the part of the critical reader to stay abreast of such developments. It is no surprise, then, that an increasing number of clinicians disregard methods of design and analysis as being "too complex" for their understanding. Similarly, a growing number of clinical investigators have become satisfied with the safe haven of familiar designs and statistical methods, despite recent advances that render such methods grossly deficient or obsolete.

The specific method in clinical research is of importance beyond being a mere intellectual exercise. The value of an investigation may be rendered worthless, despite skillful design and thoughtful attention to detail during the course of a study, if the data analysis is flawed, incomplete or irrelevant.[1] Equally nonbeneficial is the elegant statistical evaluation of a data set produced by faulty protocol.[2] In both of these cases the results may serve to obfuscate, rather than uncover, the "truth."

Although much attention has been afforded these issues in such fields as epidemiology and internal medicine, the discipline of reproductive endocrinology and infertility is nearly devoid of such discussion. This is unfortunate, because the clinician must be capable of effectively evaluating the literature, realizing its assets and shortcomings, and applying these new facts to his or her clinical practice.[3] The purpose of this review is to survey those methods of design and analysis that are commonly used in the investigation of fertility enhancement and to illustrate clearly the biases and limitations inherent in each technique.

STUDY DESIGN

TYPES OF CLINICAL TRIALS

A wide variety of study designs can and has been used in the assessment of therapy for infertility. Before proceeding with a discussion of their merits, however, terms must be clearly established.

Research design may be divided into two categories: descriptive, such as delineation of prognostic factors or the clinical course of a disease; and analytic, in which an interventional cause-effect relationship is being investigated.[4, 5] The latter encompasses those studies evaluating therapeutic maneuvers to enhance fertility. Within the category of analytic research there are two basic structures: the experimental trial and the observational survey.[4, 5] A study design qualifies as experimental when attempts are made for unbiased allocation into study groups; thus the randomized, controlled clinical trial is an experiment. If the therapeutic maneuver in question was assigned without a plan for unbiased allocation, the research is an observational survey.

The observational survey can take a variety of forms. In the past, the terms "prospective" and "retrospective" were widely used to describe the subtypes, but these terms can be ambiguous.[6-8] An example is an investigation of women identified as having endometriosis from 1975 to 1980. If in 1985 the researcher contacts these women to determine their rate of conception, is this a prospective or a retrospective study? In fact, it is retrospective in real time, but the research pursuit direction is prospective in that the women were first selected based on pelvic disease, and their rate of conception was subsequently determined. Obviously, such simplistic terminology is inadequate to designate clearly a mode of design.

A preferable approach to classifying observational surveys would be to have distinct terms for both real time and research pursuit direction. Studies with data accumulated in past real time can be called "retrolective," whereas those performed in current real time can be termed "prolective."[6, 9] In addition, study designs using the antecedent-to-outcome direction are called "cohort," and those in the reverse direction (outcome-to-antecedent) are referred to as "trohoc."[6] In the investigation of infertility, trohoc studies are nearly always retrolective studies; this is henceforth assumed in this review.

The primary advantage of a study design that occurs in present real time (the randomized clinical trial and the prolective cohort study) is the ability to collect data in a complete and dependable fashion. In the retrolective approach, data are gleaned from medical records or patient recall; both can be significantly unreliable to the point of severely prejudicing the conclusions. In a properly planned trial with concurrent data collection, the presence or absence of a variable can be determined uniformly and without bias.[9]

In addition, a retrolective study is limited to those methods of evaluation recorded in the chart. In the prolective or experimental trial, means of evaluation are determined before initiation of the data collection. Thus questions regarding preexisting conditions, thoroughness of initial evaluation, and degree of observation are less likely to arise if the trial was thoroughly planned before the study began.[9]

Table 1. *Twelve Standards for Retrolective Trohoc (Case-Control) Studies*

1. Predetermined method of patient selection
2. Specification of what is meant by *exposure* to suspected therapeutic agent
3. Unbiased data collection
4. Anamnestic equivalence between cases and controls
5. Avoidance of constrained cases
6. Avoidance of constrained controls
7. Equal diagnostic examination for cases and controls
8. Equal prehospital surveillance for cases and controls
9. Equal demographic susceptibility for cases and controls
10. Equal clinical susceptibility for cases and controls
11. Avoidance of protopathic bias
12. Avoidance of Berkson's bias

Finally a word about the retrolective trohoc study (also known as case-control).[10] This design is popular in the investigation of disorders of low incidence, for which a cohort study or randomized clinical trial would be too costly and time-consuming.[11] It may also be useful as a scouting method to uncover previously unknown effects, which can then be explored further by other methods.[12] Twelve standards have been delineated for such protocols to ensure confidence in the results (Table 1).[13] Horwitz and Feinstein[13] reviewed 85 such studies in which conflicts had been noted with other published reports, and in no case did a study fulfill all 12 standards. Thus, although the trohoc study does have a role in clinical investigation, the protocol must be scrutinized carefully for violations of these criteria.

Table 2 is a summary of these types of study designs, with examples. A more thorough description of these methods and a detailed listing of other types of protocols uncommon in fertility studies can be found elsewhere.[4, 5, 9, 10, 14-21]

CONTROL GROUP

To determine the value of a therapeutic maneuver on fertility status, it must be clear what would have happened had the therapy not been administered. This concept, the determination of baseline values as a source of comparison, is termed "control."[6] A study design may be controlled in a variety of ways,[22] or it may remain uncontrolled; the decision if and how to control a trial can impact greatly on the value of a clinical investigation.

The observational survey may be either uncontrolled or controlled. If it is controlled, the comparison group may consist of data collected simultaneously to the group under study (concurrent nonrandomized controls) or a group of patients

Table 2. *Types of Analytic Study Designs*

Type	Real-time events occur	Research direction		Example
Experimental				
Randomized therapeutic trial	Current	Antecedent-to-outcome		Random samples selected; treatments randomly assigned
Observational				
Prolective	Current	Antecedent-to-outcome	(Cohort)	Endometriosis patients enrolled at diagnosis; pregnancy rate followed
Retrolective	Past	Antecedent-to-outcome	(Cohort)	Chart review comparing stage of endometriosis to pregnancy rate
		Outcome-to-antecedent	(Trohoc)	Women with spontaneous abortions reviewed to detect history of luteal phase defect

previously accumulated (historical controls). Observational surveys, by their very nature, cannot have a randomized control group.

UNCONTROLLED TRIALS

In the uncontrolled survey, a new treatment is studied without any direct comparison to a different treatment group. This may be appropriate if the disorder in question produces an absolute effect, such as sterility resulting from bilateral salpingectomy. It would be pointless to include a control group of untreated patients—all successful pregnancies after a therapy (such as in vitro fertilization) clearly can be attributed to the treatment protocol. The situation is not nearly so clear, however, when the disorder to be treated merely produces a relative decrease in fertility.[23] In this case, pregnancies occurring after therapy must be shown to occur more commonly than the background pregnancy rate.[8] If no control group is used, the tendency is to attribute all pregnancies to successful therapeutic intervention. Thus, in the case of *relative* fertility reduction, the uncontrolled survey, as opposed to a properly controlled survey, is much more likely to lead to an enthusiastic recommendation of the treatment.[24] For example, a review of 52 published uncontrolled therapeutic trials in psychiatry found 85% reporting a therapeutic success, whereas in 20 trials with a control group only 25% reported therapeutic success.[25] Similarly, Grace et al.[26] reviewed 53 studies of portacaval shunt operation for portal hypertension; 32 were uncontrolled and 75% of these gave a markedly enthusiastic conclusion, while none of the six well-controlled trials led to such a level of support.

Thus the indications for an uncontrolled therapeutic trial are narrow indeed. This is supported by data from the *New England Journal of Medicine* showing a sharp decline in the proportion of published uncontrolled therapeutic trials from 1953 to 1978.[27]

HISTORICAL CONTROLS

Although many researchers recognize the need for a control group in their observational surveys, they are often reluctant to withhold treatment or administer standard therapy to a concurrent patient population, preferring instead to apply the experimental therapy to all new subjects. The most common approach in this situation is to compare the study patients with previously analyzed or published patients receiving the alternative therapy. This device is termed "the historical control." The major difficulty with historical controls is in ensuring that the comparison is fair. If the treatment and control groups differ with respect to variables other than the treatment itself, it cannot be guaranteed that any apparent improvement in fertility rate is actually due to the new treatment.

Historical control groups for prolective studies face many potential problems. Concern must be expressed for each of the following possibilities delineated by Pocock[28]:

(1) A retrolective historical control group is less likely to have clearly defined criteria for patient inclusion, since they were not known to be in a study when their treatment began.
(2) Historical controls may differ from the experimental group in the type of patient available for selection.

(3) The researcher may be more restrictive in the selection of patients for a new treatment.
(4) The quality of recorded data for retrolectively surveyed historical controls is inferior, due to its retrolective nature.
(5) The criteria for response may differ between the two groups. In looking at pregnancy rates, serum pregnancy testing may be used in the current experimental group, while less sensitive urine testing may have been employed for the controls.
(6) Patient observation may change between groups. Subjects known to be involved in a study are generally observed more closely than those reviewed retrolectively. For example, in the therapeutic fertility trial, patients in the experimental group may be suspected of and tested for pregnancy earlier than the control population.
(7) There is a tendency to invalidate more patients on a new treatment than among historical controls. If an experimental patient fares badly, a more persistent inquiry often will reveal a protocol violation; such thorough evaluation is difficult in a retrolectively accumulated control.

When retrolective surveys are compared with historical controls, the initial shortcomings of the retrolective approach are merely compounded.[18] Therefore not only must concern be expressed regarding the reliability with which data were recorded for each group, but the possibility of inconsistent record keeping *between* the two groups must be entertained. Questions arise, too, regarding similarity in initial evaluation, degree of follow-up evaluation, and criteria for inclusion in the study. Differences between the experimental subjects and the historical controls in any of these categories merely serve to magnify the lack of reliability inherent in a retrolective trial.

The end result of these problems in design is that studies with historical controls tend to exaggerate the value of an experimental treatment. Examples of this principle are well illustrated by Grage and Zelen,[29] Ingelfinger,[30] and Grace and colleagues.[26] In addition, Chalmers and Schroeder[27] demonstrated an impressive decline in the use of this technique in the internal medicine literature. Many authors have suggested statistical adjustments for the use of historical controls.[31-34] However, no amount of statistical manipulation can remedy an obvious flaw in study design, and the use of the historical control must be viewed in any instance with extreme trepidation.[28]

CONCURRENT NONRANDOMIZED CONTROLS

Investigators wishing to avoid randomization but who desire a concurrent control group have often used other methods of selection. In general, the control subjects are selected based on the judgment of the investigator or systematic assignment.[28] Both methods are fraught with difficulty.

If the clinician is allowed to exercise judgment in assigning one of several treatment options, it is obvious that considerable bias can be introduced.[35, 36] For instance, in a study evaluating the use of hysteroscopic metroplasty, compared with an abdominal approach, a clinician may decide to use the hysteroscope on those patients thought to be less complex surgically. Such manipulation by the investigator makes any conclusions tenuous at best.

A common method of "pseudorandomization" is the systematic assignment of patients to a control or experimental group based on date of birth or date of presentation or even by alternate assignment. Unfortunately, the investigator has prior knowledge of the criteria; this knowledge may affect the decision regarding entry. Numerous reports from the literature confirm this, demonstrating marked imbalances in study groups when such methods were used.[37-39] These disproportions in size bring into question the comparability of the treatment and control groups and, hence, the validity of the results.

RANDOMIZED CONTROLS

The experimental clinical trial differs from prolective surveys by the random allocation of patients into either the experimental or control group. This removes several sources of bias. The possibility of selective choices of treatment based on clinical judgment is eliminated. Also, any important prognostic factors affecting outcome should be expected to distribute randomly between the two groups.[40] Thus the randomized trial is the hallmark of the scientific clinical experiment.

Although this study design is preferable to all of those previously discussed, there are specific caveats with this type of approach. Random allocation does not necessarily mean equal allocation, and with random assignment of patients to control or treatment groups, a disproportionate prognostic factor may be found in one of the two.[41] This chance occurrence is analogous to "the luck of the draw" in a poker game: although the chances of being dealt four aces is unlikely, it certainly can be done! A thorough discussion of this concept is beyond the scope of this article, but other authors have presented methods that guard against these adverse effects of chance.[41]

A second potential flaw in the randomized clinical trial is variation in observation after treatment intervention. For instance, in a study analyzing the ovulation rate in oligoovulatory women with two dosage schedules of clomiphene citrate, the value of randomization is negated if the experimental group is followed with basal body temperatures, luteal phase progesterone levels, endometrial biopsy, and ultrasound, while the controls are evaluated by temperature alone. Care must always be taken to provide equivalent follow-up study of each subject.

A third danger in randomized trials is the use of the wrong control.[40] This does not invalidate the results, but it alters the conclusions drawn from the study. An example would be a randomized trial evaluating conservative surgery versus danazol in the enhancement of fertility in women with mild endometriosis. To demonstrate danazol to be more effective than surgery in promoting fertility would be interesting, but it would not demonstrate efficacy, because neither therapy has been proven effective when compared with expectant management. The principle is a simple one: although it is valid to use a control group receiving standard therapy (rather than no therapy), to state that a therapeutic modality is of value requires the prior demonstration that the standard therapy was in fact efficacious.

Although randomized clinical trials remain the gold standard for clinical research, they often cannot be easily accomplished because of a low rate of consent by potential subjects. Furthermore, the value of extrapolating the results of a randomized trial to the general patient population is doubtful when only a small proportion of those asked to participate are willing to consent.[42] For these situations, Zelen[43, 44] proposed alternative experimental study designs that may be deemed more acceptable by the investigator and may prove more desirable in specific situations. In addition, Begg[45] proposed a quantitative method to estimate the potential magnitude by which the reported efficacy of a treatment might be inflated. This quantity, to be applied when only nonrandomized studies have been performed, is called the "publication bias." The value of these alternatives is yet to be determined.

Many investigators have concerns regarding the ethics of the randomized clinical trials.[46] These doubts have been responded to by various authors who point out that, in essence, it is unethical to use a therapeutic approach that has not been clearly demonstrated to be of value and may, in fact, be harmful.[47, 48] It should not be forgotten that there was considerable controversy regarding the need for the University of Chicago randomized trial on diethylstilbestrol and spontaneous abortion,[49] because diethylstilbestrol had been well demonstrated to be efficacious in case reports and observational surveys![50] Space limitations prevent a detailed discussion of this issue, but the reader is referred to several excellent essays on the subject.[47, 51]

STUDY DESIGN IN THERAPEUTIC FERTILITY TRIALS

The fertility investigator is faced with difficult choices in the selection of a research protocol. Although there is an overabundance of therapeutic questions in need of data, the clinician is faced with few patients with "pure" disorders. Furthermore, he or she may feel compelled to try some empiric therapy, for this is, in fact, why the patient was referred. However, simply to report uncontrolled data for most fertility disorders can be grossly misleading, because the couples are, for the most part, subfertile rather than sterile.[52-57] Leridon and Spira[23] pointed out that in a group of subfertile couples unable to conceive for 3 years, the proportion spontaneously achieving pregnancy in the fourth year will be as high as 41% to 48%. Nevertheless, fertility investigators have apparently failed to appreciate this fact fully.

I performed a survey of therapeutic fertility trials published in *Fertility and Sterility* from 1953, 1963, 1973, and 1983. The results can be seen in Table 3. No controlled trials were seen in 1953, but a decade later, historical controls were used in two of seven studies. There was one nonrandomized, concurrently controlled prolective study in 1973. In 1983, there were 27 such trials, more than the other 3 years combined. However, only three could be construed as having an experimental design, and 40% were totally uncontrolled. These data contrast sharply with the much more prevalent use of appropriately controlled trials in internal medicine.[4]

Table 3. *Review of Study Designs in Therapeutic Fertility Trials Published in* Fertility and Sterility, *1953 to 1983*

	Study type	Randomized	Controls		
			Nonrandomized concurrent	Historical	None
1953	Experimental	0	—	—	—
	Prolective	—	0	0	2
	Retrolective cohort	—	0	—	4
	Retrolective trohoc	—	0	0	0
1963	Experimental	0	—	—	—
	Prolective	—	0	2	0
	Retrolective cohort	—	0	0	4
	Retrolective trohoc	—	0	0	1
1973	Experimental	0	—	—	—
	Prolective	—	1	0	0
	Retrolective cohort	—	0	0	3
	Retrolective trohoc	—	0	0	0
1983	Experimental	3[a]	—	—	—
	Prolective	—	2	1[b]	3
	Retrolective cohort	—	3	7[b]	8
	Retrolective trohoc	—	0	0	0

[a]Includes one cross-over trial.
[b]Two studies with historically analyzed controls from the author's patient population, the remainder with controls from the published literature.

Thus, although there has been a gradual evolution in study design over the past three decades in therapeutic fertility trials, the acceptance of the need for more rigorously planned and executed investigations has been slow. It is hoped that appropriate construction of a study protocol, the province of the clinician rather than the statistician, will become a greater priority in future investigations. Until then, the reader must be urged to temper therapeutic claims with the utmost caution.

DATA ANALYSIS

Regarding the clinical response (conception) to treatment, there are a variety of ways to evaluate and report success rates. Each has its place in the fertility literature, but each also has limitations inherent to the method. As with study design, a thorough knowledge of the methods of measuring the effectiveness of therapy is critical to evaluating the therapeutic fertility trial.

PREGNANCY RATES

The most common calculation in fertility trials is the simple (or crude) pregnancy rate. This value is defined merely as the number of pregnancies divided by the number of patients treated. Of all methods of analysis, it is the easiest to perform. However, there are a number of major drawbacks.

First, this approach does not adjust for sample bias; that is, confounding variables that may affect fertility. If the purpose of a study is to glean the value of tetracycline in enhancing conception rates among women with cervicitis, a drastically different picture might evolve if women with other infertility factors were eliminated from the calculation.

Second, it is dependent on length of follow-up study. The data pictured in Figure 1 illustrate this point. In this example, ten women were fol-

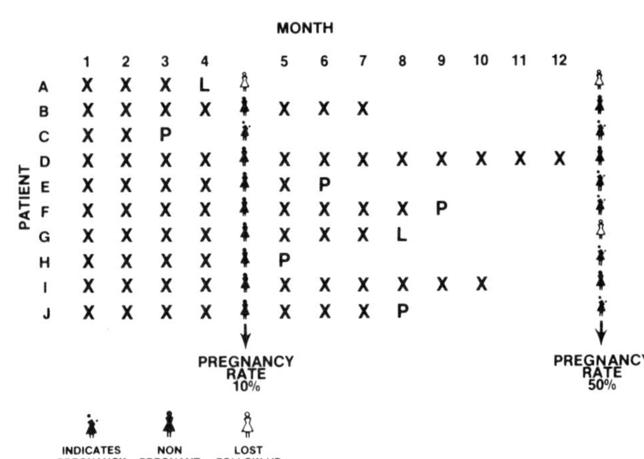

Figure 1
Variation in pregnancy rate as a function of length of follow-up study. A trial of these ten women ended at 4 months' follow-up would have yielded a pregnancy rate of 10%; the same ten women followed up for 12 months provide a 50% pregnancy rate. X, cycle without conception; P, cycle with conception; L, lost to follow-up.

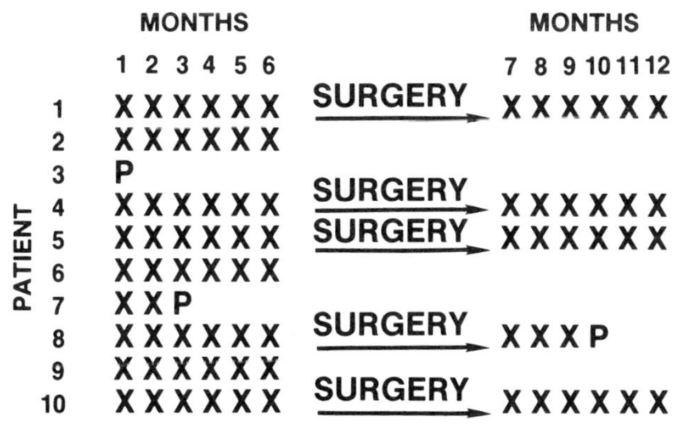

Figure 2
Overestimation of pregnancy rate because of removal of treatment failures. A trial of expectant management in ten women is illustrated, with two achieving pregnancy. Five of the eight women without conceptions then undergo surgery, with one pregnancy resulting. An erroneous conclusion would be that expectant management results in a pregnancy rate of 40% (2 of 5). X, cycle without conception; P, cycle with conception.

lowed after therapy for as long as 12 months. Over the course of follow-up study, five achieved pregnancy, two were lost to follow-up, two were begun in the study less than 12 months before completion, and one was followed 1 full year without conception. The simple pregnancy rate was thus 50%. However, if the study had been halted after 4 months of follow-up, the pregnancy rate would have been only 10%. Furthermore, suppose a diligent medical student finds the two women who had been lost to follow-up and discovers that both achieved pregnancy within 1 year of treatment. Also suppose that the two women begun less than 1 year from the study completion date were followed a full 12 months anyway, and one conceived. By increasing the follow-up, we have now increased the pregnancy rate to 80%. Thus the duration of follow-up and number of censored participants (the women not completing the full follow-up period) can both radically effect simple pregnancy rates.

Some authors have argued that the simple pregnancy rate will provide at least a *minimum* rate of success with a therapeutic agent.[58] However, even this claim may not be true. Suppose, as in Figure 2, that ten women undergo expectant management for mild endometriosis. Two women achieve pregnancy within the first 6 months, but the others fail to conceive during the interval. Five of those who did not become pregnant then elect to undergo conservative resection (three refuse), with one pregnancy resulting. In retrolective analysis of the data, it might be erroneously concluded that two of five (40%) expectantly managed women conceived and one of five surgical patients become pregnant. The fact that only two of the *ten* who had *initially* attempted expectant management actually conceived is easily overlooked, victimized by faulty analytic methods. Thus the true value of a therapy may be underestimated because of a too-brief study interval, or it may be overestimated by removing treatment failures and intervening with a second therapeutic method, selecting out the women with poor outcomes.

In the clinical trial in which all patients enroll for the entire investigative period and none are lost to follow-up, the simple pregnancy rate may provide a rapid means of comparing study groups. However, for analyzing data with censored patients or comparing groups with variable durations of follow-up, the simple pregnancy rate is a poor standard.

Corrected pregnancy rates are calculated similarly, except that couples with additional infertility factors are excluded from the statistics. Thus a more homogeneous patient population is obtained. However, the same problems with variable follow-up seen with crude pregnancy rates make this analytic approach of little value to the clinical investigator. Furthermore, there is an additional difficulty: a lack of standardization among researchers as to what defines a confounding factor in the infertile couple. For instance, many authors suggest that husbands with sperm counts $< 20 \times 10^6$/ml should be excluded on the basis of the male factor, yet others define this threshold as 60×10^6/ml. Another example is the diagnosis of luteal phase defect, with criteria including short luteal phase on basal body temperature, serum progesterone level < 10 ng/ml, progesterone < 15 ng/ml, endometrial biopsy delayed by 2 days or more, and endometrial biopsy delayed by more than 2 days on two consecutive biopsies. Clearly, the phrase "corrected for additional infertility factors" can have different meanings with different researchers, making comparisons between reports with this method virtually impossible.

LIFE-TABLE ANALYSIS

Although pregnancy rates are clearly inadequate in describing the outcome of trials with

Table 4. *Data Set for Couples Attempting Pregnancy with Diagnosis of Unexplained Infertility*

Patient	Months of follow-up	Outcome
A	2	Pregnant
B	4	No pregnancy, study ended
C	7	Lost to follow-up
D	1	Pregnant
E	3	No pregnancy, study ended
F	2	Pregnant
G	6	Pregnant
H	6	Lost to follow-up
I	4	No pregnancy, study ended
J	12	Pregnant
K	8	No pregnancy, study ended
L	1	Pregnant
M	11	Lost to follow-up
N	10	Pregnant
O	12	No pregnancy, study ended
P	5	Lost to follow-up
Q	4	Lost to follow-up
R	2	Lost to follow-up
S	6	Pregnant
T	8	Pregnant

variable follow-up, a method of graphic display called the life table compensates well for this.[59-62] Life-table analysis has become a fixture in the evaluation of survival data,[63] yet application to fertility trials has been sorely limited.[8]

The purpose of a life table in therapeutic fertility trials is to estimate the percentage of study subjects who will conceive at any given period of follow-up. Table 4 provides a data set for couples attempting pregnancy after a diagnosis of unexplained infertility, with nine women conceiving, five failing to conceive before termination of the study, and six lost to follow-up study during the course of the investigation. The data can be rearranged by months of follow-up into the form seen in Table 5. For each month of follow-up, a certain number of women achieved pregnancy and others are censored (lost to follow-up or electively terminated because the protocol is ended). These pregnant or censored patients thus do not enter the next month of follow-up, for they have already achieved a terminal event in the evaluation. In the next month, only the women who have not conceived but are still followed are "at risk" for becoming pregnant, and calculations for each monthly interval are based only on the at-risk patient pool.

For the above example, 20 patients entered the first month of follow-up, with 2 becoming pregnant. The cumulative pregnancy rate at 1 month is, therefore, 2 of 20 = 10%. In the second month, 2 of the remaining 18 women conceived, for a pregnancy rate of 2 of 18 = 11.1%. However, in this second month only 90% of the women originally enrolled in the study were still at risk to conceive (18 of 20). Thus the contribution to the cumulative pregnancy rate is the proportion at risk multiplied by the proportion conceiving, or 0.90 × 0.111 = 0.10. The cumulative pregnancy rate at 2 months is then the rate at 1 month plus this new contribution at 2 months: 10% + 10% = 20%. This same series of calculations can be repeated at 3 months. Here, only 15 women began the month at risk (4 pregnancies and 1 censored patient had previously been recorded). However, no pregnancies occurred at 3 months, and the cumulative pregnancy rate remained at 20%. The same holds true for the fourth and fifth months.

At the onset of month 6, only ten women remain in the study. We have already seen a 20% cumulative pregnancy rate calculated through 5 months; thus the remaining ten women serve to represent the additional 80% of the population who would have entered the sixth month attempting to conceive. Two became pregnant, for a pregnancy rate of 20%. The addition of the cumulative pregnancy rate will now be the pregnancy rate for month 6 (0.20) multiplied by the cumulative nonpregnancy rate through 5 months (0.80), for a value of 0.16. The 6-month cumulative pregnancy rate is then 0.20 + 0.16 = 0.36. This same series of calculations can be carried out for months 7 through 12 (Table 6). By then plotting the cumulative pregnancy rate across the entire duration of the study, a graphic representation can be created for pregnancies as a function of time after diagnosis (Fig. 3). With large patient numbers, the life table often takes on the appearance of a relatively smooth curve.[64] As the number of pa-

Table 5. *Data Set for Couples with Unexplained Infertility by Length of Follow-up*

Months of follow-up	No. of patients	No. of patients pregnant	No. of patients censored
1	20	2	0
2	18	2	1
3	15	0	1
4	14	0	3
5	11	0	1
6	10	2	1
7	7	0	1
8	6	1	1
9	4	0	0
10	4	1	0
11	3	0	1
12	2	1	1
> 12	0	—	—

Table 6. *Life-Table Calculations for Couples with Unexplained Infertility*

Month	Proportion not pregnant	Pregnancies/couples followed	Addition to cumulative pregnancy rate	Cumulative pregnancy rate
1	1.00	2/20	0.1 × 1.0 = 0.10	0.10
2	0.90	2/18	0.11 × 0.9 = 0.10	0.20
3	0.80	0/15	0	0.20
4	0.80	0/14	0	0.20
5	0.80	0/11	0	0.20
6	0.80	2/10	0.2 × 0.8 = 0.16	0.36
7	0.64	0/7	0	0.36
8	0.64	1/6	0.17 × 0.64 = 0.11	0.47
9	0.53	0/4	0	0.47
10	0.53	1/4	0.25 × 0.53 = 0.13	0.60
11	0.40	0/3	0	0.60
12	0.40	1/2	0.5 × 0.40 = 0.20	0.80

tients decrease with increasing length of follow-up, the variance for each data point increases (Fig. 4).

Although the life table represents a tremendous improvement over the simple calculation of pregnancy rates, there is one potentially misleading facet of the technique. Note that in the above example, when patients were censored, those that remained for follow-up (nonpregnant) were presumed to represent all patients who had failed to conceive. That is, women who are lost to follow-up are assumed to be identical to those who continue to be followed up. Unfortunately, this premise is often untrue. Take, for example, the following hypothetic study. A physician has decided to evaluate the effects of laser fimbrioplasty on fertility rates and enrolls 50 women for the study. All patients are followed for 12 months, with 20 pregnancies occurring, for a cumulative rate of 40%. At this point, follow-up becomes more sporadic, but over the next 12 months the physician sees or hears from 10 of the women, 8 of whom are pregnant. According to the method previously illustrated, the 2-year cumulative pregnancy rate would be 0.40 + (0.8 × 0.60) = 0.88. But did the 10 women the investigator "heard from" in the second year represent the 30 women who were not pregnant at the onset of year 2? Of course not; these women were much more likely to notify the physician in the event of pregnancy and much more likely not to if the surgery had failed. The principle is clear: when using life-table analysis, there must be reasonable assurance that censored patients do not differ substantially from noncensored patients.

Finally, the life table is merely a visual device for estimating cumulative pregnancy rates. To use the life table for comparative purposes, it is generally necessary to create a mathematic model that describes the curve and provides parameters for comparison.

METHODS OF COMPARING LIFE TABLES

The visual comparison of two life tables is subjective. Therefore, it is necessary to provide a more objective mechanism for describing the curve and testing the significance of any difference between two life tables. Historically, investigators have tended to compare percentages of women conceiving after some fixed time period (i.e., 12 months). This approach is unsatisfactory for several reasons: (1) the choice of time period is often arbitrary; (2) it may be tempting to exaggerate the treatment difference by selecting post hoc the time point with the largest difference between pregnancy curves; and (3) full use is not being made of the precise data for each patient.

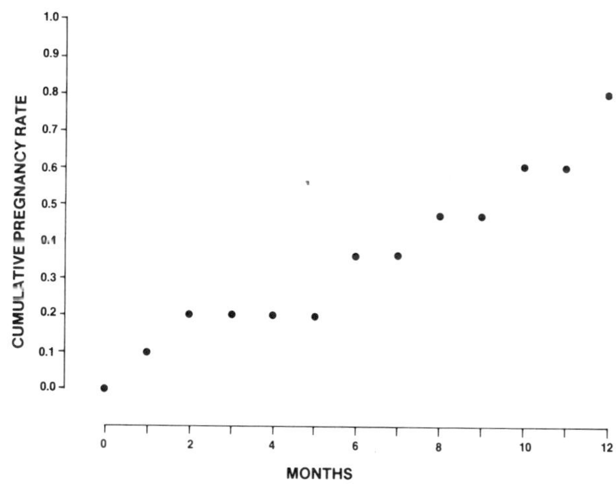

Figure 3
Graphic representation of a life table based on the conception rate of 20 infertile couples.

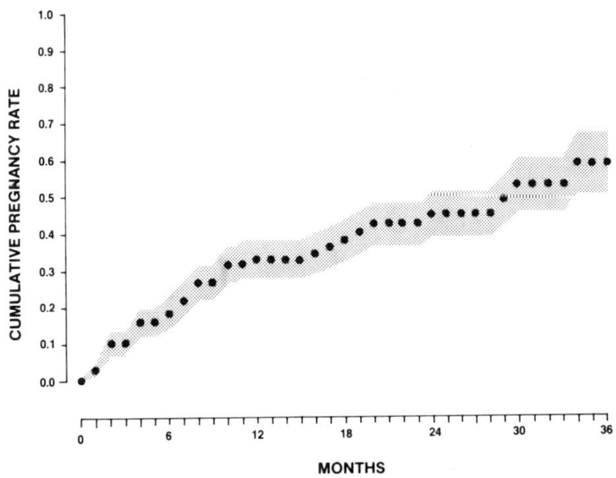

Figure 4
Graphic representation of a life table based on the conception rate of 88 women undergoing conservative surgery for endometriosis-associated infertility. The *shaded area* indicates the variance at each time point.

A more valid comparison of two curves can be achieved by fitting a mathematic model to the observed data and then statistically testing the model's parameters in an appropriate fashion. Cramer et al.,[65] described a single-parameter exponential model with a calculation of what we may term the "monthly fecundity rate" (MFR). This calculation is made by dividing the number of pregnancies by the number of cycles of follow-up after treatment. All patients, even those eventually lost to follow-up, are included for the total number of cycles during which they were followed (Fig. 5). This approach represents a powerful tool for describing a cumulative pregnancy curve, because it is simple to calculate the MFR, the confidence limits, and the statistics for comparison. However, there are major drawbacks to the routine use of this device. First, because the model is based on a single-parameter exponential function, the MFR is assumed to remain fairly constant throughout the posttreatment interval (Fig. 6). This, unfortunately, may not be valid; a therapeutic modality may have a brief, limited effect on fertility enhancement after intervention.[64] Conversely, a treatment protocol may initially demonstrate no effect, only later to produce delayed efficacy. In either case, the single-parameter exponential model is inappropriate for describing and evaluating the data.

A second shortcoming is the implicit assumption of 100% pregnancy given an infinite amount of follow-up. Although this condition may be approximated for many different infertile subtypes (such as parous women undergoing artificial insemination),[66, 67] the model fails to hold for others. As an example, Guzick and Rock[68] clearly demonstrated the MFR to severely underestimate initial cumulative pregnancy rates but to overestimate at time points greater than 4 years in women with surgically treated endometriosis. Thus the MFR must be applied with caution as an analytic method in life-table analysis, with care taken to demonstrate that the above assumptions have been met.

Recently, a two-parameter exponential model was developed to describe the fertility trial life table.[68] The underlying assumption of this model is that the observed cumulative pregnancy curve is really a weighted average of two curves, one for cured patients and the other for uncured patients. In the latter instance, the curve is a horizontal line at 0%. As time advances and women from the cured group achieve pregnancy, the uncured group represents a larger and larger proportion of those remaining in the study; thus, the cumulative pregnancy curve appears to plateau well before 100% conception is achieved (Fig. 7). Two clinically meaningful parameters describe this model: the "cure rate," which represents the percentage of women who conceive (found in the cured group) given an infinite length of follow-up;

STUDY A

PATIENT	MONTHS 1	2	3	4	5	6
A	X	X	X	P		
B	X	X	X	X	X	X
C	X	P				
D	X	X	X	X	X	X
E	X	X	X	X	X	X
F	P					

STUDY B

PATIENT	MONTHS 1	2	3	4	5	6	7	8	9	10	11	12
A	X	X	X	X	X	X	X	X	X	X	X	X
B	X	X	X	P								
C	X	X	X	X	X	X	X	X	X	P		
D	X	X	X	X	X	X	X	X	X	X	X	X
E	X	X	X	X	X	X	X	X	X	X	X	X
F	X	X	X	X	X	X	P					

Figure 5
MFR and simple pregnancy rates for two studies. Both studies have a simple pregnancy rate of 50%. However, study A has an MRF of 12% and study B has an MFR of only 5.3%. X, cycle without conception; P, cycle with conception.

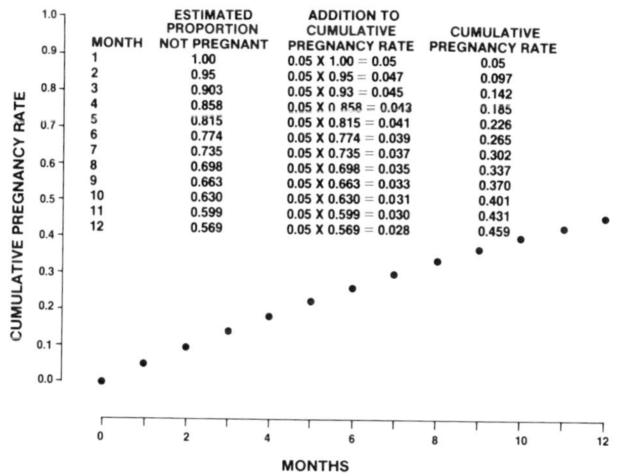

MONTH	ESTIMATED PROPORTION NOT PREGNANT	ADDITION TO CUMULATIVE PREGNANCY RATE	CUMULATIVE PREGNANCY RATE
1	1.00	0.05 X 1.00 = 0.05	0.05
2	0.95	0.05 X 0.95 = 0.047	0.097
3	0.903	0.05 X 0.93 = 0.045	0.142
4	0.858	0.05 X 0.858 = 0.043	0.185
5	0.815	0.05 X 0.815 = 0.041	0.226
6	0.774	0.05 X 0.774 = 0.039	0.265
7	0.735	0.05 X 0.735 = 0.037	0.302
8	0.698	0.05 X 0.698 = 0.035	0.337
9	0.663	0.05 X 0.663 = 0.033	0.370
10	0.630	0.05 X 0.630 = 0.031	0.401
11	0.599	0.05 X 0.599 = 0.030	0.431
12	0.569	0.05 X 0.569 = 0.028	0.459

Figure 6
Cumulative pregnancy graphic representation based on the single-parameter exponential model. The above estimation has an MFR of 5%. Note that although the MFR remains constant, the addition to the cumulative pregnancy rate decreases steadily each month.

and the monthly probability of pregnancy (MPP) for those who do achieve conception. This model has been shown to fit well the life table generated by treated infertile endometriosis patients.[68]

An early version of the two-parameter model used the Marquardt method for nonlinear regression to determine, given the data points, the value of the cure rate and the MPP.[68] Unfortunately, this method of calculation gives equal weight to all data points, despite the fact that the cumulative pregnancy rate at 3 months may be based on 200 women and the rate at 30 months may be based on only 20. To remedy this, a method was developed with an iterative computer program that appropriately weights all data points in assigning parameter values.[69] This technique is easily the most sophisticated attempt at modeling the success rates of a therapeutic fertility trial thus far developed. Furthermore, a likelihood ratio method has been described that allows easy comparison of two cumulative pregnancy curves modeled by these parameters.[69]

There are, however, several difficulties. The assumption of an exponential change in pregnancy rate over time is inherent, and should the data not fit this model with precision, the parameters used to describe the population of patients is meaningless. Also, this method of analysis requires large numbers (at least 30 to 40 per category) to provide interpretable results. Thus its applicability may be limited, despite the obvious power of the technique.

Other sophisticated methods of describing and comparing life tables have been developed. The Cox proportional hazards model[70] is an analog of the multiple linear regression model; it takes into account the overall structure of the pregnancy curve.[71] Its primary advantage is its independence from the traditional exponential model for life tables; i.e., data that do not conform to the prerequisite of a constant rate of pregnancy after therapeutic intervention can be analyzed in this way. The major disadvantage is the greater sensitivity of this model to rate of pregnancy rather than cure rate. Thus the Cox model would be

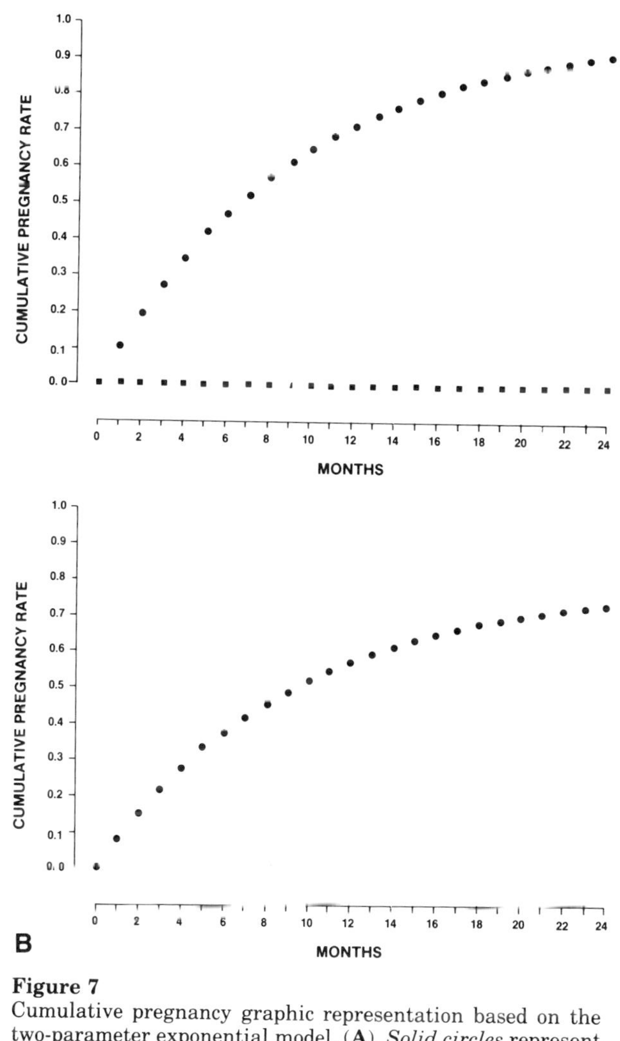

Figure 7
Cumulative pregnancy graphic representation based on the two-parameter exponential model. (**A**), *Solid circles* represent the cumulative pregnancy curve for the "cured" couples, who comprise 80% of the total sample. *Solid squares* represent the cumulative pregnancy rate for the "uncured" couples, who comprise 20% of the sample. (**B**), A weighted average, combining the two curves in panel **A**. Note the apparent plateau at a cumulative rate of 0.8.

optimal in those trials in which *rate* of success, rather than the ultimate proportion of pregnancy, is the primary question.[72]

Several methods independent of modeling and based entirely on evaluating differences in life tables have been described. These include the log-rank test[63, 73] and the Breslow formulation[74] of the Kruskal-Wallis test.[75] These methods are valuable for comparing two data sets within the same trial.[76] However, they are not based on a modeling process and thus do not present a clear picture of what the life table is attempting to illustrate. These methods function well within a given study design but have virtually no value in comparing a series of uncontrolled or poorly controlled trials to develop an overall clinical concept from the literature.

ANALYSIS OF SEQUENTIAL TREATMENT PROTOCOLS

The evaluation of comparative pregnancy data in clinical studies is subject to a variety of biases. One such bias commonly encountered when treated patients are retrospectively compared with untreated controls results from the fact that the institution of therapy may be delayed for several months after diagnosis. A treated patient must have remained infertile from diagnosis to the onset of treatment; the untreated control has no such requirement. Thus poor pregnancy rates for a particular treatment entity may reflect an unfavorable selection bias because of the "weeding out" of the most fertile women during the diagnosis-to-treatment interval. A similar bias is encountered in analyzing patients who transfer from one treatment group to another or even back and forth between two or more treatment groups.

The Mantel-Byar analysis method,[77] an approach for constructing and comparing modified life tables that reflect sequential changes of treatment status, is applicable to just these types of situations. The method eliminates the time-to-treatment bias and can compensate for patient transfer from one comparison group to another (or even back and forth between groups). The analysis is nearly assumption free, and stratification of patients to increase homogeneity can be accommodated. The Mantel-Byar approach has been applied recently to a trial involving conservative surgery and expectant management, and the results are encouraging.[78] A thorough description of the analysis is beyond the scope of this article, but it is believed that the Mantel-Byar method may offer increased power in analyzing clinical fertility trials.

ANALYTIC TECHNIQUES IN CLINICAL FERTILITY TRIALS

Before the 1970s, fertility researchers were clearly limited in their methods available for describing and testing clinical data. This changed, however, with the advent of life-table analysis and the myriad of potential statistical approaches applicable. It is correct that an analysis is only as good as its study design, but it is similarly true that a good design can be damaged severely by inadequate or misleading analysis.[79]

Virtually all reports in *Fertility and Sterility* before 1980 made use of simple or corrected pregnancy rates, as might be anticipated. With an abundance of evidence demonstrating the clear superiority of the life-table approach, it would be expected that this mode of analysis would become a fixture of the modern clinical fertility trial. This has not been the case, however. The results of a review of therapeutic investigations from five recent volumes of *Fertility and Sterility* (excluding the predominantly descriptive in vitro fertilization trials) are shown in Table 7. Of 50 such studies, only 15 made use of life-table analysis. Of these, five failed to analyze statistically the life tables further; they were used purely for descriptive purposes. Of the remaining trials, seven used a one-parameter model, three used a two-param-

Table 7. *Analytic Methods of Therapeutic Fertility Trials in* Fertility and Sterility, *Volumes 37–41*

Volume	Year	Pregnancy rate method	Life-table method	One-parameter exponential model	Two-parameter exponential model	Other analysis
37	1982	16	5	2	2	0
38	1982	6	0	0	0	0
39	1983	6	2	2	0	0
40	1983	12	5	2	1	1
41	1984	10	3	1	0	0
Total		50	15	7	3	1

eter model, and one used a statistical method independent of modeling. Thus, even in the 1980s, the predominant mode of analysis remains the critically flawed crude pregnancy rate.

As rigor is slowly increasing in the design phase of clinical fertility trials, the sophistication of descriptive and analytic methods appears to be lagging. Although some of the above studies may represent specific situations in which life-table analysis is less essential (such as complete follow-up, small numbers, or a randomized design of brief duration), this is surely not the case for most published studies. It is hoped that this deficiency of analysis can be remedied in the future, because the critical reviewer must insist on appropriate analytic methods to allow the full potential of a trial to emerge.

CONCLUSION

Clinical research is by its very nature different from laboratory experiments. It is less precise, less easily controlled, and more time-consuming.[80] In addition, the results of some clinical trials cannot always be extrapolated to a significant proportion of the patient population. For these reasons, the value of the well-planned and -constructed clinical trial is unquestioned.

If a study is to prove beneficial to the clinical practitioner, however, the tools must be readily available for a critical analysis of the report. By understanding biases, flaws, distortions, and limitations, the clinician may adequately evaluate each fertility trial and assess its applicability to his or her practice. In doing so, the goal of clinical studies may be achieved: to elevate the level of patient care from the anecdotal to the scientific.

In assessing the value of a clinical fertility trials, many issues not discussed in this review may become important; sample stratification[11, 41, 81-83] and sample size determination and statistical power[84-88] are two of the many complex issues facing the clinical trial architect. However, none are as basic or as critical to a study's value as the design and data analysis. Furthermore, in the recent literature there are serious shortcomings of both aspects in almost all clinical fertility trials. For these reasons, I have attempted to focus on these two concepts, providing both a historical perspective and an update of recent advances. My intent has been to provide the necessary insight for critical evaluation of the therapeutic literature. For clinicians to untangle the morass of data confronting them, it is essential to insist on studies that are appropriately designed, thoroughly analyzed, and meaningfully discussed. Fertility research has enough limitations at the outset; it is our responsibility as clinicians and investigators to minimize additional flaws by insisting on the use of the finest techniques at our disposal.

REFERENCES

1. Feinstein AR: Clinical biostatistics. LI. Quantitative significance and statistical indexes for a contrast of two groups. Clin Pharmacol Ther 27:567, 1980
2. Altman DG: Statistics and ethics in medical research. VII. Interpreting results. Br Med J 281:1612, 1980
3. Feinstein AR: Clinical biostatistics. VI. Statistical "malpractice"—and the responsibility of a consultant. Clin Pharmacol Ther 11:898, 1970
4. Feinstein AR: Clinical biostatistics. XLIV. A survey of the research architecture used for publications in general medical journals. Clin Pharmacol Ther 24:117, 1978
5. Feinstein AR: Clinical biostatistics. XLVII. Scientific standards vs. statistical associations and biologic logic in the analysis of causation. Clin Pharmacol Ther 25:481, 1979
6. Feinstein AR: Clinical biostatistics. LVII. A glossary of neologisms in quantitative clinical science. Clin Pharmacol Ther 30:564, 1981
7. Brown GW: 2 × 2 tables. Am J Dis Child 139:410, 1985
8. Olive DL, Haney AF: Endometriosis-associated infertility: a critical review of therapeutic approaches. Obstet Gynecol Surv. In press
9. Feinstein AR: Clinical biostatistics. XLVIII. Efficacy of different research structures in preventing bias in the analysis of causation. Clin Pharmacol Ther 26:129, 1979
10. Feinstein AR: Clinical biostatistics. XX. The epidemiologic trohoc, the ablative risk ratio, and 'retrospective' research. Clin Pharmacol Ther 14:291, 1973
11. Feinstein AR, Horwitz RI: Double standards, scientific methods, and epidemiologic research. N Engl J Med 307:1611, 1982
12. Mantel N, Haenszel W: Statistical aspects of the analysis of data from retrospective studies of disease. JNCI 22:719, 1959
13. Horwitz RI, Feinstein AR: Methodologic standards and contradictory results in case-control research. Am J Med 66:556, 1979
14. Feinstein AR: Clinical biostatistics. III. The architecture of clinical research. Clin Pharmacol Ther 11:432, 1970
15. Feinstein AR: Clinical biostatistics. IV. The architecture of clinical research (continued). Clin Pharmacol Ther 11:595, 1970
16. Feinstein AR: Clinical biostatistics. V. The architecture of clinical research (concluded). Clin Pharmacol Ther 11:755, 1970
17. Feinstein AR: Clinical biostatistics. X. Sources of 'transition bias' in cohort statistics. Clin Pharmacol Ther 12:704, 1971

18. Feinstein AR: Clinical biostatistics. XI. Sources of 'chronology bias' in cohort statistics. Clin Pharmacol Ther 12:864, 1971
19. Ederer F: Practical problems in collaborative clinical trials. Am J Epidemiol 102:111, 1975
20. Feinstein AR: Clinical biostatistics. XLII. The architecture of cross-sectional research (part 1). Clin Pharmacol Ther 23:81, 1978
21. Feinstein AR: Clinical biostatistics. XLIII. The architecture of cross-sectional research (conclusion). Clin Pharmacol Ther 23:481, 1978
22. Feinstein AR: Clinical biostatistics. XIX. Ambiguity and abuse in the twelve different concepts of 'Control.' Clin Pharmacol Ther 14:112, 1973
23. Leridon H, Spira A: Problems in measuring the effectiveness of infertility therapy. Fertil Steril 41:580, 1984
24. Metzger DA, Olive DL, Stohs GF, Franklin RR: Association of endometriosis and spontaneous abortion: effect of control group selection. Fertil Steril 45:18, 1986
25. Foulds GA: Clinical research in psychiatry. J Ment Sci 104:259, 1958
26. Grace ND, Muench H, Chalmers TC: The present status of portal hypertension in cirrhosis. Gastroenterology 50: 684, 1966
27. Chalmers TC, Schroeder B: Controls in 'Journal' articles. N Engl J Med 301:1293, 1979
28. Pocock SJ: Clinical Trials: A Practical Approach. New York, John Wiley & Sons, 1983
29. Grage TB, Zelen M: The controlled randomized trial in the evaluation of cancer treatment—the dilemma and alternative designs. UICC Tech Rep Ser 70:23, 1982
30. Ingelfinger FJ: The randomized clinical trial. N Engl J Med 287:100, 1972
31. Gehan EA: Adjustment for prognostic factors in the analysis of clinical studies. UICC Tech Rep Ser 36:35, 1978
32. Gehan EA, Freireich EJ: Non-randomized controls in cancer clinical trials. N Engl J Med 290:198, 1974
33. Byar DP, Simon RM, Freidwald WT, Schlesselman JJ, DeMets DL, Ellenberg JH, Gail MH, Ware JH: Randomized clinical trials: perspectives on some recent ideas. N Engl J Med 295:74, 1976
34. Armitage P, Gehan EA: Statistical methods for the identification and use of prognostic factors. Int J Cancer 13:16, 1974
35. Smithells RW, Sheppard S, Schorah CJ, Seller MJ, Nevin NC, Harris R, Read AP, Fielding DW: Possible prevention of neural-tube defects by peri-conceptional vitamin supplementation. Lancet 1:339, 1980
36. Student: The Lenarkshire milk experiment. Biometrika 23:398, 1931
37. Wright IS, Marple CD, Beck DF: Report of committee for evaluation of anticoagulants in treatment of coronary thrombosis with myocardial infarction. Am Heart J 36:801, 1948
38. Ehrenkranz RA, Bonta BW, Ablow RC, Warshaw JB: Amelioration of bronchopulmonary dysplasia after vitamin E administration. N Engl J Med 299:564, 1978
39. Cockburn F, Belton NR, Purvis RJ, Giles MM, Brown JK, Turner TL, Wilkenson EM, Forfar JO, Barrie WJM, McKay GS, Pocock SJ: Maternal vitamin D intake and mineral metabolism in mothers and their newborn infants. Br Med J 281:11, 1980
40. Feinstein AR: Clinical biostatistics. XXIV. The role of randomization in sampling, testing, allocation, and credulous idolatry (conclusion). Clin Pharmacol Ther 14:1035, 1973
41. Feinstein AR: Clinical biostatistics. XXII. The role of randomization in sampling, testing, allocation, and credulous idolatry (part 1). Clin Pharmacol Ther 14:601, 1973
42. Kramer MS, Shapiro SH: Scientific challenges in the application of randomized trials. JAMA 252:2739, 1984
43. Zelen M: Statistical options in clinical trials. Semin Oncol 4:441, 1977
44. Zelen M: A new design for randomized clinical trials. N Engl J Med 300:1242, 1979
45. Begg CB: A measure to aid in the interpretation of published clinical trials. Stat Med 4:1, 1985
46. Hofmenn F: Misuse of randomized clinical trials. Man Med 4:138, 1979
47. Bryce RL, Enkin MW: Six myths about controlled trials in perinatal medicine. Am J Obstet Gynecol 151:707, 1985
48. Hill AB: Statistical Methods in Clinical and Preventive Medicine. Edinburgh, Churchill Livingstone, 1962
49. Dieckmann WJ, Davis ME, Rynkiewicz LM, Pottinger RE: Does the administration of diethylstilbestrol during pregnancy have therapeutic value? Am J Obstet Gynecol 66:1062, 1953
50. Smith OW: Diethylstilbestrol in the prevention and treatment of complications of pregnancy. Am J Obstet Gynecol 56:821, 1948
51. Schafer A: The ethics of the randomized clinical trial. N Engl J Med 307:719, 1982
52. Barnea ER, Holford TR, McInnes DRA: Long-term prognosis of infertile couples with normal basic investigations: a life-table analysis. Obstet Gynecol 66:24, 1985
53. Collins JA, Wrixon W, Janes LB, Wilson EH: Treatment-independent pregnancy among infertile couples. N Engl J Med 309:1201, 1983
54. Grant A: The spontaneous cure rate of various infertility factors or post hoc and propter hoc. Aust NZ J Obstet Gynaecol 9:224, 1969
55. Lamb EJ: Prognosis for the infertile couple. Fertil Steril 23:320, 1972
56. Bernstein D, Levin S, Amsterdam E, Insler V: Is conception in infertile couples treatment related? A survey of 309 pregnancies. Int J Fertil 24:65, 1979
57. Lenton EA, Weston GA, Cooke ID: Long-term follow-up of the apparently normal couples with a complaint of infertility. Fertil Steril 28:913, 1977
58. Jones HW Jr, Rock JA: Reparative and Constructive Surgery of the Female Generative Tract. Baltimore, Williams & Wilkins, 1983
59. Lamb EJ, Cruz AL: Data collection and analysis in an infertility practice. Obstet Gynecol 23:310, 1972
60. Berkson J, Gage RP: Calculation of survival rates for cancer. Mayo Clin Proc 25:270, 1950
61. Katayama KP: A method of analyzing data with incomplete follow-up. Am J Obstet Gynecol 123:214, 1975
62. Cutler SJ, Ederer F: Maximum utilization of the life-table method in analyzing survival. J Chronic Dis 8:699, 1958
63. Peto R, Pike MC, Armitage P, Breslow NE, Cox DR, Howard SV, Mantel N, McPherson K, Peto J, Smith PG: Design and analysis of randomized clinical trials requiring prolonged observation of each patient. II. Analysis and examples. Br J Cancer 35:1, 1977

64. Katayama KP, Ju K-S, Manuel M, Jones GS, Jones HW Jr: Computer analysis of etiology and pregnancy rate in 636 cases of primary infertility. Am J Obstet Gynecol 135:207, 1979
65. Cramer DW, Walker AM, Schiff I: Statistical methods in evaluating the outcome of infertility therapy. Fertil Steril 32:80, 1979
66. Hammond MG, Halme JK, Talbert LM: Factors affecting the pregnancy rate in clomiphene citrate induction of ovulation. Obstet Gynecol 62:196, 1983
67. Peek JC, Godfrey B, Matthews CD: Estimation of fertility and fecundity in women receiving artificial insemination by donor semen and in normal fertile women. Br J Obstet Gynaecol 91:1019, 1984
68. Guzick DS, Rock JA: Estimation of a model of cumulative pregnancy following infertility therapy. Am J Obstet Gynecol 140:573, 1981
69. Guzick DS, Bross DS, Rock JA: A parametric method for comparing cumulative pregnancy curves following infertility therapy. Fertil Steril 37:503, 1982
70. Cox DR: Regression models and life-tables. J R Stat Soc [B] 34:187, 1972
71. Lee KL, McNeer JF, Starmer CF, Harris PJ, Rosati RA: Clinical judgement and statistics. Lessons from a simulated randomized trial in coronary artery disease. Circulation 61:508, 1980
72. Olive DL, Stohs GF, Metzger DA, Franklin RR: Expectant management and hydrotubations in the treatment of endometriosis-associated infertility. Fertil Steril 44:35, 1985
73. Mantel N: Evaluation of survival data and two new rank order statistics arising in its consideration. Cancer Chemother Rep 50:163, 1966
74. Breslow N: A generalized Kruskal-Wallis test for comparing K samples subject to unequal patterns of censorship. Biometrika 57:579, 1970
75. Kruskal WH, Wallis WA: Use of ranks in one-criterion variance analysis. J Am Stat Assoc 47:583, 1952
76. Federation CECOS, Schwartz D, Mayaux MJ: Female fecundity as a function of age. N Engl J Med 306:404, 1982
77. Mantel N, Byar DP: Evaluation of response-time data involving transient states: an illustration using heart-transplant data. J Am Stat Assoc 69:81, 1974
78. Olive DL, Lee KL: Analysis of sequential treatment protocols for endometriosis associated infertility. Presented at the 41st Annual Meeting of The American Fertility Society, September 28 to October 2, 1985, Chicago, IL. Published by The American Fertility Society in Abstr Suppl, p 78. Abstract P-39
79. Feinstein AR: Clinical biostatistics. XXV. A survey of the statistical procedures in general medical journals. Clin Pharmacol Ther 15:97, 1974
80. Feinstein AR: Clinical biostatistics. II. Statistics versus science in the design of experiments. Clin Pharmacol Ther 11:282, 1970
81. Feinstein AR: Clinical biostatistics. XIV. The purposes of prognostic stratification. Clin Pharmacol Ther 13:285, 1972
82. Feinstein AR: Clinical biostatistics. XV. The process of prognostic stratification (part 1). Clin Pharmacol Ther 13:442, 1972
83. Feinstein AR: Clinical biostatistics. XVI. The process of prognostic stratification (part 2). Clin Pharmacol Ther 13:609, 1972
84. Young MJ, Bresnitz EA, Strom BL: Sample size monograms for interpreting negative clinical studies. Ann Intern Med 99:248, 1983
85. Freiman JA, Chalmers TC, Smith H Jr, Kuebler RR: The importance of beta, the type II error and sample size in the design and interpretation of the randomized control trial: survey of 71 "negative" trials. N Engl J Med 299:690, 1978
86. Detsky AS, Sackett DL: When was a 'negative' clinical trial big enough? How many patients you needed depends on what you found. Arch Intern Med 145:709, 1985
87. Feinstein AR: Clinical biostatistics. XXXIV. The other side of 'statistical significance': alpha, beta, delta, and the calculation of sample size. Clin Pharmacol Ther 18:491, 1975
88. Hulka BS: When is the evidence for 'no association' sufficient? JAMA 252:81, 1984

Chapter 7

The psychological component of infertility

Patricia P. Mahlstedt, Ed.D.

Psychologist, Private Practice, Houston, Texas

"I can't be all things to all people," is the frustrated response of physicians who conscientiously focus their attention on the many aspects of infertility. Concerned about providing the most comprehensive medical care possible for their infertility patients, they keep abreast of the evolving research in this relatively new field of medicine. They work with dozens of couples every day, each with unique medical histories and physiological makeups to be analyzed in determining the cause(s) of their infertility. And they interact hourly with men and women who are in varying degrees of emotional distress over their failure to conceive. Attending to all of this is often a burdensome task. What more could patients expect?

"We needed acknowledgement from the beginning of treatment that there are common emotional responses," said a disillusioned couple who were so alarmed by the intensity of their anger and depression that they avoided many of their friends. Until joining a support group and learning about others' similar responses, they thought they were crazy. "Assurance that I had my physician's respect would have made the testing and treatment easier," said one upset patient who despondently stopped treatment. Her physician did not provide information which would have enabled her to understand the spectrum of functions that he would be examining and possibly treating so that she and her husband could participate in the process. He expected her to follow his treatment without questioning the rationale. "I felt excluded from the entire process," said one irate husband who never fully understood why his wife was still having tests (after 3 years of treatment), why she was not pregnant (after multiple operations and drugs), and why the physician did not need his input. Feeling that his wife had been a guinea pig, he wanted to "get back at" the physician.

Patients often expect more from physicians than physicians themselves believe they can give; and frustrated, angry patients sometimes want to get back at their physicians. These are not new dilemmas in medicine, nor are they unique to infertility. "We are only human," say doctors, "and can do only so much." "But it is *our* humanness that we want *you* to notice and respond to," say patients. With all the pressures to be experts on the medical aspect of infertility, should physicians further concern themselves with patients' personal and psychological needs?

To answer this question, one must decide whether (1) the emotional consequences of infertility represent a significant struggle for many patients, (2) the patients' feelings and attitudes toward their infertility and the physician have an influence on the treatment process, and (3) the patients' feelings and attitudes toward the physician affect their evaluation of the physician's competence. Anecdotal data and available research support affirmative responses to these statements.[1-10] Unlike some diagnoses, infertility has definite medical and psychological components, which are inseparable.[2, 5, 6, 9] It is one symptom of a medical problem which, by its very definition, has lasted for at least 1 year. The stresses of trying and failing to conceive for that long have significant effects on individuals, relationships, and even careers. Patients often report that no part of their lives—including, and most importantly, the treatment itself—is untouched by the disheartening experience of being infertile.

Therefore, it is recommended that specialists in infertility *know about* and *attend to* the psychological component of their patients' medical problem. It seems self-evident that doing so would be in the best interest of the patients both medically and psychologically. The problem involves defining specifically and reasonably what *knowing about* and *attending to* mean for physicians who often have little training or time for dealing with their patients' emotional needs.

This article will present a model for conceptualizing the psychological component of infertility. It then offers reasons why this aspect of infertility is often avoided by both physicians and couples. Concluding the article are recommendations for physicians and for couples to consider when challenged by infertility's intense and surprising emotional consequences.

THE PSYCHOLOGICAL COMPONENT

The process of diagnosing and treating infertility has a profound impact on the lives of those couples who encounter it. Even though this impact is usually far greater when the treatment process is prolonged and unsuccessful, the psychological component begins to develop when a couple realizes they are not conceiving according to their plan. They begin to "try harder," to contact physicians, and to worry. They wonder what is *wrong* with them that they cannot do something as natural and as simple as getting pregnant.

If they try unsuccessfully for a year, couples learn that their problem of getting pregnant now has a medical diagnosis: infertility. They become patients, and their lives begin to revolve around conceiving by following a physician's game plan. They focus their attention on what they have failed to accomplish and soon start neglecting other goals and needs in their lives. In most cases, this type of focusing leads to losses of self-esteem, confidence, security, health, close relationships, and even hope. Some patients lose sexual potency or interest in sexual intercourse, losses that interfere with treatment goals and put significant stress on marriages. There is no balance in their lives. There is, instead, hope one week, grief the next. This cycle creates a very confusing roller coaster with depression, anger, and guilt as part of its down side.

DEPRESSION

Depression, characterized by a sense of hopelessness and despair, is a very common consequence of the diagnosis and treatment of infertility. For some, depressive episodes are periodic and brief, often related to a sense of failure created by a rise in temperature and subsequent onset of menstruation. For others, depression—with occasional respites—is a daily curse throughout the entire process. Depression is for some incapacitating and for others heavy emotional baggage that they learn to carry. However it is experienced, depression is a response to both the excessive losses and the prolonged stresses created by infertility.

Loss

Barbara Berg has entitled the account of her own infertility *Nothing To Cry About.*[10] This title represents an illuminating aspect of infertility—its accompanying sense of profound loss. In one sense, it is wrong. There is much to cry about: the problem itself, its implications in the lives of infertile couples, and the reality that they may never have a child. But in another sense, the title is accurate. Who can mourn the loss of someone who has never been born or possibly conceived? The fact that there is nothing tangible to represent the loss actually intensifies the pain and makes the loss more difficult to understand. There is much to cry about, and there is nothing to cry about. Everything is lost, and nothing is lost.

All theories concerning factors which contribute to depression mention the concept of loss. The loss may involve a love object, a variety of reinforcers, power and control over the environment, or positive and hopeful developments in one's life. These losses usually involve a crucially important source of security, which, when lost, leads to a depressed condition and a sense of helplessness and hopelessness.

Recent research categorized the losses in adulthood which are of greatest clinical importance as etiologic factors in depression. They are as follows: (1) loss of a relationship; (2) loss of health; (3) loss of status or prestige; (4) loss of self-esteem; (5) loss of self-confidence; (6) loss of security; (7) loss of a fantasy or the hope of fulfilling an important fantasy; and (8) loss of something or someone of great symbolic value.[11] Any *one* of these losses could precipitate a depressive reaction in an adult. The experience of infertility involves them *all*.

Loss of a Relationship with an Emotionally Important Person Because of Death, Divorce, the Waning of Affection, or Separation. Ending a relationship may be an actuality or just an unspoken fear of many infertile couples. In fact, a couple may divorce or may sever relationships with friends and family. These breaks usually occur because of well-intentioned but insensitive remarks by others which leave the infertile person feeling unacceptable, misunderstood, unloved, or ashamed. As one infertility patient explained:

> Many of us even consciously isolate ourselves from friends or family because we come to the point of *having* to protect ourselves from their platitudes. While withdrawing from others usually is not the answer, we often do so in desperation—when our privacy, our dignity, and our self-esteem are threatened.

More often, however, the loss of significant relationships is an unspoken fear.[5] Will my spouse leave me if we cannot have our own natural children? Should I leave my spouse so that he/she can marry a fertile person? Am I acceptable to my in-laws? Is my depression driving my spouse and friends away? Will our relationship survive this ordeal?

Because both the man and the woman are hurting, tired, and under great pressure, they feel depleted of physical and emotional energy. They may become less able to fulfill each other's needs and thereby suffer a loss of closeness, to the point of feeling worlds apart.

Couples sometimes become polarized because infertility *affects* them differently or because they *cope* differently. In other words, one partner may actually be in greater despair than the other (effect), or one may feel betrayed by the other's frankness or desire to discuss their problem with family and friends (way of coping). Men, for example, often cope with their pain by keeping it to themselves and focusing on their wives. Women often cope by talking continually about their pain with their husbands, who, feeling powerless to take away the pain, sometimes stop listening. In order to get him involved, she escalates her complaints and he, in response, retreats even further and may even cease participating in the treatment process. In these cases, the woman feels abandoned when she needs her husband most, and he feels overwhelmed because she needs him so much. They begin to resent each other and become depressed not only by their failure to conceive but also by their loss of closeness and ability to understand.

Loss of Health, Important Body Functions, or Physical Attractiveness Due to Disease, Injury, Aging—In Other Words, Some Loss of an Acceptable Self or Body Image. The diagnosis and medical procedures relating to infertility influence how one feels both physically and sexually. Regardless of the causes of infertility, men and women believe their bodies are damaged or defective—something is not functioning as it should. Some people who pride themselves on taking care of their bodies find the diagnosis of infertility incompatible with their image of robust health. Uncomfortable and sometimes unsuccessful treatments, undignified positions, and even experimental medications can make the couple feel especially vulnerable and can contribute to a poor body image.

Another aspect of this loss is the loss of sexual spontaneity.[6, 7, 9] Since the course of treatment often requires scheduled sexual intercourse, sex becomes divided into "sex for love" and "sex for doctor." Each month the medical evaluation probes into the couple's sex life and evaluates the frequency and timing of intercourse, thus violating a deep sense of privacy. Constant intrusion into the most intimate aspects of one's sex life can cause men and women to feel less sexual, avoid sexual activity, and fail to respond sexually in fertile times. One man reported the following experience:

> My wife was scheduled to have a postcoital test late one afternoon. Because of our work schedules and a 30-mile distance between our home and the doctor's office, we met at a motel close to the doctor's office to have sexual intercourse. At first, I could not maintain an erection, and when I finally achieved that, I could not ejaculate. We tried everything we knew, and after no success, we dressed, checked out, and went home . . . where we tried unsuccessfully again. This whole charade was so humiliating and painful for me that I could not imagine attempting such a thing again.

Frustrated and unable to perform in the most critical time makes a woman feel inadequate, too. How does one get out of such a situation? What can anyone say? As a result of these humiliating encounters, making love becomes a mechanical chore and a painful reminder of the failure to conceive—far removed from earlier loving sexual relationships.

Finally, there may indeed be a true loss of health. The cumulative effect of the entire process of diagnosis and treatment can lead to physical illness. Stress can contribute to headaches and irritability. Some medications can cause cramping, nausea, and other negative side effects. Surgery patients must recover from anesthesia and the procedure itself. One man said:

> With all the medications and surgeries, I began to think of myself as a "sick" person. I came to depend on the doctor to make me "well" and when nothing seemed to be working, those feelings of being unhealthy or ill were intensified. I even have a scar as a reminder of my "illness."

A physically and emotionally healthy person enters the treatment process and, in no time, finds her/himself taking medication, having surgery, and becoming depressed. Men and women may enter the hospital for diagnostic or corrective surgery feeling good, and then leave the hospital physically debilitated—and all for an "illness" that others do not understand. Good health and a positive body image enhance people's opinion of themselves. Losing either can create a void, diminish that opinion, and lead to a depressed state.

Loss of Status or Prestige (in the Eyes of Others). Society places eminent value on parenthood, thereby safeguarding and reinforcing behavior that relates to procreation and child rearing. From the inevitable "How many children do you have?" to religious exhortations to "Multiply and replenish the earth," childless couples are duly reminded of society's expectations that they have children. Infertility does not reinforce this value. The stigma attached to it is great. Some couples believe that divorce would be more socially acceptable than infertility. Others think that their worth to society is lessened by their inability to produce children.

Childless couples may feel that being infertile jeopardizes their individual sexual identities. Because fertility and virility become intertwined for the infertile, a man who is unable to father a natural child may feel that others question his masculinity. For many women, having children is central to their identity. Society has been structured so that from the time they are very young, women think of themselves as—and others expect them to be—mothers. A woman's family and friends may be unfairly critical when this does not happen and sometimes imply that her identity as a woman is incomplete. She is different; she does not fit it.

> I feel like I don't belong, like a second-class citizen with no place to go. Without a child, I don't belong in the group with kids who play in the park. Without a child, my husband and I don't fit in with our friends who do.

Feeling awkward about their own children, friends and relatives may avoid the infertile couple and isolate them even more. Feelings of inadequacy and injured pride result. Couples who felt well-liked, accepted, and respected by others prior to their infertility lose the certainty that others appreciate them. Attention and respect are given to those who have children. The infertile couple now feels different, less acceptable, and left out.

Loss of Self-Esteem (or Pride in Oneself). Making the decision to consult with an infertility specialist is, for some, similar to making the decision to see a psychologist or psychiatrist. Before making that decision, a person must acknowledge that there is a problem—that something is *wrong*.

> I wanted to think I was just having trouble getting pregnant. When I went for the first appointment with the infertility specialist, I sat in the corner away from the other patients, who were probably infertile. In my mind, I was *not* one of them.

Being infertile was an insult to this woman's self-esteem.

For adults, self-esteem is enhanced by the accomplishment of basic personal, academic, and professional tasks as well as by the perceptions of how others see them. For some couples, failure to complete such an important personal life task as procreation is likely to diminish their pride in themselves both as a unit and individually.

> Never in my wildest dreams did I ever imagine that I would be infertile. The question around having children had always been "when," not "if." So when I discovered I was infertile, I felt damaged. Why couldn't I accomplish something as "natural" as conceiving a baby? Suddenly my sense of self-worth was shaken. I felt defective and very much a failure. Infertility was more than a medical problem. It was an attack on my self-esteem.

Others suffer intensely when they find that validation from family and friends gets harder and harder. As one patient said: "No one asks me about my accomplishments; it's only 'How many children do you have?' "

Self-esteem is also damaged when a couple notices the flood of emotions that overtakes them, emotions they are not accustomed to. They are especially upset by their negative attitudes toward others, particularly their anger and jealousy.

> I am experiencing feelings that are very foreign to me. I find myself *hating* the pregnant women I see at school, in the grocery store, and even in church. I have never had such intense negative feelings toward others, and I despise myself for having them.

Because many couples have been taught that "good" people do not feel angry, jealous, or resentful, and "good" people do not have "these kinds of problems," the infertile couple may temporarily accept the image of being "bad." They have daily reminders *from others* of their inability to handle their problems more effectively, *from the thermometer* of their failures to conceive, and *from themselves* of their failure to live up to their own expectations. Moreover, the temperature chart becomes a graphic representation of the cycle of hope, frustration, and failure they face. Their self-respect and pride get lost in that vicious cycle, leading some to wonder whether they are not good enough to be parents and perhaps that is why God made them infertile. Such negative self-statements are often followed by a sense of hopelessness and despair.

Loss of Self-Confidence or an Adequate Sense of Competence or Control. People who have been self-directed, been in control of their lives, and believed that hard work leads to success in all tasks are devastated by the infertility experience.[12, 13] Despite the enormous price they pay in terms of money, time, persistence, commitment to a schedule, and sacrifice to self and marriage, they cannot do what everyone else can do with little effort: get pregnant. Competence in this task is beyond their grasp—no matter what they do or how hard they try. This failure invades all aspects of their lives. Appointments with the physician take precedence over normal, day-to-day activities. They are unable to plan even a week's vacation, much less make major career decisions. Professionally, men and women have trouble concentrating on long-term goals when they are taking medication, recuperating from surgery, dealing with the emotional consequences of infertility, and hoping *daily* that the process will end soon. They have become controlled by the drive to achieve their goal to conceive.

Infertility also involves innumerable decisions concerning the medical treatment and the alternatives to continuing treatment, which are adopting or accepting childlessness. Couples struggle with the questions: "Should I go back to school, to work?" "Should we move?" "When do I stop taking medication, having surgery, or keeping the temperature chart? Am I a quitter if I do?" "Should we change physicians? How do we know who is best for us?" "Should we adopt . . . or consider artificial insemination?" Unfortunately, there are no definitive answers to these questions and no certainty that one decision is best. It seems as though the whole process of trying to conceive takes over one's life, eliminating the sense of self-confidence, competence, and control which comes from familiarity with success and in accomplishing a particular challenge.

Loss of Security (Occupational, Financial, Social, or Cultural). Job security and advancement are often affected by infertility procedures. Men and women turn down promotions which involve relocating because they have so much invested in infertility treatment with a particular physician. Women avoid career changes which might interfere with the freedom to leave the work place for medical appointments and carefully scheduled sexual encounters with their husbands. Moreover, taking time off for physicians' visits may strain the support of an employer or co-worker.

Couples may become insecure about the financial burden of repeated appointments, operations, and medications. The changes which may occur in their social relationships and cultural commitments also leave them less confident about their positions in these groups.

On a deeper level, there is a loss of security about the fairness and predictability of life.[10] Couples struggle to determine what they have done to deserve being infertile and how they could have prevented it from happening. They often fear that if this could happen, so could anything else.

Loss of a Fantasy, or More Precisely, the Loss of Hope of Fulfilling an Important Fantasy. After years of trying unsuccessfully to conceive, many couples experience great despair. They are both frustrated and sad that they have been unable to have a child and at times hopeless that they will be able to do so in the future. They may never be parents and thus never experience all that accompanies parenthood socially, personally, and religiously: from being pregnant and giving birth, to preparing for baptism and later selecting a school, to escorting a daughter down the aisle in matrimony—and so beginning again the continuous cycle of life. Having a child is tantamount for some to growing up and becoming an adult. Without this experience, individuals may not believe they have accomplished that unique psychological passage to adulthood. Being a parent is a part of one's vision of an idealized adult self; losing that vision hurts deeply.

Loss of Something or Someone of Great Symbolic Value. Paradoxically, the couple yearns for the child that may never be and mourns over the child that never was. Because there is no tangible or clearly defined loss for family and friends to see—no sense of finality as in death or divorce—it is difficult for others to truly empathize. Even the couple finds it hard to comprehend this intangible loss; but they ache nevertheless. Children acutely remind them of the children they do not have. Pregnant women remind them of the mysteries of pregnancy they may never experience. The stings come again and again as they watch giggling toddlers on television commercials, receive birth announcements from old friends, buy birthday presents for nieces and nephews, and notice their friends with children slipping away and developing different interests. They long for the sense of family that children embody.

Stress

As described above, infertility creates many simultaneous and complex losses. In this regard, it is comparable only to death and divorce. The ritual of a wake and a funeral provides support for the bereaved. For the infertile couple, there are no rituals. They are not considered bereaved. So they suffer alone. This phenomenon—that there are so many simultaneous losses and no ritualized support or outlet for the grief—leads to intense stress.

Like loss, stress depletes people of psychological energy ordinarily used to enjoy life and to solve problems of all magnitude. Less able to cope, people become depressed.

Opinions differ about what causes stress. Some define stress as a major life experience which creates the need for change in a person's life; others see it as a prolonged series of everyday hassles.[14, 15] What makes infertility stressful is that it is *both*. As a major life event, it involves the eight losses (discussed above) which contribute to depression. As a prolonged series of everyday hassles, infertility involves temperature charts, medication schedules, countless physicians appointments, programmed sexual acts, time away from work, and expensive treatment. Career and vacation plans are often thrown into chaos. The old adage "hurry up and wait" typifies the couple's routine: long delays in waiting and examination rooms and seemingly endless weeks between perfectly timed sexual intercourse or insemination and the determination of success or failure in conceiving—like the announcement of a grade weeks after taking the final examination.

The medical treatment itself is a source of stress. Some people experience great anxiety and fear about surgery, anesthesia, and even blood tests. The treatment is often painful. Others worry about the long-term and still unknown effects of hormonal therapy upon both the mother and the child. Many find that the process isolates them from family and friends, creates financial drains, and imposes a nagging hope which pushes them into more surgery and new drugs long after they have reached their limit. These stresses leave them depleted and depressed.

ANGER

The multiple losses and stresses of infertility leave couples not only depressed but angry. In particular, losing control over when or whether one becomes a parent—a loss most people never even consider, much less face—enrages many couples. How could they be deprived of something so basic and yet so significant to their lives as having children? The question "why" gets asked over and over; and when there is no answer, anger is conceived instead.

As daily lives become fragmented by personal and work obligations and treatment demands, anger grows. It is fed by other people's insensitivity, criticism from families, limited treatment options, inconclusive diagnoses, and the violation of an internal sense of justice. "What did I do to deserve this?" is a common question for couples who feel misunderstood and humiliated. "I was furious," one man said, "when I got to the lab to give a sperm sample and was directed to a bathroom with a sign on the door reading 'Sperm Count in Progress.' *No one* considered how a public notice like that would affect the men entering and leaving that room."

What is an ordinary procedure in the medical community (sperm count, artificial insemination, hysterosalpingogram, or ultrasound) is extraordinary to most patients. Events far less dramatic than the preceding illustration are distressing to emotionally frazzled patients. For example, a physician or nurse who minimizes the impact of a procedure may inadvertently leave the patient unprepared for what is to follow.

> I think the doctor was trying to alleviate my fears when he told me the procedure wouldn't hurt. But it did hurt . . . a lot. He was trying to help; but I felt deceived. It was an infuriating experience.

Unfortunately for the physician, patients are frequently unable or unwilling to discuss these occurrences or their feelings. Instead, they leave upset and postpone their next visit.

Anger, both expressed and repressed, has significant effects on individuals and on their relationships with others. In the case of the following patient, her anger almost destroyed her marriage.

> My husband told me he hated what the past few years had done to me. He said he watched me turn into an angry, bitter, hateful person. It was a long time before I realized how angry I was. I was *consumed* with anger before I understood what was eating me up inside. Then my problem was finding what to do with my anger—how at least to channel it, if not resolve it.

This internal rage may be repressed because there is no one to blame. It may manifest as depression, or it may build until it eventually is unleashed on the physician, the spouse, family, friends, and God.

GUILT

Many patients feel a tremendous sense of guilt for being infertile, for living on such an emotional roller coaster, for upsetting their spouses, for disrupting so many aspects of their own lives, and for disappointing their families. One woman said that sometimes she hopes her husband will leave her so that she will no longer have to worry about not getting pregnant or burdening him with her negative feelings. An infertile man felt such guilt about depriving his wife of a "normal pregnancy" that he filed for divorce; this was his way of coping. Other patients wonder: "Will the family name end with me?" "Did I fail to take care of my body properly?" "Did I wait too long?" "Is my infertility due to indiscretions early in my life? Did I bring this on myself? Is God punishing me?" The irrational belief that they *must* have caused their infertility imposes tremendous guilt on many innocent couples.

Guilt is also a futile attempt to gain control of the question "why." If there were an understandable reason, many would feel less frustrated, less angry, less depressed.

SUMMARY

Both the diagnosis and the treatment of infertility have a profound impact on people's lives. It is a process which invades one's body, one's personality, one's job, and one's mind. Diagnoses are often vague and inconclusive, and treatment is painful, intrusive, and time-consuming. Common emotional responses are depression due to multiple losses and prolonged stress; anger at the confusion, ambiguity, and unfairness of it all; and intense guilt for being infertile and for being up set about it. The grief associated with infertility has been compared with the grief caused by the death of a child. But it is the child who was never born, and there is no funeral. In most cases, the intense emotional responses are appropriate; there is a lot to cry about. To what extent the emotional responses incapacitate depends on many factors, including the couple's ability to communicate, the importance of the child to the couple's identity, the attitudes of others involved, particularly physicians and their support staff, and the understanding of family and friends.

WHY IS THE PSYCHOLOGICAL COMPONENT OF INFERTILITY AVOIDED?

Neither physicians nor infertile couples may fully recognize how disruptive the diagnosis and treatment of infertility can be. Physicians focus on the medical aspect of infertility, concentrating on its causes and cures and not its psychologic consequences. Discussion between physician and patient revolves around temperature charts, timed sexual intercourse, medication, and progress toward achieving the goal of pregnancy. Patients focus on the medical issues as they try hard to understand their medical problems and to do what their physicians recommend—until an emotional crisis occurs, leaving the patient impaired. As physicians and patients then try to understand and attend to the psychological needs, they encounter special complications that make that process difficult.

MEDICAL PERSONNEL

By the time a couple decides to seek medical help, they are already frustrated and worried about their failure to conceive. They wonder *why* they have failed to conceive, *what* the physicians will do, and *when* or *whether* they will achieve a pregnancy.

From the beginning of the diagnostic process, physicians and their staff have opportunities to assist the couple in handling the emotional stresses they are experiencing. It is important to note, however, that the couple's need for support may not be evident, because patients often hide emotional pain from physicians and nurses. Patients are self-conscious about their feelings and sensitive about the medical staff's opinion of them. They are afraid of being criticized for being troublesome or of being seen as crazy; so they avoid bringing their feelings to anyone's attention.

Even when infertility patients reveal that they are distressed, medical personnel may avoid their distress for a number of reasons. First of all, those specializing in the diagnosis and treatment of infertility are trained and responsible for managing a complex, multifaceted physical problem, not its psychological component. Seeing patients is only one part of the treatment process; staying abreast of the literature on detection and remediation of physical problems, refined treatment modalities, and pharmacologic developments is also necessary. Further, the physician may have responsibilities within the medical community, a medical school faculty appointment, and independent research to direct. In addition to a large case load of infertility patients in their practices, infertility specialists often treat patients with other conditions.

Second, the brief period of time physicians have with each patient makes it difficult to develop the rapport needed to discuss the despair and confusion in their lives. Patients often see the lack of time as a lack of interest in their total problem or as a narrow focus on their "blocked tubes." Furthermore, painful feelings and frustration about the lack of success with the treatment create dissonance between the patient and physician and inhibit such personal discussion.

Since the emotional consequences are very complicated, physicians sometimes believe that the means of responding effectively vary according to the needs of each patient, in the same way as the medical treatment does. Because they cannot treat the psychological component as competently as the medical component, physicians may choose to avoid it rather than make a mistake and hurt the patient.

Finally, some physicians simply do not believe that the psychological component of infertility is important enough to merit their attention. They genuinely believe that their *only*—as opposed to their *primary*—responsibility is to attend to the medical aspect of the problem.

Can nurses, receptionists, and physician assistants help patients with the psychological component of infertility? Many do, and this sensitive attention has far-reaching positive consequences on the attitudes and feelings of the patients. Those who do not often have limitations similar to those of physicians: they are trained and responsible for specific tasks, which take up most of their time; and they, like others, are uncomfortable with the patients' emotions. Unless providing emotional support is an objective of the office or clinic, staff do not focus on this process.

COUPLE

It is also difficult for a couple to handle their feelings about infertility. Many encounter infertility early in their married life, when everything has gone rather smoothly; they are healthy, and their professional and social lives are developing well. Thus, they have not developed the skills necessary for coping with such a complex problem. They are unsure about how to help each other and how to deal with physicians, parents, and friends.

Furthermore, there are so many losses and other dilemmas created by infertility that couples feel overwhelmed. They are unsure about where to begin. The medical problems themselves are frightening and painful. Then there is the depression, anger, and guilt—and the enormous task of integrating these negative feelings into a positive sense of self. The many indefinite aspects of infertility create anxiety and make coping more difficult, especially when no physical problem can be found to explain why there has been no pregnancy, when test findings are inconclusive, and when the time limit of treatment is unknown or indefinite.

Infertile couples are usually isolated from each other and so know very little about how others respond to infertility or how they communicate when there is so much stress in their lives. They assume that others are handling the stresses more effectively than they. As a result, they become critical of themselves, disillusioned, and angry—and have trouble talking about it with each other and with their physicians.

Grieving and other coping strategies are complicated when couples are not sure that they have anything about which to grieve. They cannot really grieve the loss of parenthood, because they are still hoping it will happen; maybe next month they will achieve a pregnancy. They cannot grieve the loss of control because they are still trying to attain control by doing everything the physician recommends. The loss of potential is harder to cry about. Grieving during the infertility process is like the process of grieving over the death of a soldier who is *missing in action* as opposed to grieving over one who was *killed*. In both processes, there is nothing definite, and hoping enables people to avoid the pain.

And finally, men and women respond differently to the problem of infertility. Said one man in great despair:

> I'm confused and distraught about so many things. We can't conceive; my wife is depressed; I'm sick with disappointment; and I can't do a thing about any of it. Nothing I have said or done has made a difference. So now I say nothing.

A man's silence sometimes confuses and upsets a woman, because she believes that the silence means that her husband is not as involved or concerned as she is. That perception might be accurate—some men do not feel the need for children as intensely as some women; boys are not as likely to grow up thinking of themselves primarily as fathers. And the woman's loss of being pregnant is not experienced by men. However, the perception that a husband is not as upset could also be inaccurate; perhaps he simply does not express his feelings as openly, as often, or as intensely as his wife.

Moreover, the responses to infertility depend to some degree on who is being treated for the medical problem. When a woman is the patient, she suffers not only from the psychological loss of being infertile but also from the personal and physical intrusions of the medical procedures. Keeping up with appointments, medications, scheduled intercourse, and rising and lowering temperatures consume large amounts of time and emotional energy. She sets about to succeed at the task of conceiving with such determination that the onset of menstruation each month triggers a crushing sense of failure. Men, in such cases, suffer both from the loss of fertility and from a loss of control over immediate and far-reaching aspects of their lives. Even the timing of intercourse is determined by a medical plan and not entirely by the husband and his wife. Although not directly affected by the treatment, men worry about their wives' physical and emotional health, question their abilities to make things better, and listen to and live with their wives' despair and anger. Having been conditioned by society to hide their own feelings and to take care of their wives, men appear to be less hurt by the diagnosis and treatment of infertility than women. As one man pointed out:

> My wife is upset about different parts of this experience with infertility than I am. She feels like a failure over being unable to conceive, losing contact with pregnant family and friends, and crying so much of the time. I hate going through all of this too, but I am most upset over what it is doing to her both physically and emotionally. As a result, when I do feel like crying about not having a child, I don't, because I'm afraid my crying would make her feel worse. And she believes I'm not upset. I'm playing a game, and we are both losing.

When a man is being treated for the medical problem, his experiences are different, and so, understandably, are his responses. In this case, he has to deal with his own physical pain, the inconveniences of medical appointments and treatment, the attitudes of others toward his infertility, as well as the emotional responses of his wife. In addition to feeling responsible for supporting her through this crisis, he feels responsible for creating the problem in the first place. She, in turn, vacillates between feeling supportive and angry toward him and depressed over her own losses.

When both are being treated for the medical problem, the issue of "responsibility" and subsequent guilt are absent from the response. However, the couple is still challenged by the different ways each responds to and copes with their infertility.

HOW CAN PHYSICIANS KNOW ABOUT AND ATTEND TO THE PSYCHOLOGICAL COMPONENT OF INFERTILITY?

Infertility is a life crisis that is difficult for all involved to handle. The Chinese symbol for crisis is composed of two words: danger and opportunity. Infertility is a crisis which involves many personal risks, and yet for some it becomes an opportunity for growth. Those who grow are probably surrounded by medical personnel, family, and friends who do what they can to support the couple and to help them through the crisis.

The initial recommendations of this article were that specialists in infertility *know about* and *attend to* the psychological component of their patients' medical problem.

WHAT DOES KNOWING ABOUT MEAN?

Knowing about the psychological component of infertility means becoming familiar with the first two sections of this article. It means developing a mind's eye understanding of patients' struggles to manage their lives, to field questions and responses from family and friends, to follow treatment recommendations explicitly, and to understand the surprising and painful emotions that overtake them.

This knowing will be appreciated by patients because it enables physicians to attend to their psychological and personal needs in a variety of ways. How they do so depends on the needs and personalities of both the physician and the patient.

WHAT DOES ATTENDING TO MEAN?

Attending to the psychological component of infertility means *communicating* with patients about it in several different ways. First and foremost, patients appreciate knowing *early* in the treatment that many others experience intense emotions such as depression, anger, and guilt during the testing and treatment process. Explaining that these types of responses are common and, in most cases, normal is comforting and validating when patients encounter them.

During the treatment process, physicians can attend to the psychological component by simply asking patients how they are feeling emotionally and then acknowledging how stressful these procedures are to most people. This type of recognition is enough for most patients. However, if a patient is extremely upset, the physician, a nurse, or a physician's assistant should make special contact with the patient before the appointment ends. Sometimes referrals for professional help can be made when patients appear to need more than the physician can offer.

Because some patients hide their emotions, physicians, nurses, and others involved with the patient need to be familiar with observed or reported symptoms which are indicative of depression and other problems in coping. They include the following: (1) change in personality (unusual withdrawal, sudden difficulty in talking with physician, extreme moodiness); (2) changes in appetite or sleep patterns; (3) unexplainable loss of friends; (4) marital or sexual difficulties; (5) excessive crying; (6) physiologic or psychologic tension; or (7) serious employment problems.

Support groups often create opportunities for patients to develop positive perceptions of themselves and for physicians to attend to the psychological component without taking time from their work to do so. Some physicians sponsor support groups for their infertility patients in the same way that they sponsor childbirth education classes for obstetric patients. These groups are often led by professionals. There are also local and national support groups composed of and directed by infertility patients, which provide counseling, education, and support to infertile couples and their families.

In order to lessen the stress of the infertility process on their patients, physicians might encourage both partners to participate in the process whenever possible. Sharing the experience doubles the patients' power to learn from the physician, to ask questions, and to help each other, thus freeing the physician from that task. Discussing the diagnosis and treatment plan with both partners can prevent one person from feeling like the cause of all the problems and the *one* responsible for fixing them—a heavy burden.

Another supportive action on the part of physicians is to encourage communication with patients about *all* aspects of their infertility. Information on the various diagnoses and treatments as well as the psychological component should be discussed along with options and the pros and cons of each. Written and verbal information could be provided by the physician or nurse with explanations of office and hospital procedures; various diagnoses, treatments, and medications; and common emotional consequences. Reprints of scientific papers of physicians and colleagues are also of interest to some patients. A well-informed patient is more responsive to input from the physician and more competent in his/her handling of the infertility. It is also helpful to be available for consultation between visits. These types of communication enable patients to feel that physicians are working *with* them. The process is a team effort.

Sensitivity to patients' psychological needs can be increased by explaining their medical problems in terms they can understand, allowing time for questions that either the physician or the nurse could answer, and avoiding well-intended remarks like "You need to relax" and "You may be trying too hard."

A final, more time-consuming way to attend to the psychological component is to discuss strategies that couples can use to help themselves. They are often upset and confused by their feelings as well as their failure to conceive, and assistance from someone who knows more about the process than they is comforting. Because an opportunity to help them in this way may arise when there is also enough time to do so, the following recommendations are included for physicians to share with their patients:

- Because infertility represents a loss of very great magnitude, *couples must grieve those losses.* In order to facilitate each other's grieving, individuals need to have permission to grieve, understanding that a loss of very great magnitude has occurred and grieving is normal, a social support system to comfort them as they grieve, and an awareness that grieving has a time-limited course. Successful resolution of the grief will enable the couple to give up the anger, depression, and resentment that cling to them before the grieving is done and to move to an acceptance of their infertility, of others' insensitivity, and of the unfairness of it all. Acceptance will enable couples to realize that their identities do not depend upon fertility.

- *Couples need to accept differences in feelings and in ways of coping.* Although few people see divorce as a consequence of infertility, many couples report increased hostility and anger. This fighting is usually about the other person's feelings or attitude: "You are crying too much." "You don't care about having a child." "It's not as important to you." "You are too sensitive." Couples argue about feelings because they make assumptions about what the other person's feelings mean, do not like the assumptions, and so try to change the other's feelings. That one person cares more than another or that one is more reserved in the expression of feelings does not have to matter. A couple is *two* individuals, and to expect both to feel the same about infertility or to express their feelings in the same way causes considerable stress.

- *Each person needs to take time to hear how the infertility process is affecting his/her spouse.* Listen carefully. If the person feels pain, show understanding. Instead of saying, "You cry all the time. What's wrong with you?" say, "You must be sad a lot lately. Infertility is a horrible experience." If necessary, couples can set aside a specific amount of time each day (10 to 30 minutes) to talk about feelings. Some may set a timer and stop when the time is over. Of course, this routine is not to be used on a day when the couple gets especially discouraging news.

- *Each person needs to take responsibility for his/her feelings,* knowing that only he can determine what kind of support he needs and when and from whom he needs it. Likewise, feeling responsible for taking away a spouse's pain is fruitless. One can only listen and be supportive. The other person must make the changes.

- *Couples must nurture their marriage.* They can learn to live for what is present and not for what is missing in their relationship. They can go out on dates and talk about the love they feel for each other. Having fun and creating a balance between the sadness of infertility and the joy of being married lessens the burden.

- *Some couples might want to take a vacation from the day-to-day struggles of infertility.* A "time-out" can make it easier to see infertility as just a part of their lives and can enable them to see times ahead when work for pregnancy will be over. A vacation can also give them new energy for meeting the tasks at hand and renewed enthusiasm for their everyday lives.

- *Couples must share with others and ask for what they need from them.* They must widen support systems and broaden their bases of information. Some join support groups in which they can share their experiences, learn about the process, and feel understood and supported.

- Very importantly, *each couple must be reasonable in their expectations.* No one can take away the realities of life that cause pain: stories about friends who accidentally get pregnant; television commercials that convey happy couples with their new babies; holidays which focus on children; child abuse; and people who make inappropriate comments like "Relax or adopt a child and then you'll get pregnant."

CONCLUSION

An infertility patient once said:

> My infertility is a blow to my self-esteem, a violation of my privacy, an assault on my sexuality, a final exam on my ability to cope, an affront to my sense of justice, a painful reminder that nothing can be taken for granted. My infertility is a break in the continuity of life. It is above all, a wound—to my body, to my psyche, to my soul.[16]

When physicians involved in the lives of infertile couples know about the wound which infertility causes and the subsequent suffering it creates, and when they can attend to this wound by communicating with their patients about it, the infertility crisis can present opportunities for growth for many couples, overshadowing the inherent psychological dangers of its treatment.

REFERENCES

1. Seibel MM, Taymor ML: Emotional aspects of infertility. Fertil Steril 37:137, 1982
2. Berger DM: Psychological assessment of the infertile couple. Can Fam Phys 20:89, 1974
3. Wilson EA: Infertile couple: interview and examination. In The Infertile Female, Edited by JR Bivens. Chicago, Yearbook Medical Publishers, 1979, p 27
4. Menning B: Counseling infertile couples. Contemp Obstet Gynecol 13:101, 1979
5. Mazor MD: Barren couples. Psychology Today 12:101, 1979
6. Rosenfeld DL, Mitchell D: Treating the emotional aspects of infertility: counseling services in an infertility clinic. Am J Obstet Gynecol 135:177, 1979
7. Walker HE: Psychiatric aspects of infertility. Urol Clin North Am 5:481, 1978
8. Mennings B: Infertility. Englewood Cliffs, NJ, Prentice-Hall, Inc., 1977
9. Mennings B: The emotional needs of infertile couples. Fertil Steril 34:313, 1980
10. Berg B: Nothing To Cry About. New York, Seaview Books, 1981
11. White RB, David HK, Cantrell WA: Psychodynamics of depression: implications for treatment. In Depression: Clinical, Biological and Psychological Perspectives, Edited by G Usdin. New York, Brunner/Mazel, 1977, p 308
12. McCormick RM: Out of control: one aspect of infertility. J Obstet Gynecol Neonat Nurs 2:205, 1980
13. Platt JJ, Ficher I, Silver MJ: Infertile couples: personality traits and self-ideal concept discrepancies. Fertil Steril 24:972, 1973
14. Holmes TH, Rahe RH: The social readjustment rating scale. J Psychosom Res 11:213, 1967
15. Wallis C: Stress: can we cope? Time, June 6, 1983, p 49
16. Jorgenson MA: On healing. Resolve Newsletter, December 1981, p 1

Chapter 8

Mollicutes (mycoplasma) in infertility

Marianne Styler, M.D.
Sander S. Shapiro, M.D.

Department of Obstetrics and Gynecology, University of Wisconsin Medical School, Center for Health Sciences, Madison, Wisconsin

In 1937, *Mycoplasma* organisms were first isolated in man.[1] Since then, there has been intense interest in determining what role these agents might play in the diseases of man, particularly in the pathogenesis of genital tract disease. Considerable data have been compiled to support the thesis that mycoplasmas can cause nongonococcal urethritis.[2-5] Conversely, the contributory role of these organisms in involuntary infertility and fetal wastage has yet to be conclusively established.[6-8] Numerous reports have appeared that document the recovery of mycoplasmas from infertile patients and the results of eradication with antibiotics. Still, the debate over the commensal versus pathogenic status of these organisms continues, leaving therapists to make their own decisions as to the value of culture and treatment.

TAXONOMY AND CHARACTERIZATION

The term "mycoplasma" has been used loosely to describe all of the self-replicating prokaryotes that lack a cell wall.[9] These organisms, once referred to as pleuropneumonia-like organisms, form the taxonomic class Mollicutes.[10] They are the smallest and simplest self-replicating prokaryotes.[9] All Mollicutes organisms have a trilaminar cell membrane similar to that of eukaryotes, but no cell wall. Their minimal reproductive units are the size of large viruses. They contain both ribosomal ribonucleic acid and double-stranded deoxyribonucleic acid. The genus *Mycoplasma* comprises in excess of 60 species, including all of the human parasitic Mollicutes except the genus *Ureaplasma*, which has a single species, *urealyticum*. *Ureaplasma urealyticum,* once called T-mycoplasma, has been separated from the genus *Mycoplasma* because of its distinctive capacity to hydrolyze urea. The so-called genital mycoplasmas include *Mycoplasma hominis, Mycoplasma genitalium, Mycoplasma fermentans,* and *U. urealyticum*. *M. fermentans* has been isolated from the genital tract too infrequently to allow adequate study of its potential as a pathogen. *M. genitalium* is of relatively recent identification and has not been studied extensively.[11] Therefore, the remainder of this contribution will deal primarily with *M. hominis* and *U. urealyticum*, the primary genital Mollicutes species (Table 1).

The fact that Mollicutes infections are known to cause reproductive problems in other mammals[12-14] and that some species can cause infection in man[6] has led to the suspicion that asymptomatic genital tract colonization may contribute to human infertility and fetal wastage. On the other hand, high rates of colonization among reproductive-age men and women make it both likely that these agents are commensals and difficult to establish that there is any pathogenic role for them.

Organisms of the Mollicutes class are fastidious, requiring special care in recovery, culture, and identification.[15] Successful recovery methods vary with the particular organ or site to be sampled and with the conditions under which specimens are transported to processing laboratories. Specimens can be inoculated directly into growth media, but in most cases a specialized transport medium is used at the time of collection. Fluid specimens such as semen and urine are put into transport media or, if the volume is great enough to prevent drying by evaporation, can be sent directly to the laboratory. Mucosal surfaces such as

Table 1. *Mollicutes Isolated from the Urogenital Tract*

Species	Frequency of isolation	Association with urogenital disease
M. hominis	Common	Yes[55]
U. urealyticum	Common	Yes[3]
M. genitalium	Rare	Yes[11]
M. fermentans	Rare	No
M. primatum	Rare	No
M. salivarum	Rare	No
M. pneumonae	Rare	No

those of the urethra, vagina, and cervix are best sampled with the use of swabs moistened in broth or saline. Attention must be paid to the type of swab used for collection because some contain ingredients that inhibit growth.[16] Aseptic conditions should be present during sampling, but antiseptics and lubricants that might adversely affect cultures must be avoided.[17] Swabs should not be allowed to dry out. Solid tissue samples can be minced or homogenized before they are introduced into transport media. Many biologicals, standard reagents, and other chemicals are known to inhibit colony growth.[18] It is, therefore, important that any nonstandard materials used for obtaining or processing samples be adequately tested before they are used in clinical sampling.

Samples placed in transport medium should be kept at 4°C if more than a few hours will elapse before inoculation into growth medium.[15] Mollicutes organisms are able to survive freezing, so that in those cases where processing must be delayed, sample maintenance at $< -20°C$ is recommended. Laboratories will use various specialized media and methods to culture, isolate, and identify *U. urealyticum* and *M. hominis*.[19] *Ureaplasma* grown on agar produces small colonies which are morphologically fairly distinctive (Fig. 1).[20] Further effort at positive identification involves subculture on urea containing medium to demonstrate the organism's urease capacity.[21] *M. hominis, M. fermentans,* and several other species grow in large colonies with a dense center that gives them a fried-egg appearance. Further identification of these large-colony species depends on differential growth in several defined media and serologic characterization.[22] Some laboratories routinely report all large-colony growth from genital tract specimens as *M. hominis*. When the presence of *M. hominis* is of interest, the laboratory should use methods that facilitate a positive identification rather than labeling all colonies that are not positive for *U. urealyticum* as being *M. hominis*. If large-colony mycoplasmas are not identified by specific means, there remains the possibility that *M. fermentans. M. genitalium,* or one of the oral mycoplasmas is the cultured agent.

There is a wide range of techniques used to serotype Mollicutes.[23] These can be used both to differentiate species and to type cultures within a species. Work with both *M. hominis* and *U. urealyticum* has resulted in the identification of multiple serotypes, at least 8 for *M. hominis* and 14 for *U. urealyticum*.[24, 25] At present, however, serotyping is not routinely performed in most culture laboratories.

M. hominis and *U. urealyticum* can frequently be isolated from urine, the urethral meatus, the vagina, and the cervix in asymptomatic women.[26, 27] The urethral meatus, coronal sulcus, urine, and semen are the common sources of genital Mollicutes organisms in men.[23, 28] The false-negative rate for single versus multiple specimens and for various sampling methods has not been clearly determined, nor have the relative rates of positive culture from different genital tract sites been firmly established. Available data suggest that urethral swabs from men are most often positive,[16, 29] and that urine sediment, vaginal samples, and cervical samples from women offer about the same frequency of positive cultures.[2, 30] Single samples from genital sites that are colonized provide about an 80% rate of positive identification for *U. urealyticum* and a 90% rate for *M. hominis*.[26] Almost all clinical investigation into the relationship between genital tract

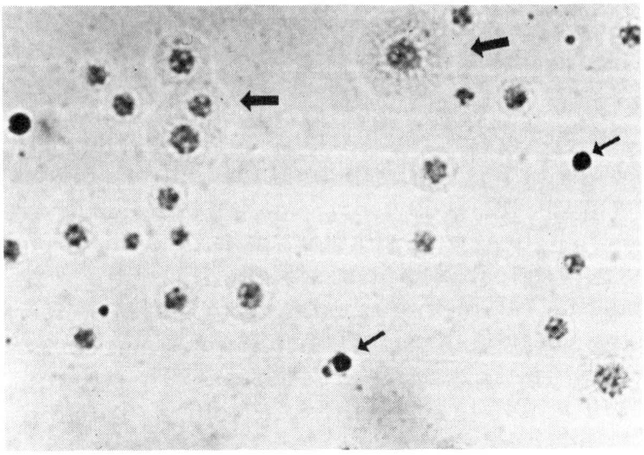

Figure 1
Photomicrograph of colonies of *M. hominis* and *U. urealyticum* on A_7 Agar ($\times$ 100). The *large arrows* show the typical "fried egg" appearance of *M. hominis*: a dense granular center with a foamy, light periphery. The *small arrows* point to the tiny spherical granular colonies of *U. urealyticum*.

colonization and infertility has involved the sampling of fresh cervical mucus and/or semen.

Both *M. hominis* and *U. urealyticum* may colonize the fetus during vaginal delivery.[31] Subsequently, there is a gradual decrease in the frequency of colonization through early childhood.[32] Recovery of these agents from prepubertal boys is rare. In groups of young girls, the frequency of recovery is about 10% for either organism. With puberty, the frequency of colonization rises. A strong correlation exists in both sexes between onset of sexual activity, frequency of sexual activity, number of partners, and the incidence of positive culture.[33, 34] In the healthy, sexually active, adult woman, *M. hominis* and *U. urealyticum* can frequently be found in the cervical opening, vagina, vestibule, and distal urethra.[26] The proximal urethra, bladder, uterus, and fallopian tubes of healthy women have rarely been found to harbor these agents.[23] Most investigators have found that the greatest incidence of genital colonization in women occurs during pregnancy.[27, 30, 35] After menopause, the incidence of carriers decreases significantly.[2, 27, 30] Studies on the frequency of intercourse and the effect of estrogens on the postmenopausal carrier are not available. Virgin adult men seldom carry either *M. hominis* or *U. urealyticum* in their urethras, whereas over 50% of males who have multiple partners may be culture-positive.[34] In both sexes, the frequency of *M. hominis* colonization is considerably lower than that of *U. urealyticum*. In the United States, there is a greater incidence of asymptomatic genital tract colonization among blacks than among whites (Table 2).[36, 37]

Table 2. *Epidemiology of Isolation Rates of Genital Mollicutes*

Factor	Appearance of Mollicutes
Age	Lowest in childhood and postreproductive age, highest during early adulthood
Sex	Greater in women than in men, of all ages
Race	Greater in black race in all groups
Socioeconomic level	Greater in lower socioeconomic groups
Sexual experience	Increases with increased sexual activity and number of partners

POTENTIAL MECHANISMS OF INDUCED INFERTILITY

There are a number of interactions between Mollicutes and eukaryotic cells, both in culture and in vivo, which suggest ways in which human infertility might occur in exposed individuals.

In rodents, the intraperitoneal or intravenous inoculation of murine *Mycoplasma* species will cause reproductive failure.[38] Exposure of murine sperm to the human pathogen *M. pulmonis* will also do this.[39] Swenson[40] found that after exposure to these organisms, the number of sperm located around each egg in the oviduct was decreased and the fraction of sperm that had organisms attached to their surface was lower in the oviduct than in the uterus. The author further reported that when exposed sperm were placed in the ovarian bursa, there was no decrease in fertilization rates. She therefore concluded that *M. pulmonis*, by attaching to sperm, caused a diminished transport through the female reproductive tract. *U. urealyticum* are known to bind to human sperm.[41, 42] A mechanism analogous to that found in the mouse might therefore result in a decreased transport of sperm across the cervix, through the uterus, and into the fallopian tubes. This theory is much like that proposed to explain the diminished transport of sperm exposed to antisperm antibodies.[43] It has not been systematically evaluated in man except in cervical mucus. At that site, the presence of *Ureaplasma* in either semen or mucus fails to inhibit sperm motility and viability.[44, 45]

The extracellular parasitism of some Mollicutes organisms may inhibit normal cell function, cause severe cell dysfunction, or stimulate specific cellular activities. Many species of *Mycoplasma*, including *M. fermentans* and *M. pulmonis*, act as mitogens, stimulating lymphocytes to undergo blast formation.[46] The immunopathologic consequences of this stimulation are not known, but an inflammatory tissue response with resultant cellular incapacity has been envisioned by some investigators. Examples of this kind of tissue response could include the endometritis and salpingitis produced in heifers inoculated with *M. bovis*[47] and the distinctive endometrial lesions described by Hertig[48] in women with genital colonization by *U. urealyticum*. In the male genital tract, colonization that induces a mitogenic reaction could produce a local immune response with the production of antisperm antibodies. Clinically, Witkin and Toth[49] have found antisperm antibodies in the semen of *Ureaplasma* carriers more often than in men who were culture-negative. Thus, the presence of these organisms might be one of a number of nonspecific stimuli that induce a form of autoimmune infertility.

Several Mollicutes species have been reported to induce chromosome changes in cells infected during culture. *U. urealyticum* will cause chromosomal damage including gaps, breaks, and even tetraploidy in cultured human lymphocytes.[50, 51] The types of alterations seem to vary with the individual *Ureaplasma* strain. Abnormal chromosome patterns have also been produced in human amnion cell cultures.[52] However, in vivo chromosomal damage in animal models infected with Mollicutes organisms has not been induced. Likewise, attempts at demonstrating similar abnormalities in human gametes have not been reported. Thus, it seems relatively unlikely that chromosomal damage as a result of otherwise asymptomatic infection is the means by which infertility or early fetal wastage originates.

The demonstration that genital Mollicutes organisms can attach to sperm has led to the suggestion of several pathogenic mechanisms besides an alteration in sperm transport.[41, 42, 53] They include abnormal sperm metabolism, masking of sperm membrane sites involved in sperm/egg recognition, and impaired ovum-penetrating ability.[8] Recently, egg-penetrating ability has been studied with the use of the hamster egg penetration assay.[54] Busolo and Zanchetta[54] reported that exposure of test sperm samples to *M. hominis* and most serotypes of *U. urealyticum* resulted in a diminished hamster ovum penetration rate. This occurred without a change in sperm motility. Neither killed organisms nor those incubated in the presence of doxycycline altered sperm penetration. Preincubation of sperm with the supernatant from *Ureaplasma* cultures decreased the penetration rate. This effect could be reversed by heating the supernatant before sperm exposure. These results led the investigators to hypothesize that genital Mollicutes organisms in the vagina produce a factor that impairs sperm function. The extent to which inhibition of penetration occurred varied considerably between *U. urealyticum* serotypes. Serotype 1 gave a penetration rate that was similar to that of controls (51%), whereas serotype 4 gave a very low (6%) rate of penetration. Unfortunately, the *M. hominis* used in these experiments was not serotyped.

Both acute infection with residual tissue destruction and reversible alterations resulting from chronic colonization have been suggested as mechanisms of Mollicutes-induced infertility. Direct infection of tissues, causing macroscopic and microscopic destruction, may result from colonization. The inoculation of *M. bovis* into heifers is known to cause salpingitis and endometritis.[47] In a series of acute human salpingitides, 4 of 50 women were found having pure cultures of *M. hominis* in their fallopian tubes.[55] Since mycoplasmas could not be isolated from a group of noninflamed tubes, the investigators who reported this suggested that tubal infection with residual damage could be caused by the organisms. The same suggestion has been made for *U. urealyticum* on the basis of two positive salpingitis cultures. A higher incidence of cervical *M. hominis* has been found in women with a past history of pelvic inflammatory disease.[41, 56] During acute salpingitis in which either *M. hominis* or *U. urealyticum* is found on the cervix, serum antibodies against these agents have been identified.[56-58] And in the general population of salpingitis patients, a rise in specific antibodies for these organisms occurs up to 25% of the time.[58] However, large-scale studies in which *Chlamydia trachomatis*, Mollicutes, and gonococcal organisms are simultaneously sought in the fallopian tube have not yet been reported. In those published cases where Mollicutes organisms have been found, no attempt was made to culture *C. trachomatis*. Thus, while there is the suggestion that acute salpingitis may be caused by *U. urealyticum* and *M. hominis* (up to 15% of the cases in the view of one author[59]), there is insufficient data to establish this as fact. Moreover, the existence of large numbers of genital Mollicutes carriers who are free of demonstrable tubal disease makes this an unlikely infertility-inducing mechanism.

Evidence that Mollicutes species can occasionally cause tissue destruction within the genital tract,[55] although they more frequently act as commensals, has caused concern about their role in postoperative healing.[48, 60] To date, however, no studies have been published that address this possibility. The discovery that primates can harbor the same genital Mollicutes species as man should facilitate the determination of these organisms' role in surgical-wound healing.[61-63]

In addition to acute and chronic salpingitis, a more subtle alteration of tubal function has been postulated. Support for this theory comes in the form of degenerative changes produced by *M. hominis* during human fallopian tube organ culture.[64] Clubbing and swelling resulted, but the insult only modestly inhibited ciliary activity. Ureaplasmas, on the other hand, have been shown to cause marked ciliostasis in cultures of bovine oviduct.[65] The inhibition of ciliary activity could be duplicated by the addition of ammonia to the cultures, which suggests a means by which these urea-hydrolyzing organisms might cause the insult.[66] Lesions like those produced during organ culture have not as yet been shown to exist in vivo after tissue colonization with either organism, and *Ureaplasma*-induced ciliostasis has not been demonstrated with the use of human fallopian tube in culture.

In men, there is substantial evidence for documenting the capacity of *U. urealyticum* to cause acute nongonococcal urethritis.[3] However, evidence for residual disease after clearance of the acute episode is scanty. There are no published studies that describe semen or sperm function after acute *Ureaplasma* urethritis. Chronic prostatitis might result from *Ureaplasma* infection; but again, residual pathology that would conceivably contribute to infertility has not been observed.[67] *Ureaplasma*-induced epididymitis has not been reported. Nevertheless, the relatively high frequency with which epididymitis passes without an established cause (20%) leaves open the possibility that this agent might infect that organ.[68] And while an infection here might alter sperm fertilizing capacity or numbers, there is presently no evidence that such is the case. With our current understanding of pathogenicity, it seems unlikely that tissue damage resulting from an acute *Ureaplasma* infection of the urethra or prostate would cause a long-term alteration resulting in male factor infertility. However, it is conceivable that minor alterations in epididymal secretions could significantly alter sperm function. Therefore, one might consider epididymal colonization as a possible means by which infertility could occur.

Colonization of the urethra by *M. hominis*, while not as frequent as *Ureaplasma*, is a relatively common event.[34] However, to date, that organism has not been firmly implicated in acute symptomatic infections of the urethra, prostate, or epididymis.[5, 69]

The uterus is more susceptible to bacterial invasion during the midluteal phase of the cycle. This vulnerability may also be true for Mollicutes invasion. Therefore, the suggestion that embryonic mortality after transfer through the cervix might result from such an inoculation has brought about the widespread practice of antibiotic treatment before in vitro fertilization and embryo transfer. At present, there is no evidence of a beneficial effect from this therapy. Moreover, if one should be demonstrated, it would still be unclear whether the result came from eradication of pathogenic bacteria or genital Mollicutes species.[70]

ASSOCIATIONS WITH INFERTILITY (ISOLATION STUDIES)

Since Mollicutes organisms were first suggested as a possible cause of infertility, studies have been carried out for determining the incidence of genital Mollicutes colonization in various defined populations (Table 3).[71-81] The fact that a large portion of the fertile adult population carries *M. hominis* and/or *U. urealyticum* in its genital tracts has confounded those who ascribe an infertility-inducing role to these organisms. In 1972, the first study on the incidence of Mollicutes organisms in a population that had experienced infertility without identifiable cause was reported by Gnarpe and Friberg.[71] Both the women (91%) and men (85%) from these couples had a greater frequency ($P < 0.001$) of *Ureaplasma* colonization than the controls (pregnant women, 23%; male partners of pregnant women, 26%). Shortly thereafter, a similar report suggesting a higher incidence of *M. hominis* in the cervices of infertile patients (19%) than in healthy nonpregnant women (4%) and pregnant women (10%) appeared.[82] Treatment of the *Ureaplasma* colonization resulted in a higher than expected rate of pregnancy (29%) for a group with more than 5 years of infertility. During follow-up, *M. hominis*-positive women became pregnant less frequently (14%) than infertile women who were not positive (25%). These two articles, with their indictment of Mollicutes species in the etiology of infertility, stimulated a number of other epidemiologic studies.

In 1974, deLouvois and co-workers[72] compared 120 infertile couples to a group of pregnant women and their partners. They failed to find a difference in the incidence of either *M. hominis* or *U. urealyticum* in the two groups. One year later, Matthews and co-workers[73] published a similar study comparing the incidence of *Ureaplasma* colonization in infertile couples with that of pregnant women and nonpregnant demonstrably fertile women. Again, there was failure to find a significant difference in incidence; the authors concluded that these organisms were not a com-

Table 3. *Frequency of* U. urealyticum *in Cervical Mucus*

Reference	Year	Infertile patients		Fertile patients	
		% explained	% unexplained	%	Type
Gnarpe and Friberg[71]	1972	—	91	23	Pregnant
deLouvois et al.[72]	1974	—	52	55	Pregnant
Matthews et al.[73]	1975	52	—	66	Pregnant and nonpregnant with proven infertility
Stray-Pedersen et al.[74]	1978	—	83	49	Nonpregnant with proven fertility
Idriss et al.[75]	1978	41	55	33	Pregnant and fertile nonpregnant[a]
Rehewy et al.[76]	1978	47	—	35	Pregnant and nonpregnant with proven fertility[a]
Khatamee and Decker[77]	1978	35	52	68	Pregnant
Koren and Spigland[78]	1978	—	59	12	Nonpregnant with proven fertility[a]
Taymor[79]	1978	41	55	33	Pregnant and nonpregnant with proven fertility
Nagata et al.[80]	1979	63	—	68	Pregnant and nonpregnant
Upadhyaya et al.[81]	1983	—	48	33	Pregnant

[a]Not further specified.

mon cause of infertility. Then Idriss et al.[75] found a significantly higher rate of cervical *Ureaplasma* among women with unexplained infertility (55%) than among those with a known cause for their infertility (32%). Similar findings (52% versus 35%) were reported by Khatamee and Decker.[77] Rehewy et al.[76] found a slightly higher rate of cervical *Ureaplasma* colonization in a population of infertile women than in a similar group who were fertile. Nagata et al.[80] failed to find a significant difference in incidence between infertile and pregnant Japanese women for both cervical *M. hominis* and *Ureaplasma*. Taymor[79] reported a significantly ($P < 0.05$) higher incidence of cervical *Ureaplasma* among women with unexplained infertility than among a mixed group with proven fertility. Cassell et al.[83] categorized a large group of infertile patients according to their postlaparoscopic diagnosis. They found a significant ($P < 0.05$) increase in the frequency of cervically isolated *Ureaplasma* among the male factor group compared with their seven other etiologic categories. More recently, a Welsh study[81] found a highly significant difference ($P < 0.001$) in the distribution of *Ureaplasma* between infertile and pregnant women, whereas Gump et al.[44] could find no causal relationship between genital Mollicutes organisms and either infertility or subsequent pregnancy. Collectively, these epidemiologic studies fail to provide persuasive evidence that either *M. hominis* or *U. urealyticum* are causally related to infertility. Poor choices for control subjects, inadequate evaluation of infertile subjects, relatively small populations in some study subsets, and a wide range of colonization frequencies may account for the variety of data and conclusions obtained from these studies. Critical analysis, however, fails to identify one single, fundamental factor to explain the contradictory data that was obtained. Definitive conclusions about the significance of cervical colonization cannot, therefore, be drawn. Large-scale prospective studies on the relationship of cervical Mollicutes colonization to infertility, containing sufficient numbers of subjects and enough detail to provide the desired information, appear impractical. However, data derived from such studies could produce information about the potential pathogenicity of these organisms. The application of methods that isolate subsets of infertile patients would be more practical and potentially productive. More intensive efforts to correctly assign patients into explained and unexplained infertility groups and to identify colonies according to serotype are likely to provide data that would clarify rather than obscure the role of these organisms. At the same time, efforts to define parameters that might contribute to the effects of colonization should be sought. The demonstration that various strains of mice carry different levels of susceptibility to murine mycoplasmas recommends this avenue of investigation.[84] For the present, one can only generalize that genital Mollicutes organisms may play a role in the induction of infertility and that, should such a role be firmly established in the future, it is more likely to involve *U. urealyticum* than *M. hominis*.

TREATMENT TRIALS

During the period in which incidence data about cervical colonization were being gathered, attempts at treatment were being undertaken in the hope that eradication of the organisms would result in more frequent pregnancies. The impetus for these trials came from Kundsin,[85] who reported a conception after tetracycline therapy in a couple who were genital-tract carriers of *Ureaplasma*. Then Friberg and Gnarpe[86] gained a 29% pregnancy rate, in the 5 months after doxycycline treatment, in infertile couples with positive cervical *Ureaplasma* cultures. Unfortunately, these investigators did not randomize their drug trial, thus leaving open the possibility of fortuitous pregnancy. Rehewy, who had found no difference in colonization rates between fertile and infertile subjects, also failed to attain an encouraging rate of pregnancy after tetracycline treatment of infertile couples with cervical *Ureaplasma*.[76] Mathews et al.[73] without formally randomizing their patients with infertility of undetermined cause, attained a 20% and 22% pregnancy rate, respectively, in the treated and untreated subsets with positive cervical *Ureaplasma* cultures. Harrison et al.[87] assigned 88 infertile couples to treatment (doxycycline), placebo, and nontreatment groups with about equal numbers of culture-positive and culture-negative individuals in each group. During the 6 months that followed treatment, there was no significant difference in the rate of pregnancy among the three groups. Hinton et al.[88] went beyond this by performing a randomized double-blind crossover study of 42 couples with genital Mollicutes. They found a significant increase ($P < 0.05$) in pregnancies after treatment, but ascribed this to psychologic effects because the pregnancies took place in the groups who were first exposed to antibiotics and not in those exposed after the crossover. Idriss et al.,[75] using tetracycline therapy, produced a higher rate of conception in a group without an identifiable cause of infertility than in those with a known cause for their infertility. This difference was not, however, statistically significant. Similarly, Taymor[79] produced a higher, but statistically nonsignificant, rate of pregnancy in women with unexplained infertility and a positive cervical *Ureaplasma* culture than in those with negative cultures. The Welsh group that had found a significantly higher rate of cervical *Ureaplasma* among their infertility patients found no difference in the rate of pregnancy between those who were or were not treated for their positive cultures.[81] Thus, the evidence from treatment studies fails to provide substantial data to support an indictment of either *M. hominis* or *U. urealyticum* as a cause of infertility. And, like the epidemiologic reports, there is an exasperating overall failure in study design that inhibits the establishment of definitive conclusions.

The ambiguous nature of the collected treatment data could be accounted for in several ways. The infertility-inducing action of the genital Mollicutes organisms might result from synergisms with bacteria that only appear infrequently. Not all strains of either *M. hominis* or *U. urealyticum* may be pathogenic. Successful antibiotic treatment, as represented by pregnancy, might result from clearance of an organism other than Mollicutes species. Most studies have failed to identify those subjects who manifest treatment resistance, thereby introducing a confounding variable into the data. And, finally, there may be no infertility-inducing action of these organisms, a null hypothesis that will be most difficult to establish.

The equivocal nature of epidemiologic and treatment data supporting a role for cervical Mollicutes-induced infertility provoked a more selective approach to the question by several groups. Reasoning that cervical colonization might be the harbinger of endometrial infection, several investigators looked for organisms in the uterus. Hertig[48] found a histologic picture in the endometrium which he believed to be pathognomonic of Mycoplasma infection. Stray-Pedersen et al.[74] found that endometrial colonization by ureaplasmas was significantly more frequent among a small group of infertile patients than among fertile, nonpregnant controls. Unfortunately, the study specimens were obtained by curettage, which made contamination from the cervix likely and the results suspect. However, Koren and Spigland[78] then reported upon patients without an etiologic diagnosis for their infertility and also found a significantly ($P < 0.01$) higher frequency of organisms in them than in fertile, nonpregnant women. Treatment with doxycycline was followed by pregnancy in 31% of those women. Subsequently, Cassell et al.[83] cultured *M. hominis* (1.0%) and *Ureaplasma* (0.05%) from the endometrium of so few patients in their infertility population that they could not implicate this agent or site in the cause of infertility. Gump et al.[44] offered similar data concerning the low frequency of Mollicutes-positive endometrial cultures. In addition to the studies on endometrial *Ureaplasma* there is one report of a significant association of *M. hominis* serum antibodies with plasma cell endometritis.[89] The discrepancy between the two former and the latter *Ureaplasma* articles mentioned above has gone unexplained. Different populations, types of specimens, sampling techniques, and methods of cleaning the cervix might account for the variation. Nevertheless, these explanations leave us without firm grounds upon which to implicate or eliminate endometrial infection as a potential means of Mollicutes-induced infertility. Certainly most observers would not consider the information contained in these reports persuasive enough to justify clinical application of endometrial culturing without supporting data from more extensive, controlled trials.

FREQUENCY OF MOLLICUTES IN MEN

There is a fairly high correlation between positive vaginal or cervical *M. hominis* and *U. urealyticum* cultures and the presence of these organisms in the semen of male partners. Thus, it is not surprising that when investigators find a higher incidence of positive genital cultures in infertile women than in controls, they also find similar differences in their male subjects. Others, looking primarily at men, have failed to identify an incidence difference between infertile men and controls.

Studies of infertile men with and without *U. urealyticum* in their semen have shown a difference in seminal quality. Semen volumes from infertile men colonized with *U. urealyticum* were significantly higher than ejaculates from those who were not colonized.[90] Sperm numbers, morphology, and motility were found to deviate from normal more among study subjects with positive cultures. Such morphologic characteristics as coiled tails, tapering heads, and spherical at-

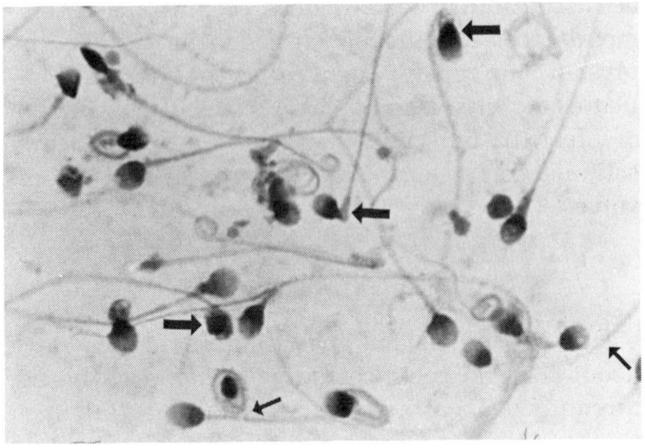

Figure 2
Photomicrograph showing morphologic changes associated with *Ureaplasma* colonization in a culture-positive semen specimen. The semen smear was stained by the Papanicolaou technique. The *large arrows* show different degrees of angulation and transition toward coiling of the tails. Most tails show a continuous fuzzy appearance. The *small arrows* denote segmental thickening of tail segments (original magnification, × 400). (Reproduced with the permission of Toth et al.[91])

tachments to the tail have been identified. In particular, a fuzzy coating over the tail segments has been described in culture-positive specimens (Fig. 2).[91] The presence of this light-microscopically observable characteristic provided a predictive indicator for the presence of *U. urealyticum* with a 10% false-negative and a 19% false-positive identification rate. Successful treatment with appropriate antibiotics is reported to result in improved sperm motility and a significant decrease in the frequency of certain abnormal morphologic characteristics.[92] Countering these studies, though, are at least two recent reports in which no significant differences were found between *Ureaplasma*-positive and -negative specimens for multiple semen parameters.[45, 93] Inspection of these various reports fails to reveal the reasons for the antithetical findings.

Two studies have been published in which couples were treated for *Ureaplasma* strictly on the basis of positive semen cultures. Rehewy et al.[94] eradicated the organism in 81% of culture-positive cases, but failed to attain any pregnancies over the following 6 months. Toth and co-workers[95] obtained a similar rate of clearance in positively cultured infertile men, but found that 60% of the *Ureaplasma*-free groups' partners became pregnant, whereas only 5% of partners became pregnant when posttherapy cultures were positive. More than half of those pregnancies occurred in the first 6 months after treatment. Thus, although there is a suggestion that semen quality and sperm function may be altered by genital Mollicutes organisms, data from clinical epidemiologic and treatment studies are collectively as ambiguous as those involving women.

MOLLICUTES IN PREGNANCY WASTAGE

Evidence implicating genital Mollicutes colonization as a cause of early pregnancy wastage has been sought by several groups. In 1969, Driscoll et al.[96] reported four of six habitual aborters cultured for cervical mycoplasmas were positive. Antibiotic treatment during early pregnancy resulted in one spontaneous abortion and five third-trimester deliveries. Subsequently, *M. hominis* was found more frequently on the cervix of febrile, spontaneous abortion patients than in those who were afebrile.[97] *Ureaplasma* organisms were not sought in that study. Mycoplasmas have also been found more frequently in the cervices of spontaneous aborters than in those whose abortions were induced.[98] The frequency with which genital Mollicutes colonization was found did not vary significantly with the number of previous pregnancy losses. In one study, endometrial *Ureaplasma* cultures from women with histories of fetal wastage had a significantly more frequent occurrence than those from women with a normal reproductive history.[99] Antibiotic treatment of those couples with positive endometrial cultures resulted in a decreased incidence of abortion. A similar diminution was found when couples with a past history of fetal wastage and positive genital *Ureaplasma* cultures were treated with doxycycline either before or during a subsequent pregnancy.[96, 100] Unfortunately, a valid control group was not included in this study. Thus, very little evidence exists to suggest that there might be an association between asymptomatic lower genital tract colonization with Mollicutes organisms and early fetal wastage.

ANTIBIOTIC TREATMENT

Long-term, serial surveillance of genital tract colonization with *M. hominis* or *U. urealyticum* has not been reported for women. Experience suggests that asymptomatic colonization may occur for extended periods of time. In men, *Ureaplasma* may persist in the urethra for several years.[101] Spontaneous clearance is, however, thought to occur.[102] Antibiotic therapy for lower genital tract Mollicutes organisms has most often been successful when tetracycline or doxycycline has been administered. A single course of either drug will clear about 90% of patients.[86, 88, 95] Because the organisms are easily passed through sexual intercourse, successful therapy requires simultaneous ingestion of the drug by both partners. Treatment in this way will result in a 90% clearance rate for both *U. urealyticum* and *M. hominis*. The most commonly used regimens are 100 mg doxycycline/day for 10 days or 2 gm tetracycline/day for 10 days. Other regimens, including 100 mg doxycycline/day for up to 28 days, have been used, but with no demonstrable advantage. Tetracycline has a significant price advantage over doxycycline. However, severe gastritis experienced by some patients can prevent completion of a therapeutic course. The appearance of resistant strains (*Ureaplasma* more frequently than *M. hominis*) has encouraged some therapists to require posttherapy cultures from all of their patients.[103-105] Erythromycin has been used in the treatment of genital *Ureaplasma* infections. Its rate of successful eradication of the organism is considerably lower than that of tetracycline, and it is not effective against *M. hominis*.[106, 107] Lincomycin has been used in the treatment of *M. hominis* with some success, but is not active against *Ureaplasma*. Neither species is sensitive to the penicillins. Up to 10% of *Ureaplasma* strains may be resistant to tetracycline. Many of these are sensitive to erythromycin.

Neither the evaluation of epidemiologic data nor the evaluation of treatment data from female members of infertile partnerships has offered substantial experimentally repeatable evidence to implicate Mollicutes organisms as etiologic agents. The same generalization can be made for male partners in infertile unions. Still, much of the literature on this subject is intriguingly suggestive. The widespread commensal distribution of these organisms and our limited access to animal models has thus far prevented a definitive determination of a role for either *M. hominis* or *U. urealyticum*. It is doubtful that the question can be resolved by attempts to fulfill Koch's postulates. Should evidence be developed to demonstrate that either organism actually causes infertility, it will, most probably, come from rigorously controlled clinical surveys and the application of new selective methods that facilitate identification of specific subsets of patients or organisms. In either case, should there be an eventual implication of this prokaryote class, it will involve no more than a small fraction of all persons who are genitally colonized. Acceptance of this limited projection, together with the very murky state of our current knowledge, leaves the clinician in a precarious position.

Physicians who currently care for infertile couples must decide whether or not to attempt identification of genital tract colonization and treat those who are culture positive. Purists will take the position that without compelling data to suggest a cause and effect relationship, the culture and treatment of Mollicutes carriers should not be undertaken.[8] Others, recognizing the benignity of treatment and having an accessible, competent culture facility, may choose to treat either universally or selectively their infertile patients and those with pregnancy wastage for Mollicutes organisms isolated in the genital tract.

REFERENCES

1. Dienes L, Edsall G: Observations on the L-organism of Klieneberger. Proc Soc Exp Biol Med 36:740, 1937
2. Csonka GW, Williams REO, Corse J: T-strain Mycoplasma in nongonococcal urethritis. Lancet 1:1292, 1966
3. Taylor-Robinson D, Csonka GW, Prentice MJ: Human intra-urethral inoculation of ureaplasmas. Q J Med 46:309, 1977
4. Bowie WR, Pollock HM, Forsyth PS, Floyd JF, Alexander ER, Wang SP, Holmes KK: Bacteriology of the urethra of normal men and men with nongonococcal urethritis. J Clin Microbiol 6:482, 1977
5. Hofstetter A: Mykoplasmeninfektionen des Urogenitaltraktes. Hautarzt 28:295, 1977
6. Taylor-Robinson D, McCormack WM: The genital mycoplasmas. N Engl J Med 302:1063, 1980
7. Friberg J: Mycoplasmas and ureaplasmas in infertility and abortion. Fertil Steril 33:351, 1980
8. Cassell GH, Cole BC: Mycoplasmas as agents of human disease. N Engl J Med 304:80, 1981
9. Razin S: Characteristics of the mycoplasmas as a group. In Methods in Mycoplasmology, Vol I, Edited by JC Tully, S Razin. New York, Academic Press, 1983, p 3
10. International Committee on Systemic Bacteriology, Subcommittee on the Taxonomy of Mycoplasmatales: Proposal for minimal standards for descriptions of new species of the order mycoplasmatales. Int J Syst Bacteriol 22:184, 1972
11. Moller BR, Taylor-Robinson D, Furr PM: Serologic evidence implicating mycoplasma genitalium in pelvic inflammatory disease. Lancet 1:1102, 1984
12. Tourtellotte ME, Lein DH: Infertility of cattle caused by mycoplasmas. Health Lab Sci 13:152, 1976
13. Taylor-Robinson D: Infections and infertility in man and animals. In Infections and Pregnancy, Edited by CR Coid. New York, Academic Press, 1977, p 141
14. Stalheim DHV, Proctor SJ: Experimentally induced bovine abortion with *Mycoplasma agalachae* subsp bovis. Am J Vet Res 37:879, 1976
15. Clyde WA Jr, McCormack WM: Collection and transport of specimens. In Methods in Mycoplasmology, Vol I, Edited by JC Tully, S Razin. New York, Academic Press, 1983, p 103
16. Poulin SA, Kundsin RB, Horne HW: Survival of *Ureaplasma urealyticum* on different kinds of swabs. J Clin Microbiol 10:601, 1979
17. Furr PM, Taylor-Robinson D: The inhibitory effect of various antiseptics, analgesics and lubricants on mycoplasmas. J Antimicrob Chemother 8:115, 1981
18. Lee Y-H, Bailey PE, McCormack WM: T-mycoplasmas from urine and vaginal specimens: decreased rates of isolation and growth in the presence of thallium acetate. J Infect Dis 125:318, 1972
19. Taylor-Robinson D: Recovery of mycoplasmas from the genitourinary tract. In Methods in Mycoplasmology, Vol II, Edited by JC Tully, S Razin. New York, Academic Press, 1983, p 19
20. Shepard MC: T-form colonies of pleuropneumonia like organisms. J Bacteriol 71:362, 1976
21. Shepard MC, Lunceford OD: Differential agar medium (A7) for identification of *Ureaplasma urealyticum* (human T mycoplasmas) in primary cultures of clinical material. J Clin Microbiol 3:613, 1976
22. Clyde WA Jr: Mycoplasma species identification based upon growth inhibition by specific antisera. J Immunol 92:958, 1964
23. Taylor-Robinson D, McCormack WM: Mycoplasma in human genitourinary infections. In The Mycoplasmas, Vol II, Edited by JC Tully, RF Whitcomb. New York, Academic Press, 1979, p 308
24. Black FT: Serological methods for classification of human T-mycoplasmas. Int Congr Infect Dis 5th Vienna Austria 1:407, 1970
25. Lin J-S, Kass EH: Serotypic heterogeneity in isolates of human genital T-mycoplasmas. Infect Immun 7:499, 1973
26. McCormack WM, Rankin JS, Lee Y-H: Localization of genital mycoplasmas in women. Am J Obstet Gynecol 112:920, 1971
27. Mårdh P, Weström L: T-mycoplasmas in the genitourinary tract of the female. Acta Pathol Microbiol Scand [B] 78:367, 1970
28. Friberg J, Gnarpe H: Mycoplasmas in semen from fertile and infertile men. Andrologia 6:45, 1974
29. Black FT, Rasmussen OG: Occurrence of T-strains and other mycoplasmata in nongonococcal urethritis. Br J Vener Dis 44:324, 1968
30. Archer JF: T-strain mycoplasma in the female urogenital tract. Br J Vener Dis 44:232, 1968
31. Klein JO, Buckland D, Finland M: Colonization of newborn infants by mycoplasmas. N Engl J Med 280:1025, 1969
32. Lee Y-H, McCormack WM, Marcy SM, Klein JO: The genital mycoplasmas: their role in disorders of reproduction and in pediatric infections. Pediatr Clin North Am 21:457, 1974
33. McCormack WM, Almeida PC, Bailey PE, Grady EM, Lee Y-H: Sexual activity and vaginal colonization with genital mycoplasmas. JAMA 221:1375, 1972
34. McCormack WM, Lee Y-H, Zinner SH: Sexual experience with urethral colonization with genital mycoplasmas: a study in normal men. Ann Intern Med 78:696, 1973

35. Jones DM: *Mycoplasma hominis* in pregnancy. J Clin Pathol 20:633, 1967
36. McCormack WM, Rosner B, Lee Y-H: Colonization with genital mycoplasmas in women. Am J Epidemiol 97:240, 1973
37. Foy HM, Kenny GE, Wentworth BB, Johnson WL, Grayston JT: Isolation of *Mycoplasma hominis*, T strains and cytomegalovirus from the cervix of pregnant women. Am J Obstet Gynecol 106:635, 1970
38. Taylor-Robinson D, Rassner C, Furr PM, Humber DP, Barness RD: Fetal wastage as a consequence of *Mycoplasma pulmonis* infection in mice. J Reprod Fertil 42:483, 1975
39. Fraser LR, Taylor-Robinson D: The effect of *Mycoplasma pulmonis* on fertilization and preimplantation development in vitro of mouse eggs. Fertil Steril 28:488, 1977
40. Swenson CE: Effect of *Mycoplasma pulmonis* on in vivo fertilization in the mouse. J Reprod Fertil 65:257, 1982
41. Gnarpe H, Friberg J: T-mycoplasmas on spermatozoa and infertility. Nature 245:97, 1973
42. Fowlkes DM, Dooher GB, O'Leary WM: Evidence by scanning electron microscopy for an association between spermatozoa and T-mycoplasmas in men of infertile marriage. Fertil Steril 26:1203, 1975
43. Cohen J, Gregson S: Antibodies and sperm survival in the female genital tract. In Spermatozoa, Antibodies and Infertility, Edited by J Cohen, WF Hendry. Oxford, Blackwell Scientific Publications, 1978, p 17
44. Gump DW, Gibson M, Ashikaga T: Lack of association between genital mycoplasmas and infertility. N Engl J Med 310:937, 1984
45. Cintron RD, Wortham JWE Jr, Acosta A: The association of semen factors with the recovery of *Ureaplasma urealyticum*. Fertil Steril 36:648, 1981
46. Naot Y: In vitro studies on the mitogenic activity of mycoplasmal species toward lymphocytes. Rev Infect Dis 4:S205, 1982
47. Hirth RS, Plastridge WN, Tourtellotte ME, Nielson SW: Genital mycoplasmosis in cattle and man. J Am Vet Med Assoc 148:277, 1966
48. Horne HW, Hertig AT, Kundsin RB, Kosasa TS: Subclinical endometrial inflammation and T-mycoplasmas: a possible cause of human reproductive failure. Int J Fertil 18:266, 1973
49. Witkin SS, Toth A: Relationship between genital tract infections, sperm antibodies in seminal fluid, and infertility. Fertil Steril 40:805, 1983
50. Allison AC, Paton GR: Chromosomal abnormalities in human diploid cells infected with mycoplasma and their possible relevance to the etiology of Down's syndrome (Mongolism). Lancet 2:1229, 1966
51. Kundsin RB, Ampola M, Streeter S, Neurath P: Chromosomal aberrations induced by T-strain mycoplasmas. J Med Genet 8:181, 1971
52. Fogh J, Fogh H: Chromosome changes in PPLO-infected FL human amnion cells. Proc Soc Exp Biol Med 119:233, 1965
53. Taylor-Robinson D, Mandill RJ: Sperm absorption and sperm agglutination by mycoplasma. Nature 215:484, 1967
54. Busolo F, Zanchetta R: The effect of *Mycoplasma hominis* and *Ureaplasma urealyticum* on hamster egg in vitro penetration by human spermatozoa. Fertil Steril 43:110, 1985
55. Mårdh P-A, Weström L: Tubal and cervical cultures in acute salpingitis with special reference to *Mycoplasma hominis* and *T-strain mycoplasmas*. Br J Vener Dis 46:179, 1970
56. Eschenbach DA, Buchanan TM, Pollock HM, Forsyth PS, Russell AE, Lin JKS, Wang SP, Wentworth BS, McCormack WM, Holmes KK: Polymicrobial etiology of acute pelvic inflammatory disease. N Engl J Med 293:166, 1975
57. Mårdh P-A, Weström L: Antibodies to *Mycoplasma hominis* in patients with genital infections and in healthy controls. Br J Vener Dis 46:390, 1970
58. Moller BR, Mårdh P-A, Ahrons S, Nussler E: *Chlamydia trachomatis, Mycoplasma hominis* and *Neisseria gonorrhoeae* in patients with signs of pelvic inflammatory disease. Sex Transm Dis 8:198, 1981
59. Sweet RL, Mills J, Hadley KW, Blumenstock E, Schachter J, Robbie MO, Draper DL: Use of laparoscopy to determine the microbiologic etiology of acute salpingitis. Am J Obstet Gynecol 134:68, 1979
60. Henry-Suchet J, Loffredo V: Chlamydiae and mycoplasma genital infection in salpingitis and tubal sterility. Lancet 1:539, 1980
61. Moller BR, Freundt EA, Black FT, Fredrikson P: Experimental infection of the genital tract of female grivet monkeys by *Mycoplasma hominis*. Infect Immun 20:258, 1979
62. Kundsin RB, Rowell T, Shepard MC, Panero A, Lunceford CD: T-strain mycoplasmas and reproductive failure in monkeys. Lab Anim Sci 25:221, 1975
63. Swenson CE, O'Leary WM: An animal model for the study of infectious human infertility. Fertil Steril 29:462, 1978
64. Mårdh P-A, Weström L, von Mecklenburg C, Hammar E: Studies on ciliated epithelia of the human genital tract. I. Swelling of the cilia of Fallopian tube epithelium in organ cultures infected with *Mycoplasma hominis*. Br J Vener Dis 52:52, 1976
65. Stalheim OHU, Proctor SJ, Gallagher JE: Growth and effects of ureaplasmas (T-Mycoplasmas) in bovine oviductal cultures. Infect Immun 13:915, 1976
66. Stalheim OHU, Gallagher JE: Ureaplasmal epithelial lesions related to ammonia. Infect Immun 15:995, 1977
67. Weidner W, Brunnertt H, Krause W: Quantitative cultures of *Ureaplasma urealyticum* in patients with chronic prostatitis or prostatosis. J Urol 124:622, 1980
68. Berger RE, Alexander ER, Harnisch JP, Paulsen CA, Monda GD, Ansell J, Holmes KK: Etiology, manifestations and therapy of acute epididymitis: prospective study of 50 cases. J Urol 121:750, 1979
69. Oriel JD: Role of genital mycoplasmas in nongonococcal urethritis and prostatitis. Sex Transm Dis 10:S263, 1983
70. Christie WB, Newcomb R, Rowson LE: Non-surgical transfer of bovine eggs: investigation of some factors affecting embryo survival. The Vet Rec 106:910, 1980
71. Gnarpe H, Friberg J: Mycoplasma and human reproductive failure. I. The occurrence of different mycoplasmas in couples with reproductive failure. Am J Obstet Gynecol 114:727, 1972

72. deLouvois J, Blades M, Harrison RF, Hurley R, Stanley VC: Frequency of mycoplasma in fertile and infertile couples. Lancet 1:1073, 1974
73. Matthews CD, Elmslie RG, Clapp KH, Svigos JM: The frequency of genital mycoplasma infection in human fertility. Fertil Steril 26:988, 1975
74. Stray-Pedersen B, Eng J, Reikman TM: Uterine T-mycoplasma colonization in reproductive failure. Am J Obstet Gynecol 130:307, 1978
75. Idriss WM, Patton WC, Taymor ML: On the etiologic role of *Ureaplasma urealyticum* (T-mycoplasma) infection in infertility. Fertil Steril 30:293, 1978
76. Rehewy MSE, Jaszczak S, Hafez ESE, Thomas A, Brown WJ: *Ureaplasma urealyticum* (T-mycoplasma) in vaginal fluid and cervical mucus from fertile and infertile women. Fertil Steril 30:297, 1978
77. Khatamee MA, Decker WH: Recovery of genital mycoplasma from infertile couples using New York City medium. Infertility 1:155, 1978
78. Koren Z, Spigland I: Irrigation technique for detection of mycoplasma intrauterine infection in infertile patients. Obstet Gynecol 52:588, 1978
79. Taymor ML: Mycoplasma infection. In Infertility, Edited by ML Taymor. New York, Grune & Stratton, 1978, p 126
80. Nagata Y, Iwasaka T, Wada T: Mycoplasma infection and infertility. Fertil Steril 31:392, 1979
81. Upadhyaya M, Hibbard BM, Walker SM: The role of mycoplasmas in reproduction. Fertil Steril 39:814, 1983
82. Love W, Jones M, Andrews B, Thomas M: Mycoplasmas in human infertility. Lancet 1:1130, 1973
83. Cassell GH, Younger BJ, Brown MB, Blackwell RE, Davis KJ, Marriott P, Stagno S: Microbiologic study of infertile women at the time of diagnostic laparoscopy. N Engl J Med 308:502, 1983
84. Cassell GH: The pathogenic potential of mycoplasmas: *Mycoplasma pulmonis* as a model. Rev Infect Dis 4:S18, 1982
85. Kundsin RB: Mycoplasma in genitourinary tract infection and reproductive failure. In Progress in Gynecology, Vol 5, Edited by SH Sturgis, ML Taymor. New York, Grune & Stratton, 1970, p 275
86. Friberg J, Gnarpe H: Mycoplasma and human reproductive failure. III. Pregnancies in "infertile" couples treated with doxycycline for T-mycoplasmas. Am J Obstet Gynecol 116:23, 1973
87. Harrison RF, Blades M, deLouvois J, Hurley R: Doxycycline treatment and human infertility. Lancet 1:605, 1975
88. Hinton RA, Egdell LM, Andrews BE, Clarke SKR, Richmond SJ: A double-blind cross-over study of the effect of doxycycline on mycoplasma infection and infertility. Br J Obstet Gynaecol 86:379, 1979
89. Paavonen J, Miettinen A, Stevens CE, Kiviat N, Kuo C-C, Stamm WE, Holmes KK: *Mycoplasma hominis* in cervicitis and endometritis. Sex Transm Dis 10:S276, 1983
90. Fowlkes DM, MacLeod J, O'Leary WM: T-mycoplasmas and human infertility: correlation of infection with alterations in seminal parameters. Fertil Steril 26:1212, 1975
91. Toth A, Swenson CE, O'Leary WM: Light microscopy as an aid in predicting ureaplasma infection in human semen. Fertil Steril 30:586, 1978
92. Swenson CE, Toth A, O'Leary WM: *Ureaplasma urealyticum* and human infertility: the effect of antibiotic therapy on semen quality. Fertil Steril 31:660, 1979
93. Desai S, Cohen MS, Khatamee M, Leiter E: *Ureaplasma urealyticum* (T-mycoplasma) infection: does it have a role in male infertility? J Urol 124:469, 1980
94. Rehewy MSE, Thomas AJ, Hafez ESE, Brown WJ, Moghissi KS, Jaszczak S: *Ureaplasma urealyticum* (T-mycoplasma) in seminal plasma and spermatozoa from infertile and fertile volunteers. Eur J Obstet Gynecol Reprod Biol 8:247, 1978
95. Toth A, Lesser ML, Brooks A, Labriola D: Subsequent pregnancies among 161 couples treated for T-mycoplasma genital-tract infection. N Engl J Med 308:505, 1983
96. Driscoll SG, Kundsin RB, Horne HW Jr, Scott JM: Infections and first trimester losses: possible role of mycoplasmas. Fertil Steril 20:1017, 1969
97. Harwick HJ, Purcell HR, Iuppa JB, Fekety RF Jr: *Mycoplasma hominis* and abortion. J Infect Dis 121:260, 1970
98. Caspi E, Solomon F, Sompolinsky D: Early abortion and mycoplasma infection. Isr J Med Sci 8:122, 1972
99. Horne HW Jr, Kundsin RB, Kosasa TS: The role of mycoplasma infection in human reproductive failure. Fertil Steril 25:380, 1974
100. Quinn PA, Shewchuck AB, Shuber J, Lie KI, Ryan E, Chipman ML, Noncilla DM: Efficacy of antibiotic therapy preventing spontaneous pregnancy loss. Am J Obstet Gynecol 145:239, 1983
101. Holmes MJ, Furr PM, Taylor-Robinson D: The persistence of ureaplasmas in the urogenital tract of men in the Antarctic. J Hyg (Lond) 72:355, 1974
102. Coufalik ED, Taylor-Robinson D, Csonka GW: Treatment of nongonococcal urethritis with rifampicin as a means of defining the role of *Ureaplasma urealyticum*. Br J Vener Dis 55:36, 1979
103. Evans RT, Taylor-Robinson D: The incidence of tetracycline-resistant strains of *Ureaplasma urealyticum*. J Antimicrob Chemother 4:57, 1978
104. Spaepen MS, Kundsin RB, Horne HW: Tetracycline-resistant T-mycoplasmas (*Ureaplasma urealyticum*) from patients with a history of reproductive failure. Antimicrob Agents Chemother 9:1012, 1976
105. Ford DK, Smith JR: Non-specific urethritis associated with tetracycline-resistant T-mycoplasma. Br J Vener Dis 50:373, 1974
106. Braun P, Klein JO, Kass EH: Susceptibility of genital mycoplasmas to antimicrobial agents. Appl Microbiol 19:62, 1970
107. Harwick HJ, Fekety RF: The antibiotic susceptibility of *Mycoplasma hominis*. J Clin Pathol 22:483, 1969

SECTION II

Reproductive Endocrinology

Endocrinologic management of reproductive problems requires a basic understanding of the interactions between the endocrine system and ovarian function. Endocrinologic aberrations can be appreciated through alterations in the appropriate function at any level along the hypothalamic-pituitary-ovarian axis as well as through their direct influences on the follicle and its enclosed oocyte. Advances in reproductive endocrinology over the past 3 years have included: (1) adaptations of the principles of hypothalamic releasing substances and their analogs; (2) knowledge of the behavior of prolactin-producing pituitary adenomas; (3) an enhanced understanding of the involvement of endogenous opioids in regulation of hypothalamic function; (4) protocols for achieving follicular and oocyte maturation; and (5) means whereby ovarian function can be assessed and monitored.

Congenital adrenal hyperplasia has been known for many years to result from a hereditary defect in one of the five enzymatic steps responsible for the conversion of cholesterol to cortisol. The clinical manifestations of a defect in any particular step in this sequence may depend upon a deficiency in cortisol biosynthesis as well as on the excessive accumulation of precursor steroids proximal to the block which are utilized for androgen biosynthesis. Many of the proteins involved in the biosynthesis of cortisol have been purified. Some of the genes responsible for enzyme production have also been isolated using principles of molecular genetics, thus enabling evaluation and treatment of certain cases of congenital adrenal hyperplasia. Brodie and Wentz have updated our perspective on congenital adrenal hyperplasia. Now because of the recognition that 21-hydroxylase deficiency is inherited as a monogenic autosomal recessive trait closely linked to the human leukocyte antigen (HLA) histocompatibility complex on chromosome 6, HLA typing can be employed to determine the carrier status of family members of the proband. Various forms of 21-hydroxylase deficiency are inherited as alleles of a single locus. Today's investigative tools enable us to establish the diagnosis prenatally and to treat the fetus by suppressing its pituitary with dexamethasone administered to the mother. These tools include: (1) determination of 17-hydroxyprogesterone in amniotic fluid; and (2) HLA typing of cells in amniotic fluid or in chorionic villus biopsy specimens, prior to the time at which masculinization of the external genitalia takes place in the affected female fetus. Testing of the nonpregnant patient with adrenocorticotropic hormone (ACTH) also enables recognition of attenuated forms of the disorder or diagnosis of adult onset adrenal hyperplasia.

A single isolated laboratory test frequently provides limited insight into the extent of the defect in endocrine disorders. When one considers that endocrine secretions demonstrate cyclic variations—long term, as in the human menstrual cycle; short term as in the diurnal variations of cortisol elaboration; and ultra-short term as in the case of oscillating levels of gonadotropins—a single measurement is certainly inadequate in assessing any endocrine function. The case of adrenal hyperplasia exemplifies this principle. Dynamic testing of endocrine function involves manipulation of the patient's hormonal milieu to evaluate the functional ability of an endocrine-secreting structure and its ability to be regulated through stimulation, suppression, or feedback. The review of dynamic testing in reproductive endocrinology in Schlaff's chapter characterizes the theory behind dynamic testing and reviews the tests currently used in the diagnosis of endocrine disorders. Protocols are provided and a discussion of the rationale, risks, and interpretation of each test serves as a convenient guide to dynamic testing in our subspecialty.

Prior to the introduction of ultrasound, detection and timing of ovulation depended primarily upon biochemical determinations of progesterone or its metabolites, histologic interpretation of uterine endometrium, and review of basal body temperature records. Ultrasound makes possible a noninvasive method of observing follicle development and detecting ovulation. This modality has achieved a prominent role in our diagnostic portfolio during the recent decade. Undoubtedly, in vitro fertilization (IVF) and related technologies have improved our skills in the use of exogenous gonadotropins for follicle maturation and for ovulation induction. Concomitantly, we now rely on sonography for guidance in establishing doses and protocols for use of these potent and expensive agents. Follicle tracking has indeed become standard operating procedure in gonadotropin therapy and useful in the appraisal of patients with unexplained infertility. Richie's chapter describes the sonographic findings associated with follicle tracking, and includes an atlas of findings. If there should be a syndrome characterized by luteinization of unruptured follicles, sonography may be the only noninvasive means for its detection. However, final proof of the existence of this proposed entity will depend upon identifying the retained oocyte within the follicle in cases in which a luteinized unruptured follicle (LUF) is suspected. Currently, although sonographic diagnosis of ovarian dysfunction is beset with many pitfalls, sonography has come to play a major role in follicle tracking. The scope of ultrasound in follicle tracking and oocyte retrieval alone can be appreciated by the current and projected sales data for ultrasound equipment. According to *The New York Times,* total sales of ultrasound equipment, including vaginal probes, are likely to rise to nearly $35 million within a few years from $5 million at present.

Three events have aided in rendering gonadotropin-releasing substances clinically useful. The identification of the biochemical structure of gonadotropin-releasing hormone (GnRH) led to the synthesis of this simple decapeptide. The recognition that GnRH is secreted into the hypothalamic-pituitary circulation in a pulsatile manner brought to light the refractory period during which the pituitary cell replenishes its receptors, a phenomenon also referred to as "down-regulation." The ability to make substitutions at active sites in the decapeptide molecule has led to the synthesis of long-acting, potent agonists and antagonists. The agonists act by causing sustained stimulation of the cell, thus leading to prolonged refractoriness; the antagonists compete with endogenous GnRH for receptor sites. The actions of GnRH and its analogs therefore depend upon the mode of their administration (pulsatile or continuous) and their duration of action. The continuous administration of long-acting agonists results in a hypoestrogenic state as a consequence of diminished luteinizing hormone (LH) and follicle-stimulating hormone (FSH) secretion. GnRH administered in a pulsatile fashion can substitute for a hypothalamic deficiency of this hormone and result in restoration of ovulation in the anovulatory patient. Zacur's chapter reviews the biochemistry of GnRH and presents practical aspects of its clinical use via portable infusion pumps. Although human menopausal gonadotropins and human chorionic gonadotropins (hMG, hCG) may induce ovulation, bypassing the pituitary and directly stimulating the ovaries, the replacement of the specific substance (GnRH) which is lacking is the most direct means to correct a deficiency state while maintaining internal controls. As Zacur points out, the use of GnRH and its analogs is not problem-free. Although hyperstimulation with GnRH is rare, multiple pregnancies have been reported with this means of ovulation induction. Attention also must be paid to optimizing the quality of the luteal phase when using GnRH.

Past volumes of *Modern Trends* trace the history of our knowledge of prolactin-secreting tumors. Archer's contribution in Volume I presented the physiologic basis for amenorrhea related to hyperprolactinemia and provided a differential diagnosis for prolactin excess.[1] In Volume 3, Barbieri and Ryan discussed the clinical pharmacology of bromocriptine.[2] The outcome of pregnancy among women treated for hyperprolactinemia was reviewed by Ruiz-Velasco also in Volume 3.[3] As data accumulate, the pathophysiology and behavior of prolactinomas have become better understood. Blackwell's contribution to this section focuses on diagnostic modalities for evaluation and management of prolactinomas. Computed tomography scans appear to provide excellent resolution of small tumors (2 mm in diameter); the schedule Blackwell proposes for radiographic follow-up of patients treated medically is helpful. Of course, two of the major questions confronting the clinician revolve around how long a patient with a prolactinoma should be treated medically and whether one can anticipate long-term arrest of tumor growth when using dopamine agonists. As Blackwell indicates in the introduction to his chapter, his objective was to summarize "the contemporary view of the diagnosis and treatment of pituitary prolactinomas." What is considered contemporary today will hopefully be viewed as a "historical milestone" within several years.

Edward E. Wallach, M.D.

REFERENCES

1. Archer DF: Current concepts of prolactin physiology in normal and abnormal conditions. In Modern Trends in Infertility and Conception Control, Vol 1, Edited by EE Wallach, RD Kempers. Baltimore, The Williams & Wilkins Co., 1979, p 134
2. Barbieri RL, Ryan KJ: Bromocriptine: endocrine pharmacology and therapeutic applications. In Modern Trends in Infertility and Conception Control, Vol 3, Edited by EE Wallach, RD Kempers. Chicago, Year Book Medical Publishers, Inc., 1985, p 206
3. Ruiz-Valasco V, Tolis G: Pregnancy in hyperprolactinemic woman. In Modern Trends in Infertility and Conception Control, Vol 3, Edited by EE Wallach, RD Kempers. Chicago, Year Book Medical Publishers, Inc., 1985, p 71

Chapter 9

Late onset congenital adrenal hyperplasia: a gynecologist's perspective

Beverly L. Brodie, M.D., F.R.C.S.C.
Anne Colston Wentz, M.D.

Center for Fertility and Reproductive Research, Department of Obstetrics and Gynecology, Vanderbilt University Medical Center, Nashville, Tennessee

Congenital adrenal hyperplasia encompasses a family of inherited disorders, involving in each instance a deficiency of one of several enzymes in the pathway required for normal adrenal steroidogenesis. In the last decade, great advances have been made in understanding this disease, particularly its genetic basis and the existence of allelic variants with their resulting phenotypic and biochemical characteristics. The literature, however, also has produced a confusing abundance of new terms and diagnostic tests, making it difficult for the clinician to decide which patients to test, what test to use, and how to interpret the results.

Several excellent reviews cover the classical forms of adrenal hyperplasia that are recognized at birth or during childhood and that present a pediatric management problem.[1–4] This article will review the current thoughts on the genetics, classification, diagnosis, and treatment of nonclassical or late-onset congenital adrenal hyperplasia (LOCAH), focusing particularly on 21-hydroxylase (21-OH) deficiency.

ANATOMY

The adrenal glands lie at the superior pole of each kidney and are composed of two distinct parts: an internal medulla and an external cortex. The adrenal medulla is functionally related to the sympathetic nervous system and secretes the hormones epinephrine and norepinephrine in response to sympathetic stimulation. The adrenal cortex, containing the zona glomerulosa, zona fasciculata, and zona reticularis, secretes three classes of steroid hormones: mineralocorticoids (e.g., aldosterone), glucocorticoids (e.g., cortisol) and sex steroids (e.g., androstenedione and testosterone) (Fig. 1).[5]

BIOSYNTHETIC PATHWAYS

Cholesterol is the biosynthetic precursor for all the steroid hormones. Plasma cholesterol and cholesterol esters are attached to low-density lipoproteins that react with receptors on the adrenal cortical cells allowing internalization of the cholesterol.[6] Some cholesterol may be formed de novo in the gland from acetate. Further conversion of the cholesterol occurs via a series of enzyme-mediated reactions involving removal of the cholesterol side chain, hydroxylation, and rearrangement of the A ring (Fig. 2). The first step in the pathway, where the side chain is cleaved from cholesterol yielding pregnenolone, is under the control of adrenocorticotropic hormone (ACTH) in the fasciculata and reticularis cells and is the rate-limiting step for cortisol biosynthesis.[7] The subsequent steps in the formation of individual steroid hormones simply require sufficient substrate and appropriate enzymes.

FEEDBACK REGULATION

A negative feedback system is operative between the adrenal gland and the anterior pituitary whereby decreased cortisol levels stimulate increased ACTH release from the pituitary and increased levels suppress it. Common to all forms of congenital adrenal hyperplasia is a relative deficiency of cortisol production secondary to a congenital enzyme deficiency, leading to increased

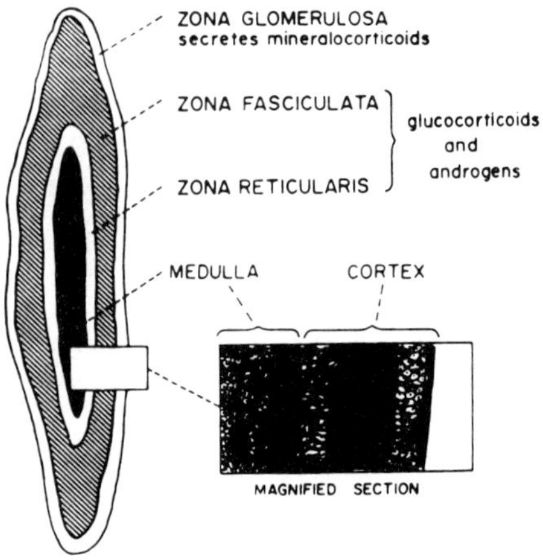

Figure 1 Secretion of adrenocortical hormones by the different zones of the adrenal cortex. (From Guyton AC.[5] Reproduced with the permission of the publisher.)

ACTH release. Depending on the severity of the enzyme defect, serum cortisol levels may or may not be normalized by the increased circulating levels of ACTH. In any case, elevated levels of the precursor hormones result in identifiable biochemical and phenotypic deviations from normal. The location of the block determines which precursors are elevated while the relative severity of the enzyme deficiency determines the extent to which an individual is affected clinically. Using 21-OH deficiency as an example, the deficit, in its mildest form, may result in a normal phenotype, normal serum cortisol levels, and precursor aberrations identifiable only with provocative testing. In its most severe form, cortisol levels are depressed, female infants are virilized by the overproduction of fetal adrenal androgens, and death may occur secondary to a salt-wasting crisis.

21-HYDROXYLASE DEFICIENCY

Historical Background

The first case compatible with congenital adrenal hyperplasia was reported in 1865 by Luigi de Crecchio, Professor of Anatomy at the University of Naples.[8] His detailed report described a patient who had the appearance of a young man, bearded, with a male pubic hair distribution and penis, but with first-degree hypospadias and the internal genital structures of a woman: uterus, vagina, fallopian tubes, and ovaries. While further case reports appeared in the literature,[9] the etiology of this intersex disease remained a mystery for many years. By the late 1930s, advances in urinary steroid chemistry allowed measurement of androgen metabolites and led to the recognition that the adrenal glands, markedly hypertrophied in patients with this disease, produced excess androgens.[10] In 1937, Butler and Marrian[11] identified 3,17,20-preganetriol, a urinary metabolite of 17-hydroxyprogesterone (17-OHP), in the urine of a group of female pseudohermaphrodites and, finally, in the 1950s,[12] the pathways necessary for biosynthesis of cortisol were detailed and the enzyme blocks demonstrated.[13]

Originally, deficiency of the 21-OH enzyme was thought to be an all-or-none phenomenon, presenting at birth with ambiguity of the genitalia (in females) secondary to increased adrenal androgen production in utero and progressing, if untreated, to include such symptoms as development of a masculine body habitus, precocious appearance of sexual hair, acne, further enlargement of the clitoris, hirsutism, oligomenorrhea, and infertility. It became apparent, however, that hyperandrogenic symptoms in a female, attributable to malfunction of the 21-OH enzyme, could appear for the first time not only at birth but later in childhood or peripubertally. Since the early 1950s, gynecologists

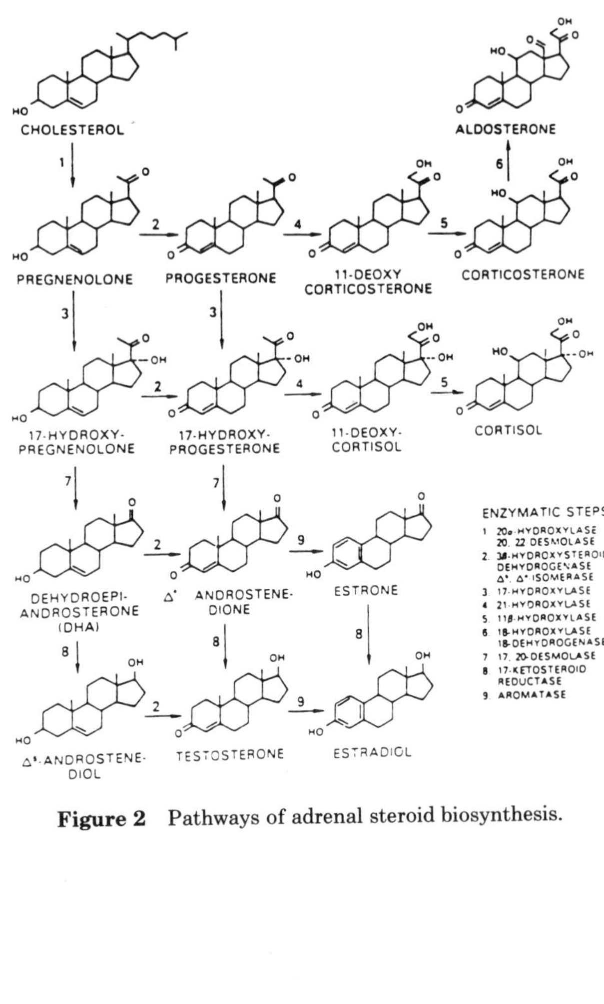

Figure 2 Pathways of adrenal steroid biosynthesis.

have suspected that some patients presenting with a polycystic ovarian picture of oligomenorrhea and hirsutism had a variant of classical congential hyperplasia.[14] Hormonal testing of affected individuals and their relatives revealed a spectrum of biochemical responses associated with varying phenotypes. The terms late-onset, partial, nonclassical, attenuated, and acquired were coined to emphasize the delayed onset of symptoms and distinguish this entity from the more severe classical form of disease with its prenatal onset. It was not until the discovery of linkage between 21-OH and the human leukocyte antigen (HLA) loci[15] that the true relationships between these apparently different forms of disease could be determined.

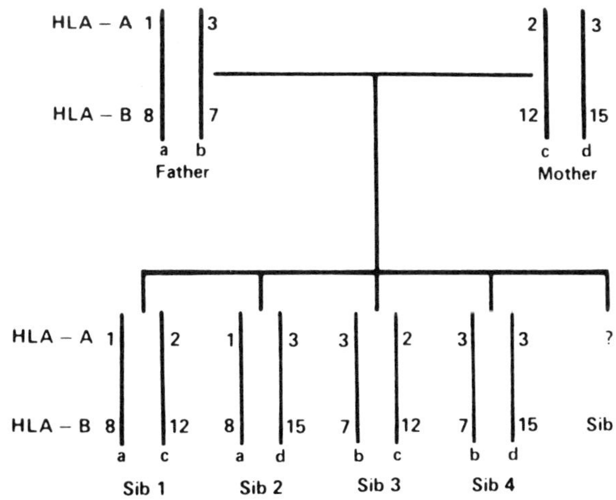

Figure 3 Segregation of HLA haplotypes in a typical Caucasian family. One of the father's number 6 chromosomes is marked by HLA-A1, B8 (*a*), and his other by HLA-A3, B7 (*b*). Similarly, the mother's number 6 chromosomes are marked by HLA-A2, B12 (*c*) and HLA-A3, B15 (*d*). *a,b,c,* and *d* are referred to as haplotypes and each child inherits only one haplotype from each parent. Barring genetic recominbation, Sib 5 must be HLA identical to one of his siblings. For clarity, only HLA-A and -B loci are included. (From Harris R.[16] Reproduced with the permission of the publisher.)

Genetics

Congenital adrenal hyperplasia is transmitted as an autosomal recessive trait with males and females equally affected.[1] Close genetic linkage between the HLA complex located on the short arm of chromosome six and 21-OH deficiency was first described by Dupont et al. in 1977.[15] The HLA complex, coding for a large number of leukocyte surface antigens important in human organ transplantation, is comprised of several closely linked loci. Four of these loci, HLA-A, HLA-B, HLA-C, and HLA-D/DR, can be defined by serologic testing and have been subdivided further on the basis of the specific tissue antigen produced by each of their multiple alleles (e.g., B14, A2, DR7, A9). One allele from each of HLA loci A, B, C, and D/DR constitutes a "haplotype." Each individual carries two haplotypes, having inherited one from the father and one from the mother. Figure 3[16] depicts the pattern of haplotype inheritance within a family, illustrating the en bloc transmission of intact haplotypes from generation to generation. Studies of families with informative recombinations clearly indicate that the 21-OH deficiency gene segregates with HLA-B, constituting genetic linkage with this locus.[4,17] The closer together two loci are on a chromosome, the less likely they will be to separate when recombination of genetic material occurs. Genetic linkage occurs with a locus, not with a particular allele at that locus. In contrast, genetic linkage disequilibrium is the nonrandom association of particular alleles of different genetic loci; in this case, a particular HLA-coded antigen in patients with 21-OH deficiency occurs more frequently than in the general population. For classical 21-OH deficiency, the most significant association is with HLA-B47.[18–20] Genetic linkage disequilibrium also has been reported for the nonclassical form of 21-OH deficiency, with a significantly increased frequency of HLA-B14, DR1 observed.[21–25]

Because 21-OH deficiency is inherited in an autosomal recessive fashion, parents of a homozygous (affected) child are obligate heterozygotes, each having contributed one 21-OH deficiency gene to the child. ACTH stimulation testing of obligate heterozygotes shows a 17-OHP response indicating a reduction of 21-OH enzyme function compared with controls.[26–32] The deficit is mild, however, and some degree of overlap exists with the general population. Testing of females with the late-onset form of disease produces a response intermediate between that of classical homozygotes and their heterozygote parents.[33–35] The response exhibited by heterozygotes for late onset 21-OH deficiency is similar to that of classical heterozygotes.[35]

By combined HLA genotyping and ACTH stimulation testing of families that contained patients with late-onset or classical disease, the concept of allelic variants at the 21-OH locus evolved.[24,36–38] Kohn et al.[36] studied ten females with symptoms of androgen excess attributable to late-onset 21-OH deficiency and their families using ACTH stimulation and HLA typing. In addition to the ten patients, eight family members exhibited an abnormal 17-OHP response to ACTH. Of these, some had clinical evidence of androgen excess whereas others were phenotypically normal, representing the so-called cryptic form of 21-OH deficiency, evidenced only on biochemical testing. Kohn and coworkers[36] concluded that the classical form of 21-OH deficiency, in linkage disequilibrium with the HLA-B47 allele, is transmitted by an allelic variant of steroid 21-OH different from that of the late-onset disease which is in linkage disequilibrium with B14. Cryptic 21-OH deficiency, also in linkage disequilibrium with B14, responds to ACTH testing in a manner that is indistinguishable from the late-onset form suggesting that, despite the absence of symptoms, it is transmitted by the same allele.[39,40]

The 21-OH gene has been cloned recently,[41] allowing better understanding of the genetic architecture underlying this enzyme deficiency. A particularly important application of this technique relates to prenatal diagnosis. Presently, amniocentesis at or after 16 weeks' gestation is required to allow measurement of amniotic fluid 17-OHP[42,43] or HLA typing of cultured amniotic fluid cells[44] to determine whether a fetus is affected with congenital adrenal hyperplasia. Since masculinization of the female fetus is thought to occur between 10 and 16 weeks' gestation,[45] genital virilization will occur before the results of diagnostic amniocentesis are available and the only decision remaining is whether to terminate the pregnancy. Using chorionic villus sampling and molecular biology techniques, it may be possible in the future to offer prenatal diagnosis to couples at risk early in the first trimester. Studies have shown that maternal ingestion of dexamethasone early in pregnancy can prevent fetal virilization.[45]

Classification

A scheme of classification has been suggested by Kohn and associates[36] (Table 1). This scheme recognizes three alleles for 21-OH deficiency (21-OH deficiency^{normal}, 21-OH deficiency^{mild}, 21-OH deficiency^{severe}). Classical disease results when an individual is homozygous for the 21-OH deficiency^{severe} allele. Simple virilizing denotes a reduction of cortisol production alone, while in salt-wasting both cortisol and aldosterone production are impaired.[2] The terms late-onset, partial, acquired, nonclassical, and attenuated are synonymous for individuals who carry either two mild alleles (homozygous mild) or one mild and one severe allele (compound heterozygote). Despite the absence of symptoms, individuals with cryptic 21-OH deficiency are biochemically indistinguishable from those with the late-onset form[39,40] and carry the same genotypes (21-OH deficiency^{mild}/21-OH deficiency^{mild} or 21-OH deficiency^{severe}/21-OH deficiency^{mild}). Finally, heterozygotes for either the mild or severe deficiency allele exhibit the mildest enzyme deficiency and are clinically asymptomatic.[40]

Incidence

Among North American and European populations, the estimated incidence of classical congenital adrenal hyperplasia (21-OH) varies between 1 in 5000 and 1 in 15,000 live births, with one out of

Table 1 Glossary of Terms for Disorders of Steroid 21-OH Deficiency[a]

Form of 21-OH deficiency	Clinical phenotype	Hormonal phenotype	21-OH genotype[b]
Classical	Virilized prenatally and symptomatic	Markedly elevated serum 17-OHP and Δ4 concentration	21-OH deficiency^{severe} / 21-OH deficiency^{severe}
Nonclassical	Symptomatic: Virilized postnatally and symptomatic Asymptomatic: Not virilized prenatally or postnatally and asymptomatic	Modestly elevated serum 17-OHP and Δ4 concentration	21-OH deficiency^{severe} / 21-OH deficiency^{mild} or 21-OH deficiency^{mild} / 21-OH deficiency^{mild}

[a] From Kohn et al.[36] Reproduced with permission of the publisher.
[b] The allelic variant that transmits severe 21-OH deficiency is in genetic linkage disequilibrium with HLA-Bw47. The allelic variant that transmits mild 21-OH deficiency is in genetic linkage disequilibrium with HLA-B14.

every 100 Caucasians being a genetic carrier.[4] An unusually high incidence is seen among the Yupik Eskimos of Alaska, where neonatal screening programs measuring the 17-OHP of heel stick capillary blood have documented a disease frequency of 1 in 684 live births.[46] In contrast to classical congenital adrenal hyperplasia, individuals with the nonclassical form have lower baseline 17-OHP, are not affected at birth, and may remain phenotypically normal throughout life. Therefore, frequency estimates for the general population cannot be based upon the results of neonatal screening programs or case surveys. Instead, frequencies obtained using genetic linkage markers and ACTH testing of affected families have been extrapolated to the general population. As in the classical form, ethnic differences have been observed. Speiser et al.[21] found the frequency of nonclassical disease and its heterozygous carrier state to be 1 in 27 and 1 in 3, respectively, for Ashkenazi Jews; 1 in 53 and 1 in 4 for Hispanics; 1 in 63 and 1 in 5 for Yugoslavs; 1 in 333 and 1 in 9 for Italians; and 1 in 1000 and 1 in 14 for other Caucasians. As Figure 4 illustrates,

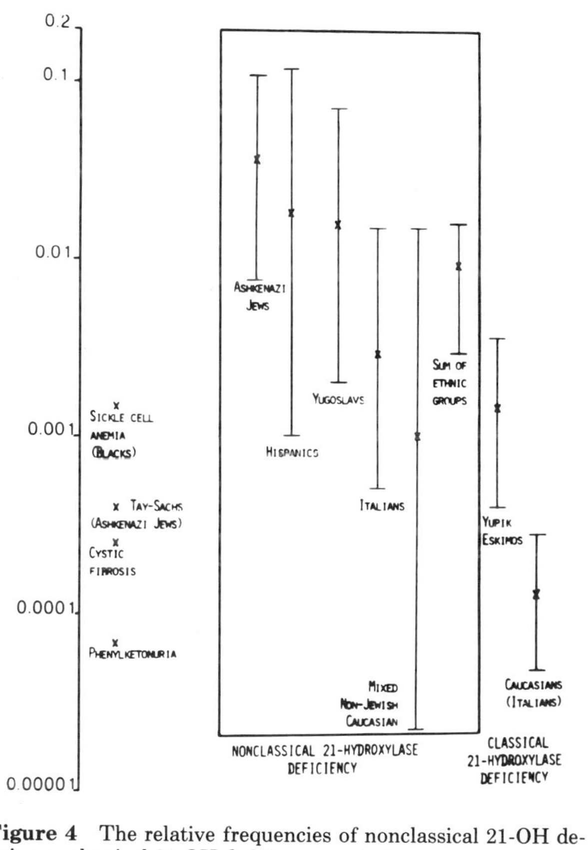

Figure 4 The relative frequencies of nonclassical 21-OH deficiency, classical 21-OH deficiency, and other autosomal recessive disorders. (From Speiser et al.[21] Reproduced with the permission of the publisher.)

Table 2 Spectrum of Clinical Features That May Affect Patients with Symptomatic Nonclassical (Late-Onset) 21-OH Deficiency

Precocious adrenarche
Advanced bone age
Acne
Oily hair
Temporal balding
Clitoromegaly
Short adult height
Hirsutism
Menstrual irregularity
Amenorrhea
Infertility

LOCAH is one of the most common autosomal recessive disorders in humans.

Based on the 17-OHP response to ACTH testing, the incidence of 21-OH deficiency among hirsute women is estimated to be between 1.2% and 20.0%.[47–53] These studies, viewed as a composite, document 40 cases of LOCAH among 804 hirsute women, or an incidence of 5.0%.

Clinical Features

Nonclassical congenital adrenal hyperplasia is a disease of extreme phenotypic diversity. Affected individuals, while normal at birth, may present in childhood, peri- or postpubertally, with symptoms referable to excess androgen production,[47–57] or, in the case of cryptic 21-OH deficiency, individuals may not manifest symptoms at all (Table 2).[36,38] Salt-wasting has never been reported in association with nonclassical disease.[4] Within a given family, late onset and cryptic 21-OH deficiency may exist in siblings who are biochemically and genotypically identical. It is not uncommon for symptoms to wax and wane during a lifetime. Cryptic patients have been reported to develop symptoms (sometimes quite rapidly) and symptomatic late-onset patients have been reported to undergo spontaneous improvement.[36] It remains uncertain why this phenotypic variability exists. Most likely, as suggested by Kuttenn et al.,[53] factors other than the degree of genetic mutation and enzyme deficiency are important, such as (1) variability in cortisol requirements among different subjects, caused by differences in environment and resulting in differences in androgen production; (2) differences in the capacity of the adrenal biosynthetic pathway, including the metabolism of 17-OHP to either androgens or pregnanetriol; and (3) individual sensitivity to androgens (exemplified by idiopathic hirsutism in the face of normal androgen levels).

Clinicians have recognized for years that, among patients presenting for evaluation of hirsutism, acne, and oligomenorrhea, a subgroup exists that has LOCAH.[33,47–59] Attempts are made to identify these women because corticosteroid therapy has proved beneficial.[48,49,55,56] Despite claims to the contrary,[52] it must be emphasized that, based on physical findings and presenting complaints alone, it is impossible to distinguish between women with LOCAH and those with symptoms of other masculinizing disorders, such as polycystic ovarian disease and idiopathic hirsutism.[47–49,53,54] Therefore, some form of diagnostic screening must be performed.

Importance of Diagnosis

Accurate identification of patients with LOCAH is important. Serum androgen levels and dexamethasone suppression testing are not helpful in distinguishing LOCAH from other causes of adrenal hyperandrogenism[48,50,57] and, whereas patients with the latter may respond satisfactorily to a 1-year course of dexamethasone therapy (some exhibiting no recurrence after discontinuation),[60] patients with the former require long-term therapy. Oral contraceptives, widely used to suppress ovarian androgen production, may also suppress adrenal function, as demonstrated by a decrease in ACTH[61] and serum dehydroepiandrosterone sulfate (DHEAS).[62] Although of benefit for the treatment of hirsutism in patients with LOCAH who require contraception, oral contraceptives are an inappropriate choice for primary therapy, especially in patients over 35, since they do not remedy the source of the problem (i.e., decreased cortisol production). Finally, it is important for the purposes of genetic counselling to determine whether a patient is affected with congenital adrenal hyperplasia. For example, if a woman's genotype is compound heterozygote ($21\text{-OH}^{severe}/21\text{-OH}^{mild}$) and her husband also happens to carry a 21-OH^{severe} allele, preconception counselling is advisable since they have a 25% chance of conceiving a child with the classical form of disease. Also, treatment with dexamethasone during the first trimester might be instituted in such a pregnancy since prenatal glucocorticoid therapy has been shown to prevent virilization of fetuses identified to be at risk.[45]

Baseline Hormone Values

Testosterone

Plasma testosterone (T) levels may be elevated or fall within the range of normal.[38,53] When compared with patients with other causes of hirsutism, the elevations of T in LOCAH are similar,[48,49,54] as illustrated in Figure 5. Treatment with dexamethasone markedly decreases serum levels.[50,55]

Androstenedione and Dehydroepiandrosterone Sulfate

Elevation of androstenedione is common,[53] but values generally fall within the 95% confidence limits established for hirsute women.[49,54] Following ACTH administration, a marked increase in serum androstenedione occurs, exceeding that observed in hirsute or normal women.[35,49] DHEAS levels overlap significantly with those of normal controls[38,50,51,53] (Fig. 6).

Cortisol and Adrenocorticotropic Hormone

Baseline serum cortisol levels are normal,[33,49,50,53,54] as are ACTH levels.[48,50,53,54] Following ACTH stimulation, blunting of the cortisol response has been observed in some patients,[34,49,53] suggesting that these patients may be susceptible to cortisol deficiency during periods of stress.

Follicle-Stimulating Hormone and Luteinizing Hormone

Follicle-stimulating hormone (FSH) to luteinizing hormone (LH) ratios are variable among patients with LOCAH. They may be normal,[50,51] slightly elevated,[54] or demonstrate the classic 3:1 pattern observed in women with polycystic ovarian disease (PCOD).[48]

17-Hydroxyprogesterone

Random plasma values in LOCAH tend to be elevated when compared with normal women in the follicular phase,[38] but overlap those of women with

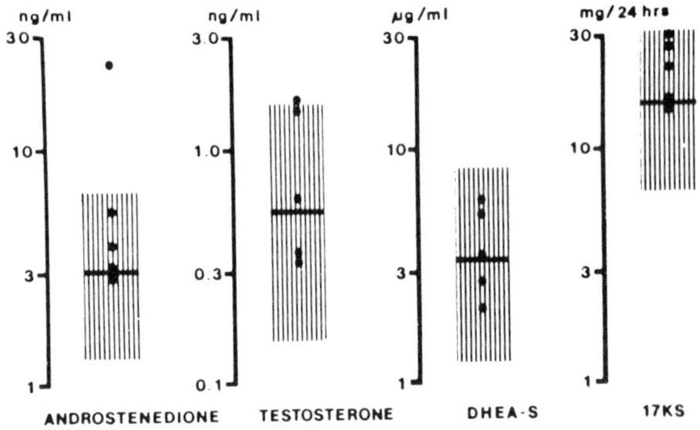

Figure 5 Serum levels of androstenedione, testosterone, DHEA-S, and urinary 17-ketosteroids (17-KS) in five patients with CAH (*dots*) as compared with the 95% confidence limits established for these steroids in 47 hirsute women (*hatched bars*). (From Lobo and Goebelsmann.[49] Reproduced with the permission of the publisher.)

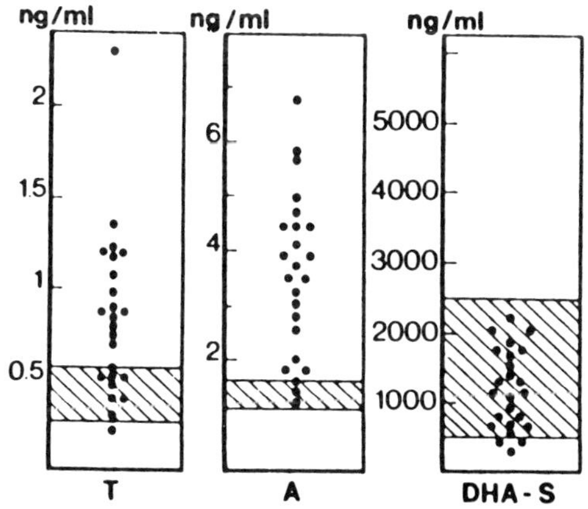

Figure 6 Androgen levels in 24 women with LOCAH. T denotes plasma testosterone; A, androstenedione; DHA-S, dehydroepiandrosterone sulfate. *Hatched areas* indicate normal ranges. (From Kuttenn et al.[53] Reproduced with the permission of *The New England Journal of Medicine* [313:224, 1985].)

other causes of hirsutism.[47,49,54] During the luteal phase, ovarian production of 17-OHP increases the basal levels in all groups,[33] making distinction more difficult. A circadian pattern of production, mimicking cortisol, has been described in LOCAH,[47,54,63] with values peaking around 6 A.M. This rhythm is not observed in normal or other hirsute women[63] and is abolished by therapeutic administration of dexamethasone.[47]

Stimulated Hormone Values

Assay of 17-OHP following ACTH stimulation is an accurate method of diagnosing LOCAH.[35,47–50] While many investigators believe that routine screening of hirsute oligomenorrheic women with ACTH is necessary,[48,50,53] others have questioned the cost-effectiveness of this approach, suggesting that stimulation testing be limited to women demonstrating particular symptoms[52] or defined elevations of 17-OHP[54] and T.[51]

A variety of methods that have been proposed to detect individuals with deficient 21-OH activity are summarized subsequently.

Method of Gutai and Associates[28]

Gutai et al.[28] examined 16 controls and 14 obligate heterozygotes before and 30, 45, and 60 minutes after a 1.0-mg intravenous (IV) bolus of Cortrosyn (ACTH 1-24, Organon, Inc., West Orange, NJ). Testing was performed during the follicular phase, but time of day was not controlled. A significant difference was observed in the rate of increase of both progesterone (P) and 17-OHP at 30, 45, and 60 minutes between controls and heterozygotes, with the greatest rate of rise seen at 30 minutes. Combining the rates of increase of P and 17-OHP resulted in the best separation between groups, and the mean value obtained for the controls plus 2 standard deviations (SD) was chosen as the upper limit of normal. This formula is defined as follows:

$$\text{Normal} = \frac{(P_{30} - P_0) + (17\text{-OHP}_{30} - 17\text{-OHP}_0)}{30 \text{ minutes}} \leq 6.5 \text{ ng/dl/min.}$$

In a later study of two affected families, Lee et al.[39] found the greatest rates of increase of 17-OHP and P for normal males and females were 6.7 and 6.8 ng/dl/min, respectively. Therefore, they amended the original value of 6.5 ng/dl/min such that heterozygosity is diagnosed if the combined rate of rise of 17-OHP and P exceed 6.8 ng/dl/min. The mean elevation of 17-OHP after ACTH stimulation in women with LOCAH is greater than that of heterozygotes[35] (Table 3); thus, these diagnostic criteria proposed for heterozygote identification will also allow detection of women with LOCAH.

Method of Krensky and Associates[27]

This study also attempted to define a method whereby heterozygote carriers of classical congenital adrenal hyperplasia could be distinguished from the general population. 17-OHP levels were measured in 14 controls and 26 obligate heterozygotes prior to and 30, 60, and 90 minutes after 25 units (0.25 mg) of Cortrosyn administered IV push. 17-OHP levels were significantly higher at 60 and 90 minutes in the heterozygotes. Using an arbitrary cut-off for normality of 200 ng/dl at 60 minutes identified 77% of the heterozygotes, but considerable overlap with controls existed. Raising the cut-off to 250 ng/dl eliminated the false-positives, but decreased heterozygote identification to 58%. Again, although stimulated levels of 17-OHP in LOCAH will markedly exceed 250 ng/dl at 60 minutes, Table 3 points out that some genotypically normal individuals may also exceed this value, resulting in incorrect assignment of diagnosis.

Method of Dewailly and Associates[54]

An attempt was made to provide guidelines that would allow more selective screening of hirsute patients, reserving ACTH stimulation for a specific subgroup. Clinical and hormonal data were analyzed from 20 adult patients in whom the diagnosis of LOCAH was established using ACTH 1-24 stimulation testing (0.25 mg IV bolus at 8 A.M.). Bloods for 17-OHP were drawn at time 0 and 60 minutes. The authors concluded that clinical diagnosis of

Table 3 ACTH Tests: 60-minute ACTH-Stimulated Hormone Concentrations of 17-OHP and Δ4-Androstenedione (Δ4) of Patients Used to Generate Nomogram in Figure 7[a]

	Classical CAH patients			Nonclassical patients			Classical hets[b]				Nonclassical hets				
	SW[c]	SV[d]	SW + SV	Late-onset	Cryptic	Cryptic + late-onset	Parents only	SW hets	SV hets	SW + SV hets	Late-onset hets	Cryptic hets	Classical and nonclassical hets	HLA normal	General population
60-min 17-OHP (ng/dl)															
n[e]	3	3	6	12	8	20	83	51	56	104	10	6	123	5	51
Average	27,520	38,276	39,457	6110	9210	7350	637	638	640	639	511	920	639	208	351
SD	14,963	13,740	12,354	3092	4006	3724	248	242	270	255	245	477	255	92	221
Minimum	16,260	23,300	16,260	2160	3290	2160	210	210	295	210	230	320	210	120	119
Maximum	44,500	50,300	50,300	12,320	16,050	16,050	1544	1490	1590	1590	960	1650	1590	350	920
60-min Δ^4 (ng/dl)[f]															
n[e]	3	4	7	12	8	20	83	43	49	92	6	4	102	2	27
Average	1987	1057	1456	586	537	567	207	205	214	210	232	169	205	181	198
SD	1903	430	1244	350	167	286	75	73	83	77	90	66	78	57	96
Minimum	480	621	480	242	295	242	49	78	105	278	147	124	78	141	61
Maximum	4126	1604	4126	1379	804	1379	396	356	411	411	393	265	411	221	538

[a] From New et al.[35] Reproduced with permission of the publisher.
[b] hets, heterozygotes.
[c] SW, salt-wasting.
[d] SV, simple virilizing.
[e] Number of tests in population described in Table 1.
[f] Except for classical and nonclassical CAH patients, only subjects in Tanner stages IV and V are included.

LOCAH was impossible, but recommended screening hirsute patients with a baseline 17-OHP assay obtained during the follicular phase at 8 A.M. They thought that, when baseline levels were below 2 ng/ml, the diagnosis was considered unlikely and, above 5 ng/ml, the diagnosis was confirmed. Only patients having basal 17-OHP values between 2 and 5 ng/ml required ACTH stimulation testing for diagnosis.

The drawback with this method is the requirement for patients to return to the office during a specific time in their menstrual cycle for screening and, if the result is equivocal (2 to 5 ng/ml), to return again for the stimulation testing.

Method of New and Associates[35]

By plotting the log of the baseline and ACTH-stimulated 17-OHP values of a genetically defined population, a nomogram was devised (Fig. 7) that provides the clinician with an easy method for diagnosing and predicting the degree of 21-OH deficiency. The population whose data generated the nomogram included affected patients, their parents (obligate heterozygotes), and other family members in whom recombination between the steroid 21-OH gene and HLA-B or DR locus was excluded. In all, 7 patients with classical congenital adrenal hyperplasia, 18 patients with nonclassical congenital adrenal hyperplasia, 120 heterozygotes, 5 family members predicted by HLA genotyping to be unaffected, and 51 subjects from the general population were examined. The ACTH-stimulated 17-OHP values of the various groups are shown in Table 3. The coordinates of their hormonal values aggregated into easily distinguishable groups, distributed on a regression line in order of descending severity: classical 21-OH deficiency, nonclassical 21-OH deficiency, heterozygotes for classical and nonclassical disease, and unaffected individuals.

Originally, nomograms using long and short ACTH stimulation tests were created. In the long test, ACTHAR 40 units (Armour Pharmaceutical, Tarrytown, NJ) or ACTH 1-24 0.4 mg was administered as a continuous IV infusion in 250 ml 5% dextrose for 360 minutes beginning at 8 A.M. In the short test, ACTH 1-24 0.25 mg was injected IV bolus at 8 A.M. Blood samples for 17-OHP were drawn at time 0 and 360 or 60 minutes, respectively. Because the results of the two correlated strongly, the shorter, more convenient test is now recommended for routine use. This 60-minute test provides an easy and reliable method of screening for late-onset 21-OH deficiency in a hirsute patient population. The advantages are numerous: testing must be performed in the morning (8 A.M.) but need not be scheduled during a particular phase of the menstrual cycle, only one visit and two 17-OHP assays are required for diagnosis, and family members also can be tested, their hormonal values

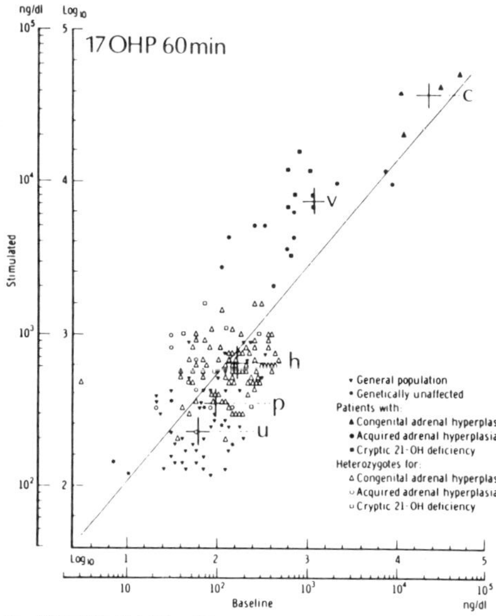

Figure 7 Nomogram relating baseline and 60-minute ACTH-stimulated serum 17-OHP concentrations. The mean values for each group are as follows: *c*, congenital adrenal hyperplasia; *v*, patients with nonclassical symptomatic (late-onset) or asymptomatic (cryptic) 21 OH deficiency; *h*, heterozygotes for classical CAH, nonclassical symptomatic CAH, and nonclassical asymptomatic CAH; *u*, family members predicted by HLA genotyping to be unaffected; and *p*, general population (not genotyped). (From New et al.[35] Reproduced with the permission of the publisher.)

plotted on the nomogram, and a genotype assigned. Classical and nonclassical 21-OH deficiencies are readily identified and minimal overlap exists between the lowest heterozygote and highest HLA "normal" populations. The considerable overlap observed between the heterozygote and "general" populations is not surprising in view of the high incidence of heterozygosity in the latter.

Method of Chrousos and Associates[24]

A method of testing was proposed to detect LOCAH in hirsute women who have been treated with glucocorticoids empirically without prior testing for 21-OH deficiency. HLA genotyping of affected families revealed two individuals who had LOCAH and were receiving empiric treatment with dexamethasone. These individuals underwent testing with 160 units cosyntropin in normal saline infused IV over 48 hours. Blood samples were drawn at 0, 8, 24, 30, 36, and 48 hours. The 17-OHP response of both patients was increased markedly compared with that of 11 young female controls on glucocorticoid therapy for nonadrenal disease such as idiopathic thrombocytopenic purpura. Compared with controls, patient plasma cortisol levels were significantly blunted during the stimulation.

Dexamethasone Pretreatment

Dexamethasone administration the evening prior to ACTH testing has been suggested to improve detection of 21-OH deficiency heterozygotes.[29,30] Some authors use overnight dexamethasone suppression when testing for LOCAH.[49,52] Theoretically, baseline fluctuation of steroid values will be diminished so that the incremental response of cortisol precursors can be evaluated precisely. Rosenfield et al.[64] examined the efficacy of dexamethasone pretreatment in ACTH testing for mild defects of 21-OH enzyme activity and believed that it offered no advantage. Simply measuring the pre- and post-ACTH 17-OHP levels seems to be an adequate way of diagnosing LOCAH.[35]

Adrenocorticotropic Hormone Dosage and Administration

A bolus IV injection of 250 μg (25 units) of ACTH 1-24 is commonly employed for adrenal function screening[35,48,51,52,54] and the cortisol response evoked compares favorably with that induced by insulin hypoglycemia testing,[65] suggesting maximal adrenal stimulation using this dose. Investigators have tried to determine what minimum dose of ACTH is required to elicit a maximum cortisol response from the adrenal. ACTH has a short half-life,[66] but this can be overcome by using either continuous administration of a small dose or bolus injection of a larger one. Chrousos and associates[67] observed that 2 units of ACTH 1-24 infused continuously over 30 minutes was as effective as 25 units administered IV bolus. Graybeal and Fang[68] reported that the pattern of cortisol secretion following 0.2 μg/kg of ACTH 1-24 infused over 10 minutes was indistinguishable from the cortisol response to insulin hypoglycemia, suggesting that the 250-μg dose used in the method of New et al.[35] and the 1000-μg dose used by Gutai et al.[28] are unnecessarily large. To date, no studies have been published that compare the 17-OHP response to smaller bolus doses of ACTH using the methods of either Gutai or New. Therefore, the original doses used to establish the standards must continue to be employed. One could argue that administration of at least 250 μg, which represents a generously supraphysiologic dose, will ensure that every patient, regardless of weight, will receive maximal stimulation.

Treatment

Expected Results

In women with LOCAH, glucocorticoid administration will decrease endogenous ACTH stimulation of the adrenals and diminish cortisol precursor production.[47,48,50,55] Expected results of treatment include return of menstrual cyclicity, decreased acne, and regression of hirsutism.[55,56,60,69] Correction of luteal phase deficiency was described in one patient following treatment with adequate doses of glucocorticoid replacement.[70] Normal fertility is possible even in women with a prolonged period of missed diagnosis or noncompliance with resulting virilization during childhood if contemporary control is adequate.[71]

Choice of Therapy and Follow-up

The aim of therapy in childhood is to achieve normal growth and sexual maturation. Replacement doses of glucocorticoids must be monitored vigorously to avoid over- or undersuppression, both of which will compromise a child's growth and development.[2,3,71] In women who have reached their ultimate adult height, iatrogenic growth retardation is no longer a problem and correction of symptoms may be achieved with larger doses of a long-acting glucocorticoid. Dexamethasone has been shown to suppress the hypothalamic-pituitary-adrenal axis better than cortisone acetate or hydrocortisone administered in equivalent doses to adults with congenital adrenal hyperplasia,[72] and may induce less fluid retention than other glucocorticoids.[60] Evening administration has proven superior.[73]

An attempt must be made to balance dexamethasone dosage such that satisfactory reversal of symptoms is achieved while iatrogenic adrenal insufficiency from oversuppression is avoided. Most side effects observed are those of hypercortisolism such as weight gain, edema, and other Cushing-like symptomatologies. A commonly prescribed regimen is 0.25 to 0.5 mg of dexamethasone nightly. Abraham et al.[74] have suggested a regimen based on a weight-related formula, but this may result in oversuppression.[75] Periodic evaluation of an A.M. serum cortisol is recommended. Boyers et al.[76] have shown that, if A.M. serum cortisol concentrations are maintained at or above 2 μg/dl, oversuppression is unlikely. Following therapy, serum T and 17-OHP values will fall to within normal range.[50]

In addition to dexamethasone, the birth control pill is a useful adjunct to therapy when contraception is required, and because the variability in clinical expression of nonclassical congenital adrenal hyperplasia seems to depend in part on the capacity of the skin to use circulating androgens,[53] antiandrogens that act directly on the target cells should be considered in resistant cases.

3β-HYDROXYSTEROID DEHYDROGENASE DEFICIENCY

Once thought to be a rare cause of hirsutism and menstrual disturbance, an increasing number of cases of 3β-hydroxysteroid dehydrogenase (3β-HSD) deficiency have been reported during the past few years.[77–80] The incidence among hirsute patients may be as high as 11.4% to 12.9%.[79–81]

3β-HSD, unlike 21- and 11-hydroxylase, is found in both adrenal and ovary,[81] and is responsible for transforming $\Delta 5$ steroids into the corresponding $\Delta 4$ compounds (Fig. 2). When a moderate deficiency exists, baseline plasma 17-hydroxypregnenolone, dehydroepiandrosterone (DHEA), and DHEAS levels will be elevated. With milder degrees of deficiency, baseline patterns may not be particularly characteristic.[82] Surprisingly, plasma elevation of T and $\Delta 4$-androstenedione are not uncommon[79] and may be due to hepatic conversion of excess circulating ovarian and adrenal precursors.[3,78,81] Evidence suggests that 3β-HSD activity in peripheral tissues (sebaceous glands, fat, hair follicles) remains intact, despite ovarian and adrenal deficiency.[78] Target tissue conversion of $\Delta 5$ precursors may be responsible for the hirsutism observed.[79]

Diagnosis of this disorder relies on the relationship of $\Delta 5$ and $\Delta 4$ steroids. Marked elevation of DHEA and DHEAS in the face of normal or mildly elevated T or androstenedione may be a signal to screen for 3β-HSD using exogenous ACTH stimulation.[80] Following administration of 0.25 mg ACTH 1-24 IV bolus, 17-hydroxypregnenolone rises significantly at 60 minutes in women with 3β-HSD compared with those with nonenzyme-deficient hirsutism. Some overlap exists between the 3β-HSD deficiency and 21-OH deficiency responses, but comparing the ratio of 17-hydroxypregnenolone with 17-OHP allows one to distinguish easily between the two. Poststimulation ratios of 17-hydroxypregnenolone to 17-OHP were found to be 4.4, 0.5, and greater than 8.0 in normals, patients with 21-OH deficiency, and 3β-HSD deficiency, respectively (Fig. 8).[80,81]

In the adrenal, the enzyme blockade and result-

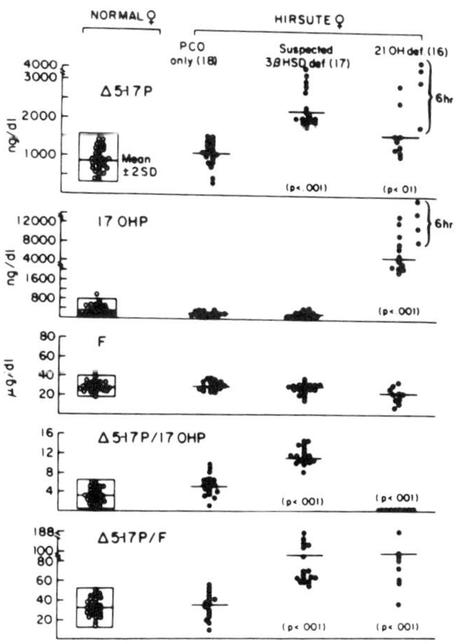

Figure 8 Serum 17-hydroxysteroid responses to ACTH stimulation (60 minutes after 0.25 mg IV bolus dose) in normal women and women with hirsutism. Cortisol = F; Δ5-17P = 17-hydroxypregnenolone; 17-OHP = 17-hydroxyprogesterone. (From Pang et al.[79] Reproduced with permission of the publisher.)

ing relative cortisol deficiency are overcome by glucocorticoid administration. Dexamethasone administration readily suppresses precursor elevation.[78,80] In the ovary, 3β-HSD deficiency should affect sex steroid synthesis and theoretically impair folliculogenesis. Reports to date, however, have indicated that dexamethasone treatment alone allows resumption of menses[78,80] and, in one patient, conception and delivery.[80]

No genetic markers for 3β-HSD deficiency are presently available.

11β-HYDROXYLASE DEFICIENCY

A relatively uncommon cause of congenital adrenal hyperplasia,[83,84] 11β-hydroxylase (11β-OH) is the enzyme responsible for conversion of 11-deoxycortisol (compound S) to cortisol, and deoxycorticosterone (DOC) to corticosterone (Fig. 2). As with 21-OH and 3β-HSD deficiency, a relative reduction of cortisol promotes increased ACTH production and compensatory overproduction of selected steroid precursors. Baseline elevation of plasma Δ4-androstenedione and testosterone are common[84,85] as well as DOC, compound S, and their urinary tetrahydrometabolites (tetrahydro-11-deoxycorticosterone and tetrahydro-11-deoxycortisol).[83] With ACTH stimulation, further increases occur,[83,85] but the method of testing and criteria for diagnosis are not well standardized.

Patients with 11β-OH deficiency may present with either a classic pattern or a mild deficiency.[83,85] Associated with the former are diagnosis at a younger age, more severe symptoms of virilization, and the frequent presence of hypertension with related cardiomyopathy and retinopathy.[83,84] In the latter, patients present with postpubertal onset of hirsutism, acne, and amenorrhea.[83,85] Although hypertension was once considered a prerequisite for the diagnosis of 11β-OH deficiency, two large studies[83,84] have revealed that elevated blood pressure is not an invariable finding, despite elevated levels of DOC. Among 50 patients described by Rosler and Leiberman[84] and Zachmann et al.,[83] a heterogeneous response to DOC was exhibited. No particular correlations were observed between specific serum levels of DOC, the degree of virilization, or the presence and severity of hypertension. In other words, when present, hypertension lends support to the diagnosis of 11β-OH deficiency, but its absence does not rule out the diagnosis.

It is unlikely that mild cases represent simple heterozygotes for 11β-OH deficiency since Pang et al.[86] have shown that parents of patients with 11β-OH deficiency do not differ from normal subjects with respect to their response to serum 17-OHP, cortisol, aldosterone, and corticosterone. Unfortunately, no linkage exists between 11β-OH and HLA loci.[87]

As with other forms of congenital adrenal hyperplasia, glucocorticoid therapy has proved beneficial.[84]

CONCLUSION

Congenital adrenal hyperplasia is an autosomal recessive disease in which there is a deficiency of one of several enzymes in the pathway required for normal adrenal steroidogenesis. 21-OH deficiency is the most common variant and has been studied extensively. Three alleles are associated with the 21-OH locus and can combine in various ways to yield individuals who are either unaffected, heterozygote carriers, or affected with classical or nonclassical disease.

Late-onset, acquired, partial, and attenuated are synonyms for nonclassical congenital adrenal hyperplasia and affected patients present with hirsutism, acne, and menstrual disturbances. They are clinically indistinguishable from patients with other causes of hyperandrogenemia. The incidence of LOCAH due to 21-OH deficiency among hirsute patients is estimated to be 5%. Diagnosis is important primarily for the purposes of genetic counselling since affected patients are at risk for conceiving affected children. Baseline androgen, cortisol, and gonadotropin values are not helpful in diagnosis. Plasma 17-OHP tends to be elevated but overlaps that of women with other causes of hirsutism. Assay of 17-OHP following ACTH stimulation is an accurate method of diagnosing 21-OH deficiency and should be employed as a routine screening procedure among hirsute patients. A variety of methods have been proposed, but the most widely used are those of Gutai et al.[28] and New et al.[35] Both methods will identify patients with deficient 21-OH activity. While the former requires 1.0 mg of ACTH and four hormone assays for diagnosis, the latter needs only 0.25 mg of ACTH and two hormone assays. 11β-OH and 3β-HSD deficiencies also may cause hirsutism and menstrual irregularity, but standards for their diagnosis are not as well established as for 21-OH deficiency. Dexamethasone suppression is the treatment of choice for all forms of LOCAH and expected results include return of menstrual cyclicity, decreased acne, and regression of hirsutism. Periodic evaluation of morning cortisols is recommended to avoid oversuppression.

Acknowledgments. We thank Carl M. Herbert, M.D., for his critical comments during the preparation of this review and Ms. Charlene McDowell for her excellent secretarial assistance.

REFERENCES

1. New MI, Dupont B, Pang S, Pollack M, Levine LS: An update of congenital adrenal hyperplasia. Recent Prog Horm Res 37:105, 1981
2. New MI: Clinical and endocrinological aspects of 21-hydroxylase deficiency. Ann NY Acad Sci 458:1, 1985
3. Savage MO: Congenital adrenal hyperplasia. Clin Endocrinol Metab 14:893, 1985
4. New MI, Speiser PW: Genetics of adrenal steroid 21-hydroxylase deficiency. Endocr Rev 7:331, 1986
5. Guyton AC: The Adrenocortical Hormones. In Textbook of Medical Physiology, Edited by D Dreibelbis. Philadelphia, WB Saunders, 1985, p 909
6. Brown MS, Kovenen PT, Goldstein JL: Receptor-mediated uptake of lipoprotein-cholesterol and its utilization for steroid synthesis in the adrenal cortex. Recent Prog Horm Res 35:215, 1979
7. James VHT, Few JD: Adrenocorticosteroids: chemistry, synthesis and disturbances in disease. Clin Endocrinol Metab 14:867, 1985
8. Bongiovanni AM: Introduction. Ann NY Acad Sci 458:ix, 1985
9. Wilkins L, Fleischmann W, Howard JE: Macrogenitosomia precox associated with hyperplasia of the androgenic tissue of the adrenal and death from corticoadrenal insufficiency. Endocrinology 26:385, 1940
10. Jones HW Jr: A long look at the adrenogenital syndrome. Johns Hopkins Med J 145:143, 1979
11. Butler GC, Marrian GE: Isolation of pregnane-3,17,20-triol from urine of women showing adrenogenital syndrome. J Biol Chem 119:565, 1937
12. Hechter O, Pincus G: Genesis of the adrenocortical secretion. Physiol Rev 34:459, 1954
13. Bongiovanni AM: In vitro hydroxylation of steroids by whole adrenal homogenates of beef, normal man and patients with the adrenogenital syndrome. J Clin Invest 37:1342, 1985
14. Jones GE, Howard JE, Langford H: The use of cortisone in follicular phase disturbances. Fertil Steril 4:49, 1953
15. Dupont B, Oberfield SE, Smithwick EM, Lee TD, Levine LS: Close genetic linkage between HLA and congenital adrenal hyperplasia (21-hydroxylase deficiency). Lancet 2:1309, 1977
16. Harris R: The HLA system. In Principles and Practice of Medical Genetics, Edited by EH Emory and DL Rimoin. Edinburgh, Churchill Livingstone, 1983, p 1127
17. Levine LS, Zachmann M, New MI, Prader A, Pollack MS, O'Neill GJ, Pang SY, Oberfield SE, Dupont B: Genetic mapping of the 21-hydroxylase deficiency gene within the HLA linkage group. N Engl J Med 299:911, 1978
18. Klouda PT, Harris R, Price DA: HLA and congenital adrenal hyperplasia. Lancet 2:1046, 1978
19. Holler W, Scholz S, Knorr D, Bidlingmaier F, Keller E, Ekkehard A: Genetic differences between the salt-wasting, simple-virilizing, and non-classical types of congenital adrenal hyperplasia. J Clin Endocrinol Metab 60:757, 1985
20. Petersen KE, Svejgaard A, Nielsen MD, Dissing J: Heterozygotes and cryptic patients in families of patients with congenital adrenal hyperplasia (21-hydroxylase deficiency): HLA and glyoxalase 1 typing and hormonal studies. Horm Res 16:151, 1982
21. Speiser PW, Dupont B, Rubenstein P, Piazza A, Kastelan A, New MI: High frequency of non-classical steroid 21-hydroxylase deficiency. Am J Hum Genet 37:650, 1985
22. Levine LS: HLA-B14 and non-classical 21-hydroxylase deficiency in a heterogeneous New York population. Ann NY Acad Sci 458:65, 1985
23. Pollack MS, Levine LS, O'Neill GJ, Pang S, Lorenzen F, Kohn B, Rondanini GF, Chiumello G, New MI, Dupont B: HLA linkage and B14, DRI, Bfs haplotype association with genes for late-onset and cryptic 21-hydroxylase deficiency. Am J Hum Genet 33:540, 1981
24. Chrousos GP, Loriaux DL, Mann D, Cutler GB: Late-onset 21-hydroxylase deficiency is an allelic variant of congenital adrenal hyperplasia characterized by attenuated clinical expression and different HLA haplotype associations. Horm Res 16:193, 1982
25. Libber SM, Migeon CJ, Bias WB: Ascertainment of 21-hydroxylase deficiency in individuals with HLA-B14 haplotype. J Clin Endocrinol Metab 60:727, 1985
26. Child DF, Bu'lock DE, Anderson DC: Adrenal steroidogenesis in heterozygotes for 21-hydroxylase deficiency. Clin Endocrinol 11:391, 1979
27. Krensky AM, Bongiovanni AM, Marino J, Parks J, Tenore A: Indentification of heterozygous carriers of congenital

adrenal hyperplasia by radioimmunoassay of serum 17-OH progesterone. J Pediatr 90:930, 1977

28. Gutai JP, Kowarski AA, Migeon CJ: The detection of the heterozygous carrier for congenital virilizing adrenal hyperplasia. J Pediatr 90:924, 1977
29. Weil J, Bidlingmaier F, Sippell WG, Butenandt O, Knorr D: Comparison of two tests for heterozygosity in congenital adrenal hyperplasia (CAH). Acta Endocrinol (Copenh) 91:109, 1979
30. Lejeune-Lenain C, Cantraine F, Dufrasnes M, Prevot F, Wolter R, Franckson JRM: An improved method for the detection of heterozygosity of congenital virilizing adrenal hyperplasia. Clin Endocrinol 12:525, 1980
31. Knorr O, Bidlingmaier F, Holler W, Kuhnle U: Diagnosis of homozygosity and heterozygosity in congenital adrenal hyperplasia (CAH) and control of treatment. J Steroid Biochem 19:645, 1983
32. Lorenzen F, Pang S, New MI, Pollack M, Oberfield S, Dupont B, Chow D, Schneider B, Levine L: Studies of the C-21 and C-19 steroids and HLA genotyping in siblings and parents of patients with congenital adrenal hyperplasia due to 21-hydroxylase deficiency. J Clin Endocrinol Metab 50:572, 1980
33. Rosenwaks Z, Lee PA, Jones GS, Migeon CJ, Wentz AC: An attenuated form of congenital virilizing adrenal hyperplasia. J Clin Endocrinol Metab 49:335, 1979
34. Bouchard P, Kuttenn F, Mowszowicz I, Schiason G, Raux-Eurin M-C, Mauvais-Jarvis P: Congenital adrenal hyperplasia due to partial 21-hydroxylase deficiency, a study of five cases. Acta Endocrinol (Copenh) 96:107, 1981
35. New MI, Lorenzen F, Lerner AJ, Kohn B, Oberfield SE, Pollack MS, Dupont B, Stoner E, Levy DJ, Pang S, Levine L: Genotyping steroid 21-hydroxylase deficiency: hormonal reference data. J Clin Endocrinol Metab 57:320, 1983
36. Kohn B, Levine LS, Pollack MS, Pang S, Lorenzen F, Levy DJ, Lerner AJ, Gian FR, Dupont B, New MI: Late-onset steroid 21-hydroxylase deficiency: a variant of classical congenital adrenal hyperplasia. J Clin Endocrinol Metab 55:817, 1982
37. Migeon CJ, Rosenwaks Z, Lee PA, Urban MD, Bias W: The attenuated form of congenital adrenal hyperplasia as an allelic form of 21-hydroxylase deficiency. J Clin Endocrinol Metab 51:647, 1980
38. Levine LS, Dupont B, Lorenzen F, Pang S, Pollack MS, Oberfield S, Kohn B, Lerner A, Cacciari E, Mantero F, Cassio A, Scaroni C, Chiumello G, Rondanini GF, Giovanelli G, Virdis R, Bartolotta E, Migliori C, Pintor C, Tato L, Barboni F, New MI: Cryptic 21-hydroxylase deficiency in families of patients with classical congenital adrenal hyperplasia. J Clin Endocrinol Metab 51:1316, 1980
39. Lee PA, Rosenwaks Z, Urban MD, Migeon CJ, Bias W: Attenuated forms of congenital adrenal hyperplasia due to 21-hydroxylase deficiency. J Clin Endocrinol Metab 55:866, 1982
40. New MI, Dupont B, Pollack MS, Levine LS: The biochemical basis for genotyping 21-hydroxylase deficiency. Hum Genet 58:123, 1981
41. White PC, New MI, Dupont B: Molecular cloning of steroid 21-hydroxylase. Ann NY Acad Sci 458:277, 1985
42. Warsos SL, Larsen JW, Kent SG, Rosenbaum KN, August GP, Migeon CJ, Schulman JD: Prenatal diagnosis of congenital adrenal hyperplasia. Obstet Gynecol 55:751, 1980
43. Forest MG, Betuel H, Goullin P, Boue A, David M, Floret R, Francois R, Guibaud P, Plauchu H, Rappaport R: Prenatal diagnosis of congenital adrenal hyperplasia (CAH) due to 21-hydroxylase deficiency by steroid analysis in the amniotic fluid of midpregnancy: comparison of HLA typing in 17 pregnancies at risk for CAH. Prenat Diagn 1:197, 1981
44. Pollack MS, Levine LS, Pang S, Owens RP, Nitowsky HM, Maurer D, New MI, Duchon M, Merkatz IR, Sachs G, Dupont B: Prenatal diagnosis of congenital adrenal hyperplasia (21-hydroxylase deficiency) by HLA typing. Lancet 1:1107, 1979
45. Chrousos GP, Evans MI, Loriaux LD, McCluskey J, Fletcher JC, Schulman JD: Prenatal therapy in congenital adrenal hyperplasia. Ann NY Acad Sci 458:156, 1985
46. Pang S, Spence DA, New MI: Newborn screening for congenital adrenal hyperplasia with special reference to screening in Alaska. Ann NY Acad Sci 458:90, 1985
47. Chrousos GP, Loriaux LD, Mann DL, Cutler GB: Late-onset 21-hydroxylase deficiency mimicking idiopathic hirsutism or polycystic ovarian disease: an allelic variant of congenital virilizing adrenal hyperplasia with a milder enzymatic defect. Ann Intern Med 96:143, 1982
48. Emans SJ, Grace E, Fleishnick E, Mansfield MJ, Crigler JF Jr: Detection of late-onset 21-hydroxylase deficiency congenital adrenal hyperplasia in adolescents. Pediatrics 72:690, 1983
49. Lobo RA, Goebelsmann U: Adult manifestation of congenital adrenal hyperplasia due to incomplete 21-hydroxylase deficiency mimicking polycystic ovarian disease. Am J Obstet Gynecol 138:720, 1980
50. Carmina E, Gagliano AM, Rosato F, Maggiore M, Janni A: The endocrine pattern of late onset adrenal hyperplasia (21-hydroxylase deficiency). J Endocrinol Invest 7:89, 1984
51. Benjamin F, Deutsch S, Saperstein H, Seltzer V: Prevalence of and markers for the attenuated form of congenital adrenal hyperplasia and hyperprolactinemia masquerading as polycystic ovarian disease. Fertil Steril 46:215, 1986
52. Chetkowski RJ, DeFazio J, Shamonki I, Judd HL, Chang J: The incidence of late-onset congenital adrenal hyperplasia due to 21-hydroxylase deficiency among hirsute women. J Clin Endocrinol Metab 58:595, 1984
53. Kuttenn F, Couillin P, Girard F, Billaud L, Vincens M, Boucekkine C, Thalabard J, Maudelorde T, Spritzer P, Mowskowitz I, Boue A, Mauvais-Jarvis P: Late-onset adrenal hyperplasia in hirsutism. N Engl J Med 313:224, 1985
54. Dewailly D, Vantyghem-Haudiquet M, Sainsard C, Buvat J, Cappoen JP, Ardaens K, Racadot A, Lefebvre J, Fossati P: Clinical and biological phenotypes in late-onset 21-hydroxylase deficiency. J Clin Endocrinol Metab 63:418, 1986
55. Blankenstein J, Faiman C, Reyes FI, Schroeder ML, Winter JSD: Adult-onset familial adrenal 21-hydroxylase deficiency. Am J Med 68:441, 1980
56. Birnbaum MD, Rose LI: Late onset adrenocortical hydroxylase deficiencies associated with menstrual dysfunction. Obstet Gynecol 63:445, 1984
57. Newmark S, Dluhy R, Williams G, Pochi P, Rose L: Partial 11- and 21-hydroxylase deficiencies in hirsute women. Am J Obstet Gynecol 127:594, 1977
58. Speiser PW, New MI: Genotype and hormonal phenotype in non-classical 21-hydroxylase deficiency. J Clin Endocrinol Metab 64:86, 1987
59. Mahesh VB, Greenblatt RB, Coniff RF: Adrenal hyperplasia: a case report of delayed onset of the congential form or an acquired form. J Clin Endocrinol Metab 28:619, 1968

60. Maroulis GB: Evaluation of hirsutism and hyperandrogenemia. Fertil Steril 36:273, 1981
61. Madden JD, Milewich L, Gomez-Sanchez C: The effect of oral contraceptive treatment on the serum concentration of dehydroepiandrosterone sulfate and ACTH. Gynecol Invest 8:16, 1977
62. Madden JD, Milewich L, Parker CR, Carr BR, Boyar RM, MacDonald PC: The effect of oral contraceptive treatment on the serum concentration of dehydroepiandrosterone sulfate. Am J Obstet Gynecol 132:380, 1978
63. Chetkowski RJ, DeFazio J, Shamonki I, Judd HL, Chang JR: Late-onset adrenal hyperplasia (Letter). N Engl J Med 314:450, 1986
64. Rosenfield RL, Helke J, Lucky AW: Dexamethasone preparation does not alter corticoid and androgen responses to adrenocorticotropin. J Clin Endocrinol Metab 60:585, 1985
65. Lindholm J, Kehlet H, Blichert-Toft M, Dinesen B, Riishede J: Reliability of the 30-minute ACTH test in assessing hypothalamic-pituitary-adrenal function. J Clin Endocrinol Metab 47:272, 1978
66. Nicholson WE, Liddle RA, Puett D, Liddle GW: Adrenocorticotropic hormone biotransformation, clearance and catabolism. Endocrinology 103:1344, 1978
67. Chrousos GP, Munabi AK, Cutler GB Jr, Loriaux DL: Diagnosis of late onset 21-hydroxylase deficiency by plasma 17-hydroxyprogesterone response to ACTH (Letter). Ann Intern Med 97:281, 1982
68. Graybeal ML, Fang VS: Physiologic dosing of exogenous ACTH. Acta Endocrinol (Copenh) 108:401, 1985
69. Rose LI, Birnbaum MD: Therapy of adrenocortical hydroxylase deficiencies in acne vulgaris. Int J Dermatol 18:386, 1979
70. Villaneuva AL, Rebar RW: Congenital adrenal hyperplasia and luteal dysfunction. Int J Gynaecol Obstet 23:449, 1985
71. Winter JSD, Couch RM: Modern medical therapy of congenital adrenal hyperplasia: a decade of experience. Ann NY Acad Sci 458:165, 1985
72. Horrocks PM, London DR: A comparison of three glucocorticoid suppressive regimens in adults with congenital adrenal hyperplasia. Clin Endocrinol 17:547, 1982
73. Nichols T, Nugent CA, Tyler FH: Diurnal variation in suppression of adrenal function by glucocorticoids. J Clin Endocrinol Metab 25:343, 1965
74. Abraham GE, Maroulis GB, Buster JE, Chang RJ, Marshall JR: Effect of dexamethasone on serum cortisol and androgen levels in hirsute patients. Obstet Gynecol 47:395, 1976
75. Wentz AC: Hypothalamic-pituitary-adrenocortical function during long-term low-dose dexamethasone therapy in hyperandrogenized women (Comment). Obstet Gynecol Surv 37:629, 1982
76. Boyers SP, Buster JE, Marshall JR: Hypothalamic-pituitary-adrenocortical function during long-term low-dose dexamethasone therapy in hyperandrogenized women. Am J Obstet Gynecol 142:330, 1982
77. Bongiovanni AM: Late-onset adrenal hyperplasia (Letter). N Engl J Med 314:450, 1986
78. Rosenfield RL, Rich BH, Wolfsdorf JL, Cassorla F, Parks JS, Bongiovanni AM, Wu CH, Shackelton CHL: Pubertal presentation of congenital Δ5-3β-hydroxysteroid dehydrogenase deficiency. J Clin Endocrinol Metab 51:345, 1980
79. Pang S, Lerner AJ, Stoner E, Levine LS, Oberfield SE, Engel I, New MI: Late-onset adrenal steroid 3β-hydroxysteroid dehydrogenase deficiency. I. A cause of hirsutism in pubertal and post-pubertal women. J Clin Endocrinol Metab 60:428, 1985
80. Lobo RA, Goebelsmann U: Evidence for reduced 3β-ol-hydroxysteroid dehydrogenase activity in some hirsute women thought to have polycystic ovarian syndrome. J Clin Endocrinol Metab 53:394, 1981
81. Bongiovanni AM: Congenital adrenal hyperplasia due to 3β-hydroxysteroid dehydrogenase deficiency. In Adrenal Diseases in Childhood, Vol 13, Edited by MI New, LS Levine. New York, S Karger, 1984, p 72
82. Bongiovanni AM: Acquired adrenal hyperplasia: with special reference to 3β-hydroxysteroid dehydrogenase. Fertil Steril 35:599, 1981
83. Zachmann M, Tassimari D, Prader A: Clinical and biochemical variability of congenital adrenal hyperplasia due to 11β-hydroxylase deficiency: a study of 25 patients. J Clin Endocrinol Metab 56:222, 1983
84. Rosler A, Leiberman E: Enzymatic defects of steroidogenesis: 11β-hydroxylase deficiency congenital adrenal hyperplasia. Pediatr Adolesc Endocrinol 13:47, 1984
85. Cathelineau G, Brerault J-L, Fiet J, Julien R, Dreux C, Canivet J: Adrenocortical 11β-hydroxylase defect in adult women with post menarchial onset of symptoms. J Clin Endocrinol Metab 51:287, 1980
86. Pang S, Levine LS, Lorenzen F, Chow D, Pollack M, Dupont B, Genel M, New MI: Hormonal studies in obligate heterozygotes and siblings of patients with 11β-hydroxylase deficiency congenital adrenal hyperplasia. J Clin Endocrinol Metab 50:586, 1980
87. Brautbar C, Rosler A, Landau H, Cohen I, Nelken D, Cohen T, Levine C, Sack J, Benderli A, Moses S, Leiberman E, Dupont B, Levine LS, New MI: No linkage between HLA and congenital adrenal hyperplasia due to 11β-hydroxylase deficiency. N Engl J Med 300:205, 1980

Chapter 10

Dynamic testing in reproductive endocrinology

William D. Schlaff, M.D.

Department of Gynecology and Obstetrics, The Johns Hopkins University School of Medicine, Baltimore, Maryland

Dynamic testing of endocrine function represents a potential powerful diagnostic tool in the clinical setting. In addition, investigation of the physiologic interactions of hormones frequently relies on such testing. Dynamic testing involves active manipulation of a patient's hormonal milieu by exogenous factors (e.g., a drug action or physical stress) in order to evaluate more completely the potential response of the patient's hormonal system. By using these techniques, subtle or insidiously developing hormonal abnormalities can be diagnosed. The fact that many different testing schemes have been presented in the literature often leads to confusion over the usefulness of any given test. It is sometimes difficult to develop an efficient and appropriate diagnostic plan in light of the many varied approaches. This article presents several concepts regarding such procedures, reviews certain dynamic tests, and presents a useful framework in which they might be used.

GENERAL CONCEPTS

The early concept of hormones, as described by Starling in 1905,[1] was that these substances acted as messengers, secreted by an endocrine gland and having distant effects. Although this concept remains tenable today, ever increasing understanding of releasing hormones, receptor physiology, and complicated hormonal interactions has caused us to modify our initial simplistic view. Similarly, early concepts of hormonal evaluation did not fully reflect the entire complex endocrine milieu. Single assays of hormones can, of course, be useful. As an example, markedly elevated serum levels of gonadotropins may be diagnostic of gonadal failure. However, acceptable baseline values do not insure than an endocrine system is functioning normally. For instance, patients with Cushing's syndrome, as well as those with adrenal insufficiency, may have normal fasting serum cortisol levels. However, by using dynamic testing, one can better characterize and differentiate these endocrine abnormalities. These dynamic studies fall into one of three general categories: stimulation tests, suppression tests, and feedback tests.

STIMULATION TESTS

Some patients with normal baseline values may have *diminished hormonal reserve*. As a first step in establishing this condition, stimulation of the gland in question may be required. Diminished reserve may occur for a number of reasons. First, local factors, such as tumor, infection, hemorrhage, or necrosis, may directly affect the gland in question. Second, immune factors may depress or interfere with the normal function of the gland. Finally, prolonged deprivation of stimulation may lead to an inadequate response to an acute stimulus. The pathology of the adrenal gland provides a good example of many of these processes. Tuberculosis, hemorrhage into the gland, or autoimmune adrenal failure may cause diminished adrenal reserve. Although the adrenal cortex so afflicted may be able to function adequately in a nonstress situation, its ability to respond to increased stress may be manifest only when provoked by exogenous adrenocorticotropic hormone (ACTH). Stimulation tests generally have the advantage of being safe and easy to perform and thus are frequently among the first diagnostic tests chosen.

SUPPRESSION TESTS

Suppression tests are frequently used to evaluate the *autonomy of hormone secretion.* The most frequent setting in which these are used is when baseline values of a hormone are elevated. A factor that normally decreases secretion of the hormone in question is administered, and hormonal levels are measured before and after its administration. Suppressibility suggests that the source of overproduction is not autonomous. A frequently employed example of the suppression test is the administration of dexamethasone to a patient suspected of having adrenal hypersecretion. Because suppression tests are generally used in settings of hormonal overproduction, their performance is usually safe. The exception to this generalization is when the suppressive drug itself conveys dangerous side effects.

FEEDBACK TESTS

Feedback tests can be used to evaluate the ability of an endocrine system to exhibit *response to maximum stress* or stress beyond that provided by simple stimulation tests. Provocative stresses are generally provided by one of two approaches. In one technique, a normal step in the synthesis of a hormone can be blocked. Consequently, absence of the end product will result in increased stimulation and ultimate production of precursor hormones, which can then be measured. The use of metyrapone to block the 11-hydroxylation step in cortisol synthesis is an example of such a feedback test. After the administration of metyrapone, secretion of ACTH, 11-deoxycortisol, and urinary 17-hydroxycorticosteroids (17-OHCS) should increase. An alternate technique involves providing a physiologic stimulus to which the system normally responds. Insulin-induced hypoglycemia exemplifies such a test. Cortisol and growth hormone are normally secreted in response to such induced hypoglycemia if the hypothalamic-pituitary-adrenal axis is intact. Thus, this type of feedback response indicates appropriate function at each level of the hormonal axis and demonstrates the patient's ability to respond to a maximal stress. Such tests, however, can be dangerous. If the patient cannot respond adequately to the induced stress, an acute state of hormonal insufficiency can be produced, which may have serious consequences.

GENERAL PRINCIPLES

The clinician's interpretation of the results of a dynamic test is the key to its usefulness. Many types of provocative testing have been subject to numerous studies involving various protocols, measuring different hormones, and citing different normal response ranges. Such lack of standardization can be confusing to the clinician. The great variety in testing protocols described provides a lesson in and of itself, leading to the conclusion that there is no single acceptable testing method, nor is there an absolute response on which we may rely. Rather, the clinician must recognize that test interpretation rests on general responses to provocation as opposed to a specific numeric range. Furthermore, it is important to recognize that any given patient may respond differently at different times. If the clinical suspicion of gland failure is high and initial results are within the quoted normal range, the patient should be tested at a later time. Strict adherence to any specific normal value ignores the fact that glandular failure may be incremental and is unlikely to be manifest as an all-or-none phenomenon.

With these caveats in mind, several general observations can be made to help characterize patterns of response. These patterns are exemplified in Figure 1, in which thyroid-stimulating hormone (TSH) response to thyrotropin-releasing hormone (TRH) administration is correlated with the cause of hypothyroidism. (1) In cases of end-organ failure or when there is a chronically increased level of a specific pituitary stimulating hormone, administration of a hypothalamic releasing factor will generally cause an exaggerated response in secretion of the appropriate pituitary hormone(s). (2) In cases of pituitary failure, there will be little or no response to hypothalamic-releasing hormone exhibited by either the pituitary or the end organ. (3) In cases of hypothalamic dysfunction, response of pituitary hormone(s) to releasing factor can vary. Generally, pituitary hormone response to the initial releasing hormone administration is delayed or absent. Repeated stimulation by a releasing factor can be used to ultimately normalize the response. This situation may reflect proliferation of receptors induced by the releasing hormone, perhaps in

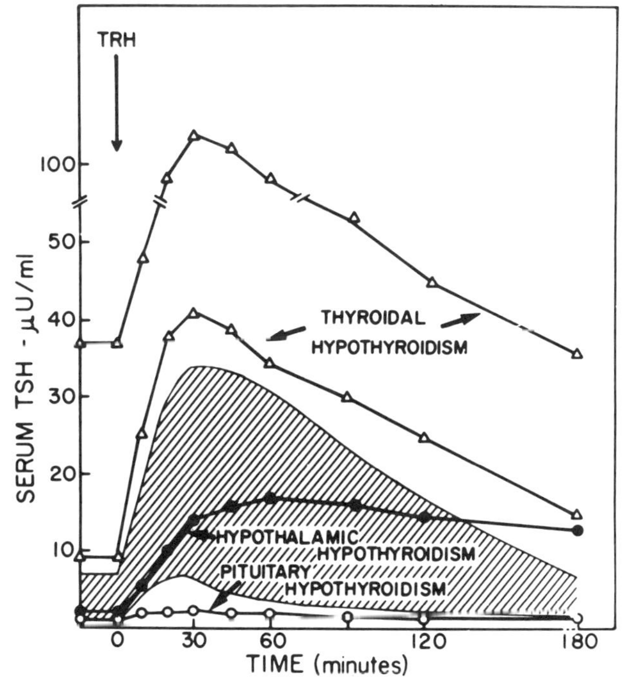

Figure 1
TSH response to TRH administration in patients with various causes of hypothyroidism (from reference 2).

concert with increasing levels of associated hormones. (4) In cases of either hypothalamic or pituitary dysfunction, a similar pattern of end organ response is common. After prolonged absence of stimulation, the end organ may not be capable of responding to the initial stimulation; only prolonged or repetitive stimulation will provoke a normal response and insure an adequately functioning end organ. These generalizations are summarized in Table 1.

INDICATIONS FOR DYNAMIC TESTING

From the outset, it is helpful to keep in mind that dynamic testing may be indicated primarily for clinical diagnosis in certain cases and for academic or research interest in others. Many of the various protocols that have been described have little impact on the management of a specific clinical problem. This statement is not meant to detract from the significance of these tests, but rather to emphasize that appropriate perspective must be maintained in ordering provocative tests.

HYPOTHALAMIC-PITUITARY TESTING

Amenorrhea is the most common manifestation of hypothalamic-pituitary dysfunction encountered by the reproductive endocrinologist. Patients who are otherwise asymptomatic should be routinely screened by a pregnancy test and measurement of serum prolactin (PRL) and gonadotropins. This step enables the clinician to exclude or detect pregnancy, PRL-secreting tumor, and gonadal failure. Thereafter, further testing may be indicated to establish a specific diagnosis. If the patient has normal or low serum gonadotropins and the PRL level is normal, some form of hypothalamic or pituitary dysfunction is likely. Pertinent history would include significant weight fluctuations, unusual stresses, drug history, psychiatric abnormalities, or onset of neurologic complaints. Counseling may be initiated to try to discover any underlying stresses that may be alleviated. Should pregnancy be the goal, ovulation induction with gonadotropin-releasing hormone (GnRH) or human menopausal gonadotropin/human chorionic gonadotropin (hMG/hCG) may be initiated. In patients not desiring pregnancy who are hypoestrogenic, estrogen replacement therapy should be considered.

The differentiation between hypothalamic and pituitary disease can be solely academic and is not always clinically necessary in patients with amenorrhea of central origin. Hypothalamic-pituitary testing should be performed if incipient hypopituitarism is suspected or if a specific diagnosis is desired. Although patients with hypothalamic dysfunction may present with no manifestations other than amenorrhea, patients with pituitary insufficiency usually have additional symptoms or signs that relate to the loss of anterior hypophyseal stimulating hormones other than gonadotropins. They might also provide a history suggestive of an acute insult such as that

Table 1. *General Responses to Hormonal Stimulation*

Diagnosis	Administration of hypothalamic hormone	Administration of pituitary hormone
Hypothalamic failure	Pituitary response variable (usually delayed or absent); end-organ response dependent on pituitary and may require priming	End-organ will respond, but may require priming
Pituitary failure	No pituitary response; no end-organ response	End-organ will respond, but may require priming
End-organ failure	Exaggerated pituitary response; no end-organ response	No end-organ response

which predisposes to hypopituitarism associated with Sheehan's syndrome. Pituitary failure is most often slowly progressive rather than abrupt and complete. Characteristically, capacity for gonadotropin secretion is lost first, followed by growth hormone (GH), TSH, ACTH, and PRL. This temporal sequence of deficiency may be related to the anatomic location of the respective secretory cells in the pituitary. If hypothalamic releasing hormones are available, pituitary hormones can be tested directly; without them, indirect tests must be used.

At this point, reference should be made to progestin withdrawal testing. Many clinicians feel that a progestin challenge is obsolete because it provides only minimal information about the degree of estrogen production, at the expense of modifying the patient's baseline hormonal status. If the patient is producing estrogen in quantities sufficient to cause endometrial proliferation, bleeding will occur after progestin administration and withdrawal. The dosage usually employed is 100 mg of progesterone (P) in oil administered intramuscularly or medroxyprogesterone acetate (Provera, The Upjohn Co., Kalamazoo, MI), 10 mg orally given daily for 5 days. Bleeding usually occurs within 1 week after progestin administration and is proportional to the degree of prior estrogen exposure. Patients whose serum estradiol (E_2) levels are below 25 to 40 pg/ml usually have no withdrawal bleeding. As E_2 levels increase, although difficult to quantitate, the amount of withdrawal bleeding would also be expected to increase. Should bleeding fail to occur, estrogen is frequently given to cause endometrial proliferation before a second course of progestin administration. Conjugated estrogens can be administered orally in a dose of 2.5 mg/day for 25 days. If bleeding fails to occur after administration of the progestin, end-organ unresponsiveness or outlet obstruction should be suspected. Many clinicians do not favor progestin withdrawal for diagnosis but instead obtain serum E_2 levels or a maturation index on epithelial cells obtained form the vaginal sidewall, thus avoiding possible confusion caused by administering exogenous hormones.

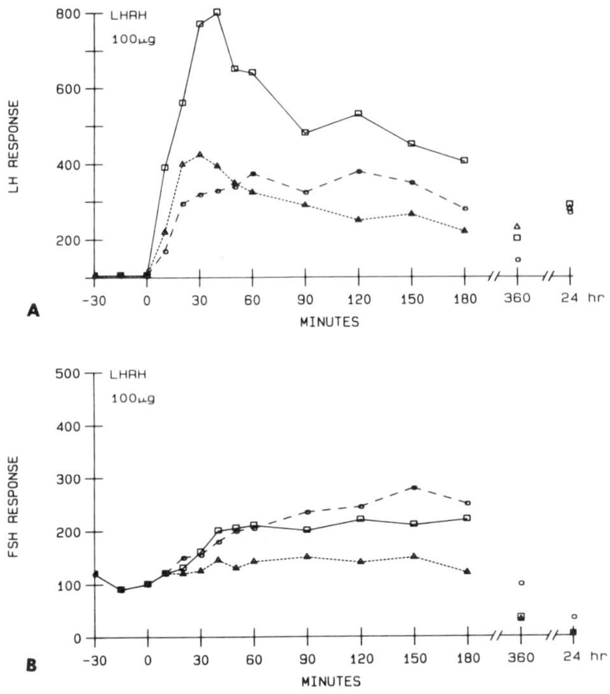

Figure 2
(**A**), Response of LH to GnRH administration in normal women at varying stages of the menstrual cycle (Δ, follicular phase; ○, preovulatory phase; □, luteal phase) (from reference 3). (**B**), Response of FSH to GnRH administration in normal women at varying stages of the menstrual cycle (Δ, follicular phase; ○, preovulatory phase; □, luteal phase) (from reference 3).

GONADOTROPINS

GnRH Stimulation Test

Pulsatile gonadotropin secretion is a reflection of episodic stimulation of gonadotropin-producing cells by hypothalamic GnRH. If the pulsatile release of GnRH is disrupted or if the gonadotropes cannot respond, oligomenorrhea or amenorrhea associated with abnormal luteinizing hormone (LH) and follicle-stimulating hormone (FSH) secretion will ensue. Pituitary failure may be distinguished from hypothalamic dysfunction with the use of a GnRH stimulation test. GnRH, 100 µg, is administered intravenously after baseline serum LH and FSH levels are obtained. Venous blood samples are obtained at 0, 30, 60, 90, and 120 minutes. The response found in the normal cycling woman is influenced by the phase of the menstrual cycle in which the test is performed. The minimal response is observed in the early preovulatory phase, characterized by at least a doubling of the LH level from baseline values and a 1.5 times increase in FSH level. The maximal response occurs in midcycle or in the luteal phase, when, presumably, availability of GnRH receptors is maximal, having been induced by the effects of both E_2 and GnRH itself. At this point, LH levels should rise to four to eight times baseline

Table 2. *Summary of Hypothalamic-Pituitary Testing*[a]

Hormone system	Agent	Expected result	Interpretation
LH/FSH	GnRH 100 μg IV	LH 2 × baseline at 30 mins; FSH 1.5 × baseline at 60 mins (proliferative phase); LH 4–8 × baseline, FSH 2 × baseline (luteal phase)	Adequate response suggests normal axis; absent response suggests pituitary failure although prolonged stimulation is required to insure absent response
	CC 100 mg/day × 7 days	LH, FSH 2 × baseline on day 8	Adequate response suggests normal axis; subnormal response suggests abnormality at hypothalamic or pituitary level
TSH	TRH 500 μg IV	TSH increases by a minimum of 5 μU/ml up to 30 μU/ml within 30 mins	Adequate response suggests normal axis; absent response suggests pituitary failure; delayed response with slow return to baseline suggests hypothalamic disease
GH	Insulin 0.10	Glucose < 40 mg/dl or decreased 50% from baseline GH > 7 ng/ml at 60 mins	Adequate response suggests normal axis; subnormal response on two tests suggests pituitary insufficiency of GH secretion; thyroid function must be normal for accurate interpretation
	GH releasing hormone; no established protocol		
	Exercise × 20 mins	GH > 7 ng/ml	
	Arginine 30 gm over 30 min	GH > 7 ng/ml at 60 min	
	L-dopa 500 mg by mouth	GH > 7 ng/ml at 90 mins	
ACTH	Insulin (as for GH)	Glucose < 40 mg/dl or 50% suppressed from baseline; cortisol increased by > 10 μg/dl; peak cortisol > 20 μg/dl at 60 mins	Adequate response suggests integrity of axis including adrenal; inadequate response suggests dysfunction at any point along axis
	Metyrapone 750 mg by mouth every 4 hrs × 6 doses	Cortisol < 7 μg/dl, 17-OHCS 2 × baseline and increased by 10–40 mg/24 hrs Deoxycortisol > 10 μg/dl at 8:00 A.M. after 24-hr metyrapone administration	
	CRF; no established protocol		
PRL	TRH (as per TSH protocol)	PRL 2 × baseline in 15–30 mins	Adequate response suggests intact axis; inadequate response suggests failure of lactotropes
	Chlorpromazine 25 mg IM or by mouth	PRL 2–3 × baseline; peak at 60 mins (IM) or 90 mins (by mouth)	
	Metoclopramide 20 mg IV	PRL 6 × baseline	

[a]IV, intravenously; IM, intramuscularly.

and FSH values to two times baseline. Maximal levels of LH usually occur 30 minutes after GnRH administration, and of FSH at approximately 60 minutes (Fig. 2).[3] Patients with pituitary failure will not respond to GnRH stimulation. Those with hypothalamic failure may have a blunted response or no response at all. Repeated administration of GnRH may be necessary to stimulate a normal response.[4] A pulsatile form of GnRH administration with the use of a pump may be necessary to evaluate the ability of the pituitary to respond, because it simulates the physiologic means by which GnRH is delivered to the gonadotrope. Absence of response to either repetitive or pulsatile infusion suggests pituitary failure. In patients with polycystic ovarian syndrome (PCO), where LH is tonically elevated, the LH response to GnRH administration is markedly increased above the normally expected values. This heightened pituitary sensitivity to GnRH is probably related to maximally induced GnRH receptors at the pituitary level.[5] No significant side effects to GnRH administration have been encountered, and no contraindications have been noted.

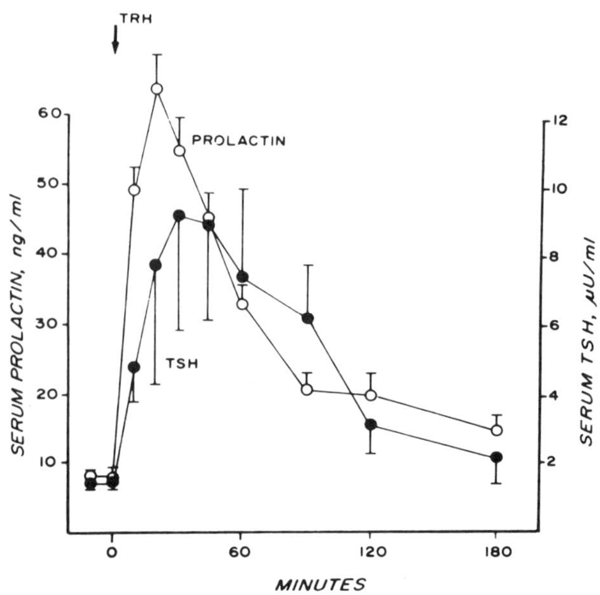

Figure 3
Response of TSH and PRL to administration of TRH in normal women (from reference 8).

Clomiphene Stimulation Test

A stimulation test using clomiphene citrate (CC) has also been described as useful when attempting to distinguish hypothalamic from pituitary amenorrhea. After baseline serum LH and FSH values are obtained, CC, 100 mg, is given by mouth daily for 7 days. Serum LH and FSH levels are expected to at least double when measured on the eighth day thereafter in the presence of a normally functioning hypothalamic-pituitary axis.[6] In patients who lack LH/FSH reserve, there would be no expected rise in LH or FSH. There can be a significant overlap in the results of such a test in patients with hypothalamic and with pituitary dysfunction; therefore, this test has limited value in differentiating between these two conditions. Tests of gonadotropin response are summarized in Table 2.

THYROID-STIMULATING HORMONE

TRH Stimulation Test

Whether hypothyroidism is primary (due to thyroid gland failure) or secondary (due to hypothalamic or pituitary dysfunction), thyroxine (T_4) levels are low. TSH levels are elevated in primary hypothyroidism and should be low in secondary thyroid disease. During incipient pituitary or thyroid gland failure, serum levels of TSH or T_4 may be within the normal range. In such instances, TRH stimulation may be indicated to evaluate TSH reserve. TRH is given intravenously, usually in a dose of 500 μg, although doses of 200 to 500 μg have been recommended. Serum levels of TSH are measured at 0, 30, 60, 90, 120, and 180 minutes. In the normal patient, TSH levels will increase a minimum of 5 μU/ml above the baseline to a maximum of 30 μU/ml and occur within 30 minutes of TRH administration (Fig. 3).[7, 8] A flat or blunted response is highly suggestive of pituitarty disease (secondary hypothyroidism). Patients with hypothalamic hypothyroidism will frequently have a higher but delayed peak value of TSH occurring at 60 to 120 minutes after receiving TRH and slowly returning to baseline levels. Side effects of TRH infusion include transient elevation of blood pressure and an urge to urinate.

GROWTH HORMONE

Adults usually lack symptoms or signs of GH deficiency. In such circumstances, blood levels of GH are usually low, but random measurements provide little useful information about pituitary insufficiency. Therefore, provocative testing must be used to evaluate GH reserve. A GH releasing hormone has recently been characterized from a human pancreatic islet cell tumor,[9] which selectively stimulates GH secretion.[10] However, the normal range of response to this releasing factor has not yet been established. Therefore, this factor cannot yet be used routinely in the evaluation of GH reserve, and the traditional methods of indirect stimulation are still indicated.

Insulin Challenge Test

Insulin-induced hypoglycemia is currently the most common and reliable method used to measure pituitary GH reserve (Table 2). Insulin (0.05 to 0.15 U/kg body weight) is administered intravenously to the fasting patient. Glucose and GH are measured at 0, 30, 45, 60, 90, and 120 minutes. To insure appropriate stimulation of GH release, the serum glucose level must decrease by 50% or to a value of < 40 mg/dl. Serum GH should increase to a level > 7 ng/ml, peaking at 60 minutes.[11] Twenty percent of patients require a second test to exhibit a response. Thyroid function must be normal in order to elicit a normal GH response. Insulin-induced hypoglycemia frequently produces major adrenergic manifestations and may also provoke adrenal crisis in patients with adrenal insufficiency. Glucose and hydrocortisone should be available for intravenous administration whenever pituitary failure is strongly suspected.

Other GH Stimulation Tests

Other tests of GH secretion not frequently used in adults have been described. Exercise stimulates GH release. After a baseline blood specimen is obtained for GH determination, the patient is asked to exercise by running up and down stairs or in place for 20 minutes. The normal GH response should be attainment of a level > 7 ng/ml.[12] Arginine and L-dopa have also been used to stimulate GH response. Arginine (30 gm intravenously) is infused over 30 minutes or L-dopa (500 mg) is given by mouth. As with exercise, serum GH should increase to a level > 7 ng/ml. The peak is usually attained approximately 60 minutes after administration of arginine or 90 minutes after receiving L-dopa. Side effects of arginine administration are uncommon, but the agent should be avoided in patients with liver or renal disease. L-dopa may cause orthostatic symptoms and nausea. Vasopressin and glucagon have also been used to stimulate GH release, but these agents have been shown to be less effective than those previously discussed.[13] It is felt that patients who exhibit an inadequate response to one of these provocative stimuli should be retested with the use of another agent. Significant pituitary dysfunction can be assumed if the response on retesting is once again considered inadequate.

ADRENOCORTICOTROPIC HORMONE

Hypopituitarism resulting in deficient ACTH secretion can cause adrenal insufficiency. Low morning serum cortisol levels may be suggestive of this diagnosis, but unfortunately these measurements are not diagnostic. Traditionally, indirect methods have been employed to evaluate the hypothatlamic-pituitary-adrenocortical axis, much as for GH secreting function.

Insulin Challenge Test

Insulin-induced hypoglycemia has been the most commonly used provocative test of ACTH and cortisol secretion. Hypoglycemia is created as described in the previous section, and glucose and cortisol values are measured at 0, 30, 45, 60, 90, and 120 minutes. If the hypoglycemic stimulus is adequate and the patient has normal pituitary-adrenal function, an increase of 10 μg/dl in plasma cortisol with a peak value ≥ 20 μg/dl should be expected within 60 minutes.[14] An inadequate cortisol response suggests some degree of failure along the hypothalamic-pituitary-adrenal axis.

Metyrapone Test

The second most common approach uses administration of metyrapone, an agent that blocks the 11-hydroxylation step in the synthesis of cortisol. When the negative feedback effect of cortisol is prevented by limiting its synthesis, ACTH secretion increases, accompanied by an increase of cortisol precursors. Many different protocols for metyrapone testing have been described.[15] The most common technique uses orally administered metyrapone. Baseline 24-hour urine specimens are collected for determination of 17-OHCS for 2 consecutive days. On the third day, metyrapone, 750 mg, is administered every 4 hours for 24 hours. On the fourth day, cortisol and 11-deoxycortisol levels are determined on a blood sample obtained at 8:00 A.M. and a final 24-hour urine is collected for determination of 17-OHCS. Post-metyrapone cortisol levels of < 7 μg/dl demonstrate appropriate blockade of cortisol synthesis. Post-metyrapone 11-deoxycortisol levels > 10 μg/dl indicate a normal response.[16] The 17-OHCS value in the 24-hour urine specimen should be twice the basal level and demonstrate an increase of 10 to 40 mg/24 hours.[17] A single standard protocol for metyrapone testing is not nearly as well established as that for insulin. Consequently, metyrapone is used less commonly for testing ACTH-adrenal responsiveness. The single most significant risk of these feedback tests for investigating hypothalamic-pituitary-adrenal reserve is the possible provocation of an adrenal crisis in patients with adrenal insufficiency or profound pituitary failure. Hydrocortisone and 50% glucose should always be available for immediate injection, if necessary, as previously noted.

If adrenal insufficiency is strongly suspected, the initial approach to hypothalamic-pituitary testing may need to be modified. The insulin dose could be reduced to 0.05 U/kg, but a more cautious approach makes use of an ACTH stimulation test as the first step rather than a feedback test using insulin or metyrapone. Chronic glucocorticoid administration should not be overlooked as a common cause of adrenal insufficiency.

ACTH Stimulation Test

Synthetic ACTH (Cortrosyn, Organon Pharmaceuticals, West Orange, NJ) is used in clinical testing to stimulate the adrenal cortex. A dose of 250 μg is administered intravenously to the fasting patient and serum cortisol is measured at 0, 30, and 60 minutes. The serum cortisol level should increase by at least 7 μg/dl to values > 18 μg/dl by 1 hour.[18]

Prolonged ACTH Stimulation Test

In cases of secondary Addison's Disease, that is, adrenal insufficiency secondary to hypothalamic or pituitary dysfunction, priming of the adrenal cortex is frequently necessary to demonstrate responsiveness of the gland. A prolonged or 3-day ACTH stimulation test is then performed. Baseline 24-hour urine specimens are initially collected for 17-OHCS determination for 2 consecutive days. On each of the next 3 days, 250 μg of Cortrosyn is given intravenously by infusion over 8 hours. Plasma cortisol levels are determined daily at 8:00 A.M. and 4:00 P.M., and 24-hour urine specimens are collected for 17-OHCS determination. Plasma cortisol levels should increase by 15 to 40 μg/dl over the baseline value by the end of the first day's infusion and should reach 30 to 60 μg/dl the following days in the presence of normal adrenal responsiveness. The 24-hour 17-OHCS levels should increase 15 to 40 mg/24 hours after the first infusion and reach values of 30 to 40 mg/24 hours by the end of the final infusion.[19] It should be stressed that specific criteria for normal values are not as important as the observation of a significant rise of glucocorticoid secretion. Once the adrenal gland has been determined to be capable of appropriate response, pituitary challenge testing can be ordered with renewed assurance.

Corticotropin-Releasing Factor Stimulation Test

The previously described indirect methods of evaluating the hypothalamic-pituitary-adrenal axis may soon be rendered obsolete by the identification and characterization of a corticotropin-releasing factor (CRF). CRF has recently been described and used to distinguish hypothalamic from pituitary disease.[20] In this approach, patients are administered 100 μg of synthetic ovine CRF intravenously, and blood specimens are obtained at 0, 15, 30, 45, 60, 90, and 120 minutes. Patients with pituitary disease have displayed either a blunted response or no response with regard to ACTH or cortisol levels. Patients with hypothalamic hypopituitarism have demonstrated an exaggerated response of both hormones. The use of CRF in this context is promising, but clinical experience with this approach is at this point limited. Therefore, the more common tests, with their well-characterized responses are still useful.

PROLACTIN

Unlike the previously mentioned pituitary hormones, PRL is primarily under constant inhibitory hypothalamic control. Pituitary tumors or neoplastic impingement on the pituitary stalk, therefore, may increase, rather than decrease, PRL elaboration. Nevertheless, with complete failure or destruction of the pituitary gland, PRL secretion can be absent. Failure of lactation may be the only symptom of hypoprolactinemia. Inability of the pituitary gland to respond to stimulation of PRL release suggests profound functional failure. Characterization of PRL response may be important in evaluating pituitary reserve or in providing a baseline for pituitary status before hypophysectomy.

TRH Stimulation Test

A number of agents and protocols have been used to provoke PRL secretion. The most commonly used approach is TRH infusion, which directly stimulates the pituitary lactotropes (Fig. 3). The test is performed in the same manner as that described for TSH testing. After 500 μg of TRH is given intravenously, serum PRL should reach levels at least double the baseline value within 15 to 20 minutes.[21]

Alternative Drug Tests

As an alternative to TRH testing, drugs that interfere with dopamine action can also be used to stimulate PRL release indirectly. Chlorpromazine is the most frequently used agent for this purpose and is administered at a dose of 25 mg. Blood is obtained at 30-minute intervals over 2 hours. Serum PRL may be expected to increase two to three times with the peak value achieved in 60 to 90 minutes with oral chlorpromazine, or at 60 minutes when chlorpromazine is administered intramuscularly.[22] Lack of response may be found in either primary pituitary failure or in hypothalamic disease. Chlorpromazine testing provides little advantage in differentiating the site of failure. Side effects of chlorpromazine administration, e.g., hypotension and dizziness, can be profound.

Metoclopramide has also been used to provoke PRL secretion. This agent is administered intravenously in a dose of 10 mg, and blood samples are obtained at 0, 15, 30, 60, and 120 minutes. The serum PRL level normally increases six times, and values may remain elevated for 4 to 6 hours after metoclopramide administration.[23] A blunted resonse may be found in patients with pituitary or hypothalamic disease.

MULTIPLE SIMULTANEOUS TESTING

Brief note should be made of multiple simultaneous testing, often referred to as a "megatest" of hypothalamic-pituitary function. The purpose of such a megatest is to derive the most possible information from one set of blood specimens obtained after incorporation of several agents into a single infusion. The megatest effectively combines several of the stimulation tests described earlier. With the patient fasting, TRH (500 μg), GnRH (100 μg), and insulin (0.10 U) are administered simultaneously by vein. Blood specimens are obtained for glucose, GH, cortisol, PRL, TSH, LH, and FSH determinations at 15-minute intervals for 180 minutes. Results are interpreted as described for each individual test. Although considerable information may clearly be gained from such testing, the financial implications are substantial. Care should be taken to insure that all tests requested are truly warranted by the clinical situation.

HYPERPROLACTINEMIA

Identifying a patient with fasting levels of serum PRL $\geq$ 25 ng/ml mandates an evaluation of the cause of hyperprolactinemia. Stress, thyroid function, history of drug ingestion, and history of chest trauma or breast stimulation are factors to consider in making an initial differentiation between a PRL-secreting adenoma or functional hyperprolactinemia. Computerized tomography (CT) scan is routinely indicated to identify a microadenoma. Pituitary tumors can be demonstrated in > 50% of those patients with serum PRL levels > 100 ng/ml. Virtually all patients with PRL levels > 300 ng/ml will have pituitary tumors.[24] When serum PRL levels fall between 20 and 100 ng/ml, dynamic testing has been advocated to distinguish patients with microadenoma from those with functional hyperprolactinemia. TRH stimulation is frequently employed. Patients with pituitary microadenomas tend to have a blunted and delayed response, with the peak PRL level more than twice the baseline value, a pattern usually considered to be a normal response.[25] Not all studies have found this test to be sufficiently specific to be diagnostically helpful.[26] Patients with PRL-secreting adenomas tend to demonstrate a flat response to chlorpromazine administration, but some patients will respond with an increase in PRL, especially when higher doses of chlorpromazine are administered.[27] Suppression of normal prolactin release has also been studied with the use of L-dopa. Approximately 85% of patients with functional hyperprolactinemia will demonstrate suppression of PRL levels in response to L-dopa, whereas suppression will occur in only 50% of patients with a microadenoma.[24] The ability of any of these tests to effectively differentiate the two groups has not been well established. Rather, the significant degree of overlap between the two groups is a characteristic finding. Therefore, any provocative test employed to differentiate those patients with pituitary microadenoma from those with functional hyperprolactinemia has limited usefulness. Ultimately, the differentiation between the two groups may be purely academic in that contemporary management of such patients would likely be identical, independent of the cause of the hyperprolactinemia.

HYPERANDROGENISM

The reproductive or medical endocrinologist investigates many patients with complaints relating to hyperandrogenism. The evaluation of such problems is frequently confusing, and dynamic testing can often prove to be a useful diagnostic tool in elucidating the cause. In women, androgens generally originate from either the adrenal cortex or the ovary. The primary diagnostic goals are to identify the organ primarily responsible for overproduction of androgens and to de-

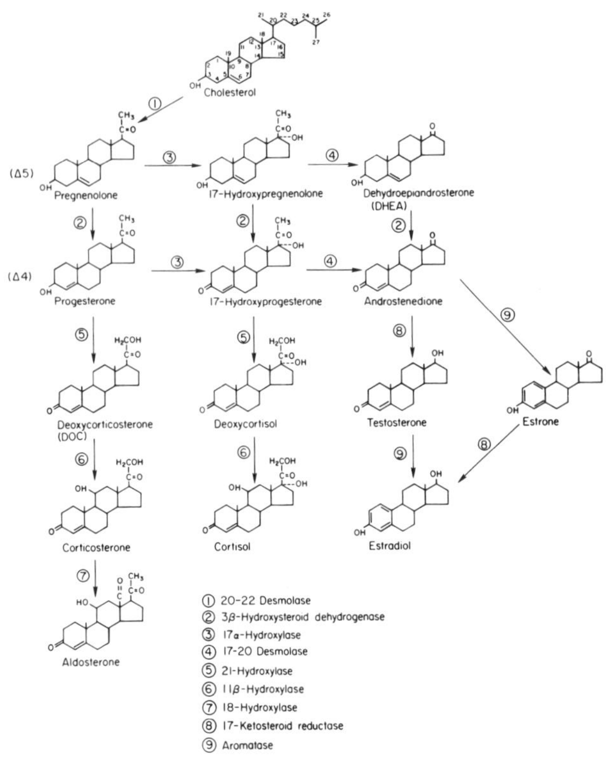

Figure 4
Steroid biosynthesis from cholesterol precursor.

termine whether a neoplasm or autonomous source of secretion is present.

Screening tests usually include measurement of the weak androgens dehydroepiandrosterone (DHEA) or more commonly its sulfated metabolite (DHEA-S) and androstenedione (Δ^4A) as well as the more potent androgen testosterone (T). DHEA-S is predominantly secreted by the adrenal cortex and thus serves as a marker for adrenal activity. Δ^4A is produced by the adrenal cortex and ovary in approximately equal proportions. T is also secreted almost equally by the adrenal cortex and ovary, although 50% of circulating T results from peripheral conversion of Δ^4A. If any of the serum androgens are elevated in the hirsute woman, more specific testing should be initiated.

MEASUREMENT OF URINARY STEROIDS

Measurement of urinary steroid including 17-OHCS, 17-ketosteroids (17-KS), and 17-ketogenic steroids (17-KGS) has long been associated with the workup of the androgenized patient. These assays measure groups of steroid hormones with similar structure. Most dynamic testing protocols define normal response ranges with the use of 24-hour urinary values. Direct assay of individual steroid hormones in peripheral blood is becoming more widely used, but until normal responses are well established, 24-hour urinary steroid levels may continue to represent the standard. The biosynthetic pathway of steroid hormones from their cholesterol precursor is reviewed in Figure 4. The structural relationship of 17-OHCS, 17-KS, and 17-KGS is summarized in Figure 5.

Twenty-four-hour urinary 17-OHCS reflect glucocorticoid production. The Porter-Silber reaction measures those steroid hormones containing a hydroxyl group on carbon numbers 17 and 21 and a ketone group at carbon 20.[28] Cortisol and its metabolites including cortisone, 11-deoxycortisol, and tetrahydrocortisol and tetrahydrocortisone are measured by this reaction (Fig. 6). The value for 17-OHCS represents only approximately 40% of the total cortisol and metabolites produced. Nevertheless, its usefulness as an indicator of glucocorticoid production stems from the fact that metabolites of steroid hormones other than cortisol contribute very little to this determination. Normal levels for 24-hour urinary 17-OHCS are 4 to 10 mg/24 hours. Our ability to measure cortisol and other glucocorticoid metabolites directly diminishes the usefulness of urinary 17-OHCS measurements. Determination of urinary 17-KS serves as an index of adrenal androgen production. The 17-KS are measured by the Zimmerman reaction and include only those steroids containing a ketone group at carbon 17.[30] Thus DHEA-S, as well as Δ^4A and its metabolites etiocholanolone and androsterone, are included in this measurement. Dihydrotestosterone (DHT) and T, the most potent androgens, lack a ketone group at carbon 17 (Fig. 7) and are not measured by the Zimmermann reaction. Therefore, determination

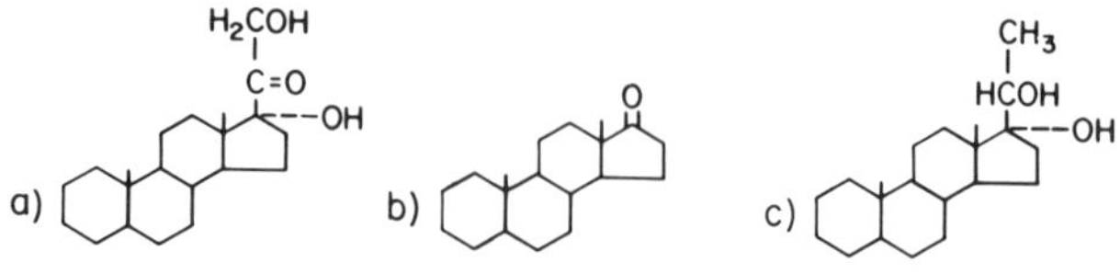

Figure 5
(a), Structure of steroids measured by Porter-Silber Chromogen reaction (17-OHCS). Hydroxyl groups must be present on C-17 and C-21 and a ketone group at C-20. (**b**), Structure of steroids measured by Zimmerman reaction (17-KS). A ketone group must be present at C-17. (**c**), Structure of 17-KGS. Hydroxyl groups must be present at C-17 and at either C-20 (shown here) or C-21.

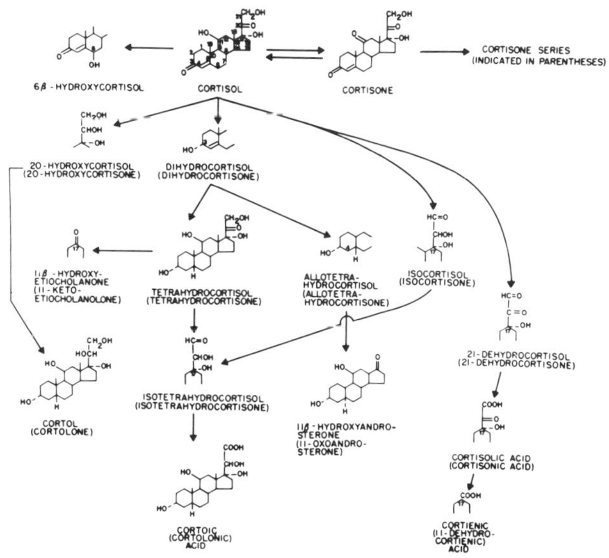

Figure 6
Structure and metabolism of cortisol and key metabolites (from reference 29).

of 17-KS as well as serum androgens may be important in evaluating the hyperandrogenized patient. Normal values for urinary 17-KS in the woman are 7 to 13 mg/24 hours.

The 17-KGS contain one hydroxyl group at C-17 and a second hydroxyl group at either C-20 or C-21. This group of steroids includes not only those measured by the Porter-Silber reaction but also other metabolites of cortisol, including cortol and cortolone. Assay of urinary 17-KGS is performed by oxidation with sodium bismuthate to yield 17-KS, which are then measured by the Zimmermann reaction. Thus the 17-KGS can be determined by comparing the net value of 17-KS obtained before and after oxidation. Normal values for urinary 17-KGS in the woman range from 8 to 20 mg/24 hours. Measurement of 17-KGS is rarely helpful because of the wide range of steroids that comprise the group.

ENZYME DEFECTS

The most common cause of hyperandrogenism in women of reproductive age is polycystic ovarian disease (PCO). This diagnosis is usually one of exclusion, made only after other endocrine or neoplastic processes have been excluded.

Partial deficiency of 21-hydroxylase, 11-hydroxylase, and 3β-ol dehydrogenase (3β-HSD) can lead to a PCO-like picture. As diagnostic criteria become more firmly established and widely used, undoubtedly more patients thought to have PCO will be identified as having a specific enzyme deficiency. It is important to identify these patients, because therapy with glucocorticoid replacement can be more specifically applied to their clinical problem. Well-established screening criteria would be helpful to determine which patients require formal testing. Because these defects are frequently genetically transmitted, patients who have a family history of PCO should probably be tested. Furthermore, one should consider testing those with uncharacteristic body habitus for PCO or severe hirsutism at a young age.

21-Hydroxylase Deficiency

Partial deficiency in 21-hydroxylase activity has been recognized since the 1970s.[31-33] Relative deficiency of the 21-hydroxylase enzyme may result in compensatory overstimulation of steroidogenesis by ACTH. Other steroid hormones in the biosynthetic schema proximal to this enzymatic step are chronically increased in the case of an absolute deficiency (Fig. 4), but baseline levels may be normal when the enzyme deficiency is only partial. ACTH stimulation can be used to accentuate the relative deficiency and make a diagnosis possible. The diagnostic criteria used at Johns Hopkins were established by testing obligate heterozygotes for 21-hydroxylase deficiency (parents of children with congenital virilizing adrenal hyperplasia).[34] Synthetic ACTH (Cortrosyn), 1.0 mg, is administered intravenously to the fasting patient after blood for baseline levels of P and 17-hydroxyprogesterone (17-OHP) is obtained. Levels of P and 17-OHP are once again determined at 30 minutes. The sum of the pre-ACTH levels of P and 17-OHP is subtracted from the sum of the post-ACTH levels and the result divided by 30 (minutes) to calculate the rate of

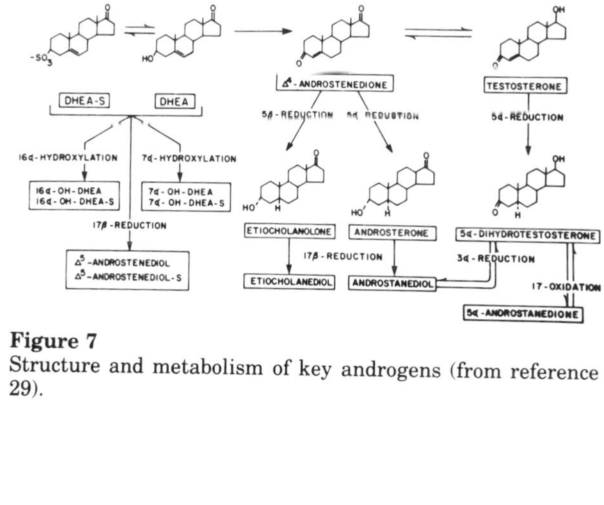

Figure 7
Structure and metabolism of key androgens (from reference 29).

rise of precursor levels. This relationship is defined by the formula

$$\frac{(P_2 - P_1) + (17\text{-OHP}_2 - 17\text{-OHP}_1)}{30}$$

Patients with deficient 21-hydroxylase activity demonstrate a greater rate of rise than those with normal enzyme function. Values < 6.5 ng/dl/minute are considered to be within normal limits.[34] In the normally cycling woman, this test should be performed during the preovulatory phase of the cycle. An adult-onset, milder form of congenital virilizing adrenal hyperplase has also been described.[35] This condition is felt to possibly be a homozygous, although attenuated, form of 21-hydroxylase deficiency. The diagnostic criteria established for testing those patients who are obligate heterozygotes are equally applicable to this latter group of patients with attenuated adrenal hyperplasia. Suppression of adrenal overstimulation by exogenous glucocorticoids will frequently decrease androgen levels and induce ovulatory menstrual cycles in affected patients. Prednisone, 5 mg, taken orally at night is the most commonly used regimen.

Routine screening with 17-OHP determinations has been advocated in order to identify patients with 21-hydroxylase deficiency. ACTH stimulation should be performed in patients with screening values of 17-OHP > 5 ng/ml.[36] Unfortunately, no clearly established minimum value assures normal enzyme activity. Therefore, the dilemma of whom to test persists, and the decision continues to rest on clinical suspicion.

11-Hydroxylase Deficiency

Late-onset 11-hydroxylase deficiency has also been postulated to cause a PCO-like picture. The cause of the hyperandrogenism in this deficiency state is similar to that for 21-hydroxylase deficiency. These patients can synthesize 11-deoxycorticosterone and may therefore be hypertensive. ACTH stimulation has been described as producing an undue elevation of precursor hormones,[37] but no specific hormone levels have been described as diagnostic. Although this syndrome may be significant, it is difficult to characterize until more patients are identified and studied and firm diagnostic criteria have been established. Patients in whom this deficiency is identified should be treated with glucocorticoids if they have symptoms of adrenal hyperstimulation.

3β-Hydroxysteroid Dehydrogenase Deficiency

Patients with presumed PCO who have elevated levels of Δ^5 steroids (DHEA-S) and normal levels of Δ^4 steroids (Δ^4A and T) may have a deficiency of 3β-HSD. A number of reports[38-40] have described such patients and have sought to characterize the defect. ACTH stimulation has been advocated if the screening serum level of DHEA-S is elevated out of proportion to Δ^4A or T. Unfortunately, specific diagnostic criteria are not well established. One study reported a higher baseline ratio of 17-hydroxypregnenolone (Δ^5 17-OHP) to 17-OHP among 24 hirsute women, compared with normal women (2.8 versus 1.2).[41] With ACTH stimulation, the ratio increased to a level as high as 14 in affected women versus 4.4 in normal women. This group estimated that 3% of women with PCO have this enzyme defect. Another recent study suggested several discriminating measures including the baseline Δ^5 17-OHP/17-OHP ratio.[42] This ratio was 1.0 + 0.6 in normal women, 3.8 + 2.9 in women felt to have 3β-HSD deficiency, and 0.6 + 0.5 in women with 21-hydroxylase deficiency. These patients were then stimulated with 25 U of Cortrosyn administered intravenously. The ratios of DHEA/Δ^4A and DHEA/T were 8 and 60, respectively. Similarly, stimulated control patients had ratios of DHEA/Δ^4A of 4 and DHEA/T of 25. The 3β-HSD defect was present in 12.9% of their population of patients with PCO. This enzyme, unlike 11- and 21-hydroxylating enzymes, is normally present in both the ovary and adrenal cortex. A difference in the expression of the deficiency between the two glands has been postulated.[43] Thus, clinical manifestations of such an enzyme defect may differ significantly among patients. Many patients will respond to glucocortoid suppression with regularization of menses and decreased androgen levels, whereas others will not. Uniform diagnostic criteria must be established in order to have an accurate understanding of the impact and therapy of this problem.

CUSHING'S SYNDROME

A frequent concern in the evaluation of the hyperandrogenized patient is the possibility that the patient has Cushing's syndrome. The clinical presentation in all types of Cushing's syndrome results from hypercortisolism. Manifestations of excessive secretion of androgens and mineralocorticoids are far more variable. Screening for Cushing's syndrome is not indicated in women whose only signs are hirsutism or oligomenorrhea and in whom signs of cortisol excess are lacking. Further studies should be initiated in patients who manifest symptoms consistent with Cushing's syndrome. The goals of the evaluation are twofold. First, patients who have hypercortisolism should be distinguished from those who do not. Second, the pathophysiologic process responsible for the excess cortisol must be identified. Fasting and 4:00 P.M. cortisol levels have not proven predictive of Cushing's syndrome. Cortisol values obtained late in the evening are frequently elevated in patients with Cushing's syndrome but are not always diagnostic.

Screening Tests

The two most frequently used screening tests for Cushing's include measurement of 24-hour urinary free cortisol and an overnight dexamethasone suppression test. Plasma cortisol circulates almost completely bound, primarily to cortisol binding globulin and, to a lesser extent, albumin. When cortisol levels exceed the binding capacity, the urinary free cortisol level increases. Values of urinary free cortisol > 100 μg/24 hours suggest a diagnosis of Cushing's syndrome.[44] A frequently used protocol for overnight dexamethasone suppression involved administration of 1 mg of dexamethasone orally at 11:00 P.M. followed by a fasting blood specimen obtained at 8:00 A.M. for determination of plasma cortisol. Glucocorticoids administered at night serve to block the normal early morning cortisol surge. Thus, fasting cortisol levels would normally be expected to be 6 μg/dl or less.[45]

Low-Dose Dexamethasone Suppression

If there is any inconsistency or uncertainty in the interpretation of the results of the two previously described tests, a standard, or low-dose dexamethasone suppression test, should be considered. Two baseline 24-hour urine specimens are collected for determination of free cortisol and 17-OHCS; then dexamethasone is given at a dosage of 0.5 mg orally every 6 hours for 2 days. Twenty-four-hour urine specimens should be collected on these days, and plasma cortisol is determined at 4:00 P.M. on the second day. A normal response entails values for 17-OHCS of < 4 mg/24 hours[46] and suppression of urinary free cortisol to < 20 μg/24 hours on the second day. The serum cortisol should be < 5 μg/dl on the afternoon of the second day.[47] These tests are sensitive in that few patients with Cushing's syndrome have normal results. However, there are a number of confounding factors that can cause abnormal, or false-positive, dexamethasone suppression tests, including obesity, depression, and alcoholism. Patients taking an estrogen preparation will have increased corticosteroid-binding globulin, thus raising the total level of plasma cortisol. In these patients, overnight dexamethasone suppression values may also be abnormal. They usually respond normally to the 2-day low-dose suppression test. Exogenous estrogen should not interfere with the interpretation of the 24-hour urinary free cortisol test. Phenytoin (Dilantin) accelerates hepatic metabolism of dexamethasone and thus can cause abnormal suppression tests. Phenytoin will not interfere with interpretation of the urinary free cortisol assays.[29]

High-Dose Dexamethasone Suppression

If hypercortisolism is established on the basis of the aforementioned criteria, the diagnosis of Cushing's syndrome is made. The remainder of the evaluation is aimed at identifying the pathophysiology of cortisol excess. Naturally occurring Cushing's syndrome is due to an ACTH-producing pituitary adenoma (Cushing's disease) in approximately 70% of cases. Adrenal adenoma or carcinoma is responsible for 15% of the cases, and ectopic ACTH produced by neoplasms accounts for another 15%. Oat cell carcinoma of lung, bronchial adenoma, thymoma, pheochromocytoma, medullary thyroid carcinoma, and islet cell tumor of the pancreas have all been associated with ACTH secretion. Most patients with Cushing's disease have at least some degree of feedback responsiveness to cortisol at the pituitary level. Therefore, high-dose or prolonged dexamethasone administration will cause suppression of pituitary ACTH and cortisol secretion in Cushing's disease. Patients with autonomous adrenal function and those with ectopic ACTH production usually do not have suppressible cortisol. The high-dose dexamethasone suppression test is performed in the same manner as the low-dose test except that 2 mg of dexamethasone is adminis-

Table 3. *Tests of Adrenal Cortical Suppression*

	Protocol	Expected result	Interpretation
Overnight dexamethasone	1 mg at 11:00 P.M.	Cortisol < 6 μg/dl	If elevated (in absence of obesity, estrogen, phenytoin, stress, alcoholism), probable Cushing's syndrome
Low-dose dexamethasone	0.5 mg by mouth every 6 hours × 2 days	17-OHCS < 4 mg/24 hrs on day 2; serum cortisol < 10 μg/dl at 4 P.M. on day 2	If elevated, probable Cushing's syndrome
High-dose dexamethasone	2 mg by mouth every 6 hours × 2 days	17-OHCS suppressed at least 40% on day 2; serum cortisol < 10 μg/dl at 4 P.M. on day 2	If appropriate suppression, probable Cushing's disease; if not, adrenal neoplasm versus ectopic ACTH syndrome

tered orally every 6 hours rather than 0.5 mg. Patients with Cushing's disease should have suppression of urinary 17-OHCS levels of 40% or more on the second day of the test[46] and an afternoon serum cortisol level on the second day < 10 μg/dl.[47] Dexamethasone suppression testing is summarized in Table 3.

Further Testing

The patient whose serum cortisol is not suppressed even by high-dose dexamethasone is likely to have either an autonomous adrenal source of cortisol or ectopic ACTH production. As assays for ACTH continue to become more reliable, these conditions will be easier to differentiate. Patients with autonomous adrenal secretion should have suppressible pituitary ACTH. Their ACTH levels should be considerably lower than 200 pg/ml, a value usually seen in patients with an ACTH-producing tumor (Fig. 8).[29, 48] Patients with low levels of ACTH should have a CT scan to evaluate the possibility of an adrenal tumor. If ACTH levels remain high despite high dose dexamethasone suppression, further diagnostic steps should be aimed at identifying an ACTH-secreting neoplasm. A notable exception to the generalized protocol outlined may be encountered in patients with nodular adrenal hyperplasia, whose source of cortisol is frequently sporadic and unpredictably suppressible. In such cases, ACTH and cortisol levels are variable, as is their response to attempts at suppression. A CT scan may sometimes demonstrate the nodular adrenal, which is frequently quite difficult to distinguish from the other entities mentioned. Although the procedures described will establish the cause of hypercortisolism in most cases, it would be unrealistic to expect that all patients would be neatly categorized by this diagnostic scheme. Further testing, such as CT scans or selective venous catheterization for hormone determination, is sometimes indicated. Above all, the clinician must consider the characteristics of the patient's presentation, which include rapidity of onset of symptoms and associated signs and severity of hypercortisolism in reaching an accurate diagnosis.

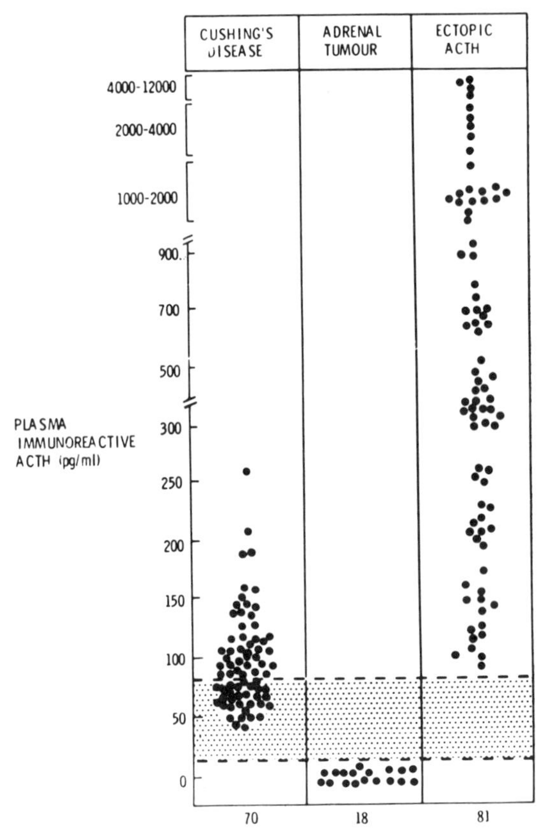

Figure 8
Plasma ACTH levels depending on cause in patients with Cushing's syndrome. *Dotted area* represents the normal range. *Numbers under panels* are numbers of patients (from reference 48).

Table 4. *Adrenal and Ovarian Contributions to Peripheral Serum Androgens*[a]

Subjects	Steroids				
	Δ^4A	T	DHT	DHEA-S	Cortisol
	ng/ml	*ng/ml*	*ng/ml*	*ng/ml*	*ng/ml*
Normal (upper limits)					
Control	1.65	0.55	0.30	2900	180
After dexamethasone (ovarian)	0.75	0.35	0.10	400	30
Control after dexamethasone (adrenal)	0.90	0.20	0.20	2500	

[a]Modified from Maroulis.[51]

Neoplasm

The ultimate goal in evaluation of the hyperandrogenic patient is the differentiation of hyperplasia from a neoplasm. A reasonable plan must be established based on the clinical presentation and results of laboratory tests. Elevated levels of DHEA-S to value > 7000 ng/ml mandate a thorough evaluation to exclude the possiblity of adrenal neoplasm. If hirsutism is rapid in onset and associated with hypercortisolism, adrenal carcinoma should be suspected. An adrenal adenoma may produce hypercortisolism but is not likely to cause elevated levels of androgens. A CT scan of the adrenal gland should be ordered. If no tumor is identified by the CT scan, suppression of adrenal androgens with glucocorticoids should be initiated. Suppression of adrenal androgens requires 4 days in normal women[49] and perhaps up to 2 weeks in certain hirsute women.[50] Dexamethasone is administered orally in dosages of 2 mg/day (patients weighing between 70 and 90 kg) to 4 mg/day (patients weighing > 90 kg) for 9 to 14 days, by which time serum DHEA-S levels should be suppressed to < 400 ng/ml. The serum cortisol value should be < 4 μg/dl to assure adequate adrenal suppression.[51] If appropriate suppression is documented, a diagnosis of adrenal hyperplasia is likely and the patient should be maintained on glucocorticoid therapy. In the absence of suppression, adrenal neoplasm or possibly nodular adrenal hyperplasia must still be suspected, and adrenal vein catheterization or surgical exploration may be considered to establish a diagnosis.

There is no consensus as to the clinical importance of identifying the source of increased T and Δ^4A. Ovulation induction or management of hirsutism can be provided without this specific information. However, there is general agreement that T values > 200 ng/dl mandate a thorough evaluation to exclude the possibility of a neoplasm. Because T may originate from either the ovary or adrenal cortex, the evaluation must include consideration of either as the potential source of the hormone. Ultrasound and/or CT of the ovaries are frequently performed first. CT of the adrenal is less commonly performed if the DHEA-S is normal and when evidence of hypercortisolism is lacking. Differential catheterization of ovarian and adrenal veins has also been used to identify the source of excess androgens. This technique is sometimes dangerous to perform, and yields results that are often difficult to interpret.[52, 53] Catheterization should therefore be reserved for those patients in whom tumor is likely and other diagnostic methods have failed to provide a diagnosis.[54]

A variety of techniques of adrenal and ovarian suppression have been used. Suppression of adrenal androgens with glucocorticoids can require up to 2 weeks. Androgen levels after adrenal suppression usually reflect ovarian contribution. Normal values are shown in Table 4. If androgen levels are not suppressed by the protocol outlined, an autonomous source, either ovarian or adrenal, is still possible. Several other inferences can be made based on glucocorticoid suppression pat-

Table 5. *Androgen Suppression Patterns*[a]

Baseline androgens	Androgens after dexamethasone	Baseline − value after dexamethasone	Androgen source
Elevated	Normal	Greater than normal adrenal contribution	Adrenal
Elevated	Elevated	Equal to normal adrenal contribution	Ovary
Elevated	Elevated	Greater than normal adrenal contribution	Ovary and adrenal

[a]Adapted from Maroulis.[51]

terns (Table 5). This scheme has been used to tailor therapy to suppress the primary source of overproduction.[55] The prolonged dexamethasone suppression test of adrenal androgens is sometimes supplemented with hCG administration. After 9 days of dexamethasone, hCG, 10,000 U intramuscularly, is administered for 1 to 3 days with evaluation of serum and/or urinary androgens thereafter. If the ovary is responsive, androgen levels will rise.

Oral contraceptive agents may be used to suppress ovarian hormone production. Androgen levels can be measured before and after at least 3 weeks of oral contraceptive administration.[56] If excess androgens originate from the ovary, suppression of ovarian function by an exogenous estrogen/progestin preparation should result in reduced elaboration of androgens by the ovaries. On the other hand, sex hormone-binding globulin levels also increase during estrogen administration, which would tend to increase the total androgen levels measured (although not the level of free hormone). In one study, five women with hirsutism and elevated androgens were given oral contraceptive agents (mestranol, 50 μg, and norethindrone, 1 mg) for 6 months. All five subjects demonstrated marked suppression of T, including two women whose baseline serum T values were 260 and 269 ng/dl.[57] Lack of suppression after therapy tends to support either an adrenal or an autonomous ovarian source of androgens. Unfortunately, interpretation may be difficult, and the effects of exogenous estrogen on sex hormone-binding globulin and thus bound androgen must be considered. There is no standard protocol with clearly established diagnostic criteria for ovarian suppression. Furthermore, suppressibility of ovarian tumors can be variable. Despite these potential drawbacks, investigation into this area of testing may prove fruitful in the future. Radioactive imaging using NP-59 (6-β^{131}I iodomethylnorcholesterol) has recently been used in identifying a lipoid cell ovarian tumor. The patient studied had prolonged adrenal suppression before administration of the radionuclide. This isotope was concentrated in the steroid-active ovarian tissue, allowing localization of the tumor on the right side of the pelvis. The use of this or related techniques in nuclear imaging holds promise for the future although present data are insufficient to document utility. If concern over the possibility of an ovarian tumor is high and hormonal testing is inadequate to exclude such a diagnosis, differential adrenal and ovarian vein catheterization may be performed, obtaining venous effluent for steroid determinations. Ultimately, laparotomy may be necessary for diagnosis.

CONCLUSION

A variety of dynamic testing protocols has been reviewed, along with the clinical situations in which the protocols might be applied and commentary on interpretation and potential side effects. As new interrelationships are discovered and hormonal substances identified, testing will likely become even more sophisticated. Ideally, invasive catheterization studies will become obsolete. Ultimately, it is hoped that new and specific tests will be developed, with normal results standardized such that specific dissection of the hormonal milieu will be made possible.

Acknowledgments. I wish to thank Edward E. Wallach, M.D., for his guidance, support, and editorial expertise, and Ms. Becky Davis for her secretarial contribution.

REFERENCES

1. Medvei VC: A History of Endocrinology. Boston, MTP Press, Ltd., 1982, p 7
2. Spaulding SW, Utiger RD: The thyroid: physiology, hyperthyroidism, hypothyroidism, and the painful thyroid. In Endocrinology and Metabolism, Edited by Felig P, Baxter JD, Broadus AE, Frohman LA. New York, McGraw-Hill Book Co., 1981, p 335
3. Wolleson F, Swerdloff RS, Odell WD: LH and FSH responses to luteinizing releasing hormone in normal fertile women. Metabolism 25:1275, 1976
4. Snyder PJ, Rudenstein RS, Gardner DF, Rothman JG: Repetitive infusion of gonadotropin-releasing hormone distinguishes hypothalamic from pituitary hypogonadism. J Clin Endocrinol Metab 48:864, 1979
5. Rebar R, Judd HL, Yen SSC, Rakoff J, Vandenberg G, Naftolin F: Characterization of the inappropriate gonadotropin secretion in polycystic ovary syndrome. J Clin Invest 57:1320, 1976
6. Paulsen CA: Short- and long-term effects of clomiphene citrate on the pituitary-testicular axis. J Clin Endocrinol Metab 33:970, 1971
7. Hershman JH: Use of thyrotropin-releasing hormone in clinical medicine. Med Clin North Am 62:313, 1978
8. Frohman LA: Diseases of the anterior pituitary. In Endocrinology and Metabolism, Edited by P Felig, JD Baxter, AE Broadus, LA Frohman. New York, McGraw-Hill Book Co., 1981, p 183
9. Rivier J, Spiess J, Thorner M, Vale M: Characterization of a growth hormone-releasing factor from a human pancreatic islet tumour. Nature 300:276, 1982
10. Thorner MO, Spiess J, Vance ML, Rogol AD, Kaiser DC, Webster JD, Rivier J, Borges JL, Bloom SR, Cronin MJ,

Evans WS, MacLeod RM, Vale W: Human pancreatic growth-hormone-releasing factor selectively stimulates growth-hormone secretion in man. Lancet 1:24, 1983
11. Lamberton PR, Jackson MD: Investigation of hypothalamic pituitary disease. Clin Endocrinol Metab 12:509, 1983
12. Johnsonbaugh RE, Bybee DE, Georges LP: Exercise tolerance test: single sample screening technique to rule out growth-hormone deficiency. JAMA 240:664, 1978
13. Eddy RL, Gilliand PF, Ibarra JD, McMurry JF, Thompson JQ: Human growth hormone release: comparison of provocative test procedures. Am J Med 56:179, 1974
14. Greenwood FC, Landon J, Stamp TCB: The plasma sugar, free fatty acid, cortisol, and growth hormone response to insulin. J Clin Invest 45:429, 1966
15. Streeten DHP, Anderson GH, Dalakos TG, Seeley D, Mallov JS, Eusebio R, Suderlin FS, Badawy SZA, King RB: Normal and abnormal function of the hypothalamic-pituitary-adrenocorticol system in man. Endocr Rev 5:371, 1984
16. Spark RF: Simplified assessment of pituitary-adrenal reserve: measurement of serum 11-deoxycortisol and cortisol after metyrapone. Ann Intern Med 75:717, 1971
17. Liddle GW, Island D, Meudor CK: Normal and abnormal regulation of corticotropin secretion in man. Recent Prog Horm Res 18:125, 1962
18. Speckart PF, Nocoloff JT, Bethune JE: Screening for adrenocorticol insufficiency with cosynthropin (Synthetic ACTH). Arch Intern Med 128:761, 1971
19. Streck WF: Adrenocorticol insufficiency. In Endocrine Diagnosis: Clinical and Laboratory Approach, Edited by WF Streck, DH Lockwood. Boston, Little, Brown & Co., 1983, p 130
20. Tsukada T, Nakai Y, Koh T, Tsujii S, Inada M, Nishikawa M, Shinoda H, Kawa I, Takezawa N, Imura H: Plasma adrenocorticotropin and cortisol responses to ovine corticotropin-releasing factor in patients with adrenocorticol insufficiency due to hypothalamic and pituitary disorders. J Clin Endocrinol Metab 58:758, 1984
21. Jackson IMD: Thyrotropin-releasing hormone. N Engl J Med 306:145, 1982
22. Friesen H, Guyda H, Hwang P, Tyson JE, Barbeau A: Functional evaluation of prolactin secretion: a guide to therapy. J Clin Invest 51:706, 1972
23. Jacobs LS: Anterior pituitary disorders: Hypopituitarism, prolactin, growth hormone. In Endocrine Diagnosis: Clinical and Laboratory Approach, Edited by WF Streck, DH Lockwood. Boston, Little, Brown & Co., 1983, p 22
24. Kleinberg DZ, Noel GL, Frantz AG: Glactorrhea: a study of 235 cases, including 48 with pituitary tumors. N Engl J Med 296:589, 1977
25. Marrs RP, Bertolli SJ, Klotzky OA: The use of thyrotropin-releasing hormone in distinguishing prolactin-secreting pituitary adenoma. Am J Obstet Gynecol 138:620, 1980
26. Klijn JGM, Lamberts SWJ, DeJong FH, Birkenhäger JC: The value of the thyrotropin-releasing hormone test in patients with prolactin-secreting pituitary tumors and suprasellar non-pituitary tumors. Fertil Steril 35:155, 1981
27. Zarate A, Jacobs LJ, Canales ES, Schally AV, DeLa Cruz A, Soria J, Daughaday WH: Functional evaluation of pituitary reserve in patients with the amenorrhea-galactorrhea syndome utilizing luteinizing hormone-releasing hormone (LH-RH), L-Dopa, and chlorpromazine. J Clin Endocrinol Metab 37:855, 1973
28. Porter CC, Silber RH: A quantitative color reaction for cortisone and related 17, 21-dihydroxy-20-ketosteroids. J Biol Chem 185:201, 1950
29. Baxter JD, Tyrrell JB: The adrenal cortex. In Endocrinology and Metabolism, Edited by P Felig, JD Baxter, AE Broadus, LA Frohman. New York, McGraw-Hill Book Co., 1981, p 412
30. Margray HW, Weicheselbaum TE: Laboratory procedures in diagnosis of adrenal cortical diseases. In The Adrenal Cortex, Edited by AB Eisenstein. Boston, Little, Brown & Co., 1967, p 405
31. Hall R, Smith PA, Harkness RA, Smart GA: A study of the parents of patients with congenital adrenal hyperplasia. Proc R Soc Med 63:1040, 1970
32. Qazi QH, Hill JG, Thompson MW: Steroid studies in parents of patients with congenital virilizing adrenal hyperplasia. J Clin Endocrinol Metab 33:23, 1971
33. Lee P, Gareis FJ: Evidence for partial 21-hydroxylase deficiency among heterozygotes carriers of congenital adrenal hyperplasia. J Clin Endocrinol Metab 41:415, 1975
34. Gutai JP, Kowarski AA, Migeon CJ: The detection of the heterozygous carrier for congenital virilizing adrenal hyperplasia. J Pediatr 90:924, 1977
35. Rosenwaks Z, Lee PA, Jones GS, Migeon CJ, Wentz AC: An attenuated form of congenital virilizing hyperplasia. J Clin Endocrinol Metab 49:355, 1979
36. Lobo RA: The role of the adrenal in polycystic ovary syndrome. Semin Reprod Endocrinol 2:251, 1984
37. Cathelineau G, Brereault JL, Fiet J, Julien R, Dreux C, Canivet J: Adrenocorticol 11-hydroxylation defect in adult women with postmenarchial onset of symptoms. J Clin Endocrinol Metab 51:287, 1980
38. Bongiovanni AM: The adrenogenital syndrome with deficiency of 3β-hydroxysteroid dehydrogenese. J Clin Invest 41:2086, 1962
39. Zachmann M, Vollmin JA, Murset G, Curtuis H-Ch, Prader A: Unusual type of congenital adrenal hyperplasia probably due to deficiency of a 3β-hydroxysteroid dehydrogenase. Case report of a surviving girl and steroid studies. J Clin Endocrinol Metab 30:719, 1970
40. Rosenfield RL, Rich BH, Wolfsdorf JI, Cassorla F, Parks JS, Bongiovanni AM, Wu CH, Shackleton CHL: Pubertal presentation of congenital 3β-hydroxysteroid dehydrogenase deficiency. J Clin Endocrinol Metab 51:345, 1980
41. Lobo RA, Goebelsmann U: Evidence for reduced 3β-hydroxysteroid dehydrogenase activity in some hirsute women thought to have polycystic ovary syndrome. J Clin Endocrinol Metab 53:394, 1981
42. Pang S, Lerner AJ, Storer E, Levine LS, Oberfield SE, Engle I, New MI: Late-onset adrenal steroid 3-β-hydroxysteroid dehydrogenase deficiency. I. A cause of hirsutism in pubertal and post-pubertal women. J Clin Endocrinol Metab 60:428, 1985
43. Bongiovanni AM: Acquired adrenal hyperplasia: with special reference to 3β-hydroxysteroid dehydrogenase. Fertil Steril 35:599, 1981
44. Eddy RL, Jones AL, Gilliland PF, Ibarra JD, Thompson JQ, McMurry JF: Cushing's syndrome: a prospective study of diagnostic methods. Am J Med 55:621, 1973

45. Crapo L: Cushing's syndrome: a review of diagnostic tests. Metabolism 28:955, 1979
46. Liddle GW: Tests of pituitary-adrenal suppressibility in diagnosis of Cushing's syndrome. J Clin Endocrinol Metab 20:1539, 1960
47. Ashcraft MW, Van Herle AJ, Vener SL, Geffner DL: Serum cortisol levels in Cushing's syndrome after low- and high-dose dexamethasone suppression. Ann Intern Med 97:21, 1982
48. Symington TS, Carter RL (Eds): Scientific Foundations of Oncology. London, Heinemann Medical Books, 1976, p 112
49. Abraham GE: Ovarian and adrenal contribution to peripheral androgens during the menstrual cycle. J Clin Endocrinol Metab 39:340, 1974
50. Maroulis GB: Comparison between the source of hyperandrogen and ovarian morphology in hirsute patients. Fertil Steril 33:239, 1980
51. Maroulis GB: Polycystic ovarian disease and dexamethasone. Semin Reprod Endocrinol 2:263, 1984
52. Kirschner MA, Jacobs JB: Combined ovarian and adrenal vein catheterization to determine the site(s) of androgen overproduction in hirsute women. J Clin Endocrinol Metab 33:199, 1971
53. Wentz AC, White RI, Migeon CJ, Hsu TH, Barnes HV, Jones GS: Differential ovarian and adrenal vein catheterization. Am J Obstet Gynecol 125:1000, 1976
54. Moltz L, Schwartz U, Sörenson R, Pickartz H, Hammerstein J: Ovarian and adrenal vein steroids in patients with nonneoplastic hyperandrogenism: selective catheterization findings. Fertil Steril 42:69, 1984
55. Abraham GE, Maroulis GB, Boyers SP, Buster JE, Magyar DM, Elsner CW: Dexamethasone suppression test in the management of hyperandrogenized patients. Obstet Gynecol 57:158, 1981
56. Givens JR, Andersen RN, Wiser WL, Fish SA: Dynamics of suppression and recovery of plasma FSH, LH, androstenedione, and testosterone in polycyctic ovarian disease using an oral contraceptive. J Clin Endocrinol Metab 38:727, 1974
57. Wiebe RH, Morris CV: Effect of an oral contraceptive on adrenal and ovarian androgenic steroids. Obstet Gynecol 63:12, 1984
58. Barkan AL, Cassorla F, Loriaux DL, Kelch RP, Marshall JC: Steroid and gonadotropin secretion in a patient with a 30-year history of virilization due to lipoid-cell ovarian tumor. Obstet Gynecol 64:287, 1984

Chapter 11

Ultrasound in the evaluation of normal and induced ovulation

William G. M. Ritchie, M.D.

Department of Radiology, Pennsylvania Hospital, Philadelphia, Pennsylvania

The detection and timing of ovulation is an important step in the evaluation and management of female infertility. Prior to the advent of ultrasound, only presumptive evidence of follicular development and ovulation was readily available. Absolute evidence of follicular maturation and ovulation required the establishment of pregnancy, recovery of an oocyte, or direct visualization of a corpus luteum with a stigma at laparoscopy or laparotomy. The latter criterion for ovulation is, however, controversial. Indirect assessment of follicular maturation was usually obtained by steroid or gonadotropic hormone assays or by observation of peripheral changes in the reproductive tract associated with ovulation. Changes in these parameters preceding, coinciding with, and succeeding the ovulatory process have been extensively documented and are widely used in the management of female infertility.

Ultrasound is a relatively new imaging technique that allows repeated noninvasive examination of the ovaries and related pelvic structures. With high-resolution real-time ultrasound equipment it is possible to obtain accurate and reproducible studies of ovarian size and follicular development. The purpose of this communication is to correlate the ultrasonographic features of normal and induced ovulatory cycles with the accepted hormonal and clinical parameters that are currently used in the management of female infertility. The sonographic features of some associated pelvic diseases commonly encountered in the practice of infertility will also be discussed.

SONOGRAPHIC TECHNIQUE AND NORMAL ANATOMY

With a distended-bladder technique it is possible to demonstrate the uterus and ovaries in the majority of women in their reproductive years. The ovaries are attached to the uterus and pelvic side walls by pliable adnexal structures, the ovarian and infundibulopelvic ligaments, respectively. As a result, the ovaries can be found in variable cephalocaudal locations, and the uterine corpus can be found in varying right-to-left and anterior-to-posterior positions. The ovaries are readily detected by their distinctive morphologic features, and measurement of size and any follicles present can be obtained in three dimensions.

The ovaries are usually identified lying against the side walls of the pelvis in both longitudinal and transverse sections (Fig. 1). The normal ovary is ellipsoid in shape with a volume of < 6 cm^3.[1] The volume may be approximated by a simplified formula for a prolate ellipsoid ($\frac{1}{2} \times$ width $\times$ thickness $\times$ length). A varying number of small (1 to 3 mm) cystic structures are often identified around the periphery of the ovary, and these represent developing antral follicles. The ovarian artery and vein can also be identified entering the ovary through the infundibulopelvic ligament (Fig. 2) and this feature may help to differentiate the ovary from the adjacent fundus of uterus or other pelvic structures which, when imaged in single section, may mimic the ovary in appearance.[2] The ovary often lies on the internal iliac

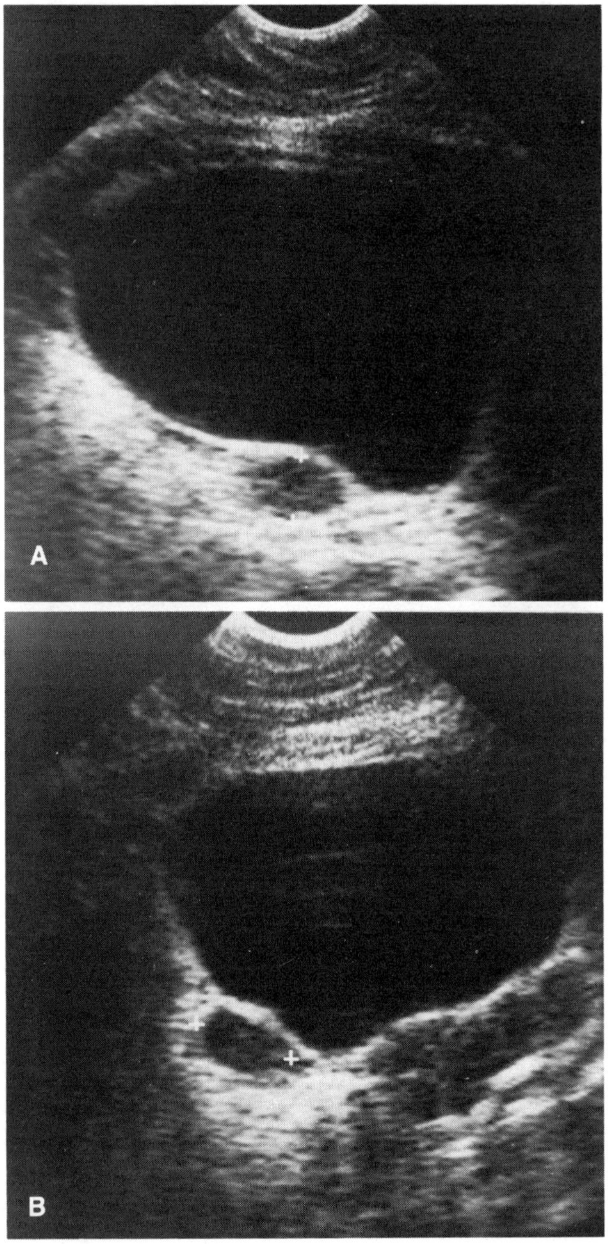

Figure 1
Sagittal (**A**) and transverse (**B**) sections through a normal ovary lying behind the distended bladder. The ovarian size is $26 \times 24 \times 16$ mm. The estimated volume is 4.9 cm^3. Multiple very small cysts (*black holes*) can be seen in the ovary, and these represent developing antral follicles.

artery and vein but does not maintain a consistent relationship with these vessels. In the presence of previous surgery, pelvic inflammatory disease, or endometriosis, the ovaries may be more difficult to identify and are often abnormally positioned within the pelvis.

NORMAL CYCLES

The development and fate of a follicle has been documented by sequential scanning throughout the normal menstrual cycle.[3-7] The process of recruitment, selection, dominance, and demise of a follicle can be observed and related to the complex hormonal changes occurring in each cycle. Cyclic changes in the uterus can also be documented. A thorough understanding of the hormonal events which control the ovulatory process is essential to appreciate the role of ultrasound and the ability to relate it to the other criteria used to predict and confirm ovulation.

PREOVULATORY FOLLICLE

Any ovarian follicle destined to ovulate is derived from a cohort of growing follicles drawn in turn from the pool of nonproliferating primordial follicles formed during fetal development. The initiation of follicular growth is a continuous process that is independent of gonadotropin influence. About 99.9% of all ovarian follicles are lost spontaneously to atresia, and only an exceptional few achieve ovulation. The primordial and preantral follicles are too small to be defined sonographically. However, as the antral follicles develop, with the accumulation of follicular fluid in the intercellular spaces of the granulosa, the developing follicles become large enough to be detected sonographically. In optimal conditions, cystic structures as small as 2 to 4 mm in diameter can be detected within the ovaries. Early in the menstrual cycle, a varying number of follicles

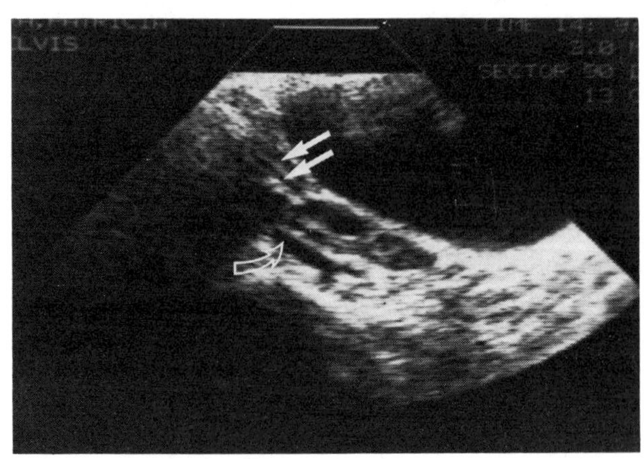

Figure 2
A sagittal section through the right ovary lying on the internal iliac vein (*open curved arrow*) with two vessels—the ovarian artery and vein entering the superior pole of the ovary through the infundibulopelvic ligament (*two solid arrows*).

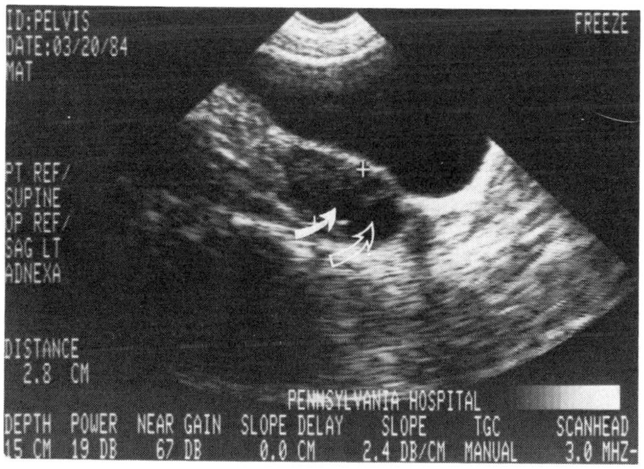

Figure 3
A sagittal section of the left ovary demonstrating a dominant follicle (*open curved arrow*) and a smaller second-order follicle (*solid arrow*).

will have been recruited and by days 5 to 7 will be readily visible. About this time, one of these follicles will be selected as the dominant follicle; and under the influence of follicle-stimulating hormone (FSH), the granulosa cells will begin to synthesize estrogens. Sonographically, the dominant follicle cannot be differentiated from its fellow follicles until days 8 to 12, at which time the size and rate of growth of the dominant follicle exceeds that of the remainder.[6] The dominant follicle can thus be recognized in the preovulatory period because its size exceeds that of the subordinate or lesser order follicles, which are doomed to become atretic. These subordinate follicles may continue to grow but rarely exceed 14 mm in diameter (Fig. 3). A follicle > 14 mm in diameter is therefore usually destined to ovulate.

The dominant and lesser order follicles are distributed randomly in both ovaries during single and sequential cycles. In > 80% of ovaries with a dominant follicle, a second follicle is present in one or the other ovary and undergoes parallel but limited development. Three or four growing follicles are found in ~ 50% and 20% of cycles, respectively. In 5% to 11%, two dominant follicles may develop.[6, 8]

The size of the dominant follicle can be followed to the time of ovulation. During the 4 to 5 days prior to ovulation, the follicle grows rapidly, in a linear manner, by ~ 2 to 3 mm a day, reaching a mean diameter of ~ 20 to 24 mm by the time of ovulation (Fig. 4). However, the range of size detected immediately prior to ovulation is great, extending from 18 to 28 mm, and this makes measurement of follicle size as an absolute predictor of the time of ovulation of limited use.[3, 4, 9]

The accuracy of ultrasonographic measurements of follicular size has been confirmed by laparoscopic studies at which time the follicles were aspirated and the follicular diameters were directly measured or estimated from the amount of aspirated fluid. Both of these techniques tend to underestimate the size, because the dominant follicle is often partly submerged below the surface

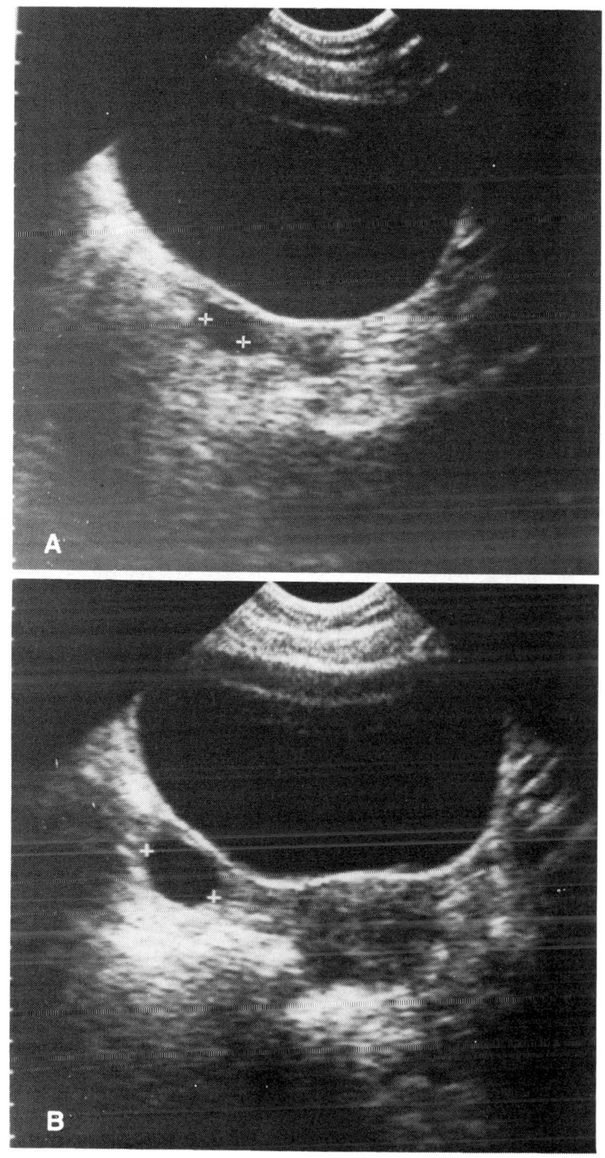

Figure 4
(**A**), Cycle day 8. A transverse section through the right ovary demonstrates a single developing follicle measuring 16 × 12 × 10 mm (average diameter, 12.7 mm). (**B**), Cycle day 11, the day before ovulation. The follicle now measures 25 × 17 × 15 mm (average diameter, 19 mm).

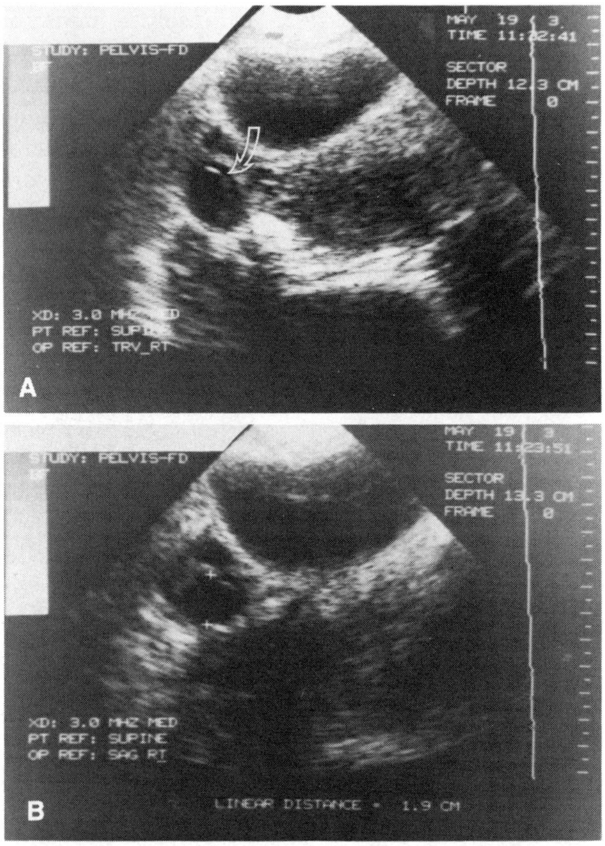

Figure 5
Preovulatory follicle. Sagittal (**A**) and transverse (**B**) sections of a right ovary demonstrating a preovulatory follicle (average diameter, 21 mm) with a sonolucent halo (*open curved arrow*) and a crenated echogenic rim.

of the ovary, and, second, aspiration of a follicle is usually incomplete, with fluid remaining in the collapsed follicle or leaking around the needle at the aspiration site.[6, 8]

Over the period of maximum follicular growth and development there is good correlation between follicular diameter and peripheral plasma 17β-estradiol (E_2) levels.[4, 6, 10] Extrapolation of the correlation line of follicular diameter and plasma E_2 shows that during the phase of rapid development the dominant follicle is the only major source of circulating E_2.[10] This supports earlier conclusions that at least 95% of the circulating E_2 emanates from the dominant follicle and that subordinate orders of follicles do not contribute significant amounts of estrogen. As the preovulatory follicle approaches maturity, increasing amounts of estrogen are produced, and the E_2 levels rise rapidly, surging to a peak approximately 24 to 36 hours before ovulation. The sustained threshold concentration of E_2 initiates the luteinizing hormone (LH) surge, which promotes luteinization of the granulosa cells, resulting in the production of progesterone (P). The onset of the LH surge appears to be a reliable indicator of impending ovulation, occurring 28 to 32 hours before follicle rupture. The LH surge is also required to initiate the resumption of meiosis in the oocyte and the synthesis of prostaglandins essential to follicle rupture.

Although the wide range in the diameter of the preovulatory follicle precludes its use as a single index for the prediction of ovulation, several other preovulatory sonographic features have been described. These reflect the hormonally induced morphologic changes occurring in the preovulatory follicle following the onset of the LH surge and, when observed, may have a predictive value. With the LH surge, the thecal tissue becomes hypervascular and edematous, and the granulosa cell layer begins to separate from the thecal cell layer. These features can be appreciated sonographically[11] and may be detected by the appearance of a line of decreased reflectivity around the follicle. This feature is consistently seen within 24 hours of ovulation and is associated with increasing plasma P levels. Advanced folding and separation of the granulosa cell layer from the underlying thecal layer produces a crenated pattern of the lining of the follicle. This latter sign is less consistently seen but occurs when ovulation is imminent, within 6 to 10 hours (Fig. 5).

Another sign of developing follicular maturity is the detection of a small echogenic area projecting into the follicle which represents the cumulus oophorus. This may be identified in $>$ 20% of follicles $>$ 18 mm in diameter[6] (Fig. 6). Identification of the cumulus oophorus confirms that a cystic structure is indeed an oocyte-containing follicle and that ovulation will occur within 36 hours.[12]

FOLLICLE RUPTURE

The changes associated with ovulation have been documented,[4, 7, 13] and actual follicular rupture has been observed sonographically.[14] When follicular rupture occurs, there is a rapid reduction in follicular size and an escape of fluid to the periovulatory area. Thereafter, the process may be variable, with complete follicular emptying taking from 1 to 45 minutes. A corpus hemorrhagicum may develop within 1 hour of ovulation and is recognized as a smaller irregular cyst con-

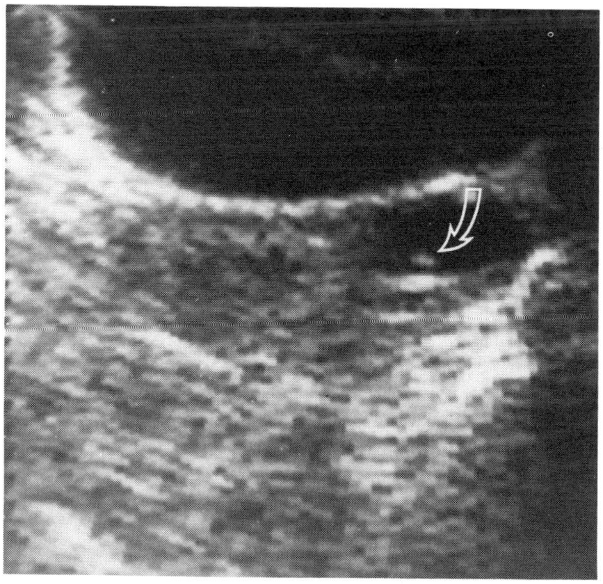

Figure 6
Cumulus oophorus. A transverse section through a preovulatory follicle in the left ovary. A small echogenic mound protrudes from the wall into the follicle (*open curved arrow*). This represents the cumulus oophorus and is only seen in the immediate preovulatory period.

taining numerous echoes (Fig. 7). The source of such echoes is probably a blood clot. While the most frequent pattern is that of an irregular cyst, containing low-level echoes, which diminishes in size over 4 to 5 days, other changes following follicular rupture are also seen. Occasionally, the corpus luteum cyst will increase in size before resolving. Infrequently, the follicle will disappear and no corpus luteum can be identified. In a few of these cases a corpus luteum will develop a few days after ovulation and grow slowly in size until it resolves spontaneously early in the next cycle.[4] With daily scanning, ovulation can be demonstrated in > 80% of cases.[3, 4, 6] Some instances will be missed when after initial rupture no marked collapse occurs or when the collapsed follicle is rapidly filled with blood within a few hours and the change in the intrafollicular echogenicity is not appreciated.

The occurrence of sonographically detectable fluid in the pouch of Douglas is also seen following ovulation in ~ 25% of patients[7, 14] (Fig. 8). While small amounts of fluid may be detected laparoscopically before ovulation, the volume increases progressively during the follicular phase, with an abrupt increase following ovulation and peak volumes detected in the early luteal phase. This has been measured by laparoscopic aspiration to be ~ 15 to 25 ml, which is greatly in excess of the amount (4 to 6 ml) released by follicular rupture.[15] While relatively small amounts of fluid (5 to 10 ml) can be detected sonographically under ideal circumstances, the sudden appearance of significant amounts of fluid in the pelvis is very suggestive of ovulation. It has been inferred that the peritoneal fluid is predominantly formed by exudation from the active ovary, and this is strongly supported by the higher concentration of ovarian steroid hormones in the peritoneal fluid than in plasma.

The occurrence of mittelschmerz is also closely associated with the process of follicular rupture and was initially thought to be due to peritoneal irritation from blood and follicular contents following ovulation. Midcycle sonographic surveillance of the ovaries has shown that in the major-

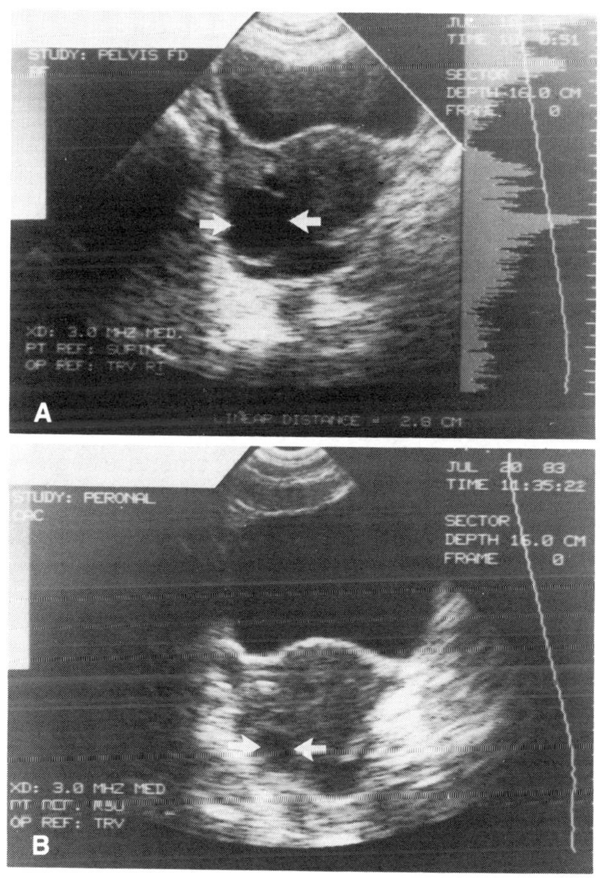

Figure 7
Preovulatory follicle and corpus hemorrhagicum. (**A**), A transverse section through the right ovary demonstrates a large preovulatory follicle (*solid arrows*). (**B**), A comparable transverse section 2 days later demonstrates a much smaller irregular cyst which contains echoes reflecting the presence of blood and cellular debris.

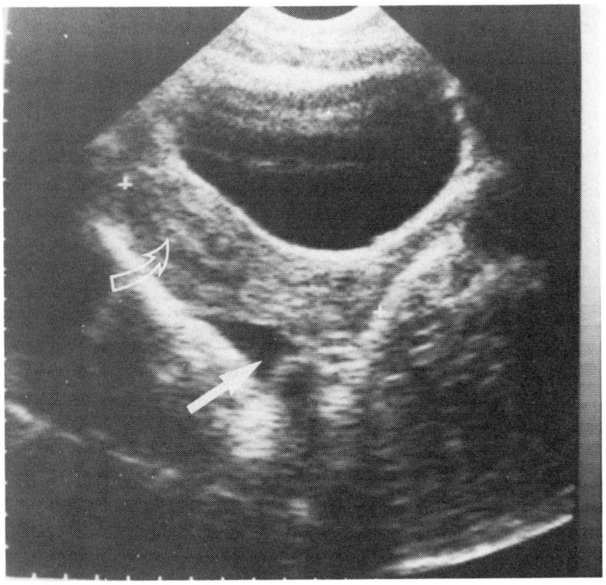

Figure 8
A longitudinal section obtained through the uterus in the immediate postovulatory period. A small sonolucent area or ring shadow (*open curved arrow*) can be seen within the echogenic endometrial canal, and fluid is seen in the cul-de-sac (*solid arrow*).

ity of cases the symptom precedes ovulation and is present on the side with the dominant follicle, suggesting local effects of the enlarging follicle.[7, 16] It has been demonstrated that 77% of women with mittelschmerz experience the symptom on the same day as the peak plasma LH, and in 97% the pain preceded follicular rupture.[16]

A significant rise in the basal body temperature (BBT) does not occur until 2 days after the LH peak, coinciding with increasing amounts of plasma P. Ovulation occurs within 36 hours of the LH peak, and sonographic correlation with the BBT has confirmed that ovulation precedes the initial rise in temperature in most subjects.[7]

UTERINE CHANGES

Cyclic changes in the endometrium can be detected by ultrasound. In the early proliferative phase, there is a thin, relatively homogeneous endometrial echo. In the late proliferative stage, the endometrial echo is much thicker, reflecting stromal and glandular hyperplasia. Stromal edema may produce a sonolucent rim around the canal (Fig. 9). Following ovulation, the endometrium shrinks slightly as the edema resolves, and the canal echo loses its lucent halo, with the occasional appearance of a ring-like echo in the canal[12] (Fig. 8).

ABNORMAL CYCLES

ANOVULATORY CYCLES

Anovulatory cycles are considered to occur in ~ 7% of cycles, but sonographic studies of apparently normal cycles with biphasic BBT curves and normal cycle lengths suggest that abnormal cycles may be significantly more frequent. In such cycles, there is asynchrony between the E_2 peak

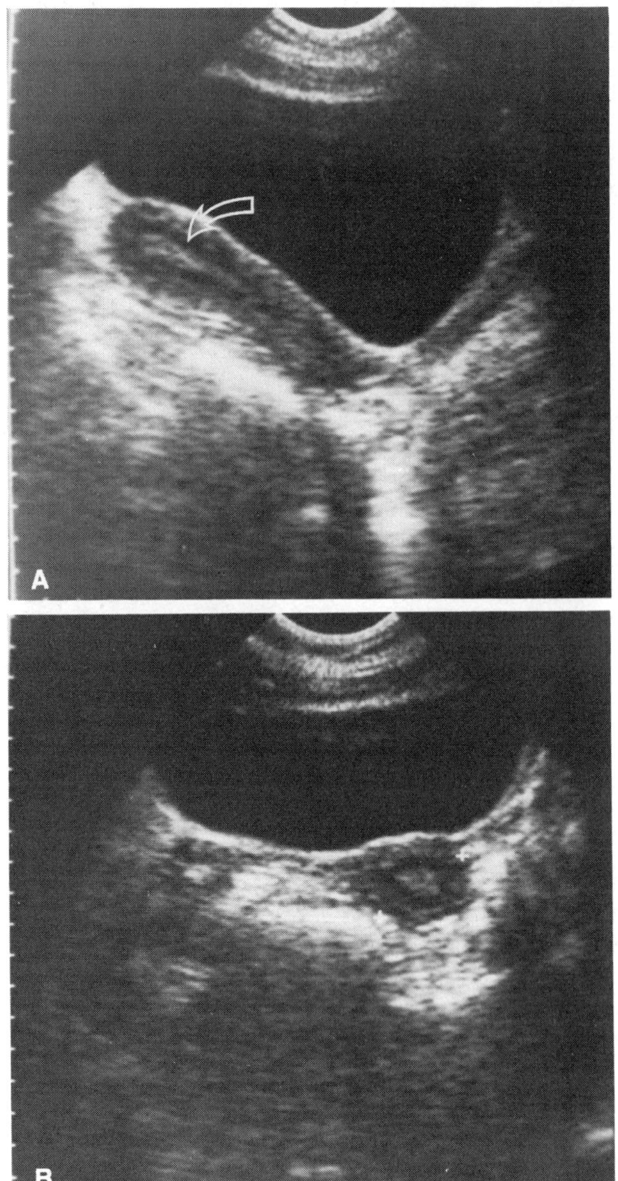

Figure 9
(**A**) Longitudinal and (**B**) transverse sections of the uterus in the immediate preovulatory period showing an echogenic endometrial canal with a sonolucent halo reflecting hyperemia (*open curved arrow*).

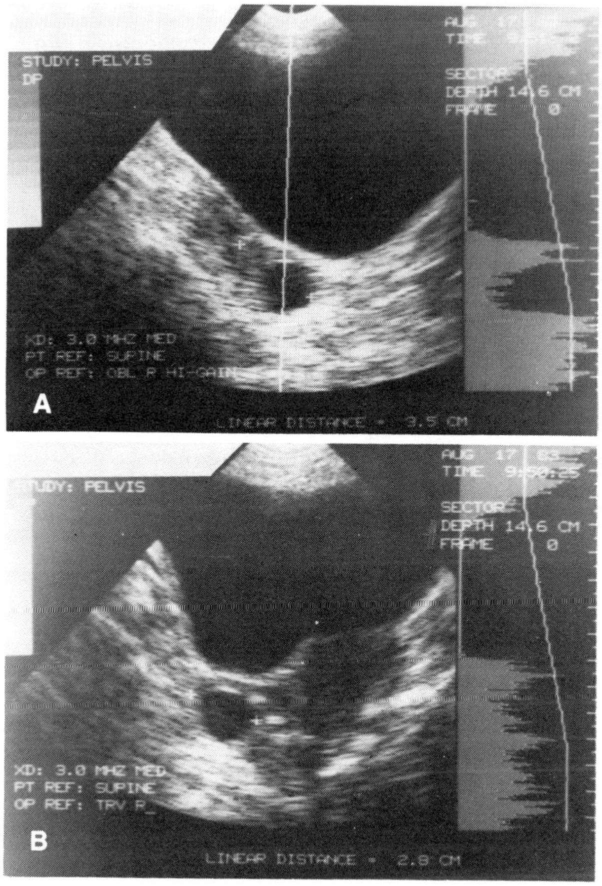

Figure 10
LUF. Sagittal (**A**) and transverse (**B**) sections through the right ovary. There is a cyst 15 mm in diameter with low-level echoes and an irregular wall. (The low-level echoes are confirmed by the accompanying A-mode recording through the cyst to the right of the image.) This cannot be differentiated from a normal corpus luteum on a single examination, but no preceding collapse or associated sonographic features of ovulation were observed, and the patient did not conceive.

and the LH surge and the growth and disappearance of ovarian follicles.[17] These cycles can only be recognized by serial sonographic observations of follicular development when the poor follicular size or premature disappearance in relation to the hormonal changes can be appreciated. In this situation, the follicle rarely reaches 14 mm in size and either ruptures prematurely or becomes rapidly atretic. A similar pattern of follicle behavior may also be seen in patients taking oral contraceptives.[4]

LUTEINIZED UNRUPTURED FOLLICLE SYNDROME

In a small number of women a luteinized follicle will fail to rupture (LUF syndrome).[18-20] In the past this diagnosis depended on the failure of laparoscopic demonstration of an ovulation stigma in a patient with apparent normal ovulatory cycles. The diagnosis was supported by the observation that peritoneal fluid volume and concentration of P and E_2 were significantly lower where the luteinized follicle failed to rupture, when these cycles were compared with normal ovulatory cycles. The presence of LUF can now be demonstrated sonographically, with a high degree of confidence,[19, 20] by sequential scanning beyond the LH peak. The persistence of a dominant follicle with an echo-free cystic appearance beyond 36 hours after the LH peak with no evidence of collapse is abnormal and may be taken as evidence of failure of ovulation. In most of these unruptured follicles, the normally sharp definition between the follicle wall and follicular fluid becomes an ill-defined gray zone due to an echogenic interface of low-density echoes. This appearance is similar to that seen in the immediate preovulatory follicle but becomes more marked in the LUF syndrome, where the sonographic gray zone may be 4 to 7 mm thick and probably reflects imaging of the hypertrophied and luteinized granulosa cells. Most of these cysts decrease in size with the peripheral echogenic zone progressively enchroaching into the central cystic area over 2 to 4 days to form an apparently normal corpus luteum (Fig. 10). The results of daily changes of LH, estrogen, and P do not differ from those in subjects ovulating normally and suggest that the LUF behaves steroidogenically as a corpus luteum with a luteal phase of normal length. This syndrome may occur continuously in all cycles or may be intermittent. The incidence of this syndrome is uncertain, having been reported in ~ 5% of cycles in fertile women.[19] It appears to be more common in the infertile patient, and persistent LUF syndrome may account for some cases of otherwise unexplained infertility.[18, 20]

INDUCED OVULATION

Disorders of ovulation are present in 15% to 25% of infertile couples. Depending on the cause, appropriate therapy can be used to induce ovulation and allow conception. In the absence of premature menopause and hyperprolactinemia, most ovulatory disorders are treated with clomiphene citrate (CC)[21-24] and gonadotropin therapy[25-30] or more recently with gonadotropin-releasing factor.[31] The aim of therapy is to induce satisfactory ovulation of one or a few follicles and to avoid

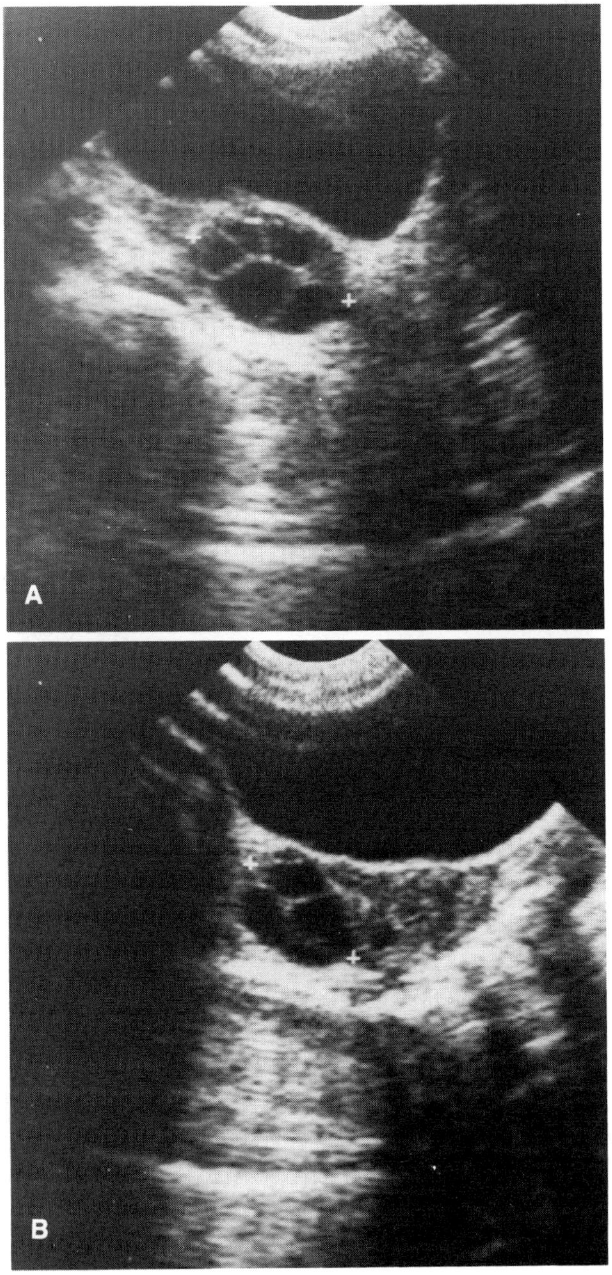

Figure 11
Sagittal (**A**) and transverse (**B**) sections through the right ovary showing multiple developing follicles of varying sizes on cycle day 10 of a menotropin-stimulated cycle.

multiple follicular development, hyperstimulation, and multiple pregnancy. In contrast to infertility programs employing ovarian stimulation followed by normal fertilization where there is significant risk of uncontrolled polypregnancy, in vitro fertilization (IVF) programs carry no such hazard because the number of embryos transferred is controlled. In fact, the aim is to produce multiple follicles, even in normally cycling women, in order to improve the pregnancy rate following IVF. The use of ultrasound monitoring has improved the results of these forms of therapy, allowing monitoring of the numbers and size of the follicles and indicating timely injection of human chorionic gonadotropin (hCG) to induce ovulation. Although the overall pattern of follicular development in each group is similar to that seen in spontaneous cycles, certain important differences exist.

CC induces endogenous FSH production and when administered early in the cycle induces a cohort of follicles to develop. The process of selection and dominance may be overridden, and multiple follicles often develop. Although preovulatory positive estrogen-LH feedback is usually preserved in CC-treated patients with an intact hypothalamus, adjuvant hCG is often given to induce ovulation. Treatment with exogenous gonadotropins, usually menotropins, does not require an intact hypothalamus or pituitary and stimulates the ovaries directly, usually overriding the process of selection and dominance, with development of multiple follicles. The dose requirements for gonadotropins are critical, the difference between nonresponse and overresponse being a dose increment of $< 50\%$, and the dose required by different individuals may differ by tenfold. hCG is given to induce ovulation of mature follicles.

Although the number of follicles developing in any cycle to a certain extent reflects the dose of each drug, it is usual to see fewer follicles developing with CC than with gonadotropins. While two follicles develop in ~ 5% to 10% of spontaneous cycles, multiple follicular development is seen in ~ 35% to 60% of CC cycles and in up to 80% of gonadotropin cycles. Furthermore, when two follicles develop in a spontaneous cycle, they are frequently in opposite ovaries; whereas in induced cycles multiple follicles frequently develop within the same ovary, reflecting overriding of the local intraovarian control of suppression of all but a single dominant follicle. Not only the frequency with which multiple follicular development occurs but also the numbers of follicles developing in these cycles tend to be greater with gonadotropins than with CC, usually averaging about four to six follicles in well-controlled cycles. In IVF programs where CC and gonadotropins are administered, the number of follicles tends to be even greater[28, 29] (Fig. 11). Hyperstimulation, with the development of many follicles, can be seen in both CC- and gonadotropin-induced cycles but is seen more frequently in the latter because of the critical ovarian response to exogenous gonadotropins. Although experience with pulsatile gonadotropin-releasing hormone treatment has been limited, apparently normal cycles have been induced with spontaneous ovulation of single follicles.[31]

Ovarian ultrasonography is usually started on about cycle day 8, by which time the induced follicles are approaching 8 to 10 mm in diameter. When many follicles develop in an ovary, the follicles may be distorted and compressed by adjacent follicles, which makes accurate measurement difficult. The rate of growth of CC- and gonadotropin-induced follicles does not differ significantly from spontaneously occurring follicles, being ~ 1 to 2 mm per day. However, because several follicles may be recruited sequentially, the developing follicles may be of varying size. This feature is seen more often with gonadotropins. In CC-induced cycles with spontaneous ovulation, the size of the mature preovulatory follicle is similar to that in spontaneous cycles.[21]

Because a spontaneous LH surge does not occur in gonadotropin-induced cycles, assessment of follicular diameter has been used to time hCG administration. hCG administration is usually deferred until at least one follicle 18 mm or more in diameter has developed. Because ovulation will not occur for about 36 hours, there will have been 2 to 3 mm further growth by the time ovulation occurs. The timing of hCG administration in relation to follicular development, however, is critical. Administering hCG too early may produce atresia, and delaying giving hCG may result in entrapment and postmaturity of the oocyte.[29] Using follicular diameter as a guide to hCG administration assumes that maturation of the oocyte can be equated with follicular size. However, oocyte retrieval in IVF programs in both spontaneous and induced cycles has shown a poor correlation, and mature oocytes can be retrieved from follicles ranging in size from 15 to 30 mm in diameter.[24] In the presence of multiple developing follicles, the largest follicle may not necessarily be the most mature follicle.[24] It has also been shown that oocytes that give rise to successful pregnancies are obtained from follicles that contain a greater concentration of E_2 and that the largest follicle is not necessarily the most estrogenic. Mature oocytes have been obtained from relatively small follicles, and aspiration from multiple follicles has confirmed that oocytes may exist at different stages of maturation in the same patient, reflecting asynchronous development.[29]

It is not surprising, then, that several studies have shown that ultrasound alone is inadequate for complete assessment of follicular development and for timing of hCG administration for ovulation induction.[24, 27-29] Simultaneous biochemical and biologic assessments of oocyte maturation are required for optimal results. The most frequently used parameter is the E_2 level and, unlike that in spontaneous cycles, the correlation of E_2 levels with follicle size is not straightforward.

In the presence of multiple follicular development there is very poor, if any, correlation between the diameter of the largest follicle and the E_2 level, but there is usually some correlation between the number of developing follicles > 10 mm in diameter and the E_2 levels.[23, 26] The rate of daily follicular growth also appears to correlate well with increasing serum E_2 levels.[6, 32] Several investigators[23, 26] have been able to obtain better correlation of E_2 with the total follicular volume in a population of cases. Correlation of individual cases, especially with many follicles, however, is less clear, because there appears to be a wide range of E_2 responses.[29] These may reflect differences in gonadotropin metabolism and E_2 clearance, differences in ovarian response (e.g., in polycystic ovaries and unstimulated ovaries of hypogonadotropic patients), and differences in the time course of developing follicles. Nevertheless, it is apparent that elevated E_2 levels can be due to multiple small follicles or to a single mature follicle. It is generally accepted that knowledge of the number and distribution of follicles is necessary for adequate interpretation of estrogen levels.

Because the E_2 levels vary from patient to patient, the biologic response as evaluated by vaginal smears and cervical mucus also needs to be reconsidered. Sonographic observation of the cervical canal in the immediate preovulatory period will often show biologic changes in response to elevated E_2 levels. These changes, however, are not consistent. Hypertrophy of the cervical mucus glands may have three appearances. The earliest noticeable change is a zone of increased echogenicity around the cervical canal. When the secretions become copious, fluid can be seen in the canal (Fig. 12). Occasionally discrete fluid-filled

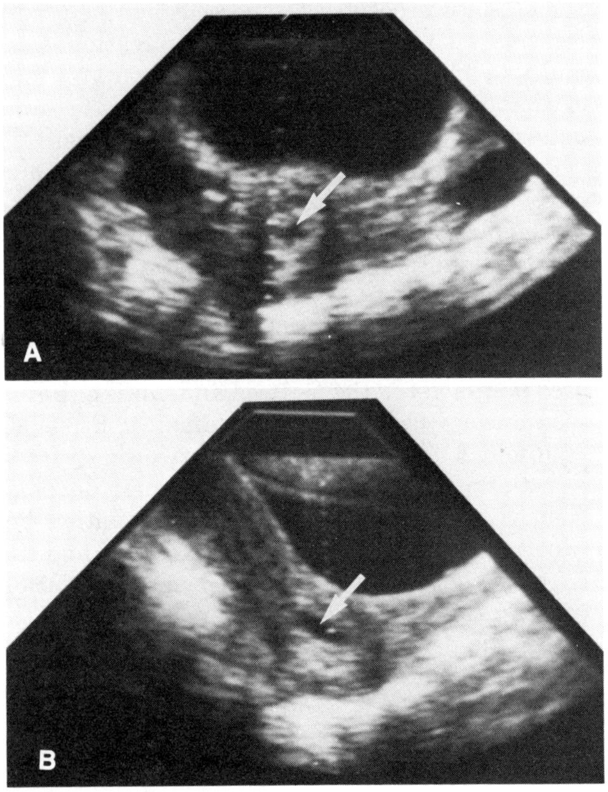

Figure 12
(**A**) Transverse and (**B**) longitudinal sections through the uterus showing fluid in the cervical canal and increased echogenicity in the cervical myometrium reflecting a strong E_2 effect in the immediate preovulatory period in a menotropin-stimulated patient.

glands can be seen as small sonolucent collections in the wall of the cervical canal (Fig. 13). These have an appearance similar to that of Nabothian cysts but disappear after ovulation.

The decision to administer hCG is usually made by a combination of sonographic observation of follicle size and numbers, level and rate of rise of E_2 levels, and vaginal cytologic and cervical mucus characteristics. The administration of hCG usually induces ovulation; but very often when several follicles are present, only one or a few will ovulate. The remainder may remain cystic,[25] which suggests that luteinization has not occurred. These cysts may persist for the remainder of the cycle but usually become absorbed in the first few days of the next cycle. Spontaneous or hCG-induced ovulation may be suspected when previously noted follicles disappear or fill in with echoes. The presence of fluid in the cul-de-sac is also suggestive, but in the presence of multiple follicles, fluid may be seen in the periovulatory period, which is presumably an exudate from the stimulated ovaries.

UNSUCCESSFUL CYCLES

The success rate for conception in induced cycles, both in vivo and in vitro, falls far short of the rate of conception in normal cycles with comparable optimal timing of fertilization. Although not all failures are attributable to failure of folliculogenesis, sonographic observations have assisted in the recognition of several patterns of abnormality. These unsuccessful cycles fall into three categories.

First, there may be poor follicular development with slow or irregular growth of follicles.[33] This phenomenon is usually associated with low or fluctuating E_2 levels and is most often seen with inadequate gonadotropin administration. If more gonadotropin is not administered, atresia will ensue.

In the second group following hCG administration, the LUF syndrome may occur.[18] This may be an expression of oocyte overexposure to human menopausal gonadotropin and may coincide with the aspiration of postmature oocytes in IVF programs.[29] This phenomenon is also seen in CC-induced cycles.[18] There are no sonographic features to allow identification of these follicles prior to hCG administration, but after hCG administration, changes similar to those occurring in spontaneous cycles may be seen, with the development of a thick gray zone around the follicle and low-level internal echoes. In the presence of multiple

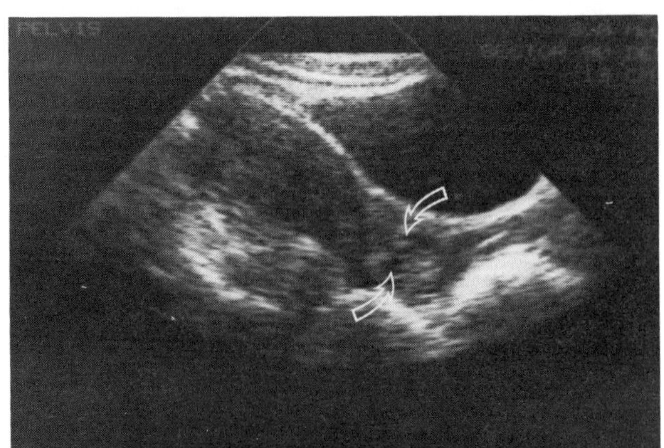

Figure 13
A longitudinal section through the uterus demonstrating distended cervical mucus glands (*open curved arrows*) reflecting increased cervical mucus production. These changes disappear shortly after ovulation.

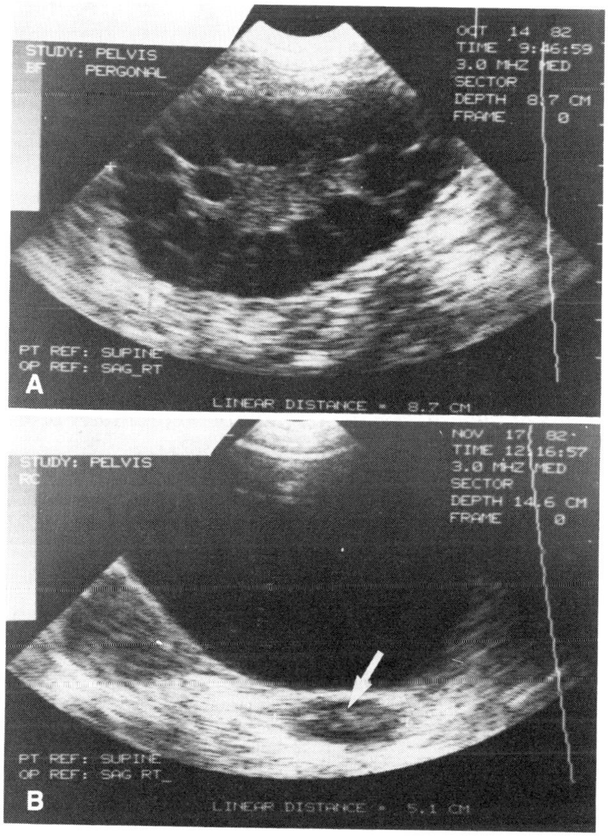

Figure 14
Ovarian hyperstimulation syndrome in a patient with PCOD. (**A**), A sagittal section through a very enlarged ovary (87 × 52 × 64 mm; estimated volume, 145 cm^3) with numerous subcapsular follicles. hCG was withheld. (**B**), The same ovary in the following cycle showing return to baseline size (51 × 21 × 22 mm; estimated volume, 11.7 cm^3).

follicles this features may not always be appreciated, and satisfactory ovulation may still occur from other mature follicles. These luteinized cysts may grow and persist into the next cycle or longer.

Third, hyperstimulation may occur.[32-34] Hyperstimulation is the most serious complication of ovulation induction. With ovarian hyperstimulation, multiple follicles are induced with the development of multiple corpus luteum cysts following ovulation. Although the ovaries can become extremely large and the estrogen levels can be very high, the full clinical syndrome of ovarian hyperstimulation does not occur unless hCG has been administered. The clinical symptoms usually appear 5 to 8 days after hCG injection, and three degrees of hyperstimulation can be distinguished clinically. Mild hyperstimulation is associated with lower abdominal discomfort but with no significant weight gain. The ovaries are enlarged but are < 5 cm in average diameter. With moderate hyperstimulation, weight gain may approach 10 pounds, and the ovaries may be enlarged up to 10 cm in average diameter. With severe hyperstimulation, the ovaries are markedly enlarged and at risk of rupture or torsion. The development of large amounts of ascites and pleural effusions leads to hemoconcentration with hypotension, oliguria, and electrolyte imbalance. In these cases, hospitalization is mandatory. The sonographic appearance of the ovaries is distinctive.[33, 34] The ovarian enlargement is mainly due to the presence of numerous large thin-walled cysts, which are often peripherally placed by may replace most of the ovary (Fig. 14). Fluid is easily detected in the pelvis and abdomen. If the patient does not become pregnant, the syndrome rapidly resolves, over 3 to 7 days, with the onset of the next menstrual cycle. It is probable that hyperstimulation is seen more commonly when a pregnancy occurs and in this situation hyperstimulation persists, with slow improvement occurring over a longer time frame of about 6 to 8 weeks.

To a certain extent, hyperstimulation, as assessed by sonographic detection of multiple follicular development and ovarian enlargement, occurs in many stimulated cycles and is just about invariably present in IVF protocols, especially those using both CC and gonadotropins. The visualization of enlarged ovaries or multiple follicular development prior to hCG administration does help to predict those patients who are at risk of developing the ovarian hyperstimulation syndrome but does not appear to be as accurate as plasma E_2 levels.[32] While mild or moderate hyperstimulation may be encountered with E_2 levels in the 1000 to 4000 pg/ml range, the risk of severe hyperstimulation becomes very significant with E_2 levels of > 4000 pg/ml at the time of hCG administration. At these levels severe hyperstimulation is particularly prone to supervene if pregnancy occurs. Because E_2 levels correlate with the number of follicles present, the sonographic observation of many (> 8 to 10) maturing follicles should suggest the possibility of potential hyperstimulation, and hCG injection should be withheld until an E_2 measurement has been obtained. Hyperstimulation is less often seen in IVF programs, because the follicles are probably damaged at the time of oocyte aspiration.

Because large cysts may persist into the next cycle, as described above, it is wise to perform a

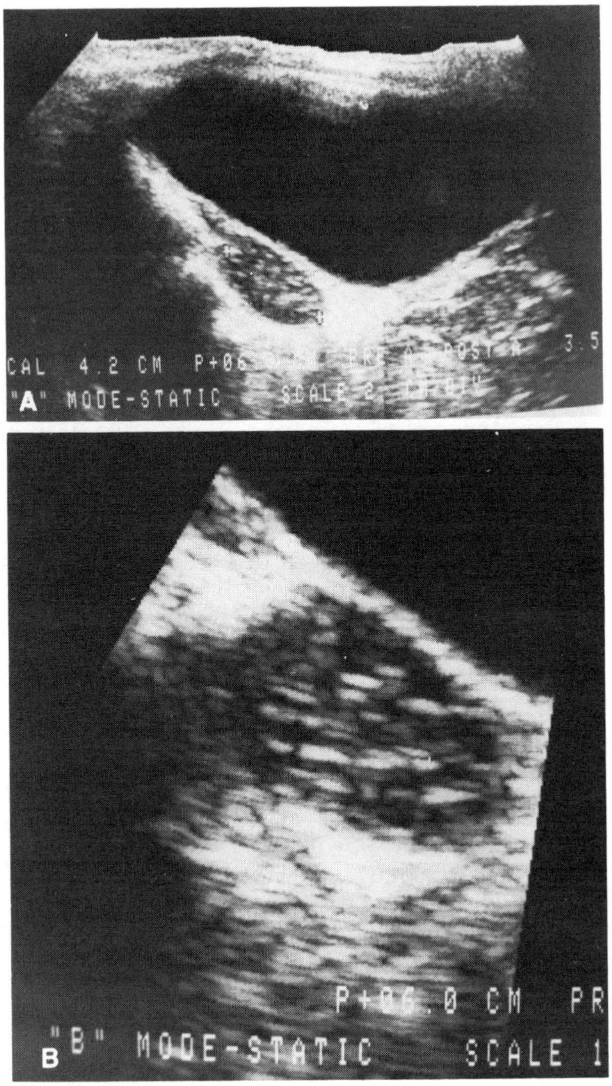

Figure 15
PCOD. (**A**), A sagittal section through the right ovary which is about twice normal size (42 × 21 × 28 mm; estimated volume, 12.3 cm^3). (**B**), An enlarged view of the ovary shows the typical features of PCOD with multiple small cysts (*black holes*) with strongly reflective back walls (*white echoes*).

baseline scan before instituting another stimulated cycle. Although the majority of these residual cysts resolve in the first few days of the cycle, some may persist, making assessment of the cohort of new follicles difficult.

PERCUTANEOUS OOCYTE RETRIEVAL

Recently, ultrasonically guided percutaneous oocyte aspiration has been suggested as an alternative approach to the inaccessible ovary.[35, 36] In skilled hands, retrieval rates approaching those of laparoscopic studies have been obtained, and this technique may offer an alternative to laparoscopy for oocyte retrieval.

POLYCYSTIC OVARIAN DISEASE

Patients with polycystic ovarian disease (PCOD) are encountered in any infertility program. In most cases, the diagnosis will have been recognized clinically and confirmed by appropriate endocrinologic studies or at laparoscopy. Sonographic detection of PCOD on a baseline study is important, because these patients are particularly sensitive to stimulation with gonadotropins and may easily become hyperstimulated. The sonographic features reflect the underlying hormonal imbalance. In PCOD, low levels of FSH continue to produce follicles but not to full maturation and ovulation. These follicles persist for several months and produce ovarian enlargement, which becomes more apparent with increasing duration of the disease. The ovarian shape becomes more spherical, rather than ellipsoid, and the ovarian diameter exceeds that of the anterior-posterior uterine diameter.[37] About a third of patients may have normal-sized ovaries, but in the remainder, the ovaries are obviously enlarged (> 6 cm^3) and are usually at least twice normal size.[38] In addition to the increase in size, multiple discrete cysts < 1 cm in size, often lying in a subcapsular position, are seen in ~ 50% of patients (Fig. 15). In some patients, the cysts are small and below the resolving power of current sonographic equipment. This may partly account for the wide spectrum of sonographic appearances of the ovaries seen in these cases. Some ovaries appear relatively sonolucent, probably reflecting many fluid-filled small follicles. Other ovaries appear more echogenic than the adjacent uterus, reflecting multiple strong interfaces produced by the back walls of many very small cysts.[38] When polycystic ovaries are incidentally detected sonographically in a group of patients referred for gynecologic ultrasound, about half of the patients will have the classic signs and symptoms associated with PCOD. Twenty-five percent will have variants of the syndrome, and in another 25% no clinical abnormality will be evident at the time of the ultrasound study.[39] Polycystic ovaries may also be associated with other clinical situations, such as Cushing's syndrome, basophilic pituitary adenoma, post-pill amenorrhea, and virilizing ovarian or adrenal tumors.

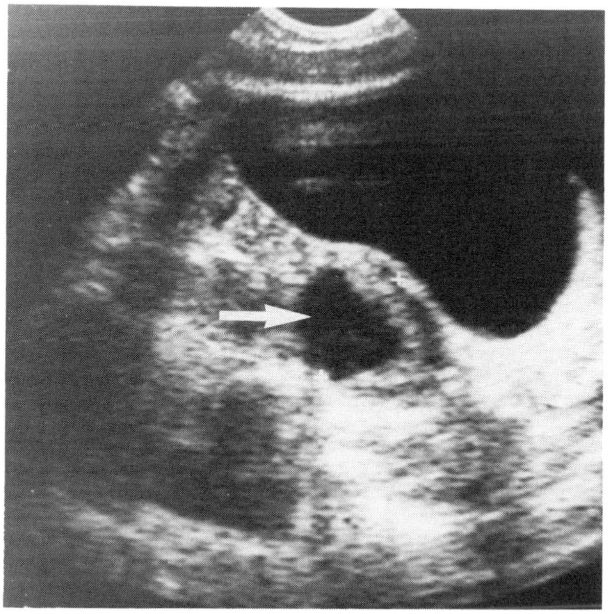

Figure 16
A sagittal section through the right ovary showing an irregularly shaped cyst with low-level internal echoes (*solid arrow*). This represents an ovarian endometrioma, which should not be mistaken for a corpus luteum.

ENDOMETRIOSIS

Unsuspected endometriosis may be found at laparoscopy in 25% to 50% of infertile patients who have otherwise normal evaluations for infertility. Sonography does not approach the ability of laparoscopy to help the physician diagnose endometriosis but may show abnormal cystic collections in the pelvis.[40] These frequently arise on the ovaries and may be mistaken for a follicle. Usually, an endometrioma contains uniform low-level echoes reflecting the hemorrhagic contents (Fig. 16) and is more likely to be mistaken for a corpus luteum, especially if first detected in the second half of the cycle. If not recognized initially, persistence or growth through several cycles, especially if stimulated, may allow recognition of these collections. It would appear that pelvic endometriosis, even in localized deposits, can effectively prevent conception despite repeated ovulation induction. The mechanism whereby conception fails under such circumstances is uncertain, although theories of the effect of increased local prostaglandins on tubal function and the inhibition of sperm survival have been proposed. An increased incidence of LUF syndrome has also been recorded. If endometriosis is suspected either sonographically or clinically, because of failure of conception, direct visualizaton via laparoscopy should be performed.

SUMMARY

In the past several years sonography has become an invaluable research tool for the investigation of spontaneous and induced ovulation and has added to the understanding of folliculogenesis and reproductive endocrinology. In practical terms, in ovulation induction sonography assists in the evaluation of the number and distribution of follicles, necessary for adequate interpretation of estrogen levels. Although there is no ideal size when it can be assumed that a follicle is mature, estimation of follicle size is of value and is a good guide to the timing of hCG administration. If the follicles are extremely small or there is evidence of hyperstimulation, these observations, together with the E_2 levels, may be used to decide whether a further ultrasonic examination is warranted for the assessment of follicular growth or whether the treatment cycle should be abandoned. Provided follicular size is within normal limits, the diameter of the largest follicle may also be used in IVF programs to determine when the patient should be admitted to the hospital for more intensive monitoring of follicular development and the administration of hCG. Ultrasound is also valuable in patients with only one ovary accessible to laparoscopy. Even if the largest follicle is in the inaccessible ovary, the treatment cycle does not have to be abandoned, provided that several follicles are developing in the contralateral ovary. If neither ovary is accessible laparoscopically, percutaneous oocyte aspiration offers the patient the opportunity of IVF and embryo transfer.

REFERENCES

1. Sample WF, Lippe BM, Gypes MT: Gray-scale ultrasonography of the normal female pelvis. Radiology 125:477, 1977
2. Hackelöer B-J, Nitschke-Dabelstein S: Ovarian imaging by ultrasound: an attempt to define a reference plane. J Clin Ultrasound 8:497, 1980
3. O'Herlihy C, de Crespigny LJCh, Robinson HP: Monitoring ovarian follicular development with real-time ultrasound. Br J Obstet Gynaecol 87:613, 1980
4. Queenan JT, O'Brien GD, Bains LM, Simpson J, Collins WP, Campbell S: Ultrasound scanning of ovaries to detect ovulation in women. Fertil Steril 34:99, 1980
5. Fleischer AC, Darnell J, Rodier J, Lindsay A, James AE Jr: Sonographic monitoring of ovarian follicular development. J Clin Ultrasound 9:275, 1981

6. Kerin JF, Edmonds DK, Warnes GM, Cox LW, Seamark RF, Matthews CD, Young GB, Baird DT: Morphological and functional relationships of graafian follicle growth to ovulation in women using ultrasonic, laparoscopic and biochemical measurements. Br J Obstet Gynaecol 88:81, 1981
7. Marinho AO, Sallam HN, Goessens LKV, Collins WP, Rodeck CH, Campbell S: Real time pelvic ultrasonography during the periovulatory period of patients attending an artificial insemination clinic. Fertil Steril 37:633, 1982
8. O'Herlihy C, de Crespigny LCh, Lopata A, Johnston I, Hoult I, Robinson H: Preovulatory follicular size: a comparison of ultrasound and laparoscopic measurements. Fertil Steril 34:24, 1980
9. Bryce RL, Shuter B, Sinosich MJ, Stiel JN, Picker RH, Saunders DM: The value of ultrasound, gonadotropin, and estradiol measurements for precise ovulation prediction. Fertil Steril 37:42, 1982
10. Hackelöer BJ, Fleming R, Robinson HP, Adam AH, Coutts JRT: Correlation of ultrasonic and endocrinologic assessment of human follicular development. Am J Obstet Gynecol 135:122, 1979
11. Picker RH, Smith DH, Tucker MH, Saunders DM: Ultrasonic signs of imminent ovulation. J Clin Ultrasound 11:1, 1983
12. Hackelöer BJ: The role of ultrasound in female infertility management. Ultrasound Med Biol 10:35, 1984
13. Nitschke-Dabelstein S, Hackelöer BJ, Sturm G: Ovulation and corpus luteum formation observed by ultrasonography. Ultrasound Med Biol 7:33, 1981
14. de Crespigny LCh, O'Herlihy C, Robinson HP: Ultrasonic observation of the mechanism of human ovulation. Am J Obstet Gynecol 139:177, 1981
15. Koninckx PR, Renaer M, Brosens IA: Origin or peritoneal fluid in women: an ovarian exudation product. Br J Obstet Gynaecol 87:177, 1980
16. O'Herlihy C, Robinson HP, de Crespigny LC: Mittelschmerz is a preovulatory symptom. Br Med J 280:986, 1980
17. Polan ML, Totora M, Caldwell BV, DeCherney AH, Haseltine FP, Kase N: Abnormal ovarian cycles as diagnosed by ultrasound and serum estradiol levels. Fertil Steril 37:342, 1982
18. Coulam CB, Hill LM, Breckle R: Ultrasonic evidence for luteinization of unruptured preovulatory follicles. Fertil Steril 37:524, 1982
19. Kerin JF, Kirby C, Morris D, McEvoy M, Ward B, Cox LW: Incidence of the luteinized unruptured follicle phenomenon in cycling women. Fertil Steril 40:620, 1983
20. Liukkonen S, Koskimies AI, Tenhunen A, Ylöstalo P: Diagnosis of luteinized unruptured follicle (LUF) syndrome by ultrasound. Fertil Steril 41:26, 1984
21. O'Herlihy C, Pepperell RJ, Robinson HP: Ultrasound timing of human chorionic gonadotropin administration in clomiphene-stimulated cycles. Obstet Gynecol 59:40, 1982
22. Hoult IJ, de Crespigny LCh, O'Herlihy C, Speirs AL, Lopata A, Kellow G, Johnston I, Robinson HP: Ultrasound control of clomiphene/human chorionic gonadotropin stimulated cycles for oocyte recovery and in vitro fertilization. Fertil Steril 36:316, 1981
23. Vargyas JM, Marrs RP, Kletzky OA, Mishell DR: Correlation of ultrasonic measurement of ovarian follicle size and serum estradiol levels in ovulatory patients following clomiphene citrate for in vitro fertilization. Am J Obstet Gynecol 144:569, 1982
24. Buttery B, Trounson A, McMaster R, Wood C: Evaluation of diagnostic ultrasound as a parameter of follicular development in an in vitro fertilization program. Fertil Steril 39:458, 1983
25. O'Herlihy C, Evans JH, Brown JB, de Crespigny LJCh, Robinson HP: Use of ultrasound in monitoring ovulation induction with human pituitary gonadotropins. Obstet Gynecol 60:577, 1982
26. Haning RV Jr, Austin CW, Kuzma DL, Shapiro SS, Zweibel WJ: Ultrasound evaluation of estrogen monitoring for induction of ovulation with menotropins. Fertil Steril 37:627, 1982
27. Marrs RP, Vargyas JM, March CM: Correlation of ultrasonic and endocrinologic measurements in human menopausal gonadotropin therapy. Am J Obstet Gynecol 145:417, 1983
28. Garcia JE, Jones GS, Acosta AA, Wright G Jr: Human menopausal gonadotropin/human chorionic gonadotropin follicular maturation for oocyte aspiration: Phase I, 1981. Fertil Steril 39:167, 1983
29. Garcia JE, Jones GS, Acosta AA, Wright G Jr: Human menopausal gonadotropin/human chorionic gonadotropin follicular maturation for oocyte aspiration: Phase II, 1981. Fertil Steril 39:174, 1983
30. Mantzavinos T, Garcia JE, Jones HW Jr: Ultrasound measurement of ovarian follicles stimulated by human gonadotropins for oocyte recovery and in vitro fertilization. Fertil Steril 40:461, 1983
31. Hurley DM, Brian RJ, Burger HG: Ovulation induction with subcutaneous pulsatile gonadotropin-releasing hormone: singleton pregnancies in patients with previous multiple pregnancies after gonadotropin therapy. Fertil Steril 40:575, 1983
32. Haning RV Jr, Austin CW, Carlson IH, Kuzma DL, Shapiro SS, Zweibel WJ: Plasma estradiol is superior to ultrasound and urinary estriol glucuronide as a predictor of ovarian hyperstimulation during induction of ovulation with menotropins. Fertil Steril 40:31, 1983
33. Coulam CB, Hill LM, Breckle R: Ultrasonic assessment of subsequent unexplained infertility after ovulation induction. Br J Obstet Gynaecol 90:460, 1983
34. McArdle C, Seibel M, Hann LE, Weinstein F, Taymor M: The diagnosis of ovarian hyperstimulation (OHS): the impact of ultrasound. Fertil Steril 39:464, 1983
35. Lenz S, Lauritsen JG: Ultrasonically guided percutaneous aspiration of human follicles under local anesthesia: a new method of collecting oocytes for in vitro fertilization. Fertil Steril 38:673, 1982
36. Wikland M, Nilsson L, Hansson R, Hamberger L, Janson PO: Collection of human oocytes by the use of sonography. Fertil Steril 39:603, 1983
37. Parisi L, Tramonti M, Derchi LE, Casciano S, Zurli A, Rocchi P: Polycystic ovarian disease: ultrasonic evaluation and correlations with clinical and hormonal data. J Clin Ultrasound 12:21, 1984
38. Hann LE, Hall DH, McArdle C, Seibel M: Polycystic ovarian disease: sonographic spectrum. Radiology 150:531, 1984

39. Swanson M, Sauerbrei EE, Cooperber PL: Medical implications of ultrasonically detected polycystic ovaries. J Clin Ultrasound 9:219, 1981

40. Birnholz JC: Endometriosis and inflammatory disease. Semin Ultrasound 4:184, 1983

Chapter 12

Ovulation induction with gonadotropin-releasing hormone

Howard A. Zacur, M.D., Ph.D.

Department of Gynecology and Obstetrics, The Johns Hopkins University School of Medicine, Baltimore, Maryland

Perhaps 20% to 25% of infertility may result from the failure to ovulate regularly.[1-3] Despite the many causes of ovulatory dysfunction (Table 1), until recently, with the introduction of gonadotropin-releasing hormone (GnRH), only three different medications have been available to treat these disorders successfully. These drugs are human menopausal gonadotropin (hMG), bromocriptine,[4] and clomiphene citrate (CC).[5]

The discovery of GnRH in 1971[6, 7] offered anovulatory patients a physiologic medication to be used in their treatment. It was felt that GnRH would eventually supplant other forms of therapy. When GnRH was initially used the results were disappointing, but it now appears that GnRH therapy may well fulfill its promised role. This review will describe the biochemistry of GnRH, past and present protocols of GnRH administration to induce ovulation, and side effects.

GONADOTROPIN-RELEASING HORMONE BIOCHEMISTRY

GnRH is a decapeptide isolated from porcine and ovine hypothalami with an amino acid sequence unchanged between these species (Fig. 1). Although first identified in the hypothalamus, GnRH or GnRH-like hormonal activity has also been discovered in extrahypothalamic sites, e.g., placenta, gonads, and pancreas[8]; but its function in these tissues remains undetermined.

In the brain, GnRH is synthesized by cell bodies in the hypothalamus and is released from these neurons into pituitary-portal blood. GnRH concentrations in pituitary-portal blood have been determined in the rat,[9] monkey,[10] and human[11] and ranged from undetectable to 130 pg/ml; undetectable to 800 pg/ml; and undetectable to 2000 pg/ml, respectively.

After its release into pituitary-portal blood, GnRH travels to the pituitary gland, where it is bound to plasma membrane receptors[12] located predominantly on gonadotropes.[13] After binding to its receptor, the hormone-receptor complex is internalized within the cell.[14] The number of receptors available for GnRH binding is increased by intermittent exposure to GnRH and represents a self-priming effect of the peptide.[15] Conversely, constant exposure of the gonadotrope to GnRH has been shown to reduce the receptor number,[16] an effect best described as down-regulation. Both effects may be modulated to some extent by the endogenous hormonal milieu.[15, 16]

After binding, GnRH stimulates pituitary release of luteinizing hormone (LH) and follicle-stimulating hormone (FSH) in amounts dependent upon the frequency and dosage of GnRH. In vivo, GnRH is believed to be secreted in a pulsatile manner. Decreasing the frequency of the GnRH pulses results in greater FSH than LH release. Increasing the GnRH pulse frequency has the opposite effect.[17] Internalization of the GnRH receptor complex is not required by the gonadotrope to release LH.[18] Adenyl cyclase mediation of gonadotropin release by GnRH was suggested initially,[19] but recent evidence favors the role of a calcium-coupled process.[19]

In the circulation, GnRH is rapidly degraded and has a half-life of only 4 minutes.[20] The susceptibility of the GnRH peptide to degradation by endopeptidases is greatest between Tyr[5] - Gly[6] and Gly[6] - Leu[7] bonds,[21] perhaps because these

Table 1. *Causes of Ovulatory Dysfunction*

Dysfunction	Causes
Hypothalamic	Stress
	Exercise
	Weight loss
	Medications
	Destructive lesions
Pituitary	Destructive lesions
	Infarcts
	Tumor
Ovarian	Resistance
	Failure
Adrenal	Enzyme defects
Prolactin disorders	Drug related
	Idiopathic
Chronic anovulatory syndrome	Polycystic ovarian disease

bonds occur at the B-turn or "kink" in the center of the peptide (Fig. 1). Degradation occurs next at the Pro^9, Gly^{10}, and NH^2 bond by a carboxyamide peptidase.[22] Prolonged activity of GnRH has been achieved by preparation of GnRH analogs, which represent amino acid substitutions of the parent molecule. Biologic activity of the analogs is maintained when the N-terminal tripeptide is retained, i.e., amino acid positions 1 to 3.[23] Analogs possessing agonistic activity are prepared by the making of substitutions at positions 6 to 7 and 9 to 10 or by deletion of the tenth amino acid. Increased biologic activity of these analogs may result from greater affinity to the receptor, greater efficacy of postreceptor effects, or diminished degradation.[23]

INITIAL ATTEMPTS TO INDUCE OVULATION WITH GONADOTROPIN-RELEASING HORMONE

After its discovery, GnRH was successfully used to induce ovulation resulting in pregnancy.[24] This initial success with GnRH was reported in a patient who also received hMG therapy to stimulate the formation of a preovulatory follicle. Acute administration of GnRH was then provided, which resulted in ovulation and pregnancy.

A single injection of GnRH to anovulatory women or daily administration of single doses of GnRH to anovulatory women in subsequent studies rarely resulted in successful ovulation induction.[25-28] Use of GnRH in conjunction with CC, human chorionic gonadotropin (hCG), or hMG was somewhat more successful, but results remained disappointing[29-32] and were far less successful than the 90% (or greater) rate of ovulation achieved with hMG and hCG.[33, 34] Lack of appropriate dosage or frequency of drug administration were explanations given for ovulatory failures with GnRH during the early 1970s.

SIGNIFICANCE OF PULSATILE ADMINISTRATION

Oscillatory changes in LH concentration during the human menstrual cycle were observed

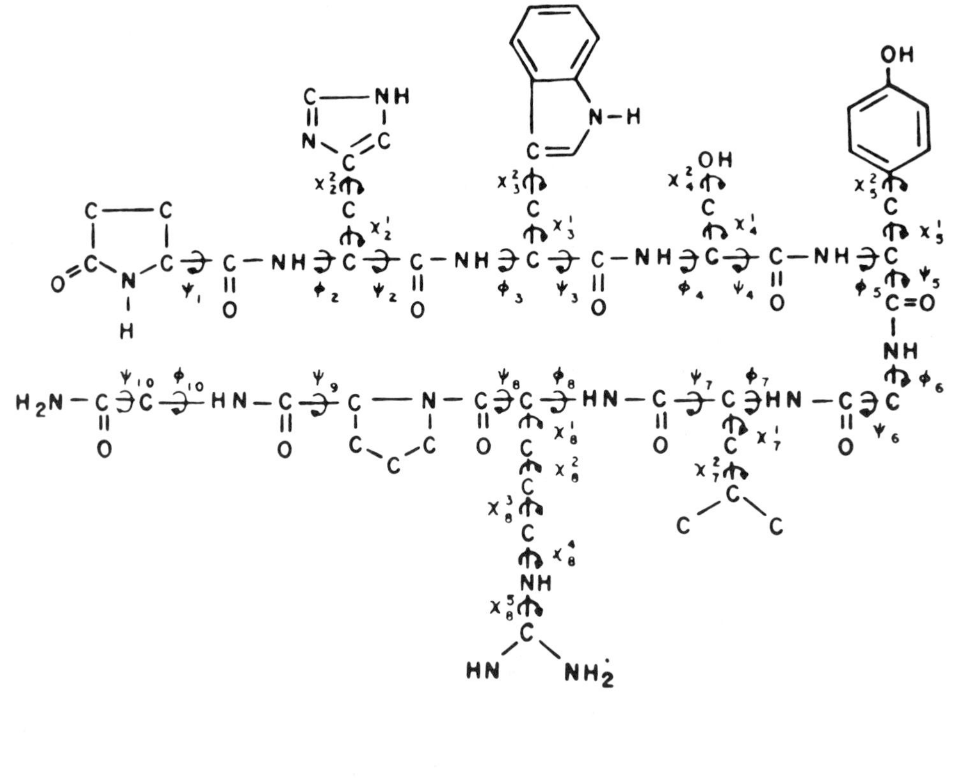

Figure 1
Primary sequence of luteinizing hormone-releasing hormone with some hydrogen atoms omitted for clarity. (From Momany FA: J Am Chem Soc 98:2990, 1976. Reproduced with the permission of the publisher.) Copyright by The American Chemical Society.

many years ago,[35, 36] but an explanation for the episodic hormonal fluctuation was not known at the time. Loss in oscillating LH concentrations was then observed in arcuate-nucleus-lesioned monkeys.[37] It was found that these oscillating concentrations could be restored by the administration of GnRH in a pulsatile manner.[38] These LH oscillations or "pulses" could therefore be directly related to the pulsed administration of GnRH. Adjustments in the administration of GnRH were followed by changes in the LH concentration in peripheral blood. For example, nonpulsatile or continuous administration of GnRH results in an initial rise in the peripheral LH concentration followed by a decline in hormone concentration, a result possibly explained by down-regulation in plasma membrane GnRH receptors.[39] Administration of GnRH intravenously at 90- to 120-minute intervals produced the typical pulsatile pattern of LH concentrations. In nonovariectomized monkeys, pulsatile GnRH administration produced pulsatile LH release followed by ovulation and a normal luteal phase.[40] If the GnRH pulse frequency was reduced, ovulation did not occur and an increase in the FSH/LH ratio occurred.[17] If the GnRH pulses were increased, LH concentrations constantly exceeded FSH concentrations,[17] a gonadotropin ratio usually seen in chronically anovulatory women with polycystic ovarian syndrome.[41, 42] As clinical investigators who had failed to induce ovulation with GnRH had suggested, the dose and frequency of administration of GnRH appeared crucial to its successful use.

HYPOTHALAMIC-PITUITARY-GONADAL RELATIONSHIP TO EXOGENOUS GONADOTROPIN-RELEASING HORMONE ADMINISTRATION

The results from subhuman primate studies suggested that ovulation induction in the arcuate-lesioned monkey could be achieved with unvarying pulsatile administration of GnRH in the presence of the pituitary gland and ovary. These findings were used to describe a permissive role for GnRH in regulating LH and FSH secretion. In this model, estrogen (E) and progesterone (P) secretion by the ovary would affect pituitary and ovarian function and not alter GnRH release.

Whereas these assumptions may be accurate with the use of an experimental model, they may not accurately reflect conditions during the normal human menstrual cycle. Changes in frequency and amplitude of LH pulses have been observed throughout the human menstrual cycle.[43, 44] LH pulses are more frequent but reduced in amplitude during the follicular phase of the cycle, whereas LH pulses have reduced frequency but increased amplitude during the luteal phase.[43] Decreased LH pulse frequency with increased amplitude has been induced during the follicular phase in normal women by exogenous administration of P.[43] These results imply that modulation of GnRH release by gonadal steroids may in fact occur in the human.

If gonadal steroids modulate GnRH secretion, may GnRH in turn directly affect gonadal steroidogenesis? Initial studies in the rat revealed that GnRH inhibited FSH-induced E and P production by granulosa cells.[45] With the use of an agonistic analog of GnRH, specific binding to rat luteal cells was demonstrated but an inhibitory effect on P production was noted.[46] Follow-up studies corroborated these findings in the rat,[47] but conflicting results have been reported in other species. GnRH had no effect on ovulation or P secretion in the in vitro perfused rabbit ovary.[48] Specific high-affinity GnRH binding has not been demonstrated in monkey,[49] human,[50] ovine,[51] bovine,[51] or porcine[51] ovaries. GnRH (or agonist) did not directly inhibit E or P production acutely in cultured human granulosa cells in one study,[52] but did when the cultured human granulosa cells were chronically exposed to the agonist.[53] Interestingly, these latter results could not be confirmed in a more recent experiment.[54] Concentrations of GnRH used in these in vitro studies (10^{-9} M to 10^{-10} M) approximated peak concentrations of GnRH measured in the peripheral plasma of women after intravenous or subcutaneous administration of this polypeptide.[55]

Existence of a negative effect on gonadal function by GnRH would be of obvious concern to clinicians who provide this drug to anovulatory patients. In view of the conflicting results reported to date, assurances that GnRH has no adverse effect on gonadal function in the human cannot as yet be given.

OVULATION INDUCTION WITH GONADOTROPIN-RELEASING HORMONE

Initial studies using GnRH to induce ovulation were largely unsuccessful. Reasons for this fail-

Table 2. *GnRH Ovulation Induction Protocol*

	Protocol
Indication	Failure to achieve repetitive ovulation with CC
Evaluation	
Endocrine	Gonadotropins, prolactin, androgens, and adrenocorticotropic hormone stimulation test when indicated
Infertility	Semen analysis, hysterosalpingogram, and diagnostic laparoscopy
Radiographic	Minimum of coned-down view of sella or computerized tomogram scan in cases categorized as hypothalamic amenorrhea
Dynamic testing	GnRH stimulation test
Therapy	Subcutaneously administered GnRH (15-µg dose) at 90-minute intervals
Monitoring	Serial plasma estradiols and pelvic sonograms; daily basal body temperatures, periodic pelvic examinations to check for changes in cervical mucus and vaginal epithelium
	Adjustment of GnRH dosage in 10 days if no change noted in hormonal or physical parameters
	Administration of vaginal P suppositories (25 mg) twice daily on the morning of the third day of basal body temperature rise following discontinuation of GnRH
	Reinstitute GnRH on third day of next menstrual cycle if needed

ure are now understandable in view of the biochemical background just reviewed. Recent clinical studies have used protocols for GnRH administration, allowing for the fact that this decapeptide must be administered in a pulsatile pattern for prolonged periods. Currently used protocols for GnRH ovulation induction are summarized below.

PATIENT SELECTION

Guidelines for the clinical evaluation of patients considered for GnRH ovulation do not currently exist. It would seem reasonable that standardized protocols should be developed before GnRH therapy is provided because (1) ovulation induction is not currently approved by the Food and Drug Administration as an indication for this drug; (2) it is relatively expensive; and (3) previous clinical experience with it has been limited.

A sample protocol for use of GnRH at our institution is provided in Table 2. It is suggested that anovulatory patients who are potential candidates for GnRH ovulation induction should have undergone a complete infertility evaluation. This would include semen analysis, hysterosalpingogram (or hysteroscopy), and diagnostic laparoscopy. Indications for this complete evaluation would be similar to those used before hMG is used for ovulation induction[56, 57]; namely, that in view of the expense and risk involved, additional causes for infertility should be sought before therapy is instituted.

Causes for anovulation in infertile patients are numerous and have already been mentioned (Table 1). It is recommended that anovulatory patients with hyperprolactinemia, premature ovarian failure, partial adrenal enzyme deficiency, and polycystic ovary syndrome (PCO) be identified. Measurement of baseline LH, FSH, prolactin, and androgen concentrations and, where indicated, adrenocorticotropic hormone stimulation testing should accomplish this. Except for patients with premature ovarian failure, induction of ovulation with the use of bromocriptine, CC, or exogenous corticosteroids should be attempted initially in women with hyperprolactinemia, PCO, and partial adrenal enzyme deficiencies, respectively. In individuals with hypothalamic amenorrhea without withdrawal bleeding after P administration, CC therapy should still be tried first because (1) this drug has been approved by the Food and Drug Administration for ovulation induction; (2) clinical experience with this medication is extensive; (3) it is relatively easy to administer; (4) it is relatively less expensive; (5) side effects are few; and (6) at least a chance (5% or greater) of successful ovulation induction exists in this type of patient.[58] Failure to induce ovulation with bromocriptine or CC is usually followed by an attempt at ovulation induction with hMG. Ovulation induction with hMG is expensive, associated with a 20% to 30% multiple pregnancy rate,[57] luteal phase defects,[59] and risk of hyperstimulation. Administration of GnRH before hMG has been advocated because GnRH is more physiologic, less expensive, and of less risk to patients. As clinical experience is gained with GnRH ovulation induction, it will become easier to determine if these assumptions concerning GnRH use are valid.

GONADOTROPIN-RELEASING HORMONE STIMULATION TESTING

Is a GnRH stimulation test required before a patient is placed in a GnRH ovulation induction program? Clinical response to intravenous administration of 100 μg of GnRH has been recommended as a screening test to identify patients with isolated deficiency of pituitary LH and FSH.[60] Obviously such individuals would not benefit from GnRH ovulation induction and should be excluded. Unfortunately, the gonadotropin response to a single dose of GnRH may not distinguish between hypothalamic and pituitary dysfunction.[61] Nevertheless, initial testing with GnRH has been used by some investigators to determine the dose of GnRH to be given during ovulation induction, with high responders receiving a lower unit dose of the releasing hormone.[62]

Because it has become clear that GnRH stimulates formation of its own membrane receptors on gonadotropes,[15] either absent or poor pituitary release of LH or FSH after initial GnRH administration may not predict the pituitary's ultimate response to prolonged pulsatile GnRH.[63] Therefore, performance of GnRH stimulation testing before attempting GnRH ovulation induction would not presently be considered an absolute requirement. It is still performed by our group for purposes of accumulating data to develop screening criteria that may be of future use in predicting patients' response to GnRH.

ADMINISTRATION AND DOSAGE OF GONADOTROPIN-RELEASING HORMONE

Oral administration of GnRH is not feasible because of the susceptibility of the decapeptide to degradation by proteolytic enzymes. Gonadotropin response to intravenous, subcutaneous, intramuscular, nasal, and sublingual GnRH administration has been reported, however.[25, 26, 64, 65] A rapid rise in LH (within 5 minutes after the onset of GnRH administration), peaking within 30 minutes and lasting for 2 to 3 hours, characterizes the response to intravenous GnRH administration in normal men.[65] The peak plasma LH concentration attained after intravenous GnRH administration is closely correlated with the dosage of GnRH given. Depending on the study, the maximal LH response in men occurs after injection of either 250 μg[65] or 150 μg[66] of the hormone. The pattern of the plasma LH response to intravenous GnRH administration in women is similar to that observed in men, with the peak LH response occurring with only 100 μg of the hormone.[67] Most dose-response studies with GnRH have been performed in men[65, 66, 68] or women with anorexia nervosa[69] or isolated gonadotropin deficiency.[70] This was done because the LH response to GnRH varies with the phase of the menstrual cycle in ovulatory women.[71] The minimal dose of intravenously administered GnRH necessary to produce a measurable increase in LH in men has ranged from 0.025 μg/kg[69] to 10 μg.[66] In women with anorexia nervosa, repetitive doses of 0.025 μg/kg of GnRH have successfully stimulated LH release.[69] Gonadotropin responses after subcutaneous or intramuscular GnRH administration are similar. In comparison to intravenous GnRH administration, the LH response after subcutaneous or intramuscular GnRH is characterized by a slower rise, decreased peak response, and slower return to baseline.[25, 26, 65] Intranasal GnRH produces an LH response similar to that obtained after intravenous GnRH, but five to ten times as much hormone is required.[64]

Lack of adequate GnRH dose-response data in women with hypothalamic amenorrhea may have contributed to early difficulties encountered in selecting the appropriate dose of GnRH to be used in inducing ovulation. For example, intravenous administration of the 0.025 μg/kg dose of GnRH determined from previous clinical studies in women with anorexia nervosa[69] or Kallman's syndrome[72] failed to induce ovulation in 19 women with CC-nonresponsive anovulatory infertility.[73] Increasing the GnRH dose to a 10- to 20-μg intravenous pulse resulted in three ovulations in 23 cycles in this study.[73] Others have also reported successful ovulation induction with intravenous GnRH given in higher dosages ranging from 10 μg[74] to 20 μg[75-77] per pulse. However, lower doses (1 to 5 μg) of GnRH given intravenously have also been successful.[78] Optimization of the GnRH dosage is of vital concern in efforts to avoid the paradoxic fall in FSH observed in the rhesus monkey when the dosage of GnRH was increased.[17, 79] Clinical response to intravenous GnRH is summarized in Table 3.

Initial studies using subcutaneous administered GnRH in dosages of 0.5 to 5 μg failed to induce ovulation,[80] but only two subjects were involved. It was suggested that this failure may have been due to the fact that slow release of GnRH from subcutaneous tissue could produce chronically elevated LH levels like those observed in anovulatory patients with PCO.[80] In subsequent investigations with larger numbers of patients, the results with subcutaneously administered GnRH have been more successful. With

Table 3. *Clinical Response to Intravenous Pulsatile Administration*

Author	Diagnosis	No. of patients	Response to CC	GnRH dose	Interval	Ovulation	Pregnancy
				μg	*min*		
Goerzen et al.[74]	Secondary amenorrhea	6	Failed	10	120	6/6	4/6
Leyendecker et al.[75]	Secondary amenorrhea	2	Not known	15–20	90	2/2	2/2
Schoemaker et al.[76]	Secondary amenorrhea	1	Failed	20	120	1/1	1/1
Miller et al.[78]	Secondary amenorrhea	8	Failed	1–5	96–120	8/8	5/8
Reid and Sauerbrei[79]	Primary amenorrhea (1); secondary amenorrhea (1)	2	Not mentioned	5	90–120	2/2	2/2
Total						19/19 (100%)	14/19 (74%)

2.5- to 20-μg doses subcutaneously every 90 to 120 minutes, successful ovulation induction and pregnancy have been reported in numerous anovulatory women.[81-86] Results are summarized in Table 4. Recently, ovulation induction and pregnancy was reported in all of 28 patients with hypothalamic amenorrhea given GnRH therapy. The dose of GnRH given subcutaneously in this study was 15 μg, and it was reported that few patients ovulated when given smaller doses.[86]

There is no argument that intravenous GnRH administration will result in a better-defined pulse of LH. However, this mode of administration requires an indwelling venous catheter, which increases the chances for morbidity (phlebitis) and failed administration due to clotting in the intravenous line or dislodgement of the catheter from the venous lumen. Intravenously administered GnRH also requires that low-dose heparin (1000 U/ml) be added to the solution to prevent clotting. Venous catheters have been left in place for 2 to 4 weeks in some studies,[77] whereas in others they have been changed every 2 to 3 days.[73] Failed drug administration with subcutaneously administered GnRH is unusual. Subcutaneously placed needles are usually left in place for 2 to 7 days.[79, 81]

PUMPS USED FOR GONADOTROPIN-RELEASING HORMONE ADMINISTRATION

Delivery of GnRH requires the use of a pulsatile pump with several models available, e.g., Autosyringe (Auto Syringe, Inc., Hooksett, NH),[81]

Table 4. *Clinical Response to Subcutaneous GnRH Administration*

Author	Diagnosis	No. of patients	Response to CC	GnRH dose	Interval	Ovulation	Pregnancy
				μg	*min*		
Seibel et al.[81]	Secondary amenorrhea	3	Failed	20	120	3/3	1/3
Hurley et al.[82]	Secondary amenorrhea	3	Failed	10	90	3/3	3/3
Skarin et al.[83]	Secondary amenorrhea	14	Failed	1, 5, 20	90	12/14	8/12
Hurley et al.[84]	Primary amenorrhea (1); secondary amenorrhea (11); oligomenorrhea (2)	14	Failed	5, 10, 15	90	14/14	4/5
Woodhouse et al.[85]	Secondary amenorrhea	5	Not mentioned	2.5–15	90	4/5	4/5
Mason et al.[86]	Secondary amenorrhea	28	Failed	10–25	90	28/28	13/28
Total						64/67 (90%)	40/67 (60%)

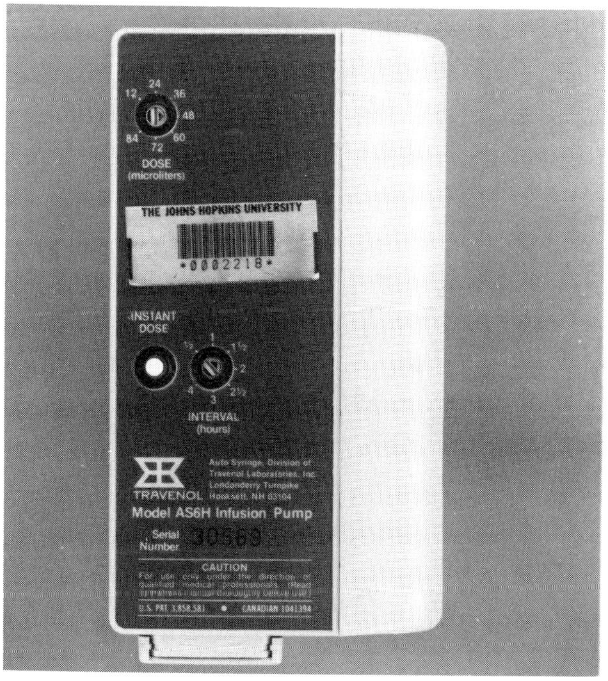

Figure 2
Auto Syringe infusion pump model AS6H supplied by Travenol Laboratories, Inc., Londonderry Turnpike, Hooksett, NH.

Zyklomat (Ferring GmbH, Kiel, FRG),[75] or Pulsamat (Ferring Laboratories, Inc., Ridgewood, NJ).[87] These pumps are relatively small (Fig. 2) and may be hidden from view, depending upon the ingenuity of the patient. Some pump models allow selection for frequency of administration as well as volume to be delivered, whereas others do not. The cost of these pumps is high ($1000 to $1500), but smaller and less expensive models are promised in the future.

DRUG AVAILABILITY

GnRH is currently available in the United States as a lyophilized powder marketed commercially as Factrel (Ayerst Laboratories, New York, NY) in 100- and 500-μg vials. The drug must be dissolved in sterile diluent before its administration. Dose is determined by the concentration of the GnRH in solution as well as by the volume of solution to be given. For example, 500 μg of GnRH dissolved in 5 ml with 50 μl of solution to be administered at each pulse represents a 5-μg dose of GnRH. Interestingly, measurements of GnRH in peripheral plasma after the subcutaneous administration of 5 μg of GnRH in different volumes of sterile saline (25, 100, and 250 μl) are the same.[55] Solubilization of GnRH may decrease its stability and thus potency if it is kept in solution for long periods.

PATIENT MONITORING

Standardized guidelines for monitoring patients receiving GnRH therapy do not currently exist. After the start of therapy, monitoring in most trials has usually consisted of periodic measurements of plasma estradiol[81, 85] or urinary E levels.[82] Ultrasonography is also used at 2- to 7-day intervals[86] initially, then more frequently when follicle growth to 10 mm is observed.[81] Pelvic examinations to detect shifts in quantity or quality of cervical mucus or changes in vaginal epithelium have not ordinarily been done. Choice of initial dose of GnRH to be used has ranged from 1 to 20 μg, with lower doses being employed when the drug is given intravenously. Fixed dosage regimens are usually successful when GnRH doses of 10 to 20 μg are used. Alternatively, doses as low as 5 μg/pulse may be tried with 5-μg increments if an increase in E is not observed within 7 to 14 days.[84] For anovulatory patients who have failed to ovulate with CC and who are not hyperprolactinemic, ovulation has generally occurred within 30 days of the start of GnRH therapy.[79, 84]

Very high LH and FSH concentrations have transiently been observed within 1 to 3 days after the start of GnRH therapy.[83] This exaggerated response in gonadotropins was followed in one case by failure to induce ovulation.[83] As previously mentioned, further studies designed to develop screening criteria to predict future response to GnRH therapy would be of benefit.

PATIENTS WITH HYPERPROLACTINEMIA AND POLYCYSTIC OVARY SYNDROME

GnRH was initially given to patients with CC-resistant secondary amenorrhea to induce ovulation. Recently, GnRH has been used to induce ovulation in patients with hyperprolactinemia or PCO. Leyendecker et al.[88] reported that 10-μg pulses of GnRH given intravenously successfully induced ovulation in an 18-year-old patient with basal serum prolactin levels in the range of 150 ng/ml. The hormonal responses were not dissimilar to those observed in other patients receiving GnRH, although a transient additional rise in prolactin occurred. Although the drug of choice for ovulation induction in hyperprolactinemic patients is bromocriptine, it appears that GnRH may represent an alternative method for those individuals unable to tolerate that medication.

Using low-dose GnRH (0.025 μg/kg) given intravenously every 90 minutes, Ory et al.[89] induced ovulation within 22 days (range, 3 to 22 days) after beginning therapy in five of six treatment cycles in four women with PCO. Burger et al.,[90] in two CC-unresponsive patients with polycystic ovary-like disease, successfully induced ovulation by giving 20-μg GnRH as intravenous pulses. These results are somewhat surprising in view of previous negative experiences with GnRH ovulation induction of PCO patients.[77] Hypothalamic dysfunction in regulating LH and FSH release has been suspected in patients with PCO, but exogenously administered GnRH may override this defect. If additional studies with larger numbers of patients confirm these successful results, a larger patient pool will become available for GnRH therapy.

SUCCESSIVE CYCLES WITH GONADOTROPIN-RELEASING HORMONE OVULATION INDUCTION

Will the same GnRH protocol used to achieve ovulation initially be similarly successful in succeeding cycles? Continued use of the same GnRH protocol results in repetitive ovulatory cycles with follicular phase lengths varying from 10 to 20 days.[73, 76, 83] Follicular phase lengths may vary more widely when anovulatory patients not diagnosed with hypothalamic amenorrhea are given repetitive GnRH therapy.[90]

LUTEAL PHASE SUPPORT

In arcuate-nucleus-lesioned monkeys, a fixed dose of GnRH given continuously results in ovulation and development of a normal luteal phase[40] even if hyperprolactinemia is present.[91] In humans, it is well-known that changes occur in LH pulse amplitude and frequency during the luteal phase[43]; it has been suggested that these changes may result from steroid-induced changes in GnRH secretion from the hypothalamus.[43]

Continued exposure of the human corpus luteum to LH has long been accepted as a prerequisite for maintaining a normal luteal phase.[92] However, corpus luteum function has been maintained without exogenous LH administration in hypophysectomized monkeys,[93] and luteinized granulosa cells in culture are capable of producing P for 14 days without the addition of gonadotropins to the culture medium.[94] Although these studies suggest that LH may not be essential for corpus luteum function, other studies have suggested that it is. Cessation of GnRH infusion during the early and midluteal phases in monkeys with radiofrequenced arcuate-nucleus lesions resulted in premature menses.[95] Administration of LH antisera during the luteal phase of the rhesus monkey menstrual cycle also resulted in premature menses.[96] Effects of GnRH administration on luteal function are therefore of obvious concern when this drug is used to treat anovulatory infertility. Cessation of pulsatile GnRH administration in anovulatory patients after ovulation is followed by a defective luteal phase,[97] whereas continuation of pulsatile GnRH at the same dose and time interval of administration during the luteal phase has also been associated with luteal phase defects.[98-100] As mentioned previously, this latter finding should not prove surprising if in humans hypothalamic release of GnRH is altered during the luteal phase. Therefore, a fixed dosage regimen of GnRH provided to induce follicular growth and ovulation may not be optimal to sustain luteal function.

Alternatively, GnRH itself could directly affect ovarian function as previously discussed or indirectly affect ovarian function through changes in gonadotropin secretion. Results consistent with this latter hypothesis have recently been reported. Sheehan et al.[101] administered a GnRH agonist during the follicular phase of the normal human menstrual cycle, which depressed FSH levels, prolonged the follicular phase, and shortened the luteal phase. Administration of GnRH or analog during the midluteal to late luteal phase in normal women resulted in diminished P levels and a shortened luteal phase length.[101-105] No effect was seen, however, if GnRH was only given at midcycle.[106]

In many of the clinical protocols with GnRH, the luteal phase has been supported by continuing pulsatile GnRH administration at the same dose and time interval of administration until pregnancy is achieved[73, 76, 86] or by stopping GnRH but giving hCG injections, 1000 to 2500 U intramuscularly every 3 to 4 days during the luteal phase.[73, 74, 82, 83, 86] Alternatively, continuation of GnRH coupled with hCG administration has also been advised.[98] Objections exist for all of these management recommendations. First, continuation of the same dose and frequency of GnRH may fail to provide optimal LH release to maintain corpus luteum P production or may directly inhibit corpus luteum P production. Second, use of hCG introduces potentially undesirable side effects, such as multiple births or hyperstimulation, which would defeat one of the original aims for using GnRH.

Cessation of the GnRH pump therapy followed by P vaginal suppository use represents an alternative approach. Vaginal suppository use of P (25 mg) begun on the third day of basal body temperature rise and given twice daily has already been successfully employed.[107] After the beginning of suppository use in the morning, GnRH therapy is discontinued in the afternoon. This method avoids the possibility of inducing luteal phase abnormalities by GnRH, decreases the risk of multiple pregnancy associated with hCG, and decreases drug cost and time required for pump use. This will be more convenient for patients and allows more women to be treated when only a small number of pumps are available.

SIDE EFFECTS

Use of GnRH to induce ovulation has been promulgated as a physiologic method that reduces the risks of side effects observed with other methods. Recent information suggests that this may not in fact be the case. Side effects from CC or hMG therapy include hyperstimulation and multiple births, and each of these side effects has now been reported with GnRH therapy.

HYPERSTIMULATION SYNDROME

This phenomenon entails varying degrees of ovarian enlargement, abdominal pain, ascites, and electrolyte disturbances. The syndrome may be classified as mild, moderate, or severe.[108, 109] Ovulation induction with CC is rarely associated with moderate to severe hyperstimulation, although mild hyperstimulation may occur in up to 13.5% of cases.[110] Use of hMG to induce ovulation has been reported to cause mild hyperstimulation in 8.4% to 23% of cycles, moderate hyperstimulation in 6% to 7% of cycles, and severe hyperstimulation in 0.8% to 2% of cycles.[109]

Mild hyperstimulation after GnRH use has now been reported in several patients.[84, 90, 111, 112] It is still too early to estimate the risk of hyperstimulation in patients receiving GnRH. Dosage, frequency of GnRH administration, and type of anovulatory patient will all probably affect the incidence of hyperstimulation. As an example, Liu et al.[113] have demonstrated that an increased dosage of GnRH will stimulate multiple follicular development.

MULTIPLE PREGNANCY

Incidence of multiple gestation after hMG induction of ovulation has been reported to range from 21% to 34%,[57] whereas a multiple pregnancy rate of 5% has been reported with CC.[58]

Use of GnRH has been advocated as a possible means to avoid a higher than normal incidence (< 1%) of multiple gestation. As experience with GnRH ovulation induction has been gained, reports have now been published of triplet[114] and quadruplet[115] pregnancies. Whereas use of hCG may have contributed to the birth of triplets,[114] intravenous pulsatile administration of only GnRH (18 μg) resulted in the birth of quadruplets.[115] As with hyperstimulation, it is still too early to estimate accurately the true incidence of multiple pregnancy occurring with GnRH ovulation induction. Variables such as dosage and type of anovulatory patient treated may no doubt affect the occurrence rate of multiple gestation.

CONGENITAL MALFORMATION AND SPONTANEOUS ABORTIONS

Abortion and malformation rates are not increased after CC-induced pregnancies,[116, 117] but a high rate of spontaneous pregnancy wastage (20% to 30%) has been noted after hMG ovulation induction.[57] Although spontaneous abortions have occurred after GnRH ovulation induction,[83, 86] insufficient data are available for statistical purposes. At the present time, no data are available concerning the incidence of congenital malformations after GnRH ovulation induction; patients should be informed of this fact before treatment is induced.

INFECTION AND HEMATOMA FORMATION

Chronic administration of GnRH by either subcutaneous or intravenous routes involves placement of indwelling catheters or needles. Infections at the site of needle placement have been reported.[73, 84] To minimize this risk, frequent inspection of the needle site with frequent changing of needles and catheters is required. Development of some degree of phlebitis occurred in almost all patients treated with GnRH in one study.[73] Low-dose heparin solutions are needed for intravenous administration of GnRH to prevent catheter occlusion due to blood clots. Heparin should not be added to GnRH solutions prepared for subcutaneous administration because this inclusion has resulted in hematoma formation at the needle site.[83]

ANTIBODY FORMATION

Theoretically, chronic administration of exogenous GnRH could result in the production of anti-GnRH antibodies in the patient's sera. Should this occur, not only would interference with the action of the drug take place, but interference with endogenous GnRH activity might occur as well.

Secondary drug failure due to antibody formation against exogenously administered GnRH has already been reported in men treated for isolated gonadotropin deficiency.[118, 119] In normal, mature male monkeys, active immunization against GnRH resulted in decreased hypothalamic GnRH content, decreased pituitary LH concentration, and decreased testicular weight and steroid production.[120]

In a large clinical study, Fraser et al.[121] were unable to demonstrate the development of antisera to either GnRH or a GnRH analog in 81 patients receiving long-term GnRH analog therapy. Although these results would suggest that antibody formation to exogenous GnRH is unlikely, a recent study has suggested otherwise. In this study, 163 patients (141 men, 22 women) received GnRH from 3 weeks to 9 months. Five patients (three men and two women) were found to have specific IgG binding to labeled GnRH, suggesting that a 3% prevalence rate of GnRH antibody formation could occur after therapy.[122] Reasons for the antibody formation were not apparent, but if the results are confirmed in future studies, the clinical usefulness of GnRH therapy could be limited.

CONCLUSION

Failure to administer GnRH in a physiologic manner accounted for the disappointing results achieved when GnRH was first used to induce ovulation. After the discovery that pulsatile rather than continuous or daily drug administration of GnRH was required, a renewed interest in using GnRH as an ovulation induction agent occurred.

Use of GnRH in the therapeutic setting must still be considered experimental because clinical experience with the drug for ovulation induction is being gained. Spontaneous abortion and congenital malformation rates with GnRH have yet to be accurately calculated. Although it has been surmised that pulsatile GnRH administration reproduces normal hypothalamic-pituitary interaction and should not therefore result in untoward results, this may not be true. Multiple pregnancies after GnRH ovulation induction have been reported, although this may relate to the dosage of drug given or concomitant use of hCG. The administration of GnRH during the luteal phase at the same dose and frequency as that given in the follicular phase may be satisfactory to maintain a normal luteal phase and pregnancy in the subhuman primate, but not in the human woman.

The exact risk to the patient for development of anti-GnRH antibodies remains to be determined. The 3% prevalence rate of antibody formation would be most worrisome if confirmed in additional investigations.

Finally, it should be stressed that not all adverse effects from clinical use of GnRH may be known. Because this decapeptide stimulates pituitary secretion of LH and FSH and may have extrahypothalamic actions as well, prolonged GnRH therapy may be found to adversely affect the pituitary gland and other extrahypothalamic target organs.

Conversely, new and exciting uses of GnRH or its analogs are being discovered, as demonstrated by its beneficial effects on endometriosis,[123] leiomyomata,[124] precocious puberty,[125] and prostatic cancer.[126] Thus, GnRH is now well on its way to fulfilling the role promised for it after its discovery. However, enthusiasm for GnRH therapy must be tempered by the knowledge that due to the still-limited clinical experience with GnRH, caution must be exercised in its use.

REFERENCES

1. Katayama KP, Ju K-S, Manuel M, Jones GS, Jones HW Jr: Computer analysis of etiology and pregnancy rate in 636 cases of primary infertility. Am J Obstet Gynecol 135:207, 1979

2. Kliger BE: Evaluation, therapy, and outcome in 493 infertile couples. Fertil Steril 41:40, 1984
3. Blasco L: Clinical approach to the evaluation of sperm-cervical mucus interactions. Fertil Steril 28:1133, 1977
4. Pepperell RJ: Prolactin and reproduction. Fertil Steril 35:267, 1981
5. Pepperell RJ: A rational approach to ovulation induction. Fertil Steril 40:1, 1983
6. Matsuo H, Baba Y, Nair RMG, Arimura A, Schally AV: Structure of the porcine LH and FSH releasing hormone. I. The proposed amino acid sequence. Biochem Biophys Res Commun 43:1334, 1971
7. Burgus R, Butcher M, Amoss N, Ling N, Monahan M, Rivier J, Fellows R, Blackwell R, Vale W, Guillemin R: Primary structure of the hypothalamic luteinizing hormone-releasing factor (LRF) of ovine origin. Proc Natl Acad Sci USA 69:278, 1972
8. Siler-Khodr T: Hypothalamic-like peptides in the placenta. Semin Reprod Endocrinol 1:321, 1983
9. Eskay RL, Mical RS, Porter JC: Relationship between luteinizing hormone releasing hormone concentration in hypophysial portal blood and luteinizing hormone release in intact, castrated and electrochemically stimulated rats. Endocrinology 100:263, 1977
10. Carmel PW, Araki S, Ferin M: Pituitary stalk portal blood collection in rhesus monkeys: evidence for pulsatile release of gonadotropin releasing hormone (GnRH). Endocrinology 99:243, 1976
11. Antunes JL, Carmel PW, Housepian EM, Ferin M: Luteinizing hormone releasing hormone in human pituitary blood. J Neurosurg 49:382, 1978
12. Spona J: LH-RH stimulated gonadotropin release mediated by two distinct pituitary receptors. FEBS Lett 35:50, 1973
13. Snyder G, Naor Z, Fawcett CP, McCann SM: Gonadotropin release and cyclic nucleotides: evidence for luteinizing hormone releasing hormone-induced elevation of guanosine 3′,5′ monophosphate levels in gonadotrophs. Endocrinology 107:1627, 1980
14. Hazum E, Cuatrecasas P, Marian J, Conn PM: Receptor mediated internalization of fluorescent gonadotropin-releasing hormone by pituitary gonadotropes. Proc Natl Acad Sci USA 77:6692, 1980
15. Frager MS, Pieper DR, Tonetta S, Duncan JA, Marshall JC: Pituitary gonadotropin-releasing hormone (GnRH) receptors: effects of castration, steroid replacement and the role of GnRH in modulating receptors in the rat. J Clin Invest 67:615, 1981
16. Clayton RN, Catt KJ: Gonadotropin-releasing hormone receptors: characterization, physiological regulation and relationship to reproductive function. Endocr Rev 2:186, 1981
17. Wildt L, Hausler A, Marshall G, Hutchinson JA, Plant TM, Belchetz PE, Knobil E: Frequency and amplitude of gonadotropin releasing hormone stimulation and gonadotropin secretion in the rhesus monkey. Endocrinology 109:376, 1981
18. Conn PM, Smith RG, Rogers DC: Stimulation of pituitary gonadotropin release does not require internalization of gonadotropin releasing hormone. J Biol Chem 256:1098, 1981
19. Conn PM, Marian J, MicMillian M, Stern J, Rodgers D, Hamby M, Penna A, Grant E: Gonadotropin releasing hormone action in the pituitary: a three step mechanism. Endocr Rev 2:174, 1981
20. Redding TW, Kastin AJ, Gonzalez-Barcena D, Coy DH, Coy EJ, Schalch DS, Schally AV: The half-life, metabolism and excretion of tritiated luteinizing hormone releasing hormone (LH-RH) in man. J Clin Endocrinol Metab 37:626, 1973
21. Koch Y, Baram T, Chobsieng P, Fridkin M: Enzymatic degradation of luteinizing hormone releasing hormone (LH-RH) by hypothalamic tissue. Biochem Biophys Res Commun 61:95, 1974
22. Marks N: Biodegradation of hormonally active peptides in the central nervous system. In Subcellular Mechanisms in Reproductive Neuroendocrinology, Edited by F Naftolin, RJ Ryan, J Davis. Amsterdam, Elsevier, 1970, p 129
23. Schally AV, Kastin AJ, Arimura A: The hypothalamus and reproduction. Am J Obstet Gynecol 122:857, 1975
24. Kastin AJ, Zarate A, Midgley AR, Canales ES, Schally AV: Ovulation confirmed by pregnancy after infusion of porcine LH-RH. J Clin Endocrinol Metab 33:980, 1971
25. Akande EO, Bonnar J, Carr PJ, Corkor CS, Dutton A, MacKinnon PCB, Robinson D: Effect of synthetic gonadotropin releasing hormone in secondary amenorrhea. Lancet 2:112, 1972
26. Keller PJ: Treatment of anovulation with synthetic luteinizing hormone-releasing hormone. Am J Obstet Gynecol 116:698, 1973
27. Breckwoldt M, Czygan PJ, Lehmann F, Bettendorf G: Synthetic LH-RH as a therapeutic agent. Acta Endocrinol (Copenh) 75:209, 1974
28. Nakano R, Katayama K, Mizuno T, Tojo S: Induction of ovulation with synthetic luteinizing hormone-releasing hormone. Fertil Steril 25:471, 1974
29. Zanartu J, Dabancens A, Kastin AJ, Schally AV: Effect of synthetic hypothalamic gonadotropin-releasing hormone (FSH/LH-RH) in anovulatory sterility. Fertil Steril 25:160, 1974
30. Zarate A, Canales ES, Soria J, Forsbach G, Kastin AJ, Schally AV: Therapeutic use of gonadoliberin (follicle-stimulating hormone/luteinizing hormone-releasing hormone) in women. Fertil Steril 27:1233, 1976
31. Casas PRF, Miechi H, Badano A, Mirkin A, Aparicio N, Turner D, Nagle C, Rosner J: Clinical and gonadotropic response of amenorrheic patients treated with clomiphene and repeated injections of luteinizing hormone-releasing hormone. Fertil Steril 28:293, 1977
32. Zarate A, Canales ES, Soria J, Gonzalez A, Schally AV, Kastin AJ: Further observations on the therapy of anovulatory infertility with synthetic luteinizing hormone-releasing hormone. Fertil Steril 25:3, 1974
33. Spadoni LR, Cox DW, Smith DC: Use of human menopausal gonadotropin for the induction of ovulation. Am J Obstet Gynecol 120:988, 1974
34. March CM, Davajan V, Mishell DR: Ovulation induction in amenorrheic women. Obstet Gynecol 53:8, 1979
35. Midgley AR, Jaffe RB: Regulation of human gonadotropins. X. Episodic fluctuation of LH during the menstrual cycle. J Clin Endocrinol Metab 33:962, 1971
36. Yen SSC, Tsai CC, Naftolin F, Vandenberg G, Ajabor L: Pulsatile pattern of gonadotropin release in subjects with and without ovarian function. J Clin Endocrinol Metab 34:671, 1972

37. Plant TM, Krey LC, Moossy J, McCormack JT, Hess DL, Knobil E: The arcuate nucleus and the control of gonadotropin and prolactin secretion in the female Rhesus monkey (*Macaca mulatta*). Endocrinology 102:52, 1978
38. Nakai Y, Plant TM, Hess DL, Keogh EJ, Knobil E: On the sites of negative and positive feedback actions of estradiol in the control of gonadotropin secretion in the Rhesus monkey. Endocrinology 102:1008, 1978
39. Belchetz PE, Plant TM, Nakai Y, Keogh EJ, Knobil E: Hypophysial responses to continuous and intermittent delivery of hypothalamic gonadotropin releasing hormone. Science 202:631, 1978
40. Knobil E, Plant TM, Wildt L, Belchetz PE, Marshall G: Control of the Rhesus monkey menstrual cycle: permissive role of hypothalamic gonadotropin releasing hormone. Science 207:1371, 1980
41. Yen SSC, Vela P, Rankin J: Inappropriate secretion of follicle stimulating hormone and luteinizing hormone in polycystic ovarian disease. J Clin Endocrinol Metab 30:435, 1970
42. Rebar R, Judd HL, Yen SSC, Rakoff J, Vandenberg G, Naftolin F: Characterization of the inappropriate gonadotropin secretion in polycystic ovary syndrome. J Clin Invest 57:1320, 1976
43. Soules MR, Steiner RA, Clifton DK, Cohen NL, Aksel S, Bremner WJ: Progesterone modulation of pulsatile luteinizing hormone secretion in normal women. J Clin Endocrinol Metab 58:378, 1984
44. Reame N, Sauder SE, Kelch RP, Marshall JC: Pulsatile gonadotropin secretion during the human menstrual cycle: evidence for altered frequency of gonadotropin-releasing hormone secretion. J Clin Endocrinol Metab 59:328, 1984
45. Hsueh AJ, Erickson GF: Extrapituitary action of gonadotropin-releasing hormone: direct inhibition of ovarian steroidogenesis. Science 204:854, 1979
46. Clayton RN, Harwood JP, Catt KJ: Gonadotropin-releasing hormone analogue binds to luteal cells and inhibits progesterone production. Nature 282:90, 1979
47. Hsueh AJ, Adashi EY, Jones PBC, Welsh TH: Hormonal regulation of the differentiation of cultured ovarian granulosa cells. Endocr Rev 5:76, 1984
48. Eisenberg E, Kitai H, Kobayashi Y, Santulli R, Wallach EE: Gonadotropin releasing hormone: effects on the in vitro perfused rabbit ovary. Biol Reprod 30:1216, 1984
49. Asch RH, VanSickle M, Rettori V, Balmaceda JP, Eddy CA, Coy DH, Schally AV: Absence of LH-RH binding sites in corpora lutea from Rhesus monkeys (*Macaca mulatta*). J Clin Endocrinol Metab 53:215, 1981
50. Clayton RN, Huhtaniemi IT: Absence of gonadotropin-releasing hormone receptors in human ovarian tissue. Nature 299:56, 1982
51. Brown JL, Reeves JJ: Absence of specific luteinizing hormone-releasing hormone receptors in ovine, bovine and porcine ovaries. Biol Reprod 29:1179, 1983
52. Casper RF, Erickson GF, Rebar RW, Yen SSC: The effect of luteinizing hormone-releasing factor and its agonist on cultured human granulosa cells. Fertil Steril 37:406, 1982
53. Tureck RW, Mastroianni L, Blasco L, Strauss JF: Inhibition of human granulosa cell progesterone secretion by a gonadotropin releasing hormone agonist. J Clin Endocrinol Metab 54:1078, 1982
54. Casper RF, Erickson GF, Yen SSC: Studies on the effect of gonadotropin-releasing hormone and its agonist on human luteal steroidogenesis in vitro. Fertil Steril 42:39, 1984
55. Handelsman DJ, Jansen RPS, Boylan LM, Spaliviero JA, Turtle JR: Pharmacokinetics of gonadotropin releasing hormone: comparison of subcutaneous and intravenous routes. J Clin Endocrinol Metab 59:739, 1984
56. Mishell DR: Selection and pretreatment evaluation of patients treated with human menopausal gonadotropins. J Reprod Med (Suppl 3) 21:191, 1978
57. Schwartz M, Jewelewicz R: The use of gonadotropins for induction of ovulation. Fertil Steril 35:3, 1981
58. Rust LA, Israel R, Mishell DR: An individualized graduated therapeutic regime for clomiphene citrate. Am J Obstet Gynecol 120:785, 1974
59. Edwards RG, Steptoe PC, Purdy JM: Establishing full term human pregnancies using cleaving embryos grown in vitro. Br J Obstet Gynaecol 87:737, 1980
60. Schally AV, Schally AMC, Kastin AJ: Present status of the use of LH-RH and its analogs in the diagnosis and therapy of infertility. In The LH-Releasing Hormone, Edited by CG Beling, AC Wentz. New York, Masson, 1980, p 1
61. Mortimer CH, Besser GM, McNeilly AS, Marshall JC, Harsoulis P, Tunbridge WMG, Gomez-Pan A, Hall R: LH/FSH-RH test in patients with hypothalamic pituitary gonadal dysfunction. Br Med J 4:73, 1973
62. Leyendecker G, Struve T, Nocke W, Hansmann M: The permissive role of Gn-RH in the regulation of the human menstrual cycle: pathophysiologic aspects and therapeutic consequences. Acta Endocrinol [Suppl 234] (Copenh) 94:157, 1980
63. Hashimoto T, Miyai K, Vozumi T, Mori S, Watanabe M, Kumahara Y: Effect of prolonged LH-releasing hormone administration on gonadotropin response in patients with hypothalamic and pituitary tumors. J Clin Endocrinol Metab 41:721, 1975
64. London DR, Butt WR, Lynch SS, Marshall JC, Owvsu S, Robinson WR, Stephenson JM: Hormonal responses to intranasal luteinizing hormone releasing hormone. J Clin Endocrinol Metab 37:829, 1973
65. Gonzalo-Barcena D, Kastin AJ, Schalch DS, Bermudez JA, Lee D, Arimura A, Ruelas J, Zepeda J, Schally AV: Synthetic LH-releasing hormone (LH-RH) administered to normal men by different routes. J Clin Endocrinol Metab 37:481, 1973
66. Rebar R, Yen SSC, Vandenberg G: Gonadotropin responses to synthetic LRF: dose response relationship in men. J Clin Endocrinol Metab 36:10, 1973
67. Newton J, Collins W, Kilpatrick M, Pyke J: Studies on synthetic LH/FSH releasing hormone. J Reprod Fertil 35:622, 1973
68. Huseman CA, Kelch RP: Gonadotropin responses and metabolism of synthetic gonadotropin-releasing hormone (GnRH) during constant infusion of GnRH in men and boys with delayed adolescence. J Clin Endocrinol Metab 47:1325, 1978
69. Marshall JC, Kelch RP: Low dose pulsatile gonadotropin releasing hormone in anorexia nervosa: a model of human pubertal development. J Clin Endocrinol Metab 49:712, 1979

70. Valk TW, Corley KP, Kelch RP, Marshall JC: Hypogonadotropic hypogonadism: hormonal responses to low dose pulsatile administration of gonadotropin-releasing hormone. J Clin Endocrinol Metab 51:730, 1980
71. Yen SSC, Vandenberg G, Rebar R, Ehara Y: Variation of pituitary responsiveness to synthetic LRF during different phases of the menstrual cycle. J Clin Endocrinol Metab 35:931, 1972
72. Crowley WF, McArthur JW: Stimulation of the normal menstrual cycle in Kallman's syndrome by pulsatile administration of luteinizing hormone-releasing hormone (LH-RH). J Clin Endocrinol Metab 51:173, 1980
73. Molloy BG, Hancock KW, Glass MR: Ovulation induction in clomiphene nonresponsive patients: the place of pulsatile gonadotropin-releasing hormone in clinical practice. Fertil Steril 43:26, 1985
74. Goerzen J, Corenblum B, Wiseman DA, Taylor PJ: Ovulation induction and pregnancy in hypothalamic amenorrhea using self-administered intravenous gonadotropin-releasing hormone. Fertil Steril 41:319, 1984
75. Leyendecker G, Wildt L, Hansmann M: Pregnancies following chronic intermittent (pulsatile) administration of GnRH by means of a portable pump ("Zyklomat"): a new approach to the treatment of infertility in hypothalamic amenorrhea. J Clin Endocrinol Metab 51:1214, 1980
76. Schoemaker J, Simons AHM, van Osnabrugge GJC, Lugtenburg C, van Kessel H: Pregnancy after prolonged pulsatile administration of luteinizing hormone-releasing hormone in a patient with clomiphene-resistant secondary amenorrhea. J Clin Endocrinol Metab 52:882, 1981
77. Loucopoulos A, Ferin M, Vande Wiele RL, Dyrenfurth I, Linkie D, Yeh M, Jewelewicz R: Pulsatile administration of gonadotropin-releasing hormone for induction of ovulation. Am J Obstet Gynecol 148:895, 1984
78. Miller DS, Reid RR, Cetel NS, Rebar RW, Yen SSC: Pulsatile administration of low-dose gonadotropin releasing hormone. JAMA 250:2937, 1983
79. Reid RL, Sauerbrei E: Evaluation of techniques for induction of ovulation in outpatients employing pulsatile gonadotropin releasing hormone. Am J Obstet Gynecol 148:648, 1984
80. Reid RL, Leopold GR, Yen SSC: Induction of ovulation and pregnancy with pulsatile luteinizing hormone releasing factor: dosage and mode of delivery. Fertil Steril 36:553, 1981
81. Seibel MM, Kamrava M, McArdle C, Taymor M: Ovulation induction and conception using subcutaneous pulsatile luteinizing hormone-releasing hormone. Obstet Gynecol 61:292, 1983
82. Hurley DM, Brian RJ, Burger HG: Ovulation induction with subcutaneous pulsatile gonadotropin-releasing hormone: singleton pregnancies in patients with previous multiple pregnancies after gonadotropin therapy. Fertil Steril 40:575, 1983
83. Skarin G, Nillius SJ, Wide L: Pulsatile subcutaneous low-dose gonadotropin-releasing hormone treatment of anovulatory infertility. Fertil Steril 40:454, 1983
84. Hurley DM, Brian R, Outch K, Stockdale J, Fry A, Hackman C, Clarke I, Burger HG: Induction of ovulation and fertility in amenorrheic women by pulsatile low-dose gonadotropin-releasing hormone. N Engl J Med 310:1069, 1984
85. Woodhouse NJJ, Niles N, Othman HO: Hypothalamic hypogonadism: induction of ovulation and pregnancy by subcutaneous pulsatile injections of gonadotropin releasing hormone. Horm Res 20:172, 1984
86. Mason P, Adams J, Morris DV, Tucker M, Price J, Voulgaris Z, Vander Spuy ZM, Sutherland I, Chambers GR, White S, Wheeler MJ, Jacobs HS: Induction of ovulation with pulsatile luteinizing hormone-releasing hormone. Br Med J 288:181, 1984
87. Sopelak VM, Williams RF, Aso T, Marut EL, Hodgen GD: A mechanical hypothalamus for ovulation induction therapy. JAMA 251:1477, 1984
88. Leyendecker G, Struve J, Plotz EJ: Induction of ovulation with chronic intermittent (pulsatile) administration of LH-RH in women with hypothalamic and hyperprolactinemic amenorrhea. Arch Gynecol 229:177, 1980
89. Ory SJ, London SN, Tyrey L, Hammond CB: Ovulation induction with pulsatile gonadotropin-releasing hormone administration in patients with polycystic ovarian syndrome. Fertil Steril 43:20, 1985
90. Burger CW, van Kessel H, Schoemaker J: Induction of ovulation by prolonged pulsatile administration of luteinizing hormone releasing hormone (LRH) in patients with clomiphene resistant polycystic ovary-like disease. Acta Endocrinol (Copenh) 104:357, 1983
91. Richard DW, Goldsmith LT, Pohl CR, Schallenberger E, Knobil E: The role of prolactin in the regulation of the private corpus luteum. J Clin Endocrinol Metab 60:501, 1985
92. Vande Wiele RL, Bogumil J, Dyrenfurth I, Ferin M, Jewelewicz R, Warren M, Rizkallah T, Mikhail G: Mechanisms regulating the menstrual cycle in women. Recent Prog Horm Res 26:63, 1970
93. Asch RH, Moustapha A-S, Braunstein G, Pauerstein CJ: Luteal function in hypophysectomized rhesus monkeys. J Clin Endocrinol Metab 55:154, 1982
94. Channing CP: Influences of the in vivo and in vitro hormonal environment upon luteinization of granulosa cells in tissue culture. Recent Prog Horm Res 26:589, 1970
95. Hutchison JS, Zeleznik AJ: The rhesus monkey corpus luteum is dependent on pituitary gonadotropin secretion throughout the luteal phase of the menstrual cycle. Endocrinology 115:1780, 1984
96. Groff TR, Raj HGM, Talbert LM, Willis DL: Effects of neutralization of luteinizing hormone on corpus luteum function and cyclicity in *Macaca fascicularis*. J Clin Endocrinol Metab 59:1054, 1984
97. Weinstein FG, Seibel MM, Taymor ML: Ovulation induction with subcutaneous pulsatile gonadotropin-releasing hormone: the role of supplemental human chorionic gonadotropin in the luteal phase. Fertil Steril 41:546, 1984
98. Nillius SJ, Wide L: Gonadotropin-releasing hormone treatment for induction of follicular maturation and ovulation in amenorrheic women with anorexia nervosa. Br Med J 3:405, 1975
99. Nillius SJ, Fries H, Wide L: Successful induction of follicular maturation and ovulation by prolonged treatment with LH-releasing hormone in women with anorexia nervosa. Am J Obstet Gynecol 122:921, 1975
100. Casas PRF, Badano AR, Aparicio N, Lencioni LJ, Berli RR, Badano H, Biccoca C, Schally AV: Luteinizing hormone-releasing hormone in the treatment of anovulatory infertility. Fertil Steril 26:549, 1975

101. Sheehan KL, Casper RF, Yen SSC: Luteal phase defect induced by an agonist of luteinizing hormone-releasing factor: a model for fertility control. Science 215:170, 1982
102. Casper RF, Yen SSC: Induction of luteolysis in the human with a long acting analog of luteinizing hormone-releasing factor. Science 205:408, 1979
103. Lemay A, Labrie F, Ferland L, Raynaud J-P: Possible luteolytic effects of luteinizing hormone-releasing hormone in normal women. Fertil Steril 31:29, 1979
104. Caldwell BV, Rotchell YE, Pang CY, Anderson CG, Kase N, Behrman HR: Comparative study of high-dose chorionic gonadotropin on the human and rat corpus luteum and effect of gonadotropin-releasing hormone on human luteal function. Am J Obstet Gynecol 136:458, 1980
105. Monroe SE, Henzl MR, Martin MC, Schriock E, Lewis V, Nerenberg C, Jaffe RB: Ablation of folliculogenesis in women by a single dose of gonadotropin-releasing hormone agonist: significance of time in cycle. Fertil Steril 43:361, 1985
106. Reindollar RH, Moretuzzo RW, Ellegood JO, Mahesh VB, McDonough PG: The effects of single-dose luteinizing hormone-releasing hormone on ovulatory menstrual function: support for a single luteinizing hormone- and follicle-stimulating hormone-releasing factor. Fertil Steril 43:185, 1985
107. Berger NG, Zacur HA: Exogenous progesterone for luteal support following gonadotropin-releasing hormone ovulation induction: case report. Fertil Steril 44:133, 1985
108. Rabau E, David A, Serr DM, Mashiach S, Lunenfeld B: Human menopausal gonadotropins for anovulation and sterility. Am J Obstet Gynecol 98:92, 1967
109. Schenker JG, Weinstein D: Ovarian hyperstimulation syndrome: a current survey. Fertil Steril 30:255, 1978
110. Kistner RW: Induction of ovulation with clomiphene citrate. In Progress in Infertility, Edited by SJ Behrman, RW Kistner. Boston, Little, Brown & Co., 1975, p 509
111. Skarin G, Nillius SJ, Wide L: Pulsatile low dose luteinizing hormone releasing hormone treatment for ovulation induction of follicular maturation and ovulation in women with amenorrhea. Acta Endocrinol (Copenh) 101:78, 1982
112. Lorcy Y, Bohec M, Allannic H: Hyperstimulation ovarienne induite par l'administration pulsatile de gonadoliberine. Presse Med 41:2517, 1984
113. Liu JH, Durfee R, Muse K, Yen SSC: Induction of multiple ovulation by pulsatile administration of gonadotropin-releasing hormone. Fertil Steril 40:18, 1983
114. Boghelmann D, Lappöhn RE, Janssens J: Triplet pregnancy after pulsatile administration of gonadotropin releasing hormone. Lancet 2:45, 1982
115. Heineman MJ, Bouckaert PXJM, Schellekens LA: A quadruplet pregnancy following ovulation induction with pulsatile luteinizing hormone-releasing hormone. Fertil Steril 42:300, 1984
116. Gysler M, March CM, Mishell DR Jr, Bailey EJ: A decade's experience with an individualized clomiphene treatment regimen including its effects on the postcoital test. Fertil Steril 37:161, 1982
117. Hack M, Brish M, Serr DM, Insler V, Salomy M, Lunenfeld B: Outcome of pregnancy after induced ovulation: follow-up of pregnancies and children born after clomiphene therapy. JAMA 220:1329, 1972
118. Van Loon CR, Brown GM: Secondary drug failure occurring during chronic treatment with LH-RH: appearance of an antibody. J Clin Endocrinol Metab 41:640, 1975
119. Lindner J, McNeil LW, Marney S, Conway M, Rivier J, Vale W, Rabin D: Characterization of human anti-luteinizing hormone-releasing hormone (LRH) antibodies in the serum of a patient with isolated gonadotropin deficiency treated with synthetic LRH. J Clin Endocrinol Metab 52:267, 1981
120. Chappel SC, Ellinwood WE, Huckins C, Hubert DC, Spies HG: Active immunization of male rhesus monkeys against luteinizing hormone releasing hormone. Biol Reprod 22:333, 1980
121. Fraser HM, Sandow J, Krauss B: Antibody production against an agonist analogue of luteinizing hormone-releasing hormone: evaluation of immunological and physiological consequences. Acta Endocrinol (Copenh) 103:151, 1983
122. Meakin JL, Keogh EJ, Martin CE: Human anti-luteinizing hormone-releasing hormone antibodies in patients treated with synthetic luteinizing hormone-releasing hormone. Fertil Steril 43:811, 1985
123. Meldrum DR, Chang RJ, Lu J, Vale W, Rivier J, Judd HL: "Medical oophorectomy" using a long-acting GnRH agonist—a possible new approach to the treatment of endometriosis. J Clin Endocrinol Metab 54:1081, 1982
124. Maheux R, Guilloteau C, Lemay A, Bastide A, Fazekas ATA: Regression of leiomyomata uteri following hypoestrogenism induced by repetitive luteinizing hormone-releasing hormone agonist treatment: preliminary report. Fertil Steril 42:644, 1984
125. Comite G, Cutter GB, Rivier J, Vale WW, Loriaux DL, Crowley WF: Short-term treatment of idiopathic precocious puberty with a long-acting analogue of luteinizing hormone-releasing hormone: a preliminary report. N Engl J Med 305:1546, 1981
126. Warner B, Worgul TJ, Drago J, Demers L, Dufau M, Max D, Santen RJ: Effect of very high dose D-Lev(6) GnRH proethylamide on the hypothalamic-pituitary testicular axis in patients with prostate cancer. J Clin Invest 71:1842, 1983

Chapter 13

Diagnosis and management of prolactinomas

Richard E. Blackwell, Ph.D., M.D.

Department of Obstetrics and Gynecology, Division of Reproductive Biology and Endocrinology, University of Alabama in Birmingham Medical Center, Birmingham, Alabama

HISTORICAL MILESTONES

Although the contemporary history of prolactinomas causing galactorrhea and/or menstrual irregularities has its origins in the early 1970s, observations as early as the mid 1800s predicted this association. Chiari et al.,[1] in 1855, reported two cases of puerperal atrophy of the uterus with amenorrhea and persistent lactation. This syndrome was redescribed by Frommel in 1882.[2] Subsequently, two papers were presented by Argonz and DelCastillo[3] and Ahumada and DelCastillo[4] describing a syndrome characterized by estrogen insufficiency, galactorrhea, and decreased urinary estrogens. Finally Forbes, working in Albright's laboratory, described a syndrome characterized by galactorrhea, amenorrhea, and low urinary follicle-stimulating hormone (FSH). These observations, made around 1954, first suggested the association between galactorrhea and the presence of pituitary tumors. However, it should be noted that in the original observations of Forbes and associates, the incidence of pituitary tumor was approximately 25%.[5] At the same time the association of galactorrhea and amenorrhea with prolactinomas was being established, Costello[6] evaluated 1000 unselected pituitary glands obtained at autopsy. He found a remarkable incidence of 25% of pituitary adenomas, the frequency being 60% for men and 40% for women. Despite these clinical observations, three events would have to occur before we gained a contemporary view of prolactinoma physiology. The first of these came in the 1950s and 1960s when Greenwood and Hunter[7] described the techniques for the iodination of protein molecules. This was accompanied by the establishment of the principles of radioimmunoassay (RIA) by Berson and co-authors,[8] which allowed us to measure small amounts of hormone in serum and urine. Also during this time, new-generation radiographic techniques were being established which would allow us to study soft tissue masses more efficiently than with traditional x-rays. Of equal importance was the separation of human prolactin (PRL) from growth hormone (GH) and the development of RIA techniques for the measurement of human PRL.[9-11]

Utilizing these historical clinical observations and new technology, we now know that prolactinomas occur with great frequency in the population and that they are associated not only with galactorrhea but with many disorders of ovulation and infertility. Therefore, it is the purpose of this review to present a summary of the contemporary view of the diagnosis and treatment of pituitary prolactinomas.

CLINICAL PRESENTATION

The prolactinoma presents most frequently with galactorrhea or disorders of ovulation. The galactorrhea may be unilateral or bilateral, continuous or intermittent, free-flowing or expressible. However, it should be pointed out that we have observed a number of patients, particularly those in the late teenage years, who will present with PRL levels of 2000 to 3000 ng/ml accompanied by amenorrhea with no galactorrhea. Although prolactinomas are frequently associated with severe ovulatory disorders such as amenorrhea, anovulation, and oligoovulation, recent observations have suggested that luteal phase defects and disorders of folliculogenesis may be associated with hyperprolactinemia 20% to 30% of the time.[12-14] As with all central nervous system tumors, headache is a common presentation of the prolactinoma. This is usually a frontal type, which patients describe as "penetrating" behind the eyes. Although one would expect that visual disturbances might be noted with great frequency, suprasellar extension is necessary for this event to occur. Many patients with large adenomas, however, will not show visual alterations. This feature might be explained by the fact that these tumors are frequently not spherical and might choose to grow along paths of least resistance. Although the prolactinoma is found most frequently in adults, it should be remembered that primary amenorrhea and delayed pubescence may be associated with prolactinomas. These will frequently be large lesions that may be described as invasive by histologic type. It should be noted that children with prolactinomas may or may not lactate, lactation being dependent upon the stage of development and the onset of tumor growth. Finally, the prolactinoma may present as a component of a polyendocrinopathy such as galactorrhea and accompanying acromegaly.

CLINICAL PATHOLOGY

Although pituitary adenomas have classically been estimated to account for 10% of intracranial tumors, it has become evident that they occur with much greater frequency. It has recently been estimated that 30% of such central nervous system tumors are of the adenoma type, the prolactinoma being the most frequent. Next in frequency is the GH-secreting adenoma, followed by lesions which produce adrenocorticotropic hormone, melanocyte-stimulating hormone, gonadotropins, or thyroid-stimulating hormone (TSH).[15] This should be expected when one considers that the galactotropes make up approximately one third of the functional cells of the pituitary gland. Because of the bilateral nature of the pituitary gland and the fact that these cells are located in the lateral wings, the lesion may expand centrally or laterally. In terms of classic histochemistry, 70% of adenomas are of the chromophobic type. The remainder would be labeled eosinophilic or mixed type by hematoxylin and eosin staining. Calcification can be seen in the pituitary adenoma, but this is a rare finding. Areas of infarction may also be seen.[16] At the electron-microscopic level, the normal PRL-producing cell is heavily granulated, as opposed to the more common form of prolactinoma cell,[17] which is sparsely granulated. However, it should be noted that there are variants which have dense granules and resemble the resting lactotrope. A distinctive feature of adenomatous cells is the large oval size and pleomorphic electron-dense secretory granules. It should be noted that pituitary tumors present with various histologic types, some of which may mimic malignant lesions such as the meningioma or malignant lymphoma. Pituitary adenomas seem to be divided into two gross morphologic types: One involves an expansile-compressive type of lesion which is usually well encapsulated. The other has been described as an invasive adenoma with extensive capsular penetration and involvement of the dura, sinus, and bone. Although bone erosion occurs with an expansile lesion, this feature is thought to be due to a compression phenomenon; the invasive lesion is actually thought to destroy bone. However, one should note that the strict diagnostic criteria applied to malignancy, that is, cellular pleomorphism, mitotic activity, and nuclear atypia, frequently do not apply in these lesions. Furthermore, most of these lesions are not autonomous and respond to therapy with dopamine agonists. This characteristic raises the question that perhaps pituitary adenomas of all types may be variants of hyperplasia, because rarely are microadenomas, macroadenomas, or invasive adenomas considered to be autonomous lesions. It has been estimated that approximately 10% of pituitary adenomas are of the invasive type; despite their infrequency, they tend to occur in a younger age group. They will frequently infiltrate the cavernous sinus and extend along dural planes. Cranial neuropathies and facial neuralgia are among the early presenting symptoms. Such a presentation again is reminiscent of the meningioma, which can dissect along the dural planes.

The origin of prolactinomas is unclear. It has been suggested that these tumors arise secondary to a neurotransmitter defect[18-20] which presumably results in a decreased central suppression of PRL secretion. Such a theory is appealing when one considers the high failure rate following surgical treatment of adenomas, and suggests that perhaps this may be a multifocal disease. Despite our lack of understanding of the origin of these lesions, their natural history has been well described. They present clinically most frequently in women 20 to 40 years of age and decrease in frequency in later life. The microadenomas tend to be slow growing and follow a much more benign course than the larger invasive lesions, which tend to occur in a younger age group and can expand rapidly.

EVALUATION OF PROLACTINOMAS

The patient who presents with galactorrhea and/or menstrual disturbance should be evaluated with a screening serum PRL level. If this value is elevated, a second and/or third sample should be obtained to demonstrate the presence of disease. Elevations in serum PRL levels are frequently found on first office visits, and it should be remembered that many physiologic events trigger the release of this hormone. This is a volatile hormone, and its release may be stimulated by stress,[21, 22] food intake,[23-25] and physical examination. It should also be remembered that PRL has a sleep-entrained secretory pattern and that samples obtained early in the morning may give a false impression of the presence of disease.[26]

Serum PRL was originally measured by the pigeon crop-sac bioassay.[27] However, now it is uniformly evaluated by RIA. The definition of hyperprolactinemia varies from laboratory to laboratory, but to qualify as hyperprolactinemia, levels generally fall outside the range of 5 to 30 ng/ml. The most common reference standards used to measure PRL are National Institutes of Health (NIH) VLS-2 and World Health Organization First International Reference Preparation (WHO 1st IRP) 75/504. These standards can be converted by the following formula: 1 ng NIH VLS-2 = 20 μU/ml WHO IRP 71/222 or WHO 1st IRP 75/504; 1 μU WHO IRP 71/222 = 1 μU WHO 1st IRP 75/504.

If multiple serum PRL determinations are found to be elevated, thyroxine and TSH should be measured to rule out compensated hypothyroidism. Here one may find low-normal thyroxine and markedly elevated TSH levels. This may be accompanied by pituitary hyperplasia, mimicking the presence of a prolactinoma. Since thyrotropin-releasing factor (TRF) stimulates the secretion of both TSH and PRL,[28, 29] treatment of these patients with Synthroid (Flint Laboratories, Deerfield, IL) will result in a resolution of both hyperprolactinemia and pituitary hyperplasia. Compensated hypothyroidism may also present with visual defects, further confusing the presentation with that of a prolactinoma.[30] Therefore, it is to be emphasized that although rare, this disorder should be accurately diagnosed with a TSH measurement to prevent inappropriate treatment with a dopamine agonist and/or pituitary exploration.

Although historically important, the visual-field examination using Goldmann-Bowl perimetry has proven to be less useful than originally anticipated. Intrasellar lesions of both macroadenoma and microadenoma classifications do not produce alterations in visual fields. One must have suprasellar extension to cause chiasmatic compression. Suprasellar adenomas present with some alteration in the visual field 68% of the time.[31] Twenty-five percent of these present with superior bitemporal hemianopsia and 16% with classic bitemporal hemianopsia (Fig. 1). Therefore, visual-field examinations are useful only in the diagnosis of suprasellar adenomas; however, they may be an effective, noninvasive way of following tumor therapy.

Traditionally, anterior-posterior and lateral plane films of the sella turcica and cone views of this area were used to diagnose large pituitary adenomas. To be detected by these techniques, the lesion had to attain a size of 10 mm (macroadenoma). Although these techniques are not useful for the diagnosis of microadenomas and some minimal sized macroadenomas, they are simple, cost-effective methods for the diagnosis of larger tumors. Sellar tomography both of the linear and hypocycloidal variety once enjoyed a place in the evaluation of patients with hyperprolactinemia. Unfortunately, a number of studies have shown that there is great variation in sellar

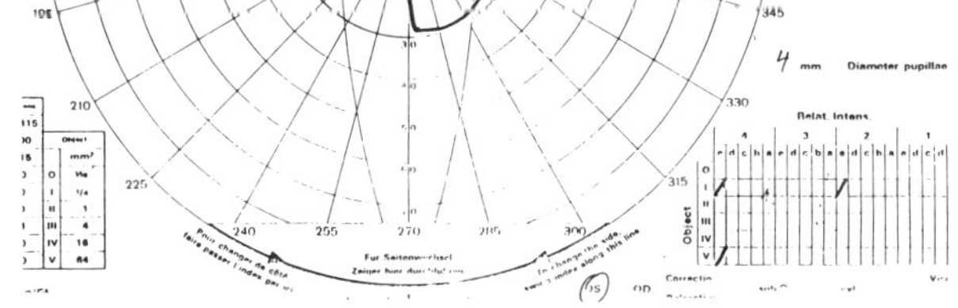

Figure 1
Visual-field deficit in a patient with a large prolactinoma. The patient lost total vision in the opposite eye.

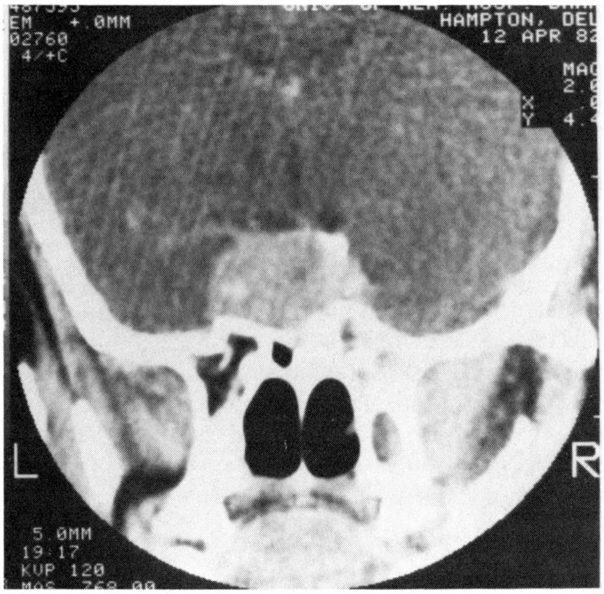

Figure 2
CAT scan of a patient with a large suprasellar macroadenoma.

architecture, resulting in a high incidence of false-positive interpretation of these studies.[32-34] It should also be remembered that sellar tomography is most effective in detecting bone erosion or invasion. Because the adenoma is a soft-tissue tumor, it may or may not involve bone compression. New-generation computed axial tomography (CAT) with metrizamide enhancement is probably the state-of-the-art technique for evaluating soft-tissue tumors[35, 36] (Fig. 2). It is sensitive enough to detect small microadenomas and, in the hands of a skilled neuroradiologist, pituitary hyperplasia. These instruments can easily measure a lesion 2 mm in diameter, which makes them effective in the diagnosis of both microadenomas and macroadenomas. Although the radiation exposure with CAT has been estimated to be nine times less than that of sella tomography, there is considerable controversy about this point. A complete study, in fact, may result in fairly equal radiation exposure, because more films are generally taken with the CAT technique. Carotid arteriography with subtraction magnification techniques was used as a diagnostic tool in the past.[37] However, its role seems to be diminished with the advent of CAT. It should be noted that carotid arteriography remains a potent tool when used prior to neurosurgical exploration of the sella to delineate critical landmarks such as the carotid arteries and possible aneurysms. The role of nuclear magnetic resonance in the diagnosis of prolactinomas remains unclear at present. This technique produces delineation of central nervous system landmarks without the side effect of radiation exposure. Whether this technique will prove superior to CAT remains to be determined.

The choice of radiologic studies is still controversial. There is some tendency to revert back to older, less complicated techniques such as the cone view of the sella turcica for initial study. There is perhaps some merit to this reevaluation, because review of the literature shows that serum PRL levels are often directly related to tumor size.[38-40] In general, if one finds a serum PRL level in the vicinity of 50 ng/ml, the incidence of detecting a microadenoma is approximately 25%. If a level of 100 ng/ml is detected, that incidence increases to nearly 50%. With a level of 200 to 300 ng/ml, there is almost a 100% incidence of finding a pituitary tumor either at the time of sellar exploration or with various radiologic studies. It could be argued that more sophisticated technology could be used for patients with markedly elevated serum PRL levels, perhaps 200 ng/ml. It should be pointed out, however, that in a number of series, a normal PRL level has been found in the patients with prolactinomas. It has been suggested that as the tumor expands, there is compression and necrosis of tissue, and the PRL level often falls in the face of a rapidly expanding lesion. In general, it is suggested that fourth-generation CAT be used as an initial study for all patients with hyperprolactinemia other than those harboring signs of androgen excess. It is believed that it is advantageous to have adequate baseline studies using state-of-the-art technology, particularly for the patient who contemplates pregnancy.

Following the isolation, structure, and synthesis of the hypothalamic-releasing factor, TRF, and luteinizing hormone-releasing factor (LRF), it was hoped that these neuropeptides could be used in the diagnosis of pituitary tumors.[41] TRF has been shown to release both TSH and PRL in vivo and in vitro, and LRF was shown to release both FSH and luteinizing hormone (LH).[42] These two tests, combined with the release of GH and cortisol following the induction of insulin hypoglycemia and the stimulation of GH and suppression of PRL following levodopa (L-Dopa; Roche Laboratories, Nutley, NJ) administration, allowed investigators to selectively test the secretory dynamics of important pituitary trophic hormones.[43] It was found that in the presence of a pituitary tumor the response of PRL to TRF stimulation was blunted, that there was an inhibition in the rate of rise of GH following the induction of insulin-induced hypoglycemia, failure of L-Dopa to inhibit PRL release in patients with these lesions, and both augmentation and suppression of the release of LH and FSH following LRF stimulation.[44-47] These tests can be performed individually, or LRF, TRF, and insulin can be administered simultaneously,[48] because there does not seem to be interaction that affects acute release of LH, FSH, TSH, PRL, cortisol, and GH. Although these differences have been described previously, the tests cannot be practically used to differentiate the presence of a prolactinoma from functional hyperprolactinemia.[49, 50] They appear to be useful only in the evaluation of residual pituitary function in the presence of large prolactinomas or in assessing the completion of neurosurgical resection of such lesions.[51, 52] If they are to be employed at all, it is suggested that they be performed on an outpatient basis with simultaneous multiple trophic stimulation.

TREATMENT OF PROLACTINOMAS

The prolactinoma may be treated by medical, surgical, or radiation therapy. Historically, primary surgical therapy was restricted to those individuals with adenomas, presenting with headache and/or visual field impairment. Surgery for smaller lesions was frequently used if fertility was desired. At first, surgical therapy was used aggressively, because no measure existed to estimate the rate of growth of the tumor, and it was unknown whether microadenomas gave rise to macroadenomas and invasive lesions. Unfortunately, these questions still remain unanswered; however, it is believed that most microadenomas grow at an extremely slow rate, and no clear-cut correlation has been found indicating that a microadenoma may become an invasive lesion. The hyperprolactinemia that accompanies prolactinomas was believed to be benign, and aggressive treatment was not recommended. Although it was known that women with hyperprolactinemia are frequently hypoestrogenic, agreement could not be reached as to whether these patients should be followed by observation, treated with low-dose estrogen replacement, or treated with dopamine agonists. In the early 1980s observations began to appear suggesting that hyperprolactinemia is associated with decreased bone density. Recently, Schlechte et al.[53] showed that hyperprolactinemia resulted in a decrease in bone density independent from the hypoestrogenic state. These investigators measured bone/mineral content of the radius by photon absorptiometry. Several groups of patients were evaluated in these studies: control subjects, women with amenorrhea and normal PRL levels, and women with PRL-secreting pituitary adenomas. These women did not differ in any parameter, including serum calcium, phosphorus, gonadotropin, testosterone, vitamin D, or parathyroid hormone concentration. The women with amenorrhea and normal serum PRL levels did not differ significantly from control subjects; however, patients with PRL-secreting pituitary adenomas studied 2 to 5 years after transsphenoidal surgery had a significant decrease in bone/mineral content whether they were cured or had persistent amenorrhea or persistent hyperprolactinemia. There was no difference in serum estradiol concentrations among the groups. If this observation is confirmed, it may indicate that women with hyperprolactinemia secondary to functional alterations or a prolactinoma might benefit from being rendered euprolactinemic permanently.

Historically, several drugs were used to treat hyperprolactinemia, including vitamin B_6, the cofactor involved in the metabolism of L-Dopa to dopamine, and L-Dopa. Several drugs are currently available for the treatment of prolactinomas. Although none are approved by the Food and Drug Administration for this purpose, two of these have been shown to be effective in the primary management of both microadenomas and macroadenomas. The drugs include Parlodel (Sandoz Pharmaceuticals, East Hanover, NJ), Pergolide (Eli Lilly & Company, Indianapolis, IN), and CU-32-085 (Sandoz) (Fig. 3). Each of these drugs is a dopamine agonist which acts at the level of the pituitary gland to inhibit PRL secretion by occupying the dopaminergic receptors.[54] Dopamine receptor blocking drugs such as metoclopramide and haloperidol antagonize the PRL-releasing inhibiting activity of dopamine agonists. Bromocriptine has been estimated in rat pituitary cell culture to be 13 times as potent as dopamine, with a slower onset of action.[55] It is metabolized in the liver and kidney, and has been found to suppress both the synthesis and secretion of PRL. Its therapeutic dose range is described as 2.5 mg twice daily to 2.5 mg four times daily in the treatment of patients with hyperpro-

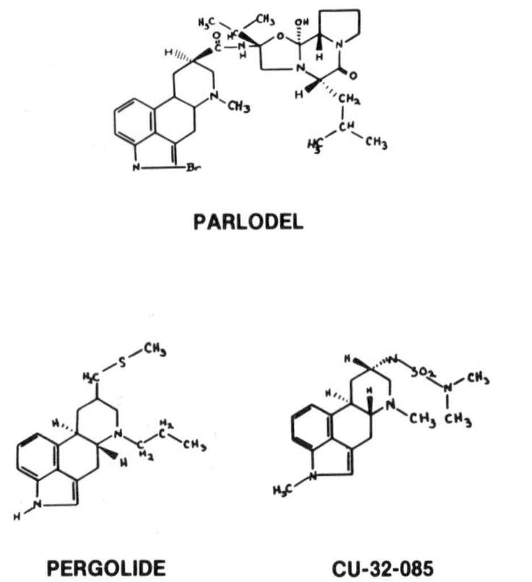

Figure 3
Structural comparison of Parlodel, Pergolide mesylate, and CU-32-085.

lactinemia. However, doses up to 80 mg/day are used in patients with Parkinson's disease. It should be noted that patients with both functional hyperprolactinemia and microadenomas and macroadenomas frequently respond to a subtherapeutic dose of Parlodel. Patients may respond to as little as 1.25 mg twice daily (Fig. 4). Also, patients whose prolactinomas have regressed to a nondetectable state by radiologic survey may be maintained on a reduced dose for long time periods. Therefore, as has recently been suggested by Soto-Albors and associates,[56] patients with various hyperprolactinemia syndromes should receive Parlodel in doses that titrate for the desired effect. It is suggested that patients be given 1.25 mg twice daily for 1 week, then 1.25 mg orally three times daily for 1 week, followed by 2.5 mg twice daily for 1 week, with increases to 2.5 mg orally three times daily to four times daily as necessary. This graded response minimizes the common side effects of nausea and vomiting, postural hypotension, and dizziness. It is suggested that patient compliance may be increased by minimizing these side effects. In addition to the adverse effects mentioned above, it might be noted that higher doses of Parlodel have been shown to produce fatal tachyarrhythmias and psychosis.

A second dopamine agonist, Pergolide mesylate (Eli Lilly & Company), has recently been shown to be effective in the treatment of patients with functional hyperprolactinemia and prolactinomas.[57-59] The agent is active orally in a dose range of 25 to 100 μg/day. It acts directly at the level of the pituitary to inhibit PRL secretion (Fig. 5). In the rat system it has a relative potency of 23 when compared with dopamine. In human monolayer culture, Pergolide and Parlodel are believed to be equally potent[60, 61] (Fig. 6). The drug's extended biologic activity may be secondary to a decreased rate of degradation or metabolism to a more active form in vivo. The side effects are similar to those demonstrated with Parlodel. The key advantage of this drug appears to be its extended half-life.

A third dopamine agonist, CU-32-085 (Sandoz), is currently under investigation. This drug appears to be equally potent or slightly more potent than Parlodel or Pergolide in vitro (Fig. 6). It inhibits PRL secretion in vivo and is, on occasion, slightly more potent than Parlodel.[62] It has been shown to inhibit PRL secretion in patients with pituitary adenomas; however, its clinical use is as yet undetermined.

The dopamine agonists, primarily Parlodel, have been shown to inhibit both the secretion of PRL from adenomas and the growth of these lesions[63-70] (Figs. 7 and 8). Because microadenomas appeared to grow at a very slow rate, observation was frequently the treatment of choice, followed by transsphenoidal hypophysectomy, if pregnancy was desired. With the suggestion that PRL seems to be directly involved in the process of bone demineralization, it seems advantageous to treat individuals with these small lesions indefinitely with first-generation dopamine agonists. It is recommended that the lowest possible dose be used, and that these lesions be monitored every 6 months with serum PRL levels as well as history-

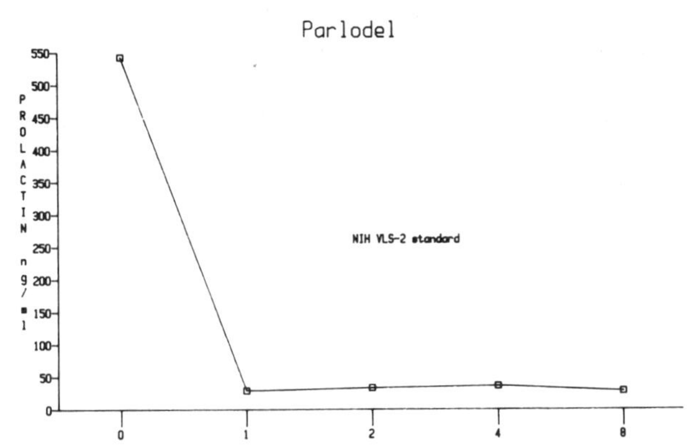

Figure 4
Inhibition of PRL production in a patient with a prolactinoma. The patient had a concomitant decrease in the size of the tumor. The dose of Parlodel administered through the first week was 1.25 mg orally twice daily. This dose was increased to 1.25 mg orally three times a day by week 2.

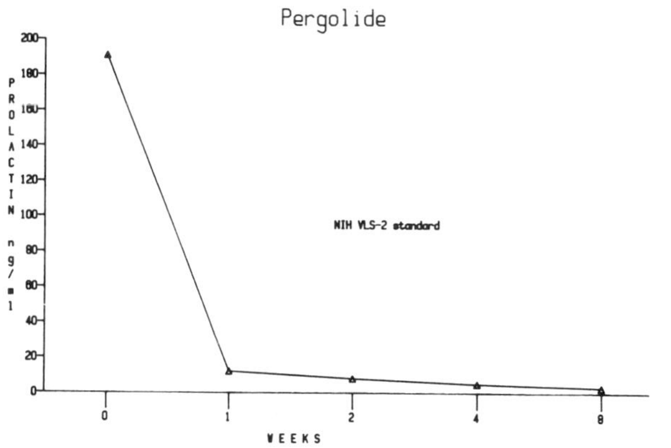

Figure 5
Decreased PRL production in a patient with a microadenoma treated with Pergolide mesylate. The patient was given 50 μg of the drug during the first week. This was increased to 100 μg by week 2.

taking and physical examination. An extensive radiologic survey is not needed in this group of patients, but a cone view of the sella every 2 years and a repeat CAT scan only in the face of resumption of amenorrhea and/or galactorrhea with an elevation in PRL level is advisable. If the patient with a microadenoma desires pregnancy, it is suggested that treatment for 1 year be carried out, followed by a repeat CAT scan. If the lesion is no longer visible by CAT scan, Parlodel therapy should be continued and pregnancy attempted. The patient should use a basal body temperature chart. Once the temperature becomes elevated and a quantitative beta-chain human chorionic gonadotropin turns positive, the drug should be discontinued and the patient followed throughout pregnancy with visual-field examinations at 2-month intervals. Although visual-field examinations, as mentioned, do not adequately evaluate microadenomas, they allow one to detect a rapidly expanding lesion. Since serum PRL levels rise during pregnancy in a linear fashion, reaching a ceiling of 200 to 300 ng/ml,[71] such determinations are not useful in the monitoring of all but the largest tumors. If one were to find a marked elevation of PRL outside this range, expansion of the tumor might be suspected.

The macroadenoma, with its invasive form, presents a challenging therapeutic problem. These lesions may be intrasellar or suprasellar and may be attached to adjacent structures such as the carotid artery. Since these lesions respond favorably to dopamine agonist therapy,[72] it is recommended that these agents be used as a primary means of treatment with neurosurgery reserved for refractory situations. Medical therapy should be continuous and at the lowest possible dose. There is controversy regarding the follow-up of the patient with a macroadenoma. It is recommended that the patient be treated with a dopamine agonist and followed by repeat CAT scan. Once the lesion has decreased to at least within the confines of the sella and galactorrhea and amenorrhea are resolved, these patients should be maintained on continuous therapy with visual-field examinations at 6-month intervals and annual cone-view evaluation of the sella turcica. A CAT scan should be carried out at approximately 2- to 4-year intervals, as a long-term surveillance mechanism. Admittedly, this is a liberal but practical follow-up scheme, and many investigators would recommend CAT scans every 6 months in patients with macroadenomas and every 2 years in patients with microadenomas. In view of our knowledge regarding the natural history of these tumors, it is believed that surveillance might be relaxed somewhat. Should the lesion escape suppression by the dopamine agonist, neurosurgical resection with or without radiation is recommended.

SURGICAL TREATMENT OF PROLACTINOMAS

In the past, neurosurgical resection of microadenomas was carried out by transsphenoidal hypophysectomy with assisted magnification. The cure rate of these lesions was described as 70% to 75%, with an operative morbidity and mortality of 10% to 15% and 0% to 1%, as described in two large series of Domingue et al.[73] and Faria and Tindall.[74] Serri et al.[75] recently reported on the follow-up of 44 patients who had been followed

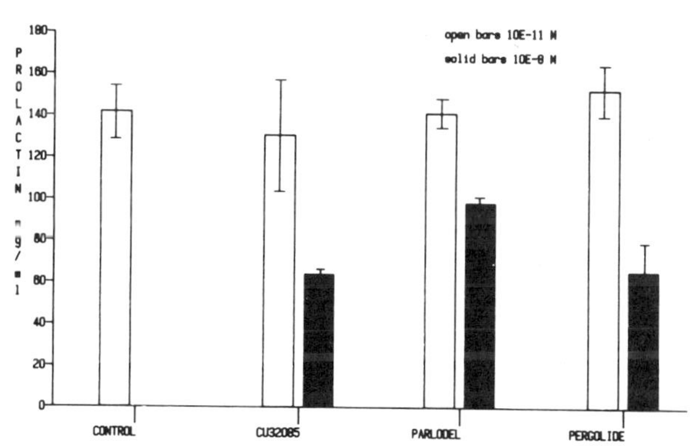

Figure 6
Inhibition of PRL production by three dopamine agonists tested in a human monolayer pituitary cell culture system.

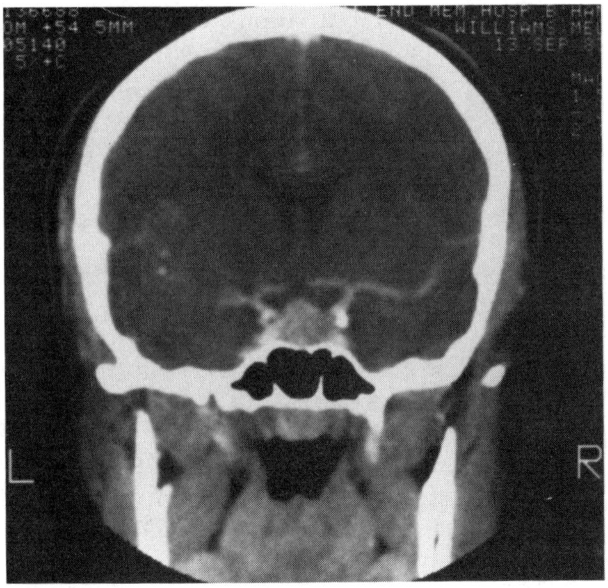

Figure 7
CAT scan showing a suprasellar PRL-secreting macroadenoma in an 11-year-old girl.

after transsphenoidal hypophysectomy for more than 6 years. Group I consisted of 28 patients. Following surgery, normalization of PRL, resumption of menstruation, and/or a cessation of galactorrhea occurred in 85% of the individuals. Hyperprolactinemia recurred in 50% of the patients, although there was no radiologic evidence for the recurrence of tumor. The experience with macroadenomas, however, was not as favorable. Normalization of PRL levels, resumption of menstruation, and cessation of galactorrhea occurred in 31% of the patients with this type of lesion, and hyperprolactinemia recurred in most of these individuals. This information is similar to that reported by Faria and Tindall.[74] Their patients were subdivided into groups 1 and 2: those with PRL levels $<$ 200 ng/ml and those with levels $>$ 200 ng/ml. In group 2, 61% remained amenorrheic, 45% continued to experience galactorrhea, and 54% had elevated PRL levels 10 days postoperatively. Likewise, Domingue et al.[73] showed that therapeutic failures tend to occur in patients who have higher preoperative serum PRL levels and in whom total tumor resection is not achieved. The failure rate with subtotal resection was 50%, but it should be noted that the failure rate did not increase as the grade of the tumor progressed from 1 to 4. In view of this high failure rate and the fact that many of these patients require permanent suppressive therapy with dopamine agonists, it is suggested that bromocriptine be used as the primary therapy for both microadenomas and macroadenomas, with neurosurgery reserved for refractory cases.

RADIATION THERAPY OF PROLACTINOMAS

In years past, multiple small doses of radiation were administered from several weeks to years to patients with prolactinomas. Currently all pituitary lesions are treated in a similar manner with therapy being given in a single course divided into four to five fractions over 5 weeks. The dose range falls between 3500 and 5500 rads at the 95% isodose line.[76] The total dose is dependent upon tumor volume. There is some radiation exposure to the eyes, optic chiasm, and hypothalamus. A number of radiation sources exist to treat prolactinomas, with radiocobalt teletherapy and 4-MEV linear accelerator being common modes of delivery. Little or no data are available on the use of radiation therapy for the primary treatment of pituitary tumors. Several small series, however, suggest that radiation therapy used for surgical failures controls symptoms in about one third of patients but only occasionally reduces serum PRL levels to normal limits.[77, 78] This is clearly a biased series, since these patients by selection probably had the most aggressive tumors. Complications following radiation therapy include epilation, optic nerve and chiasm injury, brain

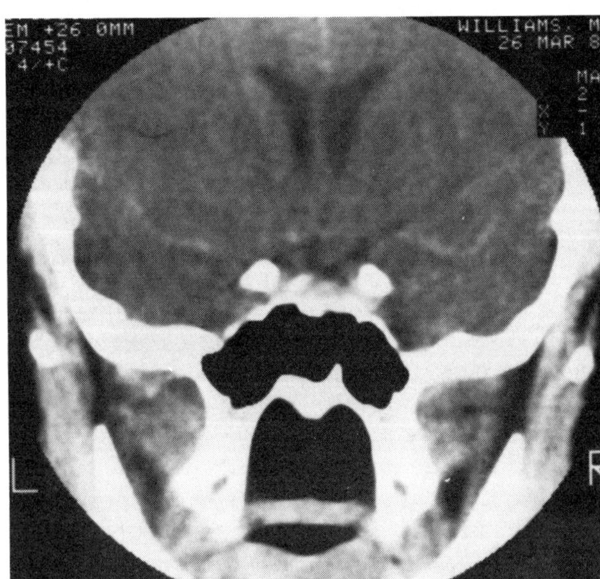

Figure 8
CAT scan of an 11-year-old girl following 1 month of treatment with Parlodel, 2.5 mg orally twice daily.

necrosis, and sarcoma formation (fibrosarcoma and osteosarcoma). Likewise, there is loss of trophic hormone secretion. Jenkins et al.[79] studied endocrine function in 22 patients with various types of pituitary adenomas treated by external radiation. One patient developed hypoadrenalism and hypothyroidism whereas several patients had increased pituitary function after therapy. It was concluded that in most cases irradiation of pituitary tumors had little effect on pituitary function.

In addition to conventional radiotherapy techniques, proton radiosurgery using open or stereotactic technique is available for the treatment of prolactinomas. This approach is effective in treating older, surgically unfit patients, as well as younger patients who are willing to risk hypopituitarism. Bragg peak proton hypophysectomy appears to have the lowest mortality rate and the greatest prospect of cure for the treatment of prolactinomas. Kjellberg and Kliman[80] treated 44 patients with proton therapy with no recurrences. If one considers all adenomas in a series of 678 patients, five recurrences or 0.7% was found. It was recommended that this form of therapy be used for large invasive lesions.

INFERTILITY

The patient who presents with infertility secondary to a prolactinoma should be evaluated as mentioned earlier. These patients may present with amenorrhea, anovulation, oligoovulation, or luteal phase defects. In general, they should be treated with low-dose bromocriptine therapy after appropriate suppression of the lesion. One tries to maintain the PRL levels in the mid-normal range, if possible. It should be remembered that both hyperprolactinemia and hypoprolactinemia will aggravate ovulatory problems, and bromocriptine has been shown to induce luteolysis either alone or in combination with estrogen.[81] Occasionally these patients will have a persistent ovulatory defect after being rendered euprolactinemic, and these individuals may be treated with cyclic early clomiphene therapy (days 2 to 6) underneath a bromocriptine umbrella.[82]

PREGNANCY IN THE MANAGEMENT OF PROLACTINOMAS

In general, the outcome of pregnancy with the treatment of prolactinomas has been excellent. Numerous reports have shown that microadenomas tend to grow slowly during pregnancy and generally do not require therapy.[83-86] Macroadenomas, on the other hand, require medical or surgical therapy about 30% of the time.[87] Divers and Yen[88] followed 54 patients with prolactinomas and had the following complications: four spontaneous abortions, one stillbirth, one premature delivery, four visual defects, and four headaches. In general, one can follow visual-field examinations at 1- to 2-month intervals and clinical symptoms such as headaches to determine whether therapy should be instituted. Bromocriptine has been successfully administered throughout the length of pregnancy and has not been associated with adverse outcome.[89-91] The report of the drug-monitoring center, Sandoz Limited, Basel, Switzerland, as reported by Turkalj et al.,[92] shows 1410 pregnancies, 197 terminations (25 induced), 1213 (86%) live births, 11.1% spontaneous abortions, 0.9% extrauterine pregnancies, 2.5% minor malformations, 1.0% major malformations, and 1.8% twins. Therefore, it appears that patients with both microadenomas and macroadenomas can achieve pregnancy and carry these gestations to term with minimum complications.

LONG-TERM FOLLOW-UP FOR PATIENTS WITH PROLACTINOMAS

Little agreement can be found regarding the appropriate follow-up of patients with prolactinomas. Weiss et al.[93] reported a 6-year follow-up of 27 patients at the University of Southern California. Ten percent developed significant growth of microadenomas. In view of information such as this, it seems appropriate to perform every 6 months a history-taking and physical examination and measurements of PRL levels for patients with evidence of microadenomas. Assuming that PRL levels are suppressed and the patient is asymptomatic, a cone view of the sella might be performed at a 1- to 2-year interval. If these remain normal, a CAT scan every 2 to 5 years would be optional. The patient with the macroadenoma presents with a more serious problem. Frequently these lesions have occurred early in life and may have produced visual impairment. The individual may have undergone one to two conservative neurosurgical procedures and failed therapy. It is suggested that a history-taking and physical examination, measurement of PRL levels, and visual-field examinations be performed at

6-month intervals, at a minimum. If the lesion appears to be clinically under control, a yearly cone view of the sella might be performed, reserving CAT scanning for situations suggestive of tumor expansion. It is suggested that CAT scanning be performed at least every 2 to 5 years for continuity. Should nuclear magnetic resonance prove to be an acceptable alternative, this technique might be substituted on a more frequent basis.

UNANSWERED QUESTIONS ABOUT PROLACTINOMAS

The prolactinoma represents a common and complex clinical entity. Many questions remain to be answered regarding the origin of these lesions, such as whether they represent a neurotransmitter defect. The natural history of these lesions needs to be better understood, so that we can determine whether all of these lesions represent hyperplasia or whether hyperplasia proceeds to microadenoma, then to macroadenoma and invasive adenoma. Agreement needs to be reached as to the treatment of prolactinomas and the method of follow-up. The relationship of hyperprolactinemia to bone metabolism needs to be further investigated. Continued investigation needs to be carried out in the area of therapeutics. Can a medical therapy be developed that is curative, and is our current medical therapy adequate to become the primary treatment mode of these lesions? These questions will be the subjects of future reviews.

REFERENCES

1. Chiari J, Braun C, Spaeth J: Report of two cases of puerperal atrophy of the uterus with amenorrhea and persistent lactation. In Klinik der Geburtshilfe und Gynaekologie. Erlangen, Enke, 1855, p 371
2. Frommel R: Ueber puerperale atrophie des uterus. Gynakologe 7:305, 1982
3. Argonz J, DelCastillo E: A syndrome characterized by estrogenic insufficiency, galactorrhea and decreased urinary gonadotropins. J Clin Endocrinol Metab 13:79, 1953
4. Ahumada J, DelCastillo E: Amenorrhea/galactorrhea. Bol Soc Obstet Ginecol (Buenos Aires) 11:64, 1932
5. Forbes A, Henneman P, Griswold G, Albright F: Syndrome characterized by galactorrhea, amenorrhea and low urinary FSH: comparison with acromegaly and normal lactation. J Clin Endocrinol Metab 14:265, 1954
6. Costello RT: Subclinical adenoma of the pituitary gland. Am J Pathol 12:205, 1936
7. Greenwood FC, Hunter WM: The preparation of ^{131}I-labelled human growth hormone of high specific radioactivity. Biochem J 89:114, 1963
8. Berson SA, Yalow RS, Bauman A, Rothschild MA, Newerly K: Insulin-I^{131} metabolism in human subjects: demonstration of insulin binding globulin in the circulation of insulin treated subjects. J Clin Invest 35:170, 1956
9. Lewis UJ, Singh RNP, Sinha YN, VanderLaan WP: Electrophoretic evidence for human prolactin. J Clin Endocrinol Metab 33:153, 1971
10. Hwang P, Guyda H, Friesen H: A radioimmunoassay for human prolactin. Proc Natl Acad Sci USA 68:1902, 1971
11. Guyda H, Hwang P, Friesen H: Immunologic evidence for monkey and human prolactin. J Clin Endocrinol Metab 32:120, 1971
12. Pepperell RJ: Prolactin and reproduction. Fertil Steril 35:267, 1981
13. Wolf AS, Musch K, Lauritzen C: Hyperprolactinemia in anovulatory women: incidence and endocrine features. J Endocrinol Invest 2:5, 1979
14. DelPozo E, Wyss H, Tolis G, Alcaniz J, Campana A, Naftolin F: Prolactin and deficient luteal function. Obstet Gynecol 53:282, 1979
15. Takei Y: Pathology of pituitary tumor and value of frozen section diagnosis. In Clinical Management of Pituitary Disorders, Edited by GT Tindall, WF Collins. New York, Raven Press, 1979, p 94
16. Scheithauer GW: Surgical pathology of the pituitary and sellar region. In Management of Pituitary Adenomas and Related Lesions with Emphasis on Transsphenoidal Microsurgery, Edited by ER Laws, RV Randall, EB Kern, CF Abboud. New York, Appleton-Century-Crofts, 1982, p 129
17. Robert F: Electron microscopy of human pituitary tumors. In Clinical Management of Pituitary Disorders, Edited by GT Tindall, WF Collins. New York, Raven Press, 1979, p 113
18. Wiebe RH, Hammond CB, Handwerger S: Treatment of functional amenorrhea-galactorrhea with 2-bromoergocryptine. Fertil Steril 28:426, 1977
19. Crosignani PG, Ferrari C, Malinverni A, Barbieri C, Mattei M, Caldara R, Rocchetti M: Effect of central nervous system dopaminergic activation on prolactin secretion in man: evidence for a common central defect in hyperprolactinemic patients with and without radiological signs of pituitary tumors. J Clin Endocrinol Metab 51:1068, 1980
20. Camanni F, Ghigo E, Ciccarelli E, Massar F, Campagnoli C, Molinatti G, Muller EE: Defective regulation of prolactin secretion after successful removal of prolactinomas. J Clin Endocrinol Metab 57:1270, 1983
21. Raud HR, Kiddy CA, Odell WD: The effect of stress upon the determination of serum prolactin by radioimmunoassay (35342). Proc Soc Exp Biol Med 136:689, 1971
22. Neill JD: Effect of "stress" on serum prolactin and luteinizing hormone levels during the estrous cycle of the rat. Endocrinology 87:1192, 1970
23. McAtee JW, Trenkle A: Effects of feeding, fasting, glucose or arginine on plasma prolactin levels in the bovine. Endocrinology 89:730, 1971
24. Carlson HE, Wasser HL, Levin SR, Wilkins JN: Prolactin stimulation by meals is related to protein content. J Clin Endocrinol Metab 57:334, 1983
25. Quigley ME, Ishizuke B, Robert JF, Yen SSC: The food-entrained prolactin and cortisol release in late pregnancy and prolactinoma patients. J Clin Endocrinol Metab 54: 1109, 1982

26. Parker D, Rossman L, VanderLaan E: Relation of sleep-entrained human prolactin release to REM-nonREM cycles. J Clin Endocrinol Metab 38:646, 1974
27. Raud HR, Odell WD: Studies of the measurement of bovine and porcine prolactin by radioimmunoassay and by systemic pigeon crop-sac bioassay. Endocrinology 88:991, 1971
28. Tashjian A, Barowsky N, Jensen D: Thyrotropin-releasing hormone: direct evidence for stimulation of prolactin production by pituitary cells in culture. Biochem Biophys Res Commun 43:516, 1971
29. Vale W, Blackwell R, Grant G, Guillemin R: TRF and thyroid hormones on prolactin secretion by rat pituitary cells in vitro. Endocrinology 93:26, 1973
30. Yamamoto K, Saito K, Takai T, Naito M, Yoshida N: Visual field defects and pituitary enlargement in primary hypothyroidism. J Clin Endocrinol Metab 57:283, 1983
31. Halle AA, Drewry RD, Robertson JT: Ocular manifestations of pituitary adenomas. South Med J 76:732, 1983
32. Pituitary Adenoma Study Group: Variation in assessing sella turcica tomograms for pituitary microadenomas. Obstet Gynecol 60:700, 1982
33. Nachtigall RD, Monroe SE, Wilson CB, Jaffe RB: Prolactin-secreting pituitary adenomas in women. Am J Obstet Gynecol 140:303, 1981
34. Burrow GN, Wortzman G, Rewcastle NB, Holgate RC, Kovacs K: Microadenomas of the pituitary and abnormal sellar tomograms in an unselected autopsy series. N Engl J Med 304:156, 1981
35. Newton DR, Witz S, Norman D, Newton TH: Economic impact of CT scanning on the evaluation of pituitary adenomas. Am J Radiol 140:576, 1983
36. Bonneville JF, Poulignot D, Cattin F, Couturier M, Mollet E, Dietemann JL: Computed tomographic demonstration of the effects of bromocriptine on pituitary microadenoma size. Radiology 143:451, 1982
37. Powell DF, Baker HL, Laws ER: The primary angiographic findings in pituitary adenomas. Radiology 110:589, 1974
38. Frantz A: Prolactin. N Engl J Med 298:201, 1978
39. Keye WR, Chang RJ, Jaffe RB: Prolactin secreting pituitary adenomas in women with amenorrhea or galactorrhea. Obstet Gynecol Surv 32:727, 1977
40. Keye WR, Chang RJ, Wilson CB, Jaffe RB: Prolactin-secreting pituitary adenomas. III. Frequency and diagnosis in amenorrhea-galactorrhea. JAMA 244:1329, 1980
41. Blackwell R, Guillemin R: Hypothalamic control of adenohypophysial secretions. Annu Rev Physiol 35:357, 1973
42. Blackwell R, Amoss M, Vale R, Burgus R, Rivier J, Monahan M, Ling N, Guillemin R: Concomitant release of FSH and LH induced by native and synthetic LRF. Am J Physiol 244:170, 1973
43. Wiebe RH, Hammond CB, Handwerger S: Prolactin-secreting pituitary microadenoma: detection and evaluation. Fertil Steril 29.282, 1978
44. Marrs RP, Bertolli SJ, Kletzky OA: The use of thyrotropin-releasing hormone in distinguishing prolactin-secreting pituitary adenoma. Am J Obstet Gynecol 138:620, 1980
45. Blackwell RE, Younger JB: Assessment of pituitary function. In Obstetric and Gynecology Annual, Vol 10, Edited by RM Wynn. New York, Appleton-Century-Crofts, 1981, p 349
46. Kletzky OA, Davajan V, Mishell DR, Nicoloff JT, Mims R, March CM, Nakamura RM: A sequential pituitary stimulation test in normal subjects and in patients with amenorrhea-galactorrhea with pituitary tumors. J Clin Endocrinol Metab 45:631, 1977
47. Lachelin GCL, Abu-Fadil S, Yen SSC: Functional delineation of hyperprolactinemia-amenorrhea. J Clin Endocrinol Metab 44:1163, 1977
48. Harsoulis P, Marshall JC, Kuku SF, Burke CW, London DR, Fraser TR: Combined test for assessment of anterior pituitary function. Br Med J 4:326, 1973
49. Chang RJ, Keye WR, Monroe SE, Jaffe RB: Prolactin-secreting pituitary adenomas in women. IV. Pituitary function in amenorrhea associated with normal or abnormal serum prolactin and sellar polytomography. J Clin Endocrinol Metab 51:830, 1980
50. Blackwell RE, Boots LR, Goldenberg RL, Younger JB: Assessment of pituitary function in patients with serum prolactin levels greater than 100 ng/ml. Fertil Steril 32:177, 1979
51. Casper RF, Rakoff JS, Quigley ME, Gilliland B, Alksne J, Yen SSC: Changes in pituitary hormones during and following transsphenoidal removal of prolactinomas. Am J Obstet Gynecol 136:518, 1980
52. Keye WR, Chang RJ, Monroe SE, Wilson CB, Jaffe RB: Prolactin-secreting pituitary adenomas in women. Am J Obstet Gynecol 134:360, 1979
53. Schlechte JA, Sherman B, Martin R: Bone density in amenorrheic women with and without hyperprolactinemia. J Clin Endocrinol Metab 56:1120, 1983
54. Barbieri RL, Ryan KJ: Bromocriptine: endocrine pharmacology and therapeutic applications. Fertil Steril 39:727, 1983
55. Delitala G, Yeo T, Grossman A, Hathway NR, Besser GM: A comparison of the effects of four ergot derivatives on prolactin secretion by dispersed rat pituitary cells. J Endocrinol 87:95, 1980
56. Soto-Albors CE, Walters CA, Riddick DH, Daly DC: Titrating the dose of bromocriptine when treating hyperprolactinemic women. Fertil Steril 41:5S, 1984
57. Blackwell RE, Bradley EL Jr, Kline LB, Duvall ER, Vitek JJ, DeVane GW, Chang RJ: Comparison of dopamine agonists in the treatment of hyperprolactinemic syndromes: a multicenter study. Fertil Steril 39:744, 1983
58. Kleinberg DL, Lieberman A, Todd J, Greising J, Neophytide A, Kupersmith M: Pergolide mesylate: a potent day-long inhibitor of prolactin in rhesus monkeys and patients with Parkinson's disease. J Clin Endocrinol Metab 51:152, 1980
59. Kleinberg DL, Boyd AE, Wardlaw S, Frantz AG, George A, Bryan N, Hilai S, Greising J, Hamilton D, Seltzer T, Sommers CJ: Pergolide for the treatment of pituitary tumors secreting prolactin or growth hormone. N Engl J Med 309:704, 1983
60. Rodgers-Neame NT, Bradley EL Jr, Blackwell RE: Long-term monolayer culture of human anterior pituitary cells: functional validation of a method. Fertil Steril 41:75, 1984
61. Rodgers-Neame NT, Blackwell RE: Culture of normal human anterior pituitary cell monolayers. J Cul Meth 7:181, 1983
62. Chang RJ: Unpublished data

63. Thorner MO, Martin WH, Rogol AD, Morris JL, Perryman RL, Conway BP, Howards SS, Wolfman MG, MacLeod RM: Rapid regression of pituitary prolactinomas during bromocriptine treatment. J Clin Endocrinol Metab 51:438, 1980
64. Bassetti M, Spada A, Pezzo G, Giannattasio G: Bromocriptine treatment reduces the cell size in human macroprolactinomas: a morphometric study. J Clin Endocrinol Metab 58:268, 1984
65. Archer DF, Lattanzi DR, Moore EE, Harger JH, Herbert DL: Bromocriptine treatment of women with suspected pituitary prolactin-secreting microadenomas. Am J Obstet Gynecol 143:620, 1982
66. Kletzky OA, Marrs RP, Davajan V: Management of patients with hyperprolactinemia and normal or abnormal tomograms. Am J Obstet Gynecol 147:528, 1983
67. Corenblum B, Hanley DA: Bromocriptine reduction of prolactinoma size. Fertil Steril 36:716, 1981
68. Chiodini P, Liuzzi A, Cozzi R, Verde G, Oppizzi G, Dallabonzana D, Spelta B, Silverstrini F, Borghi G, Luccarelli G, Rainer E, Horowski R: Size reduction of macroprolactinomas by bromocriptine or lisuride treatment. J Clin Endocrinol Metab 53:737, 1981
69. Spark RF, Baker R, Bienfang DC, Bergland R: Bromocriptine reduces pituitary tumor size and hypersecretion: requiem for pituitary surgery? JAMA 247:311, 1982
70. Corenblum B, Taylor PJ: Long-term follow-up of hyperprolactinemic women treated with bromocriptine. Fertil Steril 40:596, 1983
71. Tyson J, Hwang P, Guyda H, Friesen H: Studies of prolactin secretion in human pregnancy. Am J Obstet Gynecol 113:14, 1972
72. Molitch M, Elton R, Blackwell RE, Caldwell B, Chang RJ, Jaffe R, Joplin G, Robbins RJ, Tyson J, Thorner MO, Bromocriptine Study Group: Bromocriptine as primary therapy for prolactin secreting macroadenomas: results of a prospective, multicenter study. J Clin Endocrinol Metab. In press
73. Domingue JN, Richmond IL, Wilson CB: Results of surgery in 114 patients with prolactin-secreting pituitary adenomas. Am J Obstet Gynecol 137:102, 1980
74. Faria MA, Tindall GT: Transsphenoidal microsurgery for prolactin-secreting pituitary adenomas: results in 100 women with the amenorrhea-galactorrhea syndrome. J Neurosurg 56:33, 1982
75. Serri O, Rasio E, Beauregard H, Hardy J, Somma M: Recurrence of hyperprolactinemia after selective transsphenoidal adenomectomy in women with prolactinoma. N Engl J Med 309:280, 1983
76. Sheline G: Conventional radiation therapy in the treatment of pituitary tumors. In Clinical Management of Pituitary Disorders, Edited by GT Tindall, WF Collins. New York, Raven Press, 1979, p 287
77. Gomez F, Reyes FI, Faiman C: Non-puerperal galactorrhea and hyperprolactinemia: clinical findings, endocrine features and therapeutic response in 56 cases. Am J Med 62:648, 1979
78. Kleinberg DL, Noel GL, Frantz AG: Galactorrhea: a study of 235 cases, including 48 with pituitary tumors. N Engl J Med 296:589, 1977
79. Jenkins J, Ash S, Bloom H: Endocrine function after external pituitary irradiation in patients with secreting and non-secreting pituitary tumors. Q J Med 41:57, 1972
80. Kjellberg R, Kliman B: Proton radiosurgery for functioning pituitary adenoma. In Clinical Management of Pituitary Disorders, Edited by GT Tindall, WF Collins. New York, Raven Press, 1979, p 315
81. Blackwell RE, Boots LR, Potter HD Jr: Evaluation of Delestrogen and Parlodel as a luteolytic agent in humans. Fertil Steril 37:213, 1982
82. Diamant YZ, Yarkoni S, Evron S: Combined clomiphene-bromocriptine treatment in anovulatory, oligomenorrheic and hyperprolactinemic women resistant to separate clomiphene or bromocriptine regimens. Infertility 3:11, 1980
83. Hammond CB, Haney AF, Land MR, van der Merwe JV, Ory SJ, Wiebe RH: The outcome of pregnancy in patients with treated and untreated prolactin-secreting pituitary tumors. Am J Obstet Gynecol 147:148, 1983
84. Corenblum B: Successful outcome of ergocryptine-induced pregnancies in twenty-one women with prolactin-secreting pituitary adenomas. Fertil Steril 32:183, 1979
85. Crosignani PG, Ferrari C, Scarduelli C, Picciotti MC, Caldara R, Malinverni A: Spontaneous and induced pregnancies in hyperprolactinemic women. Obstet Gynecol 58:708, 1981
86. Lamberts SWJ, Klijn JGM, deLange SA, Singh R, Stefanko SZ, Birkenhäger JC: The incidence of complications during pregnancy after treatment of hyperprolactinemia with bromocriptine in patients with radiologically evident pituitary tumors. Fertil Steril 31:614, 1979
87. Magyar DM, Marshall JR: Pituitary tumors and pregnancy. Am J Obstet Gynecol 132:739, 1978
88. Divers WA, Yen SSC: Prolactin-producing microadenomas in pregnancy. Obstet Gynecol 61:425, 1983
89. Griffith RLW, Turkalj I, Braun P: Outcome of pregnancy in mothers given bromocriptine. Br J Clin Pharmacol 5:227, 1978
90. Skrabanek P, McDonald D, Meagher D, de Valera E, Carroll C, Lanigan O, Powell D: Clinical course and outcome of thirty-five pregnancies in infertile hyperprolactinemic women. Fertil Steril 33:391, 1980
91. Maeda T, Ushiroyama T, Okuda K, Fujimoto A, Ueki M, Sugimoto O: Effective bromocriptine treatment of a pituitary macroadenoma during pregnancy. Obstet Gynecol 61:117, 1983
92. Turkalj I, Braun P, Krupp P: Surveillance of bromocriptine in pregnancy. JAMA 247:1589, 1982
93. Weiss MH, Teal J, Gott P, Wycoff R, Yadley R, Apuzzo MLJ, Giannotta SL, Kletzky O, March C: Natural history of microprolactinomas: six-year follow-up. Neurosurgery 12:180, 1983

SECTION III

Developmental Abnormalities and Reproductive Potential

The foundation for an individual's reproductive potential has truly been established during the earliest phases of that individual's embryonic and fetal existence, for that is when genetic sex is established and the reproductive tract formed. This section provides reviews on current concepts of disorders in which developmental and physiological variations in early stages of embryonic development and maturation may result in limitations in subsequent reproductive performance.

Uterovaginal anomalies associated with obstetrical complications were first described 300 years ago, but it was not until 1907 when the first successful unification of a bicornuate uterus was performed and reported by Strassmann. These are a heterogeneous group of congenital anomalies which are the consequences of arrested development, abnormal formation, or incomplete fusion of the Müllerian ducts. Rock and Schlaff in their review note that congenital anomalies of the reproductive tract are found in 0.1% to 0.5% of all deliveries. Patients with transverse vaginal septa experience decreased fertility, but once the septa are repaired, pregnancy rates approach 50%, with living children born to 36% of patients. Lateral fusion defects may be obstructive, such as a rudimentary horn, or nonobstructive, such as uterus unicornis. The rudimentary horn should be removed prior to pregnancy to prevent conceptions which may occur from transperitoneal migration of sperm. Rupture and hemorrhage are among the serious risks in these pregnancies. Symmetrical defects such as didelphic, bicornuate, or septate uteri are the most common uterovaginal anomalies. Infertility does not seem to be a common problem in these patients, and most have no obstetrical difficulty. Surgical correction of all defects is not indicated. Those who perform poorly with respect to reproduction do so repetitively. Uterine unification procedures may be indicated in such patients. Contemporary management may include hysteroscopic resection of the uterine septum. Of patients who have undergone metroplasty and conceive, those operated through the hysteroscope may anticipate vaginal delivery, rendering this new procedure more attractive than abdominal metroplasty. There is a clear association between diethylstilbestrol (DES) usage and reproductive tract anomalies in female offspring. These authors detail the incidence of each and the poorer obstetrical outcome for many of these women. They stress timely and accurate diagnoses to provide the best possible outcome for these patients.

The anatomic defects which have been implicated in DES exposed women have been well described. However, the mechanism whereby DES exposure in utero causes these anomalies awaits elucidation. Ways and coauthors are the first to report on the possible alteration in the immunological status of DES exposed women.[1] A hyperreactive immune response in these women such as they describe could influence such mechanisms as rejection of the fetus and the production of antisperm antibodies.

Simpson reviews the evidence for genetic factors, especially mutant genes which play a role in the more common causes of infertility. Aplasia of the Müllerian ducts, which leads to absence of the uterine corpus, uterine cervix, and upper vagina, may be inherited in polygenic/multifactorial fashion. However, a single mutant gene could explain some cases. Incomplete Müllerian fusion with rudimentary or bicornuate uteri has been seen in familial aggregates with multiple affected siblings and is best explained on a polygenic/multifactorial basis. A similar mechanism has been proposed to explain possible heritable tendencies in leiomyomas.

Polygenic/multifactorial factors seem a likely explanation for familial endometriosis, but genetic heterogeneity is another possible genetic explanation. As Simpson points out, the fact that endometriosis is familial and possibly genetic has important clinical implications. An affected sibling or mother has a 7% chance of also having endometriosis. This knowledge could affect clinical decisions. For example, the awareness of endometriosis in a first degree relative might influence recommendations for timing of child bearing. In considering theories of the pathogenesis of endometriosis such as reflex menstruation, some inherited factor which confers susceptibility toward developing endometriosis also must be considered.

Patients with polycystic ovary disease have heritable tendencies. Amenorrhea due to gonadotropin resistance may also be inherited, but the mechanism involved in this condition is most likely a single mutant gene. Studies of patients with ovarian and gonadal dysgenesis reveal that in over one half of the cases the X-chromosome is completely or partially absent. Of the remainder most have a mutant X-linked recessive (XY gonadal dysgenesis) or autosomal recessive gene (XX gonadal dysgenesis). These processes sometimes cause only partial ovarian dysfunction, and clinically these patients may present with anovulation or oligomenorrhea. These and several other entities discussed in this chapter illustrate clearly how genes and chromosomes can be implicated in the pathogenesis of female infertility. It is clear that a strong fundamental knowledge of genetics is essential for gynecologists or urologists dealing with problems of infertility in order to be able to counsel their patients appropriately.

Current concepts and recent advances in isosexual precocity or precocious puberty are examined by Root and Schulman. Precocious puberty implies the appearance of phenotypically appropriate primary or secondary sexual characteristics before the ages of 8 in girls and 9 in boys. Under normal circumstances with advancing age through childhood, hypothalamic maturation progresses to the point where episodic secretory pulses of gonadotropin releasing hormone (GnRH) increase in frequency and amplitude sufficient to stimulate pituitary gonadotropin release of luteinizing hormone (LH) and follicle stimulating hormone (FSH). During childhood the hypothalamic pituitary unit is particularly sensitive to the suppressive effects of sex hormones. In addition, during puberty there is a "central restraint" manifested by higher central nervous system centers upon hypothalamic stimulation of pituitary gonadotropin secretion. Removal of the inhibitory influences which normally "restrain" results in early maturation of the hypothalamic-pituitary gonadal unit manifested by central precocious puberty. Although this condition may occur sporadically, familial, idiopathic, and central isosexual precocity has been reported in families, suggesting a dominant mode of inheritance.

Root and Schulman provide a complete tabulation of the etiologics of isosexual precocity. The etiologies fall into the main subgroups of true or complete isosexual precocity, such as certain tumors of the central nervous system; pseudoprecocious puberty, such as functioning tumors of the ovary and adrenal; and incomplete isosexual precocity, such as premature thelarche. Surgical removal or radiation of central nervous system tumors or drainage of cysts when associated with central precocious puberty may have variable results. In the past, medical therapy for children with true and complete isosexual precocity consisted of such agents as medroxyprogesterone acetate, danazol, and cyproterone acetate. While these preparations were generally successful in causing cessation of menses and occasional regression of secondary sexual characteristics, they had little effect upon the rates of linear growth or upon adult height. More recently treatment has been dramatically altered by the availability of long acting analogs of GnRH. Potent GnRH agonistic analogs may initially stimulate, but subsequently inhibit secretion of LH and FSH.

Pseudoprecocious puberty implies that the process of sexual development is not under the control of an intact hypothalamic-pituitary unit. Estrogen-secreting granulosa cell tumors of the ovaries are the most common ovarian neoplasm associated with this condition in girls, while feminizing adrenal tumors are quite unusual in prepubertal girls. Incomplete isosexual precocity, such as premature thelarche, is probably related to estrogen secretion by the prepubertal ovary. Occasionally this condition may be the consequence of exposure to exogenous estrogens either through the nursing mother who may be taking an estrogen-containing oral contraceptive or through estrogen-contaminated foods. This premature breast development may either regress, persist unchanged, or advance, but often remains unchanged for prolonged periods of time. An unanswered question is why most girls with premature thelarche do not have associated menstrual periods. The authors provide a scheme for evaluation of children presenting with isosexual precocity and stress the need for radiographic studies of the brain for all patients with central precocious puberty. While GnRH agonists are the treatment of choice at the present, it is anticipated that GnRH antagonists will replace them. Antagonists should exert a more immediate effect than the agonists which require several weeks to become fully effective.

Roger D. Kempers, M.D.

REFERENCE

1. Ways SC, Mortola JF, Zvaifler NJ, Weiss RJ, Yen SSC. Alterations In Immune responsiveness in women exposed to diethylstilbestrol in utero. Fertil Steril 48:193, 1987

Chapter 14

The obstetric consequences of uterovaginal anomalies

John A. Rock, M.D.
William D. Schlaff, M.D.

The Division of Reproductive Endocrinology and Infertility, Department of Gynecology and Obstetrics, The Johns Hopkins Hospital, Baltimore, Maryland

The patient with a uterovaginal anomaly often relies on her physician to clarify the reproductive consequences associated with her diagnosis. The couple is usually apprehensive about attempting pregnancy, especially if they have experienced prior pregnancy wastage. Thus, the physician may allay anxiety by a prompt evaluation and accurate description of the reproductive implications and obstetric consequences of a uterovaginal anomaly.

Anomalies of the reproductive tract may lead to obstetric emergencies. While certain anomalies preclude pregnancy, many are first diagnosed during pregnancy. An accurate evaluation and diagnosis are mandatory for appropriate patient care. This review will discuss diagnosis and classification of uterovaginal anomalies as well as obstetric considerations in their management.

INCIDENCE

The incidence of congenital defects of the reproductive tract is unknown. Many patients with uterovaginal anomalies are undiagnosed because they never have obstetric or gynecologic difficulty. Diagnosis is frequently made inadvertently at the time of pelvic or abdominal surgery or at autopsy. In one large series, an attempt was made to diagnose anomalies in all patients who presented with premature labor or abnormal fetal presentation. Uterine exploration was performed at delivery, and hysterosalpingography was performed 6 to 8 weeks postpartum. The authors found an incidence of reproductive tract anomalies in 0.25% of all deliveries.[1] Most estimates of the incidence of such anomalies range from 0.1% to 0.5% of all deliveries.[2-5] The most common malformations are variations of the double uterus (i.e., septate, bicornuate, didelphic). It has further been observed that vaginal anomalies make up only about 10% of the total of reproductive tract abnormalities, suggesting an incidence of 0.01%.[6] The overall incidence is directly related to the clinical interest and awareness of the attending obstetrician.[1, 7] Reproductive tract anomalies may be associated with renal anomalies in up to 20% of cases, according to some estimates.[4, 8]

DIAGNOSIS

Descriptions of uterine abnormalities associated with obstetric complications appeared in the early 15th century. In 1699, Mauriceau and Vassal reported a pregnancy occurring in a rudimentary horn.[9] Most cases described in the early literature were diagnosed at postmortem examination following maternal death.

During this century, physicians have been increasingly aware of the implications of developmental anomalies. Consequently, diagnosis has been made antenatally more frequently. Nevertheless, diagnosis is made antepartum, even in recent years, in only 32% to 65% of cases.[5, 10, 11] In all patients with premature labor or abnormal lie, contemporary management should include consideration of a uterine anomaly. Semmens[12] and Hay[13] have suggested several characteristic physical signs. These include a high presenting part in an abnormal presentation. A very broad uterus, especially with a fundal notch, is also suggestive, as is the presence of fetal limbs pushing far into the maternal flank (Fig. 1). More specific methods of diagnosis today should include ultrasonography. At the time of vaginal delivery or cesarean section, uterine exploration should be attempted. In these patients, as well as those with

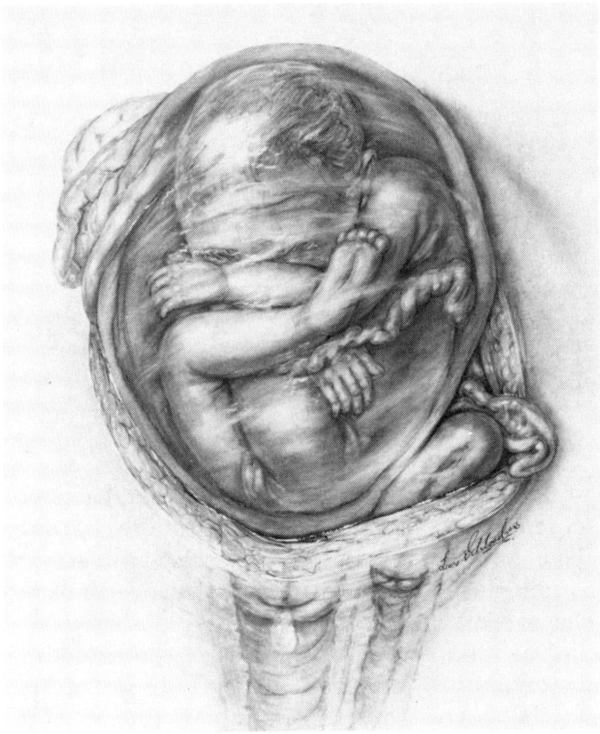

Figure 1
Malpresentation of a fetus conceived in a didelphic uterus with a longitudinal vaginal septum.

a history of retained placenta requiring manual removal, retained products of conception, or repeated miscarriages, hysterosalpingography and/or hysteroscopy should be considered after uterine involution. If a double uterus or a variant is suspected on hysterosalpingography, hysteroscopy or laparoscopy may be indicated to confirm the diagnosis.

CLASSIFICATION

During embryogenesis, the Müllerian ducts appear at about 5 weeks' gestation. The site of invagination of the coelomic epithelium to become the Müllerian duct will be the abdominal opening of the tube. The Müllerian ducts then descend medially within the mesenchyme to fuse with the duct of the opposite side. The fused septum ultimately is resorbed, which produces a single cavity, which meets the upward growing urogenital sinus at its caudal tip. Abnormalities can thus result from failure of descent, failure of lateral fusion, failure of resorption, or failure of vertical fusion. A variety of classification systems has been proposed to categorize reproductive tract anomalies.[9, 14, 15] An adaptation of these will be used in the following discussion and is represented in Figures 2 and 3.

VERTICAL FUSION DEFECTS

A transverse vaginal septum results from failure of vertical fusion between the down-growing Müllerian tubule and the urogenital sinus or from failure of canalization of the vaginal plate.

Delaunay first described this rare condition in 1877. The reported incidence varies between 1 and 5 per 70,000 patients.[16] Transverse septa can be observed high in the vagina (46%), in the mid vagina (35%), or low in the vagina (19%)[17] (Fig. 4). Patients with a transverse vaginal septum will usually present in the teenage years with cryptomenorrhea and pelvic pain.

Repair of such a septum can frequently be accomplished vaginally. However, with a thick septum high in the vagina, a combined vaginal and abdominal approach may be necessary. The abdominal surgeon may need to pass a probe through the fundus and cervix to identify the septum for the vaginal surgeon (Fig. 5). If the septum

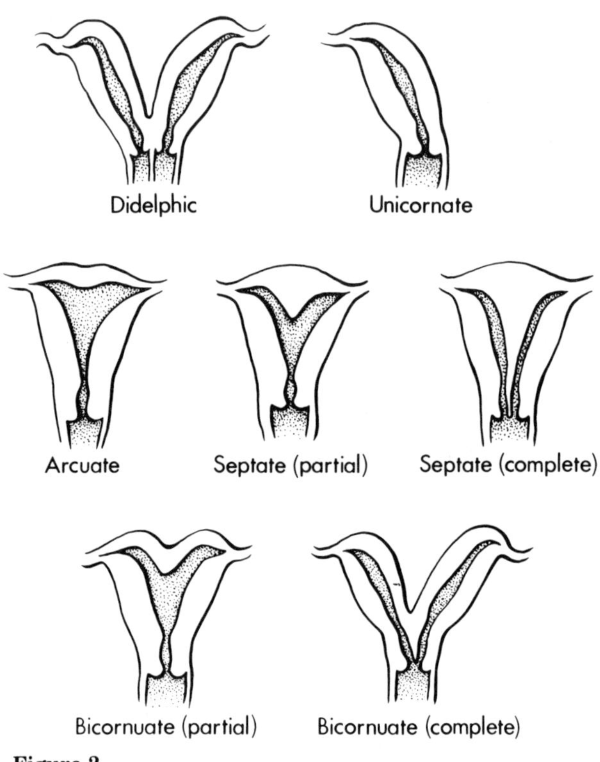

Figure 2
The classification of nonobstructive uterine anomalies (disorders of lateral fusion). From Rock JA: Diagnosing and repairing uterine anomalies. Contemp Obstet Gynecol 17:44, 1981. (Reproduced with the permission of the publisher.)

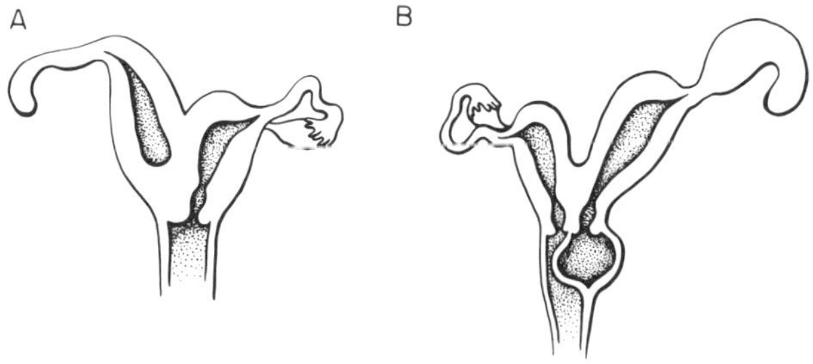

Figure 3
Unilateral obstruction (**A**) of a horn and (**B**) of the vagina. From Rock JA: Diagnosing and repairing uterine anomalies. Comtemp Obstet Gynecol 17:44, 1981. (Reproduced with the permission of the publisher.)

is so thick that its removal results in a large open space, anastomosis of vaginal mucosa is not possible. A Lucite form with a central canal to permit menstrual outflow is inserted and remains in place for 6 months to allow reepithelialization. Once corrected, the pregnancy rate approaches 50% with living children born to only approximately 36% of patients. The etiology of decreased fertility in this population is not clear, although endometriosis is common in cases of complete obstruction and may interfere with conception. Increased difficulty achieving and maintaining pregnancy is observed among patients with a high vaginal septum (Table 1). Once pregnancy reaches term there seems to be no serious obstetric difficulty, although soft tissue dystocia from a constricted vagina is possible. A more common complication is a lateral vault laceration through existing scar tissue.

Imperforate Hymen

The imperforate hymen is not truly an abnormality of vertical fusion. Rather, it represents a failure of degeneration of epithelial cells in the junctional membrane between the caudal end of the Müllerian duct and the invaginated urogenital sinus. This diagnosis is included because of the importance of distinguishing it from the transverse vaginal septum. Patients with an imperforate hymen will frequently present in a similar fashion, i.e., as teenagers with cryptomenorrhea and pelvic pain. These patients are easily treated by a cruciate incision and excision of the hymen. Their subsequent fertility and obstetric

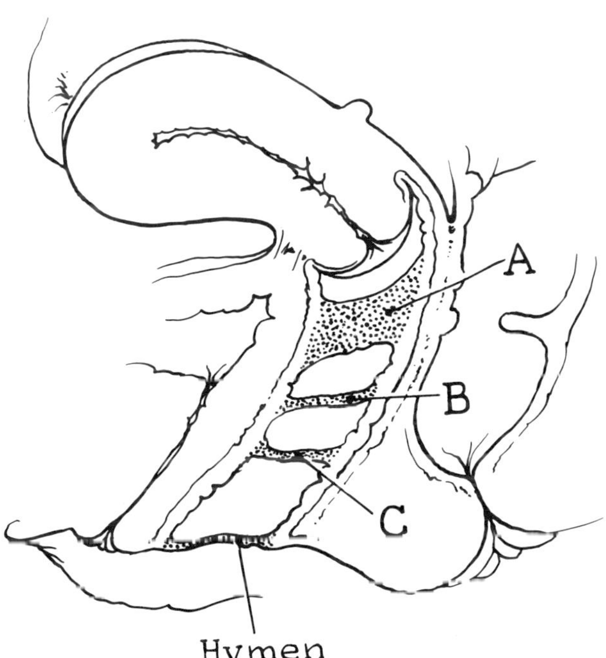

Figure 4
Positions of septa responsible for complete vaginal obstruction. *A*, A high transverse vaginal septum is in most instances thicker than a septum in the middle or lower vagina. *B*, Transverse septum in the middle third of the vagina. *C*, Transverse septum in the lower third of the vagina.[17]

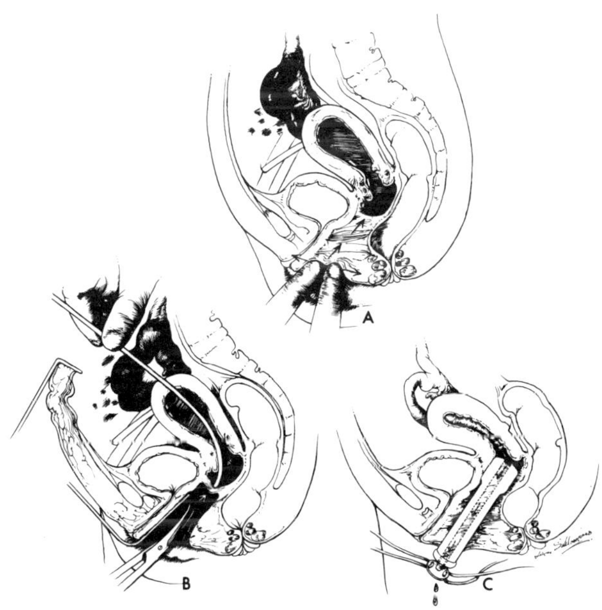

Figure 5
The surgical management of a high transverse vaginal septum where the upper vagina cannot be safely entered without risk of damage to the bladder or the rectum. (**A**), Creation of a neovaginal space. (**B**), If unable to enter the vagina from below, a sound may be passed through the uterine fundus to tent the upper vagina. (**C**), A Lucite form may be placed in the neovagina, the tip of which occupies the upper vaginal space. From Rock JA: Surgical correction of uterovaginal anomalies. In Gynaecology and Obstetrics, Vol I, 49th Revision, Edited by J Sciarra. Philadelphia, Harper & Row, 1984. (Reproduced with the permission of the publisher.)

Table 1. *Pregnancy Success After Surgical Correction of Complete Transverse Vaginal Septum*[a]

Site of septum	Lower third	Middle third	Upper third	Total
Patients	5	9	12	26
Adequate follow-up	5	8	9	22 (84%)
Patients attempting pregnancy	4	7	8	19 (73%)
Patients pregnant	4	3	2	9 (47%)
Patients with a living child	4	2	1	7 (35%)

[a]Adapted from Rock et al.[17]

management are no different from those of the general population[17] (Table 2).

Congenital Absence of the Uterine Cervix

Congenital absence of the cervix with a uterus present is uncommon. Only about 20 cases have been reported. Several surgical approaches have been advocated, including anastomosis or creation of a fistulous tract between a vagina and uterus. However, the reobstruction rate is high, and many surgeons have suggested primary hysterectomy. There have been two general configurations described. The first is characterized by small bits of endocervical buds within the endocervical stroma (Fig. 6), and the second, by attenuation of the uterine cavity within the stroma with no evidence of any cervical or endocervical tissue (Fig. 7). There has been only one reported case of a pregnancy following any procedure to correct this maldevelopment.[18] Because attempts at establishing a fistulous tract can produce ascending infection (and death from sepsis, as shown in at least one case), and because conception is so unlikely, hysterectomy is probably indicated in these patients. Therefore, an obstetric management problem is unlikely.

Table 2. *Pregnancy Success After Surgical Correction of an Intact Hymen Versus Correction of a Complete Transverse Vaginal Septum*[a]

	Hymen	Transverse septum	Total
Patients	22	26	48
Adequate follow-up	18	22	40
Patients attempting pregnancy	15	19	34
Patients pregnant[b]	13 (86%)	9 (47%)	22 (65%)
Patients with a living child	10 (66%)	7 (36%)	17 (50%)

[a]Adapted from Rock et al.[17]
[b]$P < 0.05$, chi-square analysis.

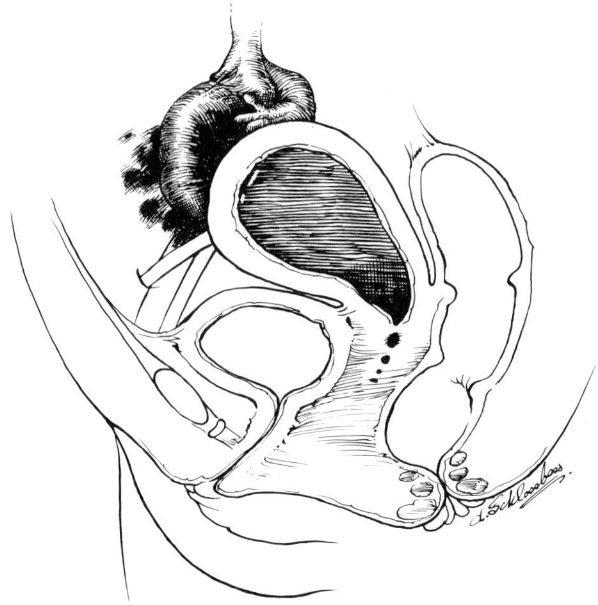

Figure 6
Congenital absence of the uterine cervix with cervical stroma. From Rock JA: The clinical management of congenital absence of the uterine cervix. Int J Gynaecol Obstet 22:231, 1984.

LATERAL FUSION DEFECTS

Lateral fusion defects are a result either of incomplete or absent fusion of the caudally directed Müllerian ducts and also include those abnormal-

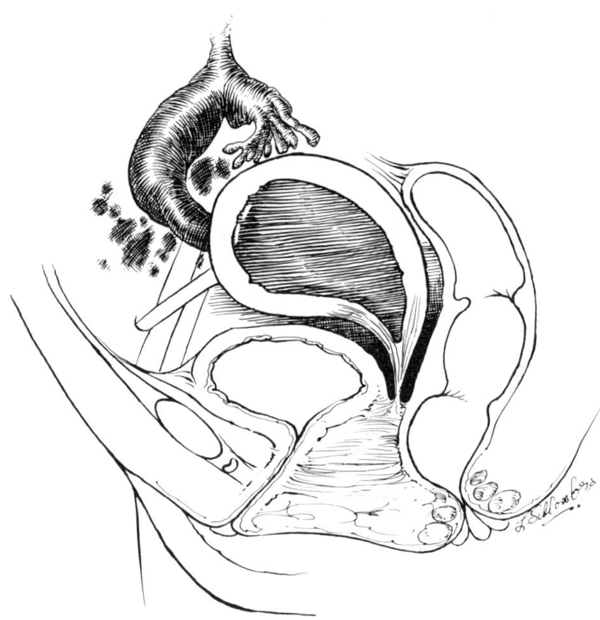

Figure 7
Cervical agenesis. A narrowing of the lower uterine segment eventually ends in a peritoneal sleeve at a point well above the vaginal apex.

ities which result from lack of degeneration of the midline septum formed by this fusion. These defects may be characterized by side-to-side duplication of all or part of the reproductive system. An asymmetric defect may occur with failure of descent of a portion of the Müllerian duct. Symmetric or asymmetric Müllerian dysgenesis may be obstructive or nonobstructive (Fig. 3).

Obstructive

Rudimentary Horn. Patients with an asymmetric uterus and a rudimentary horn constitute 5% to 10% of those with uterovaginal anomalies. Such a rudimentary horn may be related to the uterus by a broad or thin fibrous band or not at all (Fig. 3B). Approximately 75% of such horns do not communicate with the normal hemiuterus.[19] This anomaly is usually associated with ipsilateral renal agenesis (67%) or ipsilateral pelvic kidney (15%).[20]

Overall, this group of patients seems to be normal in their ability to conceive. Their fertility rate in a large series of patients was 94.9%, with 163 pregnancies occurring in 59 patients.[7] The outcome depends on whether the pregnancy is in the normal hemiuterus or in the rudimentary horn. The former group does relatively well. The overall fetal wastage rate ranges between 15%[7] and 36%.[20] Management of labor is no different from that of normal patients. In vertex presentations, labor will proceed normally in 70% to 85% of cases. Fetal malpresentation is common; thus, a need for cesarean section is frequent.

The patient whose pregnancy occurs in the rudimentary horn, however, poses an obstetric emergency. Pregnancy usually occurs by transperitoneal migration of sperm. Some investigators feel that a tiny channel may provide a communication between the rudimentary horn and the normal hemiuterus. Once implantation has occurred, the myometrium will hypertrophy as in any pregnancy, and rupture may result. Rupture has been reported as early as the tenth week and as late as at term. Most reports suggest that rupture is most likely to occur around 20 weeks. A high rate of rupture (89%) has been observed.[21] If rupture does occur, massive hemorrhage may ensue. Kehrer reported a maternal mortality in 1900 of 47.6%.[20] Contemporary management makes maternal death unlikely. A great variety of obstetric outcomes has been described, including deliveries at term by incision of the uterine horn as well as delivery of abdominal pregnancies felt initially to have implanted in the rudimentary horn. Third-trimester antepartum diagnosis may be suggested by an abnormal lie, with the presenting part well out of the pelvis. A spherical uterine enlargement is sometimes described, accompanied by extreme flexion of the fetal neck.[22] The overall fetal survival rate is 1% to 2%,[21] although this figure may well be improved by contemporary technology.

Missed abortion may be a confounding diagnosis in these patients. If the fetus dies within the rudimentary horn in the second trimester, the diagnosis is frequently missed, and attempts to induce delivery are unsuccessful. Ultrasound may help to define this anomaly. One must maintain a high index of suspicion to make an early diagnosis and reduce morbidity.

Contemporary management of the uterus with a rudimentary horn would dictate surgical removal of the horn prior to pregnancy, which would thereby prevent all of the aforementioned risks. At the time of elective surgery, the normal hemiuterus and adnexa should not be disturbed, because successful pregnancy after removal of the rudimentary horn is the rule rather than the exception.

Uterine Duplication with Unilateral Vaginal Obstruction. The double uterus with unilateral vaginal obstruction and ipsilateral renal agenesis is an infrequent anomaly (Fig. 3B). Patients will frequently have cyclic abdominal pain but can be asymptomatic. Vaginal obstruction is associated with a perivaginal mass, but cyclic menstrual flow may be present because of the normally functioning opposite side. The obstructed vagina is usually lined with columnar epithelium. Therefore, there is sometimes an inordinate mucoid discharge which is likely secondary to a small perforation in the partially obstructed vagina. If the vaginal septum is diagnosed prior to pregnancy, it should be excised. The obstetric management thereafter would depend solely on the configuration of the uterus. If a complete obstructed septum is discovered during pregnancy, excision may be necessary. However, a generous pedicle should be left so that bleeding can be avoided if the vaginal mucosa retracts. Ultrasound may be helpful in distinguishing whether the pregnancy is ipsilateral or contralateral to the obstructed side.

Nonobstructive

Asymmetric: Uterus Unicornis. Uterus unicornis is an uncommon abnormality constituting 1%

Table 3. *Distribution of Anomalies in Different Centers*[a]

Author	% Malformations					
	Fenton and Singh (New York)	Baker et al. (North Carolina)	Philpott and Ross (Montreal)	MacGregor (Bristol)	Way (Newcastle)	Blair (Glasgow)
Uterus didelphys	30.0	39.3	12.2	—	—	2.9
Uterus bicornis bicollis	5.2	1.6	—	—	—	11.8
Uterus bicornis unicollis	26.0	46.5	48.8	43.7	58.3	30.8
Uterus septus	6.2	4.7	4.9	—	—	1.5
Uterus subseptus	5.2	4.7	12.2	18.7	41.6	11.8
Uterus arcuatus	7.2	0.8	19.5	37.5	—	25.0
Uterus unicornis	—	3.2	2.4	—	—	—
Septate vagina	11.4	—	—	—	—	16.2
Stricture of vagina	8.3	—	—	—	—	—
Total no. of cases	96	127	41	16	12	68

[a]From Blair.[10]

to 2% of uterovaginal anomalies.[1, 6, 7] As such, large series of cases have not been compiled to provide an accurate understanding of the obstetric implications. Achieving a pregnancy does not seem to be a problem. The incidence of miscarriage, overall fetal wastage, and abnormal presentation, however, are all increased. Estimates of spontaneous abortion range between 21% and 48%,[23] while overall fetal wastage has been calculated by Semmens to be 31%.[7] A recent report of five patients and six pregnancies has suggested that growth retardation and intrapartum fetal distress are both increased in such patients.[24] The authors hypothesize that increased morbidity in three of six pregnancies was due to the absence of uterine arteries and utero-ovarian anastomosis on the undeveloped side, which resulted in decreased blood flow. The small number of patients in this study does not allow us to reach a conclusion but mandates that pregnancy in such a patient should be aggressively managed to provide the optimum chance for adequate fetal growth and development.

Symmetric: Didelphic Uterus, Bicornuate Uterus, and Septate Uterus. Symmetric defects of the uterus are the most common uterovaginal anomalies (Table 3). They result from abnormal fusion of the Müllerian ducts or lack of degeneration of the fused septum. The uterine abnormalities are frequently accompanied by vaginal septa. Uterus didelphys is associated with a septum in 75% of cases, septate uteri in 25%, and bicornuate uteri in less than 5%.[23] Concomitant renal anomalies are also frequent, occurring at least 15% of the time. The incidence of renal agenesis alone has been quoted as 9%[11] to 20%.[4]

There seems to be little doubt that the double uterus is associated with compromised obstetric outcome. The literature is replete with reports which document an increased risk of abortion, vaginal bleeding, malpresentation, premature

Table 4. *Pregnancy Associated with Genital Abnormalities and "Normal" Pregnancy Compared*[a]

	Pregnancy associated with congenital abnormalities of the genital tract	"Normal" incidence (from Sloane Hospital, 1933–1942)
	%	%
Corrected abortion rate	16.5	5.6
Viable birth rate	66.4	93.1
Term birth rate	56.1	85.0
Abruptio placentae	5.5	1.2
Unexplained vaginal bleeding	7.4	1.9
Toxemia	11.1	14.2
Hydramnios	0.8	0.6
Breech and transverse presentations	17.5	3.9
Premature rupture of membranes	44.0	26.2
Premature labor	15.2	6.8
Precipitate labor	9.2	6.5
Intrapartum uterine inertia	20.3	3.2
Cervical dystocia	2.5	0.8
Operative deliveries	50.0	20.0
Uterine inertia, third stage	9.0	1.9
Postpartum hemorrhage	5.2	0.4
Curettage for retained secundines	12.9	0.8
Corrected fetal mortality	8.5	0.9

[a]From Fenton AN, Singh BP: Pregnancy associated with congenital abnormalities of the female reproductive tract. Am J Obstet Gynecol 63:744, 1952. (Reproduced with the permission of the publisher.)

Table 5. *Outcome of Pregnancies in Women with Uterine Anomalies Before Seeking Evaluation*[a]

	Patients	Total conceptions	Wastage		Success	
			No.	%	No.	%
Didelphic	11	35	15	43	20	57
Septate	14	46	39	85	7	15
Bicornuate	12	31	28	90	3	10
Unicornuate	1	5	2	40	3	60
Arcuate	3	5	4	80	1	20
Total	41	122	88	72	34	28

[a]From Musich and Behrman.[26]

labor, operative delivery, and postpartum hemorrhage (Table 4). Other literature further suggests an increased incidence of twins, at least in uterus didelphys.[25] Infertility does not seem to be a common association. However, one must evaluate older literature very carefully, in that the data frequently lump all these anomalies into the category of "double uterus"; therefore, it may be inaccurate in describing the true situation. For example, it is necessary to distinguish between the bicornuate and septate uterus, the latter being more frequently associated with reproductive failure.[11] The distinction is made on the basis of the external configuration of the uterus; hysterosalpingography alone is inadequate. Recent studies have shown that a much higher percentage of double uteri are septate and not bicornuate (Table 5) when compared with the older literature. As the accuracy of diagnosis and careful evaluation of such anomalies improves, a more accurate prognosis may emerge.

Most patients with symmetric uterine abnormalities have no obstetric difficulty. A review of patients between 1953 and 1964 at the Mayo Clinic revealed that 70 patients were found to have uterine malformations at the time of abdominal or pelvic surgery performed for other reasons.[2] Of those patients who were candidates for pregnancy, 83% bore living children (Table 6). Their data continue to be supported by more recent authors.[11] This observation clearly implies that surgical correction of all uterine defects is not indicated. While most patients do quite well, those who do poorly seem to do so on a repetitive basis. The etiology of their poor reproductive performance is not clear. Hypotheses have included insufficient blood flow due to the less vascular

Table 6. *Uterine Malformations Incidentally Discovered in 70 Surgical Patients*[a]

	Uterus			Total
	Didelphys	Bicornis	Septus	
Patients	13	36	21	70
Candidates for pregnancy	9	30	16	55
Actually pregnant[b]	7	22	11	40
Total pregnancies	14	56	32	102
Successful pregnancies	13	47	25	85
Success rate (%)	93	84	78	83

[a]From Thompson et al.[2]

[b]All those achieving pregnancy carried at least one infant to term.

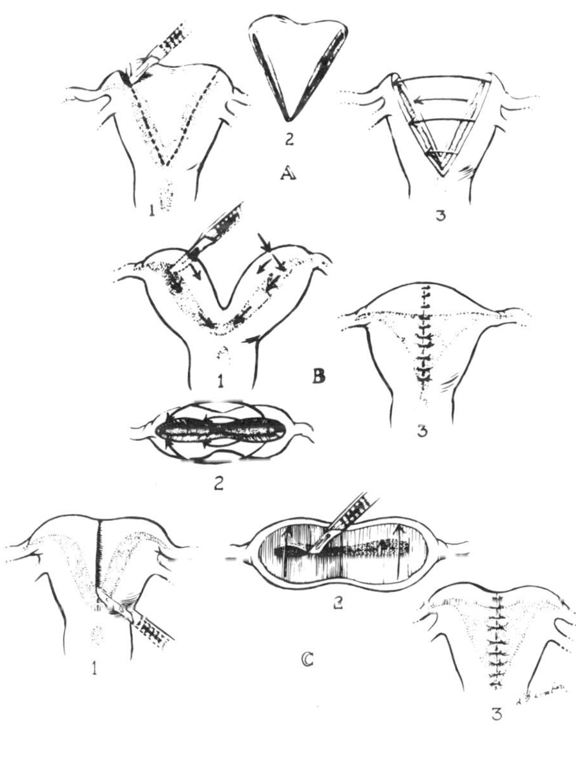

Figure 8
Techniques for uterine unification. (**A**), Wedge technique of Jones and Jones. (**B**), Transverse fundal incision of Strassmann. (**C**), Median bivalving technique from Rock and Jones.[11]

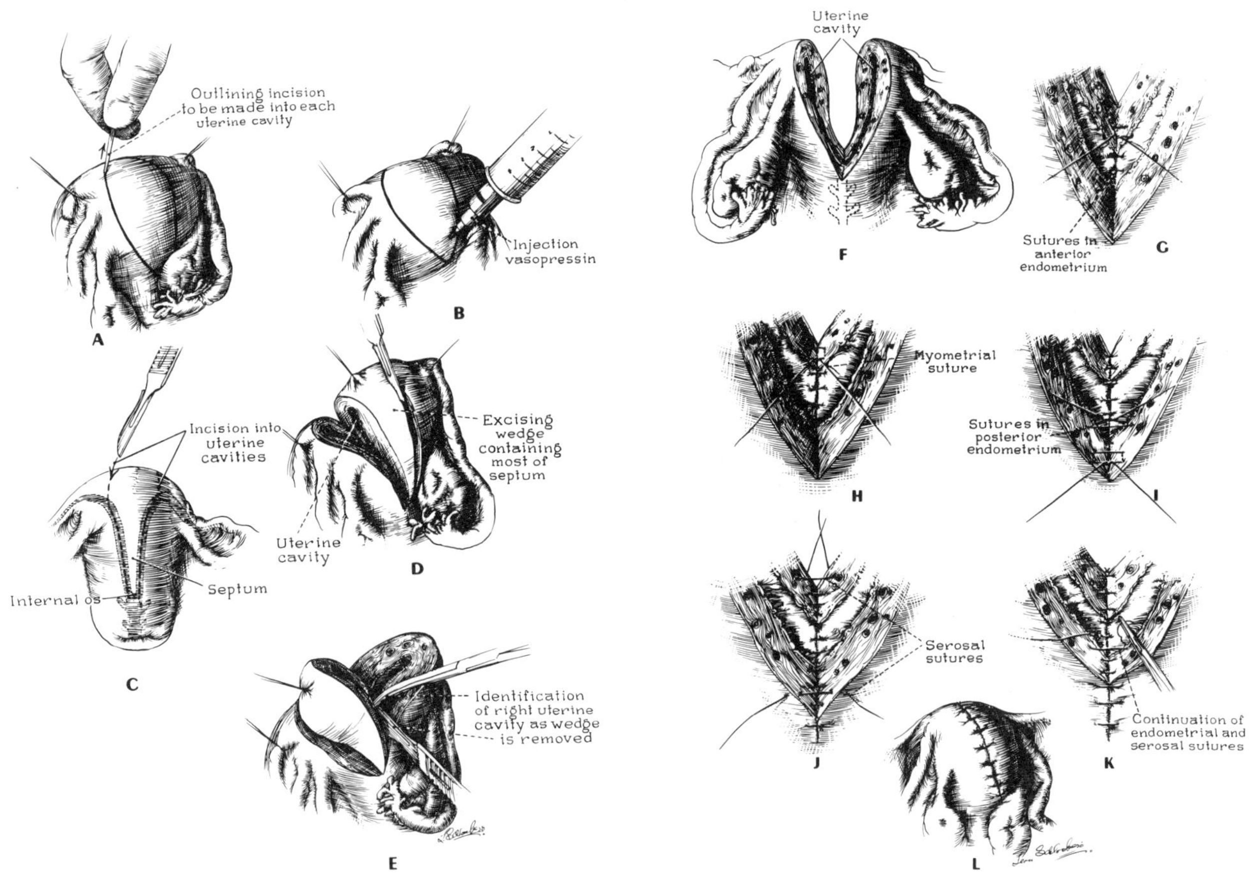

Figure 9
The wedge metroplasty for unifying the uterus. From Jones HW Jr, Rock JA: Reparative and Constructive Surgery of the Female Generative Tract. Baltimore, Williams & Wilkins, 1983.

septum or disruption of intrauterine pressure causing abnormalities or prematurity of labor. Prior to reconstructive surgery, all potential factors which may be responsible for repeated pregnancy wastage should be considered. An evaluation should include studies to determine the genetic complement, adequacy of the luteal phase, the presence of reproductive tract or systemic infection, and the presence of medical illness. If all these factors are normal, surgical correction may then be planned.[27]

There are several procedures which have been recommended for uterine reconstruction (Fig. 8). The wedge metroplasty has been used at The Johns Hopkins Hospital since 1953; thus, a large number of patients have been carefully selected and treated. The overall term birth rate with this technique is 83% (Table 7; Fig. 9). Recently, hysteroscopic resection of a uterine septum has been performed with good success and minimal morbidity.[28]

In patients who have not undergone metroplasty, several important obstetric factors must be recognized. The incidence of malpresentation is clearly increased, making cesarean section more likely. The surgical approach, i.e., low vertical/classical versus low transverse, has not been specifically discussed in the literature. It is clear, however, that low transverse incisions have been frequently performed with no mention of morbidity. Therefore, low transverse cesarean section is the preferred approach, at least in the term uterus. Preterm uteri with a narrow lower uterine segment may well require delivery through a vertical incision. Individualization of the surgical approach is indicated.

Once the patient is in labor, there may be an increased incidence of obstruction by a rotated

Table 7. *Reproductive Performance with Double Uterus: Before and After Wedge Metroplasty*[a]

Patients	Before	After
No. with adequate follow-up	62	58
No. pregnant	62 (100%)	56 (96%)
No. with living children	4 (6%)	47 (82%)
Total pregnancies	165	77
Term	0 (0%)	59 (77%)
Premature	9 (5%)	4 (5%)
Abortion	156 (95%)	14 (18%)
Living children	4 (2%)	58 (75%)

[a]Johns Hopkins Hospital (1936 to 1982). From Rock and Zacur.[27]

rudimentary horn or a hemiuterus. This problem should be managed expectantly, and cesarean section is indicated when such an obstruction prevents appropriate descent.

The management of an associated longitudinal vaginal septum in pregnancy is not clear. Whereas certain authors[7, 29] advocate an excision of such a septum prior to or during early pregnancy, most authors believe that such a septum should be left undisturbed unless it presents an obstructive problem in labor. Review of several series would suggest that this problem occurs in only about 13% of cases.[5, 10, 30]

Contemporary management of patients who have undergone metroplasty mandates cesarean section to avoid the possibility of uterine rupture in labor. Patients who have had hysteroscopic resection of the uterine septum have the advantage of never having had the full thickness of the uterine wall incised. Therefore, cesarean section has not been advocated, which renders this new procedure even more attractive.

Metroplasty does not appear to predispose to the development of cervical incompetence. Nevertheless, it would be prudent to carefully follow all such patients for evidence of premature cervical dilatation.

CHANGES ASSOCIATED WITH DIETHYLSTILBESTROL EXPOSURE IN UTERO

Diethylstilbestrol (DES) is a synthetic estrogen which was used from 1949 until 1971 in some locations in cases of threatened abortion or poor obstetric history. It is estimated that 2 to 3 million women were prescribed DES during their pregnancy.[31] In the 1970s a clear association was established between DES usage and reproductive tract anomalies in female offspring. Such anomalies included vaginal adenosis as well as vaginal ridges or transverse septa. Apical funneling was also described. Cervical abnormalities included hypoplasia, hoods, collars, and pseudopolyps. It is estimated that 50% to 75% of female offspring exposed in utero to DES have adenosis and that 22% to 58% of exposed individuals have other structural anomalies of the cervix.[32] In 1971, an infrequent association between DES exposure and clear-cell adenocarcinoma of the vagina was described by Herbst et al.[33] In 1977, Kaufman et al.[34] described upper tract lesions, including hypoplastic uterus, T-shaped uterus, and constriction within the uterine body, as demonstrated by hysterosalpingography (Fig. 10). Such findings prompted further study, and it is becoming clear that DES exposure has similar deleterious effects on reproductive performance.

Present data have not been adequate to clearly implicate DES exposure as a factor in infertility. The National Cooperative Diethylstilbestrol Adenosis (DESAD) project compared fertility in 618 DES-exposed females with that of 618 control subjects and found no difference in the number of pregnancies achieved.[35] This finding was further supported by a study at the University of California at San Diego.[36] Conversely, a study of 160 DES-exposed women at the University of North Carolina revealed 31 infertile for 1 to 8 years, which suggested an infertility rate of 29.2%.[37] Herbst et al.,[38] in 1980, observed the same increased risk of infertility.

While an increase in infertility is not clearly established, present data do implicate DES as a

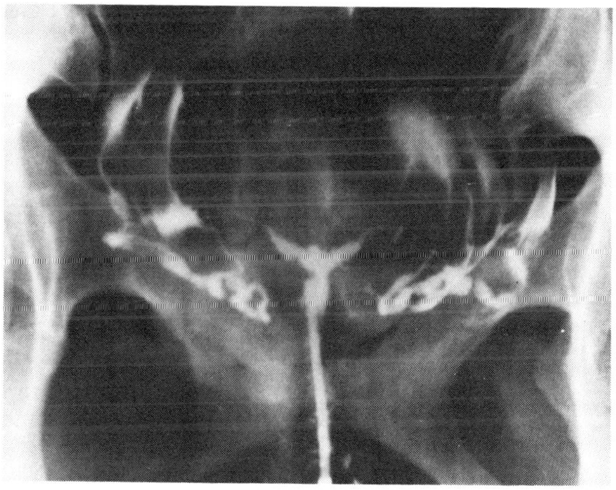

Figure 10
A typical hysterogram of a woman whose mother used DES during pregnancy.[27]

Table 8. *Summary of Pregnancy Experience, DES-Exposed Versus Unexposed Patients*[a]

	Exposed		Unexposed	
	No. of women with outcome	No. of pregnancies	No. of women with outcome	No. of pregnancies
Full-term birth	40	57[b]	79	129
Premature live birth (excluding twins)	18	19	5	5
Premature nonviable (excluding twins)	7	9	2	2
Subtotal—women with premature births	24[c]		7	
Premature twins	2	2	3	3
Miscarriage				
One only	13	13	12	12
More than one	4	12	3	8
Ectopic pregnancy	4	4	0	0
Elective abortion	19	21	35	42
Current pregnancy	12	12	11	11
Total pregnancies		149 (38%)		212 (60.8%)

[a]From Herbst et al.[38]
[b]One full-term neonatal death.
[c]One woman had both a premature live birth and a stillbirth.

significant risk factor in pregnancy outcome. The literature suggests that both spontaneous abortion and ectopic pregnancies may be increased, although no one study is able to demonstrate statistical significance to support this conclusion.[35, 38] Incompetent cervix, in association with DES changes, has further been described.[39] The most troublesome data have been those which have demonstrated an increased risk of premature labor and perinatal loss in DES-exposed women. Such an increase in prematurity has been described in a number of studies and has ranged between 13% and 40% of live births.[36-38, 40] Not surprisingly, perinatal loss is increased in the same studies, presumably as a result of prematurity (Table 8). The etiology of the observed poor reproductive outcome has not been specifically identified. Decreased uterine volume and cervical and connective tissue abnormalities have all been suggested as the most significant factors. There has been no description of abnormalities of labor, cesarean section, or delivery-related problems in DES-exposed patients who reach term.

Kaufman et al.[34] have sought to correlate the presence of DES-related upper-tract abnormalities with poor obstetric outcome. Hysterosalpingography was performed on 267 women who had been exposed to DES. They found upper-tract abnormalities—small or T-shaped cavities with or without uterine constriction—in 185 patients (69%).[34] In their series, 118 patients (44%) had gross structural changes of the cervix, including an anterior cervical ridge, a cervical collar or pseudopolyp, or a hypoplastic cervix.[34] Of those with cervical structural changes, 86% had upper-tract abnormalities, and 56% of those with normal cervices had upper-tract abnormalities (Table 9). Those patients with upper-tract abnormalities had poorer outcomes in every area of reproductive performance when compared with those with normal upper tracts. Similar results were observed by Cousins et al.[36] Once pregnant, DES-

Table 9. *Types of Hysterosalpingography Findings After DES Exposure in Utero*[a]

	Hysterosalpingography findings										
Structural changes	No. of women	Normal findings	T shape	Small cavity	Constriction	T shape plus small cavity	T shape plus constriction	Small cavity plus constriction	T shape plus small cavity plus constrictions	Other abnormality	Total abnormal findings
Present	118	17	12	15	3	34	7	7	16	7	101 (86%)
Absent	149	65	24	10	4	23	4	3	9	7	84 (56%)
Total	267	82 (31%)	36 (19%)	25 (13%)	7 (4%)	57 (31%)	11 (6%)	10 (5%)	25 (13%)	14 (8%)	185 (69%)

[a]From Kaufman RH, Adam E, Binder GL, Gerthoffer E: Upper genital tract changes and pregnancy outcome in offspring exposed in utero to diethylstilbestrol. Am J Obstet Gynecol 137:299, 1980. (Reproduced with the permission of the publisher.)

exposed patients should be closely followed to ensure early diagnosis of ectopic pregnancies, cervical incompetence, or premature labor.

SUMMARY

Congenital uterovaginal anomalies can have adverse effects on pregnancy outcome. Early diagnosis and an aggressive evaluation of any patient presenting with mid-trimester abortion, premature labor, malpresentation, or retained placenta may prevent additional pregnancy wastage and maternal morbidity. With more timely and accurate diagnosis, appropriate management is likely to provide the best possible outcome for all such patients.

REFERENCES

1. Green LK, Harris RE: Uterine anomalies—frequency of diagnosis and associated obstetric complications. Obstet Gynecol 47:427, 1976
2. Thompson JP, Smith RA, Welch JS: Reproductive ability after metroplasty. Obstet Gynecol 28:363, 1966
3. Strassman EO: Plastic unification of double uterus. Am J Obstet Gynecol 64:25, 1952
4. Capraro VJ, Chuang JT, Randall CL: Improved fetal salvage after metroplasty. Obstet Gynecol 31:97, 1968
5. Fenton AN, Singh BP: Pregnancy associated with congenital abnormalities of the female reproductive tract. Am J Obstet Gynecol 63:744, 1952
6. Lewis BV, Brant HA: Obstetric and gynecologic complications associated with Müllerian duct abnormalities. Obstet Gynecol 28:315, 1966
7. Semmens JP: Congenital anomalies of female genital tract: functional classification based on review of 56 personal cases and 500 reported cases. Obstet Gynecol 19: 328, 1962
8. Woolf RB, Allen WM: Concomitant malformations of the reproductive and urinary tracts. Obstet Gynecol 2:236, 1953
9. Jarcho J: Malformations of the uterus. Am J Surg 71:106, 1946
10. Blair RG: Pregnancy associated with congenital malformations of the reproductive tract. Br J Obstet Gynaecol 67:36, 1980
11. Rock JA, Jones HW Jr: The clinical management of the double uterus. Fertil Steril 28:798, 1977
12. Semmens JP: Abdominal contour in the third trimester—an aid to diagnosis of uterine anomalies. Obstet Gynecol 25:779, 1965
13. Hay D: Uterus unicollis and its relationship to pregnancy. J Obstet Gynaecol Br Commonw 68:361, 1961
14. Jones HW Jr, Wheeless CR: Salvage of the reproductive potential of women with anomalous development of the Müllerian ducts: 1868-1968-2068. Am J Obstet Gynecol 104:348, 1969
15. Buttram VC Jr, Gibbons WE: Müllerian anomalies: a proposed classification (an analysis of 144 cases). Fertil Steril 32:40, 1979
16. Suidan FG, Azoury RS: The transverse vaginal septum: a clinicopathological evaluation. Obstet Gynecol 54:278, 1979
17. Rock JA, Zacur HA, Dlugi AM, Jones HW Jr, Telinde RW: Pregnancy success following surgical correction of imperforate hymen and complete transverse vaginal septum. Obstet Gynecol 59:448, 1982
18. Zarou GS, Esposito JM, Zarou DM: Pregnancy following the surgical correction of congenital atresia of the cervix. Int J Gynaecol Obstet 11:143, 1973
19. Mulsow FW: Pregnancy in a rudimentary horn of the uterus. Am J Obstet Gynecol 49:773, 1945
20. Rolen AC, Choquette AJ, Semmens JP: Rudimentary uterine horn: obstetric and gynecologic implications. Obstet Gynecol 27:806, 1966
21. O'Leary JL, O'Leary JA: A rudimentary horn pregnancy. Obstet Gynecol 22:371, 1963
22. Jarrell J, Effer SB, Mohide PT: Pregnancy in a rudimentary horn with fetal salvage. Am J Obstet Gynecol 127:676, 1977
23. Buttram VC Jr: Müllerian anomalies and their management. Fertil Steril 40:159, 1983
24. Andrews MC, Jones HW Jr: Impaired reproductive performance of the unicornuate uterus: intrauterine growth retardation, infertility, and recurrent abortion in five cases. Am J Obstet Gynecol 144:173, 1982
25. Brown DC, Nelson RF: Uterus didelphys and double vagina with delivery of a normal infant from each uterus. Can Med Assoc J 96:675, 1967
26. Musich JR, Behrman SJ: Obstetric outcome before and after metroplasty in women with uterine anomalies. Obstet Gynecol 52:63, 1978
27. Rock JA, Zacur HA: The clinical management of repeated early pregnancy wastage. Fertil Steril 39:123, 1983
28. Daly DC, Walters CA, Soto-Albors CE, Riddick DH: Hysteroscopic metroplasty: surgical technique and obstetric outcome. Fertil Steril 39:623, 1983
29. Hanzlik H: Double uterus with vaginal delivery of term pregnancy: review of the literature and report of a case. Obstet Gynecol 27:214, 1966
30. Miller NF: Clinical aspects of uterus didelphys. Am J Obstet Gynecol 4:398, 1922
31. Richmond JB: Physician Advisory: health effects of the pregnancy use of diethylstilbestrol. DES Task Force Summary Report, United States Department of Health, Education and Welfare, October 4, 1978, Washington, D.C.
32. Stillman RJ: In utero exposure to diethylstilbestrol: adverse effects on the reproductive tract and reproductive performance in male and female offspring. Am J Obstet Gynecol 142:905, 1982
33. Herbst AL, Ulfelder H, Poskanzer LC: Adenocarcinoma of the vagina: association of maternal stilbestrol therapy with tumor appearance in young women. N Engl J Med 284:878, 1971
34. Kaufman RH, Adam E, Binder GL, Gerthoffer E: Upper genital tract changes and pregnancy outcome in offspring exposed in utero to diethylstilbestrol. Am J Obstet Gynecol 137:299, 1980
35. Barnes AB, Colton T, Gundersen J, Noller K, Tilley BC, Strama T, Townsend DE, Hatab P, O'Brien PC: Fertility

and outcome of pregnancy in women exposed in utero to diethylstilbestrol. N Engl J Med 302:609, 1980
36. Cousins L, Karp W, Lacey C, Lucas WE: Reproductive outcome of women exposed to diethylstilbestrol in utero. Obstet Gynecol 56:70, 1980
37. Schmidt G, Fowler WC Jr, Talbert LM, Edelman DA: Reproductive history of women exposed to diethylstilbestrol in utero. Fertil Steril 33:21, 1980
38. Herbst AL, Hubby MM, Blough RR, Azizi F: A comparison of pregnancy experience in DES-exposed and DES-unexposed daughters. J Reprod Med 24:62, 1980
39. Goldstein DP: Incompetent cervix in offspring exposed to diethylstilbestrol in utero. Obstet Gynecol (Suppl) 52:735, 1978
40. Berger MJ, Goldstein DP: Impaired reproductive performance in DES-exposed women. Obstet Gynecol 55:25, 1980

Chapter 15

Genes and chromosomes that cause female infertility

Joe Leigh Simpson, M.D.

Section of Human Genetics, Department of Obstetrics and Gynecology, Northwestern University Medical School, Chicago, Illinois

The genetic causes of gonadal failure are well-known.[1, 2] Absence of all or most of an X chromosome in women results in ovarian dysgenesis, and an additional X chromosome in men results in Klinefelter's syndrome. One mutation on the X causes androgen insensitivity and another, gonadal dysgenesis.

Yet, all these disorders are relatively rare and seldom encountered in otherwise normal women who consult physicians only after realizing they are infertile. If disorders such as those cited above were the only genetic disorders that cause female infertility, the infertility specialist would be justified in concluding that genetic factors were less than immediately relevant. Do genetic factors, especially mutant genes, play roles in the more *common* causes of infertility? Indeed, there is evidence for genetic factors in such conditions. The evidence has accumulated more slowly than has evidence for genetic causes in many other organ systems. One reason for the slow progress is that gynecologic and urologic disorders often involve internal organ systems that are visualized only infrequently. A second reason is that such disorders occur in members of only one sex; thus, familial aggregates would be rarer than if both sexes were affected. Third, progress has been delayed by the relative scarcity of gynecologists or urologists interested in genetics.

Despite these caveats, several common disorders show heritable tendencies. In this communication these disorders will be identified, and those genetic mechanisms most likely to explain familial tendencies will be considered.

MUTANT GENES, POLYGENIC/ MULTIFACTORIAL INHERITANCE, AND GENETIC HETEROGENEITY

Few of the conditions discussed will show simple Mendelian modes of inheritance. This can be deduced because the proportion of affected relatives will usually prove to be lower than expected on the basis of autosomal dominant (50%) or autosomal recessive (25%) inheritance. Likewise, a chromosomal cause can easily be disproved. Recurrence risks in first-degree relatives (siblings, parents, offspring) usually will be 1% to 7%.

For recurrence risks of this magnitude, several explanations can be postulated. First, the familial aggregates might merely reflect the tendency of near relatives to be similar in socioeconomic status and life-style. That is, a disorder could be familial but not genetic. This possibility is especially reasonable in disorders like endometriosis, which is known to be influenced by life-style and socioeconomic factors. However, in endometriosis as well as other disorders, a strictly nongenetic explanation for an increased prevalence in relatives will be shown to be unlikely because the frequency of symptomatic endometriosis is much higher than in either the general population or relatives of the husband.

Second, a genetic cause must be proposed. At least three genetic causes are consistent with recurrence risks of 1% to 7%: (1) polygenic/multifactorial inheritance; (2) a single mutant gene, but one of low penetrance or varied expressivity; or (3) a single mutant gene, yet one occurring in

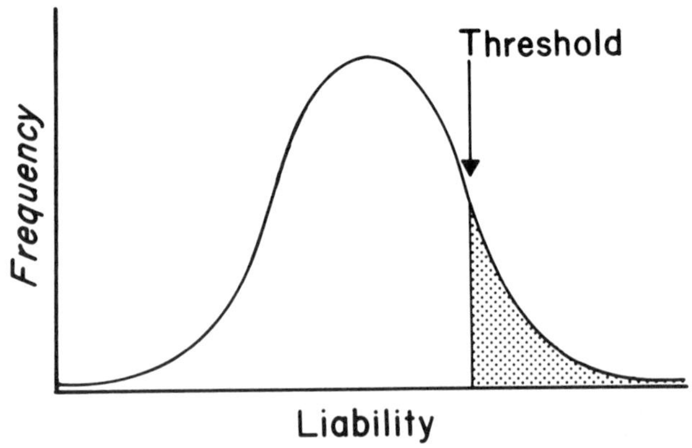

Figure 1
Schematic diagram illustrating the threshold model of polygenic/multifactorial inheritance. Beyond a certain point, the genetic liability is so great that a trait is manifested. (From Simpson et al.[1, 2])

only a small subset of patients with a given disorder (genetic heterogeneity).

The first genetic explanation is polygenic/multifactorial inheritance, discussed in detail elsewhere by the author and colleagues.[1, 2] This mechanism of inheritance assumes that a given trait is influenced either by (1) several different genes, each with small individual effects (polygenic), or (2) interaction between genetic and environmental factors (multifactorial). It can be shown that even a small number of genes (or factors) can produce enough genotypes to yield a continuous distribution of genotypic liabilities in the population.[1, 2] Beyond a given threshold, the liability becomes so great that an abnormality is manifested (Fig. 1). For polygenic/multifactorial traits, recurrence rates among first-degree relatives (siblings, offspring, parents) are usually 1% to 5%.[1] Unlike Mendelian traits, polygenic/multifactorial inheritance is compatible with discordance among monozygotic twins; however, concordance rates are still higher in monozygotic than in dizygotic twins.

Second, a single autosomal or X-linked gene may exist in some relatives in nonpenetrant form. Other relatives may have such a mildly expressed form of a disorder that they pass detection. In fact, in most gynecologic disorders, the frequency of clinically affected relatives must be considered minimal, because aggressive diagnostic efforts (e.g., laparoscopic visualization) cannot be performed routinely on asymptomatic or even mildly symptomatic relatives. Recall, as well, that clinical appearance may be only a very indirect measure of the activity of a mutant gene. If the gene's product could be measured directly in first-degree relatives, the frequencies might approximate 25% or 50%. Thus, existence of single autosomal dominant or autosomal recessive genes can never be excluded, although it remains unlikely, with the low (5% to 10%) recurrence risks we will often be observing.

A third possibility is that a disorder could represent not just one but rather several different entities (i.e., heterogeneity). Some entities could be inherited as a result of a single mutant gene, whereas others could result from a different gene or from nongenetic factors[3] (Fig. 2). Pooling nongenetic and genetic cases would result in intermediate recurrence risks (e.g., 6.5% in Fig. 2) that would obscure recognition of a Mendelian mutant. Heterogeneity of the type described is difficult to establish unless genetic and nongenetic cases differ with respect to a distinctive qualitative marker, such as a human leukocyte antigen (HLA) type. Absence of a distinctive marker would not, of course, exclude the existence of such a single gene.

NORMAL ANATOMIC AND PHYSIOLOGIC VARIATION

In view of the many unknown causes of infertility (male and female), it seems relevant to recall that polygenic/multifactorial mechanisms are

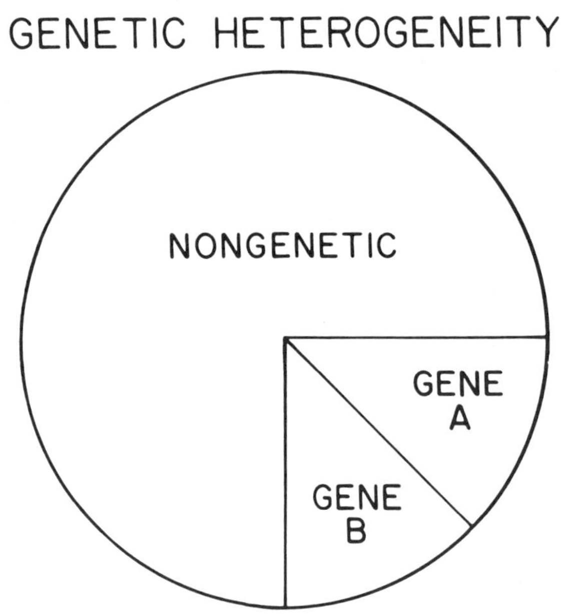

Figure 2
Schematic diagram illustrating the concept of etiologic and genetic heterogeneity. If genes A and B are autosomal recessive, the overall recurrence risk would be 6.5%, i.e., the risk is 25% for one-fourth of cases but 0% for three-fourths.

usually responsible for normal anatomic and physiologic variation.

One illustrative example concerns age of menarche. Social and environmental factors complicate human studies, but it is clear that the mean age of menarche differs less between monozygotic twins (2 months) than between dizygotic twins (12 months).[4, 5] The mean differences are even greater among unrelated women. The magnitude of the observed differences is consistent with polygenic/multifactorial mechanisms. Knowledge of relatives' age of menarche might permit a clinician to predict an individual's age of menarche. Probably the same conclusion exists with respect to age of menopause.

Inbred strains of mice display heritable tendencies in many aspects of ovarian development.[6] Ovarian weight, number of follicles per ovary, age of onset of estrus, ovarian response to gonadotropins, rate of follicular atresia relative to age, and sperm morphologic features differ between strains. These differences imply genetic and probably polygenic control. None of these variables has been studied well in humans. However, there is every expectation that genetic factors will prove to be important.

MÜLLERIAN APLASIA

Aplasia of the Müllerian ducts leads to absence of the uterine corpus, uterine cervix, and upper vagina.[2] A blindly ending 1-cm to 2-cm vagina exists, presumably derived exclusively from invagination of the urogenital sinus. Uterine remnants may persist in the form of bilateral cords. Some investigators prefer the term Rokitansky-Kuster-Hauser syndrome, especially if remnants persist. Renal anomalies (pelvic kidney, renal ectopia, and unilateral aplasia) are frequently (20% to 40%) associated with Müllerian aplasia. The frequency of skeletal anomalies, especially vertebral anomalies, is also increased. Secondary sexual development is normal, except of course for lack of uterine enlargement. Müllerian aplasia occurs in 46,XX individuals, the chromosomal status readily distinguishing affected individuals from those with 46,XY androgen insensitivity syndrome (testicular feminization). Müllerian aplasia is the more common cause of absence of the uterus.

Familial aggregates of Müllerian aplasia are well documented. In particular, affected siblings have been reported by several investigators.[7-11] Such reports initially raised the formal possibility of an autosomal recessive cause, but in 1973 Lischke et al.[12] reported three families in which monozygotic twins were discordant. Thus, autosomal recessive inheritance seemed an unlikely explanation for all cases.

Dominant factors were next proposed. Shokeir[11] studied 16 Saskatchewan families in which the proband had Müllerian aplasia. In 13 families, the proband showed complete absence of the uterine cervix and corpus; in the remaining three subjects, uterine remnants persisted. None of the 3 subjects with uterine remnants had an affected relative, but 10 of the 13 subjects with complete absence of the uterine cervix and corpus did. Two of these ten subjects showed only affected siblings, whereas the other eight subjects had affected paternal relatives (aunts, first cousins, second cousins, or great aunts). These observations suggested sex-limited (i.e., female-limited) autosomal dominant inheritance. Women with the postulated mutant gene would manifest Müllerian abnormalities, but men would show no deleterious effect because they have no important Müllerian derivatives.

In contrast to expectations based on the work of Shokeir[11] were results of a study of 23 families by Carson et al.[13] Studying subjects ascertained in both Chicago (Northwestern University) and Houston (Baylor College of Medicine), we failed to observe a single affected relative. The absence of affected relatives among 30 postpubertal sisters, 30 paternal aunts, and 41 maternal aunts makes sex-limited autosomal dominant inheritance an unlikely explanation in our sample. Of course, dominant genes could exist in Saskatchewan but not in other populations, and fresh dominant mutations can never be excluded. The latter will be difficult to prove, because women with Müllerian aplasia are sterile. Thus, there will be no opportunity to observe affected offspring. On the other hand, absence of affected siblings and absence of parental consanguinity exclude autosomal recessive inheritance, even on the basis of a small sample.

A logical explanation for extant data is that Müllerian aplasia is inherited in polygenic/multifactorial fashion. Indeed, this is the usual mode of inheritance for anomalies affecting either a single organ system or a single embryologically related organ system. Müllerian aplasia obviously fulfills these characteristics. Relevant as well is knowledge that after the birth of one child with a polygenic/multifactorial disorder, the recurrence risk for first-degree relatives approximates the square root of the incidence of the trait in the population. Because Müllerian aplasia is rare, the absolute recurrence risks in siblings should be low. Thus, our failure to observe affected siblings in a relatively small sample is not surprising, remaining consistent with a low (1% to 2%) recurrence risk for first-degree relatives.

Another possible explanation is genetic (etiologic) heterogeneity. A dominant or recessive gene could explain some cases, whereas nongenetic factors or polygenic/multifactorial inheritance could explain most. Genetic heterogeneity would explain discrepancies between our data and that of Shokeir.[11] Shokeir's sample was derived from a different population, in which a different gene could have been segregating. Genetic heterogeneity could be deduced if a distinctive somatic anomaly were present in one patient subset. Renal and vertebral anomalies are not unexpected in Müllerian aplasia, for they involve embryologically related systems. Of note, however, is the coexistence of Müllerian aplasia and the Klippel-Feil anomalad, sometimes also in association with middle-ear anomalies.[14-16] This triad could signify an entity distinct from the common form of Müllerian aplasia, and thus an example of genetic heterogeneity. A further observation that suggests either heterogeneity or varied expressivity is the occasional patient with an unusual degree of persistence of Müllerian remnants. Sometimes a large solid uterine remnant that contains foci of endometrial tissue persists.

In conclusion, a single mutant gene is an unlikely explanation for all cases of Müllerian aplasia, but heritable tendencies clearly exist.

TRUE DUPLICATION OF THE MÜLLERIAN DUCTS

True duplication of the uterus is a rare anomaly that probably results from division of one or both Müllerian ducts early in embryogenesis.[2] Affected individuals have two separate uteri, each of which may have two fallopian tubes. One or both uteri may be rudimentary or bicornuate. True duplication should be distinguished from incomplete Müllerian fusion, the much more common condition in which each of two hemiuteri is associated with only a single fallopian tube. The frequent clinical practice of referring to a bicornuate uterus as a "double uterus" thus constitutes a misnomer.

INCOMPLETE MÜLLERIAN FUSION

During early embryonic development, the Müllerian ducts are paired. Later they fuse and canalize to form the upper vagina, cervix, uterus, and fallopian tubes. Failure of fusion results in two hemiuteri, each associated with no more than one fallopian tube. Sometimes one of the two Müllerian ducts fails to contribute to the definitive uterus, which leads to a rudimentary horn. Renal anomalies frequently coexist. If one uterine horn is atretic, ipsilateral renal agenesis is especially common.

Several familial aggregates of incomplete Müllerian fusion have been reported. These include multiple affected siblings,[17-20] as well as affected mother and daughter.[21-24] Analogous to Müllerian aplasia, few formal genetic studies exist. In addition, the ideal genetic study can be planned but probably not performed. Such a study would necessitate subjecting asymptomatic relatives to hysterosalpingography or hysteroscopy.

Not unaware of experimental pitfalls, a small pilot study was attempted by our group.[20] We studied 24 patients ascertained from a private infertility practice. Only 1 of 37 (2.7%) sisters had a clinically *symptomatic* uterine anomaly. Not a single mother (0 of 24), maternal aunt (0 of 44), or paternal aunt (0 of 50) was affected. Of course, the 2.7% frequency of affected siblings represents merely the minimum number of affected relatives; those with minor uterine anomalies would not have been recognized. In fact, some adult women had not yet attempted pregnancy, which thus further limited the opportunity to manifest symptoms indicative of an anomaly.

Irrespective of shortcomings in experimental design, the relatively low frequency of first-degree female relatives with incomplete Müllerian fusion is not without significance. The findings are surely incompatible with an autosomal dominant or autosomal recessive etiology. That approximately 3% of female siblings were affected remains consistent with a polygenic/multifactorial cause.

HAND-FOOT-GENITAL SYNDROME AND OTHER MULTIPLE MALFORMATION SYNDROMES

The hand-foot-genital (HFG) syndrome is an

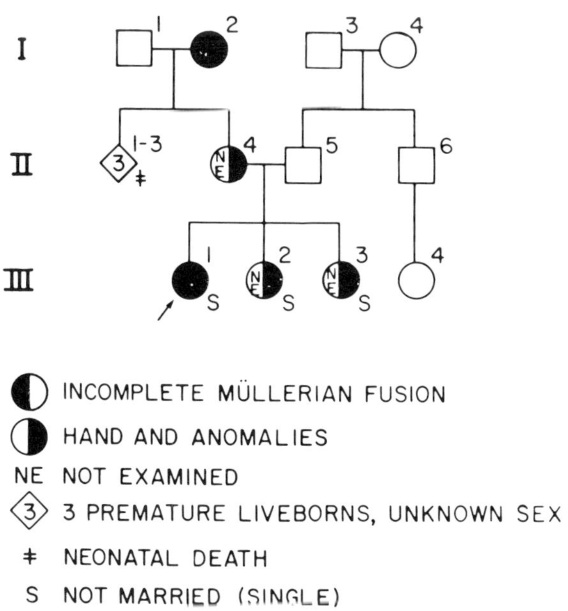

Figure 3
Partial pedigree of a family in which several members had the HFG syndrome (From Verp et al.[19])

autosomal dominant disorder characterized by skeletal (hand, foot) malformations and either incomplete Müllerian fusion in women or hypospadias in men. Coexisting urologic anomalies include urinary incontinence in women, displaced urethral meatus in either men or women, and ureteral-vesicular malposition in women.

Four families have been reported.[19, 25-27] In each, the mutant gene segregates in autosomal dominant fashion[19, 25-27] (Fig. 3). Variable expression occurs, as expected for a dominant trait. This observation is particularly relevant to gynecologists, because some women having the HFG gene may manifest only uterine anomalies or only skeletal anomalies.

Furthermore, there are several additional multiple malformation syndromes in which incomplete Müllerian fusion is only one of several components (Table 1).[19] Some syndromes result from chromosomal imbalance; others result from a single mutant gene, and in yet others the cause is unknown. Other syndromes have been claimed, but often it is not certain whether the proposed condition[28] is truly distinct from the HFG syndrome.

LEIOMYOMATA

Leiomyomas are common tumors of smooth muscle origin, well-known to physicians. Their relationship to infertility is arguable, but there seems to be a consensus that at least occasionally a correlation exists.

Most clinicians have the impression that leiomyomas are more common in blacks than in whites, although definitive studies have not been reported. Differences in racial prevalences suggest that genetic factors are important in the cause of uterine leiomyomata. Indeed, our group not infrequently observes multiple affected family members. Formal studies are limited by the inability to subject asymptomatic relatives to examinations that would detect small leiomyomas.

The one formal genetic study was questionnaire in nature, subject to inherent limitations. In 1938, Winkler and Hoffman[29] compared the prevalence of leiomyomas in relatives of 356 subjects to that in relatives of 356 control subjects. Sixty-two relatives of women with leiomyomas were said to be affected, compared with only 19 relatives of control subjects. A proband's near relative (defined by Winkler and Hoffman[29] as siblings, mother, daughters, grandmother, and granddaughters) had leiomyomas affected four times more often than did relatives of control subjects; more distant relatives were affected twice as often. Such data are consistent with a polygenic/multifactorial cause.

In conclusion, a formal study would probably confirm heritable tendencies in leiomyomas. The likely mechanism would be polygenic/multifactorial. The ideal study will be very difficult to perform, because asymptomatic relatives would need to be assessed.

ENDOMETRIOSIS

Endometriosis is an accepted explanation for female infertility, even if its precise mechanism is sometimes unclear. The disorder has long been suspected to have familial tendencies. In addition to earlier reports of familial aggregates,[30, 31] there are now several formal studies. Ranney[32] confirmed familial tendencies in a questionnaire study, and later our group[33, 34] in collaboration with colleagues at Baylor College of Medicine performed a more formal study.

In our study we ascertained 123 probands with histologically verified endometriosis. Nine of 153 (5.9%) female siblings over 18 years of age were considered similarly affected, based upon reviews of relatives' medical records. Ten of 123 (8.1%)

Table 1. *Multiple Malformation Syndromes with Anomalies of the Uterus or Vagina*[a]

Syndrome	Uterine or vaginal anomaly	Prominent somatic features	Cause
Beckwith Wiedemann	Bicornuate uterus	Macroglossia, omphalocele, macrosomia	Unknown
Donohue (Leprechaunism)	Bicornuate uterus	Elfin facies with thick lips, large low-set ears, prominent breasts and external genitalia, hirsutism, abnormal carbohydrate metabolism (hypoglycemia, hyperinsulinism, hyperplasia of islets of Langerhans), failure to thrive, motor and mental retardation	Autosomal recessive
Edwards and Gale	Longitudinal vaginal septum	Urinary incontinence due to bladder neck abnormality, flexion contractions of distal interphalangeal joints, brachydactyly, syndactyly, polydactyly	Autosomal dominant
Exstrophy of cloaca	Bicornuate uterus; short septate, or atretic vagina	Omphalocele, hydromyelia, exstrophy of cloaca, rudimentary hindgut with imperforate anus, failure of fusion of pubic rami and genital tubercles, cryptorchidism in men	Unknown
Fraser	Bicornuate uterus, vaginal atresia (absence of lower vagina with intact upper vagina)	Cryptophthalmos, external ear anomalies, syndactyly	Autosomal recessive
Hand-Foot-Genital	Bicornuate uterus	Metacarpal and metatarsal anomalies, malformed thumbs, hypospadias in men	Autosomal dominant
Johanson-Blizzard	Longitudinal vaginal septum	Deafness, hypoplastic alae nasi, primary hypothyroidism, mental retardation	Probably autosomal recessive
McKusick-Kaufman	Transverse vaginal septum	Congenital heart defect, postaxial polydactyly	Autosomal recessive
Laryngeal atresia	Bicornuate uterus	Hydrocephaly, complete or partial laryngeal obstruction, tracheoesophageal fistula and/or atresia, renal hypoplasia, pedal varus deformity	Unknown
Meckel	Bicornuate uterus, longitudinal vaginal septum	Microcephaly, posterior encephalocele, eye anomalies, cleft palate, polycystic kidneys, polydactyly	Autosomal recessive
Müllerian aplasia, middle ear anomalies, Klippel-Feil anomaly	Absence of uterus and upper vagina	Malformation of malleus, incus, stapes; Klippel-Feil anomaly	Unknown
Renal agenesis, bilateral	Absence of uterus and upper vagina	Oligohydramnios, flattened (Potter) facies, pulmonary hypoplasia, absent kidneys; anal, esophageal, duodenal atresia; lower limb deformities	Unknown
Roberts	Bicornuate uterus	Sparse silvery blond hair, midfacial hemangioma, cleft lip with or without cleft palate, hypomelia, intrauterine growth retardation	Autosomal recessive
Rudiger	Bicornuate uterus	Coarse facies, absent ear cartilage, hydronephrosis secondary to ureterovesical stenosis, short digits	Possibly autosomal recessive
Thalidomide embryopathy	Bicornuate uterus, longitudinal vaginal septum, aplasia of uterus and vagina	Nasal hemangioma, neurosensory hearing loss, congenital defects, phocomelia, and other limb reduction defects	Teratogen
Trisomy 18	Bicornuate uterus	Prominent occiput, malformed ears, micrognathia, short sternum, cardiac defects, horseshoe kidney and other renal anomalies, overlapping fingers, intrauterine growth retardation, severe developmental retardation	Chromosomal
Trisomy 13	Bicornuate uterus with or without septate vagina	Microcephaly, microphthalmia, malformed ears, cleft lip and palate, cardiac anomalies, polydactyly, intrauterine growth retardation	Chromosomal
Winter	Vaginal atresia (absence of lower vagina)	Middle ear anomalies, renal hypoplasia or agenesis	Autosomal recessive

[a]Other possible multiple malformation syndromes have been claimed (e.g., Bernhisel et al.[28]). However, these "syndromes" have not been verified as independent entities. (This table is modified from Verp et al.[19])

mothers were affected. Only 1% of the patient's husband's first-degree relatives (control subjects) had endometriosis. The magnitude of the increased risk (7% for first-degree relatives) suggests polygenic/multifactorial tendencies. Of course, other relatives could have had unrecognized disease, which would make our 7% recurrence risk spuriously low. In fact, the frequency of affected relatives would surely be higher if one could directly measure a mutant gene's product. Thus, single-gene (dominant) inheritance is not formally excluded. Since our original study, we have encountered at least five additional familial aggregates,[34] which has helped to minimize the possibility of selection bias in our original sample.

Relevant to the mode of inheritance is our observation that patients with an affected sibling or an affected mother are especially likely to have severe endometriosis. In our study, severe endometriosis was present in 11 of the 18 probands (61%) who had an affected first-degree relative.[34] By contrast, severe endometriosis was present in only 25 of the 105 subjects (23%) who did not have an affected first-degree relative. The higher frequency of severe endometriosis in familial cases is consistent with predictions based upon a polygenic/multifactorial model, because an axiom of this model is the prediction that the greater a disease's severity, the greater its genetic liability for near relatives. Our observations concerning severity also lessen the likelihood that endometriosis was detected in one family member merely because a similar diagnosis had already been made in another.

Although polygenic/multifactorial factors seem a likely explanation for familial endometriosis, another genetic explanation, genetic (etiologic) heterogeneity, cannot be excluded. That both familial and nonfamilial endometriosis cases differ only with respect to quantitative phenomena (e.g., severity of disease) provides some evidence against heterogeneity. We later sought evidence for genetic heterogeneity by separately studying familial and nonfamilial subjects for HLA associations. Neither familial nor nonfamilial probands could be distinguished on the basis of HLA studies.[35, 36] Likewise, no particular HLA antigen proved increased in frequency, based on 53 subjects.

The fact that endometriosis is familial and probably genetic has important clinical implications. First, the likelihood that an affected patient's female sibling or mother will be similarly affected is 7%. Although our studies did not formally determine the likelihood that daughters of affected individuals would be affected, one would expect the risk for all first-degree relatives (siblings, parents, and offspring) to be similar, because in each relationship the percentage of genes shared is 50%. More distant relatives (e.g., cousins, nieces) should be affected much less often, perhaps 1% or less. Second, knowledge that a first-degree relative has endometriosis may influence several clinical decisions. What is the recommended timing of childbearing? A positive family history might favor early rather than delayed childbearing. What form of contraception is most advisable? Oral contraceptives would seem to be preferable to intrauterine contraceptive devices.

Finally, the existence of genetic factors should be weighed when the pathogenesis of endometriosis is considered. The thesis that endometriosis is caused by menstrual reflex seems less tenable than previously. Some inherited factor must in addition confer increased susceptibility toward development of endometriosis. Perhaps the pathogenesis involves tubal dyskinesia predisposing to reflux or increased susceptibility of coelomic epithelium to metaplasia as a result of exposure to menstrual fluid.

POLYCYSTIC OVARY SYNDROME AND CHRONIC ANOVULATION

Polycystic ovary syndrome (PCO) is a common disorder that has traditionally been characterized by polycystic ovaries, hirsutism, and anovulation. Secondary amenorrhea is not uncommon, but primary amenorrhea is unusual. Gonadotropin secretion is altered, showing elevated luteinizing hormone/follicle-stimulating hormone (LH/FSH) ratios. Whether an alteration in the LH/FSH ratio is the primary defect is arguable.

The pathogenesis is surely heterogeneous. Increased body fat alone could lead to increased estrone, as a result of increased peripheral conversion from androstenedione. Anovulation might then arise secondarily, leading to an elevated LH/FSH ratio. In nonobese women, the LH/FSH ratio could be elevated for other (primary) reasons. The initial defect might involve increased secretion of bioavailable androgens or hypothalamic dysfunction. In still other cases, completely different causes exist.

Let us first consider a cause of polycystic ovarian disease (PCOD) that is rare but whose genetics is known: adult-onset and cryptic 21-hydroxylase deficiency. These two defects are probably caused by alleles at the same locus as that responsible for congenital adrenal hyperplasia. The locus is on chromosome 6, closely linked to HLA.[37, 38] Women with adult-onset 21-hydroxylase show hirsutism and anovulation.[37, 39-44] Women who show elevated 17α-hydroxyprogesterone but no clinical symptoms are believed to have one congenital-onset and one cryptic allele[37, 38]; however, other explanations are possible.

Women with adult-onset 21-hydroxylase deficiency may be indistinguishable from hirsute women who have other causes, which include PCOD. In fact, relatively high proportions of hirsute women have been claimed to have 21-hydroxylase deficiency.[39-44] However, Chetkowski et al.[45] found only one case of adult-onset 21-hydroxylase deficiency among 83 unselected hirsute women (1.2%), as determined by exaggerated response of serum 17α-hydroxyprogesterone to adrenocorticotropic hormone. One confounding variable in determining relative frequency is that adult-onset (attenuated) 21-hydroxylase deficiency occurs more often in women with HLA-B-14.[38, 46, 47] In addition, combined 21- and 11β-hydroxylase deficiency also may produce hirsutism as its only symptom.[48] (Although Hurwitz et al.[48] showed linkage of combined deficiency to HLA, adult-onset hirsutism associated with 11β-hydroxylase alone is clearly not linked to HLA.[49] This same holds true for 3β-ol dehydrogenase deficiency.[50]) Overall, the contribution of these enzyme deficiencies to hirsutism and PCOD is uncertain. A primary pathogenic relationship may exist, but in some cases anovulatory women may manifest an enzyme deficiency secondary to suppression induced by anovulation. The frequency with which primary adrenal enzyme defects cause PCOD thus remains uncertain.

Do heritable tendencies exist in those forms of PCOD in which LH/FSH ratios are increased and in which adrenal hyperplasia can be excluded? Indeed, familial aggregates are commonly reported. There are reports of affected siblings,[51, 52] concordant monozygotic twins,[53-55] and affected mother and daughter.[56-58] There are fewer systematic genetic studies.

The first formal study was conducted in 1968 by Cooper et al.,[59] who studied 18 women with the "Stein-Leventhal syndrome." Oligomenorrhea existed in 4 mothers of 13 subjects but in none of 13 control mothers. Oligomenorrhea similarly occurred much more commonly in sisters of subjects (9 of 19) than in sisters of control subjects (1 of 18). Hirsutism was likewise more common in relatives. Under culdoscopy, eight cases of Stein-Leventhal syndrome were detected among 12 relatives of affected women. Male relatives also showed an increased prevalence of pilosity. (We shall see below that another study showed opposite findings in men.) Irrespective, these data suggested autosomal dominant inheritance with decreased penetrance. Indeed, autosomal dominant genes are characterized by varied expressivity, a phenomenon well established in PCOD.

Investigators at the University of Tennessee later concluded that PCOD, especially hyperthecosis, was inherited in X-linked dominant fashion.[60-62] In this study, many female relatives showed oligomenorrhea or hirsutism; some male relatives were infertile and showed large testes. Elevated LH/FSH ratios were observed in various family members in a pattern suggestive of dominant inheritance. Overall, 47% of female offspring of affected women were considered affected on the basis of elevated LH/FSH ratios; 89% of female offspring of affected men (i.e., men with elevated LH/FSH ratios) were affected. That almost all daughters of affected men were affected is consistent with X-linked dominant inheritance. In fact, X-linked tendencies had previously been suggested by Netter et al.[63] and Ginsberg and Havard.[64]

Ferriman and Purdie[65] determined the frequency of oligomenorrhea and infertility among first-degree relatives of 284 hirsute French women. The control group consisted of 179 normal women. Hirsutism, oligomenorrhea, and evidence for ovarian enlargement were sought in relatives. Frequencies of affected relatives were tabulated separately for subjects with or without hirsutism as well as with or without enlarged ovaries. In particular, the status of relatives of women with enlarged ovaries but no hirsutism was sought. Table 2 summarizes the findings. Familial tendencies were greatest among hirsute women with enlarged ovaries; however, far fewer than 50% of relatives were similarly affected. In addition, premature male baldness was significantly more frequent in relatives of hirsute women than in either relatives of control subjects or relatives of nonhirsute women with enlarged

Table 2. *Prevalence of Hirsutism and Oligomenorrhea in Relatives of Women with Specific Clinical Features*[a]

Clinical features	No. of subjects	Affected first-degree relatives: Hirsutism No.	Hirsutism %	Oligomenorrhea No.	Oligomenorrhea %
Hirsutism					
Ovarian enlargement	188	38	20	30	16
No ovarian enlargement	96	13	14	15	16
No hirsutism					
Ovarian enlargement	45	1	2	8	18
No ovarian enlargement	45	1	2	7	16

[a]From Ferriman and Purdie.[65]

ovaries. Ferriman and Purdie[65] concluded that a modified dominant disorder exists in some families. This disorder is characterized by hirsutism, oligomenorrhea, infertility, and sometimes polycystic ovaries (women) or premature balding (men). By contrast, a second group of women was considered to show oligomenorrhea, infertility, and sometimes enlarged ovaries; however, neither hirsutism nor premature male baldness was common.

The studies cited above make it clear that heritable tendencies are indeed detected in PCO. On the other hand, the mode or modes of inheritance remains unclear. In most studies, far fewer than 50% of first-degree relatives are usually affected. Indeed, symptomatic disease occurs in only perhaps 5% to 10% of first-degree relatives. Either of several genetic mechanisms could exist, especially dominant factors or polygenic/multifactorial factors. For various reasons it will be difficult to distinguish between these possibilities. One reason is the inevitable selection bias. What is the population base of a given sample? How representative is the sample? Indeed, some of the confusion concerning the role of genetic factors in PCO is probably the inevitable result of unwittingly pooling subjects with diverse causes.

Identification of the primary defect would enable the gene product to be measured in all relatives, which would thus provide more precise statements. (Elevated LH/FSH ratios may or may not reflect the primary defect.) Even in the absence of a primary gene product, analysis of subgroups separated according to clinical criteria (e.g., obese or nonobese) might be enlightening. One study sought to demonstrate linkage between HLA and nonadrenal PCO. Mandel et al.[52] studied HLA types in 23 probands. Included in the sample were four families in each of which two siblings showed PCO. Neither linkage nor HLA association was observed.

One final issue is the uncertain relationship between PCO and X-chromosomal abnormalities. Many authors have reported polycystic changes in women with X-chromosomal abnormalities such as 45,X/46,XX or 46,XX/46,X,del(Xq).[66-68] Parker et al.[68] provide a recent review. Our group has studied a fertile 45,X/46,X,i(Xq) woman who had a left polycystic ovary and a right streak gonad.[69] The above observations might merely reflect coincidence, biases of reporting, or ascertainment. Consistent with this possibility is the failure of Stenchever et al.[70] to detect X abnormalities among one group of 41 PCO patients. The potential relationship thus remains arguable, although a logical claim can be made for PCO and X abnormalities being pathogenically related.[66]

OVARIAN UNRESPONSIVENESS OF GONADOTROPINS

Primary as well as secondary amenorrhea may result from gonadotropin resistance. Gonadotropin levels are elevated. Breast development and pubic hair growth occurs. Thus, affected women are generally normal in appearance. Their ovaries may be longer and thinner than normal (fat streaks), but ovarian follicles are present. Possible mechanisms include functionally abnormal FSH or LH, autoimmunity, or receptor abnormalities. FSH and LH seem normal by both immunoassay and bioassay, and autoimmunity does not seem to be of primary pathogenic importance. Deoxyribonucleic acid (DNA)-sequencing studies are awaited with interest.

Although familial aggregates of gonadotropin resistance have not been reported, receptor defects involving other organ systems invariably prove to be genetic. Usually the mechanism involves a single mutant gene, as exemplified by X-linked androgen insensitivity. Because women with gonadotropin resistance do not usually reproduce, dominant inheritance may prove difficult to recognize. A somatic marker (e.g., associated skeletal defect) would be helpful, and linkage analysis and cloning studies might eventually be informative. Recessive factors would be evident by affected siblings, an observation not yet recorded.

X-CHROMOSOMAL ABNORMALITIES, XX GONADAL DYSGENESIS, AND FAMILIAL PREMATURE OVARIAN FAILURE

More than half of all women with ovarian failure (ovarian or gonadal dysgenesis) show complete or partial absence of the X chromosome.[2, 71, 72] Most of the remainder have a mutant X-linked recessive or autosomal recessive gene, respectively, XY gonadal dysgenesis or XX gonadal dysgenesis.[73] Nongenetic factors also cause ovarian failure,[74] but segregation analyses by our group indicate that nongenetic explanations for XX gonadal dysgenesis constitute a minority.

Although the sex chromosome abnormalities and mutant genes mentioned above more often cause primary amenorrhea and complete ovarian failure, it is becoming increasingly evident that these same etiologic processes may sometimes be responsible for only partial ovarian dysfunction. In other words, these processes may cause anovulation, oligomenorrhea, and later *premature* ovarian failure. Thus, sex chromosomal abnormalities and XX gonadal dysgenesis must be entertained as possibilities in women with infertility.

Discussing the genetic causes of female infertility will thus require our briefly reviewing three seemingly disparate but actually interrelated topics: (1) X-chromosomal abnormalities, (2) 46,XX gonadal dysgenesis, and (3) familial premature ovarian failure.

X-CHROMOSOME ABNORMALITIES

Approximately 50% of all patients with gonadal dysgenesis have a 45,X complement, and 25% have sex chromosomal mosaicism without a structural abnormality (e.g., 45,X/46,XX).[2] Far fewer have a structurally abnormal X or Y. In those 45,X patients who survive until adulthood, the normal gonad is usually replaced by a white fibrous streak 2 to 3 cm long and about 0.5 cm wide. The streak is located in the position ordinarily occupied by the ovary. Of clinical relevance are observations that absence of oocytes in monosomy X is the result of increased oocyte atresia, not failure of oocyte formation. 45,X embryos and 45,X neonates have germ cells.[75, 76] It is thus not too surprising that an occasional 45,X patient menstruates spontaneously and even becomes pregnant.[77, 78]

45,X/46,XX women have fewer anomalies than 45,X women. In one survey by this author, 12% of 45,X/46,XX women menstruated; only 3% of 45,X women menstruated.[2] Probably many mosaic women are so mildly affected that they are never even detected. 45,X and especially 45,X/46,XX women may thus be encountered during infertility evaluations.

DELETIONS OF THE X SHORT ARM [del(Xp)] AND X LONG ARM [del(Xq)]

Deletion of the X short arm may be associated with complete ovarian failure (primary amenorrhea), but less severe abnormalities (premature ovarian failure) may also occur. Spontaneous menstruation, albeit often leading to *secondary* amenorrhea, occurs in almost 40% of 46,X,del(X)(p11) women.[71, 72] Almost all 46,X,del(X)(*P*21 or 22) individuals are fertile.[71, 72] In addition, there have been reports of siblings showing del(X)(p11) or del(X)(p21). Usually, their mother had an X-autosome translocation, transmitting the deleted (Xp) chromosome but not the autosome to the daughters.

Analogous to del(Xp), many women with deletion of the X long arm never menstruate.[71, 72] Deletions or X-autosomal translocations involving the region Xq13 to Xq26 seem especially likely to be associated with sterility.[71, 72, 79, 80] This indicates that either (1) important ovarian determinants exist in this region, or (2) the entire region must remain unperturbed (critical) for ovarian function. However, menstruation and breast development *do* occur in some 20% of del(X)(q13,22 or 24) women.[71, 72] Those with more distal deletions, namely Xq26, menstruate even more commonly; however, they may show premature ovarian failure. A 46,X,del(X)(q26) deletion has been transmitted from a mother to her two daughters; all three had premature ovarian failure.[81]

X-chromosomal abnormalities (monosomy X; 45,X/46,XX; 46,X,del(Xp); 46,X,del(Xq)) thus do not always produce complete ovarian failure. Premature ovarian failure or merely anovulation may occur. Cytogenetic examination should not be restricted to women with primary amenorrhea but should be considered when examining infertile women.

Table 3. *Multiple Malformation Syndromes in Which 46,XX Patients Show Streak Gonad*

Author	Somatic findings
Maximilian et al.[89]	Short stature, microcephaly, mental retardation, arachnodactyly
Hamet et al.[90]	Neurosensory deafness, adrenal hyperplasia, renal failure, decreased spermatogenesis in men
Skre et al.[91]	Cerebellar ataxia
Lundgren[92]	Mental retardation, myopathy

XX GONADAL DYSGENESIS

The external genitalia and the streak gonads of patients with XX gonadal dysgenesis are morphologically indistinguishable from those of patients who have gonadal dysgenesis because of an abnormal chromosomal complement. Likewise, the endocrine profile in XX gonadal dysgenesis does not differ from that of other patients with streak gonads. However, patients with XX gonadal dysgenesis are usually normal in stature.

In 1960, De Court and associates[82] were the first to report a patient with gonadal dysgenesis and an apparently normal female (46,XX) complement. By 1971, Simpson and colleagues[83] had tabulated 61 patients with XX gonadal dysgenesis. They concluded that the disorder was inherited in an autosomal recessive fashion, based upon frequent occurrence of multiple affected siblings and the presence of increased parental consanguinity. Available data have since continued to support autosomal recessive inheritance.

Although the typical patient with XX gonadal dysgenesis is of normal stature and lacks somatic anomalies, neurosensory deafness has been observed in some families (siblings).[84-88] The coexistence of XX gonadal dysgenesis and neurosensory deafness suggests the existence of a mutant autosomal recessive allele differing from that producing XX gonadal dysgenesis without deafness. Alternatively, pleiotropy for a single mutant gene is possible. In at least four other families, there exist mutant genes responsible for gonadal dysgenesis.[89-92] Unique genes can in each family be assumed to exist, based upon presence of distinctive multiple malformation patterns (Table 3). In addition, individuals with galactosemia, an autosomal recessive trait, may show gonadal dysgenesis.

Of great relevance for our current discussion is evidence that varied expressivity may occur in XX gonadal dysgenesis. Evidence centers around dissimilar gonadal development in siblings. An example is the family reported by Guisti and coworkers.[93] One affected sibling had streak gonads, whereas another had primary amenorrhea and extreme ovarian hypoplasia (a few ova were detected). Boczkowski[94] described a family in which one sibling had streak gonads, whereas another menstruated spontaneously despite increased gonadotropins. Malkova et al.[95] reported further examples, and this author has encountered a family in which one sibling showed streak gonads and another sibling showed small rounded rudimentary ovaries without functioning ova. In conclusion, women carrying the recessive XX gonadal dysgenesis mutant need not have *complete* absence of oocytes, but rather less severe pathologic features. Logically, the mutant gene may be responsible for familial premature ovarian failure, especially in siblings.

FAMILIAL PREMATURE OVARIAN FAILURE

It is already evident that multiple pathogenic mechanisms are responsible for premature ovarian failure. A recent endocrine review is that of Rebar,[96] who defined the entity as menopause before age 35. Among postulated mechanisms are autoimmune factors, infiltrative diseases (e.g., sarcoidosis), environmental toxins,[74] and genetic factors. Genetic mechanisms include X deletions and XX gonadal dysgenesis, as already discussed.

Familial aggregates that ostensibly result from other causes have also been reported. Smith et al.[97] reported premature ovarian failure in three Greek siblings (one male, two female) of consanguineous parents. Coulam et al.[98] observed the same phenomenon in two affected siblings who had an affected mother and aunt. Relatives in more than one generation were also reported by Starup and Sele[99] and by Austin et al.[100] Mattison et al.[101] reported five families in which relatives in more than one generation manifested ovarian failure before age 40. Ovarian antibodies were not detected, and the authors believed their data were best explained on the basis of a mutant autosomal or X-linked dominant gene. However, the families could have been drawn from a very large population base, with familial aggregates observed by chance or on the basis of polygenic factors.

If a single gene were the cause of ovarian failure, a likely mechanism would be meiotic abnormalities. Although meiotic abnormalities associated with chromosomal abnormalities (e.g., translocations) are well-known, almost no attention has been devoted to meiotic abnormalities in cytogenetically normal men or women. This is actually not surprising, because investigations are formidable. In women, meiotic preparations are possible only by obtaining oocytes, a task requiring surgical intervention. In men, definitive meiotic studies require testicular biopsy, although sperm analysis can indirectly provide data.

In contrast to the scarcity of information in human beings is a wealth of evidence concerning meiotic mutants in plants and animals. Plant and *Drosophila* mutants were reviewed by Baker et al.[102] and mammalian mutants by Chaganti et al.[103] In addition, spermiogenesis mutants are well-known, especially in bulls. In general, meiotic mutants interfere with synapsis, that process by which homologous chromosomes become apposed during meiosis. Failure of synapsis (or desynapsis) produces meiotic breakdown. In men, the result is azoospermia. In women, the outcome is uncertain because such mutants have not been confirmed. Possible outcomes include streak gonads and 46,XX gonadal dysgenesis, rudimentary ovaries, or merely normal ovaries with decreased numbers of follicles (premature ovarian failure).

An illustrative report is that of Chaganti et al.[103] A 36-year-old Iranian man was ascertained because of azoospermia. Meiotic studies on testicular biopsy revealed asynapsis, defective synaptonemal complexes, chiasma failure, and degenerating prophase spermatocytes. His sibling had a decreased sperm count; their parents were consanguineous, which suggests autosomal recessive inheritance. The authors[103] reviewed the cases of 16 similar patients, several of whose parents were consanguineous. In view of animal models that show similar phenotypes, it is indeed reasonable to conclude that this abnormality results from one or more recessive genes.

A second meiotic mutant has been described by German et al.[104] and by Carson and Rao.[105] The former observed an infertile man of consanguineous parents. His sperm showed large heads with multiple tails; DNA content was increased fourfold (4C). Carson and Rao[105] observed an apparently identical phenomenon in each of three siblings. A maternal uncle was also infertile but could not be studied. The logical explanation for this second mutant is existence of an autosomal or X-linked recessive gene interfering with meiotic reduction. The mutant must act in both meiosis I and in meiosis II.

These few examples of human meiotic mutants represent merely exceptional reports of a surely not uncommon phenomenon. In women, analogous conditions most certainly cause infertility.

REFERENCES

1. Simpson JL, Golbus MS, Martin AO, Sarto GE: Genetics in Obstetrics and Gynecology. New York, Grune & Stratton, 1982
2. Simpson JL: Disorders of Sexual Differentiation: Etiology and Clinical Delineation. New York, Academic Press, 1976
3. Simpson JL: Abnormal sexual differentiation in humans. Annu Rev Genet 16:193, 1982
4. Petri E: Untersuchungen zur Erbbedingtheit der Menarche. Z Morphol Anthropol 33:43, 1934
5. Tisserant-Perrier M: Etude comparative de certains processus de croissance chez les jumeaux. J Genet Hum 2:87, 1953
6. Land RB, Falconer DS: Genetic studies of ovulation rates in the mouse. Genet Res 13:25, 1969
7. Kupperman HJ: Human Endocrinology, Vol 1. Philadelphia, F. A. Davis Co, 1963, p 261
8. Angel D, Hamet J, Ensel J: Forme familiale du syndrome de Rokitansky-Kuster-Hauser. Bull Féd Soc Gynecol Obstet Lang Fr 18:229, 1966
9. Jones HW Jr, Mermut S: Familial occurrence of congenital absence of the vagina. Am J Obstet Gynecol 114:1100, 1972
10. Griffin JE, Edwards C, Madden JD, Harrod MJ: Congenital absence of the vagina. The Mayer-Rokitansky-Kuster-Hauser syndrome. Ann Intern Med 85:224, 1976
11. Shokeir MHK: Aplasia of the Müllerian septum: evidence for probable sex-limited autosomal dominant inheritance. Birth Defects 14(6c):147, 1978
12. Lischke JH, Curtis CH, Lamb EJ: Discordance of vaginal agenesis in monozygotic twins. Obstet Gynecol 41:920, 1973
13. Carson SA, Simpson JL, Malinak LR, Elias S, Gerbie AB, Buttram VC Jr, Sarto GE: Heritable aspects of uterine anomalies. II. Genetic analysis of Müllerian aplasia. Fertil Steril 40:86, 1983
14. Park IJ, Jones HW Jr: A new syndrome in two unrelated females: Klippel-Feil deformity, conductive deafness, and absent vagina. Birth Defects 7(6):311, 1971
15. Baird PA, Lowry RB: Absent vagina and the Klippel-Feil anomaly. Am J Obstet Gynecol 118:290, 1974
16. Mecklenburg RS, Krueger PM: Extensive genitourinary anomalies associated with Klippel-Feil syndrome. Am J Dis Child 128:92, 1974
17. Tyler GT: Didelphys in sisters. Am J Surg 45:337, 1939
18. Polishuk WZ, Ron MA: Familial bicornuate and double uterus. Am J Obstet Gynecol 119:982, 1974
19. Verp MS, Simpson JL, Elias S, Carson SA, Sarto GE, Feingold M: Heritable aspects of uterine anomalies. I.

Three familial aggregates with Müllerian fusion anomalies. Fertil Steril 40:80, 1983
20. Elias S, Simpson JL, Carson SA, Malinak LR, Buttram VC Jr: Genetic studies in incomplete Müllerian fusion. Obstet Gynecol 63:276, 1984
21. Way S: The influence of minor degrees of failure of fusion of the Müllerian ducts on pregnancy and labour. J Obstet Gynaecol Br Emp 52:325, 1945
22. Holmes JA: Congenital abnormalities of the uterus and pregnancy. Br Med J 1:1144, 1956
23. Stevenson AC, Dudgeon MY, McClure HI: Observations on the results of pregnancies in women resident in Belfast. II. Abortions, hydatidiform moles, and ectopic pregnancies. Ann Hum Genet 23:395, 1959
24. Hay D: Uterus and unicollis and its relationship to pregnancy. J Obstet Gynaecol Br Emp 68:361, 1961
25. Stern AM, Gail JC Jr, Perry BL, Simpson CW, Weitkamp LR, Poznanski AK: The hand-foot-uterus syndrome. J Pediatr 77:109, 1970
26. Poznanski AK, Kuhns LR, Lapides J, Stern AM: A new family with the hand-foot-genital syndrome. A wider spectrum of the hand-foot-uterus syndrome. Birth Defects 11(4):127, 1975
27. Giedion A, Prader A: Hand-foot-uterus (HFU) syndrome with hypospadias. The hand-foot-genital (HFG) syndrome. Pediatr Radiol 4:96, 1976
28. Bernhisel MA, London SN, Haney AF: Unusual Müllerian anomalies associated with distal extremity abnormalities. Obstet Gynecol 65:291, 1985
29. Winkler H, Hoffman W: Zur Frage der Veriebbarket des Uterusmyom. Deutsch Med Wochenschr 64:253, 1938
30. Gardner GH, Greene RR, Ranney B: The histiogenesis of endometriosis. Obstet Gynecol 1:615, 1953
31. Frey GH: The familial occurrence of endometriosis. Am J Obstet Gynecol 73:418, 1957
32. Ranney B: Endometriosis. IV. Hereditary tendency. Obstet Gynecol 34:734, 1971
33. Simpson JL, Elias SE, Malinak LR, Buttram VC Jr: Heritable aspects of endometriosis. I. Genetic studies. Am J Obstet Gynecol 137:327, 1980
34. Malinak LR, Buttram VC Jr, Elias S, Simpson JL: Heritable aspects of endometriosis. II. Clinical characteristics of familial endometriosis. Am J Obstet Gynecol 137:332, 1980
35. Simpson JL, Malinak LR, Elias S, Carson SA, Radvany RA: HLA associations in endometriosis. Am J Obstet Gynecol 148:395, 1984
36. Elias S, Simpson JL, Malinak LR, Carson SA, Radvany RA: HLA studies in familial endometriosis. Surg Forum 34:497, 1983
37. New MI, DuPont B, Grumbach K, Levine LS: Congenital adrenal hyperplasia and related conditions. In The Metabolic Basis of Inherited Disease, Fifth edition, Edited by JB Stanbury, JB Wyngaarden, DS Frederickson, JL Goldstein, MS Brown. New York, McGraw-Hill, 1983, p 93
38. Pollack MS, Levine LS, O'Neill GJ, Pang S, Lorenzen F, Kohn B, Rondanini GF, Chiumello G, New MI: HLA linkage and B14, DR1, BFS haplotype association with the genes for late onset and cryptic 21-hydroxylase deficiency. Am J Hum Genet 33:540, 1981
39. Migeon CJ, Rosenwaks Z, Lee PA, Urban MD, Bias WB: The attenuated form of congenital adrenal hyperplasia as an allelic form of 21-hydroxylase deficiency. J Clin Endocrinol Metab 51:647, 1980
40. Newmark S, Dluhy RG, Williams GH, Pochi P, Rose LI: Partial 11- and 21-hydroxylase deficiencies in hirsute women. Am J Obstet Gynecol 127:594, 1977
41. Lobo RA, Goebelsmann U: Adult manifestation of congenital adrenal hyperplasia due to incomplete 21-hydroxylase deficiency mimicking polycystic ovarian disease. Am J Obstet Gynecol 138:720, 1980
42. Chrousos GP, Loriaux DL, Mann DL, Cutler GB: Late-onset 21-hydroxylase deficiency mimicking idiopathic hirsutism or polycystic ovarian disease. Ann Intern Med 96:143, 1982
43. Gibson M, Lackritz R, Schiff I, Tulchinsky D: Abnormal adrenal responses to adrenocorticotropic hormone in hyperandrogenic women. Fertil Steril 33:43, 1980
44. Ayers JWT: Differential response to adrenocorticotropin hormone stimulation in polycystic ovarian disease with high and low dehydroepiandrosterone sulfate levels. Fertil Steril 37:645, 1982
45. Chetkowski RJ, DeFazio J, Shamonki I, Judd HL, Chang RJ: The incidence of late-onset congenital adrenal hyperplasia due to 21-hydroxylase deficiency among hirsute women. J Clin Endocrinol Metab 58:595, 1984
46. Holler W, Scholz S, Knorr D, Bidlingmaier F, Keller E, Albert ED: Genetic differences between the salt-wasting, simple virilizing, and nonclassical types of congenital adrenal hyperplasia. J Clin Endocrinol Metab 60:757, 1985
47. Libber SM, Migeon CJ, Bias WB: Ascertainment of 21-hydroxylase deficiency in individuals with HLA-B14 haplotype. J Clin Endocrinol Metab 60:727, 1985
48. Hurwitz A, Brautbar C, Milwidsky A, Wecsei P, Milewicz A, Navot D, Rosler A: Combined 21- and 11β-hydroxylase deficiency in familial congenital adrenal hyperplasia. J Clin Endocrinol Metab 60:631, 1985
49. Gabrilove JL, Sharma DC, Dorfman RI: Adrenocortical 11β-hydroxylase deficiency and virilism first manifest in the adult woman. N Engl J Med 272:1189, 1965
50. Pang S, Lerner AJ, Stoner E, Levine LS, Oberfield SE, Engel I, New MI: Late onset adrenal steroid 3β-hydroxysteroid dehydrogenase deficiency. I. A cause of hirsutism in pubertal and postpubertal women. J Clin Endocrinol Metab 60:428, 1985
51. Evans TM, Riley GM: Polycystic ovarian disease. Am J Obstet Gynecol 77:873, 1960
52. Mandel FP, Chang RJ, DuPont B, Pollack MS, Levine LS, New MI, Lu JKH, Judd HL: HLA genotyping in family members and patients with familial polycystic ovarian disease. J Clin Endocrinol Metab 56:862, 1983
53. Goldzieher JW, Green JA: The polycystic ovary. I. Clinical and histological features. J Clin Endocrinol 22:325, 1962
54. Jeffcoate TNA: The androgenic ovary, with special reference to the Stein-Leventhal Syndrome. Am J Obstet Gynecol 88:143, 1964
55. McDonough PG, Mahesh VB, Ellegood JO: Steroid, follicle-stimulating hormone, and luteinizing hormone profiles in identical twins with polycystic ovaries. Am J Obstet Gynecol 113:1072, 1972
56. Scully RE: Cited in Case Records of the Massachusetts General Hospital (Case 43481). N Engl J Med 257:1086, 1957

57. Suzor R, Falloux P: Is the Stein-Leventhal syndrome hereditary? Bull Féd Soc Gynecol Obstet Lang Fr 13:12, 1961
58. Judd HL, Scully RE, Herbst AL, Yen SSC, Ingersol FM, Klinman B: Familial hyperthecosis: comparison of endocrinology and histologic findings with polycystic ovarian disease. Am J Obstet Gynecol 117:976, 1973
59. Cooper HE, Spellacy WN, Prem KA, Cohen WD: Hereditary factors in the Stein-Leventhal syndrome. Am J Obstet Gynecol 100:371, 1968
60. Cohen PN, Givens JR, Wiser WL, Wilroy RS, Summitt RL, Coleman SA, Andersen RN: Polycystic ovarian disease, maturation arrest of spermiogenesis, and Klinefelter's syndrome in siblings of a family with familial hirsutism. Fertil Steril 26:1228, 1975
61. Wilroy RS Jr, Givens JR, Wiser WL, Coleman SA, Andersen RN, Summitt RL: Hyperthecosis: an inheritable form of polycystic ovarian disease. Birth Defects 11(4):81, 1975
62. Givens JR, Wiser WL, Coleman SA, Wilroy RS, Andersen RN, Fish SA, Watson BS: Familial ovarian hyperthecosis: a study of two families. Am J Obstet Gynecol 110:959, 1971
63. Netter A, Bloch-Michel H, Solomon Y, Thervet F, deGrouchy J, Lamy M: Etude du caryotype dans la maladie de Stein-Leventhal. Ann Endocrinol (Paris) 22:841, 1961
64. Ginsberg J, Havard CWH: Polycystic ovary disease. Br Med J 2:737, 1976
65. Ferriman D, Purdie AW: The inheritance of polycystic ovarian disease and a possible relationship to premature balding. Clin Endocrinol (Oxf) 11:291, 1979
66. Givens JR, Wilroy RS, Summitt RL, Andersen RN, Wiser WL, Fish SA: Features of Turner's syndrome in women with polycystic ovaries. Obstet Gynecol 45:619, 1975
67. Gardo S, Papp Z, Smid I, Borsos A: Cytogenetic studies in Stein-Leventhal syndrome. Arch Gynecol 216:311, 1974
68. Parker R, Ming P-ML, Rajan R, Goodner DM, Reme G: Clinical and cytogenetic studies of patients with polycystic ovary disease. Am J Obstet Gynecol 137:656, 1980
69. Elias S, Martin AO, Simpson JL: Longitudinal stability of sex chromosome mosaicism. Am J Obstet Gynecol 136:509, 1980
70. Stenchever MA, MacIntyre MN, Jarvis JL, Hempel JM: Cytogenetic evaluation of 41 patients with Stein-Leventhal Syndrome. Obstet Gynecol 32:794, 1968
71. Simpson JL, LeBeau MM: Gonadal and statural determinants on the X chromosome and their relationship to in vitro studies showing prolonged cell cycles in 45,X; 46,X,del(X)(p11): 46,X,del(X)(q13) and (q22) fibroblasts. Am J Obstet Gynecol 141:698, 1981
72. Simpson JL: Ovarian dysgenesis and related genetic disorders. In Gynecologic Endocrinology, Fourth edition, Edited by JJ Gold, JM Josimovich. Philadelphia, Plenum. In press
73. Simpson JL: Genetic forms of gonadal dysgenesis in 46,XX and 46,XY individuals. Semin Reprod Endocrinol 1:93, 1983
74. Verp MS: Environmental causes of ovarian failure. Semin Reprod Endocrinol 1:101, 1983
75. Singh RP, Carr DK: The anatomy and histology of XO human embryos and fetuses. Anat Rec 155:369, 1966
76. Jirasek J: Principles of reproductive embryology. In Disorders of Sexual Differentiation, Edited by JL Simpson. New York, Academic Press, 1976, p 51
77. Simpson JL: Pregnancies in women with chromosomal abnormalities. In Genetic Diseases in Pregnancy, Edited by JD Schulman, JL Simpson. New York, Academic Press, 1981, p 439
78. Dewhurst J: Fertility in 47,XXX and 45,X patients. J Med Genet 15:132, 1978
79. Mattei M, Mattei JF, Vidal I, Giraud F: Structural anomalies of the X chromosome and inactivation center. Hum Genet 56:401, 1981
80. Madan K: Balanced structural changes involving the human X: effect on sexual phenotype. Hum Genet 63:216, 1983
81. Fitch N, DeSaint Victor J, Richer CZ, Pinsky L, Sitahal S: Premature menopause due to a small deletion in the long arm of the X chromosome: a report of three cases and a review. Am J Obstet Gynecol 142:968, 1982
82. DeCourt J, Michaud JP, Delzant G: Syndrome de Turner avec caryotype feminin normal. Rev Fr Endocrinol Clin Nutr Metab 1:321, 1960
83. Simpson JL, Christakos AC, Horwith M, Silverman FS: Gonadal dysgenesis in individuals with apparently normal chromosomal complements: tabulation of cases and compilation of genetic data. Birth Defects 7(6):215, 1971
84. Perrault M, Klotz P, Housset E: Deux cas de syndrome de Turner avec surdi-mutite dans une meme fratrie. Bull Soc Med Hop (Paris) 67:79, 1951
85. Christakos AC, Simpson JL, Younger JB, Christian CD: Gonadal dysgenesis as an autosomal recessive condition. Am J Obstet Gynecol 104:1027, 1969
86. Greenblatt RB, Byrd JR, McDonough PG, Mahesh VB: The spectrum of gonadal dysgenesis. Am J Obstet Gynecol 98:151, 1967
87. Perez-Ballester B, Greenblatt RB, Byrd JR: Familial gonadal dysgenesis. Am J Obstet Gynecol 107:1261, 1970
88. Pallister PD, Opitz JM: The Perrault syndrome: autosomal recessive ovarian dysgenesis with facultative, non-sex-limited sensorineural deafness. Am J Med Genet 4:239, 1979
89. Maximilian C, Ionescu B, Bucur A: Deux soers avec dysgenesie gonadique majeure, hypotrophic staturale, microcephalie, arachnodactylie et caryotype 46,XX. J Genet Hum 18:365, 1970
90. Hamet P, Kuchel O, Nowacinski W, Rojo-Ortega JM, Sasaki C, Genest J: Hypertension with adrenal, genital, renal defects, and deafness. Arch Intern Med 131.563, 1973
91. Skre H, Bassöe HH, Berg K, Frövig AG: Cerebellar ataxia and hypergonadotropic hypogonadism in two kindreds. Chance concurrence, pleiotropism or linkage? Clin Genet 9:234, 1976
92. Lundgren PO: Hereditary myopathy, oligophrenia, cataract, skeletal abnormalities and hypergonadotropic hypogonadism: a new syndrome. Eur Neurol 10:261, 1973
93. Guisti G, Borghi A, Salti M, Bigozzi U: "Disgenesia gonadica pura," con cariotipo 44A + XX in sorelle figlie di cugini. Acta Genet Med Gemellol (Roma) 15:51, 1966
94. Boczkowski K: Pure gonadal dysgenesis and ovarian dysplasia in sisters. Am J Obstet Gynecol 106:626, 1970

95. Malkova J, Chrz R, Motik K, Starka L, Kobilkova J, Silinkova-Malkova E: 46,XX gonadal dysgenesis and ovarian hypoplasia. Humangenetik 23:205, 1974
96. Rebar RW: Premature menopause. Semin Reprod Endocrinol 1:161, 1983
97. Smith A, Fraser IS, Noel ML: Three siblings with premature gonadal failure. Fertil Steril 32:528, 1979
98. Coulam CB, Stringfellow S, Hoefnagel D: Evidence for a genetic factor in the etiology of premature ovarian failure. Fertil Steril 40:693, 1983
99. Starup J, Sele V: Premature ovarian failure. Acta Obstet Gynecol Scand 52:259, 1973
100. Austin GE, Coulam CB, Ryan RJ: A search for antibodies to luteinizing hormone receptors in premature ovarian failure. Mayo Clin Proc 54:394, 1979
101. Mattison DR, Evans MI, Schwimmer WB, White BJ, Jensen B, Schulman JD: Familial premature ovarian failure. Am J Hum Genet 36:1341, 1984
102. Baker BS, Carpenter ATC, Esposito MS, Esposito RE, Sandler L: The genetic control of meiosis. Annu Rev Genet 10:53, 1976
103. Chaganti RSK, Jhanwan SC, Ehrenbard LT, Kourides IA, William JJ: Genetically determined asynapsis, spermatogenic degeneration and infertility in men. Am J Hum Genet 32:833, 1980
104. German J, Rasch EM, Huang CY, MacLeod J, Imperato-McGinley J: Human infertility due to production of multiple-tailed spermatozoa with excessive amounts of DNA. Am J Hum Genet 33:64A, 1981
105. Carson SA, Rao R: Mutant gene causing large sperm heads with multiple tails. In Abstracts of the Thirtieth Annual Meeting of the Society for Gynecologic Investigation, Washington, D.C., March 17 to 20, 1983, p 271

Chapter 16

Isosexual precocity: current concepts and recent advances

Allen W. Root, M.D.
Dorothy I. Shulman, M.D.

Department of Pediatrics, University of South Florida College of Medicine, Tampa, and All Children's Hospital, St. Petersburg, Florida

Isosexual precocity (precocious puberty) is the appearance of phenotypically appropriate primary or secondary sexual characteristics before the age of 8 years in girls and the age of 9 years in boys.[1] Common findings in girls with isosexual precocity include rapid linear growth, development of breasts (thelarche), pubic and axillary sexual hair (pubarche), and menses (menarche). In the sexually precocious boy, deepening of the voice, acne, phallic, scrotal, and testicular enlargement, and pubic and axillary hair may be present. In this section we will discuss newer developments and concepts concerning the diagnosis and management of children with true and complete (central) isosexual precocity, the newly described entity of gonadotropin-independent isosexual precocity ("testotoxicosis," which, we will learn, is too restricted a term), and the evolving entity of premature adrenarche, which in some patients may represent variant forms of congenital adrenal hyperplasia.

Many hormonal changes accompany the physical signs of puberty. With advancing age through childhood, hypothalamic maturation progresses to the point where episodic secretory pulses of gonadotropin-releasing hormone (GnRH) increase to a frequency (and perhaps amplitude) sufficient to stimulate pituitary gonadotroph release of luteinizing hormone (LH) and follicle-stimulating hormone (FSH). These are glycoproteins with alpha and beta subunits. Biologic activity of the gonadotropin depends upon the specificity of the beta subunit and the degree of glycosylation of the molecule. The more glycosylated and basic the LH species is the greater is the biologic activity.[2] The mechanism by which the frequency of GnRH secretory pulses increase with advancing age is unknown; there may be waning of intrahypothalamic or extrahypothalamic inhibitory neural signals which impinge upon the cells and neural processes in the anterior and basomedial hypothalamus which synthesize, transport, store, and secrete GnRH. The hypothalamic-pituitary unit is quite sensitive to the suppressive effects of sex hormones during childhood; but, in addition, there is "central restraint" of puberty in these years.[3] The earliest hormonal change in puberty is increase in sleep-associated secretion of immunoreactive (i) LH (and testosterone [T] in the male), which appears in the late childhood-early pubertal period. By 10 to 11 years of age diurnal serum concentrations of iLH and iFSH begin to increase, followed by progressive increase in serum T and/or estradiol (E_2) levels. The radioimmunologic characteristics of iLH alter during puberty, probably reflecting an increase in the glycosylation of the LH molecule. Total serum biologic (b) LH activity also increases during puberty, but the basal bLH/iLH (b/i) ratio does not change.[2] In both sexes the secretion of LH becomes clearly episodic during puberty; in girls cyclic release of LH and FSH can be demonstrated. There is increased sensitivity of the gonadotrophs to the LH-releasing effects of GnRH, seen in both early pubertal boys and girls. FSH secretion in response to GnRH does not change greatly with the onset of puberty in males, but declines in females. The inhibitory effect of sex hormones upon gonadotropin secretion declines, and a positive or stimulatory effect of estrogens upon LH release is demonstrable in girls by midpuberty. The stimulatory effect of human chorionic gonadotropin (hCG) upon Leydig cell secretion of T increases with advancing maturation in males. Serum concentrations of the adrenal androgens dehydroepiandrosterone (DHEA) and its sulfated product (DHEA-S) increase by 6 to 8 years of age in both sexes. The mechanism of the adrenarche remains enigmatic (see section on premature adrenarche). In the female, prolactin (PRL) levels also increase because of the increase in E_2 secretion. Somatomedin C/insulin-like growth factor-I (SmC/IGF-I) concentrations rise dramatically during puberty, and correlate quite closely with the (Tanner) stages of sexual maturation.[4-6] Administration of T or E_2 is followed by increased SmC/IGF-I levels in peripubertal subjects.[7-9]

The hypothalamic-pituitary-gonadal unit begins to function in utero. In midgestation, after development of the hypophysial-portal vasculature, hypothalamic GnRH stimulates secretion of pituitary LH and FSH, which is more marked in the female than in the male fetus, possibly because of delayed ovarian formation and function relative to the testis. In the newborn male infant there is an increase in the secretion of LH and T beginning at 1 month of age and continuing for the next 2 to 4 months, followed by gradual decline to prepubertal values by 6 to 12 months. In female infants serum concentrations of LH and particularly FSH are higher than in male infants for the first several years of life, declining to prepubertal values by 2 to 4 years of age. At approximately 2 months of age there is a transient increase in serum concentrations of E_2.[10] Basal gonadotropin concentrations and the secretory response to GnRH are increased in infants with primary hypogonadism but decline spontaneously between 4 and 10 years of age.[3, 11] The decline in serum gonadotropin concentrations in midchildhood is a manifestation of the "restraint" exercised by higher central nervous system centers upon hypothalamic stimulation of pituitary gonadotropin secretion.

Table 1. *Etiology of Isosexual Precocity*

- True and complete isosexual precocity
  - Idiopathic
    - Familial
  - Congenital anomalies
    - Septooptic dysplasia
    - Hydrocephalus
  - Tumors of the central nervous system
    - Glioma of optic nerve or hypothalamus (neurofibromatosis)
    - Astrocytoma
    - Ependymoma
    - Germinoma/pinealoma
    - Teratoma
    - Hamartoma
    - Craniopharyngioma
    - Cysts
    - Sarcoid granuloma
  - Postinflammatory: Meningitis, encephalitis, brain abscess
  - Posttraumatic
  - Other
    - Following late treatment of congenital adrenal hyperplasia, or virilizing/feminizing adrenal or gonadal tumor
    - Chronic renal failure
    - Post cranial radiation
    - Primary hypothyrodism (?)
    - Isolated LH secretion (?)
- Pseudoprecocious puberty
  - hCG-secreting tumors
    - Hepatoma
    - Chorioepithelioma (gonadal, extragonadal)
    - Teratoma
  - Gonadal
    - Ovarian
      - Granulosa or theca cell tumor
      - Follicular luteal cysts
    - Testicular
      - Leydig cell tumor
      - Adrenal rest tumor
  - Adrenal
    - Congenital adrenal hyperplasia
    - Adrenal neoplasm—virilizing or feminizing
  - Iatrogenic, surreptitious, or drug-contaminated sex hormone or hCG administration
  - Gonadotropin-independent
    - Sporadic
    - Male limited familial
    - McCune-Albright
    - Tuberous sclerosis
- Incomplete isosexual precocity
  - Premature thelarche
  - Premature adrenarche
  - Premature menarche
- Other
  - Adolescent male gynecomastia
  - Vaginitis, foreign body
  - Vaginal or uterine neoplasm

CLASSIFICATION OF ISOSEXUAL PRECOCITY

The causes of isosexual precocity are listed in Table 1. True and complete isosexual precocity (central precocious puberty [CPP]) denotes the early maturation of the hypothalamic-pituitary-gonadal unit due to removal of the inhibitory influences which normally "restrain" the function of this system. Other forms of isosexual precocity involve secretion of gonadotropins and/or sex hormones independently of hypothalamic-pituitary control (isosexual pseudoprecocity or pseudoprecocious puberty) and isolated manifestations of sexual development (incomplete isosexual precocity). This classification is subject to modification as further data clarify the pathogenesis of various disorders; entities classified in one group may actually belong in another category. For instance, it had been assumed that patients with polyostotic fibrous dysplasia (McCune-Albright syndrome) and tuberous sclerosis had CPP. Yet recent studies[12, 13] indicate that at least some of these patients have a gonadotropin-independent process, possibly associated with derangement of intragonadal regulation of steroidogenesis. In sexual precocity secondary to hypothyroidism, gonadotropin excess is more likely due to decreased catabolism of LH/FSH rather than to excessive gonadotropin secretion under physiologic hypothalamic regulation.

Intermittent or unsustained puberty in the female is defined[14] as the association of thelarche with at least one other physical sign of sexual development which is nonprogressive or which may spontaneously regress and relapse. Basal E_2 levels are intermittently elevated, basal gonadotropin values are low, and the gonadotropin secretory response to GnRH is suppressed. Estrogen-secreting ovarian follicles and cysts in prepubertal females result in a wide spectrum of clinical findings, including premature thelarche and premature menarche (*vide infra*).

TRUE AND COMPLETE ISOSEXUAL PRECOCITY

True and complete isosexual precocity is present when there has been activation of the intact hypothalamic-pituitary-gonadal axis. This is presumably due to interruption or waning of physiologic inhibitory restraint upon hypothalamic GnRH secretion, resulting in gonadotropin and subsequently gonadal sex steroid secretion. CPP is more prevalent (4 to 8 times) in girls than in boys. Although CPP usually occurs sporadically, familial idiopathic central isosexual precocity has been reported in a brother, sister, and father who developed signs of puberty by 5 years of age, which suggests a dominant mode of inheritance.[15] Rosenfeld et al.[16] described a brother and sister with isolated LH secretion who presented with isosexual and heterosexual precocity, respectively. The boy developed testicular enlargement and pubic hair by 1.5 years; his sister presented with clitoral hypertrophy and pubic hair growth at 4 years of age—findings consistent with LH stimulation of androgen secretion from the preovulatory ovarian follicle. Although it had long been considered that in the majority of children (particularly in girls) CPP was "idiopathic," computerized tomographic (CT) and magnetic resonance imaging (MRI) scans have revealed a surprisingly large number of central nervous system lesions in both boys and girls with this disorder. Thus Hung et al.[17] described three children with CPP in whom clinically unsuspected intracranial neoplasm (1) or cysts (2) were found by computed tomography. In the series of Cacciari et al.[18] hypothalamic hamartomas were present in 33% of children with CPP. In addition several individual reports have documented the frequency of this lesion.[19-21] Therefore, radiographic scanning of the central nervous system is indicated in all children with CPP.

CPP has been reported in children with septo-optic dysplasia, hydrocephalus, and the primary empty sella syndrome, in whom diffuse hypothalamic dysfunction may occur.[22-25] A number of hypothalamic tumors have been associated with CPP, including gliomas, astrocytomas, ependymomas, germinomas, teratomas, and hamartomas. In a child with neurofibromatosis and CPP, an optic nerve or hypothalamic glioma must be strongly considered.[26] Hypothalamic tumors, particularly those involving the posterior hypothalamus, may interrupt inhibitory input into the medial basal hypothalamus, thereby permitting increased secretion or more frequent pulsatile release of GnRH and increased gonadotropin secretion.[27] Immunoreactive GnRH has been identified in hypothalamic hamartomas, which suggests that this structure may function as an autonomous accessory hypothalamus responsible for pituitary stimulation.[19, 20] Hamartomas are most commonly found in children in whom isosexual precocity occurs before 3 years of age.[18, 19, 21] Other perisellar masses, such as suprasellar cysts, sarcoid granulomas, and pinealomas, have been associated with precocious puberty. (However, pinealomas or germinomas may also secrete hCG, which may result in pseudoprecocious puberty [*vide infra*] or a sequence of pseudoprecocity leading to true and complete isosexual precocity.) CPP may follow central nervous system infections, including meningitis, encephalitis, and brain abscess. It may also occur after severe head trauma or cranial irradiation for neoplasia.[28, 29]

Primary hypothyroidism may present with isosexual precocity and growth failure. Frequently, serum gonadotropin concentrations are increased in these patients. There are several possible explanations for this observation: (1) excessive hypothalamic function in the primary hypothyroid state may result in "hormonal overlap" with increased secretion of both gonadotropins and thyroid-stimulating hormone (TSH); (2) decreased catabolism of LH and FSH may lead to prolonged and enhanced biologic gonadotropin activity[30]; (3) hyperprolactinemia may lead to increased gonadal steroidogenesis by a direct effect[31]; or (4) altered sex steroid metabolism in hypothyroidism may result in prolonged biologic activity. Because treatment with thyroid hormone causes regression of sexual development, hypothalamic maturation is incomplete. Transient precocious puberty has been described in a 7.5-year-old boy with chronic renal failure, which resolved following peritoneal dialysis.[32] He had testicular enlargement, pubic hair, and galactorrhea. Basal LH, FSH, and T levels were in the pubertal ranges, while thyroxine, triiodothyronine, and TSH concentrations were low, and the basal PRL level was elevated. The pathophysiology of sexual precocity in this boy is unclear, but may relate to the hyperprolactinemic state, which may have affected LH secretion and testicular LH receptors.[33] The Russell-Silver syndrome, an entity characterized by asymmetry of the limbs, trunk, and face, growth retardation of prenatal onset, and a triangular face, is only occasionally associated with early puberty.[34]

True and complete isosexual precocity may follow successful treatment of children with pseudoisosexual precocity such as congenital adrenal hyperplasia[35] or virilizing tumors of the adrenal gland.[36] If the bone age of such patients has advanced beyond 12 to 13 years of age, mechanisms that are poorly understood result in activation of the hypothalamic-pituitary-gonadal axis after treatment has decreased pathologic sex hormone production.

Thelarche is usually the first sign of CPP in the female, but a growth spurt may precede or accompany breast development. Pubic hair often appears within 6 to 12 months of the onset of thelarche. In males, testicular enlargement occurs initially, followed by phallic growth, acceleration of linear growth rate, increased musculature, pubic and axillary hair growth, acne, and deepening of the voice. The bone age is usually quite advanced in children with true and complete isosexual precocity. Random basal concentrations of iLH and iFSH may be normal or slightly elevated for chronologic age, but in children with hypothalamic hamartomas basal LH and FSH concentrations are often higher than in patients with idiopathic CPP.[18] LH and FSH concentrations increase at night during sleep in children with CPP. Bioactive LH concentrations as measured by the rat Leydig cell bioassay are increased in patients with CPP but not in patients with premature thelarche or adrenarche, or non-hCG-associated pseudoisosexual precocity.[37] Urinary gonadotropin excretion is also increased in children with true and complete isosexual precocity.[38] Basal serum concentrations of E_2 and T in children with CPP are elevated for chronologic age but usually appropriate for the stage of sexual maturation.[39] Greatly elevated basal serum E_2 or T concentrations are more common in children with pseudoprecocious puberty associated with gonadal cysts or adrenal/gonadal neoplasms. The pubertal gonadotropin secretory response to GnRH is helpful in differentiating true and complete isosexual precocity from pseudoprecocity or incomplete forms in which the response is suppressed or quantitatively prepubertal.[40, 41] If true and complete isosexual precocity is confirmed, studies to determine its cause are warranted. CT or MRI of the brain with contrast enhancement should be performed in all patients.

In children with CPP treatment of the underlying cause should be undertaken. In addition to the psychosocial disadvantage of this disorder, adverse emotional problems, such as aggressive or withdrawn behavior, may be observed in affected children and warrant intervention. Compromised adult stature secondary to premature closure of epiphyses is a significant long-term complication of CPP.[42, 43]

Surgical removal or radiation of central nervous system tumors or drainage of cysts associated with CPP has had variable results, depending upon the site, size, and type of lesion and upon the extent of the surgery. Because hypothalamic hamartomas are common, usually small, and grow slowly if at all, close observation of children with such lesions is recommended unless associated with significant neurologic symptoms.[18]

Until recently, medical therapy for children with true and complete isosexual precocity relied upon agents such as medroxyprogesterone acetate (MPA), danazol, and cyproterone acetate. These drugs often resulted in cessation of menses and occasional regression of secondary sexual characteristics, but had little effect upon the rates of linear growth or skeletal maturation or upon adult height. Lee[42] reported a long-term follow-up study of 13 girls who had received MPA for idiopathic CPP. When compared with 15 girls with CPP who were untreated, the mean adult stature of each group was similar to that of the other (treated, 155.6 cm; untreated, 155.4 cm), and in both groups adult heights were significantly less than adjusted midparental heights. Resumption of menses was delayed 0.1 to 4.9 (mean, 1.2) years after cessation of MPA; the interval between cessation of treatment and resumption of menses was directly related to the dosage of the drug and the duration of treatment. Untoward side effects of MPA include Cushingoid features, excessive weight gain, adrenal suppression, and chromosomal damage. Danazol, a 19-nor-testosterone derivative, has limited use in the treatment of girls because of its androgenic effects. Cyproterone acetate is an antiandrogenic steroid analog which when given in doses of 100 mg/m^2/day suppresses the LH response to GnRH and results in regression of breasts and cessation of menses. A beneficial effect on linear growth has not been clearly demonstrated. This drug also suppresses adrenal function.[44-46]

Recent development of long-acting analogs of GnRH has dramatically altered the treatment of children with CPP. The rationale for the use of this agent is based upon data demonstrating that continuous infusion of GnRH or intermittent administration of potent agonist analogs of GnRH initially stimulate but subsequently inhibit secretion of LH and FSH. This phenomenon appears to reflect prolonged occupancy of pituitary GnRH receptors by the analogs or loss (down-regulation) of receptors, thereby rendering the gonadotrophs unresponsive to endogenous GnRH.[47] In rodents the analogs also interfere with gonadal receptors for gonadotropins.

In 1981, several investigators[48-50] reported suppression of gonadotropin and E_2 concentrations in girls with idiopathic true and complete isosexual precocity using the long-acting GnRH analogs D-Trp^6-GnRH or D-Trp^6-Pro^9-NEt-GnRH (GnRH-a). Short-term (8-week) studies demonstrated that gonadotropin secretory responses to acute administration of GnRH were suppressed throughout the treatment period with subcutaneous dosages of 4 to 8 μg/kg/day of the latter analog.[48] Breast development regressed in most girls, and menses ceased in all subjects. Emotional lability was noted to decrease. E_2 concentrations fell, and vaginal maturation indices declined. The effects of GnRH-a are rapidly reversible. Within 8 weeks after stopping therapy, hormonal parameters return to pretreatment values, and menses resumes. Long-term administration of GnRH-a results in prolonged suppression of the pituitary-gonadal unit in children with CPP. Decrease in sex steroid levels is followed by decline in rates of linear growth and skeletal maturation and improved prognosis for adult stature. Mansfield et al.[51] reported that after 18 months of treatment with GnRH-a, growth velocity in nine girls declined from a mean rate of 9.3 cm/year before to 4.6 cm/year during therapy. Bone age advanced 9.4 months during the 18-month treatment period, which suggests a potential increase in adult height with therapy. Similar experiences have been reported by other investigators[52, 53] over periods of treatment as long as 36 months. Intranasal as well as subcutaneous administration of GnRH-a has been reported[53] to be effective, although the latter route is preferred by the present authors. Mild local reactions occur occasionally at the injection site. Styne et al.[52] reported that hot flashes developed in 3 girls following suppression of E_2 secretion; in 6 of 19 patients cutaneous reactions to GnRH-a were associated with the development of immunoglobulin E antibodies directed toward the analog. After desensitization a second course of the analog could be given without adverse effects. SmC/IGF-I concentrations are increased relative to chronologic age in children with CPP and decline to levels appropriate for bone age (but not for chronologic age) during administration of GnRH-a.[4]

The GnRH-a has been used effectively in boys and girls with true and complete isosexual precocity due to hypothalamic hamartomas[54, 55] and in children with optic nerve gliomas associated with neurofibromatosis.[26] It has also proven effective in suppressing gonadotropin and sex steroid levels in CPP complicating congenital adrenal hyperplasia and virilizing adrenal tumors where early maturation of the hypothalamic-pituitary-gonadal axis has occurred after treatment of the underlying disorder.[35, 36]

There is a high incidence of behavioral problems and moodiness in children with CPP as well as other forms of precocious puberty.[56] These children display both aggressive and withdrawal behavior relative to their peers because of age/appearance dyssynchrony and the environmental response to this discrepancy. Frequently these behavioral patterns will improve when sex steroid levels decrease during GnRH treatment.

Long-term follow-up studies of children with CPP are relatively few. Sigurjonsdottir and Hayles[43] surveyed 96 patients with isosexual precocity followed over 30 years at the Mayo Clinic. In six men with idiopathic precocious puberty adult height ranged from 145 to 171 cm; in only two was adult height 160 cm or greater. In 30 women adult height ranged between 136 and 171 cm and was 150 cm or greater in 21 subjects. Lee[42] reported that menstrual cycles were regular in a group of MPA-treated girls with CPP within 2 years after completion of therapy; one patient had two pregnancies, which terminated prematurely because of cervical incompetence. Murram et al.[57] reported that 40 of 42 adult women with idiopathic CPP had regular menstrual patterns (in 2 women menses was infrequent and irregular); 8 of 9 married women and 3 unmarried women had had 17 normal pregnancies. The evolution of girls with apparent CPP into adolescents with the hyperandrogenism/polycystic ovarian syndrome has been recorded.[43, 58]

Case Report

K. O. (birthdate, January 10, 1978), a girl with myelomeningocoele, hydrocephalus, paraplegia, and a seizure disorder, developed thelarche at 5.25 years followed by menses at 5.7 years. At 5.75 years, bone age was 7 years; the gonadotropin and estrogen secretory responses to GnRH were pubertal. The basal LH, FSH, and E_2 concentrations were 14.5 mIU/ml, 5.6 mIU/ml, and 58 pg/ml, respectively, and reached peak values of 53.5 mIU/ml, 10.7 mIU/ml, and 89 pg/ml, respectively, after administration of GnRH.

Therapy with the GnRH-a (10 μg/kg/day subcutaneously (D-Ser(TBU)^6-GnRH-[1-9]EA^{10}, Buserelin, Hoechst-Roussel Inc., Somerville, NJ) was initiated at 7 years, by which point bone age had advanced to 11 years. Within 4 weeks serum E_2 concentrations were within the prepubertal range (< 20 pg/ml) and the LH secretory response to GnRH had declined (Fig. 1). The LH secretory response to GnRH-a persisted within the high prepubertal range after the second month of therapy. Menses ceased, and the breasts regressed. After 6 months of treatment with GnRH-a bone age was still 11 years of age.

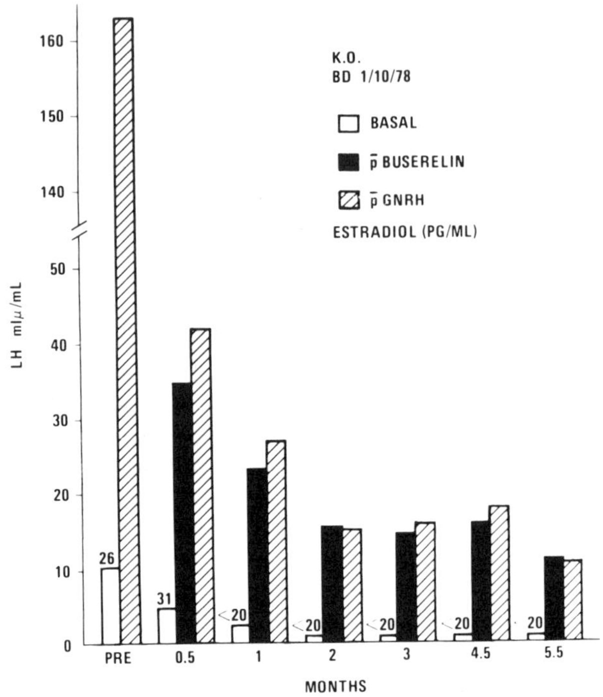

Figure 1
LH secretory response to GnRH and GnRH-a (Buserelin) prior to and during treatment of K. O., a girl with true and complete isosexual precocity. Prior to administration of GnRH-a, the LH responses to both GnRH and GnRH-a (Buserelin) were exaggerated and E_2 values increased. Within 2 weeks after initiation of treatment with GnRH-a the basal LH concentration fell and the LH secretory response to GnRH was inhibited; E_2 concentrations declined to prepubertal values (< 20 pg/ml). The LH secretory response to GnRH-a persisted at a prepubertal value.

Case Report

I. K. (birthdate, December 11, 1978) was found to have pseudoisosexual precocity because of 21-hydroxylase-deficient congenital adrenal hyperplasia at 4.9 years of age, at which point bone age was 13 years. Despite suppression of adrenal androgens with cortisol, by 6 years of age it was apparent that endogenous hypothalamic-pituitary-testicular function had begun because testicular size had increased substantially, T values remained elevated, and there were pubertal LH and T secretory responses to GnRH. The basal LH (9 mIU/ml), FSH (3.5 mIU/ml), and T (94 ng/dl) concentrations achieved peak values of 62.0 mIU/ml, 7.4 mIU/ml, and 460 ng/dl after administration of GnRH.

Thus, I. K. had developed true and complete isosexual precocity. Within 2 days after beginning GnRH-a (10 μg/kg/day subcutaneously) at 6.3 years the LH secretory response to GnRH was depressed, and within 1 month T values fell into the prepubertal range (< 10 ng/dl). There was a marked improvement in I. K.'s general behavior with therapy, and the rates of linear growth and skeletal maturation declined.

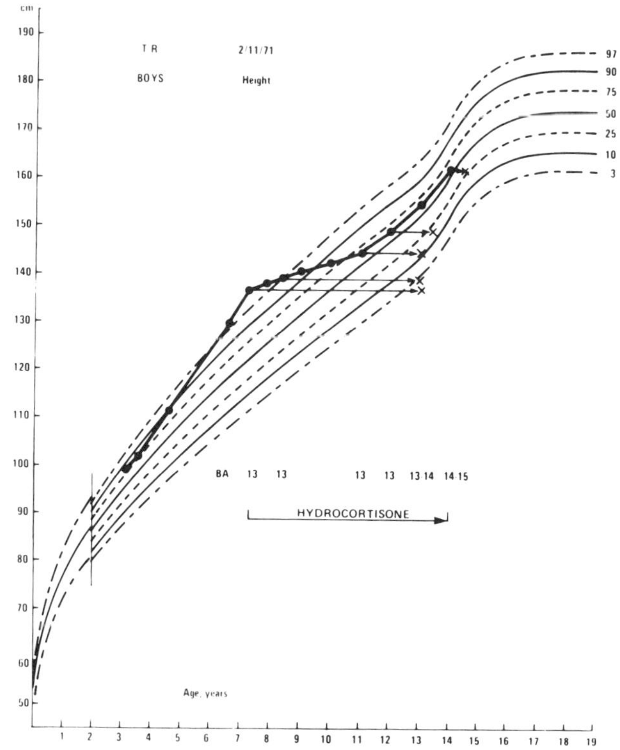

Figure 2
Growth pattern of T. R., a boy with congenital adrenal hyperplasia and advanced bone age (13 years) at diagnosis. With adequate suppression of adrenal androgens, the rate of linear growth declined, there was no advancement in skeletal maturation, and hypothalamic-pituitary-testicular development did not occur until 11 years. Chronologic, bone, and height ages were approximately equal by 14 years, which indicated a good prognosis for height. Thus, CPP did not follow adrenal suppression in this patient.

Case Report

In T. R. (birthdate, February 11, 1971) the diagnosis of pseudoisosexual precocity due to 21-hydroxylase-deficient congenital adrenal hyperplasia was established at 7.3 years, when his bone age was 13 years. With cortisol therapy there was adequate suppression of adrenal function and a marked decline in the rates of growth and skeletal maturation (Fig. 2). Normal adolescent sexual development (testicular enlargement) occurred at 11 years; by 14 years height and bone ages were equivalent and height was at the 50th percentile, indicating an excellent height potential.

This patient is presented in relation to I. K. to illustrate that despite an advanced bone age in T. R., endogenous pituitary testicular function did not follow adrenal suppression. Thus, the use of GnRH-a in patients with congenital adrenal hyperplasia or other forms of pseudoisosexual precocity, the treatment of which results in CPP, should not be considered until there is clinical and laboratory evidence that CPP has occurred in the specific child.

PSEUDOPRECOCIOUS PUBERTY

Pseudoprecocious puberty (pseudoisosexual precocity) implies that the process of sexual development is not under the control of an intact hypothalamic-pituitary unit. It can be due to gonadotropin-secreting tumors or to iatrogenic administration of gonadotropins; estrogen- or androgen-secreting neoplasms of the ovary, testes, or adrenals; exposure to exogenous sex hormones; ovarian cysts; or autonomously functioning ovaries or testes apparently regulated by intragonadal factors incompletely characterized at this time.

Secretion of a glycoprotein with immunologic, physicochemical, and biologic characteristics of hCG is a cause of pseudoisosexual precocity more commonly in boys than in girls.[59, 60] Immunoreactive hCG is present normally in small quantities in human liver, colon, testes, lung, and pituitary, and in normal human serum and urine.[61] HCG-secreting hepatic, pineal, intracranial, retroperitoneal and thoracic tumors have caused sexual precocity in children. The predominance of sexually precocious males with hCG-secreting tumors is explained by the fact that hCG has primarily LH-like biologic activity.[59] Thus, hCG is able to stimulate testicular Leydig cell function and T secretion. Ovarian estrogen synthesis requires both LH and FSH. Because some FSH-like activity is intrinsic to the hCG molecule,[62] sexually precocious girls with an hCG-secreting tumor have been observed occasionally.[59] Several boys with 47,XXY testicular dysgenesis (Klinefelter syndrome) and hCG-secreting neoplasms causing sexual precocity have been recorded, which suggets more than a casual association between the two disorders.[63] Patients with hCG-secreting neoplasms usually have very high serum concentrations of "LH" in routine radioimmunoassays for LH, because the alpha subunit is common to all of the glycoprotein hormones (hCG, LH, FSH, TSH). The presence of high concentrations of the beta subunit of hCG in a specific assay identifies the circulating gonadotropin. The source of hCG secretion may then be localized by appropriate radiographic and sonographic techniques. Surgical removal of the tumor is the treatment of choice.

Pseudoisosexual precocity due to an LH-secreting tumor of the pituitary is unusual. Faggiano et al.[64] described a 4.7-year-old body with increased somatic growth, pubarche, testicular and phallic enlargement, and galactorrhea. Serum concentrations of LH, PRL, and T were increased. After removal of a pituitary chromophobe adenoma there was rapid normalization of all hormonal values.

Estrogen-secreting granulosa cell tumors of the ovaries are the most common ovarian neoplasms associated with pseudoisosexual precocity in girls.[65] Because these tumors secrete estrogens and androgens, affected children often develop both breast and pubic/axillary hair. The average diameter of the juvenile granulosa cell tumor at diagnosis is 12 cm, but it may be as small as 3 cm; it is composed of follicles of various sizes. In 80% of children the tumor is functional and associated with isosexual precocity. Usually only one ovary is involved with the tumor, but a neoplasm may develop in the contralateral ovary, and therefore, prolonged follow-up of affected children is necessary. Five percent of juvenile granulosa cell tumors are malignant. Mixed sex cord tumors (granulosa/Sertoli/theca cell) may produce a similar picture in girls and gynecomastia and pubic hair growth in the male. Patients, particularly girls, with the Peutz-Jehgers syndrome are at high risk for the development of such neoplasms.[66]

Feminizing adrenal tumors in prepubertal girls are quite unusual. Comite et al.[67] described a 2.8-year-old girl with breast, pubic, and axillary hair development of 5 months' duration. Clinical signs of the hyperglucocorticoid state or of virilization were absent. Within the adrenal carcinomatous tissue there were low 3β-hydroxysteroid dehydrogenase (3β-HSD) and 21-hydroxylase activities which resulted in very high serum concentrations of DHEA and DHEA-S and modestly increased T and E_2 values, probably because of peripheral conversion of the adrenal androgens; all values returned to normal after excision of the tumor. Such tumors may also cause gynecomastia, virilization, or Cushing's syndrome in boys. Leydig cell tumors of the testes, adrenal rests, and congenital adrenal hyperplasia associated with absence of 21- or 11-hydroxylase activities are significant causes of pseudoisosexual precocity in boys.

Familial male isosexual precocity is an autosomal dominant, sex-specific form of precocious puberty occurring at 2 to 4 years of age, characterized by phallic and testicular enlargement, pubic hair growth, rapid linear growth, advanced bone age, elevated T concentrations, low diurnal and nocturnal basal LH and FSH concentrations, absent or minimal LH and FSH secretory responses to GnRH, early spermatogenesis, and hyperplasia of the interstitial cells of the testes.[68-70] It was Schedewie et al.[71] who demonstrated that increased T secretion in this disorder is independent of endogenous gonadotropin secretion and associated with increased Leydig cell number. T secretion in these boys may fluctuate, at times falling spontaneously to low levels.[70] Basal diurnal and nocturnal gonadotropin concentrations and GnRH-provoked LH and FSH secretion are low when compared with normal pubertal boys and boys with true and complete isosexual precocity, but within normal limits for prepubertal boys. The GnRH-a that inhibits endogenous gonadotropin secretion is of no therapeutic usefulness in these children, confirming the gonadotropin independence of T secretion. With advancing age the LH and FSH secretory responses to GnRH increase into the adult range, and there is increased secretion of the alpha glycoprotein subunit.[69] In older boys basal and post-GnRH concentrations of FSH are elevated, which suggests seminiferous tubular dysfunction.[68, 69]

Testicular biopsy reveals an increased number of mature Leydig cells relative to that expected for the patient's age. Adjacent to the Leydig cells, the seminiferous tubules display varying degrees of spermatogenesis to the spermatid stage,[71] a response to the locally high intragonadal levels of T.[72] Testicular biopsies from older patients reveal still further increase in Leydig cell numbers, but relatively little evidence of advanced stages of spermatogenesis. Semen analysis may reveal a low sperm count.[68] Most affected men are fertile, but reproductive capacity may decline with age.

The mechanism of autonomous T secretion in this disorder is not known. Bioactive LH levels are low and Leydig cell-stimulating immunoglobulins have not been identified in the serum of young patients.[73] In older subjects, basal and post-GnRH levels of bLH measured by the rat interstitial cell T assay are detectable.[69-71, 73] It has been suggested that an intratesticular mechanism that either stimulates or inhibits stimulation of Leydig cell function may be deranged.[73]

The nature of this factor(s) is unknown, but both GnRH and hCG have been identified in testicular extracts.

This form of sexual precocity may also occur as an autosomal recessive disorder or sporadically.[70, 71] In the male siblings described by Schedewie et al.[71] who presented with isosexual precocity at 2 years, follow-up study revealed later development (5 to 6 years) of mental retardation and spastic paraplegia.[74] The relationship of Leydig cell hyperplasia to the neurologic disorder in these brothers is unclear.

We have studied a boy with tuberous sclerosis and isosexual precocity due to autonomous Leydig cell function.

Case Report

A. L. (birthdate, February 23, 1980) presented at 4.2 years with the chief complaints of phallic enlargement present for 1 year and pubic hair growth of several weeks' duration. In the preceding 2 years the growth rate had accelerated (his height had increased from the 50th percentile at 2 years to the 75th percentile at 3 years and was above the 97th percentile at 4 years). Upon examination A. L. was a tall, muscular, mature boy with a height age of 5.1 years; there was a papillary rash over the bridge of the nose initially thought to be acne and a 5 × 2-cm hypopigmented area on the medial aspect of the left thigh which was accentuated under a Wood's lamp. The phallus measured 8 × 2.6 cm in the relaxed state, and the testes measured 3.5 × 1.7 cm bilaterally (Tanner stage III). There was Tanner stage II pubic hair. Bone age was 7 years at 4.2 years. T concentrations were elevated (125 to 321 ng/dl); serum levels of 17-hydroxyprogesterone (17-OHP), androstenedione (Δ^4A), Δ^5-17-hydroxypregnenolone (17-OHPreg), DHEA, and DHEA-S were normal for a prepubertal boy. Serum concentrations of LH and FSH were undetectable (< 1 mIU/ml) in basal specimens and increased only to 2.7 and 2.8 mIU/ml, respectively, after administration of GnRH (normal prepubertal male responses). After hCG administration the T concentration increased from 125 to 755 ng/dl. Testicular sonogram revealed no discrete masses; skeletal survey and a CT scan of the abdomen were normal; the CT scan of the brain revealed subependymal calcifications but no masses; the electroencephalogram revealed generalized bursts of polyspike and slow wave activity. The clinical diagnosis of tuberous sclerosis was made; by 4.5 years seizures developed. This child's mental development and school performance have been normal.

Administration of the antiandrogen spironolactone, 75 mg daily, did not return serum T concentrations to normal; rapid linear growth and advanced skeletal maturation persisted (Fig. 3). At 5.6 years therapy with ketoconazole (200 mg twice daily) was initiated, causing a rapid decline in T values.

Autonomous gonadal secretion of sex hormones in patients with tuberous sclerosis has not been described previously. It has been assumed that these patients had true and complete isosexual precocity. In a 12-year-old boy reported by Cummings et al.,[75] basal LH and FSH values were in the adult male range, but bone age was 14 years and maturation of endogenous hypothalamic gonadotropin secretory function may have occurred by this age. In another disorder, polyostotic fibrous dysplasia (McCune-Albright syndrome), ovarian function in young girls with isosexual precocity is gonadotropin-independent. E_2 secretion is episodic and associated with cyclic growth and regression of ovarian follicles documented by pelvic sonography. With advancing skeletal maturation the gonadotropin secretory response to GnRH increases, as it does in the familial male-limited form of isosexual precocity.[12, 13, 70, 76] The association of neurologic, cutaneous, and gonadal abnormalities is of interest, but unexplained at present.

Treatment of gonadotropin-independent autonomous gonadal function has been unsatisfactory. It is unresponsive to the GnRH-a; MPA has been reported to be useful,[73] but in the experience of the present authors this drug has been unsatisfactory. The antiandrogen spironolactone has not been useful (Fig. 3). Netzloff and Wilson[77] reported that cyproterone acetate caused regression of secondary sexual characteristics, rapid (within 24 hours) lowering of serum T values, and a decreased rate of skeletal maturation. Recently Holland et al.[78] reported that the antifungal agent ketoconazole effectively lowered T levels, reduced the rates of linear growth and skeletal maturation and improved behavior in three boys with this disorder, a response we have confirmed in short term observations. Ketoconazole inhibits 17-hydroxylase and 17,20-desmolase activities, thereby inhibiting adrenal and gonadal steroidogenesis.[79] Transient glucocorticoid insufficiency

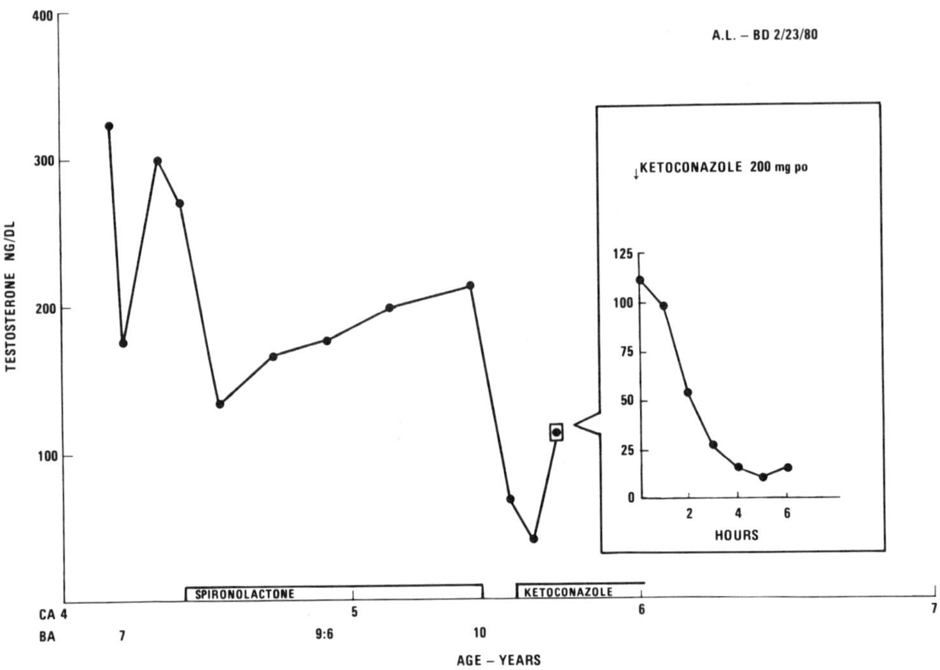

Figure 3
Serum T concentrations in A. L., a boy with tuberous sclerosis and gonadotropin-independent isosexual precocity. T values fluctuated erratically during administration of spironolactone, but fell after ketoconazole administration. The inserted graph depicts the rapid decline in serum T concentrations that followed ingestion of 200 mg of ketoconazole.

may occur in ketoconazole-treated patients but this was of no clinical significance in the patients reported by Holland et al.,[78] nor have we observed this complication. It is suggested that ketoconazole may also be useful in girls with autonomous ovarian estrogen secretion (McCune-Albright syndrome); alternatively, estrogen antagonists may also be of value in these subjects. The GnRH-a is not useful in young girls with this syndrome.[13, 76]

INCOMPLETE ISOSEXUAL PRECOCITY

Premature Thelarche

Premature thelarche is defined as isolated development of breast tissue in a girl less than 8 years of age. Breast tissue is often present in the normal neonate. McKiernan and Hull[80] observed that 90% of newborn boys and girls had breast tissue palpable within the first 2 days of life. Neonates without palpable breast tissue tended to be preterm (< 36 weeks' gestation) or to be products of complicated pregnancies and/or deliveries. Breast diameter increased during the first 2 weeks of life in both sexes and then regressed but was still palpable in many infants at 10 months of age, after which time it disappeared. Between 5 and 8 months of age breast diameter was wider in female than in male infants. In most patients with premature thelarche breast development begins in the first year of life and in 30% to 40% is present from birth.[81, 82] It is thus apparent that in many infant girls referred for evaluation of premature thelarche, the presence of breast tissue is a normal finding for the age of the child. Premature thelarche might better apply to those infants in whom breast growth begins after previously documented regression or persists after 10 months of age. The pathogenesis of premature thelarche is probably related to estrogen secretion by the prepubertal ovary, which normally develops small follicles to the preantral and large antral stages; these may enlarge to a size sufficient to be identified by ultrasonography.[83] Because gonadotropins stimulate ovarian follicle development and estrogen secretion, serum concentrations of LH and FSH are high in female infants,[10] and the FSH (but not the LH) secretory response to GnRH is normally highest in the infant female,[84] these gonadotropins may stimulate early ovarian follicle development. Under usual circumstances the production rate of estrogens by the prepubertal ovary is low, but in some children it apparently exceeds the tissue resonse threshold and breast growth (or even menses) occurs. The peak age incidence of girls with premature thelarche is between 4 and 12 months,[81] whereas the peak incidence of true and complete isosexual precocity is 4 to 5 years of age.[85]

Often vaginal smears of girls with premature thelarche reveal an estrogenic effect, and occasionally serum estrogen concentrations may be slightly and intermittently elevated.[82, 86] (In more exteme instances ovarian cysts secrete sufficient estrogen to elevate significantly serum E_2 concentrations.) Basal and post-GnRH serum concentrations of LH and FSH may be within the female prepubertal range,[87] although several investigators[40, 82, 86, 88] have reported exaggerated FSH secretory responses to GnRH in girls with this disorder. Linear growth is normal or increased,[82] and bone maturation relatively appropriate for chronologic age in girls with premature thelarche.

Mills et al.[81] reported that in girls with premature thelarche breast development may regress (30%), persist unchanged in size (50%), increase in size (10%), or regress and reappear. In those children in whom breast growth ultimately regressed, periods of 3 to 60 months (mean 23 months) elapsed before resolution. Breast growth often remained unchanged for prolonged periods (up to 113 months) in the report of Mills et al.,[81] but further clinical signs and laboratory evidence of puberty did not appear. The age of onset of the breast growth does not predict whether breast tissue will regress, persist, or enlarge. The association of premature thelarche with prematurity was pointed out by Nelson.[89] She reported that in 6 of 68 (8.7%) surviving very-low birth weight (VLBW $<$ 1000 gm) infant girls breast tissue first developed between 11 and 14 months of age with no further signs of puberty. In this population vaginal smears revealed only minimal or no estrogen effect. This investigator noted that the VLBW infants who developed premature thelarche were gestationally more immature, of lower birth weight, and had a higher incidence of significant central nervous system dysfunction than did those infants who did not experience breast growth.

Premature thelarche may also be the consequence of exposure to exogenous estrogens, either through the nursing mother (who may herself be exposed to estrogen-containing oral contraceptives or creams or other environmental estrogen-like agents) or through estrogen-contaminated foods, drugs, or vitamins that the infant may ingest. Epidemic outbreaks of premature thelarche due to estrogen-contaminated baby foods have been reported in Italy[90] and Puerto Rico.[85, 91] In Puerto Rico, Comas[85] examined 118 girls with premature thelarche over a 10-year period. Saenz de Rodriguez et al.[91] examined 482 girls with premature thelarche in 8.7 years. In addition, both investigators reported an increase in other forms of isosexual precocity in children on that island.[85, 91] Elevated serum and/or urine estrogen levels were found in approximately 30% of patients so tested. Contamination of food supplies, particularly poultry, beef, pork, eggs, and milk, with estrogenic (and possibly androgenic) compounds is strongly suspected as the cause of this epidemic of isosexual precocity, although the exact compound(s) has not been identified. Utilizing a cytosol receptor assay for estrogen, Saenz de Rodriguez et al.[91] demonstrated that an estrogen like compound could be found in extracts of chicken, pork, beef, and milk not only of Puerto Rican origin, but also from Philadelphia. Loizzo et al.[92] reported that diethylstilbestrol could be detected in baby meat products in Italy. Contamination of meat supplies with anabolic steroids might arise by direct administration of these agents to the animals or by contamination of the grain these animals are fed.[93] Follicular cysts of the ovary were often noted in children reported by Saenz de Rodriguez et al.,[91] who attributed them to the effects of environmental estrogens.

Premature Menarche

Vaginal bleeding in young girls not associated with estrogen secretion may be due to trauma, self-manipulation, foreign bodies, sexual abuse, prolapse of the urethral mucosa, vulvovaginitis, or vulvovaginal tumors.[94] In the newborn, vaginal bleeding often occurs within the first few weeks of life because of withdrawal of maternal/placental estrogens. Vulvovaginitis may be due to bacterial, parasitic, mycotic, viral, or mycobacterial infections or to local allergic reactions. Neoplasms of the genital tract of young girls are unusual but often highly malignant. Polyps, sarcomas, mixed mesodermal tumors, and adenocarcinomas have been reported in this age range.

Vaginal bleeding of uterine origin without evidence of excessive estrogen secretion or disease of the vulva or vagina was reported by Heller et al.[95] and termed premature menarche. These investigators described four girls, 3 months, 10 months, 1.6 years, and 2.2 years of age, who experienced recurrent vaginal bleeding for several years without clinical evidence of estrogenization, with normal serum gonadotropin and estrogen values and bone ages commensurate with chronologic ages. Estrogenized vaginal smears were occasionally recorded. In a later report Murram et al.[96] described 12 patients with isolated premature menarche beginning between 9 months and 9 years, which recurred cyclically for 1 to 6 years and ceased by age 10. Thereafter, normal sexual development and regular monthly menstrual periods occurred at the anticipated ages. Fertility was normal in the married women of this series. Blanco-Garcia et al.[97] described 17 prepubertal girls, 1 to 8 years of age, with a history of vaginal bleeding of uterine origin without evidence of estrogenization. Six children experienced only one menstrual period, eight had two to three, and individual patients had four, five, or ten, usually in the winter months. Linear growth, bone maturation, and basal and post-GnRH-stimulated gonadotropin levels were normal for chronologic age and prepubertal state, but plasma E_2 concentrations were slightly but significantly elevated above prepubertal values. Ultrasonography revealed prepubertal size ovaries; in 7 of 15 children small cysts were seen. The presence of small follicular cysts in normal prepubertal girls is common, however.[83] Follow-up studies revealed that menses ceased spontaneously in all subjects, and none experienced further sexual development until the appropriate pubertal age.

Blanco-Garcia et al.[97] reported that over the 12-year period in which the 17 children with premature menarche were observed, their pediatric endocrinology clinic also examined 61 girls with premature thelarche and 120 girls with true and complete (central) isosexual precocity. Thus, girls with premature menarche represented 8.6% of this patient population, a much higher number of children than is the reported experience of American investigators. The pathogenesis of isolated premature menarche is probably not too dissimilar from that of premature thelarche in many patients. That is, small follicular cysts of the prepubertal ovary secrete sufficient estrogen to stimulate endometrial growth; when estrogen production declines or ceases, the endometrium is shed. An unanswered question is why in most girls thelarche occurs and in only a few do menstrual periods develop in response to slightly elevated estrogen secretion.

Premature Adrenarche

Adrenarche refers to the increase in adrenal androgen secretion that accompanies sexual maturation. The major androgens of adrenal origin are DHEA and DHEA-S. (In adult females approximately 90% of serum DHEA-S is attributable to secretion by the adrenal cortex; in adult males the testes also contribute substantial amounts of this androgen to the circulation.) Adrenal androgen secretion usually begins by 6 to 7 years of age in both sexes and is related to the development of the zona reticularis, the only adrenal cortical zone with DHEA-sulfotransferase activity.[98, 99] Adrenarche usually precedes onset of pubertal activity of the hypothalamic-pituitary gonadal axis.[100, 101] "Pubarche" is a term applied to the appearance of pubic hair, which usually occurs several years after the adrenarche. An adult axillary odor and/or axillary hair growth are also clinical signs of adrenal androgen secretion. Pubarche usually occurs after 8 years of age in girls and after 10 years of age in boys.[101] Premature pubarche is present when pubic hair develops before these ages. It is attributable to premature adrenarche when accompanied by serum concentrations of DHEA and/or DHEA-S that are increased for the chronologic age of the child, but appropriate for the stage of sexual hair growth in the absence of more complete sexual development. Although premature pubarche is most often due to premature adrenarche, other causes of pseudoisosexual precocity to be considered include simple virilizing and variant forms of congenital adrenal hyperplasia, autonomous gonadotropin- or androgen-secreting neoplasms, administration of exogenous androgens or gonadotropins, and Cushing's syndrome. Premature adrenarche is far more common in girls than in boys; in boys it is frequently associated with obesity or central nervous system insults.[101] It is more common in black than in white girls.[102]

Clinically, in patients with premature adrenarche, the signs of puberty are pubic or axillary hair growth or axillary odor and a modest increase in height age relative to chronologic age. Bone age may be equal to or slightly in advance of chronologic age (1 to 2 years). There is considerable variability in the relationship between serum concentrations of DHEA-S and the appearance of pubic hair. In normal subjects pubic hair usually develops when the DHEA-S level exceeds 40 μg/dl;[98] in boys DHEA-S concentrations are higher than in girls at comparable (Tanner) stages of pubic hair growth. Thus, Rosenfield et al.[101] reported that at pubic hair stage II, the mean DHEA-S level in boys was 170 μg/dl (range, 40 to

474 μg/dl), whereas in girls the mean DHEA-S value was 80 μg/dl (range, 35 to 180 μg/dl). These absolute values are somewhat higher than those reported by other investigators. Although mean DHEA-S concentrations increase with advancing pubic hair stages, there is considerable overlap between stages and within the sexes. Thus, there is significant individual sensitivity to the biologic effects of these androgens.

Increase in DHEA and DHEA-S secretion during adrenarche is accompanied in vivo by a maturational decrease in 3β-HSD activity and increase in 17,20-lyase activity in the adrenal cortex. These changes result in increased conversion of 17-OHPreg to DHEA and subsequently to DHEA-S. Rich et al.[103] demonstrated that in female subjects in response to adrenocorticotropic hormone (ACTH) there is a significant increase with age of the product/precursor (substrate) ratios of DHEA/17-OHPreg and Δ^4A/17-OHP, indicating more efficient 17,20-lyase activity; they also observed significant decrease with age in the 17-OHP/17-OHPreg and Δ^4A/DHEA ratios, evidence of decreasing 3β-HSD activity. In girls with premature adrenarche the response ratios are intermediate between prepubertal and adult women, but closer to the latter. Schiebinger et al.[104] studied human adrenal microsomal activity in vitro and found that quantitatively 17-hydroxylase and 17,20-lyase activities increased between childhood (2 to 9 years) and adulthood (20 to 60 years), but that 3β-HSD activity did not change, an observation in conflict with the in vivo data cited above. Dickerman et al.[105] reported that human adrenal cortical concentrations of 17-OHPreg, DHEA, 17-OHP, and Δ^4A increased in late childhood and adolescence; further, the concentrations of these steroids increased from the outer to the inner layers of the gland. Analysis of these data in terms of product/substrate ratio confirmed the in vivo findings—that is, the ratios of Δ^4A/DHEA and 17-OHP/17-OHPreg declined between childhood and adulthood, which implies decreased 3β-HSD activity; the ratio of DHEA/17-OHPreg and Δ^4A/17-OHP rose, which suggests increased 17,20-lyase activity. The concentrations of steroids present in the adrenal cortex are of a magnitude (10^{-6} M) that could affect the respective enzyme activities which govern their metabolism. Byrne et al.[106] observed that the kinetics of human adrenal 3β-HSD activity did not change with age or substrate, which indicates the presence of a single species of 3β-HSD isozyme.

The mechanism of the adrenarche and its control are poorly understood. Cortisol secretion remains reasonably constant (relative to body surface area) through childhood and adolescence, whereas adrenal androgen secretion increases during late childhood and puberty. It has been suggested that ACTH may be responsible for the adrenarche, but there are no significant changes in plasma ACTH concentrations during childhood; in children with hyperadrenocorticotropism and hypercortisolemia, DHEA and DHEA-S concentrations are not elevated, but are appropriate for chronologic and/or bone age.[107] Furthermore, in patients with ACTH deficiency and in hypophysectomized chimpanzees, ACTH is able to stimulate and maintain cortisol secretion but not adrenal androgen secretion.[108, 109] A pituitary principle with specific adrenal androgen-stimulating activity has been postulated, and a 60,000 molecular weight glycoprotein with this property isolated from human pituitaries, but definitive identification of this material has not yet been accomplished.[98, 110] If such an agent exists, it is thought not to be a fragment of the proopiomelanocortin molecule.[104] Estrogens, gonadotropins, PRL, cortisol, prostaglandins, and angiotensin have also been postulated to influence adrenal androgen secretion, but evidence of their importance is equivocal.[98] Dickerman et al.[105] and Byrne et al.[106] suggest that the adrenarche is the natural consequence of increasing adrenal gland mass and thickness, which parallels increase in body size. As intraadrenal steroid concentrations increase during the growth process, they achieve levels capable of inhibiting 3β-HSD activity; in order to maintain cortisol secretion, ACTH increases substrate flux and the activity of various steroidogenic enzymes (21-hydroxylase, 11-hydroxylase, 17,20-lyase), which results in increased DHEA and DHEA-S secretion. In this view, premature adrenarche represents a normal response to the increased body size of such patients. Indeed, boys and girls with premature adrenarche are frequently obese. In adult women with anorexia nervosa, basal and ACTH-stimulated serum concentrations of DHEA and DHEA-S are low and increase after long-term weight gain.[111] Nevertheless, premature adrenarche does occur in children who are not tall or heavy for their age. Therefore, body type (and presumably adrenal

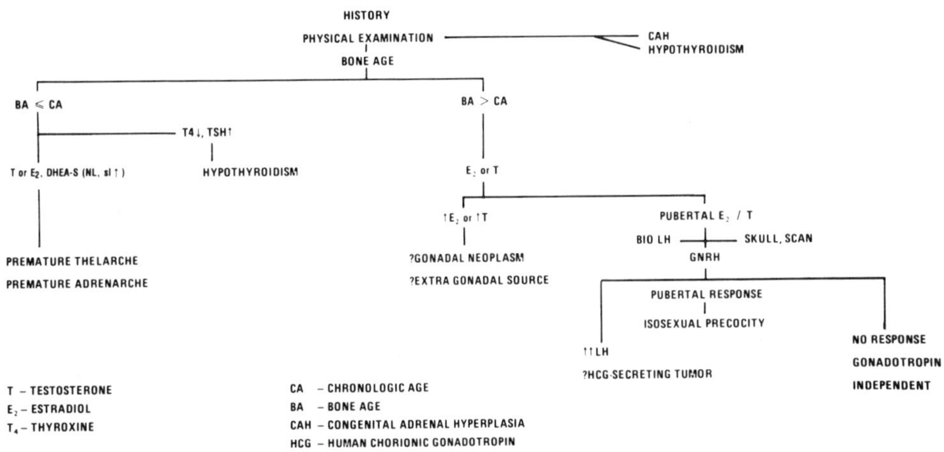

Figure 4
Outline for evaluation of the child with isosexual precocity.

gland size) plays a limited role in the development of premature adrenarche.

The long-term consequences of premature adrenarche are unknown. Follow-up of 24 children with this anomaly through the third decade of life revealed normal growth, sexual development, and fertility[112]; but more prolonged observation is a large group of patients has not been reported. In the experience of some investigators, some children with premature adrenarche have developed the hirsutism/polycystic ovarian syndrome. Whether these are children with a variant form of congenital adrenal hyperplasia or heterozygous carriers of the gene for 21-hydroxylase deficiency is unknown. Temeck et al.[113] reported that 10 of 25 children with premature adrenarche were partially deficient in 21-hydroxylase or 3β-HSD activities. Granoff et al.[114] noted that the 17-OHP secretory response to ACTH in children with premature adrenarche was similar to that of obligate heterozygotes for 21-hydroxylase deficiency, a finding distinct from that of Rosenfield et al.[101] and Rich et al.[103] Further studies are required to define the incidence of subtle forms of 21-hydroxylase, 3β-HSD, and 11-hydroxylase deficiencies in premature adrenarche, the natural history of this anomaly, and whether intervention (adrenal cortical suppression) is warranted and helpful.

DIAGNOSIS AND MANAGEMENT

A scheme for the evaluation of the child with isosexual precocity is outlined in Figure 4. In most subjects careful historical, review, physical examination (including rectal examination in the girl), assessment of bone age, and a few hormonal measurements are sufficient for categorizing the form of sexual precocity and determining whether more extensive studies are required. All children with CPP should undergo structural radiographic studies of the brain. It is unclear whether all patients with premature adrenarche should undergo testing with ACTH in a search for subtle abnormalities in cortisol biosynthesis. Present data do not suggest that this is indicated. However, the present authors do measure basal serum 17-OHP levels in all such children, searching for variant forms of 21-hydroxylase-deficient congenital adrenal hyperplasia. Treatment of children with isosexual precocity requires specific diagnosis and careful follow-up. The parents of children with premature thelarche and premature adrenarche can usually be reassured and the child followed. Patients with pseudoisosexual precocity associated with gonadotropin or sex hormone-secreting neoplasms require surgical attention; in those with congenital adrenal hyperplasia adrenal suppressive therapy with glucocorticoids is necessary; in children with autonomous gonadal sex hormone secretion, agents that interfere with sex hormone synthesis or antagonize its peripheral action may be helpful.

When the diagnosis of true and complete isosexual precocity has been established (and its primary cause eliminated or treated if possible), the GnRH-a is clearly the treatment of choice at present, having supplanted MPA, cyproterone, danazol, and similar agents. In the future, it is anticipated, GnRH antagonists will replace GnRH agonists, because the former agents are likely to have more immediate effects than the agonists, which often require several weeks to become fully effective. Inasmuch as these drugs are proteins, antibody formation to the structures may occur and in some instances may neutralize their activities. Neutralizing antibodies to native GnRH have developed in patients treated with this material.[30] The development of agonists or antagonists of neurotransmitters that regulate the secretion of endogenous GnRH and that maybe useful in the treatment of children with true and complete isosexual precocity may be anticipated.

Acknowledgment. The authors thank Ms. Sue Fine for competent, dedicated, and cheerful secretarial assistance.

REFERENCES

1. Diamond FB Jr, Root AW: Delayed sexual maturation and sexual precocity. In Current Diagnosis, 7th edition, Edited by R Conn. Philadelphia, W. B. Saunders Co., 1985, p 1252
2. Burstein S, Schaff-Blass E, Blass J, Rosenfield RL: The changing ratio of bioactive to immunoreactive luteinizing hormone (LH) through puberty principally reflects changing LH radioimmunoassay dose-response characteristics. J Clin Endocrinol Metab 61:508, 1985
3. Conte FA, Grumbach MM, Kaplan SL, Reiter EO: Correlation of luteinizing hormone releasing factor-induced luteinizing hormone and follicle-stimulating hormone release from infancy to 19 years with the changing pattern of gonadotropin secretion in agonadal patients: relation to the restraint of puberty. J Clin Endocrinol Metab 50:163, 1980
4. Harris DA, Van Vliet G, Egli CA, Grumbach MM, Kaplan SL, Styne D, Vainsel M: Somatomedin C in normal puberty and in true precocious puberty before and after treatment with a potent luteinizing hormone-releasing hormone agonist. J Clin Endocrinol Metab 61:152, 1985
5. Luna AM, Wilson DM, Wibbelsman CJ, Brown RC, Nagashima RJ, Hintz RL, Rosenfeld RG: Somatomedins in adolescence: a cross-sectional study of the effect of puberty on plasma insulin-like growth factor I and II levels. J Clin Endocrinol Metab 57:268, 1983
6. Rosenfield RL, Furlanetto R, Bock D: Relationship of somatomedin-C concentrations to pubertal changes. J Pediatr 103:723, 1983
7. Craft WH, Underwood LE: Effect of androgens on plasma somatomedin C/insulin-like growth factor I responses to growth hormone. Clin Endocrinol 20:549, 1984
8. Parker MW, Johanson AJ, Rogol AD, Kaiser DL, Blizzard RM: Effect of testosterone on somatomedin-C concentrations in prepubertal boys. J Clin Endocrinol Metab 58:87, 1984
9. Rosenfield RL, Furlanetto R: Physiologic testosterone or estradiol induction of puberty increases plasma somatomedin-C. J Pediatr 107:415, 1985
10. Sizonenko PC: Endocrinology in preadolescents and adolescents. I. Hormonal changes during normal puberty. Am J Dis Child 132:704, 1978
11. Conte FA, Grumbach MD, Kaplan SL: A diphasic pattern of gonadotropin secretion in patients with the syndrome of gonadal dysgenesis. J Clin Endocrinol Metab 40:670, 1975
12. D'Armiento M, Reda G, Camagna A, Tardella L: McCune-Albright syndrome: evidence for autonomous multiendocrine hyperfunction. J Pediatr 102:584, 1983
13. Foster CM, Ross JL, Shawker T, Pescovitz OH, Loriaux DL, Cutler GB Jr, Comite F: Absence of pubertal gonadotropin secretion in girls with McCune-Albright syndrome. J Clin Endocrinol Metab 58:1161, 1984
14. Lightner ES, Kelch RP: Treatment of precocious pseudopuberty associated with ovarian cysts. Am J Dis Child 138:126, 1984
15. Hopwood NJ, Kelch RP, Helder LJ: Familial precocious puberty in a brother and sister. Am J Dis Child 135:78, 1981
16. Rosenfeld RG, Reitz RE, King AB, Hintz RL: Familial precocious puberty associated with isolated elevation of luteinizing hormone. N Engl J Med 303:859, 1980
17. Hung W. August GP, Brallier DR, Milhorat TH: Computerized tomography in the evaluation of isosexual precocity. Am J Dis Child 134:25, 1980
18. Cacciari E, Frejaville E, Cicognani A, Pirazzoli P, Frank G, Balsamo A, Tassinari D, Zapulla F, Begamaschi R, Cristi GF: How many cases of true precocious puberty in girls are idiopathic? J Pediatr 102:357, 1983
19. Hochman HI, Judge DM, Reichlin S: Precocious puberty and hypothalamic hamartoma. Pediatrics 67:236, 1981
20. Price RA, Lee PA, Albright AL, Ronnekleiv OK, Gutai JP: Treatment of sexual precocity by removal of a luteinizing hormone-releasing hormone secreting hamartoma. JAMA 251:2247, 1984
21. Zuniga OF, Tanner SM, Wild WO, Mosier HD: Hamartoma of CNS associated with precocious puberty. Am J Dis Child 137:127, 1983
22. Costigan DC, Daneman D, Harwood-Nash D, Holland FJ: The empty sella in childhood. Clin Pediatr 23:437, 1983
23. LaFranchi S: Sexual precocity with hypothalamic hypopituitarism. Am J Dis Child 133:739, 1978
24. Margalith D, Tze WJ, Jan JE: Congenital optic nerve hypoplasia with hypothalamic-pituitary dysplasia. Am J Dis Child 139:361, 1985
25. Shulman DL, Martinez CR, Bercu BB, Root AW: Hypothalamic-pituitary dysfunction in the primary empty sella syndrome in childhood. J Pediatr 108:540, 1986
26. Laue L, Comite F, Hench K, Loriaux DL, Cutler GB Jr, Pescovitz OH: Precocious puberty associated with neurofibromatosis and optic gliomas: treatment with luteinizing hormone releasing hormone analogue. Am J Dis Child 139:1097, 1985
27. Terasawa E, Noonan JJ, Nass TE, Loose MD: Posterior hypothalamic lesions advance the onset of puberty in the female rhesus monkey. Endocrinology 115:2241, 1984
28. Shaul PW, Towbin RB, Chernausek SD: Precocious puberty following severe head trauma. Am J Dis Child 139:467, 1985
29. Brauner R, Czernichow P, Rappaport R: Precocious puberty after hypothalamic and pituitary irradiation in young children. (Letter) N Engl J Med 311:920, 1984
30. Root AW, Diamond F: The pituitary gland. In Pediatrics, Edited by VC Kelley. Philadelphia, Harper & Row, 1982, p 1
31. Hemady ZS, Siler-Khodr TM, Najjar S: Precocious puberty in juvenile hypothyroidism. J Pediatr 92:55, 1978

32. Geffner ME, Kaplan SA, Lippe BM, Fine RN: Precocious puberty and chronic renal failure. Am J Dis Child 137: 956, 1983
33. Zipf WB, Payne AH, Kelch RP: Prolactin, growth hormone and luteinizing hormone in the maintenance of testicular luteinizing hormone receptors. Endocrinology 103:595, 1978
34. Saal HM, Pagon RA, Pepin MG: Reevaluation of Russell-Silver syndrome. J Pediatr 107:733, 1985
35. Pescovitz OH, Comite F, Cassorla F, Dwyer AJ, Poth MA, Sperling MA, Hench K, McNemar A, Skerda M, Loriaux DL, Cutler GB Jr: True precocious puberty complicating congenital adrenal hyperplasia: treatment with luteinizing hormone-releasing hormone analog. J Clin Endocrinol Metab 58:857, 1984
36. Pescovitz OH, Hench K, Green O, Comite F, Loriaux DL, Cutler GB Jr: Central precocious puberty complicating a virilizing adrenal tumor: treatment with a long-acting LHRH analog. J Pediatr 106:612, 1985
37. Lucky AW, Rich BH, Rosenfield RL, Fang VS, Roche-Bender N: Bioactive LH: a test to discriminate true precocious puberty from premature thelarche and adrenarche. J Pediatr 97:214, 1980
38. Kulin HE, Santner SJ: Timed urinary gonadotropin measurements in normal infants, children, and adults, and in patients with disorders of sexual maturation. J Pediatr 90:760, 1977
39. Bidlingmaeir F, Butenandt O, Knorr D: Plasma gonadotropins and estrogens in girls with idiopathic precocious puberty. Pediatr Res 11:91, 1977
40. Reiter EO, Kaplan SL, Conte FA, Grumbach MM: Responsivity of pituitary gonadotropes to luteinizing hormone-releasing factor in idiopathic precocious puberty, precocious thelarche, precocious adrenarche, and in patients treated with medroxyprogesterone acetate. Pediatr Res 9:111, 1975
41. Zipf WB, Kelch RP, Hopwood NJ, Spencer ML, Bacon GE: Suppressed responsiveness to gonadotropin-releasing hormone in girls with unsustained isosexual precocity. J Pediatr 95:38, 1979
42. Lee PA: Medroxyprogesterone therapy for sexual precocity in girls. Am J Dis Child 135:443, 1981
43. Sigurjonsdottir TJ, Hayles AB: Precocious puberty: a report of 96 cases. Am J Dis Child 115:309, 1968
44. Editorial: Adrenal suppression by cyproterone acetate. Lancet 2:290, 1981
45. Kauli R, Prager-Lewin R, Keret R, Laron Z: The LH response to LH-releasing hormone in children with true isosexual precocious puberty treated with cyproterone acetate. Clin Endocrinol 4:305, 1975
46. Neumann F: Review: Pharmacology and potential use of cyphoterone acetate. Horm Metab Res 9:1, 1977
47. Clayton RN, Catt KJ: Gonadotropin releasing hormone receptors-characterization, physiologic regulation and relationship to reproductive function. Endocrinol Rev 2:186, 1981
48. Comite F, Cutler GB Jr, Rivier J, Vale WW, Loriaux DL, Crowley WF Jr: Short-term treatment of idiopathic precocious puberty with a long acting analogue of luteinizing hormone-releasing hormone. N Engl J Med 305: 1546, 1981
49. Crowley WF Jr, Comite F, Vale W, Rivier J, Loriaux DL, Cutler GB Jr: Therapeutic use of pituitary desensitization with a long-acting LHRH agonist: a potential new treatment for idiopathic precocious puberty. J Clin Endocrinol Metab 52:370, 1981
50. Laron Z, Kauli R, Ben Zeev Z, Comaru-Schally AM, Schally AV: D-Trp^6-analogue of luteinising hormone releasing hormone in combination with cyproterone acetate to treat precocious puberty. Lancet 2:955, 1981
51. Mansfield MJ, Beardsworth DE, Loughlin JS, Crawford JD, Bode HH, Rivier J, Vale W, Kushner DC, Crigler JF, Crowley WF Jr: Long-term treatment of central precocious puberty with a long-acting analogue of luteinizing hormone-releasing hormone. N Engl J Med 309:1286, 1983
52. Styne DM, Harris DA, Egli CA, Conte FA, Kaplan SL, Rivier J, Vale W, Grumbach MM: Treatment of true precocious puberty with a potent luteinizing hormone-releasing factor agonist: effect on growth, sexual maturation, pelvic sonography and the hypothalamic-pituitary-gonadal axis. J Clin Endocrinol Metab 61:142, 1985
53. Luder AS, Holland FJ, Costigan DC, Jenner MR, Wielgosz G, Fazekas ATA: Intranasal and subcutaneous treatment of central precocious puberty in both sexes with a long-acting analogue of luteinizing hormone-releasing hormone. J Clin Endocrinol Metab 58:966, 1984
54. Comite F, Pescovitz OH, Rieth KG, Dwyer AJ, Hench K, McNemar A, Loriaux DL, Cutler GB Jr: Luteinizing hormone-releasing hormone analog treatment of boys with hypothalamic hamartomas and true precocious puberty. J Clin Endocrinol Metab 59:888, 1984
55. Pescovitz OH, Comite F, Hench K, Barnes K, McNemar A, Foster C, Kenigsberg D, Loriaux DL, Cutter GB Jr: The NIH experience with precocious puberty: diagnostic subgroups and response to short-term luteinizing hormone releasing hormone analogue therapy. J Pediatr 108:47, 1986
56. Sonis WA, Comite F, Blue J, Pescovitz OH, Rahn CW, Hench KD, Cutler GB Jr, Loriaux DL, Klein RP: Behavior problems and social competence in girls with true precocious puberty. J Pediatr 106:156, 1985
57. Murram D, Dewhurst J, Grant DB: Precocious puberty: a follow-up study. Arch Dis Child 59:77, 1984
58. Root AW, Moshang T Jr: Evolution of the hyperandrogenism-polycystic ovarian syndrome from isosexual precocious puberty: report of two cases. Am J Obstet Gynecol 149:763, 1984
59. Demura R, Kubo O, Kitamura K, Jibiki K, Odagiri E, Demura H, Shizume K: Puberty due to ectopic hCG production in a girl with suprasellar ectopic pinealoma associated with panhypopituitarism. Endocrinol Jpn 31:71, 1984
60. Sklar CA, Conte FA, Kaplan SL, Grumbach MM: Human chorionic gonadotropin-secreting pineal tumor: relation to pathogenesis and sex limitation of sexual precocity. J Clin Endocrinol Metab 53:656, 1981
61. Root AW, Diamond FB Jr, Duncan JA: Ectopic and entopic peptide hormone secreting neoplasms of childhood. Adv Pediatr 32:369, 1985
62. Bosu WTK, Johansson EDB: Effect of hCG on plasma levels of estrogens and progesterone during the luteal phase of the menstrual cycle in rhesus monkeys (*Macaca mulatta*): stimulation of sex steroid production in rhesus monkeys. Int J Fertil 19:28, 1974
63. Chaussain JL, Lemerle J, Roger M, Canlorbe P, Job JC: Klinefelter syndrome, tumor, and sexual precocity. J Pediatr 97:607, 1980

64. Faggiano M, Criscuolo T, Perrone L, Quarto C, Sinisi AA: Sexual precocity in a boy due to hypersecretion of LH and prolactin by a pituitary adenoma. Acta Endocrinol 102:167, 1983
65. Case records of the Massachusetts General Hospital: Juvenile granulosa-cell tumor of ovary with sexual precocity. N Engl J Med 308:1279, 1983
66. Solh HM, Zaoury RS, Najjar SS: Peutz-Jeghers syndrome associated with precocious puberty. J Pediatr 103:593, 1983
67. Comite F, Schiebinger RJ, Albertson BD, Cassorla FG, VanderVen K, Cullen TF, Loriaux DL, Cutler GB Jr: Isosexual precocious pseudopuberty secondary to a feminizing adrenal tumor. J Clin Endocrinol Metab 58:435, 1984
68. Elgi CA, Rosenthal SM, Grumbach MM, Montalvo JM, Gondos B: Pituitary gonadotropin-independent male-limited autosomal dominant sexual precocity in nine generations: familial testotoxicosis. J Pediatr 106:33, 1985
69. Reiter EO, Brown RS, Longcope C, Beitins IZ: Male limited familial precocious puberty in three generations: apparent Leydig-cell autonomy and elevated glycoprotein hormone alpha subunit. N Engl J Med 311:515, 1984
70. Wierman ME, Beardsworth DE, Mansfield MJ, Badger TM, Crawford JD, Crigler JF Jr, Bode HH, Loughlin JS, Kushner DC, Scully RF, Hoffman WH, Crowley WF Jr: Puberty without gonadotropins: a unique mechanism of sexual development. N Engl J Med 312:65, 1985
71. Schedewie HK, Reiter EO, Beitins IZ, Seyed S, Wooten VD, Jimenez JF, Aiman EJ, DeVane GW, Redman JF, Elders MJ: Testicular Leydig cell hyperplasia as a cause of familial sexual precocity. J Clin Endocrinol Metab 52:271, 1981
72. Steinberger E, Root A, Ficher M, Smith KD: The role of androgens in the initiation of spermatogenesis in man. J Clin Endocrinol Metab 37:746, 1973
73. Rosenthal SM, Grumbach MM, Kaplan SL: Gonadotropin-independent familial sexual precocity with premature Leydig and germinal cell maturation (familial testotoxicosis): effects of a potent luteinizing hormone-releasing factor agonist and medroxyprogesterone acetate therapy in four cases. J Clin Endocrinol Metab 57:571, 1983
74. Raphaelson MI, Stevens JC, Elders J, Comite F, Theodore WH: Familial spastic paraplegia, mental retardation and precocious puberty. Arch Neurol 40:809, 1983
75. Cummings JL, Oppenheimer EY, Hochman HI: Tuberous sclerosis. Am J Dis Child 132:1215, 1978
76. Comite F, Shawker TH, Pescovitz OH, Loriaux DL, Cutler GB Jr: Cyclical ovarian function resistant to treatment with an analogue of luteinizing hormone-releasing hormone in McCune-Albright syndrome. N Engl J Med 311:1032, 1984
77. Netzloff ML, Wilson BE: Benign Leydig cell hyperplasia: treatment with cyproterone acetate. (Abstr) Pediatr Res 17:167A, 1983
78. Holland FJ, Fishman L, Bailey JD, Fazekas ATA: Ketoconazole in the management of precocious puberty not responsive to LHRH-analogue therapy. N Engl J Med 312:1023, 1985
79. Sikka SC, Swerdloff RS, Rajfer J: In vitro inhibition of testosterone biosynthesis by ketoconazole. Endocrinology 116:1920, 1985
80. McKiernan JF, Hull D: Breast development in the newborn. Arch Dis Child 56:525, 1981
81. Mills JL, Stolley PD, Davies J, Moshang T Jr: Premature thelarche: natural history and etiologic investigation. Am J Dis Child 135:743, 1981
82. Ilicki A, Lewin RP, Kauli R, Kaufman H, Schacter A, Laron Z: Premature thelarche: natural history and sex hormone secretion in 68 girls. Acta Paediatr Scand 73:756, 1984
83. Rosenfield RL: The ovary and female sexual maturation. In Clinical Pediatric and Adolescent Endocrinology, Edited by SA Kaplan. Philadelphia, W. B. Saunders Co., 1982, p 217
84. Suwa S, Maesaka H, Matsui I: Serum LH and FSH responses to synthetic LH-RH in normal infants, children and patients with Turner's syndrome. Pediatrics 54:470, 1974
85. Comas AP: Precocious sexual development in Puerto Rico. (Letter) Lancet 1:1299, 1982
86. Pasquino AM, Piccolo F, Scalamandre A, Malvaso M, Ortolani R, Boscherini B: Hypothalamic-pituitary-gonadotropic function in girls with premature thelarche. Arch Dis Child 55:941, 1980
87. Caufriez A, Wolter R, Govaerts M, L'Hermite M, Robyn C: Gonadotropins and prolactin pituitary reserve in premature thelarche. J Pediatr 91:751, 1977
88. Job JC, Guilhaume B, Chaussain JL, Garnier PE: Le development premature isole des seins chez les fillettes: resultats de l'epreuve a la LH-RH. Arch Fr Pediatr 32:39, 1975
89. Nelson KG: Premature thelarche in children born prematurely. J Pediatr 103:756, 1983
90. Fara GM, Del Corvo G, Bernuzzi S, Bigatello A, DiPietro C, Scaglioni S, Chiumella G: Epidemic of breast enlargement in an Italian school. Lancet 2:295, 1979
91. Saenz de Rodriguez CA, Bongiovanni AM, Conde de Borrego L: An epidemic of precocious development in Puerto Rican children. J Pediatr 107:393, 1985
92. Loizzo A, Gatti GL, Macri A, Moretti G, Ortolani E, Palazzesi S: Italian baby food containing diethylstilbestrol: three years later. (Letter) Lancet 1:1014, 1984
93. Schoental R: Precocious sexual development in Puerto Rico and oestrogenic mycotoxins (Zearalenone). (Letter) Lancet 1:537, 1983
94. Widholm O: Genital bleeding during childhood. Ann Pediatr 10:170, 1981
95. Heller ME, Dewhurst J, Grant DB: Premature menarche without other evidence of precocious puberty. Arch Dis Child 54:472, 1979
96. Murram D, Dewhurst J, Grant DB: Premature menarche: a follow-up study. Arch Dis Child 58:142, 1983
97. Blanco-Garcia M, Evain-Brion D, Roger M, Job JC: Isolated menses in prepubertal girls. Pediatrics 76:43, 1985
98. Parker LN, Odell WD: Control of adrenal androgen secretion. Endocrinol Rev 1:392, 1980
99. Kennerson AR, McDonald DA, Adams JB: Dehydroepiandrosterone sulfotransferase localization in human adrenal glands: a light and election microscopic study. J Clin Endocrinol Metab 56:786, 1983

100. Reiter EO, Fuldauer VG, Root AW: Secretion of the adrenal androgen, dehydroepiandrosterone sulfate, during normal infancy, childhood, and adolescence, in sick infants, and in children with endocrinologic abnormalities. J Pediatr 90:766, 1977
101. Rosenfield RL, Rich BH, Lucky AW: Adrenarche as a cause of benign pseudo-puberty in boys. J Pediatr 101: 1005, 1982
102. Kaplowitz PB, Cockrell JL: Premature adrenarche: clinical and diagnostic features. (Abstr) Pediatr Res 19: 186A, 1985
103. Rich BH, Rosenfield RL, Lucky AW, Helke JC, Otto P: Adrenarche: changing adrenal response to adrenocorticotropin. J Clin Endocrinol Metab 52:1129, 1981
104. Schiebinger RJ, Albertson BD, Cassorla FG, Bowyer DW, Geelehoed GW, Cutler GB Jr, Loriaux DL: The developmental change in plasma adrenal androgens during infancy and adrenarche are associated with changing activities of adrenal microsomal 17-hydroxylase and 17,20-desmolase. J Clin Invest 67:1177, 1981
105. Dickerman Z, Grant DR, Faiman C, Winter JSD: Intraadrenal steroid concentrations in man: zonal differences and developmental changes. J Clin Endocrinol Metab 59:1031, 1984
106. Byrne GC, Perry YS, Winter JSD: Kinetic analysis of adrenal 3β-hydroxysteroid dehydrogenase activity during human development. J Clin Endocrinol Metab 60: 934, 1985
107. Hauffa BP, Kaplan SL, Grumbach MM: Dissociation between plasma adrenal androgens and cortisol in Cushing's disease and ectopic ACTH-producing tumor: relation to adrenarche. Lancet 1:1373, 1984
108. Cutler GB Jr, Davis SE, Johnsonbauch RE, Loriaux DL: Dissociation of cortisol and adrenal androgen secretion in patients with secondary adrenal insufficiency. J Clin Endocrinol Metab 49:604, 1979
109. Albertson BD, Hobson WC, Burnett BS, Turner PT, Clark RV, Schiebinger RJ, Loriaux DL, Cutler GB Jr: Dissociation of cortisol and adrenal androgen secretion in the hypophysectomized, adrenocorticotropin-replaced chimpanzee. J Clin Endocrinol Metab 59:13, 1984
110. Parker LN, Lifrak ET, Odell WD: A 60,000 molecular weight human pituitary glycopeptide stimulates adrenal androgen secretion. Endocrinology 113:2092, 1983
111. Winterer J, Gwirtsman HE, George DT, Kaye WH, Loriaux DL, Cutler GB Jr: Adrenocorticotropin-stimulated adrenal androgen secretion in anorexia nervosa: impaired secretion at low weight with normalization after long-term weight recovery. J Clin Endocrinol Metab 61:693, 1985
112. Sigurjonsdottir TJ, Hayles AB: Premature pubarche. Clin Pediatr 7:26, 1968
113. Temeck JW, Pang S, New MI: Premature adrenarche resulting from symptomatic non-classical congenital adrenal hyperplasia. (Abstr.) Pediatr Res 18:178A, 1984
114. Granoff AB, Chasalow FI, Blethen SL: 17-hydroxyprogesterone responses to adrenocorticotropin in children with premature adrenarche. J Clin Endocrinol Metab 60:409, 1985

SECTION IV

Female Reproductive Tract Surgery

Modern medicine has progressively become procedure-oriented. The evolution of methodology has been abetted by technologic developments applicable to both diagnosis and treatment. In reviewing developments in infertility surgery over the last 3 years, the expression "we have both good news and bad news" is appropriate. First, the good news! As this section of the text demonstrates, we currently can boast of exciting new modalities for reconstructive reproductive tract surgery. Operative endoscopy has become a widely utilized entity, and laser surgery continues to generate significant enthusiasm among reproductive surgeons. The bad news, however, is that despite the potential for dramatically improving the outlook for infertile couples with tubal and peritubal disease, many of the new techniques have yet to demonstrate marked superiority over conventional methodology. Not intended to denigrate these novel approaches to infertility surgery, this statement is based upon a deficiency of comparable data on which to draw valid conclusions. In vitro fertilization (IVF), as an alternative to these surgical techniques, has already established itself as a vital component of infertility services. We now are positioned to compare the results of new and conventional methods of reconstructive surgery to what IVF can offer. In the evaluation of pharmacologic agents, randomized and double blinded studies are prerequisites for comparing the efficacy of various treatment modalities. In contrast, overzealous conclusions and enthusiastic claims regarding elective surgery for correction of infertility outnumber carefully prepared studies designed to determine whether a specific procedure using a new approach produces superior results to those using an established method. In this section the reader should note each author's clear proclamation that the data available to us are as yet insufficient to document superiority, primarily due to the lack of appropriate clinical trials.

Operative laparoscopy has truly come of age over the past 15 years. Operative laparoscopy, which had its origin as a means for tubal sterilization in the early 1970s, has been used for ever-increasing indications. Substantial data have accumulated to justify its use in many of these situations. The range of laparoscopic procedures described by Murphy in her chapter now encompasses ectopic pregnancy, endometriosis, tuboplasty, lysis of adhesions, ovarian cystectomy, oophorectomy, and myomectomy. These applications are in addition to the well-established technique of oocyte retrieval by follicle aspiration. What are the advantages of operative laparoscopy? The potential decrease in duration of hospital stay and reduction in hospital costs represent significant benefits in the cost-conscious field of medicine. Increasing expertise with these laparoscopic procedures and experience with new instruments should also diminish the amount of operating time. Instruments have already been designed to suture, coagulate, grasp, cut, irrigate, morcellate, and provide hemostasis. Just as the vaginal approach to hysterectomy reduces operating time and morbidity as compared to abdominal hysterectomy, operative laparoscopy could convey similar benefits. It is important to appreciate, however, that the goal of infertility-related surgery is attainment of a functional result. The mere ability to carry out a given procedure does not guarantee satisfactory results. Definitive conclusions await, as Murphy clearly states, carefully conducted clinical trials on which to base an evaluation of functional results.

The incidence of ectopic pregnancy has increased dramatically over the past decade. In 1970, the rate of ectopic pregnancy was 4.5 per 1,000; by 1978 it had reached 9.4 per 1,000 pregnancies. Translated into actual numbers, 17,800 ectopic pregnancies were reported in the United States in 1970 and 42,400 by 1978. More than half the ectopic pregnancies occurred in the 25- to 34-year age range, but a rising incidence has also been noted in the 15 through 19 age group (2.7 per 1,000 in 1976; 5.7 per 1,000 in 1981). Implications with regard to future reproductive potential are obvious. New modes of management and therapy have had a dramatic influence on morbidity and future fertility. The four most prominent factors in making this possible have been: (1) introduction of sensitive pregnancy testing; (2) the widespread use of diagnostic laparoscopy; (3) increasing experience with diagnostic sonography; and (4) development of microsurgical techniques. Early diagnosis of ectopic pregnancy has paved the way for a more conservative approach to its management.

Ironically, the acceptance of conservative surgery for ectopic pregnancy as well as a heightened increase in reconstructive tubal surgery have led to an increase in the iatrogenic etiology of ectopic pregnancy. Lavy, Diamond, and DeCherney have carefully reviewed the world's literature and point out that a history of tubal surgery places the patient in a "higher-risk group for ectopic pregnancy." Of patients undergoing reconstructive tubal surgery, 3% to 20% will ultimately experience an ectopic pregnancy. The reality of these figures should be considered whenever tubal reconstructive surgery is contemplated or recommended. The last table in this chapter summarizes the range in risk for ectopic pregnancy following five distinct surgical procedures. Individual rates are cited for each type of procedure depending on whether microsurgical or macrosurgical techniques were used. The bottom line tells us that overall the ranges for viable pregnancies and ectopic pregnancies do not differ dramatically in the microsurgical and macrosurgical groups.

Since the mid 1970s when surgical lasers were introduced, we've witnessed an expansion in their use from several experimental programs to widespread popularity. The term "laser surgery" has become considered synonymous with the ultimate in high technologic expertise. The word *laser* is an acronym for "light amplification by stimulated emission of radiation." With this technique, electrical energy is converted to light; the light energy released is manipulated by optical and mechanical means to achieve its effect on tissues. Currently, the lasers most frequently used in female reproductive tract procedures are carbon dioxide, argon, and neodymium:yttrium-aluminum garnet (YAG). At present, the laser is more widely used for cervical, vaginal, and vulvar surgery than for intra-abdominal procedures associated with correction of infertility or treatment of endometriosis. Its less frequent use for intra-abdominal purposes is based in part on potential for injury to underlying structures by misdirection of the laser beam. Possible injury to adjacent or underlying structures, damage to the eyes of operating room personnel, and irritating effects of the smoke (vaporized plume) on the respiratory tract of the surgical team represent the major hazards. Long-term implications of the residue of intra-abdominal laser use remain unknown. Despite these potential risks, the safety record with lasers has been good. As a new tool for patients with surgically correctable infertility problems, lasers offer many potential advantages. Accurate and carefully directed hemostasis, reduced adhesion formation, and less tissue injury are among the presumed benefits over conventional microsurgical techniques. In Daniell's chapter each of these advantages is subjected to review and evaluation. The conclusions to be drawn from both animal experimentation and clinical experience are that we need more hard data, and that specific indications and long-term results are still undefined. Vaporization of endometriosis may be the major exception in that with both laparoscopic or open surgical use of the CO_2 laser, the percentage of patients with endometriosis achieving term pregnancy seems high. The range of results within the data cited is too wide, however, to justify a final conclusion as to the superiority of laser approaches to infertility surgery. Daniell carefully emphasizes these considerations, concluding that at present we are still in the developmental stage. Daniell's statement ". . . in spite of claimed improvements in surgical results with the use of the CO_2 laser for difficult reconstructive pelvic procedures, the true benefits of the laser are still unproven in infertility surgery," appears to sum up the lack of sufficient, comparative control data necessary to enable definitive conclusions. Those centers which have the expert reconstructive surgeons, the proper facilities and instruments, a large volume of patients requiring infertility surgery, and an investigative spirit will undoubtedly provide answers to the question raised by the chapter's title, "The role of lasers in infertility surgery."

Although lasers offer an additional tool for reproductive surgeons in their pursuit of restoring tubal function, the maximum potential of the damaged tube following its repair is important in understanding our limitations. In this light, Bateman and his associates have inquired as to whether we've progressed in the surgical management of distal tubal obstruction. His comprehensive chapter outlines the physiologic components of tubal function and describes the means whereby injury distorts oviductal anatomy and function of the oviducts. The major question is whether these changes, once established, are reversible. Ciliary function, tubal muscular activity, and endosalpingeal secretions all cooperate in providing the optimum environment for gamete transport, fertilization, and early embryonic development. Are these functions restorable by anatomic reconstruction once they've been disrupted? Over the past 10 years, chlamydia infections have rivalled gonococcal disease as a cause of tubal and peritubal disease. That chlamydial infections can be asymptomatic is of special concern, since silent salpingitis defies treatment of the active phase. Bateman and colleagues have outlined the spectrum of procedures which have been performed on the distal tube. Use of laparoscopic procedures, laser, prostheses, microsurgical technique, hydrotubation, and adjuvants are among the variables which need to be considered. The tables in the Bateman chapter are extremely valuable in comparing various techniques and reported series. The range in the results of surgery is reminiscent of the data cited by Daniell and by Murphy in their chapters in this section. In addition to viable pregnancy rates, the increased incidence of ectopic pregnancy following reconstructive surgery must be considered for each modality of therapy. Following correction of distal tubal occlusion, a long latent period usually precedes resumption of tubal function. As Bateman points out, a minimum of 1 year is usually required until post-salpingostomy pregnancies begin to appear.

In the previous volume of *Modern Trends,* Muse and Wilson[1] reviewed the mechanism(s) whereby endometriosis leads to infertility. Schmidt revisits this question in her chapter, reappraising pathogenesis and treatment of endometriosis. Over the past 3 years our knowledge about danazol and its effectiveness has increased.[2] During the same time period a revised classification system for endometriosis has also been developed by The American Fertility Society, enabling better comparisons among different groups.[3] This type of standardization is a sine qua non for evaluation of therapeutic results. Gonadotropin releasing hormone and the availability of IVF have become promising additions to our therapeutic arsenal of what we can now offer infertile patients with endometriosis. We have not yet found the answer to endometriosis, but at least we're currently able to select from among a variety of approaches the appropriate therapy to meet the needs of individual patients. Once measures are developed to prevent this disease, which is being encountered with increasing frequency, the dilemma of endometriosis may be a thing of the past.

Rounding out this section, the chapter of Syrop and Halme reviews the function of peritoneal fluid in the reproductive process. With its constituents—steroids, protein hormones, prostaglandins, plasminogen activator, and macrophages—peritoneal fluid has the potential for aiding or impeding reproductive function. The steroid milieu is thought to reflect ovulation and corpus luteum function; peritoneal prostaglandin levels may correlate with ovulatory or tubal dysfunction; the presence of plasminogen activator in peritoneal fluid may serve as an index of ovulation. Syrop and Halme cite evidence to suggest that macrophages in peritoneal fluid are instrumental in endometriosis-related infertility. Their presence may alter sperm migration and/or function. The realization that peritoneal fluid is readily obtainable and has the potential for supplying important diagnostic or prognostic information opens new vistas for investigation in the province of reproductive failure.

Edward E. Wallach, M.D.

REFERENCES

1. Muse K, Wilson E: How does mild endometriosis cause infertility? In Modern Trends in Infertility and Conception Control, Vol 3, Edited by EE Wallach, RD Kempers. Chicago, Year Book Medical Publishers, Inc., 1985, p 264
2. Dmowski W: Endocrine properties and clinical application of danazol. In Modern Trends in Infertility and Conception Control, Vol 3, Edited by EE Wallach, RD Kempers. Chicago, Year Book Medical Publishers, Inc., 1985, p 162
3. The American Fertility Society: Revised American Fertility Society Classification of Endometriosis. Fertil Steril 43:351, 1985

Chapter 17

Operative laparoscopy

Ana Alvarez Murphy, M.D.

Department of Gynecology and Obstetrics, Division of Reproductive Endocrinology, The Johns Hopkins University School of Medicine, Baltimore, Maryland

Operative laparoscopy is a powerful technique in the armamentarium of the reproductive and gynecologic surgeon. By definition, the technique refers to a large number of procedures that can be carried out through the laparoscope. A distinction is made between the use of the laparoscope for diagnostic purposes and its use in performing surgical procedures. This section will review the prerequisites for safe endoscopic surgery, the instrumentation available, and the pelvic reconstructive and gynecologic procedures that can be carried out through the laparoscope. Although laparoscopic female sterilization may be considered an operative procedure, much has been written on the subject and it will not be covered here.

The evolution of endoscopy has been rapid in the various medical fields, and gynecology is no exception. In 1901, Kelling published, in Hamburg, an experimental study of endoscopy of the abdomen in dogs.[1] Nine years later, Jacobaeus, of Sweden, recorded the first visualization of the human peritoneal cavity.[2] He used a trocar with a cannula to create pneumoperitoneum and introduced a German cystoscope through the cannula. Bernheim,[1] in America, described peritoneal "cystoscopy" in 1911.

In 1937, Ruddock, in the United States, reported 500 cases with a mortality of 0.2% and introduced a biopsy forceps with diathermy coagulation.[1] In 1939, TeLinde[1] attempted endoscopy through the cul-de-sac but abandoned it because of difficulty with the presence of the small intestine. Decker, in 1944,[1] introduced the "pneumoperitoneum" by creating a negative pressure with the genupectoral position. Palmer[1] of France in 1946 used the lithotomy Trendelenberg position and created a "gaseous distention." He also used a uterine cannula to elevate the uterus.

An important breakthrough was made when Fourestier, Gladu, and Vulmiere[2] developed a cool method of transmitting intense light in 1947. That same year, Hopkins and Kampany[2] of England introduced fiber optics. The first English language laparoscopic monograph was written by Steptoe[2] in 1967 and the first American one by Cohen[2] in 1968.

In 1962, Palmer[1] published his initial experience with destruction by unipolar electrosurgery of the isthmic and proximal ampulla of the tube. Since the early 1970s the quest for safe, effective methods of sterilization led to bipolar electrocautery, thermocoagulation, clips, and rings.

Semm of Germany[3] reported the performance of salpingectomy, adnexectomy, myomectomy, oophorectomy, ovarian cystectomy, and salpingostomy through the laparoscope as early as 1974. In 1977, Gomel[4] reported sharp dissection and neosalpingostomies in nine patients, eight with previous tuboplastics. Of note is the achievement by four of these patients of an intrauterine pregnancy. More recent contributions will be discussed in the text. In essence, however, the future of operative laparoscopy remains to be written.

GENERAL CONSIDERATIONS

Many gynecologic surgical procedures can be achieved safely and effectively by laparoscopy. However, prior to operative laparoscopy, an appropriate workup is essential, whether for infertility, pelvic pain, ectopic pregnancy, or a variety of other disorders. The indications for the procedure must be carefully reviewed, as for any surgical procedure.

The contraindications to operative laparoscopy are the same as for diagnostic laparoscopy. Absolute contraindications include bowel obstruction, ileus, abdominal hernia, peritonitis, brisk intraperitoneal bleeding, diaphragmatic hernia, and severe cardiorespiratory disease.[5, 6] The first four contraindications take into consideration the unacceptably high risk of bowel perforation in patients with distended bowel and of strangulation of hernial contents. Patients with diaphragmatic hernias and cardiorespiratory disease may experience intraoperative distress induced or exacerbated by the pneumoperitoneum raising the diaphragm, the Trendelenburg position, and decrease in venous return from gaseous compression of the large vessels.

Relative contraindications include extremes of body weight, inflammatory bowel disease, previous surgery, the presence of a large intraabdominal mass, and advanced intrauterine pregnancy.[5, 6] Massive obesity should be an absolute contraindication because it is nearly impossible to manipulate instruments through the second puncture site even if trocars are long enough to enter the peritoneal cavity. Small, thin patients are also at risk because the distance between the anterior abdominal wall and the abdominal aorta is often quite small. The Verres needle should be inserted almost parallel to the abdominal wall.

Adhesive bowel disease and fistula formation increase the risk of laparoscopy in patients with inflammatory bowel disease such as regional enteritis. Obviously, previous surgery and subsequent adhesions increase the risk of perforating bowel, bladder, or other pelvic organs. A large intraabdominal mass and advanced pregnancy make visualization difficult through the laparoscope and increase the risk of puncturing the mass. Exploration, when indicated, should probably be approached through a laparotomy incision in both cases.

TECHNIQUE OF OPERATIVE LAPAROSCOPY

Regardless of the operative procedure performed, general anesthesia with good muscle relaxation is a must. Although sterilization under local anesthesia with sedation can be performed without much difficulty, operative cases are long by comparison and are associated with continued painful stimuli. Good muscle relaxation is necessary to facilitate introduction of trocars and manipulation of instruments. In essence, it offers greater comfort to patient and surgeon as well as increased safety.

Most, if not all, operative laparoscopists place the patient in the dorsal lithotomy position with the table broken at the perineum to facilitate uterine manipulation. Frequently it is necessary to depress the uterine manipulator sharply, and this can only be done with the patient's buttocks protruding slightly from the table. Multiple rigid cannulas are available for manipulation of the uterus and chromotubation. Manual manipulation is not advisable in extensive operative cases.

Laparoscopy should be performed with the patient's bladder empty. For diagnostic laparoscopy we ask the patient to void immediately before proceeding to the operating room. Because patients undergoing operative laparoscopy have often undergone previous laparotomies and the operating time is increased over diagnostic cases, an indwelling Foley catheter is generally inserted and removed immediately postoperatively.

Pneumoperitoneum is achieved, as in diagnostic laparoscopy, with great care. This step is critical in avoiding major complications. A Verres needle is usually introduced at the inferior rim of the umbilicus; however, in patients with previous scars, alternate sites for achieving pneumoperitoneum should be considered. These include all the sites for "second puncture," as well as above the umbilicus in the midline and below the costal margin, and to the left approximately 2 fingerbreadths.[7] Insufflation has also been approached vaginally.

The primary trocar is introduced through the same incision once adequate pneumoperitoneum has been achieved. Gomel[7] and Semm[8] have advocated testing for free space under the umbilicus with a glass syringe containing a small amount of saline. If there is adequate space, gas bubbles will be seen in the saline and the plunger will elevate. The limits of the space may be defined by gradually moving the needle up and down and from side to side. Alternatively, one may inject saline and withdraw. If fluid returns into the syringe, one may conclude that the fluid inside the peritoneum is not free-flowing and may be contained in bowel or bladder. One may again define the limits of free space under the umbilicus in this manner.

Many manufacturers offer a wide range of laparoscopes with corresponding trocars and cannulas, which, unfortunately, are often not interchangeable. Laparoscopes may be changed during the operation. Many operators prefer to begin with a small 6.5-mm scope. The larger 11-mm scope with twin fiber bundles or an operative channel can later be introduced for better visualization and/or photographic documentation. Small diameter laparoscopes ranging from 5 to 10 mm are available and are adequate for diagnostic and operative cases. Theoretically, these instruments are safer because less force is required to penetrate the abdomen, and the smaller tip of the trocar will decrease the depth of penetration.[9] Different angles of view, either straightforward or oblique (45 degrees), are available. We prefer the former, but the choice, in essence, belongs to the surgeon. Several operating laparoscopes are available and are, by necessity, of greater diameter. The Jacob Palmer instrument, which has an offset eyepiece but a viewing system that allows a "straight on" view identical to that of a diagnostic laparoscope, works well. The proximity of instruments to the operator's head is a disadvantage; however, this is offset by the advantage of an angle for operation not offered by ancillary operating equipment inserted through second, third, and even fourth puncture sites.

Many apparatuses for pneumoperitoneum have been specifically designed that deliver carbon dioxide. The insufflators employed for laparoscopy and hysteroscopy are not interchangeable, because the volume and flow rates are significantly different in these two procedures. Laparoscopy units generally permit insufflation at 1 l/minute. Those with "high or fast flow" can insufflate at 3 l/minute. This is particularly helpful to have when one is performing operative laparoscopy and changing instruments frequently.

Fiber optic technology has provided the ability to transmit light through the laparoscope and into the abdominal cavity. Most endoscope manufacturers produce light sources that are adequate for operating purposes. A high-powered light source is necessary for photography. The light delivered is a function of the power of the external source and the diameter of the cable (number of fibers). The laparoscope with twin fiber bundles allows photodocumentation with clarity and sharpness. It is also very useful for video recording.

Proper placement of the second, third, and even fourth puncture site is necessary to manipulate, cut, and suture pelvic tissues. One should transilluminate the abdominal wall in an effort to locate large vessels prior to insertion of a second puncture lateral to the midline. The course of the inferior epigastric artery, which comes up over the semicircular fold of Douglas and enters the rectus sheath, should be kept in mind. Hypotensive collapse of a patient from inferior epigastric vessel trauma is not unknown.[10] Punctures should also be performed under direct visualization so that the bladder is not inadvertently punctured and other pelvic organs are also protected. Feasible puncture sites are illustrated in Figure 1. Generally we use two or three ancillary puncture sites. The midline site is usually used for stabilizing the adnexa. The side punctures are placed slightly anterior and to either side of the operative site where the abnormality is located. If the puncture site is not lateral to the area of interest, the instrument may originate from an angle of poor visibility. These recommendations are, of course, generalizations, and the surgeon's approach must always be tailored to the individual patient.

Persistent bleeding from an anterior wall puncture site is uncommon. Usually coagulation solves the problem. On the rare occasions when

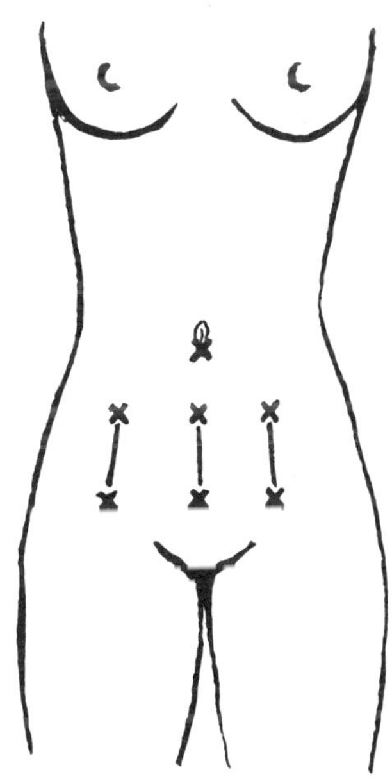

Figure 1
Ancillary puncture sites.

bleeding persists, the surgeon can enlarge the puncture site and locate the specific cause. Alternatively, the Kiel group[8] uses a very large "abdominal wall needle" that transfixes the abdominal wall on either side of the bleeding site and is tied externally. This "pressure suture" is then removed in 48 hours. No significant bleeding has been noted after the suture removal.

ANCILLARY INSTRUMENTS

Almost all manufacturers produce a complete line of ancillary instruments to be used through a second puncture site or through the operating channel of a laparoscope. The use of both types of instruments provides much versatility in an endoscopy system. A myriad of instruments are produced by several companies. Because of limitations in the length of this text, all instruments will not be discussed; nevertheless, the broad categories of instrumentation will be considered.

PROBES

A blunt probe is probably the most commonly used instrument. It is often essential for visualization of structures that require manipulation, such as the lateral sides of both ovaries. These probes are usually marked in centimeters, a useful adjunct because the magnification of the laparoscopic lens can make estimation of size difficult. Probes are also useful in immobilizing structures atraumatically for operative laparoscopy.

GRASPER/FORCEPS

A range of forceps is an essential part of an operative laparoscopy set. The ability to stabilize a structure atraumatically is the key to many procedures. The small forceps can also be used to dilate the ampulla when performing a salpingostomy. Large traumatic forceps are used to stabilize structures for the purpose of morcellation (Fig. 2).

SCISSORS

These come in many designs, including toothed, "micro," and hooked. It is essential that they be kept in good repair. Some scissors can be combined with unipolar electrocoagulation. The hooked scissors which have overlapping tips

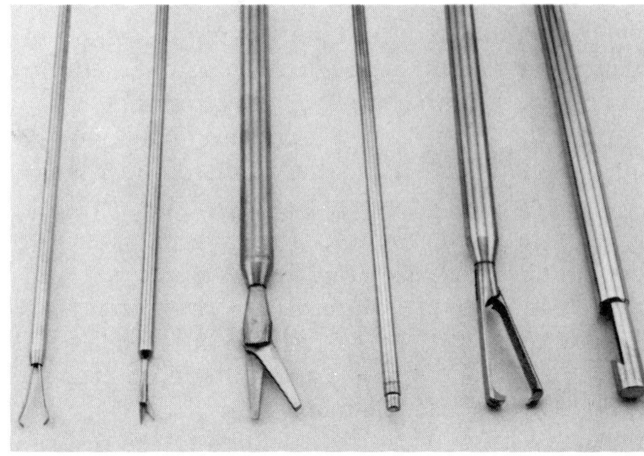

Figure 2
Ancillary instruments. From left to right: atraumatic grasper, microscissors, large scissors, point endocoagulator, traumatic forceps, morcellator. All instruments made by Wisap Co., Sauerlach, FRG.

should be used very cautiously, because even when closed they may cause inadvertent damage.[9]

BIOPSY

Biopsy forceps that are sharp and overlap slightly when closed provide the best biopsy specimens. Instruments that are not sharp tear tissue, and bleeding is usually greater than with a clean cut. These instruments come in various sizes, with one or two movable jaws. The biopsy forceps with a small hook in its upper and/or lower jaw is helpful in obtaining a biopsy from "hard" tissue. It keeps the tissue from slipping out of the jaw before it can be cleanly cut.

ASPIRATORS

With the advent of in vitro fertilization (IVF), aspirators have become an important part of our instrumentation. The cannula should have a large tip, permitting clean penetration. Some operators prefer a beveled tip, and others believe that the sharp tip is traumatic to the oocyte. Aspiration may be regulated manually with suction provided by a large syringe or by mechanical means, depending upon the surgeon's preference. A combined irrigation aspiration instrument is useful, especially after an operation for lavage and also to pinpoint bleeding sites.[11] A combination bipolar electrocoagulator and irrigation/aspiration instrument is also available, permitting irrigation or aspiration of a specific site to facilitate localization and coagulation of a bleeding point.[9]

TISSUE REMOVAL

Large pieces of tissue may be removed from the abdomen by cutting them into pieces small enough to be grasped and removed through the laparoscope. Alternatively, a tissue punch is available for morcellation with an automatic device for obtaining multiple tissue specimens, which are stored in the sheath[11] (Fig. 2). In either case, the pathologist may question mincing of the specimen before submitting it. The surgeon may also choose to make a small suprapubic incision for removal of the specimen.

HEMOSTASIS

Methods of achieving hemostasis include unipolar or bipolar electrocautery, endocoagulation, laser, and intraabdominal suturing. The ability to achieve hemostasis is integral to any endoscopic procedure. The method selected usually depends on instrument availability and the degree of familiarity the surgeon has with a particular method.

ELECTROCAUTERY

Most modern electrosurgical units can be employed in both unipolar and bipolar modes. In a unipolar system the current passes from the generator through the instrument to a ground plate and then back to the generator. The bipolar system uses the two insulated jaws of the instrument to carry the current to and from the generator. The tissue between the jaws completes the circuit, and tissue is heated (coagulated) by passage of the current. Both unipolar and bipolar units are available for use through the laparoscope. Many instruments, especially scissors, can be combined with electrocautery. The complications inherent in electrocautery, especially unipolar, when used at laparoscopy and the means of preventing these accidents have been reviewed.[12, 13]

THERMOCOAGULATION/ENDOCOAGULATION

This technique, developed by Semm in 1962 for the treatment of "benign lesions of the cervix," has since been successfully extended to laparoscopy.[14] Endocoagulation achieves hemostasis by heating the tissue to 100° to 140°C. It is thought that denaturing of proteins and dessication cause coagulation. The temperature can be monitored visually and by a changing tone which indicates that the temperature is in the correct coagulating range. There are two instruments available to deliver the heat, a crocodile forceps and a point coagulator.[15] Unfortunately the point coagulator is fairly large and difficult to use in microsurgical work (Fig. 2), but is quite useful for endometriotic implants.

LASER

Endoscopic laser technology is evolving rapidly and provides a new technique for both coagulation and cutting. The power density is directly proportional to the power level (selected by the surgeon) and inversely proportional to the surface area hit by the beam. The ability of the target tissue to absorb the beam determines the area of destruction.[9] Special modification of the operating channel allows the focusing lens and gas to flow through the same channel.[16] The laser is focused to a small spot beyond the end of the laparoscope. A channel is also available for plume evacuation. The need to evacuate the plume represents a drawback, and a pneumoperitoneum may be difficult to maintain. The laser energy can also be carried by a second puncture with a 1-mm spot size, 2 cm beyond the probe tip. Three types of lasers have been used in endoscopy: carbon dioxide (CO_2), argon, and neudymium/yttrium/aluminum garnet (YAG). The CO_2 laser is the most commonly used. Its energy is converted to heat and adsorbed, resulting in vaporization of the tissue. Measurements of the velocity at which steam expands reveal that the pressure exerted on adjacent tissue by cell disruption is small. Fine focusing (high power density) results in cutting, whereas a defocused beam (low power density) has coagulating properties. Its use in endometriosis is becoming more common and will be discussed later in the text.

Unfortunately, the four methods of coagulation have not been compared, except as techniques of sterilization. Riedel and Semm[17] performed CO_2 laparoscopies on New Zealand white rabbits and used either unipolar or bipolar high-frequency current or the endocoagulation technique for sterilization. Laparotomies were performed for sterilization with the CO_2 laser. The area of destruction around the coagulated area was found to be greatest with unipolar followed by bipolar and endocoagulation. The CO_2 laser had the smallest area of peripheral tissue destruction. Follow-up study revealed that the extent of coagulation could not be correlated with surgical experience but rather was correlated with the maximum temperature in the tissue and the coagulation time.[18] Our microsurgical laboratory is presently examining these four modalities with respect to ability to achieve hemostasis and consequent tissue damage and healing.

SUTURE

The ability to suture intraabdominally has certainly widened our horizons. The Roeder loop (Ethibinder, Ethicon, Somerville, NJ) is a Semm modification of the loop developed by Roeder in the early 1900s for tonsillectomy in children.[19] Soderstrom and Smith,[20] in 1971, also described a modification of a rectal polyp snare for laparoscopic tubal ligation which resulted in a Pomeroy type of sterilization. This loop can be placed around the structure and tightened, thereby ligating the tissue and its blood vessels. The loop is introduced with an applicator, and forceps are used to hold the tissue until the loop is tightened. At present the loop is only available in 1 plain and 0 chromic catgut. Only one suture is usually placed for omental bleeding points. In adnexectomy, salpingectomy, and ovariectomy, three sutures are usually placed.[21] The Kiel group has not had a bleeding complication with the Roeder loop following the above recommendation.[22] Intraabdominal suturing is also possible with a straight needle (ST-3) and suture of 2 plain catgut (Ethi-endo-naht) or 4-0 polydioxanone suture (PDS) with a double arm taper (ST-4) which can be introduced through a second puncture. Needle holder and forceps allow appropriate manipulation of the tissue and needle[12] (Fig. 3). Tying is accomplished either by an instrument tie intraabdominally or extracorporeally with a Roeder knot tied outside the abdomen but tightened intraabdominally (Figs. 4 and 5).

The pelvis should always be copiously lavaged at the end of surgery and any blood removed from the cul-de-sac if present. One may also instill a solution of choice—dextran, hydrocortisone and heparin, or promethazine at the end of surgery.

The assistant is an integral part of the team. The surgeon may have both hands occupied using ancillary instruments, in which case the assistant must hold the laparoscope or other instruments steadily. His/her role is greatly facilitated by a teaching attachment or video. Unfortunately, especially with the teaching attachment, visualization is decreased because of diminution of illumination. An ancillary puncture site may be used for insertion of a small laparoscope. An assistant may observe all or part of an operation. A light source for the second laparoscope is not necessary.

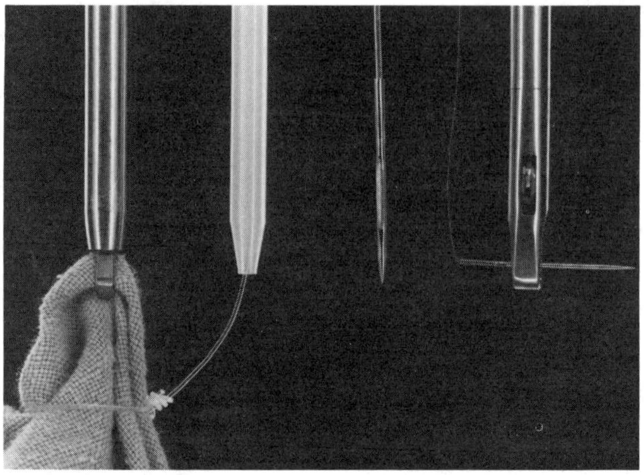

Figure 3
Intraabdominal sutures. From left to right: Ethibinder, Ethi-endo-naht, needleholder with a taper needle and 4-0 PDS.

Laparoscopic surgery should not be attempted by surgeons who have not mastered the technique of diagnostic laparoscopy. Further training can be

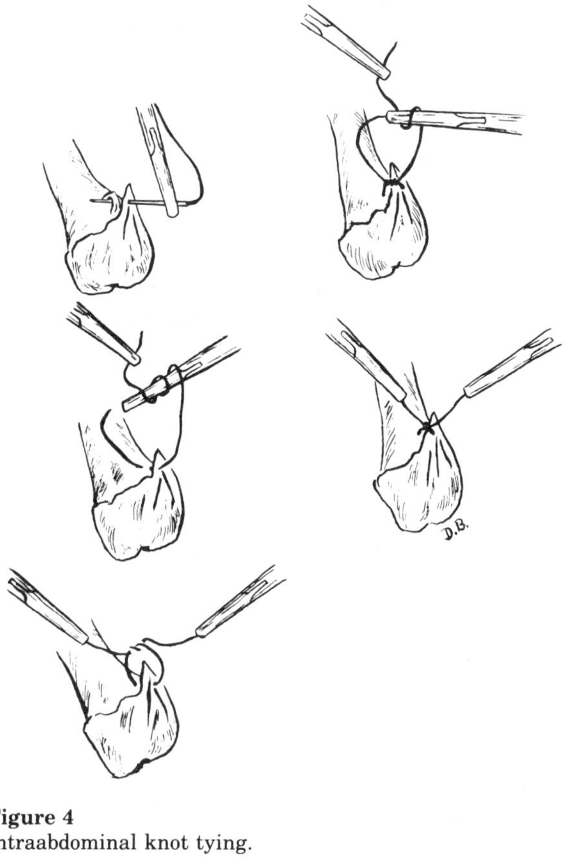

Figure 4
Intraabdominal knot tying.

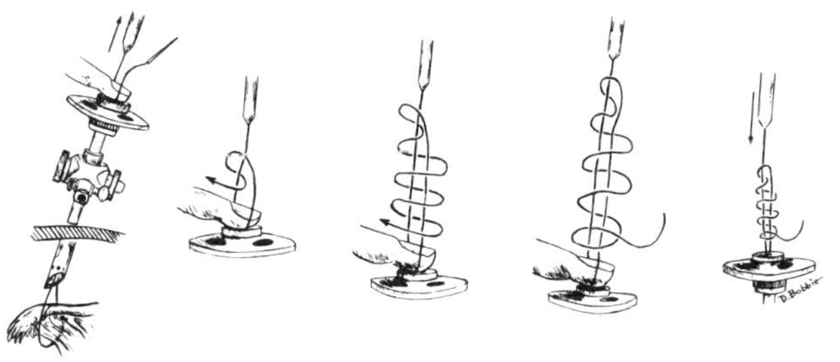

Figure 5
Extracorporeal knot tying. Adapted from Semm.

achieved by assisting a trained laparoscopic surgeon and operating under supervision with the teaching attachment. Recently a "pelvic trainer," developed by Semm,[23] has become available as a commercial product (Pelvi Trainer, Wisap Co., Sauerlach, FRG). This apparatus consists of a Plexiglass rectangular box with rubber puncture sites for laparoscope and ancillary instrumentation on its upper side (Fig. 6). A hysterectomy specimen or other material (even a sponge) may be placed in the trainer for practice in using the instruments and the various suturing techniques. As operative laparoscopy has become more popular, many practice courses have become available. Operative laparoscopy is not for the novice, but for a well-trained gynecologic or reproductive surgeon.

SURGICAL PROCEDURES

Indication for laparoscopic procedures are varied. The laparoscope has a clearly defined role in sterilization as well as IVF and gamete intrafallopian transfer. These procedures are beyond the scope of this section.

ECTOPIC PREGNANCY

The clinical presentation of a patient with an ectopic pregnancy is well known. With the availability of the rapid quantitative β-human chorionic gonadotropin titers and more accurate sonograms (to rule out early intrauterine pregnancy) the diagnosis of probable ectopic pregnancy is being made earlier and often before tubal rupture. The laparoscope is an essential tool in making the diagnosis and, given certain criteria, can be useful for management as well. In a surgically stable patient, especially with an unruptured, accessible tube, several laparoscopic procedures are available, depending on the patient's desire for maintaining fertility. Both conservative and radical procedures have been described.

Gomel and Taylor[24] and others[25] have described a sterilization type of technique for small (< 1.5 cm) ectopic pregnancies either in the isthmus or proximal ampulla. The tube is grasped to the mesosalpinx, and the segment containing the ectopic is coagulated. That segment of oviduct is destroyed.

Segmental resection of a small (< 3 cm) tubal pregnancy in the isthmus or proximal ampulla may be accomplished with electrocautery, endocoagulation, and laser, as well as a Roeder loop.[26-29] Shapiro and Adler[29] reported the first ectopic pregnancy removed solely through the laparoscope. Thorough coagulation of the tube proximal and distal to the ectopic pregnancy is achieved. The tube is incised in the area of coagulation and grasped with forceps and elevated. A series of burns and cuts are placed progressively along the mesosalpinx, beneath the tubal segment being excised. The mesosalpinx is inspected carefully, and any bleeding area can be recoagulated. Soderstrom and Smith[20] described a technique for tubal sterilization (Pomeroy type) with a rectal polyp snare and in a similar manner excised five ectopic pregnancies by partial tubal resection. Tubal anastomosis may be performed with the use of standard microsurgical techniques at a later date. In the future, tubal anastomosis under laparoscopic visualization may be possible, as suggested by DeCherney, who has begun this work using clip approximation over a stent approach.[30]

Conservative procedures that preserve the affected tube were attempted as early as the 19th

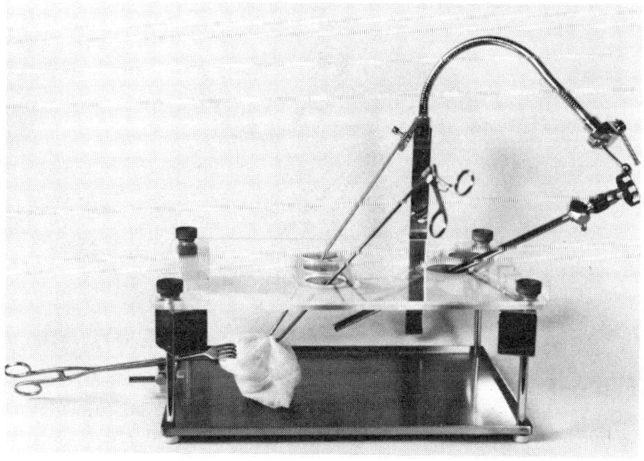

Figure 6
Pelvi Trainer. According to Semm. Made by Wisap Co.

century. Stromme et al.[31] and others[32] have shown that the major argument against this approach (the risk of recurrent ectopic pregnancy in the same tube) is unfounded. Ectopic pregnancy will recur with the same frequency regardless of the procedure. Bruhat et al.[33] reported the technique of linear salpingostomy through the laparoscope using multiple punctures. An incision is made along the antimesenteric border of the tubal ectopic with a "diathermy cutter." The conceptional debris is removed with an aspirator or forceps. If bleeding is observed after aspiration, hemostasis is achieved by compression or electrocoagulation. The fallopian tube is left open (Fig. 7). Semm[11] suggests approximating the tubal edges using endosuture technique. Bruhat et al.[33] reported 43 cases with "no failures" (need for laparotomy at a later date). Of 25 women who later desired pregnancy, 18 conceived; the recurrence rate was 12%. DeCherney et al.[34] reported 18 patients with unruptured ectopic pregnancies < 3 cm in diameter who underwent laparoscopic linear salpingostomy in a manner very similar to Bruhat's. The following criteria were met by all patients: (1) normal pelvic anatomy other than ectopic pregnancy; (2) ampullary, unruptured pregnancy < 3 cm in diameter; (3) < 8 weeks by dates; (4) stable vital signs; (5) preoperative diagnosis of ectopic strongly suggested. All tubes were found to be patent at the time of postoperative hysterosalpingography. Fifty percent of those actively trying to achieve pregnancy conceived. There were no repeat ectopic pregnancies or abortions. There were no immediate or long-term postoperative complications. The only failure was a 5-cm ectopic pregnancy that could not be removed through the second puncture site. This patient was not included in the above figures.

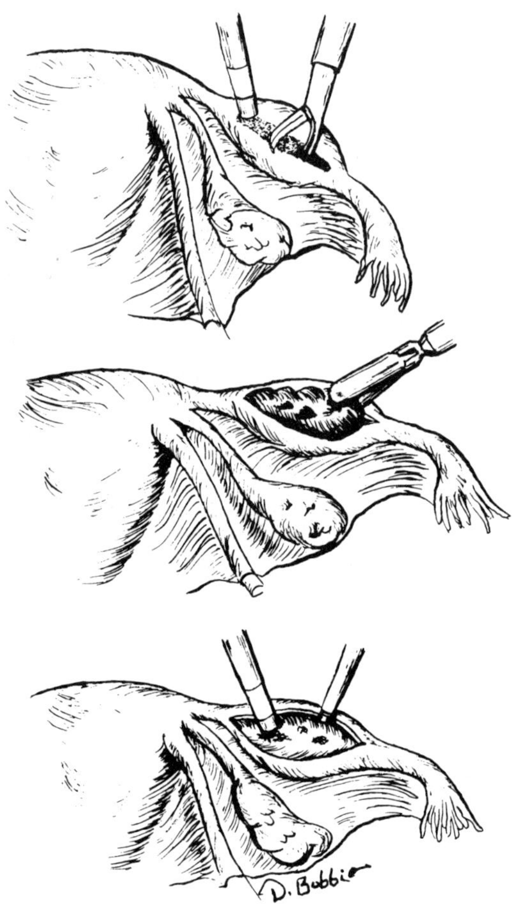

Figure 7
Linear salpingostomy. After coagulation of the antimesenteric border, an incision is made. The contents of the tube are removed, and the tubal lumen is coagulated to achieve hemostasis. The tube is left to heal by secondary intention or sutured.

The figures of Bruhat et al.[33] and DeCherney et al.[34] compare favorably with those of other studies utilizing conservative surgical methods. Pregnancy rates for conservative surgery (laparotomy) range from 40% to 70% with a 4% to 16% repeat ectopic pregnancy rate.[34-37]

A subtotal or total salpingectomy may be performed when preservation of fertility is not a concern or when the pregnancy has ruptured, with marked destruction of the tube. Of course, the criteria for safe laparoscopic surgery must be met: i.e., the patient's condition is stable with no brisk intraperitoneal bleeding. The procedure may be performed by successive coagulation and cutting of the mesosalpinx, beginning at the fimbriated end. The tube is transsected proximal to the ectopic gestation after adequate coagulation[24] (Fig. 8). The tube is removed by any of the previously discussed methods. Schwartz and Martin[38] have also described a similar method using bipolar cautery and transection of the tube with systematic fulguration and cutting of mesosalpinx toward the fimbriated end. Both of these methods are modifications of the procedure described by Tarasconi for salpingectomy by electrocoagulation.[39] In this series salpingectomy was performed for chronic pelvic pain, adnexal tenderness on examination, and enlarged or hyperemic tubes on laparoscopy. The report consists of 100 cases with only 1 case of late (day 7) postoperative bleeding requiring laparotomy.

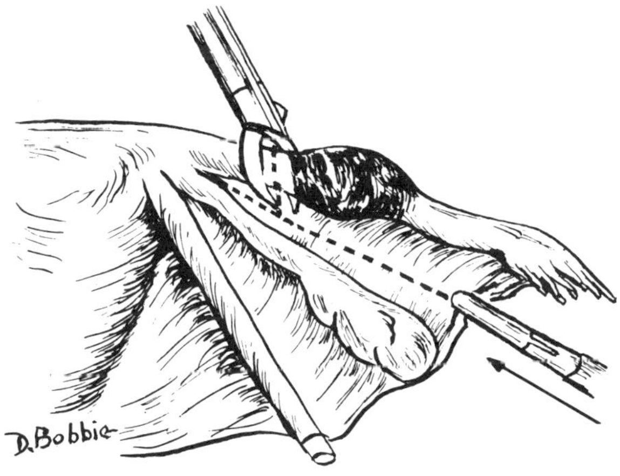

Figure 8
Salpingectomy by coagulation. The mesosalpinx is coagulated and cut in stepwise fashion to just beyond the ectopic gestation. The tube is coagulated and cut proximal to the ectopic.

Soderstrom,[28] in 1975, reported the use of the "snare" technique in five partial salpingectomies for ectopic pregnancy. Semm[11] has also advocated the use of the Roeder loop for partial salpingectomy. Three loops are placed proximal to the ectopic pregnancy. The tube is then transected and removed (Fig. 9). The loop can usually be placed without difficulty. Occasionally one may need to dissect the mesosalpinx partially to facilitate placement of the loop.

Tubal aspiration has been proposed for terminal ampullary ectopic pregnancies. The procedure has been abandoned because of an unacceptably high risk of subsequent laparotomy. Bruhat et al.[33] performed 17 tubal aspirations through the laparoscope with three failures. If tubal conservation is desired, the patient is best treated by terminal salpingostomy or a conservative partial salpingectomy. If conservation is not an issue, partial salpingectomy should be performed.

ENDOMETRIOSIS

Laparoscopy, with visualization of the internal genitalia, has enabled the gynecologist to make the diagnosis of endometriosis with relative ease. Its importance is unquestioned in diagnosis and staging, but whether endometriosis can be adequately treated through the laparoscope remains to be answered. The evidence for its efficacy is very suggestive. Surgical procedures may be performed during the initial diagnostic laparoscopy with little increase in the morbidity of the procedure. This procedure offers the advantage of surgery performed simultaneously with the initial laparoscopy and potentially avoids further surgical or medical therapy. An endoscopic procedure may also be performed later, after options have been thoroughly discussed with the patient. A second-look laparoscopy combined with surgical endoscopy may be used in assessing past treatment as well as providing further treatment.

Endometriotic implants may be coagulated with unipolar or bipolar modalities. The use of unipolar cautery has been questioned because of its potential risk; however, for deeper lesions where greater penetration of current is necessary, unipolar may be more effective than bipolar. Bipolar cautery is very effective for superficial implants. Particular attention needs to be paid to adjacent structures such as ureters, bowel, bladder, and vessels. Endocoagulation also may be used. Because the area of destruction around the

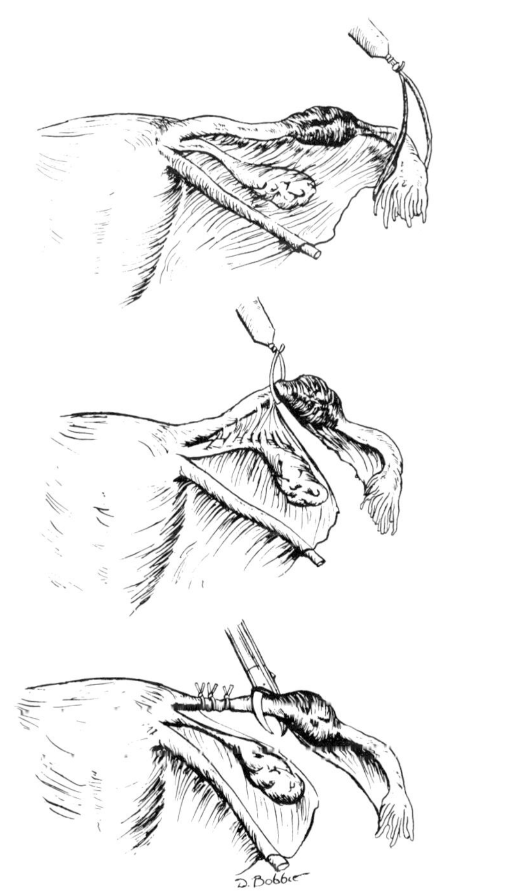

Figure 9
Salpingectomy using the Roeder loop. Three loops are placed proximal to the gestation. The tube is then sharply excised. The tubal stump is coagulated if necessary.

coagulation point is smaller, this may be safer than electrocautery. Laser surgery is effective and may provide greater safety in the treatment of such lesions. The accuracy of the CO_2 laser in depth of penetration permits safe vaporization, particularly when vital structures are nearby.[40] Histologic examination of sections from laser wounds has shown that cellular damage occurs up to 500 μm from laser impact, but the depth of thermal necrosis is usually < 100 μm for the CO_2 laser.[41] Rapid beam movement or pulse mode is employed at low power density until the implant is "erased." Because of its selective absorption by hemoglobin-pigmented tissues and its ability to be transmitted through a flexible fiber, the argon laser appears promising for endometriosis.[42, 43]

The adhesions associated with endometriosis can be vascular and very dense, with structures intimately adherent to one another. It is especially important to follow the guidelines for safe endoscopic surgery, which include the ability to recognize the involved structures and sufficient space between structures to permit safe division of adhesions.[24] Severe cases ("frozen pelvis") are not amenable to safe laparoscopic lysis.

Endometriomas may be removed through the laparoscope. Small (< 2 to 3 cm) surface endometriomas can be "decapitated" at the ovarian endometrioma junction and the base coagulated or vaporized. The resulting defect is usually not closed. Bellina and Bandieramonte[16] have observed at the time of second-look laparoscopy that the defect closes spontaneously and rarely adheres to adjacent structures when the CO_2 laser is used. Larger endometriomas can be similarly approached. With a CO_2 laser or endocoagulator, the cyst is unroofed. The contents are drained and the cyst lining is either dissected or destroyed by vaporization with a defocused CO_2 laser beam or endocoagulator.[14, 40] Most defects are not closed, but can be closed by the previously described suturing technique.

Martin[44] recently published photographs documenting laser treatment of endometriosis in the ovary, as described above. Reich and McGlynn[45] reported 79 cases of ovarian endometrioma treated through the laparoscope. The technique reported gradually evolved from drainage alone to fulguration and finally to excision of the endometrioma cyst wall. Bipolar forceps were used for hemostasis. After 25 laparoscopic endometrioma procedures on 23 women with infertility, there were 12 term pregnancies with no further treatment, 3 following infertility laparotomy and 1 following 6 months of pseudopregnancy. Thirty-three laparoscopic endometrioma procedures were performed for pain, with 19 patients reporting symptomatic relief.

Electrocoagulation of pelvic endometriotic lesions under laparoscopic control was reported in the late 1970s.[46, 47] Hasson,[48] in 1979, reported 19 patients who underwent fulguration of endometriosis for pain and infertility. Seven of the 11 patients noted relief of pain, and 6 of 8 became pregnant postoperatively. Sulewski et al.[49] studied 100 consecutive patients with mild to moderate endometriosis treated with laparoscopy and reported a 40% pregnancy rate (35% live-born pregnancy rate). Daniell and Christianson[50] looked at combined laparoscopic surgery and postoperative danazol therapy in 60 patients. Fifty-seven percent of patients with mild and 56% with moderate endometriosis conceived without further therapy. Cohen[51] obtained similar results with combined therapy.

Daniell and Brown[52] reported their initial experience with the CO_2 laser in patients with mild to moderate endometriosis. With only a 5-month follow-up interval, a 30% pregnancy rate was reported. Kelly and Roberts[53] reported similar results with only a 6-month follow-up interval. More recently, Martin[54] reported 50 patients who underwent initial or second-look laparoscopies with American Fertility Society stage I, II, or III endometriosis.[55] Eleven pregnancies are reported at 7 to 19 months' follow-up, with a 60% estimated long-term pregnancy rate, with laser vaporization. Fifty-eight patients with stage I and II endometriosis who underwent vaporization and adhesiolysis were reported by Feste.[56] At 1-year follow-up a 72% pregnancy rate was seen in patients without other factors and 31% in patients with multiple factors. Interestingly, a laser neurectomy was also performed on patients with dysmenorrhea. This procedure was first described by Doyle and Des Rosiers[57] and consists of excising the uterosacral ligaments adjacent to the cervix. Laser vaporization of the ligament at its attachment to the posterior portion of the cervix will destroy a significant number of sensory nerve fibers to the cervix and lower uterine segment. A 1.0- to 5.0-cm diameter crater is created in the avascular portion of the ligament. Of the 42 patients treated with laser neurectomy for dysmenorrhea, 71% had minimal or no dysmenorrhea after 1 year.

The above studies suffer from few patients, short follow-up intervals, and no randomization. Comparison with published pregnancy rates for conservative surgery and danazol is not ideal. However, the pregnancy rates with laparoscopic surgery in stage I and II endometriosis compare favorably with those for danazol therapy alone[58] and conservative surgery.[59] Thus, firm conclusions cannot be drawn, but these studies suggest a place for laparoscopic surgery in endometriosis.

TUBOPLASTY/SALPINGOSTOMY

Fertility-enhancing laparoscopic surgery was reported as early as 1975 by Gomel,[60] who described salpingolysis and salpingostomy by laparoscopy. Other fertility-enhancing procedures include adhesiolysis and fimbrioplasty.

Pelvic adhesions may differ widely, from thin, filmy, avascular to multilayered, dense, and vascular adhesions, making adherent structures difficult to define. Most adhesions are amenable to laparoscopic surgery, but the latter type may not be. In adhesiolysis, it is key to recognize all structures before cutting, coagulating or vaporizing.[24] There should be sufficient space between adhesions, especially vascular ones, permitting safe coagulation prior to dividing them. Although it is preferable to lyse adhesions sharply, occasionally a blunt probe is safer when one is dividing closely adherent structures. Adhesions should be incised at both ends and removed from the cavity. This step may not always be possible. Multilayered adhesions should be divided one layer at a time for prevention of trauma to underlying structures that may not have been well recognized before.

Adhesiolysis is best accomplished by putting the adhesion on stretch. By manipulating the uterus and/or using a blunt probe or forceps through a second incision, one can achieve satisfactory visualization. The scissors are then introduced through a separate small incision or the operating channel, if appropriate. The defocused beam of a CO_2 laser also may be used. Vascular adhesions should be coagulated prior to incising. It is important to consider the surrounding area of tissue damage associated with the various methods of achieving hemostasis, especially when one is dissecting near the bowel, ureter, bladder, and other pelvic structures.

Phimotic or clubbed fimbria may be treated with laparoscopy. More proximal obstruction makes the patient ineligible. After salpingolysis, the tube is distended (chromopertubation) and stabilized with atraumatic forceps. If the fimbria are agglutinated, forceps may be introduced into the opening in a closed position and then opened and gently withdrawn. This is carried out several times with variation in the direction of the jaws. Gentleness is necessary if one is to avoid bleeding.

As with release of phimotic fimbria, a neosalpingostomy requires that the end of the tube be free of adhesions. The area of the dimple is coagulated and cut in a radial manner so the edges can be everted. This can be accomplished by grasping the luminal surface gently and using another forceps to evert the edges. The edges may be gently coagulated or intraabdominal suturing may be employed to hold the edges back. A CO_2 laser also can be used in performing a laparoscopic salpingostomy. A linear incision is made at a 90-degree angle to the obstructed tube from anterior to posterior. The tubal edges are grasped and the incisions radially extended with the uterus as a backdrop.[61] Eversion is accomplished with a defocused, less powerful beam aimed approximately 1 cm from the cut edge. The beam is moved continuously over the serosal area to limit damage to the tube. The absorption of water causes contraction of the serosal surface of the tube, exposing more mucosal area (Fig. 10).

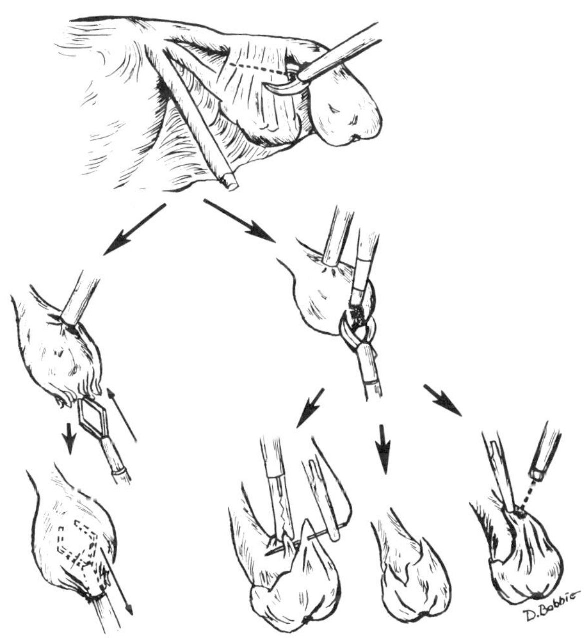

Figure 10
Lysis of adhesions, fimbrioplasty and neosalpingostomy. The everted edges may be sutured, left alone, or gently vaporized.

Some have interpreted the laparoscopic surgical treatment of infertility as crude when compared with microsurgery; however, there is evidence suggesting that these procedures can restore pelvic anatomy. Mettler et al.[47] published one of the first series of ovariolysis, salpingolysis, fimbrioplasty, and salpingostomy with an overall pregnancy rate of 29.3%. Gomel[62] performed lysis of periadnexal adhesions in 92 infertile patients, who were subsequently followed for at least 9 months. The adhesions were graded severe in most cases and moderate in the remainder. Only those cases where ovum pickup was deemed impossible or greatly hampered were included. Fifty-seven (62%) achieved at least one intrauterine pregnancy, 54 (58.7%) had one or more full-term pregnancies, and 5 (5.4%) had ectopic pregnancies. There were no significant postoperative complications. Fayez[63] performed laparoscopic ovariolysis, salpingolysis, and salpingo-ovariolysis on a total of 30 patients. Pregnancy rates were 72%, 67%, and 50%, respectively. Success rates for salpingo-ovariolysis range from 30% to 60% in the literature.[64, 65] The pregnancy rates seen above compare favorably with these results.

Salpingostomy by laparoscopy was reported by Gomel[4] in nine patients, eight of whom had had previous reconstructive surgery. Five had unilateral salpingostomy. Two patients who underwent bilateral salpingostomy had reocclusion of three tubes. Four patients had intrauterine term pregnancies. Fayez[63] also reported patency in 64% and 31% of patients with fimbrioplasty and neosalpingostomy. Pregnancy rates were, respectively, 35% and 10%. Gomel[62] reported a 47.5% (19 of 40) viable birth rate in patients undergoing laparoscopic fimbrioplasty and a 5% ectopic pregnancy rate. Mettler et al.[47] noted a 31% and 26% pregnancy rate for fimbrioplasty and salpingostomy, respectively. Daniell and Herbert[61] recently reported a series of 22 patients with 1-year follow-up who underwent CO_2 laser terminal salpingostomy with the laparoscope. Patency was 75% at follow-up hysterogram, and the pregnancy rate was 14% in this series made up of patients with at least one prior tuboplasty. Tulandi et al.[66] compared reconstructive surgery of hydrosalpinx with microdiathermy needle and CO_2 laser in a laparotomy setting. Intrauterine pregnancy rate following laser salpingostomy was 21.7% and 22.7% following the use of the microdiathermy needle. Gomel,[67] using standard microsurgical techniques, reported a 29% intrauterine pregnancy rate and 27% live birth rate in 41 patients. The ectopic gestation rate was 12%. Although the results reported above are comparable to those reported for laparotomy, no randomized study has been published comparing these two modalities.

IN VITRO FERTILIZATION AND EMBRYO TRANSFER

The role of laparoscopic adhesiolysis in an IVF program has expanded with the realization that the laparoscope can be used to optimize ovarian access. It may be performed prior to or at the time of oocyte recovery, depending on the extent of disease, thus greatly decreasing the need for laparotomy for adhesiolysis. Mettler et al.[68] performed 142 laparoscopies on 114 patients with long-standing tubal factor infertility. Operative procedures were performed in all cases and follicular puncture was attempted in all but 16 patients where adhesions prevented access to the ovaries. Daniell et al.[69] evaluated laparoscopic adhesiolysis in 129 laparoscopies (82 patients) for an IVF program. Fifty-five women (67%) had lysis during the first laparoscopic attempt, and 20 of the 129 laparoscopies (16%) required lysis for identification and aspiration of follicles. In 11 women who had a second laparoscopy, 69% of the ovaries had improved access. With the use of laparoscopic lysis, only 3 of 82 women (4%) had insufficient ovarian access, preventing recovery of at least one oocyte. Keye et al.[70] reported the use of the argon laser to treat endometriosis and vaporize periovarian and/or omental adhesions, dramatically improving the chances of oocyte recovery. These findings support the efficacy of laparoscopic adhesiolysis and indicate that it has an important role in assuring initial access for oocyte recovery and in improving access for subsequent attempts. We have noted several pregnancies after failed IVF-embryo transfer (ET) in patients with long standing infertility who underwent operative laparoscopy at the time of IVF-ET.

SECOND-LOOK LAPAROSCOPY

Operative laparoscopy may be combined with second-look laparoscopy after reconstructive surgery. Results of second salpingostomy and tuboplasty were presented earlier. These "second tuboplasties" are generally performed after 1 year or more. Some investigators[71-74] have recently suggested early second-look laparoscopy with lysis of adhesions as early as 8 days to 12 weeks. Raj and Hulka[71] suggest that lysis of reformed adhesions may have prognostic and therapeutic benefit after laparotomy for lysis of adhesions. Trimbos-Kemper et al.[74] found that fewer than 50% of patients (104 of 188) had adhesions on the eighth postoperative day. More than half of the adhesions that were separated at "first look" did not recur. The incidence of ectopic pregnancy after salpingostomy was significantly lower in those who underwent second-look laparoscopy than in those who did not. It should be clear that there is disagreement regarding the role of second-look laparoscopy following tubal surgery. Gomel and Taylor[24] state that they have abandoned the practice after a 2-year trial because there was no improvement in the pregnancy rate.

OVARIAN BIOPSY/CYSTECTOMY

Biopsy may be necessary to confirm or identify suspicious lesions on ovary, omentum, or peritoneum. A punch biopsy usually provides the necessary information. Forceps with teeth are useful in providing accurate control of biopsy size, because the tissue is held within the jaws. Drill forceps may be used on the antimesenteric border of the ovary to provide a biopsy specimen of approximately 1 cm. Bleeding sites may be coagulated. Many believe this is an accurate reflection of the ovarian tissue present and sufficient when ruling out resistant ovary syndrome in those with premature ovarian failure. Others believe that only a true wedge section is an accurate reflection of the histologic features of the ovary. Portuondo et al.[75] reported 12 patients with bilateral wedge resection and adhesion formation in 92%. Twenty-four with laparoscopic ovarian biopsy were found to be free of periovarian adhesions during a second-look ovarian visualization.

Ovarian cystectomy is performed in the same manner as that previously described for endometriomas. It is important to obtain frozen section interpretation if there is any question of malignancy and then to proceed accordingly. Paraovarian cysts are also easily removed. The cyst may be aspirated after the pedicle is identified. The pedicle is coagulated and cut, and the deflated cyst is easily removed through a trocar.

ADNEXECTOMY/OOPHORECTOMY

Although infrequently used, Semm and Mettler[14] have described a technique for adnexectomy/oophorectomy using the Roeder loop (Ethibinder) (Fig. 11). The adnexa/ovary must be free of adhesions before the loops can be placed. Incisions in the mesosalpinx are usually not necessary. Three loops are placed before cutting the pedicle. With this precaution no bleeding problems have been encountered. We have performed bilateral oophorectomy in patients with recurrent breast cancer positive for estrogen receptors.

MYOMECTOMY

Techniques for resection of pedunculated myomas have been described as well as for intramural myomas by the Kiel group.[11] A pedunculated myoma is easily resected if the pedicle can be coagulated with forceps (Fig. 12). The myoma is then morcellated and removed. Hemostasis is easy to obtain with the endocoagulator, and the defect is usually not closed. Semm reports minimal adhesion formation in the operative site.[76] Intramural myomas are resected by first coagulating over the

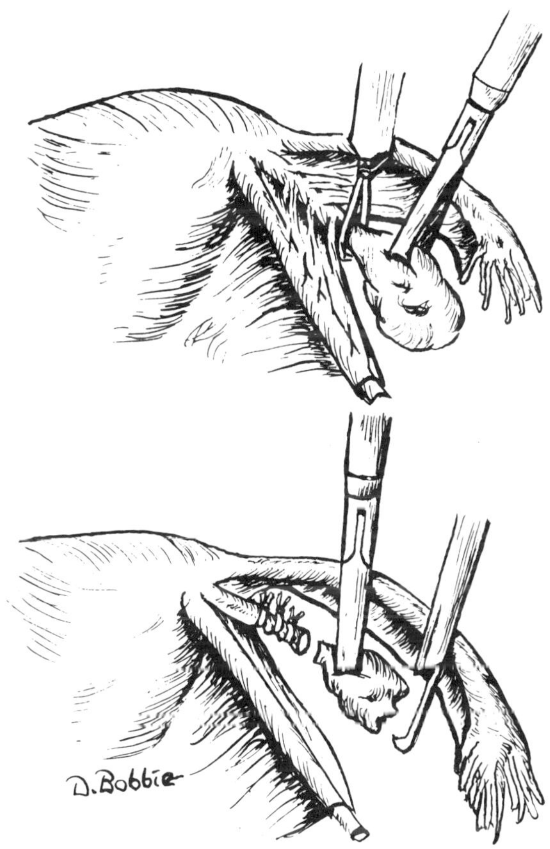

Figure 11
Oophorectomy. Three Roeder loops are placed. The ovarian pedicle is cut and coagulated if necessary. The ovary is morcellated. An adnexectomy is performed in the same manner.

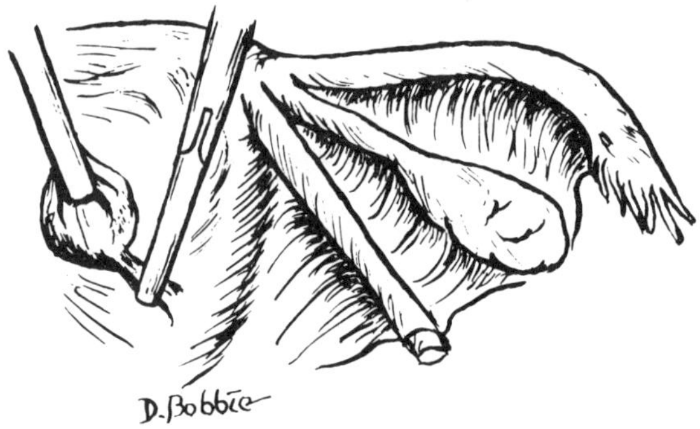

Figure 12
Resection of pedunculated myoma. The base is coagulated and cut. The myoma is removed by morcellation.

incision site. The incision is made with scissors, and the edges are held open with forceps. One grasps the myoma and resects, using the endocoagulator for both dissection and hemostasis. After complete removal of the myoma, bleeding points are coagulated. The defect may then be closed by the intraabdominal suturing technique described earlier. Most often, the defect is left open (Fig. 13).

UTERINE SUSPENSION

Steptoe[77] described the modern technique of laparoscopic ventrosuspension in 1967. Patterson et al.[78] described the technique and results of 100 ventrosuspensions, performed usually for pain. Bilateral incisions 3 cm in length are made lateral to the inferior epigastric vessels and above the inguinal ligament. Forceps are then used to grasp the round ligament and bring it out anteriorly. The round ligament is sutured to the abdominal fascia with Prolene. After a 40-month follow-up interval all but 11% of the uteri were anteverted. Two bleeding complications from avulsion of the ligament were encountered; one required laparotomy and transfusion with two units of blood. The experience of Mann and Stenger[79] was quite similar to that of Patterson et al.[78] Uterine suspension has become an infrequent primary operation for most gynecologic services; however, it is still occasionally used and may be performed laparoscopically.

COMPLICATIONS

Complications of diagnostic laparoscopy are well known and of course pertinent to operative laparoscopy as well. But operative laparoscopy has complications unique to it, which include mechanical trauma, electrical, heat- or laser-induced injury, and bleeding.

All structures within the pelvis and even extraperitoneal structures may be damaged during operative laparoscopy by scissors, a blunt probe, faulty forceps, and other ancillary instruments. Cutting poorly visualized or identified structures may inadvertently damage them. Blunt probes can produce damage to bowel, bladder, cysts, etc., when too much force is used. Ureters are especially vulnerable during dissection of ovaries adherent to the pelvic side wall.

Trauma may cause bleeding. Tears to the oviduct, mesosalpinx, and infundibulopelvic ligament from rough manipulation may bleed profusely. Biopsy and lysis of adhesions may also cause bleeding, especially when adhesions are

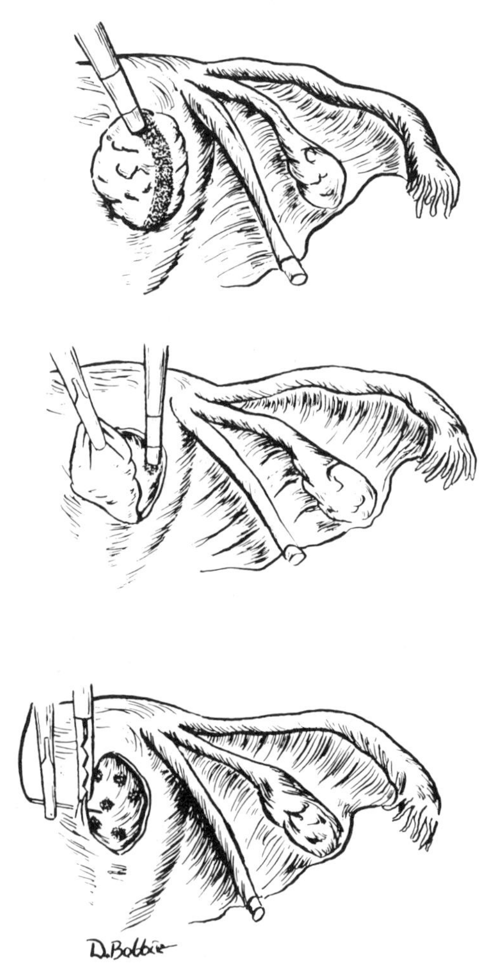

Figure 13
Resection of intramural myoma. The overlying myometrium is coagulated and incised. The myoma is dissected bluntly by coagulation. The defect may be left open or sutured, depending on its size and the surgeon's preference.

vascular and coagulation has not been adequate. Minor bleeding is usually self-limited. More significant bleeding can usually be managed by electrocautery, endocoagulation, laser, or suturing techniques. Laparotomy to control bleeding is rarely necessary.

Abdominal wall hemorrhage is a well-recognized complication of laparoscopy. Operative laparoscopy which places ancillary puncture sites outside the midline increases this risk. Hypotensive collapse secondary to inferior epigastric vessel trauma is not unknown.[10]

The complications of unipolar and bipolar cautery are well known. Burns may occur at any site in contact with a noninsulated portion of the electrical circuit. These burns are painful and slow to heal. Internal damage may be caused by unipolar and bipolar current, endocoagulation, or laser. The most common sites are large and small bowel. The bladder, ureter, and other pelvic structures are also vulnerable. The damage may be from inadvertent grasping or contact with the tissue or from the spread of current or heat from adjacent tissue. Damage to bowel is most serious and needs to be assessed carefully. Minor injury may be observed, but frank perforation usually leads to bowel resection and colostomy in cases of large bowel damage. Unrecognized damage will later present as acute peritonitis.

Semm[11] reported a 0.28% overall complication rate in 8943 laparoscopies, of which 6114 were operative cases. The complications consisted of 13 cases of vessel damage, 9 cases of bowel or stomach puncture, 1 case of ureteral damage, and 2 cases of cardiac arrest. Ten laparotomies were performed because of complications (0.11%). No deaths were reported.

Operative laparoscopy is a safe technique when guidelines are observed and the surgeon is aware of the limitations of the technique. We take the precaution of having a laparotomy table available in the operating room for each case. The patients understand the risks and complications of the procedure and have also consented to a possible exploratory laparotomy in every case. Operative laparoscopy should not be performed in an outpatient surgicenter if full operating room capabilities are not available. In almost all cases the patients are admitted overnight for observation. We have seen two cases of postoperative ileus that resolved spontaneously in 2 to 5 days. Both patients had extensive bowel adhesions that were lysed. One case was abandoned becuase of extremely dense adhesions that could not be safely lysed. No other bowel, bladder, ureter, bleeding, or infectious complications have been encountered.

WHY DO OPERATIVE LAPAROSCOPY?

Patient acceptance of this procedure is high. Levine[80] evaluated the economic impact of operative laparosocpy, as compared with more traditional surgery, for endometriosis, lysis of adhesions, oophorectomy, salpingo-oophorectomy, and myomectomy. The average postoperative length of stay was 0.5 to 2 days for operative laparoscopy versus 5 to 5.7 days for laparotomy. An average reduction of 69% was observed. Women who would normally have had to wait 4 to 6 weeks to return to full activity after conventional surgery can recover fully in 7 to 10 days after laparoscopic surgery. There is a significant savings in wage loss and recovery time.

The health care system may realize a substantial reduction in expense. Levine[80] matched operative laparoscopy records with those for conventional surgery for diagnosis, difficulty, and procedure performed during the same time period. An average reduction of 49% in overall hospital costs was observed with operative laparoscopy. The largest percentage of economic savings was in the use of drugs and other medical supplies (79%).

Operative time appears to be equivalent or shorter for operative laparoscopy.[80] As we become more adept at using the new instruments, operative time will probably decrease even more. It has been suggested that operative laparoscopy represents surgical gymnastics that only a few can perform with great effort. Given adequate training and practice, most trained gynecologic and reproductive surgeons can use these techniques well and in less time than through a laparotomy incision.

The advantages of a laparoscopic procedure are obvious. There is decreased morbidity after operative laparoscopy, and the risks and complications appear to be at least equivalent. A substantial reduction in expense is seen. The crucial question, however, is whether the results are equivalent to those of laparotomy. Some studies have been presented that suggest that operative laparoscopy is as effective as the more conventional laparotomy. Studies comparing endoscopy with laparotomy, the same procedure and the same surgeon still need to be done. Randomized, clinical trials are needed to address adhesion formation and subsequent pregnancy success. To determine whether the endoscopic procedures are as successful will certainly require time.

There is general agreement that operative laparoscopy is an important technique in the armamentarium of the reproductive and gynecologic surgeon. It has earned its place in IVF and gamete intrafallopian transfer. Second attempts at lysis of adhesions, neosalpingostomies, and coagulation of endometriosis should be performed through the laparoscope at the time of second-look laparoscopy. Laparotomy for these "second time" procedures has not proven fruitful.[81, 82] The evidence for effectiveness of the laparoscope in primary procedures, while suggestive, is not conclusive. Only carefully designed clinical trials will identify procedures that can be performed safely with increased effectiveness. Appropriate clinical trials and time will determine the extent to which reproductive and gynecologic surgery will be performed with the laparoscope in the future.

Acknowledgments. I would like to thank Diana Bobbie for the illustrations and George Cook for the photography.

REFERENCES

1. Steptoe PC: Laparoscopy in Gynecology. Edinburgh, E & S Livingstone, 1967, p 1
2. Taylor PJ, Gomel V: Introduction. In Laparoscopy and Hysteroscopy in Gynecologic Practice, Edited by V Gomel, PJ Taylor, AA Yuzpe, JE Rioux. Chicago, Year Book Medical Publishers, 1986, p 1
3. Semm K: Endocoagulator: new possibilities for tubal surgery via pelviscopy. Excerpta Medica 370:242, 1974
4. Gomel V: Salpingostomy by laparoscopy. J Reprod Med 18:265, 1977
5. Corson SL: Use of the laparoscope in the infertile patient. Fertil Steril 32:359, 1979
6. Gomel V, Taylor PJ, Yuzpe AA, Rioux JE: Indications, contraindication, complications. In Laparoscopy and Hysteroscopy in Gynecologic Practice, Edited by V Gomel, PJ Taylor, AA Yuzpe, JE Rioux. Chicago, Year Book Medical Publishers, 1986, p 56
7. Gomel V, Taylor PJ: The technique of endoscopy. In Laparoscopy and Hysteroscopy in Gynecologic Practice, Edited by V Gomel, PJ Taylor, AA Yuzpe, JE Rioux. Chicago, Year Book Medical Publishers, 1986, p 32
8. Semm K: Operations Lehre fur Endoskopiche Abdomical-Chirugie. Stuttgart, F. K. Schattauer Verlag, 1984, p 271
9. Yuzpe AA, Gomel V, Taylor PJ, Rioux JE: Instruments for laparoscopy and hysteroscopy. In Laparoscopy and Hysteroscopy in Gynecologic Practice, Edited by V Gomel, PJ Taylor, AA Yuzpe, JE Rioux. Chicago, Year Book Medical Publishers, 1986, p 7
10. Pring DW: Inferior epigastric haemorrhage, an avoidable complication of laparoscopic clip sterilization. Br J Obstet Gynaecol 90:480, 1983
11. Semm K: Endoscopic Intraabdominal Surgery. Kiel, Christian-Albrects-Universitat, 1984, p 4
12. Esposito JM: The laparoscopist and electro-surgery. Am J Obstet Gynecol 126:633, 1976
13. Bahig CS: Electrosurgical burn injuries and their prevention. JAMA 204:1025, 1968
14. Semm K, Mettler L: Technical progress in pelvic surgery via operative laparoscopy. Am J Obstet Gynecol 138:121, 1980
15. Semm K: Diagnostic tools: instruments and techniques for endoscopic ovarian surgery. In The Ovary, Edited by GB Serra. New York, Raven Press, 1983, p 159
16. Bellina JH, Bandieramonte G: Principles and Practice of Gynecologic Laser Surgery. New York, Plenum Medical Book Co, 1984, p 6
17. Riedel HH, Semm K: An initial comparison of coagulation techniques of sterilization. J Reprod Med 27:261, 1982
18. Riedel HH, Cordts-Kleinwordt G, Semm K: Endocrine findings in rabbits after sterilization with electrocoagulation. J Reprod Med 28:665, 1983
19. Semm K: Tissue-puncher and loop ligation: new aids for surgical-therapeutic pelviscopy. Endoscopy 10:119, 1978
20. Soderstrom RM, Smith MR: Tubal sterilization—a new laparoscopic method. Obstet Gynecol 38:152, 1971
21. Semm K: New methods of pelviscopy for myomectomy, ovariectomy, tubectomy and adnectomy. Endoscopy 2:85, 1979
22. Mettler L: Personal communication.
23. Semm K: Endoscopic appendectomy. Endoscopy 15:59, 1983
24. Gomel V, Taylor PJ: Surgical endoscopy. In Laparoscopy and Hysteroscopy in Gynecologic Practice, Edited by V Gomel, PJ Taylor, AA Yuzpe, JE Rioux. Chicago, Year Book Medical Publishers, 1986, p 140
25. Esposito JM: Ectopic pregnancy management. In Laparoscopy, Edited by JM Phillips. Baltimore, Williams & Wilkins, 1977, p 120
26. Stangel JJ, Gomel V: Techniques in conservative surgery for tubal gestation. Clin Obstet Gynecol 23:1221, 1980
27. Daniell JF, Pittaway DE: Use of the CO_2 laser in laparoscopic surgery: initial experience with the second puncture technique. Infertility 5:15, 1982
28. Soderstrom RM: Unusual uses of laparoscopy. J Reprod Med 15:77, 1975
29. Shapiro HI, Adler DH: Excision of an ectopic pregnancy through the laparoscope. Am J Obstet Gynecol 117:290, 1973
30. DeCherney AH: The leader of the band is tired. Fertil Steril 44:299, 1985
31. Stromme WB, McKelvery JL, Adlans CD: Conservative surgery for ectopic pregnancy. Obstet Gynecol 19:294, 1962
32. DeCherney AH, Kase N: The conservative management of unruptured ectopic pregnancy. Obstet Gynecol 54:451, 1979
33. Bruhat MA, Manhes H, Mage G, Pouly JL: Treatment of ectopic pregnancy by means of laparoscopy. Fertil Steril 33:411, 1980
34. DeCherney AH, Romero R, Naftolin F: Surgical management of unruptured ectopic pregnancy. Fertil Steril 35:21, 1981

35. Bukowsky I, Lauger K, Herman A, Caspi E: Conservative surgery for tubal pregnancy. Obstet Gynecol 53:709, 1979
36. Stromme WB: Conservative surgery for ectopic pregnancy. Obstet Gynecol 41:215, 1973
37. Timonen S, Nieminen V: Tubal pregnancy: choice of operative method of treatment. Acta Obstet Gynecol Scand 46:327, 1967
38. Schwartz RO, Martin JB: Laparoscopic salpingectomy for ectopic pregnancy. South Med J 78:1341, 1985
39. Tarasconi JC: Endoscopic salpingectomy. J Reprod Med 26:541, 1981
40. Yuzpe AA, Gomel V, Taylor PJ: Endoscopy in the patient with endometriosis. In Laparoscopy and Hysteroscopy in Gynecologic Practice, Edited by V Gomel, PJ Taylor, AA Yuzpe, JE Rioux. Chicago, Year Book Medical Publishers, 1986, p 111
41. Daniell JF: The role of lasers in infertility surgery. Fertil Steril 42:815, 1984
42. Keye WR Jr, Watson GA, Dixon J: The use of the argon laser in the treatment of experimental endometriosis. Fertil Steril 39:26, 1983
43. Keye WR Jr, Dixon J: Photocoagulation of endometriosis by the argon laser through the laparoscope. Obstet Gynecol 62:282, 1983
44. Martin D: Avoid laparotomy using laser laparoscopy. Contemp Obstet Gynecol 25:101, 1985
45. Reich H, McGlynn F: Treatment of ovarian endometriomas using laparoscopic surgical techniques. J Reprod Med 31:577, 1986
46. Edward RD: Cauterization of stage I and II endometriosis and resulting pregnancy rate. In Endoscopy and Gynecology, Edited by JM Phillips. Downey, Calif, American Association of Gynecologic Laparoscopists, 1978, p 276
47. Mettler L, Giesel H, Semm K: Treatment of female infertility due to tubal obstruction by operative laparoscopy. Fertil Steril 32:384, 1979
48. Hasson HM: Electrocoagulation of pelvic endometriotic lesions of endometriosis at laparoscopy for infertility. Am J Obstet Gynecol 135:115, 1979
49. Sulewski JM, Curcio FD, Bronitsky C, Stenger VG: The treatment of endometriosis at laparoscopy for infertility. Am J Obstet Gynecol 138:128, 1980
50. Daniell JF, Christianson C: Combined laparoscopic surgery and danazol therapy for pelvic endometriosis. Fertil Steril 35:521, 1981
51. Cohen MR: Laparoscopy in the diagnosis and management of endometriosis. J Reprod Med 27:240, 1982
52. Daniell JF, Brown DH: Carbon dioxide laser laparoscopy: initial experience in experimental animals and human. Obstet Gynecol 59:761, 1982
53. Kelly RW, Roberts DK: CO_2 laser laparoscopy: a potential alternative to danazol in the treatment of stage I and II endometriosis. J Reprod Med 28:638, 1983
54. Martin DC: CO_2 laser laparoscopy for the treatment of endometriosis associated with infertility. J Reprod Med 30:409, 1985
55. American Fertility Society: Classification of endometriosis. Fertil Steril 32:633, 1979
56. Feste JR: Laser laparoscopy—a new modality. J Reprod Med 30:413, 1985
57. Doyle JB, Des Rosiers JJ: Paracervical uterine denervation for relief of pelvic pain. Clin Obstet Gynecol 6:742, 1963
58. Barbieri RL, Evans S, Kistner RW: Danazol in the treatment of endometriosis: analysis of 100 cases with a 4-year follow-up. Fertil Steril 37:737, 1982
59. Buttram VC Jr: Conservative surgery for endometriosis in the infertile female: a study of 206 patients with implications for both medical and surgical therapy. Fertil Steril 31:117, 1979
60. Gomel V: Laparoscopic tubal surgery in infertility. Obstet Gynecol 46:47, 1975
61. Daniell JF, Herbert CM: Laparoscopic salpingostomy utilizing the CO_2 laser. Fertil Steril 41:558, 1984
62. Gomel V: Salpingo-ovariolysis by laparoscopy in infertility. Fertil Steril 40:607, 1983
63. Fayez JA: An assessment of the role of operative laparoscopy in tuboplasty. Fertil Steril 39:476, 1983
64. Gomel V: Microsurgery in Female Infertility. Boston, Little, Brown & Co, 1983, p 80
65. Jones HW Jr, Rock JA: Reparative and Constructive Surgery of the Female Generative Tract. Baltimore, Williams & Wilkins, 1983, p 72
66. Tulandi T, Farag R, McInness BA, Gelfand MM, Wright CV, Vilos GA: Reconstructive surgery of hydrosalpinx with and without the carbon dioxide laser. Fertil Steril 42:839, 1984
67. Gomel V: Salpingostomy by microsurgery. Fertil Steril 29:380, 1978
68. Mettler L, Seki M, Baukloh V, Semm K: Human ovum recovery via operative laparoscopy and in vitro fertilization. Fertil Steril 38:30, 1982
69. Daniell JF, Pittaway DE, Maxson WS: The role of laparoscopic adhesiolysis and an in vitro fertilization program. Fertil Steril 40:49, 1983
70. Keye WR, Paulson AM, Worley RJ: Application of simplified laser laparoscopy to preparation of the pelvis for in vitro fertilization. J Reprod Med 30:418, 1985
71. Raj SG, Hulka JF: Second-look laparoscopy in infertility surgery: therapeutic and prognostic value. Fertil Steril 38:325, 1982
72. Surrey MW, Friedman S: Second-look laparoscopy after reconstructive pelvic surgery for infertility. J Reprod Med 27:658, 1982
73. Diamond MP, Daniell JF, Martin DC, Feste J, Vaughn WK, McLaughlin DS: Tubal patency and pelvic adhesions at early second-look laparoscopy following intraabdominal use of the carbon dioxide laser: initial report of the intraabdominal laser study group. Fertil Steril 42:717, 1984
74. Trimbos-Kemper TCM, Trimbos JB, van Hall EV: Adhesion formation after tubal surgery: results of the eighth-day laparoscopy in 188 patients. Fertil Steril 43:395, 1985
75. Portuondo JA, Melchor JC, Neyro JL, Alegre A: Periovarian adhesions following ovarian wedge resection or laparoscopic biopsy. Endoscopy 16:143, 1984
76. Semm K: Personal communication
77. Steptoe PC: Laparoscopy in Gynecology. Edinburgh, E & S Livingstone, 1967, p 73
78. Patterson MEL, Jordan JA, Logan-Edwards R: A survey of 100 patients who had laparoscopic ventro suspension. Br J Obstet Gynaecol 85:468, 1978
79. Mann WJ, Stenger VG: Uterine suspension through the laparoscope. Obstet Gynecol 51:563, 1978
80. Levine RL: Economic impact of pelviscopic surgery. J Reprod Med 30:655, 1985

81. Kistner RW: Management of endometriosis in the infertile patient. Fertil Steril 26:1151, 1975

82. Lauritsen JG, Pagel JD, Vangsted P, Starup J: Results of repeated tuboplasties. Fertil Steril 37:68, 1982

Chapter 18

Ectopic pregnancy: its relationship to tubal reconstructive surgery

Gad Lavy, M.D.
Michael P. Diamond, M.D.
Alan H. DeCherney, M.D.

Department of Obstetrics and Gynecology, Division of Reproductive Endocrinology, Yale University, School of Medicine, New Haven, Connecticut

The passage of the fertilized ovum through the fallopian tube has been compared to a perilous journey.[1] Indeed, only too frequently, this journey terminates in disaster. Failure of the fertilized egg to gain access into the uterine cavity may lead to a catastrophic event in which the fertilized egg implants outside of the uterine cavity proper. Ectopic pregnancy is, indeed, a reproductive disaster, compromising the woman's life and frequently leading to a permanent loss of reproductive function.

Most ectopic pregnancies occur in the fallopian tube, usually in its distal portion. Both mechanical and hormonal factors, by interfering with the successful transport of the ovum through the fallopian tube, can lead to an ectopic implantation.

The association of tubal surgery and ectopic pregnancy is well recognized. This "iatrogenic" etiology of ectopic pregnancy is of particular concern to the reproductive surgeon. The risk of ectopic pregnancy after tubal surgery varies greatly and depends on the prior condition of the tube, the nature of the surgical procedure performed, the technique employed, and the surgeon's skill.

This section reviews the various aspects of the association between tubal surgery and ectopic pregnancy. The impact of the improvement in surgical technique and the availability of in vitro fertilization and embryo transfer (IVF-ET) as an alternative to tubal surgery is also evaluated.

INCIDENCE

The incidence of ectopic pregnancy in the United States is approximately 1 in 120 pregnancies. The incidence varies greatly in different populations and can be as high as 1 in 80 pregnancies in some large urban centers. A steep rise in the incidence of ectopic pregnancy in this country has been observed over the past several decades. From 1965 to 1977 the number of ectopic pregnancies in the United States almost tripled.[2] The increase in incidence is linked to the rise in the incidence of sexually transmitted diseases, and, paradoxically, to the improvement in early antibiotic therapy for these diseases. Aggressive antibiotic therapy results in damaged but partially functional tubes, which, in turn, can give rise to an ectopic pregnancy.

Ectopic pregnancy is one of the leading causes of maternal mortality and a major etiologic factor in infertility. In the United States, the mortality associated with ectopic pregnancy is approximately 1 in 1000 cases, contributing to 10% to 12% of maternal deaths.[3, 4] An improvement in the early diagnosis and therapy of this disease has resulted in a decrease in mortality rates and has offset the rise in incidence of this disease. After an ectopic gestation, approximately 50% of women will be unable to conceive, and in a substantial number of patients, the condition will recur in a future pregnancy, representing a constant threat to the woman's health and well-being.[5]

THE TUBAL ETIOLOGY OF ECTOPIC PREGNANCY

The most common etiologic factors for ectopic pregnancy are related to abnormalities of the fallopian tube resulting from prior pelvic inflammatory disease (PID), tubal and abdominal surgery, or a combination of these factors. In more than 50% of patients with ectopic pregnancy one or more of these factors is present. Less common, ectopic pregnancy occurs in morphologically normal tubes. An abnormal endocrine milieu leading to abnormal tubal transfer may be the underlying factor in these cases.

The two major "tubal" etiologies of ectopic pregnancy, tubal surgery and PID cannot be readily separated, because a substantial number of patients undergoing tubal surgery have underlying tubal disease resulting from prior PID.

The association between ectopic pregnancy and PID is well established. A six- to seven-fold increase in the incidence of ectopic pregnancy after acute salpingitis was demonstrated by Westrom and colleagues.[6] The exact nature of the association between the two conditions is, however, difficult to determine, because only poor correlation exists between a clinical history of PID and histopathologic evidence for its existence. In various reports, a history of PID can be elicited in 10% to 50% of patients presenting with an ectopic pregnancy. Morphologic evidence for prior PID was found in up to 50% of patients at the time of surgery for ectopic pregnancy.[5]

An association between ectopic pregnancy and tubal surgery is also evident. Among 195 patients with ectopic pregnancy, DeCherney et al.[7] have reported 27% to have had prior abdominal surgery and 9% prior tubal surgery. Other authors[8, 9] have reported a history of prior abdominal surgery in 15% to 30% of patients presenting with an ectopic pregnancy. The association between appendectomy and right-sided tubal pregnancy has also been proposed.

It appears, therefore, that only a relatively small proportion of patients with ectopic pregnancy have prior tubal surgery as the likely etiologic factor. The presence of such historical data, however, should place these patients at a higher-risk category for encountering an ectopic pregnancy because its occurrence is more common in these patients than in the general population.

PATHOPHYSIOLOGY

NORMAL TUBAL ULTRASTRUCTURE AND FUNCTION

A delicate balance of structure and function governs tubal transport. The oviduct actively participates in the transport of sperm and the egg to the site of fertilization, and of the preembryo from the tube into the uterine cavity. Tubal function is affected by the contraction of the smooth muscle in the tubal wall, and by the constant beat of the cilia that line some of the tubal mucosal cells. Tubal contractile activity in the periovulatory phase of the cycle, and under the influence of estrogen, is regular and well coordinated. Under the influence of progesterone (P), in the early luteal phase, this pattern is replaced by one of irregular and "random" contractions. These contraction patterns facilitate sperm transport in the periovulatory phase and preembryo transport in the early luteal phase.[10, 11]

Tubal ultrastructure is also under direct influence of ovarian estrogen and P. The mucosa of the fallopian tube is lined by ciliated and mucus-secreting cells. Both cell types demonstrate structural changes related to circulating levels of these hormones. The growth of the cilia and their beat frequency are enhanced by estrogen and inhibited by P.[12-14] Similarly, the nonciliated mucus-secreting cells of the tubal mucosa secrete thick tenacious mucus under the influence of estrogen. This mucus is responsible, in part, for retaining the fertilized egg in the ampulla after fertilization.[15]

Tubal surgery or infection can disrupt this balance of structure and function and thus predispose the patient to an ectopic pregnancy.

TUBAL SURGERY, TUBAL DISEASE, AND ECTOPIC PREGNANCY

Ectopic pregnancy results from a delay in the passage of the preembryo through the fallopian tube. This delay can be caused by anatomic defects (e.g., constriction, false passage formation) or by tubal dysfunction (altered contractility or abnormal ciliary activity). Tubal anatomy and function can both be altered by either tubal surgery or prior PID. The relative importance of these two factors is difficult to determine because they are often both present in the same individual.

The study of ectopic pregnancy is limited by the absence of an animal model. Our understanding of the pathophysiology of this condition is, therefore, derived mostly from observations made in patients presenting with this disease. The association between ectopic pregnancy and other gynecologic conditions, such as PID, and tubal surgery, also helps in understanding its pathophysiology. Animal models can be used, however, to assess the degree of tubal dysfunction that is caused by surgery. Tubal dysfunction can be determined by the "nidation index" (the ratio of embryos implanted in the uterine horn to the number of corpora lutea in the homolateral ovary); this measure of tubal dysfunction can serve indirectly to study the effect of tubal surgery on tubal function and thus can help in the understanding of the pathophysiology of ectopic pregnancy.

TUBAL ANATOMY AND FUNCTION AFTER SURGERY

The tubal dysfunction that follows tubal surgery is exemplified by the discrepancy that exists between the rates of tubal patency after surgery and the rates of pregnancy,[16] and by the increased incidence of both ectopic pregnancy and spontaneous abortions after tubal surgery.[17]

Tubal anatomy can be readily disrupted as a result of surgery. Even with the use of magnification in relatively "healthy" tubes, it is often difficult to restore normal anatomy. Animal studies have demonstrated the difficulty in achieving proper alignment of the mucosal folds at surgery for tubal anastomosis.[18] Women who have undergone tubal anastomosis after a simple tubal ligation may be the human counterpart of this condition. Imperfect surgical repairs may also lead to the formation of blind mucosal pouches, which in turn could entrap the ovum and thus predispose the patient to an ectopic pregnancy.

Tubal function can also be disrupted after surgery; peritubal adhesions, which are a common sequel of surgery, may restrict tubal motility and thus interfere with ovum pickup and transport. It appears that the partial denervation of the tube, which accompanies some surgical procedures, does not have a significant impact on tubal function. Disruption of the rich adrenergic nerve supply of the tubal isthmus does not cause a significant impairment in tubal function.[19]

The operator's skill determines, to a large extent, the anatomic and functional integrity of the tube after surgery. Gomel[20] and Paterson and Wood[21] have demonstrated that simple transection and anastomosis of the fallopian tube in the rabbit, with microsurgical technique, do not result in a reduction in fertility. Oelsner et al.,[22] however, have clearly demonstrated the effect of training on the outcome of microsurgical procedures in the rabbit. In human beings, under normal circumstances, one can expect some degree of tubal dysfunction to follow tubal surgery, because in most cases tubal surgery involves more than the repair of a simple tubal transection. In addition, the surgery is not uncommonly performed by surgeons lacking in experience.

The surgical technique used in performing the surgery also has an effect on the incidence of ectopic pregnancy, as will be demonstrated in the next section. The introduction of microsurgical technique has resulted in a reduction in the rate of ectopic pregnancy. This may be due to better restoration of normal tubal function that can be achieved with microsurgery.

TUBAL FUNCTION AFTER TUBAL DISEASE

Pelvic infections can lead to disruption of the normal tubal anatomy and function. The peritubal and intratubal adhesions that are a common sequel of PID can also interfere with tubal motility and ovum transport and thus predispose the patient to an ectopic pregnancy. Even more important, the destruction of the endosalpinx by the infectious process can be a source of major tubal dysfunction.

The effect of tubal disease on the structure and function of the cilia has been demonstrated. In the human being, a significant reduction in the concentration of the ciliated cells was observed after infections. The ciliary beat frequency in these diseased tubes is also abnormally low. Ultrastructural studies of fallopian tubes obtained from patients at the time of surgery for ectopic pregnancy demonstrate a decrease in cell height and an early onset of deciliation.[23, 24] This reduction in the number and function of the cilia may explain the persistence of infertility after tuboplasty even in the face of tubal patency, and the occurrence of tubal pregnancy.

In animals, by use of microsurgical techniques, structural changes simulating tubal disease have been created and correlated with tubal function.

Vasquez et al.[25] have demonstrated the process of deciliation that accompanies the development of hydrosalpinx. In addition to the loss of cilia, these structurally altered tubes may lose their steroid receptors, thus impairing their ability to respond to hormones. The deciliation process may not be reversible even after surgical restoration of patency, thus leading to a permanent loss of tubal function.[26]

SPECIFIC TUBAL SURGERY

Various types of tubal surgery are associated with different rates of ectopic pregnancy. It is often difficult to separate the contribution to the creation of the ectopic pregnancy by the surgical procedure itself from that of the underlying tubal disease process, because each procedure is performed to correct a specific tubal lesion.

The success of surgery is measured by a high rate of intrauterine pregnancy, a low rate of ectopic pregnancy, and a short delay from the procedure to conception. These reflect the extent to which normal tubal function has been restored. Restoration of anatomic and functional integrity depends on the severity of the mucosal damage present before surgery, and on the surgical technique used for the repair.

SURGICAL TECHNIQUE AND ECTOPIC PREGNANCY

The use of magnification and of microsurgical technique for surgery of the female reproductive tract has introduced new hopes for higher reproductive success after surgery (i.e., an increase in the rate of intrauterine pregnancy and a reduction in the incidence of tubal pregnancy). As will be demonstrated later in this section, such an improvement in outcome has, indeed, occurred. Some drawbacks to the improved surgical technique do exist, however. The reproductive surgeon is now able to achieve patency of severely damaged tubes. These patent but functionally abnormal tubes may predispose the patient in some cases to an increased risk of ectopic pregnancy.

The impact of the newer operative techniques such as the operative laparoscopy and the use of the CO_2 laser will also be discussed with reference to the incidence of ectopic pregnancy associated with their use in performing the various surgical procedures.

MUCOSAL DAMAGE AND ECTOPIC PREGNANCY

A good correlation exists between the degree of tubal mucosal damage and the occurrence of ectopic pregnancy. Surgery often cannot reverse the mucosal damage and the abnormal function that resulted from prior tubal disease. The surgically repaired tube is therefore functionally abnormal and predisposes the patient to an ectopic pregnancy. For this reason, even a skilled surgeon using the most meticulous of techniques will not be able to eliminate completely the occurrence of ectopic pregnancy. An exception to this rule can be found in patients with severe tubal disease. In some patients with severe hydrosalpinx the incidence of both intrauterine and ectopic pregnancy is low, reflecting the complete loss of the functional capacity of the tube, and precluding the occurrence of intrauterine or extrauterine pregnancy.

SALPINGOLYSIS AND OVARIOLYSIS

These procedures involve the removal of peritubal and/or periovarian adhesions. The adhesions are usually caused by extragenital disease such as appendicitis, and the endosalpinx is, therefore, usually spared. The disruption of normal tubal anatomy and function in these patients is only minimal, and as a result, one can expect a high rate of intrauterine pregnancy, and a low rate of ectopic pregnancy. Patients with thicker, more vascular, and more extensive adhesions fare worse after surgery. In these patients, the pregnancy rates are reduced, and the ectopic pregnancy rates are increased.[27-29]

The outcome of these procedures is represented in Table 1. As can be seen in the table, the use of microsurgical technique has led to a substantial reduction in the rate of ectopic pregnancy and to a modest increase in the overall pregnancy rates associated with this procedure. The use of magnification for simple lysis of periadnexal adhesions does not seem necessary. Meticulous microsurgical technique is, however, recommended to prevent adhesion reformation and to improve the outcome.

The role of operative laparoscopy in the lysis of periadnexal adhesions is still to be determined. Fayez[35] has reported a pregnancy rate of 50% to 72% in 24 patients. The incidence of pregnancy was dependent on the extent of the adhesions found at laparoscopy. The ectopic pregnancy rate in this group was 8% for patients who underwent

Table 1. *Salpingolysis and Ovariolysis — Macrosurgery Versus Microsurgery*

Author	Surgery	Year	Patients	Pregnancies	%	Ectopic	Ectopic	
							% patients	% pregnancies
Siegler and Kontopoulos[27]	Macr[a]	1979	15	6	40	3	20	50
Wallach et al.[30]	Macr	1983	94	48	52	3	3.2	6.2
Bronson and Wallach[31]	Macr	1977	35	22	65	1	2.8	4.5
Diamond[32]	Macr	1979	220	77	35	8	3.6	10.3
Caspi and Halperin[28]	Macr	1981	101	45	45	1	1	2.2
Diamond[32]	Micr[b]	1979	140	85	61	1	0.7	1.1
Hulka[29]	Micr	1982	47	14	31	1	2	7.1
Siegler and Kontopoulos[27]	Micr	1979	6	3	50	1	16	33
Frantzen and Schlosser[33]	Micr	1982	49	20	41	2	4.1	10
Betz et al.[34]	Micr	1980	29	20	69	0	0	0
Total			736	340	46	21	2.8	6.1
Macr			465	198	42	16	3.4	8
Micr			271	142	52	5	1.8	3.5

[a]Macr, macrosurgery.
[b]Micr, microsurgery.

lysis of both periovarian and peritubal adhesions. None of the 26 patients undergoing either ovariolysis or salpingolysis alone had an ectopic pregnancy. Similar results have been reported by Gomel.[36] These reports suggest that operative laparoscopy may have a role in the treatment of this condition (Table 2).

The functional integrity of the tube in these patients with peritubal and periovarian adhesions seems to be relatively intact resulting in high pregnancy rates, and in low rates of ectopic pregnancy. The occurrence of ectopic pregnancy seems to be related to the nature and extent of the adhesive disease and to the surgical technique used for its repair.

FIMBRIOPLASTY

Fimbrial agglutination interferes with ovum pickup and conception in these patients. Tubal occlusion if present is only partial. PID is the underlying process in the majority of cases, and involvement of the endosalpinx is, therefore, common. The pregnancy rates after fimbrioplasty (50% to 60%) are similar to those observed after salpingolysis or ovariolysis. The rate of ectopic pregnancy, however, is slightly higher and may reflect a higher degree of tubal dysfunction in these patients. Table 3 demonstrates the pregnancy rates in patients undergoing fimbrioplasty by either microsurgical or macrosurgical techniques. The use of microsurgical technique in this group results in both an increase in intrauterine pregnancy (from 42% to 59%) and a decrease in the rate of ectopic pregnancy (from 14% to 6%).

The use of operative laparoscopy in these patients was reported by Fayez[35] in his series. A pregnancy rate of 35% and an ectopic pregnancy rate of 14% were obtained in a group of 14 patients. Despite the small number of patients, the results seem inferior to those achieved by laparotomy and microsurgical repair. The role of operative laparoscopy in these instances should therefore be carefully reevaluated.

NEOSALPINGOSTOMY

Distal tubal occlusion and varying degrees of dilatation of the distal tubal segment are characteristic of this situation and are usually a result of PID. The endosalpinx is often severely affected as a result of the underlying disease process, and the long-standing dilatation of the tube that follows obstruction. Tubal function in these patients

Table 2. *Operative Laparoscopy*

Author	Surgery	Year	Patients	Pregnancies	%	Ectopic	Ectopic	
							% patients	% pregnancies
Fayez[35]	Lap[a]	1983	24	12	50	2	8	16
Gomel[36]	Lap	1983	92	60	65	3	3.2	5

[a]Lap, operative laparoscopy.

Table 3. *Fimbrioplasty*

Author	Surgery	Year	Patients	Pregnancies	%	Ectopic	Ectopic	
							% patients[a]	% pregnancies[b]
Palmer[37]	Macr[c]	1969	10	5	50	1	10	20
Siegler and Kontopoulos[27]	Macr	1979	11	4	36	2	18	50
Siegler and Kontopoulos[27]	Micr[d]	1979	9	6	66	1	11	16
Audebert et al.[38]	Micr	1980	76	34	45	3	4	9
Patton[39]	Micr	1982	40	27	68	2	5	7
Frantzen and Schlosser[33]	Micr	1982	9	13	26	2	4	15
Fayez[35]	Lap[e]	1983	14	5	35	2	8	40
Total (Macr and micr)			155	89	57	11	7	12
Macr			21	9	42	3	14	33
Micr			134	80	59	8	6	10

[a]Percent of all patients with ectopic pregnancy.
[b]Percent of pregnant patients with ectopic pregnancy.
[c]Macr, macrosurgery.
[d]Micr, microsurgery.
[e]Lap, laparoscopy.

is usually severely affected. The outcome of surgical repair is determined by the size of the hydrosalpinx and its thickness, the extent of disruption to the tubal mucosa, and the presence or absence of peritubal adhesions. Table 4 describes the overall pregnancy rates and the ectopic pregnancy rates in patients undergoing salpingostomy. The variability in pregnancy rates after surgical repair (17% to 44%) represents, at least in part, the varying degrees of tubal destruction associated with this condition and the varying length of follow-up.[50]

In addition to an overall low pregnancy rate, the risk of ectopic pregnancy in these patients is higher than that seen with most other procedures. Paradoxically, patients with either mild or severe disease have lower ectopic pregnancy rates than those with moderate disease. The degree of tubal dysfunction determines the rate of both intrauterine and ectopic pregnancy. Severe dysfunction interferes with both intrauterine and ectopic pregnancy, whereas moderate dysfunction allows for higher rates of ectopic pregnancy.

Paradoxically, the use of microsurgical technique for salpingostomy has resulted in a surprisingly high rate of ectopic pregnancy (Table 4). The total pregnancy rate in the two groups appears not to be different. The reason for this difference is not entirely clear. Possibly, the partial restoration of tubal function, made possible by the new surgical technique, allows for ovum pickup. The abnormal tube, however, is unable to transport the embryo into the uterus properly, and an ectopic pregnancy results.

The use of the CO_2 laser for salpingostomy, as can be seen in Table 5, does not offer any clear advantages over electrocautery in either increasing the incidence of pregnancy or reducing the incidence of ectopic pregnancy.[51, 53] Similarly, the use of operative laparoscopy in 20 patients resulted in a pregnancy rate of 10% and in an ectopic pregnancy rate of 10%,[30] offering no clear advantage over conventional techniques.

In some patients distal tubal occlusion results from previous fimbriectomy, usually performed for the purpose of sterilization. Neosalpingostomy in these patients is associated with a pregnancy rate of 44% to 57% and an ectopic pregnancy rate of 0% to 14%. Two such reports are represented in Table 6.

TUBAL ANASTOMOSIS

Tubal anastomosis is performed to overcome an area of blockage. The block can be a result of prior tubal sterilization, previous PID, or even a segmental resection, which is occasionally used in the treatment of an ectopic pregnancy.

Tubal dysfunction often follows an anastomosis. Causes for dysfunction may include the sterilization procedure itself, the damage caused by prolonged tubal occlusion that follows obstruction, the effect of prior tubal infection, and the anastomosis procedure itself. Abnormal tubal function is manifested by a prolongation of the interval from reversal to conception, and by the occurrence of ectopic pregnancies in these operated tubes.

Table 4. *Neosalpingostomy*

Author	Surgery	Year	Patients	Pregnancies	%	Ectopic	% patients	% pregnancies
O'Brien et al.[40]	Macr[a]	1969	57	14	24	1	2	7
Horne et al.[41]	Macr	1973	52	20	38	2	4	10
Marik[42]	Macr	1977	52	12	23	1	2	8
Cognat and Rochet[43]	Macr	1977	118	28	20	5	4	18
Siegler and Kontopoulos[27]	Macr	1979	15	5	33	3	20	60
DeCherney and Kase[44]	Macr[b]	1981	9	2	22	0	0	0
Wallach et al.[30]	Macr	1983	24	5	20	2	8	40
Swolin[45]	Micr[c]	1966	33	8	24	1	18	12
Rock et al.[46]	Micr	1978	99	26	26	6	6	23
Gomel[47]	Micr	1978	41	12	29	4	12	33
Siegler and Kontopoulos[27]	Micr	1979	23	8	34	3	13	37
Gomel and Swolin[48]	Micr	1980	72	21	30	7	10	33
Audebert et al.[38]	Micr	1980	96	29	30	5	5	17
Winston[26]	Micr	1980	241	42	17	23	10	54
DeCherney and Kase[44]	Micr	1981	54	24	44	4	7	16
Larsson[49]	Micr	1982	54	21	39	0	0	0
Frantzen and Schlosser[33]	Micr	1982	85	16	18	3	4	18
Russell et al.[50]	Micr	1986	68	28	41	12	17	42
Total (macr and micr)			1193	325	27	82	6.9	25
Macr			327	86	26	14	4.3	17
Micr			866	239	27	68	7.8	28

[a]Macr, macrosurgery.
[b]Rock-Mulligan Hood prosthesis.
[c]Micr, microsurgery.

The effect of prolonged occlusion on tubal ultrastructure was demonstrated by Vasquez and coworkers[55] in patients after surgical sterilization. A variety of lesions could be demonstrated at the time of the anastomosis. Those lesions included deciliation, flattening of the mucosal folds, and mucosal polyps and were found to progress with time after the original sterilization procedure. The anastomosis procedure itself can lead to tubal malfunction because constriction at the site of anastomosis and malalignment of the mucosal folds can result in a delay in ovum transport and can predispose the patient to an ectopic pregnancy.

The outcome of tubal anastomosis is determined by a variety of factors, including the location of anastomosis along the tube, a residual tubal length of greater than 3 to 4 cm,[56, 57] the presence of coexisting tubal disease, the method used for sterilization, and whether or not microsurgical technique was used for the repair. Some sterilization procedures carry a higher rate of ectopic pregnancy than others when reversal is attempted. The reversal of tubes treated with unipolar cautery carries a notoriously high incidence of ectopic pregnancy.[58] Table 7 summarizes the outcome of tubal anastomosis after sterilization by a variety of methods. As is clearly evident from this table, the use of simple ligation and of the Falope ring (Cooper Medical, Langhorne, PA) is associated with a higher overall pregnancy rate, and a low rate of ectopic pregnancy, whereas the use of cautery is associated with lower overall pregnancy rates and higher ectopic pregnancy rates. Anastomosis of one versus two tubes can also alter the rate of ectopic pregnancy. Repair of one tube is associated with lower overall pregnancy rates and ectopic pregnancy rates than the

Table 5. *Neosalpingostomy—Laparoscopy and Laser*

Author	Surgery	Year	Patients	Pregnancies	%	Ectopic	Ectopic % patients	Ectopic % pregnancies
Fayez[35]	Lap[a]	1983	20	2	10	2	10	100
Tulandi et al.[51]	Laser[b]	1984	23	5	22	0	0	0
Daniell et al.[52]	Laser	1986	48	10	21	1	2	10

[a]Lap, operative laparoscopy.
[b]Laser, CO_2 laser.

Table 6. *Neosalpingostomy—Postfimbriectomy*

Author	Surgery	Year	Patients	Pregnancies	%	Ectopic	Ectopic % patients	Ectopic % pregnancies
Novy[54]	Fimb[a]	1980	9	4	44	0	0	0
Betz et al.[34]	Fimb	1980	7	4	57	1	14	25

[a]Fimb, postfimbriectomy.

anastomosis of both tubes[60] (pregnancy rate of 55% versus 64% and ectopic pregnancy rate of 10% versus 15%).

The effect of surgical technique on the outcome of midsegment tubal anastomosis is presented in Table 8. The figures demonstrate the superiority of the microsurgical technique in improving the outcome of surgery and reducing the rate of ectopic pregnancy.

Tubocornual anastomosis is performed in cases of cornual occlusion. The outcome of this procedure was shown to be dependent on the etiology of the cornual block. Lavy et al.[59] have reported on the outcome of tubocornual anastomosis. In 8 patients with cornual occlusion secondary to PID and in 17 patients with obstruction secondary to sterilization, the ectopic pregnancy rate was 40% and 11%, respectively. Of the 17 patients with cornual occlusion secondary to surgical sterilization who conceived, ectopic pregnancy occurred in 16%. In the group of six patients sterilized by tubal ligation and requiring tubocornual anastomosis, no ectopic pregnancies were reported. Table 9 represents some of the available data on pregnancy outcome after tubocornual anastomosis for reversal of sterilization and correction of the sequel of tubal disease.

RECURRENT ECTOPIC PREGNANCY

Patients with a history of prior ectopic pregnancy are at significant risk for recurrence. This risk is related to the underlying tubal disease that led to the initial ectopic pregnancy and to the surgical procedure performed for its removal. The procedures aimed at removing the ectopic pregnancy can be classified as either radical (salpingectomy) or conservative (e.g., salpingostomy, segmental resection). The choice of procedure usually depends on the condition of the patient, the location of the ectopic pregnancy within the tube, its size, and whether or not tubal rupture has already occurred. In general it is desirable to attempt to preserve the involved tube at the time of surgery, because recurrence of an ectopic pregnancy in the contralateral tube may necessitate salpingectomy, rendering the patient without tubes.

Radical Surgery

Salpingectomy is indicated in the case of tubal pregnancy, uncontrollable bleeding, or multiple recurrences in the same tube.

In a literature review that included 1083 women, Oelsner et al.[73] have calculated the risk of

Table 7. *Tubal Anastomosis for Reversal of Sterilization—Outcome by Procedure*

Author	Year	Method	Patients	Pregnant	%	Ectopic	%
Rock et al.[58]	1982	Caut uni[a]	48	25	52	4	8.3
		Pomeroy[b]	31	22	71	1	3.2
		Falop ring[c]	22	18	82	0	0
		Irving[d]	6	4	66	0	0
Seiler[59]	1983	Caut uni	22	15	67	2	9
		Pomeroy	40	25	62	0	0
		Falop ring	6	3	50	0	0
		Irving	4	3	75	0	0
Total		Pomeroy	71	47	66	1	1.4
		Caut uni	70	40	57	6	8.5
		Falop ring	28	21	75	0	0
		Irving	10	7	70	0	0

[a]Caut uni, unipolar cautery.
[b]Pomeroy, Pomeroy's tubal ligation.
[c]Irving, Irving's tubal ligation.
[d]Falop ring, Falope ring sterilization.

Table 8. *Midsegment Tubal Anastomosis*

Author	Surgery	Year	Patients	Pregnancies	%	Ectopic	% patients	% pregnancies
Siegler and Perez[61]	Macr[a]	1975	46	16	39	4	8.6	25
Diamond[62]	Macr	1977	12	8	66	0	0	0
Jones and Rock[63]	Macr	1978	12	10	83	1	8.3	10
Siegler and Kontopoulos[27]	Macr	1979	20	5	25	3	15	60
Wallach et al.[30]	Macr	1983	18	9	50	2	11.1	22
Siegler and Kontopoulos[27]	Micr[b]	1979	16	9	56	1	6.2	11
Gomel[64]	Micr	1980	118	76	64	1	1	1.3
Wilson[65]	Micr	1980	41	16	35	2	5	12.5
Silber and Cohen[56]	Micr	1980	25	14	56	1	4	7
Winston[66]	Micr	1980	126	73	57	3	2.3	4
Grunert et al.[67]	Micr	1981	40	22	55	1	2.5	4
Meldrum[68]	Micr	1981	25	14	56	1	4	7
Gomel[1]	Micr	1983	118	92	78	2	1.7	2
DeCherney et al.[69]	Micr	1983	124	92	74	8	6.4	8.6
Total			607	364	59	22	3.6	6
Macr			108	48	44	10	9.2	22
Micr			509	316	62	12	2.3	3.7

[a]Macr, macrosurgery.
[b]Micr, microsurgery.

ectopic pregnancy after salpingectomy in women desiring pregnancy. Ectopic pregnancy occurred in 15.4% of the women and intrauterine pregnancy in 36.5%. Similar results have been reported by other authors and are represented in Table 10.

Conservative Surgery

Conservative procedures are performed to remove the ectopic pregnancy and preserve the tube. The choice of technique is determined by the location of the pregnancy within the tube and by the presence or absence of active bleeding. These surgical procedures include linear salpingostomy, expression of the pregnancy through the distal tubal ostium, and segmental resection followed by an end-to-end anastomosis.

Linear salpingostomy has become the procedure of choice for the treatment of ectopic pregnancy. The pregnancy is removed through a linear incision on the antimesenteric surface of the tube, bleeding is controlled, and the incision is left open to prevent scarring. Indications for this procedure include a hemodynamically stable patient with an unruptured tubal pregnancy who desires to preserve her reproductive potential. The recurrent ectopic pregnancy rates following this procedure are listed in Table 10. The rates of recurrence in these patients are not different from those achieved after salpingectomy. A group of special interest consists of patients with one remaining patent oviduct after salpingostomy for ectopic pregnancy. The recurrence rate of ectopic pregnancy in these patients is unusually high. In 15 patients with a sole patent oviduct, DeCherney

Table 9. *Tubocornual Anastomosis—The Effect of Etiology of Obstruction*

Author	Year	Lesion	Patients	Pregnancies	%	Ectopic	% patients	% pregnancies
Winston[70]	1977	TS[a]	16	11	69	1	6	9
Winston[66]	1980	TS	43	26	61	1	2	4
Henderson[71]	1981	TS	8	NA[b]	NA	2	25	NA
Lavy et al.[57]	1986	TS	17	9	53	1	6	11
McComb and Gomel[72]	1980	TD[c]	38	22	58	2	5	9
Gomel[20]	1977	TD	14	7	50	0	0	0
Meldrum[68]	1981	TD	7	5	71	0	0	0
Lavy et al.[57]	1986	TD	8	5	62	2	25	40

[a]TS, tubal sterilization.
[b]NA, not available.
[c]TD, tubal disease.

Table 10. *Surgical Management of Ectopic Pregnancy*

Procedure	Author	Year	Patients	% pregnancies	% ectopic
Salpingectomy					
	Vehaskari[74]	1960	219	48	8
	Polman and Wicksell[75]	1960	92	38	7
	Timonen and Nieminen[76]	1967	558	49	11
	Kucera et al.[77]	1969	106	34	17
	DeCherney and Kase[78]	1979	50	42	12
Salpingostomy					
	Vehaskari[74]	1960	88	49	16
	Tomonen and Nieminen[76]	1967	185	53	12
	Jarvinen et al.[79]	1972	43	60	9
	Bukovsky et al.[80]	1979	23	70	4
	DeCherney and Kase[78]	1979	48	39	8
	DeCherney et al.[81a]	1982	15	73	20
	Patton[82a]	1986	17	53	11
	DeCherney et al.[83b]	1980	9	55	0
"Milking"					
	Timonen and Nieminen[76]	1967	24	24	
	Swollin[84]	1972	5	—	
Operative laparoscopy	DeCherney et al.[85]	1981	18	50	0
	Bruhat et al.[86]	1980	25	72	12

[a]Single remaining tube.
[b]Microsurgical technique.

et al.[81] have reported a 53% intrauterine pregnancy rate and a 20% recurrent ectopic pregnancy rate.

Segmental resection is recommended for patients with isthmic ectopic pregnancies and for those with ruptured ectopic pregnancies who are hemodynamically stable. An anastomosis at the resection site can be performed either at the time of the original operation or later. Swolin and Fall[84] have reported a series of 42 patients who underwent a segmental resection and anastomosis. Intrauterine pregnancy was achieved in 10 (23.8%) and an ectopic pregnancy in 6 patients (14.3%). In another report, elective tubal reconstruction in 6 patients after segmental resection resulted in an intrauterine pregnancy in 4 (66%), with one of the pregnancies ectopic (16%).[87]

Expressing the ectopic pregnancy through the distal tubal ostium (milking) results in an extremely high rate of ectopic pregnancy and in a low rate of intrauterine pregnancy,[76, 84] suggesting possible damage to the tube at the time of the procedure.

The use of microsurgical technique for removal of an ectopic pregnancy can reduce the incidence of recurrence. With microsurgical technique, intrauterine pregnancy was achieved in five of nine patients. No ectopic pregnancies occurred in this group.[84] Similar results have been reported by other authors.[80, 88] These reports clearly demonstrate the advantage of microsurgical technique over conventional surgery in these patients.

Operative laparoscopy can be used for removal of an ectopic pregnancy. A linear salpingostomy with unipolar cautery is usually performed. For best results and fewer complications, preselection of patients is advisable. The patient must be hemodynamically stable, and the tubal gestation should be unruptured and < 3 cm in size. Encouraging results have been reported with this technique in preselected patients (Table 10).

Special consideration should be given to patients who have had multiple ectopic pregnancies. The recurrence in this group is high and the rate of intrauterine pregnancy is low. DeCherney et al.[89] have followed 13 patients actively attempting to conceive after two previous ectopic pregnancies. Only 4 of 13 patients were able to conceive (39%), and one had a recurrent ectopic pregnancy (20% of conceptions). Halat[90] has reported repeat ectopic pregnancy in 4 of 7 patients conceiving after two ectopic pregnancies (57% of conceptions). The high rate of repeat ectopic pregnancy and the low rates of intrauterine pregnancy should suggest the use of other methods, such as salpingectomy or in vitro fertilization and embryo transfer in order to avoid recurrence in these patients.

THE ALTERNATIVE

IVF-ET is rapidly becoming an alternative mode of therapy for patients with a variety of infertility disorders. Tubal factor infertility remains the major indication for IVF-ET, accounting for up to 80% of the patients.[91] In this procedure, ova are aspirated from the ovaries and fertilized in vitro, and the resulting preembryo(s) are then placed in the uterine cavity approximately 48 hours later. The fallopian tube is thus bypassed.

The success achieved with IVF-ET as reported by multiple centers is modest at best. Factors associated with success include the method of ovarian stimulation, the etiology of infertility, the woman's age, the quality of the semen, and many others. The pregnancy rate per treatment cycle ranges from 7% to 17%.[91]

Ectopic pregnancy, although uncommon, was reported in the World Collaborative report in 1.7% of pregnancies (19/1084), and in 0.23% of embryo transfers (19/7993).[91] In fact, the first pregnancy achieved through IVF-ET was ectopic.[92] A higher incidence, up to 11% of the pregnancies, was reported by others.[93] Ectopic pregnancy occurring in IVF-ET cycles is the result of reflux of the embryo from the uterine cavity into the tube after embryo transfer. Yovich and coworkers[94] have reported an increased incidence of ectopic pregnancy, which appeared to be associated with high fundal transfers of the embryos. The embryos refluxed into the tubes are not able to return into the uterine cavity because of mechanical interference caused by tubal disease. Martinez et al.[95] have reported 10 ectopic pregnancies after IVF-ET. Nine of the patients had tubal factor infertility. No other association could be demonstrated between the occurrence of ectopic pregnancy and the ovarian stimulation protocol, the method of ova recovery, or the number of embryos transferred.

Although in most cases the pregnancy rates achieved with tubal surgery are superior to those of IVF-ET, several exceptions exist. Some surgical procedures, such as repeat tubal surgery after an unsuccessful attempt, carry a low rate of pregnancy even when compared with IVF-ET. IVF-ET is an attractive alternative to tubal surgery in these patients. In conditions that predispose the patient to an unacceptably high rate of ectopic pregnancy, such as multiple previous ectopics or a significant hydrosalpinx, IVF-ET should also be considered as an alternative to surgery as the risk of ectopic pregnancy can be significantly reduced.

SUMMARY

Ectopic pregnancy is the shady companion of tubal surgery. Among patients with ectopic pregnancy, relatively few have a history of tubal surgery as their underlying etiologic factor when compared with other etiologies such as PID. Nevertheless, a history of tubal surgery should place the patient at a higher-risk group for ectopic pregnancy; 3% to 20% of these patients will encounter an ectopic pregnancy after the corrective surgery.

Table 11. *Summary: Ectopic Pregnancy After Tubal Surgery*

Procedure	Technique	% Total pregnancy	Pregnancy range	% Ectopic	Ectopic range
Salpingostomy	Macr[a]	42	35–65	3.4	1–20
	Micr[b]	52	31–69	1.8	0–16
Fimbrioplasty	Macr	42	36–50	14	10–18
	Micr	59	26–68	6	4–11
Neosalpingostomy	Macr	27	20–38	4.2	2–20
	Micr	26	17–44	7.7	0–18
Tubal anastomosis	Macr	44	25–83	9.2	0–15
	Micr	62	35–78	2.3	1–6.2
Removal of ectopic pregnancy					
	Salpingectomy	42	38–49	12	8–17
	Salpingostomy	57	39–73	11	0–20

[a]Macr, macrosurgery.
[b]Micr, microsurgery.

The incidence of ectopic pregnancy after tubal surgery is extremely variable and is closely linked to the degree of restoration of normal functional and anatomic integrity after the surgical procedure. This depends, to a large extent, on the amount of previous damage to the tube and its potential reversibility. Major improvements in surgical technique can, therefore, have reduced, but not eliminated, the occurrence of tubal pregnancy.

The incidence of ectopic pregnancy associated with any given tubal surgical procedure should be taken into consideration when surgery is contemplated. When the risk of ectopic pregnancy is unacceptably high, or when the patient is reluctant to be exposed to a high risk of ectopic pregnancy, IVF-ET could be offered as an alternative. Table 11 represents the incidence of ectopic pregnancy associated with the various surgical procedures. The figures demonstrate the wide variation in outcome for the same procedure.

REFERENCES

1. Gomel V: An odyssey through the oviduct. Fertil Steril 39:144, 1983
2. Rubin GL, Peterson HB, Dorfman SF: Ectopic pregnancy in the United States. JAMA 249:1725, 1983
3. Schiffer MA: A review of 268 ectopic pregnancies. Am J Obstet Gynecol 86:264, 1963
4. Dorfman SF: Death from ectopic pregnancy, United States, 1979 to 1980. Obstet Gynecol 62:334, 1983
5. Bronson RA: Tubal pregnancy and infertility. Fertil Steril 28:221, 1977
6. Westrom L, Bengtsson L, Mordh PA: Incidence, trends and risks of ectopic pregnancy in a population of women. Br Med J 282:15, 1981
7. DeCherney AH, Minkin MJ, Spanger S: The contemporary surgical management of unruptured ectopic pregnancy. J Reprod Med 26:519, 1981
8. Crawford E, Hutchinson H: A decade of reports on tubal pregnancies condensed from the literature plus three hundred consecutive cases without a death. Am J Obstet Gynecol 67:568, 1954
9. Fielding WL, Kennedy RK, Gillies RW: Extrauterine pregnancy: statistical review of 160 cases. Obstet Gynecol 26:702, 1965
10. Blandau RJ: The mechanism of ovulation and how eggs and sperm reach the site of fertilization. In Hormonal Contraceptives, Estrogens, and Human Welfare, Edited by MC Diamond, CC Korenbrot. New York, Academic Press, 1978, p 31
11. Settlage DSF, Motoshima M, Tredway DR: Sperm transport from the external cervical os to the fallopian tubes in women: a time and quantitation study. Fertil Steril 24: 655, 1973
12. Verhage HG, Bareither ML, Jaffe RC, Akbar M: Cyclic changes in ciliation, secretion and cell height of the oviductal epithelium in women. Am J Anat 156:505, 1979
13. Jansen RPS: Endocrine responses in the fallopian tube. Endocr Rev 5:525, 1984
14. Critoph FN, Dennis KJ: Ciliary activity in the human oviduct. Br J Obstet Gynaecol 84:216, 1978
15. Jansen RPS: Cyclic changes in the human fallopian tube isthmus and their functional importance. Am J Obstet Gynecol 136:292, 1980
16. Crane M, Woodruff JD: Factors influencing the success of tuboplastic procedures. Fertil Steril 19:810, 1968
17. Jansen RPS: Abortion incidence following fallopian tube repair. Obstet Gynecol 56:499, 1980
18. Patton DL, Halbert SA: Electron microscopic examination of the rabbit oviductal ampulla following microsurgical end to end anastomosis. Fertil Steril 32:691, 1979
19. Winston RML, McLure M, Browne JC: Pregnancy following autograft transplantation of the fallopian tube and ovary in the rabbit. Lancet 2:294, 1974
20. Gomel V: Tubal reanastomosis by microsurgery. Fertil Steril 28:59, 1977
21. Paterson P, Wood C: The use of microsurgery in the reanastomosis of the rabbit fallopian tube. Fertil Steril 25: 757, 1974
22. Oelsner G, Boeckx W, Verhoeven H, Koninckx Ph, Brosens I: The effect of training in microsurgery. Am J Obstet Gynecol 152:1054, 1985
23. Peretz BA, Lindenbaum ES, Beach D: Ectopic pregnancy effects on the ipsilateral fallopian tube epithelium—an ultrastructural study. Eur J Obstet Gynecol Reprod Biol 17:19, 1984
24. Vasquez G, Winston RML, Brosens IA: Tubal mucosa and ectopic pregnancy. Br J Obstet Gynaecol 90:468, 1983
25. Vasquez G, Winston RML, Brosens I, Boeckx W: La microanatomie de la trompe de Fallope. In Oviducte et Fertilite, Edited by I Brosens, M Cognat, A Constantin, M Thieber. Paris, Masson, 1979, p 17
26. Winston RML: Microsurgery of the fallopian tube: from fantasy to reality. Fertil Steril 34:521, 1980
27. Siegler AM, Kontopoulos V: The analysis of macrosurgical and microsurgical techniques in the management of the tuboperitoneal factor in infertility. Fertil Steril 32: 377, 1979
28. Caspi E, Halperin Y: Surgical management of periadnexal adhesions. Int J Fertil 26:49, 1981
29. Hulka JF: Adnexal adhesions: a prognostic staging and classification system based on a five-year survey of fertility surgery results at Chapel Hill, North Carolina. Am J Obstet Gynecol 144:141, 1982
30. Wallach EE, Manara LR, Eisenberg E: Experience with 143 cases of tubal surgery. Fertil Steril 39:609, 1983
31. Bronson RA, Wallach EE: Lysis of periadnexal adhesions for correction of infertility. Fertil Steril 28:613, 1977
32. Diamond E: Lysis of postoperative pelvic adhesions in infertility. Fertil Steril 31:287, 1979
33. Frantzen C, Schlosser HW: Microsurgery and postinfectious tubal infertility. Fertil Steril 38:397, 1982
34. Betz G, Engel T, Penney LL: Tuboplasty—comparison of the methodology. Fertil Steril 34:534, 1980
35. Fayez JA: An assessment of the role of operative laparoscopy in tuboplasty. Fertil Steril 39:476, 1983

36. Gomel V: Salpingo-ovariolysis by laparoscopy in infertility. Fertil Steril 40:607, 1983
37. Palmer R: Salpingostomy: a critical study of 396 personal cases operated upon without polyethylene tubing. Proc R Soc Lond (Biol) 53:357, 1960
38. Audebert AJM, Laure-Charlus S, Emparaire JC: Aspects actuels de la chirurgie tubaire pour infertilite. Rev Fr Gynecol Obstet 75:427, 1980
39. Patton GW: Pregnancy outcome following microsurgical fimbrioplasty. Fertil Steril 37:150, 1982
40. O'Brien JR, Arrenet GH, Eduljee SY: Operative treatment of fallopian tube pathology in human fertility. Am J Obstet Gynecol 103:520, 1969
41. Horne HW, Clyman M, Debrovner C, Griggs G, Kistner RW, Kosasa T, Stevenson CS, Taymor M: The prevention of postoperative pelvic adhesions following conservative operative treatment for human infertility. Int J Fertil 18:109, 1973
42. Marik J, Microsurgical repair of hydrosalpinx. In Microsurgery in Infertility, Edited by JM Phyllips. St. Louis, St. Louis Board of Publication, 1977, p 147
43. Cognat M, Rochet Y: Notre experience de la salpingoplastie. J Fr Gynecol Obstet 6:839, 1977
44. DeCherney AH, Kase N: A comparison of treatment for bilateral fimbrial occlusion. Fertil Steril 35:162, 1981
45. Swolin K: Electromicrosurgery and salpingostomy long term results. Am J Obstet Gynecol 121.418, 1974
46. Rock JA, Katayama KP, Martin EJ, Woodruff JD, Jones HW Jr: Factors influencing the success of salpingostomy techniques for distal fimbrial occlusion. Obstet Gynecol 51:591, 1978
47. Gomel V: Salpingostomy by microsurgery. Fertil Steril 29:380, 1978
48. Gomel V, Swolin K: Salpingostomy: microsurgical technique and results. Clin Obstet Gynecol 23:1203, 1980
49. Larsson B: Late results of salpingostomy combined with salpingolysis and ovariolysis by electromicrosurgery in 54 women. Fertil Steril 37:156, 1983
50. Russell JB, DeCherney AH, Laufer N, Polan ML, Naftolin F: Neosalpingostomy: comparison of 24 and 72 month follow-up time shows increased pregnancy rate. Fertil Steril 45:296, 1986
51. Tulandi T, Farag R, McInnes RA, Gelfand MM, Wright CV, Vilos GA: Reconstructive surgery for hydrosalpinx with and without the carbon dioxide laser. Fertil Steril 42:839, 1984
52. Daniell JF, Diamond MP, McLaughlin DS, Martin DC, Feste J, Surrey MW, Friedman S, Vaughn WK: Clinical results of terminal salpingostomy with the use of the CO_2 laser: report of the intraabdominal laser study group. Fertil Steril 45:175, 1986
53. Mage G, Bruhat M-A: Pregnancy following salpingostomy: comparison between CO_2 laser and electrosurgery procedures. Fertil Steril 40:472, 1983
54. Novy MJ: Reversal of Kroener fimbriectomy sterilization. Am J Obstet Gynecol 137:198, 1980
55. Vasquez G, Winston RML, Boeckx W, Brosens I: Tubal lesions subsequent to sterilization and their relation to fertility after attempts at reversal. Am J Obstet Gynecol 138:86, 1980
56. Silber SJ, Cohen R: Microsurgical reversal of female sterilization: the role of tubal length. Fertil Steril 33:598, 1980
57. Lavy G, Diamond MP, DeCherney AH: Pregnancy following tubocornual anastomosis. Fertil Steril 46:21, 1986
58. Rock JA, Bergquist CA, Zacur HA, Parmley TH, Guzick DS, Jones HW Jr: Tubal anastomosis following unipolar cautery. Fertil Steril 37:613, 1982
59. Seiler JC: Factors influencing the outcome of microsurgical tubal ligation reversals. Am J Obstet Gynecol 146: 292, 1983
60. McCormick WG, Torres J, McCane LR: Tubal reanastomosis: an update. Fertil Steril 31:689, 1979
61. Siegler AM, Perez RJ: Reconstruction of fallopian tubes in previously sterilized patients. Fertil Steril 26:383, 1975
62. Diamond E: Microsurgical reconstruction of the uterine tube in sterilized patients. Fertil Steril 28:1203, 1977
63. Jones HW Jr, Rock JA: On the reanastomosis of the fallopian tubes after surgical sterilization. Fertil Steril 29: 702, 1978
64. Gomel V: Microsurgical reversal of female sterilization: a reappraisal. Fertil Steril 33:587, 1980
65. Wilson PCM: Reversing female sterilization. Population reports, Vol VIII, No. 5, Series C. Population Information Program. Baltimore, The Johns Hopkins University, 1980, p C-97
66. Winston RLM: Reversal of tubal sterilization. Clin Obstet Gynecol 23:1261, 1980
67. Grunert GM, Drake TS, Takaki NK: Microsurgical anastomosis of the fallopian tubes for reversal of sterilization. Obstet Gynecol 58:148, 1981
68. Meldrum DR: Microsurgical tubal reanastomosis: the role of splints. Obstet Gynecol 57:613, 1981
69. DeCherney AH, Mezer HC, Naftolin F: Analysis of failure of microsurgical anastomosis after midsegment, non-coagulation tubal ligation. Fertil Steril 39:618, 1983
70. Winston RML: Microsurgical tubocornual anastomosis for reversal of sterilization. Lancet 1:284, 1977
71. Henderson SR: Reversal of female sterilization: comparison of microsurgical and gross surgical techniques for tubal anastomosis. Am J Obstet Gynecol 139:73, 1981
72. McComb P, Gomel V: Cornual occlusion and its microsurgical reconstruction. Clin Obstet Gynecol 23:1229, 1980
73. Oelsner G, Tarlatzis BC: Radical surgery for extrauterine pregnancy. In Ectopic Pregnancy, Edited by AH DeCherney. Rockville, MD, Aspen Publishers, 1986, p 127
74. Vehaskari A: The operation of choice for ectopic pregnancy with reference to subsequent fertility. Acta Obstet Gynecol Scand 39 (supple 13):3, 1960
75. Polman L, Wicksell F: Fertility after conservative surgery in tubal pregnancy. Acta Obstet Gynecol Scand 39: 143, 1960
76. Timonen S, Nieminen U: Tubal pregnancy: choice of operative method of treatment. Acta Obstet Gynecol Scand 46:327, 1967
77. Kucera E, Mack F, Novak J, Andrasova V: Fertility after operations of extrauterine pregnancy. Int J Fertil 14:127, 1969
78. DeCherney AH, Kase N: The conservative surgical management of unruptured ectopic pregnancy. Obstet Gynecol 54:451, 1979
79. Jarvinen PA, Nummi S, Pietila K: Conservative operative treatment of tubal pregnancy with postoperative daily hydrotubations. Acta Obstet Gynecol Scand 51:169, 1972

80. Bukovsky I, Langer R, Herman A, Caspi E: Conservative surgery for tubal pregnancy. Obstet Gynecol 53:709, 1979
81. DeCherney AH, Maheaux R, Naftolin F: Salpingostomy for ectopic pregnancy in the sole patent oviduct: reproductive outcome. Fertil Steril 37:619, 1982
82. Patton WP: Conservative surgery for ectopic pregnancy. In Ectopic Pregnancy, Edited by AH DeCherney. Rockville, MD, Aspen Publishers, 1986, p 105
83. DeCherney AH, Polan ML, Kort H, Kase N: Microsurgical technique in the management of tubal ectopic pregnancy. Fertil Steril 34:324, 1980
84. Swollin K, Fall M: Ectopic pregnancy. Acta Eur Fertil 3:147, 1972
85. DeCherney AH, Romero R, Naftolin F: Surgical management of unruptured ectopic pregnancy. Fertil Steril 35:21, 1981
86. Bruhat M-A, Manhes H, Mage G, Pouly JL: Treatment of ectopic pregnancy by means of laparoscopy. Fertil Steril 33:411, 1980
87. DeCherney AH, Boyers SP: Isthmic ectopic pregnancy: segmental resection as the treatment of choice. Fertil Steril 44:307, 1985
88. Sherman D, Langer R, Sadovsky G, Bukovsky I, Caspi E: Improved fertility following ectopic pregnancy. Fertil Steril 37:497, 1982
89. DeCherney AH, Silidker JS, Mezer HC, Tarlatzis BC: Reproductive outcome following two ectopic pregnancies. Fertil Steril 43:82, 1985
90. Halatt JG: Repeat ectopic pregnancy: a study of 123 consecutive cases. Am J Obstet Gynecol 122:520, 1975
91. Seppälä M: The world collaborative report on in vitro fertilization and embryo replacement: current state-of-the-art in January 1984. In Annals of the New York Academy of Sciences, Vol 442: In Vitro Fertilization and Embryo Transfer, Edited by M Seppälä, RG Edwards. New York, The New York Academy of Sciences, 1985, p 558
92. Steptoe PC, Edwards RG: Reimplantation of a human embryo with subsequent tubal pregnancy. Lancet 1:880, 1976
93. Lopata A: Concepts in human in vitro fertilization and embryo transfer. Fertil Steril 40:289, 1983
94. Yovich JL, Turner SR, Murphy AJ: Embryo transfer technique as a cause of ectopic pregnancies in in vitro fertilization. Fertil Steril 44:318, 1985
95. Martinez F, Trounson A: An analysis of factors associated with ectopic pregnancy in a human in vitro fertilization program. Fertil Steril 45:79, 1986

Chapter 19

The role of lasers in infertility surgery

James F. Daniell, M.D.

The Women's Health Group, Nashville, Tennessee

Since the first reported use of the CO_2 laser intraabdominally for female reconstructive pelvic surgery in 1974,[1] much has been written about the use of lasers for infertility surgery both in medical journals and in lay publications. The media publicity given to the visually impressive moving beam of a CO_2 laser bloodlessly vaporizing human tissues is to be expected, considering the high interest in technology by today's journalists. Unfortunately, many patients have too easily accepted some of the glowing claims made for infertility surgery performed with lasers, while too many surgeons not personally familiar with surgical lasers have been quick to make negative statements concerning lasers. It is normal for skepticism to exist in the minds of many infertility surgeons concerning the real benefits of laser surgery, considering the expense of the hardware, the lack of available data, and the small numbers of surgeons that have as yet had an opportunity to gain hands-on experience in either laboratory animals or clinically with lasers. As more long-term follow-up becomes available and respected researchers begin to critically and unemotionally investigate the various surgical lasers that are available today, meaningful data will be forthcoming from both animal and clinical studies. Thus, the real role of lasers in infertility surgery is not yet determined and must await the results of future and ongoing investigations. The goal of this article is to review the various surgical lasers that have been used in infertility surgery and report briefly the methods of use and results reported from both research and clinical investigations.

TYPES OF LASERS IN INFERTILITY SURGERY

Of the many lasers that have been used in various surgical fields, three have been used in gynecology—the CO_2, the argon, and the neodymium:yttrium-aluminum-garnet (Nd:YAG). Each of these lasers has a specific wave length and, thus, different characteristics and tissue effects. These properties are listed in Table 1. As can be seen, both the Nd:YAG laser and the argon laser can be delivered via flexible fibers and passed through fluids, which are advantages over the CO_2 laser with regard to the ease of delivery. The amount of scattering of the beam and the depth of penetration also vary for these lasers. Only the CO_2 laser can allow vaporization and precise incision of tissue with any degree of effectiveness. Thus, the CO_2 laser has been, and will continue to be, the primary laser used for female infertility surgery.

BIOPHYSICS OF THE CO_2 LASER

Radiation from the CO_2 laser has three special qualities: it is coherent, collimated, and monochromatic. Coherent radiation is when the waves are exactly in step (phase) with each other in both time and space. Monochromatic waves have exactly the same wavelength (or color if they are visible). Collimated rays are parallel to each other.

The radiation of the CO_2 laser occurs at a wavelength of 10.6 μm in the infrared portion of the spectrum, which is invisible to the human eye. Carefully placed mirrors, one at each end of the laser resonator chamber, allow the 10.6-μm co-

Table 1. *Different Properties of Surgical Lasers*

	CO_2	Nd:YAG	Argon
Wave length of laser	10.6 μm	1.06 μm	0.5 μm
Primary tissue effect	Vaporization	Coagulation	Coagulation
Color-dependent	No	Yes	Yes
Scattering of beam	None	Moderate	Slight
Effect on water	Beam strongly absorbed	Beam slightly absorbed	Beam not absorbed
Passed through fibers	No	Yes	Yes
Depth of tissue effect[a]	0.1 mm	4 mm	0.5 mm

[a]In comparison studies in rat and rabbit bladders.

herent waves to reflect back and forth many times along the axis of the tube, thus amplifying the radiant energy emitted. The power of an unfocused CO_2 laser beam is relatively low when compared with the beam surface area. By a system of optics, using special focusing lenses, the emitted column of laser energy must first be focused further so that it can be applied for use surgically.

The selection of a lens for a specific application is a function of minimum spot size and depth of focus. Due to their high degree of coherence, laser beams can be focused to a very small spot, with an energy power density considerably higher than in the parallel beam. The importance of coherence and collimation can be illustrated by comparing a 60-watt electric bulb with a CO_2 laser producing 60 watts. Trying to focus the white light from a bulb with lenses will yield only a fraction of the emitted light energy at the focus because the bulb is emitting light in all directions. But the coherent beam from the CO_2 laser can be focused onto a tiny spot and generate enough energy to easily burn a hole in a block of wood.

There are certain properties of the CO_2 laser that make it advantageous for surgical procedures: (1) The energy is highly absorbed by nonreflective solids and liquids, notably water (the major constituent of most cells). In water this radiant energy is absorbed almost completely at a depth of 100 μm from the surface. (2) The absorption of the beam is similar on tissues of any color. (3) The energy does not cause genetic mutation of the cells. The effect of the waves from the CO_2 laser in any absorbing material is by conversion of radiant energy to heat. (4) There is minimal scattering from the point of impact. (5) The energy destroys tissue (including bacteria) by instantaneous boiling of the cellular water at 100°C. (6) The energy of the laser can be efficiently reflected by the user with mirrors of highly polished metals. (7) The energy of the CO_2 laser may be focused to a spot diameter < 1 mm with minimal energy loss by using special lenses. (8) CO_2 laser systems delivering enough power for intraabdominal surgery are compact and will operate from an ordinary electrical outlet.

ACTION ON TISSUES BY THE CO_2 LASER

The laser destruction of tissue is by vaporization of cellular elements. The tissue is incised by the boiling of intracellular and extracellular water to form steam, which expands explosively and disrupts tissue (carrying cellular debris out of the wound). Some of the debris is charred as it passes through the beam, and some ignites and burns. The actual area of laser impact does not show any sign of tissue combustion; the laser appears to destroy by vaporization of cellular water at a temperature of only 100°C at the impact point.

Measurements of the velocity at which steam expands from the point of laser impact reveal that the pressure exerted on adjacent tissue by cell disruption is small and unlikely to cause damage by shock waves or scatter of materials to adjacent sites. Histologic examination of sections from laser wounds on various organs has shown that some cellular damage occurs up to 500 μm from the laser impact but that the depth of thermal necrosis is usually < 100 μm. With normal blood flow in vessels, veins and arteries up to 0.5 mm in diameter can be sealed by the laser. If the flow is first stopped, vessels up to 2.0 mm can be sealed, as compared with vessels 0.5 to 1.0 mm in the case of cutting diathermy.

METHODS OF DELIVERING THE CO_2 LASER TO THE TISSUE

Acquiring confidence and skill in the use of the CO_2 laser for infertility surgery requires adaptation to a whole new "no-touch" form of operating. The tissue effect of the laser for incising, vaporizing, and coagulating tissue is a hands-off technique with the operator merely directing the beam and controlling the time and power density of the impact of the laser on the tissue. The beam can be delivered either at open surgery or under laparoscopic control for clinical use in female infertility operative procedures. At laparotomy, the

Table 2. *Comparison of Methods of Use for Infertility Surgery*

	Laparoscopy	Microscope	Hand-held scalpel
Avoid major surgery	Yes	No	No
Requires extra hardware	Yes	Yes	No
Easy to use deep in pelvis	Yes	Yes	No
Mirror use possible	No	Yes	Yes
Easy to vary spot size	No	No	Yes
Magnified tissue view is possible	Yes	Yes	Yes, with loupes
Good light visibility	Yes	Yes	Yes, with fiberoptic headlight
Fine control of beam with micromanipulator	Yes	Yes	No
Simple assembly	No	No	Yes

CO_2 laser can either be used with a simple hand-held probe attached to an articulated arm or via an operating microscope with a laser micromanipulator attached. There are obvious advantages, disadvantages, and differences in each method of laser beam delivery. These are outlined in Table 2. The overall goals of the surgeon and patient, the amount and type of disease present, the availability of delivery systems, and the level of experience and training of the operator will all influence the specific method of use of the CO_2 laser for an individual case. The hardware for delivery of the CO_2 laser beam for surgical uses is constantly being improved. At this writing this hardware includes easily usable, sterilizable hand pieces with focal lengths from 125 to 50 mm, variable spot size lenses for microsurgery (with excellent focusing and fine control of the beam by micromanipulators), and both second puncture and operative channel laparoscopic delivery systems.

LABORATORY EVALUATION OF THE CO_2 LASER

As with any emerging technology, the CO_2 laser has been the subject of many studies investigating the tissue effects of the beam and the results of various animal experiments.

The question of carcinogenic risks of the CO_2 laser beam was the subject of a study by Apfelberg et al.[2] in which mouse fibroblasts in tissue culture were exposed to the CO_2 laser. These cells were grown for nine generations and studied for their malignant transformation potential. This study did not show any increased incidence of malignant transformation of the cells when compared with normal, nontreated control mice.

Early animal studies of surgical intraabdominal CO_2 laser procedures included those of Klink et al.,[3] who in 1978 reported a technique of laser welding of the uterine cornua of 40 rabbits and in an unspecified number of surgically removed human fallopian tubes. They suggested that CO_2 laser welding might be a quick and effective technique for tubal anastomosis in humans. Baggish and Chong,[4] however, looked more closely at this suggested welding technique both in seven rabbits and in four patients with obstructed tubal segments. They found that laser welding did nothing to hold the anastomosis together structurally and concluded that the technique had little value for human tubal surgery. They did, however, comment favorably on the hemostatic properties of using the CO_2 laser as a cutting tool during pelvic reconstructive surgery.

Fayez et al.[5] reported, in rabbits, that they were unimpressed with laser welding of the tube. In addition, they compared needle cautery of the tube versus laser transection prior to anastomosis with 8-0 nonreactive sutures. They found the laser transection group of rabbits to be less fertile. They concluded that the CO_2 laser in the TM_{oo} mode with a 1.8 mm spot size had no place in tubal reanastomosis. However, Baggish,[6] in the "Editor's Corner" of the same journal, noted that this study was done with an older laser with lower power densities and thus probable greater thermal damage potential. Choe et al.,[7] in a more recent study, compared conventional microsurgical reanastomosis with laser microsurgical techniques of ligated uterine rabbit horns. Using the same CO_2 laser and techniques similar to those of Fayez et al.,[5] they concluded that laser microsurgery produced significantly less adhesion formation and comparative patency rates in rabbits. Other studies designed to evaluate postoperative intraperitoneal adhesion formation following CO_2 laser surgery included those of Pittaway et al.[8] and Bellina et al.[9] In the first study,[8] 31 rabbits received standard injury to the uterine horns and ovaries; then hemostasis was obtained either with the CO_2 laser or with bipolar cautery. The animals were sacrificed 5 weeks later, and the adhesions were graded in a blinded fashion. The results indicated no difference in the number of

Table 3. *Reported Clinical Results of Infertility Surgery with CO_2 Laser (Laparotomy)*

Author	Type of surgery	Length of follow-up	No. of patients	Results		
				Term pregnancy	Abortion	Ectopic
		mo				
Bellina[13]	All types of microsurgery:	24	230	91 (36%)	NS[a]	4 (4%)
	Initial procedure	24	102	44 (43%)	NS	NS
	Repeat procedure	24	114	37 (32%)	NS	NS
	Reversal of sterilization	24	14	10 (71%)	NS	NS
Mage and Bruhat[14]	Salpingostomy	21	38	9 (24%)	4 (10%)	3 (8%)
Tulandi[15]	Salpingostomy	10	11	3 (27%)	0	0
Kelly and Roberts[16]	Salpingostomy	12	28	2 (7%)	0	1 (5%)
	Adhesion vaporization	12	21	4 (19%)	1 (5%)	0
	Reversal of sterilization	12	12	8 (67%)	0	0
	Anastomosis of pathologic tubal blockage	12	8	2 (25%)	1 (13%)	0
Chong and Baggish[17]	Conservative endometriosis surgery (AFS stages: II to IV)	6	23 13 (stage II) 8 (stage III)	14 (61%) 11 (85%) 3 (38%)	NS	NS
Diamond et al.[18]	Salpingostomy, adhesion vaporization, and endometriosis surgery	12	106	38 (36%)	2 (2%)	2 (20%)
McLaughlin[19]	Myomectomy	12	5	2 (40%)	0	1 (20%)

[a]NS, not stated.

adhesions formed and the investigators suggested that the ovaries were more prone to develop postoperative adhesions than the uterine horns. In the second report,[9] comparative incisions on six rabbit peritoneums were made with the CO_2 laser and electrosurgical microneedles. The animals were sacrificed on days 5, 10, 15, 20, and 25; and the incisions were studied grossly and histologically. The investigators found adhesions to be absent in all the laser incisions but present in all the electrocautery sites. They concluded that the CO_2 laser caused less tissue injury both immediately and throughout the healing phase.

There have been fewer reports investigating use of the CO_2 laser under laparoscopic control in animal models. Daniell and Brown[10] tested a prototype system for aiming and firing a CO_2 laser beam down the operative channel of a modified laparoscope in four rabbits. They reported success in vaporizing target areas on the peritoneal sidewalls without complications but had problems with visibility of the orange helium neon target laser due to intraperitoneal smoke accumulation. Maintaining an adequate pneumoperitoneum and lens fogging was also an initial problem, but this was eventually solved by developing a special lens coupler and by using a regular laparoscope and a special second puncture probe to introduce the laser beam.[11] Tadir et al.[12] also recently reported their animal studies in Israel with both operative channel and separate puncture delivery of the CO_2 laser beam intraperitoneally under laparoscopic control. From their pioneering work evolved a system of equipment that is now clinically very effective.

CLINICAL EXPERIENCE WITH CO_2 LASERS IN INFERTILITY SURGERY

The CO_2 laser has been used for procedures encompassing almost the entire field of female reproductive surgery. The list includes cornual reimplantation, tubal transection for anastomosis, adhesiolysis, fimbrioplasty, neosalpingostomy, metroplasty, myomectomy, vaporization of ectopic gestation, conservative surgery for endometriosis, ovarian wedge resection, and uterosacral ligament vaporization. Unfortunately, most reports have been anecdotal and uncontrolled, and the number of subjects has been small. Thus, the basic question of true efficacy remains unanswered. The reported clinical results presently available for review are listed in Table 3 for open infertility surgery and in Table 4 for laparoscopic CO_2 laser surgery.

Table 4. *Reported Results of Laparoscopic Use of the CO_2 Laser*

Author	Type of surgery	Length of follow-up	No. of patients	Results		
				Term pregnancy	Abortion	Ectopic
		mo				
Daniell and Brown[10]	Vaporization of endometriosis	5	10	3 (30%)	0	0
Tadir et al.[12]	Sterilization	24	12	1 pregnancy (8% failure rate)		
	Vaporization of endometriosis	12–18	7	NS[a]		
	Adhesiolysis	12–18	14	NS		
Kelly and Roberts[21]	Vaporization of endometriosis	6	10	3 (30%)	3 (30%)	0
Martin[22]	Vaporization of endometriosis (AFS scores 1-20)	12	52	17 (33%)	NS	0
Feste[23]	Vaporization of endometriosis	24	21	16 (76%)	5 (24%)	0
Daniell and Herbert[24]	Terminal salpingostomy	9	21	3 (14%)	1 (5%)	1 (5%)
Nezhat[20]	Terminal salpingostomy	6–18	25	4 (16%)	1 (4%)	1 (4%)
	Vaporization of endometriosis	6	23	12 (56%)	3 (13%)	0

[a]NS, not stated.

RESULTS OF OPEN INFERTILITY SURGERY

Bellina[13] reported 230 cases of tubal reconstructive surgery with 2 years' follow-up. Unfortunately, he did not report his data in such a way that specific procedures could be accurately analyzed. He did, however, report a 37% conception rate for correction of bipolar tubal disease and a 32% pregnancy rate for repeat procedures, which are extremely impressive.

Mage and Bruhat[14] reported a comparative series in which terminal salpingostomy using microsurgical techniques was performed in 30 cases with electrosurgery and then, following that series, in 38 cases with the CO_2 laser. They noted a 24% term pregnancy rate with less follow-up time in the laser group, compared with 17% in the electromicrosurgery series. They stated that use of a short focal length hand piece was superior to a micromanipulator laser beam delivery system, and suggested that the laser might be a safe and effective alternative to electrosurgery in tubal surgery for correction of distal disease.

Tulandi,[15] in a prospective randomized study, compared the CO_2 laser with microdiathermy needle salpingostomy. The pregnancy rates at 10 months were similar (27% to 25%), but the surgery-to-conception time was less in the laser group. He felt this might reflect more rapid healing of the tube after laser surgery.

In yet another study, Kelly and Roberts,[16] with 1-year follow-up, reported only a 7% pregnancy rate for CO_2 laser terminal salpingostomy. However, with a second year of follow-up, this group of patients achieved a 30% pregnancy rate. This underscores the need for longer follow-up before conclusions can be drawn regarding the efficacy of CO_2 laser surgery for salpingostomy or other tubal reconstructive surgery.

Although many surgeons are now using the CO_2 laser intraabdominally for endometriosis vaporization, there have been few clinical reports to date. Chong and Baggish[17] reported the cases of 23 patients with stage II to stage IV disease (according to The American Fertility Society classification) who underwent conservative surgery for endometriosis with the use of the CO_2 laser both via the micromanipulator and the freehand piece of the laser's articulated arm. They described techniques for vaporization of implants, lysis of adhesions, and ovarian excision procedures. Their 6-month pregnancy rate of 61% included 85% for stage II and 38% for stage III, but no pregnancies in two cases of stage IV disease. In addition, 78% of these patients received danazol postoperatively in an unrandomized fashion. They concluded that the CO_2 laser offered the technical advantages of a bloodless field, precision destruction by vaporization, and the ability to treat poorly accessible areas. They recommended that further evaluation of the CO_2 laser in a randomized, collaborative, prospective study was needed before any conclusions concerning efficacy for major endometriosis surgery could be drawn.

A prospective multicenter study that involved use of early second-look laparoscopy to evaluate postoperative adhesion formation after CO_2 laser infertility surgery has recently been published.[18] This study was not randomized and had no control subjects. In spite of those deficiencies, the report was the first to accurately assess the occurrence of postoperative adhesions following intra-abdominal female infertility surgery using the CO_2 laser. These investigators found postoperative adhesion formation to be significant (91 of 106 patients) and concluded that the CO_2 laser was not a panacea for the treatment of tuboperitoneal causes of infertility.

The CO_2 laser has also been used for performing abdominal myomectomies. McLaughlin[19] reported his technique and results in eight patients, with a 40% term pregnancy rate in the five patients attempting conception. He believed that his laser technique was superior for performing myomectomies by providing improved hemostasis, better precision for removing the myomata while preserving normal uterine tissue, and by the ability to reach previously inaccessible areas. He believed that due to improved wound healing, postoperative adhesions appeared to be reduced. Unfortunately, he had no control subjects, small numbers, and only 8 months' follow-up.

CLINICAL RESULTS OF CO_2 LASER LAPAROSCOPY

The use of the CO_2 laser through a laparoscope was first reported by Bruhat et al.[25] for operative channel techniques and by Tadir et al.[26] for second puncture use with a diagnostic laparoscope. These authors initially investigated use of the CO_2 laser to perform tubal sterilization procedures. However, Tadir and associates[12] now state that "This procedure cannot be recommended for sterilization" because of tubal recanalization.

Numerous laparoscopic operative procedures have now been reported to have been performed with the CO_2 laser. Some of these are listed in Table 5. Several authors[10-12, 21-23] have now reported successful use of the CO_2 laser to vaporize endometrial implants under laparoscopic control with safety and efficiency. All these investigators indicate satisfaction with this new innovative method of selectively destroying visible areas of endometriosis without damaging adjacent tissues.

Table 5. *Operations That Have Been Performed with the CO_2 Laser Laparoscope*

1. Vaporization of endometriosis
2. Terminal neosalpingostomy
3. Uterosacral ligament ablation
4. Pelvic adhesiolysis
5. Vaporization of small uterine fibroids
6. Ovarian cystotomy
7. Ablation of hydatid cysts
8. Vaporization of ovarian fibromas

Laparoscopic salpingostomy, which has been performed with classic operative laparoscopic techniques, has certain risks, especially if cautery is used.[27-29] Daniell and Herbert[24] have recently reported a series of 22 patients with 1-year follow-up who underwent CO_2 laser terminal salpingostomy with the CO_2 laser laparoscope. The postoperative patency rate was 75% at follow-up hysterogram, and the term pregnancy rate was 14% in this series, made up of patients who had already undergone at least one previous tuboplasty. The authors believed the technique warranted further investigation with longer follow-up in a larger group of patients before any conclusions could be drawn.

INVESTIGATIONS OF THE OTHER SURGICAL LASERS FOR INFERTILITY SURGERY

Both the argon laser and the Nd:YAG laser have now been used investigationally for treatment of pelvic endometriosis. Keye and associates reported laparoscopic use of the argon laser both in rabbits[30] and in a small group of patients with endometriosis.[31] Their technique involves passing a 0.6-mm flexible quartz fiber through a second-puncture laparoscopic instrument with a steerable tip and firing the beam at endometrial implants. The argon laser, which is selectively absorbed by the hemoglobin of endometriosis implants, is much easier to deliver to the planned impact site under laparoscopic control than is the CO_2 laser. This new form of therapy for endometriosis seems very promising and is being investigated further. Preliminary results suggest that the argon laser can be safe, effective, and easy to use laparoscopically. Unfortunately, the argon laser cannot be used for vaporizing or incising tissues; so its use seems limited to photocoagulation of pigmented lesions such as endometriosis, either laparoscopically or at open surgery.

The Nd:YAG laser, which has a delivery system similar to that of the argon laser, but a greater depth of penetration of tissue, has also recently been investigated by Lamano[32] for use laparoscopically to photocoagulate endometriosis. This work, although preliminary, indicates that visible implants of endometriosis can be coagulated without complications using the powerful Nd:YAG beam. The depth of tissue destruction that occurs (3 to 4 mm beneath the surface) and the lateral beam-scattering theoretically makes this laser more dangerous, especially when used near vital structures. A particular danger also exists for the surgeon, who must use special protective lenses to guard against retinal damage from the penetrating beam's backscatter.

SAFETY OF LASERS

CO_2 lasers have been used intraabdominally for over a decade on thousands of patients. There has been a very respectable safety record, the number of reported documented injuries being $<$ 0.5%. Since CO_2 lasers concentrate such a large amount of energy into a very small, collimated beam, they are definitely capable of doing significant damage if aimed and fired inappropriately.

The types of immediate accidents that can occur include direct and indirect (e.g., a reflected beam) damage to tissues not planned to be the target of the beam, fires from ignition of flammable drapes or sponges, and anesthetic gas explosions. In addition, there is the problem of irritation to the surgeon's lungs from the vapor plume itself or vaporization of some chemical that may have been used in the operative field. These accidents can be avoided by use of protective glasses, nonreflective instruments, moist drapes and sponges, and proper venting systems.

The Nd:YAG and argon lasers present more serious safety hazards because of the properties of backscatter of the beam (reflection back toward the operator from the impact site) and the ability of these lasers to pass through clear fluids (e.g., the vitreous). Thus, very high standards of safety and special lenses must be used with these specific lasers.

Unfortunately, as more and more surgeons begin to use these various lasers, the number of accidents is sure to increase even if the rate remains the same. Therefore, all present and future users of surgical lasers must follow meticulous standards to ensure the highest level of safety for patients, physicians, and other medical personnel. Instrument manufacturers must also accept their share of responsibility for promoting safe use of medical lasers. Increasingly sophisticated lasers are becoming available, and thus manufacturers must constantly educate the medical community about the safe operation of their products. Failure to maintain adequate standards for the safe application of surgical lasers will result in increased governmental and institutional intervention and restrictions on both the development and the use of lasers for surgery.

ACQUIRING TRAINING IN LASER SURGICAL TECHNIQUES

One unique feature of undertaking to learn laser surgery for infertility problems is the difficulty in obtaining adequate hands-on clinical experience. Most residency programs do not yet offer intraabdominal laser surgery training. Thus, the interested gynecologist who desires to learn the special techniques unique to laser surgery must either attend organized courses or workshops or make arrangements to observe surgeons already active in the field. In addition, hospital committees are now setting strict credentialling guidelines that must be met by potential users of the surgical laser. This seems very appropriate, because the techniques used for CO_2 laser surgery intraabdominally require the understanding and application of a whole new technology—focused laser light. The minimal requirements should include exposure to didactic lectures on basics, safety, tissue effects, and delivery systems. In addition, "hands-on" activities that allow observation of tissue effects on laboratory animals are invaluable for learning the effects of the laser beam when used for coagulating, vaporizing, or incising tissues.

A final requirement should be some sort of preceptorship arrangement where the interested gynecologist can observe actual surgical procedures similar to those he plans to undertake. These phases of learning in various combinations should provide the neophyte ample opportunity to acquire the knowledge and technical skills needed to perform safe intraabdominal laser surgery with open surgery or via laparoscopy. For the infertility surgeon already skilled in operative laparoscopic and microsurgical techniques, it should not be difficult to become an "expert" laser surgeon in a very short period of time once the hardware is available.

FUTURE OF LASERS IN INFERTILITY SURGERY

Just as the true, present role of surgical lasers is undefined,[33] their future status for infertility surgical procedures remains unclear. Some things are certain. More technically advanced lasers will soon be available in more operating rooms. These will include small portable CO_2 lasers with smaller spot sizes and more easily used delivery systems. Flexible fibers that can safely and efficiently allow passage of the CO_2 laser may become a reality. Other, as yet undetermined, sources of laser energy may become available and replace today's CO_2 lasers. For those involved in research and development of surgical lasers, there has been an increase in funding and a resurgence in investigation that may lead to exciting new lasers for clinical use in the future. In the final analysis, skilled surgeons knowledgeable in techniques of laser surgery and the combination of advanced laser technology may produce very favorable operative results.

WHAT IS THE PRESENT ROLE OF SURGICAL LASERS IN RECONSTRUCTIVE PELVIC SURGERY?

The intraperitoneal use of lasers in gynecology must, when considering the present available knowledge, be considered still to be in the developmental stage, because the present numbers of valid investigative studies are limited. Certainly, the precision of tissue destruction that is obtainable exceeds that possible by other surgical modalities when the present state-of-the-art laser delivery systems are properly applied.

Thus, in spite of claimed improvements in surgical results with the use of the CO_2 laser for difficult reconstructive pelvic procedures, the true benefits of the laser are still unproven in infertility surgery. There are certain advantages, but also disadvantages, that may result from undertaking a laser surgery program. The advantages, suggested by laser surgery investigators, include shorter operating time, less intraperitoneal bleeding, less touching of tissue, and less tissue injury. The probable, but as yet unproven, advantages are reduced postoperative adhesion formation and improved chances of pregnancy.

Finally, it is certainly fair to say that the CO_2 laser is not a panacea for the prevention of postoperative adhesions or an automatic guarantee of high pregnancy rates. The laser is just another surgical tool whose true use needs to be further defined and applied by skilled, thoughtful surgeons. It probably already has appropriate usefulness for specific procedures such as neosalpingostomy and will, with future technological developments, be used increasingly by trained surgeons for intraabdominal operations.

It is a complicated apparatus with precise functions that requires reasonable skill and definite training time to acquire the ability for effective clinical use. Failure to accurately and adequately explore the uses of lasers in infertility surgery would be unscientific and counterproductive to true progress in our field.

REFERENCES

1. Bellina JH: Gynecology and the laser. Contemp Obstet Gynecol 4:24, 1974
2. Apfelberg DB, Mittelman H, Chadi B: Carcinogenic potential of in vitro carbon dioxide laser exposure of fibroblast. Obstet Gynecol 61:493, 1983
3. Klink F, Grosspietzsch R, von Klitzing L, Endell W, Husstedt W, Oberheuser F: Animal in vivo studies and in vitro experiments with human tubes for end-to-end anastomotic operation by a CO_2 laser technique. Fertil Steril 30:100, 1978
4. Baggish MS, Chong AP: Carbon dioxide laser microsurgery of the uterine tube. Obstet Gynecol 58:111, 1981
5. Fayez JA, McComb JS, Harper MA: Comparison of tubal surgery with the CO_2 laser and the unipolar microelectrode. Fertil Steril 40:476, 1983
6. Baggish MS: Status of the carbon dioxide laser for infertility surgery. Fertil Steril 40:442, 1983
7. Choe JK, Dawood MY, Andrews AH: Conventional versus laser reanastomosis of rabbit ligated uterine horns. Obstet Gynecol 61:689, 1983
8. Pittaway DE, Maxson WS, Daniell JF: A comparison of the CO_2 laser and electrocautery on postoperative intraperitoneal adhesion formation in rabbits. Fertil Steril 40:366, 1983
9. Bellina JH, Hemmings R, Voros JI, Ross LF: Carbon dioxide laser and electrosurgical wound study with an animal model: a comparison of tissue damage and healing patterns in peritoneal tissue. Am J Obstet Gynecol 148:327, 1984
10. Daniell JF, Brown DH: Carbon dioxide laser laparoscopy: initial experience in experimental animals and humans. Obstet Gynecol 59:761, 1982
11. Daniell JF, Pittaway DE: Use of the CO_2 laser in laparoscopic surgery: initial experience with the second puncture technique. Infertility 5:15, 1982
12. Tadir Y, Kaplan I, Zuckerman Z, Edelstein T, Ovadia J: New instrumentation and technique for laparoscopic carbon dioxide laser operations: a preliminary report. Obstet Gynecol 63:582, 1984

13. Bellina JH: Microsurgery of the fallopian tube with the carbon dioxide laser: analysis of 230 cases with a two-year follow-up. Lasers Surg Med 3:255, 1983
14. Mage G, Bruhat M-A: Pregnancy following salpingostomy: comparison between CO_2 laser and electrosurgery procedures. Fertil Steril 40:472, 1983
15. Tulandi T: Hydrosalpinx: comparison of electrosurgery and laser surgery. Fertil Steril 41:73S, 1984
16. Kelly RW, Roberts DK: Experience with the carbon dioxide laser in gynecologic microsurgery. Am J Obstet Gynecol 146:585, 1983
17. Chong AP, Baggish MS: Management of pelvic endometriosis by means of intraabdominal carbon dioxide laser. Fertil Steril 41:14, 1984
18. Diamond MP, Daniell JF, Martin DC, Feste J, Vaughn WK, McLaughlin DS: Tubal patency and pelvic adhesions at early second-look laparoscopy following intraabdominal use of the carbon dioxide laser: initial report of the intraabdominal laser study group. Fertil Steril 42:717, 1984
19. McLaughlin DS: Micro-laser myomectomy technique to enhance reproductive potential: a preliminary report. Lasers Surg Med 2:107, 1982
20. Nezhat C: Unpublished data
21. Kelly RW, Roberts DK: CO_2 laser laparoscopy: a potential alternative to danazol in the treatment of stage I and II endometriosis. J Reprod Med 28:638, 1983
22. Martin DC: Interval use of the laser laparoscope for endometriosis following danazol therapy. Fertil Steril 41:74S, 1984
23. Feste JR: Laser laparoscopy: a new modality. Fertil Steril 41:74S, 1984
24. Daniell JF, Herbert CM: Laparoscopic salpingostomy utilizing the CO_2 laser. Fertil Steril 41:558, 1984
25. Bruhat M, Mage C, Manhes M: Use of the CO_2 laser via laparoscopy. In Laser Surgery III, Proceedings of the Third International Society for Laser Surgery, Edited by I Kaplan. Tel Aviv, International Society for Laser Surgery, 1979, p 275
26. Tadir Y, Kaplan I, Zuckerman Z, Ovadia J: Laparoscopic CO_2 laser sterilization. In Human Reproduction, Edited by K Semm, L Mettler. Amsterdam, Excerpta Medica, 1981, p 429
27. Gomel V: Salpingostomy by microsurgery. Fertil Steril 29:380, 1978
28. Fayez JA: An assessment of the role of operative laparoscopy in tuboplasty. Fertil Steril 39:476, 1983
29. Mettler L, Giesel H, Semm K: Treatment of female infertility due to tubal obstruction by operative laparoscopy. Fertil Steril 32:384, 1979
30. Keye WR Jr, Matson GA, Dixon J: The use of the argon laser in the treatment of experimental endometriosis. Fertil Steril 39:26, 1983
31. Keye WR Jr, Dixon J: Photocoagulation of endometriosis by the argon laser through the laparoscope. Obstet Gynecol 62:383, 1983
32. Lamano JM: Photocoagulation of early pelvic endometriosis by the Nd:YAG laser through the laparoscope. J Reprod Med. In press
33. Daniell JF: The CO_2 laser in infertility surgery. J Reprod Med 28:265, 1983

Chapter 20

Surgical management of distal tubal obstruction—are we making progress?

Bruce G. Bateman, M.D.
Wallace C. Nunley Jr., M.D.
James D. Kitchin III, M.D.

Department of Obstetrics and Gynecology, University of Virginia Hospital, Charlottesville, Virginia

"Tubal occlusion is still the greatest bugbear of all infertility clinics."

V. B. Green-Armytage, November 1959

Early efforts at surgical correction of distal tubal obstruction were decidedly unsuccessful. Reports from the preantibiotic era of the 1930s typically noted term pregnancy rates ranging from 0% to 5%. Frustration with poor results related to proximal tubal obstruction led to the remarkable ovarian implantation operation of Estes.

In 1936, Greenhill[1] read the results of a questionnaire on tubal surgery at the annual meeting of the Chicago Gynecologic Society. One hundred seven surgeons performed 818 procedures with a cumulative 4.4% live birth rate. Fifty-six percent of the respondents were "definitely opposed" to salpingostomies and tubal implantations. Since that time, a gradual improvement has been observed; however, continued failure to achieve a satisfactory result has fostered the development of in vitro fertilization (IVF). To date, Mr. Green-Armytage's quotation is still quite appropriate.

The study of tubal dysfunction related to distal obstruction has improved our understanding of normal oviduct physiology. Whether further study of the pathophysiology of hydrosalpinges will affect continued improvement in surgical results remains to be seen. Few clinical studies of this topic are truly comparable; there is little progress toward a uniform approach to grading tubal disease and authorities in the field fail to agree on a classification system for distal tubal surgery. With this discouraging preface, we offer (1) an overview of normal tubal function and anatomy as they relate to changes observed in distal tubal obstruction, (2) pertinent experimental animal studies, and (3) a review of surgical results.

FALLOPIAN TUBE FUNCTION

Mammalian oviduct physiology shows considerable species-specific variation. The rabbit oviduct has been studied extensively, due in part to considerations of economy and convenience. In several important areas there are major differences in rabbit and primate oviduct function. This brief review will emphasize species-specific information. With due respect for the numerous scholarly studies of this subject, it is not our intent to oversimplify the complex, and in some ways poorly understood, subject of tubal physiology, but rather to note the aspects of tubal function that are apparently affected by hydrosalpinx formation in humans.

Ovum Capture

In the classic concept, the fimbriae sweep over the ovarian surface at the time of ovulation and pick up the oocyte with its investment of granulosa cells. The anatomy of the tubo-ovarian relationship shows considerable species variation. In the rabbit, a smooth muscle membrane, the mesotubarium superies, approximates the fimbriae and ovary at ovulation. Through direct observation, Blandau[2] documented a complex series of movements at ovulation resulting in repeated contact of the fimbriae with the surface of the ovary.[2] The mesotubarum, like the tubal musculature, is primarily responsive to alpha-adrenergic stimulation.[3] The human correlate of the mesotubarium is the mesotubarium ovarica (fimbria ovarica) formed by

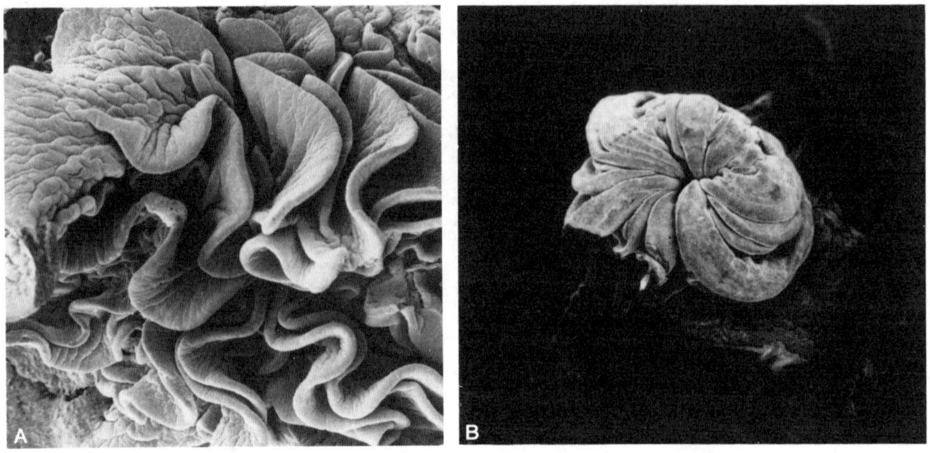

Figure 1 Scanning electron micrographs of normal rabbit fimbria (**A**) and distal ampullary neostomy (**B**) emphasizing the loss of surface area and complexity in the surgical neofimbria (original magnification was ×17).

a bridge of collagen and smooth muscle cells from the ovarian stroma to the wall of the fimbriae and tube.[4] In vitro studies suggest cyclic variation in muscle activity with maximum activity at the time of ovulation perhaps serving to facilitate contact between the fimbriae and the gonad.[5] Ovum capture in the cul-de-sac may occur, but the importance of this mechanism in the human is unknown.

With initial contact, the oocyte-cumulus mass adheres to the mucosa of the fimbriae and is swept into the tube by the cilia with their prouterine beat. Suction created by fluid currents does not seem to be a factor in oocyte capture.[6] Studies in the rhesus monkey suggest that failure of ovum pickup may occur with some frequency.[7] This suggestion is supported by relatively low ovum recovery rates from flushed oviducts and ovum recovery from the cul-de-sac as late as 72 hours after ovulation. The overall efficiency of ovum capture in the human is unknown. It may be low. In a study of salpingectomy specimens in normal women during the immediate postovulatory period, an oocyte was recovered in 44% of cases.[8]

The fallopian tube mucosa is composed of ciliated and secretory cells. In rabbits, nonhuman primates, and humans, ciliated cells predominate at the fimbriae—at least 65% in humans—and then decrease in number in the proximal ampulla.[9] Fimbrial and ampullary ciliated cells in the rabbit possess ciliary crowns that probably aid in oocyte transport. Primates lack these special cellular processes.[10] In humans, the fimbrial cilia beat approximately seven times per minute with a metachronal rhythm (not in unison).[11] Both the percentage of ciliated cells and the surface area of the distal oviduct are important factors in ovum pickup. A direct correlation between efficiency of ovum capture and degrees of fimbrial deciliation in ovariectomized rabbits has been demonstrated.[12] Halbert and Patton[13] performed a series of experiments to assess the effects of loss of the fimbriae on ovum capture, retention, and transport.[13] Fimbriectomy and microsurgical infundibular salpingostomies were performed using the rabbit model. Sixty-three percent of naturally ovulated oocytes were captured in the infundibular salpingostomy group compared with 80% in control oviducts. Using the Blandau chamber technique[13] for direct observation of the oviduct, movement of cumulus-surrogate masses across the fimbriae was found to be normal in most cases. Surrogates were normally adherent to the mucosa of the neostomy and were not dislodged, even by gentle traction with surgical forceps. Scanning electron microscopy (SEM) of the neostomy resembled the distal ampulla with regard to cell populations.

In a similar study, with resection of the fimbriae and distal one half of the ampulla, 29% of oocytes were captured in neostomy tubes versus 77% in controls[14] (Fig. 1). Surrogate transport times across the neostomy and retention of oocytes were normal. Resection of the fimbriae and more than 50% of the ampulla (52% to 95%), with microsurgical neostomy, resulted in complete failure of ovum capture and defective surrogate adherence with increased transport times.[15]

Taken together, these studies seem to indicate that loss of the fimbriae in the absence of other tubal damage might affect only minimal interference with ovum capture or retention and that the percentage of ciliated cells is of fundamental importance with regard to these functions. Even with histologically normal oviducts, neostomies in the proximal ampulla would not be expected to restore fertility. These observations seem to parallel clinical experience with neostomies in the proximal ampulla and reports of fertility subsequent to microsurgical neostomy after fimbriectomy for sterilization.

Ovum Transport in the Ampulla

Ovum transport in the ampulla has been studied extensively in the rabbit. Because of the thin wall of the tubal ampulla, movement of supravitally stained cumulus-egg masses or surrogates may be observed directly. In this species, the freshly ovulated oocyte passes through the ampulla in approximately 15 minutes.[16] Although an increase in activity of the myosalpinx has been documented at ovulation, coordinated peristalsis does not occur. Oocytes move in a to-and-fro fashion with steady progress toward the ampullary isthmic junction (AIJ).[10] Pharmacologic blockade of the myosalpinx results in the abolition of to-and-fro movement, but does not affect transit time through the ampulla, suggesting that the cilia are responsible for oocyte transport in this region.[17] Microsurgical manipulation of the oviduct also supports the import of ciliary transport. Reversed ampullary segment tubes demonstrate obstruction of oocyte transport at the site of anastomosis, apparently due to the pro-ovarian beat of the cilia in the reversed region.[18]

Direct observation of human oviducts confirms the importance of ciliary activity in the ampulla. Extirpated oviducts in physiologic solution show rapid transfer of microsphere surrogates in a pro-uterine direction.[19] Ciliary activity in the ampulla is probably greatest at midcycle. Findings in salpingectomy specimens suggest that oocytes remain in the human ampulla for approximately 72 hours.[8]

Although all of this information seems to emphasize clearly the importance of ciliary activity in ovum capture and ampullary transport, the apparent contradiction of normal fertility in women with immotile cilia syndrome is frequently cited as a disclaimer.[20] Perhaps this should be viewed as an example of the extreme redundancy of tubal transport systems. One might also comment that the overall fertility of women with Kartagener's triad is unknown; perhaps it is low.

A pause in oocyte transport at the AIJ occurs in several animal species and perhaps in humans. Although a sphincter effect exists, there is no anatomic basis for a sphincter at the AIJ. Experimental resection of the AIJ in the rabbit has no effect on ovum retention in this area and ampullary-isthmic reanastomosis following segmental resection for sterilization is capable of restoring fertility.[21] The AIJ may not be physiologically unique, but, rather, it may represent the juncture of two regions of different activity and function.

Transport in the Isthmus

The mechanisms of tubal function in the isthmus are much less clear. Blandau noted that factors in the paradox of sperm transport in one direction and egg transport in the other include the following: peristalsis, activity of the myosalpinx, antiperistalsis, ciliary activity in oviducts, function of the AIJ, and intrinsic sperm activity.[2]

The lumen of the isthmus is considerably smaller than the ampulla, with four characteristic folds of the epithelial surface in close apposition to one another. The myosalpinx is prominent and the epithelium is composed of 75% to 80% secretory cells, in contrast to the ampulla.[22] SEM of the human isthmus demonstrates cyclic changes in morphology related to the ovarian cycle. In early and midfollicular phases, secretory cells are dome-shaped, with secretions around the microvilli. In the periovulatory period, the lumen is filled with tenacious secretion and the folds of the isthmic mucosa become closely approximated. This condition persists through the immediate postovulatory period. The thick secretions of the isthmus may blanket the cilia to allow sperm to ascend to the ampulla.[23] In the postovulatory period, there is a marked change in the isthmic lumen with relative dilatation and clearing of the mucus, perhaps allowing the prouterine beat of the cilia to affect movement of the embryo.

Episodic, segregated activity in the isthmic myosalpinx affects oocyte movement, but true peristaltic waves are absent. The muscular layers of this region have heavy adrenergic innervation. With some exceptions, alpha receptors are excitatory and beta are inhibitory. The hormonal environment modifies receptor activity. In general, progesterone dominance increases beta influence.[24] The effect of estrogen on ovum transport shows considerable species and dose-related variation. A study in women undergoing salpingectomy demonstrated no effect of estradiol (E_2) on ovum transport.[25] Adrenergic denervation or pharmacologic blockade does not alter ovum transport in the rabbit and transplanted rabbit oviducts with presumed absence of adrenergic effect show normal function.[26] Prostaglandins may also play a role in isthmic transport. A complex interrelationship between the hormonal environment and adrenergic responsiveness prevents a simple unifying hypothesis of isthmic function.

Hodgson and Talo[27] have demonstrated "spike bursts" of electrical activity related to muscle contractions in the isthmus of the rabbit oviduct. Activity has been shown to correlate with increases in intraluminal pressure and surrogate ovum movement. This theory holds that ova are moved along the isthmus by tubal contractions in the sense that they move away from an active region and into inactive areas. Progesterone (P) may shorten the inactive proximal region of the isthmus and increase the frequency of muscle contractions. This would alter the otherwise random movement of the oocyte and cause a prouterine bias.

There is an unusual species-specific divergence of ciliary function in the isthmic region. Isthmic cilia in the rabbit beat in a pro-ovarian direction, while a prouterine beat is observed in humans and in nonhuman primates.[28] Information on isthmic transport in the human is limited. Extirpated human oviducts show prouterine transport of surrogate ova by ciliary activity.[19] Human oocytes can be recovered from the isthmic region 96 hours after luteinizing hormone (LH) peak and apparently remain in the isthmus for a relatively brief time.[8]

ANATOMY AND PATHOPHYSIOLOGY OF THE HUMAN HYDROSALPINX

According to Novak, a hydrosalpinx (sactosalpinx in European literature) is characterized by an accumulation of fluid in the tubal lumen due to distal tubal obstruction.[29] In some patients, fimbriae may be present after incision of the oviduct; however, they are absent in most. Hydrosalpinx usually is a consequence of infectious salpingitis and is associated with intrinsic tubal disease. Distal tubal obstruction occasionally occurs because of endometriosis or a ruptured appendix, with minimal intrinsic tubal damage.

Hydrosalpinx may be associated with massive tubal enlargement in the absence of symptoms, with the exception of the rare circumstance of tubal torsion. Histologically, two general types of hydrosalpinx are recognized with regard to effects on the lumen.[29] Hydrosalpinx simplex is characterized by the presence of a single lumen. In hydrosalpinx follicularis, trabeculations or septa created by fusion of the tubal plicae form compartments in the lumen. Chronic interstitial salpingitis is characterized by thickening of the tubal wall and usually is associated with distal tubal obstruction. The lumen frequently exhibits the trabecular pattern of hydrosalpinx follicularis. The fimbria ovarica commonly is damaged or destroyed in association with hydrosalpinx formation.

David et al.[30] noted pleomorphism in the histologic appearance of the tubal mucosa in a series of nine cases of human hydrosalpinx. Areas with loss of the tubal plicae exhibited low cuboidal and flattened cells, while relatively normal ciliated cell populations were noted in regions of intact plicae. Recent SEM studies have shown conflicting findings with regard to the appearance of the tubal mucosa in human hydrosalpinges. Vasquez et al.[9] found significant deciliation in most patients with hydrosalpinx. They reported a reduction in the mean percentage of ciliated cells in biopsies from the distal ampulla of thin-walled hydrosalpinges from 64.9% in controls to 32.4% in affected tubes. The most severe deciliation was noted in tubes with the fewest plicae. Figure 2 illustrates severe deciliation observed in a thin-walled human hydrosalpinx.

Donnez and Casanas-Roux[31] documented similar findings in a series of women undergoing terminal salpingostomies with a decreased percentage of ciliated cells in ampullary biopsies and a positive correlation with the degree of tubal dilatation. Twenty-eight percent ciliated cells were noted in the ampulla of tubes larger than 2.5 cm in diameter, 55% ciliated cells were noted in tubes with distal obstruction of normal caliber, and 63% were noted in control biopsies from the same region.

Patek and Nilsson[32] reported flattened epithelial cells in human hydrosalpinges, but no evidence of deciliation and tubal mucosa that did "not differ conspicuously" from normal. Differences in these observations may be accounted for by the sampling site. Biopsies in the later study were from "the ampullary isthmic region."[32] In addition to anatomic alterations, important new data suggest that ciliary function may be defective. Laser light scanning spectroscopy reveals a significant reduction in beat frequency of ampullary cilia in human hydrosalpinges.[33]

Light and transmission electron microscopy (TEM) of the tubal wall reveal atrophy of the muscle layers in the isthmus and ampulla and replacement with fibrous tissue associated with a proportional loss of vascular channels. Tissue levels of estrogen receptors and P receptors also are affected. Homogenates of human hydrosalpinx tissue show a decrease in cytosol and nuclear estrogen receptors and a decrease in cytosol P receptors.[34] Binding affinities are normal. Thick-walled

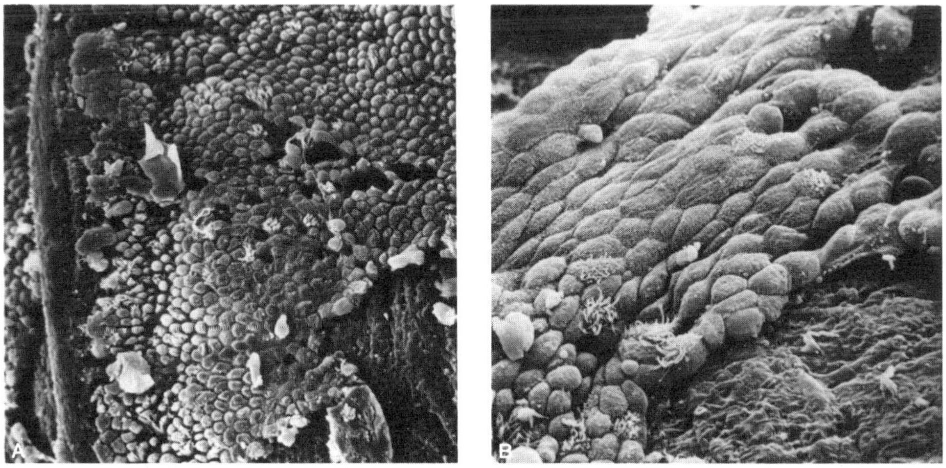

Figure 2 Scanning electron micrograph of human ampullary mucosa from a thin-walled hydrosalpinx illustrating deciliation and desquamation (**A,** ×480; **B,** ×1300). (Vasquez and Brosens)

hydrosalpinges have the lowest levels of estrogen receptors.

Fluid of the hydrosalpinx is either a transudate from the vascular bed or a product of epithelial secretion; both may be factors, with decreased absorption from the tubal wall. The constituents of human hydrosalpinx fluid are as follows: proteins with a profile similar to but in significantly lower concentrations than serum, electrolytes in concentrations similar to serum, and relatively low bicarbonate with variable pH.[30]

It seems likely that the sperm-carrying function of the human hydrosalpinx is normal. Studies in human hydrosalpinges and control oviducts 60 to 100 hours after intercourse reveal comparable densities of motile sperm.[35] This does not necessarily imply normal fertilization. Actually, some reports have documented higher concentrations of sperm in hydrosalpinges relative to normal oviducts. Theoretically, this situation might increase the risk of polyspermia.

Most of the observations described are anatomic and, although their functional import seems apparent, there is little direct information on the pathophysiology of tubal dysfunction in human hydrosalpinx. It is attractive to speculate that infertility in this setting is due to deciliation and/or cilia dysfunction in the distal oviduct with resultant failure of ovum capture or transport. This mechanism might also account for the frequency of ectopic pregnancies in the ampulla.

EXPERIMENTAL HYDROSALPINX

Elements of tubal function addressed in experimental studies of hydrosalpinges include how the structural changes in the tube evolve and to what extent these changes are reversible.

Studies of the effect of chronic distention on the oviductal epithelium have yielded discrepant results. Halbert and Patton[36] and Patton and Halbert[37] ligated the distal oviduct in rabbits and nonhuman primates, resulting in distention of the ampulla. Chronic studies of up to 52 weeks' duration revealed progressive loss of the tubal plicae, but minimal changes in the epithelial architecture and normal ciliation (Fig. 3). TEM of the tubal wall revealed generally normal morphologic features. Surrogate and cumulus-egg transport rates were normal.

Conversely, Vemer et al.[38] and Donnez et al.[39] investigated doubly ligated oviducts with findings of significant epithelial damage. Chronic studies over 1- to 6-month periods revealed loss of plicae, deciliation in the ampulla, and a marked decrease in capillary number and volume. TEM revealed disruption of normal intracellular architecture. In general, these effects were less evident in the isthmus or the isthmus was spared. Transport studies were not performed. These differences in findings may have been methodologic. With some exceptions, the induced hydrosalpinges in studies showing mucosal changes were of greater diameter than those with normal mucosa. The cause of the mucosal changes is not entirely clear. Vascular insufficiency or occult infection may have been factors.

Adrenergic innervation of the myosalpinx also is affected by hydrosalpinx formation. After 8 weeks, doubly ligated rabbit oviducts show loss of adrenergic innervation with a decrease in catecholamine histofluorescence in the isthmic region.[40] Normal

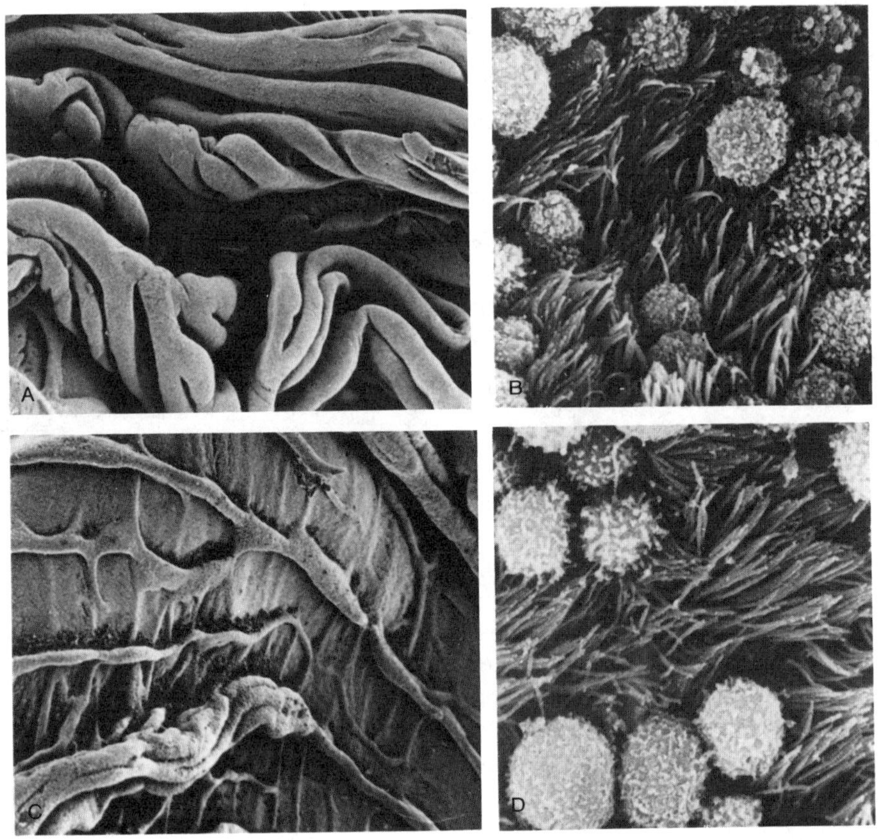

Figure 3 Scanning electron micrographs of monkey ampullary mucosa. *Top:* Normal control ampullary mucosa. (**A**) Normal longitudinal folds (original magnification was ×15). (**B**) Normal ciliated and secretory cell populations (original magnification was ×1900). *Bottom:* Five-month-old hydrosalpinx. (**C**) Loss of longitudinal folds (original magnification was ×15). (**D**) Normal ciliated and secretory cell population (original magnification was ×1900). (From Halbert and Patton.[36] Reproduced with the permission of the publisher.)

ampullae show such sparse innervation that comparison with the experimental tube in this region is not meaningful.

A question of basic importance is whether observed changes are reversible. Information in this area is limited. Neostomies performed on induced hydrosalpinx in the rabbit model result in spontaneous ciliogenesis by 2 to 3 weeks after surgery, and restoration of normal ciliation by 8 weeks.[41] Yussman[42] observed enhanced ciliogenesis in the estrogen-treated rat hydrosalpinx. Although these findings may be encouraging, the experimental and human hydrosalpinx differ fundamentally in the absence of infection. Ampullary biopsies in salpingostomy patients who do not conceive show continued evidence of deciliation more than 1 year after surgery.[31] The concept of regeneration of the tubal endothelium subsequent to salpingostomy may be spurious. Information on the reversibility of vascular changes, loss of adrenergic innervation, and disruption of the myosalpinx is lacking. A promising model for the study of tubal dynamics is the induction of hydrosalpinx in the nonhuman primate with *Chlamydia trachomatis.* Patton recently reported development of distal tubal obstruction in a pig-tail macaque after tubal inoculations with *C. trachomatis.*[43]

BACTERIOLOGIC ORIGINS OF DISTAL TUBAL OBSTRUCTION

Recent studies challenge the traditional concept that gonorrhea is the principle pathogen in pelvic inflammatory disease. There is compelling serologic and culture evidence of the importance of chlamydia as a primary agent in salpingitis. Significant immunoglobulin (IgG) antibody titers have been reported in as high as 62% of patients with acute salpingitis and have been correlated with the severity of infection.[44]

The animal model supports the theory of canalicular spread of chlamydia through the reproductive tract. Inoculation of the cervix in nonhuman primates causes an ascending infection affecting the endometrium and fallopian tubes, with resultant salpingitis. Proximal ligation of the oviducts prevents the development of salpingitis. Primary infection in pig-tailed monkeys by inoculation of the ampulla also results in acute salpingitis.[45] Progressive endothelial damage occurs with deciliation and cytoplasmic vacuolization. Areas of extensive damage are interspersed with normal epithelium. By the 35th day after inoculation, the inflammatory response has subsided, but areas of permanent cellular injury are evident with TEM. The close association of lymphocytes with intracellular degeneration of tubal epithelial cells suggests lymphocyte-mediated cytotoxicity as observed with other strains of chlamydia. Experimental studies confirm that untreated chlamydia salpingitis may show resolution of symptoms in the face of progressive tubal damage. Repeat chlamydia infections may be a key factor in the genesis of the human hydrosalpinx. Serial inoculations of the fallopian tube in pig-tailed monkeys result in intratubal adhesions, deciliation, and distal tubal obstruction.[43]

In recent years, careful culture techniques have recovered chlamydia more commonly than any other organism associated with acute salpingitis in humans. Chlamydia may be asymptomatic and carrier states are common. Progressive tubal damage may be associated with asymptomatic infections and silent salpingitis may progress to distal tubal obstruction. Chlamydia has been cultured from the tubal fluid and antibodies to *C. trachomatis* have been identified in silent salpingitis patients with tubal obstruction. Recent data suggest that the degree of tubal damage in asymptomatic patients parallels findings in patients with a history of acute pelvic inflammatory disease.[33]

Gonorrhea is cultured from a highly variable number of patients with acute salpingitis (5% to 65%). Most reports show an incidence of 50% or less. The gonococcus also exhibits a canalicular spread pattern and probably attacks the secretory cells of the tubal endothelium.[40]

Mycoplasma hominis and ureaplasma urealyticum have been cultured in a relatively small percentage of patients with acute salpingitis. Experiments in nonhuman primates suggest that mycoplasma hominis causes a primary parametritis rather than salpingitis.[47] Henry-Suchet et al.[48] failed to identify mycoplasma hominis in any of 63 patients with acute salpingitis or distal tubal obstruction. Improved culture techniques have demonstrated anaerobes in acute and chronic salpingitis. Anaerobic and facultative anaerobic bacteria of endogenous origin are thought to be secondary invaders in damaged tubes and are frequently recovered from tubo-ovarian abscesses.

Genital tuberculosis (TB) is uncommon in the western world. Hematogenous spread of the tubercule bacillus may lead to salpingitis and tubercule bacilli show a predisposition for the fallopian tube region of the genital tract. TB salpingitis is frequently asymptomatic and damage to the tubes is usually extensive. Plastic surgery for tuberculosalpingitis is almost uniformly unsuccessful, runs a risk of reactivation of tubal infection, and is associated with a significant risk of tubal pregnancy.[49]

CLASSIFICATION OF PROCEDURES

The most commonly referenced classification system for distal tubal surgery was proposed at the Ninth World Congress of Fertility and Sterility in 1977. This system defines fimbrioplasty and salpingostomy as follows: *Fimbrioplasty*—a) deagglutination and/or dilatation of the fimbriae, b) by incision of peritoneal ring, c) by incision of tubal wall. *Salpingoneostomy* (*Salpingostomy*)—a) terminal, b) midampullary (medial), c) isthmic (including linear salpingostomy).

Controversy exists regarding the classification of tubes with complete distal obstruction found to have remnants of the fimbriae after incision of the tubal wall. Authorities differ on whether this surgery constitutes a fimbrioplasty or a salpingostomy. The majority of publications in this review apply the term salpingostomy to this situation. To add a bit more confusion, the Tenth World Congress (1980) of Fertility and Sterility modified this system, defining fimbrioplasty under section C as follows: "with serosal incision (for completely occluded tube)."

In the subsequent discussion, we intend the term fimbrioplasty to apply to cases of partial tubal obstruction with fimbriae present and salpingostomy as complete tubal obstruction, regardless of the findings after incision.

SURGICAL TECHNIQUE

Salpingostomy

Several operative techniques are of historical interest. Descriptions of surgical procedures to evert

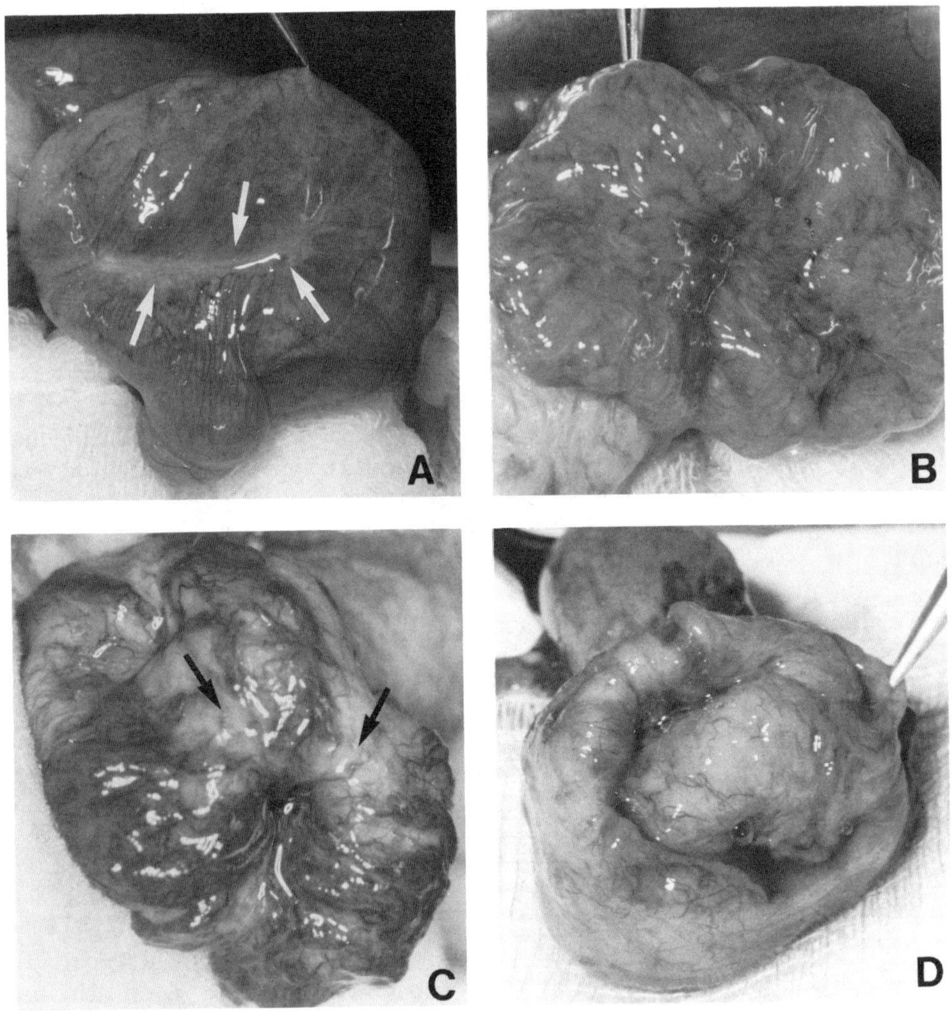

Figure 4 Human hydrosalpinx surgical specimens. (**A**) Intact hydrosalpinx illustrating central avascular area (*arrows*). (**B–D**) Tubes postsalpingostomy illustrating varying degrees of mucosal damage. (**B**) Mucosal folds intact. (**C**) Moderate damage with patches of flattened epithelium (*arrows*). (**D**) Complete loss of tubal plicae. (This tube was excised.)

the edges of the obstructed oviduct were reported in the late 1800s. In 1932, Holden and Sovak[50] published one of the first clear accounts of this procedure in the American literature. Amputation of the distal oviduct with eversion of the edges was illustrated. Postoperative pregnancy rates with this approach were quite low.

Another procedure of historical interest is lateral salpingostomy. This technique, promoted around the turn of the century, was used when the distal oviduct and ovary were densely adherent. A linear incision was made in the medial aspect of the ampulla near the ovary. Again, the results were unsatisfactory, with low postoperative patency and pregnancy rates. Incision of the entire length of the oviduct also has been reported.[51] Actually, this procedure was promoted by Israel to prevent hydrosalpinx formation when laparotomy was performed on a patient with acute salpingitis.[51] Surprisingly, several intrauterine pregnancies were reported after total linear salpingostomy.

"Conventional" surgery for terminal salpingostomy, as performed over the past 10 to 20 years, was described by Kistner and Patton in 1975.[52] Fluid distention of the oviduct allows identification of the central point in the distal tube, usually the thinnest region. A cruciate incision with the scalpel or scissors creates several flaps and the edges are sutured to the tubal serosa using fine suture material with attention to careful hemostasis.

In the late 1960s, magnification with fine-tipped electrocautery for dissection was applied to this procedure. Subsequently, a microsurgical technique related to tubal surgery evolved. Magnification aids in identification of avascular areas (Fig. 4). Glass rods are used to manipulate the oviduct, continuous irrigation prevents tissue-drying, care is taken to repair peritoneal defects, and meticulous hemostasis is emphasized. Dissection is sometimes aided by folding the incised oviduct inside out to view the mucosa. The neostomy is created by suturing the cut edge of the tube to the serosa of the ampulla with interrupted, fine, nonreactive sutures.

Microsurgical technique also emphasizes a reduction in tissue injury through the use of fine-tipped instruments, gentle tissue handling, and minimizing tension in suture lines. Although some of the principles of microsurgery are innovative, others must be regarded as traditional concepts of good surgical technique. Holden and Sovak[50] emphasized the importance of gentle tissue handling in their 1932 report. References to meticulous hemostasis, delicate instrumentation, and careful tissue handling can be found in the literature of the early 1950s.

The carbon dioxide (CO_2) laser has been used as an alternative to needlepoint electrocautery for incision of the tube in distal tubal obstruction and division of associated adhesions. With this technique, the approach to tubal incision is similar to that described for microsurgical technique. The neostomy is either sutured, "welded," or the edges everted with the defocused laser beam. Laser technique offers the theoretical advantage of decreased injury to adjacent tissue.

Prosthetic Devices

In the early 1950s, there were several publications related to the use of prosthetic devices for terminal salpingostomy. These devices were intended to maintain patency of the new ostium and/or provide protection from adhesions. The initial Mulligan prosthesis was prepared by melting polyethylene into the desired form. In 1955, polymeric silicone was adopted for the Mulligan hood because of its improved handling properties.[53] A recognized disadvantage of the Mulligan hood is the need for a second major surgery, although lysis of adhesions can be performed at the time of that procedure. Several innovative prosthetic devices have been proposed to avoid a second major surgery, including a spiral Teflon stent (Marco and Son, Oakhurst, NJ) and a pliable Silastic cone.[54,55] Both of the devices were removed by way of an abdominal extension of the prosthesis and, although the principle of this approach had obvious appeal, with the exception of the initial reports, little information exists on its effectiveness. The technique of hood application has been discussed and illustrated by Kistner and Patton.[52]

Fimbrioplasty

Fimbrioplasty is performed by division of adhesions between fimbrial folds. This is accomplished bluntly by "dilating" the fimbriae or with the identification of individual adhesions and division under direct visualization. The various surgical techniques previously described have been applied to this situation with division of adhesions by scissors, needlepoint electrocautery, or CO_2 laser with or without magnification.

Follow-up Laparoscopy

Early follow-up laparoscopy for lysis of adhesions, subsequent to salpingostomy, has been reported by several groups.[56,57] With this approach, adhesions can be lysed while still friable and gelatinous. Trimbos-Kemper et al.[56] performed follow-up laparoscopy on postoperative day 8 in a series of patients undergoing salpingostomy, fimbrioplasty, or lysis of adhesions, with no improvement in intrauterine pregnancy rate relative to patients who did not have follow-up laparoscopy.[56] Interestingly, a lower incidence of ectopic pregnancy was observed in salpingostomy patients with follow-up laparoscopy. Raj and Hulka[57] reported a series of patients with follow-up laparoscopy at varying intervals and concluded that the ideal time for this procedure was 4 to 8 weeks after surgery. Comparative data were not offered.

RESULTS OF SURGERY

We have reviewed 65 series of distal tubal surgery.[50–115] Representative studies are displayed in Tables 1 to 5. With a few exceptions, results are expressed in terms of percent viable pregnancies and percent tubal pregnancies. Tubal patency is not discussed because its assessment may be subjective and it does not represent the real goal of this procedure. The bases for selection of the studies displayed are: (1) operative procedures limited to fimbrioplasties or salpingostomies with the specific exclusion of mixed procedures; (2) relatively large numbers of patients; (3) adequate follow-up intervals (intervals displayed are minimum follow-up time unless otherwise noted); and (4) clearly expressed results.

Most surgical series reported over the past 15 years have employed the principles of microsurgery

Table 1 Conventional Surgery Salpingostomy Results: Summary of the Literature

References	Patients	Pregnancy: Term	Pregnancy: Ectopic	Follow-up	Comments
		%	%	yr	
Palmer[58] (1960)	295[a]	18[b]	7	1–17	Systemic steroids (34%)
Hanton et al.[59] (1964)	32	3	3	—	—
Arronet et al.[60] (1969)	85	24[b]	2	5	Hydrotubation
Siegler[61] (1969)	22[c]	9	0	—	—
Jessen[62] (1971)	25	20	12	—	—
Grant[63] (1971)	217	15	2	—	Hydrotubation (24%)
Rock et al.[64] (1978)	69	16	6	5.2 (mean)	Some hydrotubated

[a] Isthmic salpingostomies and tubal tuberculosis patients excluded.
[b] Intrauterine pregnancy rate, including term pregnancies and spontaneous abortions.
[c] Isthmic salpingostomies excluded.

to varying degrees. In this sense, they have become a blend of surgical techniques and a simple classification differentiating conventional surgery from microsurgery is not meaningful. The use of magnification is a common, although perhaps overemphasized, point of distinction in this regard.

In some series, data have been displayed selectively to promote a fair comparison of studies from different time periods. When possible, tubal tuberculosis and isthmic salpingostomy cases have been excluded from analysis. These procedures are criteria for exclusion from surgery in most recent reports.

Conventional Surgery

The results of representative studies performed by conventional (macrosurgical) surgery are displayed in Table 1.[59–64] Magnification was not used in these studies and most did not emphasize the other aspects of microsurgical technique. Term pregnancy rates in this group are quite variable and are generally less than 20%. Tubal pregnancy rates are generally less than 10%.

Microsurgery

The results of several series of microsurgical salpingostomies are displayed in Table 2.[65–71] All pro-

Table 2 Microsurgery Salpingostomy Results: Summary of the Literature

References	Patients	Pregnancy: Term	Pregnancy: Ectopic	Follow-up	Comment
		%	%		
Winston[65] (1980)	241	18	10	6 mo	IP steroids[a] Systemic steroids
Gomel[66] (1980)	72	29	10	1 yr	IP steroids Hydrotubation
Decherney and Kase[67] (1981)	54	26	7	1 yr	IP steroids Systemic steroids
Larrson[68] (1982)	54	31	0	4 yr	IP steroids Systemic steroids Hydrotubation
Verhoeven et al.[69] (1983)	82	24	4	8 mo	IP steroids Systemic steroids
Boer-Meisel et al.[70] (1986)	108	22	18	1 yr	IP steroids
Kitchin et al.[71] (1986)	81	23	12	1 yr	IP steroids Systemic steroids Hydrotubation (75%)

[a] Intraperitoneal steroids.

Table 3 Results of Salpingostomy with Prosthesis: Summary of Literature

References	Patients	Pregnancy Term	Pregnancy Ectopic	Follow-up	Comments
		%	%	yr	
Mulligan[53] (1966)	45	21	8	—	Silastic hood
Garcia[72] (1968)	25	28	8	—	Silastic hood
Rock et al.[64] (1978)	18	17	6	5.2 (mean)	Silastic hood Teflon splint Polyethylene splint
Decherney and Kase[67] (1981)	9	22	0	2	Silastic hood
Wallach et al.[73] (1983)	24	21	8	1–2	Silastic hood

cedures were performed using magnification (loupes or the operating microscope) and microsurgical technique. These studies tend to be more recent than conventional surgery series and almost uniformly have employed antiadhesion adjuvants. Term pregnancy rates are somewhat less variable than in other groups and most are in the 20% to 30% range. Ectopic pregnancy rates show a wide variation from 0% to 18%.

Prosthesis

Table 3 displays the results of studies using the Silastic hood of Rock and Mulligan (or splints) and employing a second laparotomy for removal of the prosthesis.[53,64,67,72,73]

Laser Surgery

Although there has been considerable interest in laser surgery of the oviduct, the number of series that clearly express salpingostomy results is low. The results of laser salpingostomies performed at laparotomy are displayed in Table 4.[74–77] In some of these procedures, the neostomy was secured with sutures and in others it was everted with the defocused laser beam.

Repeat Salpingostomies

Repeat salpingostomies have a generally low success rate (Table 5).[65,69,78–80] This is probably due to the severity of the initial tubal disease and shortening of the ampullary segment. Laparoscopic surgery in this setting has the appeal of not requiring a second major operation. The unusually high term pregnancy rate in Gomel's small series is striking and is inconsistent with most other data on this procedure.[78] Daniell and Herbert[80] performed repeat salpingostomies by laser laparoscopy on a selected group of patients with a 10% term pregnancy at 6 to 18 months follow-up. They continue to follow these patients, now more than 2 years postsurgery, and note encouraging results.[81] Ectopic pregnancy rates in repeat salpingostomies as a whole are surprisingly low.

Fimbrioplasty

The results of fimbrioplasty series are displayed in Table 6.[82–86] Two of these series were compari-

Table 4 Laser Surgery Salpingostomy Results: Summary of the Literature

References	Patients	Pregnancy Term	Pregnancy Ectopic	Follow-up	Comments
		%	%		
Kelly and Roberts[74] (1983)	28	7	6	1 yr	Systemic steroids Hydrotubation
Mage and Bruhat[75] (1983)	38	24	8	18 mo	Systemic steroids
Tulandi and Vilos[76] (1984)	37	24[a]	3	2 yr	—
Daniell et al.[77] (1986)	48[b]	19	10	3–13 mo (mean = 19)	IP dextran Hydrotubation

[a] Intrauterine pregnancy rate.
[b] Second-look laparoscopy performed.

Table 5 Repeat Salpingostomy Results: Summary of Literature

References	Patients	Pregnancy Term	Pregnancy Ectopic	Follow-up	Procedure
		%	%		
Gomel[78] (1977)	9[a]	33	0	—	Laparoscopy
Winston[65] (1980)	59	8.4	7	6 mo	Microsurgery
Lauritsen et al.[79] (1982)	23	9	9	1–6 yr	Microsurgery
Verhoeven et al.[69] (1983)	23	13	0	8 mo	Microsurgery
Daniell and Herbert[80] (1984)	21	10	5	6–18 mo	Laser laparoscopy

[a] One primary procedure.

sons of conventional surgery and microsurgery, as noted. Pregnancy rates, when any portion of the fimbria is present, are generally higher than when it is absent.

Laparoscopic Surgery

There is minimal information on the effectiveness of operative laparoscopy as a primary procedure for distal tubal obstruction. Mettler et al. reported a large series of laparoscopic surgeries, including 38 salpingostomies and 51 fimbrioplasties, with overall pregnancy rates of 26 and 31%, respectively.[87] They emphasize that the safety and effectiveness of laparoscopic salpingostomy is enhanced by the use of endocoagulation (local heat production without high-frequency electrical current). In this study, patients were hospitalized for 2 to 3 days following surgery.

Fayez[88] reported 10% tubal pregnancies and no intrauterine pregnancies in 19 patients undergoing laparoscopic salpingostomy. Fimbrioplasty was performed in 14 patients with a 21% term pregnancy rate and 14% tubal pregnancies. Interestingly, all conceptions in both groups occurred during the second year of a 2-year follow-up.

Unilateral Distal Tubal Surgery

In most series, a few unilateral salpingostomies have been performed when the contralateral oviduct was absent or irreparable and left in situ or removed. In our review, there were 136 unilateral salpingostomies with term pregnancy rate of 14% and tubal pregnancy rate of 3%.[61,68,69,71,89,90,91] These data were derived from seven surgical series using differing techniques and must be interpreted with caution, but in general show relatively low term and tubal pregnancy rates. This may be useful information in advising patients on planned repair of a solitary hydrosalpinx. Removal of a normal ovary with an irreparable oviduct has been promoted by some authors and is a matter of controversy. With IVF as an option, ovarian conservation is our approach.

Table 6 Fimbrioplasty Results: Summary of the Literature

References	Patients	Pregnancy Term	Pregnancy Ectopic	Follow-up	Comments
		%	%		
Siegler and Kontopoulos[82] (1979)	20[a]	35	15	—	Systemic steroids (50%)
Fayez and Suliman[83] (1982)	25[b]	40	4	2–9 yr	Systemic steroids Hydrotubation
Frantzen and Schlosser[84] (1982)	49	22	4	2–6 yr	Microsurgery Systemic steroids
Patton[85] (1982)	35	60[c]	3	1–24 mo	Microsurgery Systemic steroids
Donnez and Casanas-Roux[86] (1986)	132	60[c]	2	1–6 yr	Microsurgery IP dextran[d]

[a] Microsurgery 11 patients, macrosurgery 9 patients.
[b] Microsurgery 7 patients, macrosurgery 18 patients.
[c] Intrauterine pregnancy rate.
[d] Intraperitoneal dextran.

FACTORS AFFECTING THE OUTCOME OF DISTAL TUBAL SURGERY

Few studies of distal tubal surgery are truly comparable. Factors to be considered include length of follow-up after surgery, severity of tubal disease, antiadhesion adjuvants, hydrotubation, and expression of data.

Length of Follow-up

Follow-up for patients who conceive (intrauterine or ectopic pregnancy) is the surgery-pregnancy interval and will vary from months to years. Follow-up on patients who fail to conceive will also vary widely. As time passes, there will be an ever-decreasing number of patients "at risk" for pregnancy. These data are not simply or easily expressed. The comment that patients were followed for more than 1 year with a 20% intrauterine pregnancy rate and that some percentage of intrauterine or ectopic pregnancies occurred during the first year of follow-up seems an inadequate expression of how many patients conceived and when they conceived.

The parameters of median and mean may be useful. The median and mean (with standard deviations) follow-up intervals, with interquartile range (25th to 75th percentile), provide information on how long patients were followed and when pregnancies ("events" in statistical parlance) occurred. This still does not deal with the problem of expressing a pregnancy rate late in the follow-up period when a significant percentage of patients have been lost to follow-up (prior to conception). The traditional technique of considering all of these patients as failures will tend to understate the real pregnancy rate. Graphic displays of cumulative pregnancy rates are influenced by this situation. In a sense, cumulative pregnancy rates versus time graphs would only be completely accurate if all patients have been followed through the entire time period in question. Practically speaking, this condition must rarely be met. Graphic displays of this type should not be confused with life tables.

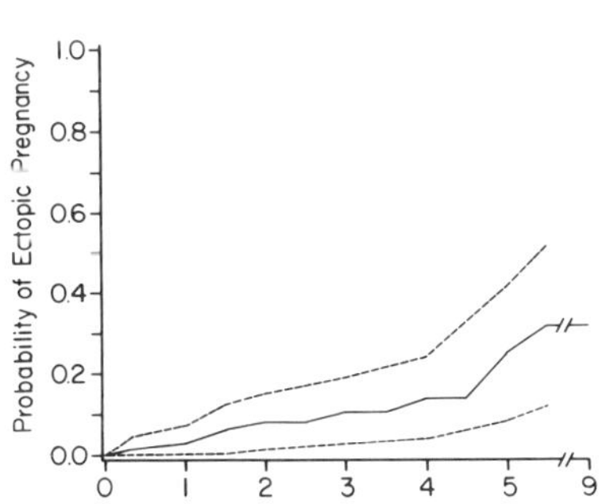

Figure 5 Kaplan-Meier display of predicted probability of ectopic pregnancy.

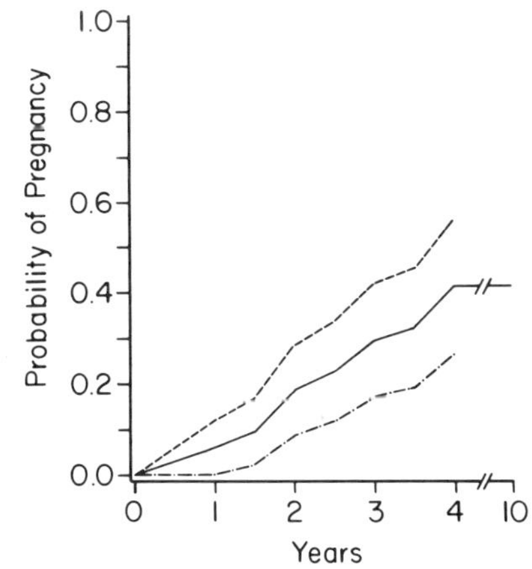

Figure 6 Kaplan-Meier display of predicted probability of term pregnancy.

Life tables (a type of survival analysis) are useful with follow-up periods of varying duration. The performance of all patients is predicted based on the follow-up information available. Therefore, in effect, patients lost to follow-up are not all considered failures. With this approach, the "probability of pregnancy" is predicted. This is not an actual pregnancy rate. There is a caution with interpretation of life-table data: as time passes and the number of patients diminish, the confidence interval will widen. In other words, life-table prediction of pregnancy probability at 1 year of follow-up will be significantly more accurate than prediction at 4 years of follow-up. The Kaplan-Meier (or product limit) method is similar to the life-table method and is perhaps a bit more accurate with this type of data in that probabilities are based on the observed surgery-event intervals rather than on predetermined fixed intervals. Figures 5 and 6 display Kaplan-Meier prediction of the probability of term and ectopic pregnancy from our data.[71]

In general, a minimum follow-up of 1 year is reported. Although convenient and academically satisfying, 1 year follow-up may not provide young patients with enough information. Even though some reports adequately document a high percentage of pregnancies occurring within the first postoperative year of a several-year follow-up period, long-term studies emphasize that many patients conceive beyond traditional follow-up intervals. In our series of 81 patients, 2 of 10 tubal pregnancies occurred within the first year. The mean surgery to tubal pregnancy interval was 2.8 ± 1.8 years (interquartile range, 1.3 to 5.0 years)[71] and the median was 2.5 years. Six of 21 intrauterine pregnancies occurred within the first year, with a mean surgery to pregnancy time interval of 2.3 ± 1.0 years (interquartile range, 1.3 to 3.0 years), and a median of 2.0 years. Patients who failed to conceive were followed for a mean of 2.3 ± 2.3 years, with a median of 2.0 years (interquartile range, 0.5 to 3.0 years). Recent long-term studies document mean surgery-pregnancy (tubal or uterine) intervals of 15 and 24 months.[92,93] Swolin[94] followed 33 patients for 8 to 13 years and, relative to a 1- to 5-year follow-up in the same group, the term intrauterine pregnancy rate increased from 18% to 24% and the tubal pregnancy rate doubled from 9% to 18%.[94] Russell et al.[95] recently reported a remarkable 42% intrauterine pregnancy rate in 68 patients, with a minimum 5-year follow-up on all patients.

All forms of long-term follow-up data are not comparable. By including only patients with a certain minimum follow-up, pregnancy rates will increase dramatically. In our series, a subgroup of patients followed for at least 2.5 years (excluding all patients with shorter follow-up) had a 39% term pregnancy rate and an 18% tubal pregnancy rate.

Table 7 Classification of the Extent of Tubal Disease with Distal Fimbrial Obstruction[a]

Extent of disease	Findings
Mild	1. Absent or small hydrosalpinx (15-mm diameter) 2. Inverted fimbria easily recognized when patency achieved 3. No significant peritubal or periovarian adhesions 4. Preoperative hysterogram reveals a rugal pattern
Moderate	1. Hydrosalpinx (15–30-mm diameter) 2. Fragments of fimbria not readily identified 3. Periovarian and/or peritubular adhesions without fixation, minimal cul-de-sac adhesions 4. Absence of a rugal pattern on preoperative hysterogram
Severe	1. Large hydrosalpinx (30-mm diameter) 2. No fimbria 3. Dense pelvic or adnexal adhesions with fixation of the ovary and tube to either the broad ligament, pelvic sidewall, omentum and/or bowel 4. Obliteration of the cul-de-sac 5. Frozen pelvis (adhesion formation so dense that limits of organs are difficult to define)

(With this classification system, the "extent of disease" is established based on the worst feature of these findings.)

[a] From Rock et al.[64] Reproduced with permission of the publisher.

Severity of Disease

Of the 61 studies reviewed, 9 applied grading systems to judge the severity of tubal disease and offered a correlation with surgical result. Collectively, the factors that compose these systems include tubal diameter, condition of the endosalpinx, tubal wall thickness, adhesions, presence or absence of fimbriae, and presence or absence of rugation on hysterogram. The system of Rock et al. has probably gained the widest acceptance[64] (Table 7). Our data show a positive correlation with this system. Patients with the most severe disease had the lowest term pregnancy rates.

When considered as an individual finding, thickening of the tubal wall shows a consistently poor prognosis, with an intrauterine pregnancy rate of 4.1% (123 patients) from our review.[69,70,78,84] This has been a consistent observation and some surgeons have considered thickening of the tubal wall a factor for exclusion. Pathologically, tubal wall thickening usually corresponds to chronic interstitial salpingitis. As previously noted, tubal tissue from thick-walled hydrosalpinges has the lowest level of estrogen receptors.

Systems based on preoperative hysterogram findings have also shown a correlation with pregnancy rate. In 1970, Young et al.[97] reported a 7.3% intrauterine pregnancy rate in patients with complete absence of rugation on hysterogram and a 60.7% pregnancy rate in patients with normal rugation. Recently, Donnez and Casanas-Roux[86] found a correlation between tubal diameter on hysterogram and postoperative fertility. Tubal diameter greater than 2.5 cm was associated with a lower pregnancy rate than normal-diameter tubes: 22 versus 48%. Increased tubal diameter correlated with a reduction in the percentage of ciliated cells on microbiopsy of the ampulla.

Bore-Meisel et al.[70] proposed a weighted system based on the predictive value of several factors. With this approach, the weights or "likelihood ratios" are multiplied to reflect any combination of findings and translated into a probability of pregnancy. Factors considered were nature and extent of adhesions, condition of the endosalpinx, and thickness of the tubal wall. Tubal diameter was not of predictive value in this study. Overall results segregated into three prognostic groups, with probability of pregnancy being 77, 21, and 3%.

The severity of tubal disease might be expected to correlate with the incidence of tubal pregnancy. In our series, four ectopic pregnancies occurred in the mild disease group, six in the moderate group, and zero in the severe group.[71] Rock et al.[64] reported similar findings with no tubal pregnancies in 42 patients with severe disease, 13% tubal pregnancies in 30 patients with moderate disease, and 6% tubal pregnancies in 15 patients with mild disease. This effect might be accounted for, in part, by a lower postoperative tubal patency rate in severely damaged tubes.

Verhoeven et al.[69] considered the factors of dilatation, mucosal damage, and tubal wall thickness individually. Patients with tubes of normal diameter exhibited no tubal pregnancies, moderate dilatation, 1.7% tubal pregnancies, and severe dilatation, a 4.2% tubal pregnancy rate. With regard to the mucosa: patients showing slight damage exhibited an 8.7% ectopic pregnancy rate, moderate damage, 1.3%, and extensive, 0. Patients with a normal thickness of the tubal wall had no ectopic pregnancies, "thickened" tubes exhibited 3.8%, and fibrotic tubes (the most severe category) had none.

Donnez and Casanas-Roux[86] also found an increase in tubal pregnancies related to dilatation. There were no ectopic pregnancies in patients with tubes of normal diameter, 6% in tubes with moderate dilatation (15 to 25 mm), and 12% in tubes greater than 25 mm in diameter. There was an inverse relationship between progressive tubal dilatation and percent ciliated cells in the distal ampulla. The tubal pregnancy rate decreased with increasing mucosal damage and thickening of tubal wall, with no ectopic pregnancies in the most severe categories. Vasquez et al.[98] also noted deciliation in tuboplasty patients who eventually developed ectopic pregnancies.

It is striking that, with one exception,[76] all grading systems show a fairly high degree of correlation with postoperative intrauterine pregnancy rates. It is more difficult to generalize about a relationship between severity of disease and tubal pregnancy. The risk of tubal pregnancy seems to increase with increasing tubal diameter. With regard to tubal wall thickness and mucosal damage, the highest rate seems to be in tubes of intermediate injury. This might be due to complete failure of ovum capture in severely damaged oviducts, a concept supported by the experimental work of Halbert and Patton,[13] Halbert et al.,[14] and Halbert and McComb.[15] There does not seem to be a parameter that defines a group of patients at high risk for ectopic pregnancy.

With the option of IVF, grading systems should be helpful to counsel patients on their best chance for a pregnancy. The most useful system would be one based solely on hysterosalpingogram findings, whereby surgery could be avoided on poor prognosis patients. Until a uniform approach is accepted, perhaps the best system will be the careful display of all findings (e.g., tubal diameter, condition of the endosalpinx) and grading of their severity with associated intrauterine and tubal pregnancy rates.

Adjuvants

Adjuvants to reduce postoperative adhesion formation or reformation have more or less become a part of "microsurgical technique." Most recent reports of microsurgical salpingostomy note the use of an antiadhesion regimen. Parenteral glucocorticoids are the most commonly used adjuvant, although controlled human data to support their utility is lacking. Harris and Daniell[99] reported no effect on the term pregnancy rate in a controlled study employing high-dose perioperative dexamethasone. Intraperitoneal glucocorticoids and intraperitoneal dextran also are widely used. Controlled human studies on the effectiveness of intraperitoneal 32% dextran 70 (Hyskon Division, Pharmacia, Piscataway, NJ) have yielded conflicting results.[100,101] Little controlled human data exist with regard to the effectiveness of intraperitoneal glucocorticoids. Prostaglandin inhibitors have been used experimentally. Animal studies in our laboratory support the effectiveness of ibuprofen in reducing de novo postoperative adhesion formation.[102] Adhesion reformation is a more significant factor clinically and is probably a very different pathologic process. Again, there are conflicting data on this issue and prostaglandin inhibitors are not widely used clinically.

Analysis of the effectiveness of antiadhesion adjuvants is beyond the scope of this article. The use of adjuvants from differing protocols adds to the difficulty in comparing various forms of therapy for distal tubal obstruction.

Hydrotubation

Postoperative hydrotubation is another form of adjuvant and has been used extensively after distal tubal surgery. Various solutions, including enzymes, steroids, antibiotics, and dextran, have been employed in a variety of treatment protocols. Grant's encouraging results of a 41% pregnancy rate in patients treated with postoperative hydrotubation using chymotrypsin and hydrocortisone have not been repeated.[63] A controlled study by

Rock et al.,[103] using lactated Ringer's or lactated Ringer's with hydrocortisone, failed to show a significant beneficial effect of hydrotubation.

Although the concept of hydrotubation has appeal and one might picture medium bursting through the neostomy to promote patency, this spillage is probably best described as a gentle ooze, as observed at intraoperative chromotubation. In our experience, hydrotubation has not improved surgical results. It represents an extra and, at times, uncomfortable procedure and we have discontinued its routine use.

Expression of Data

The expression of data affects the interpretation of results. Surgical series that group results of dissimilar procedures (e.g., salpingostomy, salpingolysis, and reanastomosis) prevent the reader from drawing conclusions about the approach employed. Results expressed in terms of intrauterine or term pregnancy rates as well as tubal pregnancy rates provide a basis for comparison. The overall pregnancy rate, applied to both intrauterine and extrauterine pregnancies, is not a meaningful parameter. Criteria for exclusion from surgery and the number of patients with other infertility factors are also of interest to the reader.

CONCLUSION

What Surgical Technique Gives the Best Result?

Related to the variables noted in Factors Affecting Results, few of the surgical series in our review are truly comparable. The most useful data in this regard may be derived from comparison studies (Table 8).[67,75,76,82,83] All of the comparisons displayed have been drawn between diathermy microsurgery and other techniques. Fayez and Suliman[83] concluded that microsurgery is superior to conventional surgery. Comparisons of diathermy microsurgical technique to hood prosthesis and laser surgery show similar results.

With regard to the studies in Tables 1 to 6, one might make the following cautious observations. Microsurgical series have more consistent and slightly higher term pregnancy rates than conventional surgical series. Microsurgical series have variable and somewhat higher ectopic pregnancy rates than conventional surgery. Term and ectopic pregnancy rates with use of the Silastic hood prosthesis are fairly consistent and compare favorably with microsurgical salpingostomy. The limited data on laser salpingostomy suggest that this procedure yields results similar to diathermy microsurgery. Comparative data on fimbrioplasties is not sufficient to draw a conclusion.

Are We Making Progress?

It seems likely that infectious tubal disease is here to stay. Recurrent, asymptomatic chlamydia infections may be the most important etiology of distal tubal obstruction. Although tissue damage is virtually pantubal, deciliation and cilia dysfunction in the distal oviduct, resulting in failure of ovum capture and/or retention, may be key factors in this form of infertility. Postsalpingostomy "regeneration" of the tubal mucosa has not been demon-

Table 8 Results of Salpingostomy: Comparison Studies

References	Patients	Procedure	Pregnancies		Conclusion
			Term	Ectopic	
			%	%	
Siegler and Kontopoulos[82] (1979)	23	Micro	22	13	—
	15	Convent	13	20	
Decherney and Kase[67] (1981)	9	Micro	44[a]	0	Procedures
	9	Hood	22	0	Comparable
Fayez and Suliman[83] (1982)	20	Micro	35	5	Micro superior
	42	Convent	17	5	
Mage and Bruhat[75] (1983)	30	Micro	17	10	Procedures
	38	Laser	24	8	Comparable
Tulandi and Vilos[76] (1985)	30	Micro	20[b]	3	Procedures
	37	Laser	24[b]	5	Comparable

[a] Micro group extended to 54 patients had 26% term pregnancy rate.

[b] Expressed as intrauterine pregnancy.

strated in the human oviduct. The severe damage to cellular ultrastructure documented on TEM and SEM, along with depletion of estrogen receptors, makes the existence of this phenomenon seem doubtful. Prolonged surgery-to-pregnancy intervals may be due to a steady state of subfertility rather than regeneration of damaged oviducts.

The single most important prognostic factor in regard to surgical result is the initial severity of tubal damage. SEM of ampullary microbiopsies shows a correlation between deciliation and tubal dysfunction as manifest by continued infertility in the most severe degrees of deciliation. Although appealing in its elegance, this parameter may not be clinically useful. Results vary widely, depending on the biopsy site, and establishing a representative sample may be quite difficult. Furthermore, deciliation correlates with the degree of tubal dilatation-tubal diameter greater than 2.5 cm defining the most severely affected oviducts.[86] In this regard, we may have come full circle to recognize Shirodkar's observation that "thumb-sized" hydrosalpinges have a poor prognosis (although we have not seen Dr. Shirodkar's thumb).[116] In the absence of a dynamic test of tubal function, tubal diameter, as noted on hysterosalpingogram, may still be the most useful screening assessment prior to major surgery.

Some combination of microsurgical technique, antiadhesion adjuvants, exclusion of poor prognosis patients, and, perhaps, hydrotubation, has resulted in a generally more consistent and slightly higher intrauterine pregnancy rate, and, in some cases, a higher tubal pregnancy rate than older reports employing conventional surgery without adjuvants. A significant percentage of postsalpingostomy pregnancies, both tubal and intrauterine, occur more than 1 year, and maybe more than 2 years, after surgery. A greater emphasis on long-term follow-up will be useful in advising young patients on treatment options.

Acknowledgments. We gratefully acknowledge the contributions of Carlton A. Eddy, Ph.D., Dorothy L. Patton, Ph.D., Gloria Vasques, M.D., Jacques Donnez, Ph.D., Donald L. Kaiser, Dr.PH., and Stan Brown, M.D., to this manuscript. We also acknowledge Ms. Mary Phillips for the preparation of the manuscript.

REFERENCES

1. Greenhill JP: Evaluation of salpingostomy and tubal implantation for treatment of sterility. Am J Obstet Gynecol 33:39, 1937
2. Blandau RJ: Observing ovulation and egg transport. In Methods in Mammalian Embryology, Edited by JC Daniel, Jr. San Francisco, WH Freeman, 1971, p 1
3. Doteuchi M, Takeda H: Adrenergic innervation and contractile activity of the mesotubarium superius of the rabbit oviduct. J Reprod Fertil 52:213, 1978
4. Okamura H, Morikawa H, Oshima M, Man-i M, Nishimura T: A morphologic study of mesotubarium ovarica in the human. Obstet Gynecol 49:197, 1977
5. Okamura H, Morikawa H, Oshima M, Man-i M, Nishimura T: A morphological and physiological study of mesotubarium ovarica in humans. Int J Fertil 22:179, 1977
6. Clewe TH, Mastroianni L Jr: Mechanisms of ovum pickup. 1. Functional capacity of rabbit oviducts ligated near the fimbria. Fertil Steril 9:13, 1958
7. Eddy CA, Garcia RG, Kraemer DC, Pauerstein CJ: Detailed time course of ovum transport in the rhesus monkey (*Macaca mulatta*). Biol Reprod 13:363, 1975
8. Croxatto HB, Ortiz ME, Diaz S, Hess R, Balmaceda J, Croxatto HD: Studies on the duration of egg transport by the human oviduct. II. Ovum location at various intervals following luteinizing hormone peak. Am J Obstet Gynecol 132:629, 1978
9. Vasquez G, Winston RML, Boeckx W, Gordts S, Brosens IA: The epithelium of human hydrosalpinges: a light optical and scanning electron microscopic study. Br J Obstet Gynaecol 90:764, 1983
10. Blandau RJ, Bourdage R, Halbert S: Tubal transport. In The Biology of the Fluids of the Female Genital Tract, Edited by FK Beller, GFB Schumacher. New York, Elsevier North-Holland, 1979, p 319
11. Critoph FN, Dennis KJ: Ciliary activity in the human oviduct. Br J Obstet Gynaecol 84:216, 1977
12. Odor DL, Blandau RJ: Egg transport over the fimbrial surface of the rabbit oviduct under experimental conditions. Fertil Steril 24:292, 1973
13. Halbert SA, Patton DL: Ovum pick-up following fimbriectomy and infundibular salpingostomy in rabbits. J Reprod Med 26:299, 1981
14. Halbert SA, McComb PF, Patton DL: Function and structure of the rabbit oviduct following fimbriectomy. I. Distal ampullary salpingostomy. Fertil Steril 35:349, 1981
15. Halbert SA, McComb PF: Function and structure of the rabbit oviduct following fimbriectomy. II. Proximal ampullary salpingostomy. Fertil Steril 35:355, 1981
16. Harper MJK: Hormonal control of transport of eggs in cumulus through the ampulla of rabbit oviduct. Endocrinology 78:568, 1966
17. Halbert SA, Tam PY, Blandau RJ: Egg transport in the rabbit oviduct: the role of cilia and muscle. Science 191:1052, 1076
18. McComb PF, Halbert SA, Gomel V: Pregnancy, ciliary transport, and the reversed ampullary segment of the rabbit fallopian tube. Fertil Steril 34:386, 1980
19. Gaddum-Rosse P, Blandau RJ, Thiersch JB: Ciliary activity in the human and macaca nemestrina oviduct. Am J Anat 138:269, 1973
20. Jean Y, Langlais J, Roberts KD, Chapdelaine A, Bleau G: Fertility of a woman with nonfunctional ciliated cells in the fallopian tubes. Fertil Steril 31:349, 1979
21. Eddy CA, Antonini R Jr, Pauerstein CJ: Fertility following

microsurgical removal of the ampullary-isthmic junction in rabbits (Abstr). Fertil Steril 28:286, 1977

22. Donnez J, Casanas-Roux F, Caprasse J, Ferin J, Thomas K: Cyclic changes in ciliation, cell height, and mitotic activity in human tubal epithelium during reproductive life. Fertil Steril 43:554, 1985
23. Jansen RPS: Cyclic changes in the human fallopian tube isthmus and their functional importance. Am J Obstet Gynecol 136:292, 1980
24. Takeda H, Doteuchi M: Adrenergic mechanisms and hormonal status of the oviduct. II. Autonomic mechanisms in ovum transport. Presented at the Symposium on Ovum Transport and Fertility Regulation, San Antonio, Texas, June 23–27, 1975. p 307
25. Croxatto HB, Ortiz ME, Diaz S, Hess R: Attempts to modify ovum transport in women. J Reprod Fertil 55:231, 1979
26. Winston RML, McClure-Brown JC: Pregnancy following autograft transplantation of fallopian tube and ovary in the rabbit. Lancet 2:494, 1974
27. Hodgson BJ, Talo A: Spike bursts in rabbit oviduct. II. Effects of estrogen and progesterone. Am J Physiol 234:439, 1978
28. Gaddum-Rosse P, Blandau RJ: In vitro studies on ciliary activity within the oviducts of the rabbit and pig. Am J Anat 136:91, 1973
29. Pelvic infection: acute pelvic inflammatory disease. In Novak's Textbook of Gynecology (8th edition), Edited by ER Novak, GS Jones, HW Jones. Baltimore, The Williams & Wilkins Co, 1970, p 348
30. David A, Garcia CR, Czernobilsky B: Human hydrosalpinx: histologic study and chemical composition of fluid. Am J Obstet Gynecol 105:400, 1969
31. Donnez J, Casanas-Roux F: Prognostic factors of fimbrial microsurgery. Fertil Steril 46:200, 1986
32. Patek E, Nilsson L: Hydrosalpinx simplex as seen by the scanning electron microscope. Fertil Steril 28:962, 1977
33. Patton DL, Moore DE, Hicks LA, Soules MR, Spadoni LR: Tubal morphology and physiology in women with silent salpingitis. Presented at the forty-second annual meeting of The American Fertility Society, and the eighteenth annual meeting of the Canadian Andrology Society, Toronto, Ontario, Canada, September 27 to October 2, 1986. Birmingham, The American Fertility Society, 1986.
34. Devoto L, Pino AM, Heras JL, Soto E, Gunther A: Estradiol and progesterone nuclear and cytosol receptors of hydrosalpinx. Fertil Steril 42:594, 1984
35. Ahlgren M: Sperm transport to and survival in the human fallopian tube. Gynecol Invest 6:206, 1975
36. Halbert SA, Patton DL: Hydrosalpinx: effect of oviductal dilatation on egg transport. Fertil Steril 35:69, 1981
37. Patton DL, Halbert SA: Mechanically induced hydrosalpinx: long-term oviductal dilatation does not impair ciliary transport function. Fertil Steril 36:808, 1981
38. Vemer HM, Boeckx WD, Vasquez G, Brosens IA: Experimental hydrosalpinx and salpingostomy in rabbits. Eur J Obstet Gynecol Reprod Biol 18:95, 1984
39. Donnez J, Caprasse J, Casanas-Roux F, Karaman Y, Ferim J, Thomas K: Morphologic study of mechanically induced hydrosalpinges in rabbits. Acta Eur Fertil 16:257, 1985
40. Donnez J, Caprasse J, Casanas-Roux F, Ferin J, Thomas K: Loss of adrenergic innervation in inducted rabbit hydrosalpinx. Gynecol Obstet Invest 21:213, 1986
41. Vasquez G, Vemer HM, Boeckx WD, Brosens IA: Ciliogenesis following salpingostomy of rabbit hydrosalpinges. Eur J Obstet Gynecol Reprod Biol 18:103, 1984
42. Yussman MA: Unpublished data
43. Patton DL, Kuo CC, Wang SP, Halbert SA: Distal tubal obstruction induced by repeated Chlamydia trachomatis salpingeal infections in pig-tailed macaques. J Infect Dis 155:1292, 1987
44. Treharne JD, Ripa KT, Mardh P-A, Svensson L, Westrom L, Darougar S: Antibodies to Chlamydia trachomatis in acute salpingitis. Br J Vener Dis 55:26, 1979
45. Patton DL, Halbert SA, Kuo C-C, Wang S-P, Holmes KK: Host response to primary Chlamydia trachomatis infection of the fallopian tube in pig-tailed monkeys. Fertil Steril 40:829, 1983
46. Ward ME, Watt PJ: Studies on the cell biology of gonorrhoea. In Genital Infections and Their Complications, Edited by D Danielsson, L Juhlin, P-A Mardh. Stockholm, Almquist & Wiksell International, 1975, p 229
47. Moller BR, Freundt EA, Mardh P-A: Experimental pelvic inflammatory disease provoked by Chlamydia trachomatis and Mycoplasma hominis in grivet monkeys. Am Obstet Gynecol 138:990, 1980
48. Henry-Suchet J, Catalan F, Loffredo V, Serfaty D, Siboulet A, Perol Y, Sanson MJ, Debache C, Pigeau F, Coppin R, DeBrux J, Poynard T: Microbiology of specimens obtained by laparoscopy from controls and from patients with pelvic inflammatory disease or infertility with tubal obstruction: Chlamydia trachomatis and ureaplasma urealyticum. Am J Obstet Gynecol 138:1022, 1980
49. Bateman BG, Nunley WC, Kitchin JD, Fechner RE: Genital tuberculosis in reproductive-age women. J Reprod Med 31:287, 1986
50. Holden FC, Sovak FW: Reconstruction of the oviducts: an improved technic with reports of cases. Am J Obstet Gynecol 24:684, 1932
51. Israel SL: Total linear salpingostomy. Fertil Steril 2:505, 1951
52. Kistner RW, Patton GW: Atlas of Infertility Surgery (1st edition). Boston, Little, Brown and Co, 1975, p 95
53. Mulligan WJ: Results of salpingostomy. Int J Fertil 11:424, 1966
54. Roland M: Spiral Teflon splint for tuboplasty involving fimbria. Obstet Gynecol 36:359, 1970
55. Cognat M: Presentation d'une prosthese-drain destince a la chirurgic tubulaire pour sterilite. Bull Fed Soc Gynecol Obstet Fr 23:4, 1971
56. Trimbos-Kemper TCM, Trimbos JB, van Hall EV: Adhesion formation after tubal surgery: results of the eighth-day laparoscopy in 188 patients. Fertil Steril 43:395, 1985
57. Raj SG, Hulka JF: Second-look laparoscopy in infertility surgery: therapeutic and prognostic value. Fertil Steril 38:325, 1982
58. Palmer R: Salpingostomy: a critical study of 396 personal cases operated upon without polyethylene tubing. Proc R Soc Med 53:357, 1960
59. Hanton EM, Pratt JH, Banner EA: Tubal plastic surgery at the Mayo Clinic. Am J Obstet Gynecol 89:934, 1964
60. Arronet GH, Eduljee SY, O'Brien JR: A nine-year survey

of fallopian tube dysfunction in human infertility: a diagnosis and therapy. Fertil Steril 20:903, 1969
61. Siegler AM: Salpingoplasty: classification and report of 115 operations. Obstet Gynecol 34:339, 1969
62. Jessen H: 45 operations for sterility. Acta Obstet Gynecol Scand 50:105, 1971
63. Grant A: Infertility surgery of the oviduct. Fertil Steril 22:496, 1971
64. Rock JA, Katayama KP, Martin EJ, Woodruff JD, Jones HW Jr: Factors influencing the success of salpingostomy techniques for distal fimbrial obstruction. Obstet Gynecol 52:591, 1978
65. Winston RML: Microsurgery of the fallopian tube: from fantasy to reality. Fertil Steril 34:521, 1980
66. Gomel V: Clinical results of infertility microsurgery. In Microsurgery in Female Infertility, Edited by PG Crosignani, BL Rubin. London, Academic Press, 1980, p 77
67. DeCherney AH, Kase N: A comparison of treatment for bilateral fimbrial occlusion. Fertil Steril 35:162, 1981
68. Larsson B: Late results of salpingostomy combined with salpingolysis and ovariolysis by electromicroscopy in 54 women. Fertil Steril 37:156, 1982
69. Verhoeven HC, Berry H, Frantzen C, Schlosser HW: Surgical treatment for distal tubal occlusion: a review of 167 cases. J Reprod Med 28:293, 1983
70. Boer-Meisel ME, te Velde ER, Habbema JDF, Kardaun JWPF: Predicting the pregnancy outcome in patients treated for hydrosalpinx: a prospective study. Fertil Steril 45:23, 1986
71. Kitchin JD, Nunley WC, Bateman BG: Surgical management of distal tubal occlusion. Am J Obstet Gynecol 155:524, 1986
72. Garcia CR: Surgical reconstruction of the oviduct in the infertile patient. In Progress in Infertility (1st edition), Edited by SJ Behrman, RW Kistner. Boston, Little, Brown and Co, 1968, p 255
73. Wallach EE, Manara LR, Eisenberg E: Experience with 143 cases of tubal surgery. Fertil Steril 39:609, 1983
74. Kelly RW, Roberts DK: Experience with the carbon dioxide laser in gynecologic microsurgery. Am J Obstet Gynecol 145:585, 1983
75. Mage G, Bruhat MA: Pregnancy following salpingostomy: comparison between CO_2 laser and electrosurgery procedures. Fertil Steril 40:472, 1983
76. Tulandi T, Vilos GA: A comparison between laser surgery and electrosurgery for bilateral hydrosalpinx: a 2-year follow up. Fertil Steril 44:846, 1985
77. Daniell JF, Diamond MP, McLaughlin DS, Martin DC, Feste J, Surrey MW, Friedman S, Vaughn WK: Clinical results of terminal salpingostomy with the use of the CO_2 laser: report of the intraabdominal laser study group. Fertil Steril 45:175, 1986
78. Gomel V: Salpingostomy by laparoscopy. J Reprod Med 18:265, 1977
79. Lauritsen JG, Pagel JD, Vangsted P, Starup J: Results of repeated tuboplasties. Fertil Steril 37:68, 1982
80. Daniell JF, Herbert CM: Laparoscopic salpingostomy utilizing the CO_2 laser. Fertil Steril 41:558, 1984
81. Daniell J: Unpublished data
82. Siegler AM, Kontopoulos V: An analysis of macrosurgical and microsurgical techniques in the management of tuboperitoneal factor in infertility. Fertil Steril 32:377, 1979
83. Fayez JA, Suliman SO: Infertility surgery of the oviduct: comparison between macrosurgery and microsurgery. Fertil Steril 37:73, 1982
84. Frantzen C, Schlosser H W: Microsurgery and postinfectious tubal infertility. Fertil Steril 38:397, 1983
85. Patton GW Jr: Pregnancy outcome following microsurgical fimbrioplasty. Fertil Steril 37:150, 1982
86. Donnez J, Casanas-Roux F: Prognostic factors of fimbrial microsurgery. Fertil Steril 46:200, 1986
87. Mettler L, Giesel H, Semm K: Treatment of female infertility due to tubal obstruction by operative laparoscopy. Fertil Steril 32:384, 1979
88. Fayez JA: An assessment of the role of operative laparoscopy in tuboplasty. Fertil Steril 39:476, 1983
89. Spadoni LR: Tubal and peritubal surgery without magnification: an analysis. Am J Obstet Gynecol 137:189, 1980
90. Lamb EJ, Moscovitz W: Tuboplasty for infertility. Int J Fertil 17:53, 1972
91. Boyd IE, Holt EM: Tubal sterility. Patency tests and results of operation. J Obstet Gynaecol Br Commw 80:142, 1973
92. Jansen RPS: Surgery-pregnancy time intervals after salpingolysis, unilateral salpingostomy and bilateral salpingostomy. Fertil Steril 34:222, 1980
93. Tulandi T, Farag, R, McInnes RA, Gelfand MM, Wright CV, Vilos GA: Reconstructive surgery of hydrosalpinx with and without the carbon dioxide laser. Fertil Steril 42:839, 1984
94. Swolin K: Electromicrosurgery and salpingostomy: Long-term results. Am J Obstet Gynecol 121:418, 1974
95. Russell JB, DeCherney AH, Laufer N, Polan ML, Naftolin F: Neosalpingostomy: comparison of 24- and 72-month follow-up time shows increased pregnancy rate. Fertil Steril 45:296, 1986
96. Donnez J: La trompe de Fallope. In Histophysiologie Normale et Pathologique, Edited by J Donnez. Leuven, Nauwelaerts Printing Publishers, 1984, p 97
97. Young DE, Egan JE, Barlow JJ, Mulligan WJ: Reconstructive surgery for infertility at the Boston Hospital for Women. Am J Obstet Gynecol 108:1092, 1970
98. Vasquez G, Winston RML, Brosens IA: Tubal mucosa and ectopic pregnancy. Br J Obstet Gynaecol 90:468, 1983
99. Harris WJ, Daniell JF: Use of corticosteriods as an adjuvant in terminal salpingostomy. Fertil Steril 40:785, 1983
100. Larsson B, Lalos O, Marsk L, Tronstad S-E, Bygdeman M, Pehrson E, Joelsson I: Effect of intraperitoneal instillation of 32% dextran 70 on postoperative adhesion formation after tubal surgery. Acta Obstet Gynecol Scand 64:437, 1985
101. Rosenberg SM, Board JA: High-molecular weight dextran in human infertility surgery. Am J Obstet Gynecol 148:380, 1984
102. Bateman BG, Nunley WC Jr, Kitchin JD III: Prevention of postoperative peritoneal adhesions with ibuprofen. Fertil Steril 38:107, 1982
103. Rock JA, Siegler AM, Boer Meisel M, Haney AF, Rosenwaks Z, Pardo-Vargas F, Kimball AW: The efficacy of postoperative hydrotubation: a randomized prospective multicenter clinical trial. Fertil Steril 42:373, 1984
104. Comninos AC: Salpingostomy: treatment of female sterility. Fertil Steril 5:334, 1954
105. Ozaras H: The value of plastic operations on the fallopian

tubes in the treatment of infertility. Acta Obstet Gynecol Scand 47:489, 1968

106. Gomel V: Laparoscopic tubal surgery in infertility. Obstet Gynecol 46:47, 1975
107. Mroueh A, Hajj SN: Tubal plastic surgery. Int J Fertil 13:215, 1968
108. Fjallbrant BL: Tubal surgery: report of 101 cases with special reference to the experience of the surgeon. Acta Obstet Gynecol Scand 54:463, 1975
109. Bellina JH: Microsurgery of the fallopian tube with the carbon dioxide laser: analysis of 230 cases with a two-year follow-up. Lasers Surg Med 3:255, 1983
110. Bellina JH: Microsurgery of the fallopian tube with the carbon dioxide laser: eighty-two cases with follow-up. Lasers Surg Med 2:129, 1982
111. Baggish MS, Chong AP: Carbon dioxide laser microsurgery of the uterine tube. Obstet Gynecol 58:111, 1981
112. Comninos AC: Salpingostomy: results of two different methods of treatment. Fertil Steril 28:1211, 1977
113. Schoysman R: Tubal microsurgery versus in vitro fertilization. Acta Eur Fertil 15:5, 1984
114. Carey M, Brown S: Fertility surgery for pelvic inflammatory disease: success rates following salpingolysis and salpingostomy. Presented at the Society of Obstetricians and Gynecologists of Canada, Charlestown, Prince Edward Island, June 11–15, 1986
115. Betz G, Engel T, Penney LL: Tuboplasty comparison of the methodology. Fertil Steril 34:534, 1980
116. Shirodkar VN: Factors influencing the results of salpingostomy. Int J Fertil 11:361, 1966

Chapter 21

Endometriosis: a reappraisal of pathogenesis and treatment

Cecilia L. Schmidt, M.D.

Division of Reproductive Endocrinology and Infertility, Department of Obstetrics and Gynecology, University of Connecticut Health Center, Farmington, Connecticut

The controversy surrounding the optimal treatment of women with endometriosis is not simply a battle between the endocrinologist and the surgeon, but is also a dilemma of the choice between expectant management and any active treatment. Obviously, the persistence of severe dysmenorrhea and chronic, disabling pelvic pain necessitates hormonal, surgical, or combined management. However, the infertility reportedly accompanying endometriosis in 30% to 40% of affected women[1] is not so decidedly approached.

First, discriminating review of earlier regimens reveals the lack of control populations. It was this multitude of retrospective studies that limited our precision in prognostication for the infertile patient with endometriosis to the unacceptably wide range of a 40% to 90% conception rate after the end of therapy. Second, the basic tenets of this evasive disease are constantly being challenged. And third, endometriosis remains a disease whose natural history has not been characterized as a single entity. Rather, it appears to represent a continuum of individual presentations and progressions.

It is the objective of this review to reevaluate diverse modalities of treatment in the light of tenable pathogenesis and critical dissection of much-quoted studies.

PATHOGENESIS OF ENDOMETRIOSIS AS A PREEMPT TO THERAPY

CLASSIC THEORIES

Since the time when Sampson first described endometriosis as a unique entity in 1927,[2] the most common locations of this disease have remained the surfaces of the most dependent intra-abdominal structures in the upright woman. It was the apparent superficial spread of endometriosis from a retrograde menstrual seeding caudally from the cul-de-sac that was first employed to explain this distribution.[2] A theory of simple implantation was followed by one of mesothelial metaplasia induced by this menstrual detritus, as proposed by Novak.[3] However, the rare finding of endometriosis in distant parenchyma of the lung and kidney elicited Halban's hypothesis of hematogenous/lymphatic involvement.[4] Furthermore, blood has been detected in peritoneal fluid in 90% of 52 women with patent tubes who were undergoing laparoscopy during the perimenstrual period.[5] Because these observations depict retrograde menstruation through fallopian tubes as a common occurrence in women with patent tubes, only additional factors can explain the subsequent development of endometriosis in some women. A familial preponderance for endometriosis has been demonstrated by a 6.9% recurrence rate for first-degree relatives of affected women and may imply that the disease has a genetic component.[6] In this study, the incidence of endometriosis in relatives of 123 patients was compared with the incidence in relatives of their husbands; 8.1% of the mothers of women with endometriosis (10 of 123) and 5.9% of sisters (9 of 153) were affected, in contrast to 0.9% of husbands' mothers (1 of 107) and 1.0% of sisters of husbands (1 of 104). Although a significant difference was noted, the documentation of disease in relatives was not detailed.[6]

IMMUNOLOGIC STUDIES

As eloquently addressed previously by Muse and Wilson,[7] immunologic and hormonal disturbances may be involved in the etiology and manifestations of endometriosis. The macrophage-mediated autoimmune phenomenon was first proposed by Weed and Arquembourg,[8] who detected the deposition of complement around the endometrial glands of women with endometriosis but were unable to identify the causative "antigen." Badawy et al.[9] later supported these findings by demonstrating that Ouchterlony immunodiffusion produced precipitation lines between autologous endometrial homogenates and serum from two of three patients with endometriosis but not from three control infertile patients. This phenomenon suggests that the immune response mounted against the "self" endometriotic debris by women with endometriosis may vary. Sera from 11 of 13 patients with endometriosis were positive for hemagglutination antibodies to the endometrium.[10] The two patients with negative titers lacked ovarian involvement. The mean ± standard error of the mean (SEM) antibody titers of these patients with endometriosis (7.08 ± 0.80) were significantly elevated over titers of 15 healthy age-matched nonpregnant female control subjects who had not undergone laparoscopy (1.60 ± 0.48). Similarly, antibody titers to ovary, thecal cells, and granulosa cells were also higher in the sera of patients found to harbor endometriosis than in sera from the normal women.[10] Most recently, Barbieri et al.[11] found that a monoclonal antibody, OC-125, prepared to a membrane antigen, CA-125, detected elevated levels of CA-125 in 80% of patients with epithelial ovarian cancer, in $< 2\%$ of normal women, and in 49% of women with endometriosis. However, only patients with stage III or IV endometriosis had significantly elevated levels, compared with 55 infertility patients without endometriosis. Hence, a 92% specificity for endometriosis is not acceptable when the antibody can alternatively detect an ovarian cancer antigen.[11] Laparoscopy or laparotomy currently remain the only definitive methods of diagnosis.

When 27 infertile endometriosis patients were compared with 26 age-matched infertile women without laparoscopic evidence of endometriosis, nonspecific parameters of immune function were not significantly different.[12] However, in vitro T-lymphocyte-mediated cytotoxicity to autologous endometrial cells was significantly reduced in these patients with endometriosis and was inversely correlated with severity of disease.[12] Concentrations of the complement components of C_3c and C_4 were significantly higher in the serum and peritoneal fluid of 23 women with endometriosis, compared with 22 control patients.[9] However, the serum levels of either component could not serve as a distinguishing marker for the presence of endometriosis because a substantial overlap existed between values in the two groups of patients.[9] Hence, no published studies have systematically investigated the relationship between the degree of autoimmune response and clinical symptoms, objective staging of endometriosis, or fertility potential.

Peritoneal fluid macrophages from women with endometriosis have been found to be both significantly more numerous and more voracious in phagocytosing sperm in vitro than those from fertile women or infertile women without endometriosis.[13] Similarly, higher proportions of the peritoneal macrophages from infertile patients with mild endometriosis have shown acid phosphatase activity than did those from fertile patients.[14] The numbers of oviductal macrophages were found to be significantly higher in patients with endometriosis who underwent conservative surgery than in either normal fertile or infertile women with tubal obstruction and appeared to be related to the number of peritoneal macrophages.[15] Unfortunately, this detectable difference in macrophage populations at the level of the pelvic cavity between patients with endometriosis and those without the disease was not reflected in the peripheral lymphocyte populations. Techniques with monoclonal immunofluorescence antibodies revealed no statistical difference in white blood cell subset counts between 31 infertile subjects with stage I or II endometriosis and 22 control infertility patients.[16] Hence, neither peripheral white blood cell typing nor complement component concentrations can feasibly be sensitive peripheral indicators of this disease.

PROSTAGLANDIN/PROSTANOID STUDIES

The role of prostaglandins (PGs) in the genesis of endometriosis symptoms and infertility has been muddied by diametrically opposed reports[17-21] of levels of these agents in peritoneal fluid (Table 1). First, the short half-life of PGs demands immediate preservation of the sample and emphasis upon the more stable metabolites. Although the PG metabolites thromboxane B_2 (TXB_2) and 6-keto-prostacyclin $F_{1\alpha}$ (6-KF) were found to be increased in both concentrations and total amounts in women with endometriosis in early studies by Drake et al.,[17] only the concentration (not total amount) of 6-KF remained significantly higher for women with endometriosis, compared with normal women, when menstrual cycle phase was incorporated into the investigations.[20] When peritoneal fluid was sampled only during the late proliferative phase of the cycle, no meaningful elevation of prostanoid concentrations (PGE_2, $PGF_{2\alpha}$, PGFM, TXB_2) was found.[19] As noted by Rock and associates,[19] the fluid volume measurements originally determined by Drake and co-workers to show a direct correlation between severity of endometriosis and peritoneal fluid volume[17] did not recognize the progressive increase in mean fluid volume throughout the proliferative phase and attainment of peak volumes in the early secretory phase.[22] Hence, it was suggested that those earlier prostanoid studies[17, 20] may have been subject to sampling errors.

Cognizant of menstrual cycle phase as a variable in quantitation of pelvic cavity PGs, DeLeon and associates[21] found that patients with endometriosis had elevated peritoneal fluid concentrations of $PGF_{2\alpha}$ and PGE_2 ($P < 0.01$), when compared with control subjects, only when the peritoneal fluid had been sampled during the secretory phase. There was no significant difference in concomitantly obtained peritoneal fluid estradiol and progesterone (P) concentrations.[21] This trend appears to hold true for 13,14-dihydro-15-keto $PGF_{2\alpha}$ (PGFM) concentrations when data presented by Badawy et al.[18] are regrouped according to reported phase of the menstrual cycle. Although the levels of PGE_2 show wide variations throughout the cycle and between patients, levels of PGFM, as depicted in Table 1, are higher in patients with endometriosis than in control subjects during the secretory phase (14.65 ± 5.94 ng/ml and 7.13 ± 3.23 ng/ml versus 2.27 ± 0.08 ng/ml). Therefore, as detailed in Table 1, the key to the controversy concerning the role of PGs and prostanoids may reside in both the timing of peritoneal fluid aspiration and the quality control of the assay systems.

ENDOMETRIOSIS TISSUE STUDIES

The classic description of ectopically placed endometrial glands and stroma appropriately responding to hormonal stimulation in proliferative and secretory modes is countered by dissimilar steroid-hormone control of these two tissues. Cyclical function mimicking hormonally responsive endometrium has been suggested by morphologic[23] and histopathologic[24] studies. However, the electron microscopic appearance[25] and nuclear estrogen binding studies[26] distinguish ectopic endometrial implants from uterine endometrium. Unlike the concentrations of cytosolic estrogen and P receptors in normal endometrium, which exhibit characteristic changes during proliferative and secretory phases, the levels of these receptors in endometriosis specimens showed no significant differences in relation to the menstrual cycle.[27] Vierikko et al.[27] also noted the failure of P treatment in vivo to induce 17β-hydroxysteroid dehydrogenase activity in endometriosis tissue measured in vitro, in contrast to the effect of P on endometrium during the luteal phase. Most strikingly, the discordant effect of danazol on these two tissues was supported by comparison of endometrial and endometriosis tissues obtained from four patients after 3 days' treatment with danazol. The endometrial specimens showed a clear induction of 17β-hydroxysteroid dehydrogenase activity and higher cytosolic estrogen and P receptors than the endometriosis tissues.[27] Furthermore, unlike luteal phase endometrium, which secretes prolactin (PRL),[28] endometriotic implants do not appear to produce PRL during the late secretory phase.[29] PRL concentrations of peritoneal fluid did not differ significantly between 27 infertile women with endometriosis, 13 infertile women without endometriosis, and 11 fertile women undergoing tubal cautery, regardless of menstrual cycle timing or stage of endometriosis.[29] Hence, our conception of endometriosis as microcosms of endometrial tissue appears to be unfounded.

PATHOLOGIC ENTITIES COEXISTING WITH ENDOMETRIOSIS

ASSOCIATION WITH INFECTION

The infrequently detected coexistence of endometriosis and salpingitis appears to underlie the even rarer entity of infected endometriotic cysts.[30] Of 48 women with salpingitis associated with endometriosis found on pathologic review, only 11 exhibited abscess formation within the endometriotic stroma.[30] Acknowledging the retrospective nature of this original investigation,

Table 1. *Summary of Studies Evaluating Peritoneal Fluid Prostanoid Concentrations in Women With Endometriosis and Women Without Endometriosis With Reference to Stage of Disease and Phase of Menstrual Cycle*

Reference	Group $(n)^a$	Diagnosis at laparoscopy $(n)^a$	No. in proliferative phase	No. in secretory phase	Mean ± SEM: PGE_2	$PGF_{2\alpha}$	TXB_2	6-KF	PGFM
							ng/ml		
Drake et al.[17]	Endometriosis (14)	Mild (2) Moderate (8) Severe (4)	?	?	—	—	2.27 ± 0.83[b] ($P < 0.025$)	44.5 ± 13.7[b] ($P < 0.01$)	—
	Control (15)	Tubal ligation (9) Infertile, no adhesions (6)	?	?	—	—	0.38 ± 0.15	3.85 ± 2.5	—
Badawy et al.[18]	Endometriosis (15)	I (10)	5		9.21 ± 4.45	—	—	—	5.98 ± 2.66
				5	7.27 ± 2.45	—	—	—	14.65 ± 5.94
		III (5)	3		7.46 ± 3.39	—	—	—	10.10 ± 3.07
				2	3.50 ± 0.10	—	—	—	7.13 ± 3.23
			Combined		7.45 ± 6.71	—	—	—	9.84 ± 8.98
	Unexplained infertile (5)	No abnormalities (5)	1		22.43	—	—	—	12.32
				4	10.85 ± 4.68	—	—	—	10.12 ± 3.61
			Combined		13.32 ± 9.46	—	—	—	10.47 ± 6.22
	Control (5)	Dysmenorrhea (2)	2	0	2.64 ± 0.50	—	—	—	4.43 ± 0.38
		Tubal reanastomosis (3)	1		3.20	—	—	—	4.72
				2	10.27 ± 2.12	—	—	—	2.27 ± 0.08
			Combined		5.80 ± 4.36	—	—	—	3.62 ± 1.27
Rock et al.[19]	Endometriosis (45)	Mild (15)	15	0	0.51 ± 0.10	0.16 ± 0.03	0.088 ± 0.011	—	0.035 ± 0.006
		Moderate (15)	15	0	0.56 ± 0.09	0.24 ± 0.04	0.095 ± 0.015	—	0.042 ± 0.008
		Severe (15)	15	0	0.44 ± 0.06	0.29 ± 0.09	0.116 ± 0.025	—	0.034 ± 0.009
	Infertile (17)	No abnormalities (17)	17	0	0.72 ± 0.12	0.23 ± 0.04	0.132 ± 0.028	—	0.052 ± 0.011
Dawood et al.[20]	Endometriosis (16)	Mild (5) Moderate (10) Severe (1)	4 Combined	12	1.43 ± 0.72	1.52 ± 0.59	1.14 ± 0.68	3.32 ± 0.71[b] ($P < 0.02$)	—
	Control (10)	Tubal ligation (10)	3 Combined	7	0.79 ± 0.26	0.60 ± 0.18	0.23 ± 0.09	0.48 ± 0.19	—
DeLeon et al.[21]	Endometriosis (31)	Endometriosis (31)	8		8.5 ± 0.9	5.7 ± 0.5	—	—	—
				23	8.0 ± 0.4[c] ($P < 0.01$)	6.2 ± 0.4[c] ($P < 0.01$)	—	—	—
	Control (14)	? No abnormalities (14)	6		7.5 ± 0.5	5.6 ± 0.7	—	—	—
				8	6.4 ± 0.3	4.3 ± 0.6	—	—	—

[a] (n), number of women in each category.
[b] P, compared with control.
[c] P, compared with control during secretory phase only. All other comparisons were not significant.

we have since found other cases that support endosalpingitis as the vehicle of microbial spread.[31] Because the infected endometriotic cyst can be readily misdiagnosed as a hemorrhagic tubo-ovarian abscess, the patient may be denied appropriate conservative surgery with antibiotic treatment. Although only one of five patients treated in this manner achieved a pregnancy,[30] the success of such therapy awaits more prospective studies.

ASSOCIATION WITH HYPERPROLACTINEMIA AND LUTEAL PHASE DEFECTS

Another relatively unexplored occurrence is the constellation of luteal phase defect (LPD), hyperprolactinemia, and endometriosis in infertile women, as summarized in Table 2.[7, 32-36] Sporadic reports have acknowledged the occurrence of galactorrhea in women with endometriosis[32, 33] but have not detected concomitant hyperprolactinemia. A propensity for significantly elevated PRL levels has been detected in women with endometriosis, when compared with control subjects, after thyrotropin-releasing hormone stimulation[7] and at 8:00 A.M. after an overnight fast preceding surgery.[36] However, the luteal phase in these subjects was not studied.[7, 36] Because luteal phase defective endometrium was neither found in a significantly higher proportion of 68 infertile women with endometriosis (8.8%), compared with 75 infertile women without endometriosis (5.3%),[35] nor had increased in the women with endometriosis in a smaller series,[34] we decided to

Table 2. *Association of Hyperprolactinemia, LPD, and Endometriosis*

Reference	No. of patients				
	Endometriosis	Galactorrhea	Elevated PRL	LPD	Diagnosis of LPD
Hirschowitz et al.[32]	9	8	2	—	—
Hargrove and Abraham[33]	14	7	3	14 (100%)	P < 16 ng/ml
Muse and Wilson[7]	14	—	14 (peak after thyrotropin-releasing hormone stimulation)	—	—
Brosens et al.[34]	20	—	0	5 (25%)	Endometrial biopsy
	14	—	0	—	—
Pittaway et al.[35]	68	—	—	6 (8.8%) (control: 4/75; 5.3%)	Endometrial biopsy
Radwanska et al.[36]	32	—	Mean (8:00 A.M. level)	—	—

explore the additional factor of hyperprolactinemia. LPD, as defined by two endometrial biopsy specimens obtained 11 to 13 days after the temperature nadir and histologically lagging by 2 or more days by subsequent menses, were detected in 65 infertile patients over an 8-year period at the University of Connecticut Health Center.[31] Only seven patients (10.8%) also were found to have elevated serum PRL levels (mean ± SEM, 45.5 ± 9.8 ng/ml). In four of five of these women who underwent laparoscopy, endometriosis had been diagnosed and treated, as depicted in Table 3. Three of our four patients conceived and were delivered of viable infants. As is true with LPD alone,[37] it is important to note that only corrected luteal phase endometrial biopsies predicted the possibility of viable pregnancies associated with each treatment regimen. Similarly obtained PRL levels in these originally hyperprolactinemic women were less predictive of either conception or outcome of pregnancies on a specific course of treatment. Although the true incidence of this triad of endometriosis, LPD, and hyperprolactinemia remains to be determined, the optimal prognosticator includes a corrected luteal phase biopsy.

CLASSIFICATION SYSTEMS AS A KEY TO INTERPRETING TREATMENT

In 1973 Acosta et al.[38] defined a simplistic method of deciphering the havoc wrought by endometriosis. These guidelines focused on the progressive enlargement of endometriotic cysts, the pervasive spread of endometriotic implants, and the increasing entanglement of adhesions in peritoneal, periovarian, and peritubal regions. It was this nomenclature of mild, moderate, and severe endometriosis[38] that allowed the design of rational protocols for treatment of the disease based

Table 3. *Stage of Endometriosis, Previous Treatment for Endometriosis, Treatment for LPD, Endometrial Biopsy, and Outcome of Pregnancy in Four Women with Hyperprolactinemia, LPD, and Endometriosis*

Patient	Stage of endometriosis, AFS classification[40]	Treatment for endometriosis after laparoscopy	Treatment for LPD during conception cycle	Biopsy status on this LPD regimen	Viable full-term delivery
1	Mild	Danazol, 800 mg daily for 4 months	Dexamethasone and P suppositories	Corrected	Singleton
2	Moderate	Conservative surgery; danazol, 800 mg daily for 6 months	Bromocriptine	Not obtained	Singleton
3	Moderate	Danazol, 800 mg daily for 5 months; repeat laparoscopy: resolved endometriosis	Bromocriptine	Not obtained	None
4	Severe	Conservative surgery; repeat laparoscopy: minimal endometriosis	Bromocriptine	Corrected	Twins

Table 4. *Comparison of Classification Systems with Reference to Endometrial Implants, Adhesions, and Endometriomas: Acosta et al.,[38] Kistner et al.,[39] and AFS[40]*

Acosta et al.[38]	Mild	Moderate	Severe
Endometrial implants	Scattered; superficial on ovary or peritoneum	Several; scarring on ovaries or peritoneum	Significant bowel or urinary tract involvement
Peritoneal adhesions	Absent	Minimal	Obliterated cul-de-sac; thickened uterosacral ligaments
Periovarian adhesions	Absent	Minimal	Ovaries bound
Peritubal adhesions	Absent	Minimal	Tubes bound or obstructed ligaments
Endometriomas	Absent	< 2 cm	> 2 cm

Kistner et al.[39]	I	IIA	IIB	III	IV
Endometrial implants	< 5 mm ---------->[a]		> 5 mm ---------->[a]		Bladder serosa covered
Peritoneal adhesions	Avascular (?) ---------->[a]		No adherent bowel ---------->[a]		Bowel adherent to cul-de-sac, uterosacral ligaments, or fixed uterus
Periovarian adhesions	Avascular ---------->[a]		Thick; ovaries adherent to posterior broad ligament	Ovaries adherent to tube or broad ligament ---------->[a]	
Peritubal adhesions	Avascular ---------->[a]		Thick; fimbria free	Fimbria covered by adhesions ---------->[a]	
Endometriomas	Absent	< 5 cm (−1) > 5 cm (−2) Ruptured (−3) ---------->[a]			

AFS classification[40]	No. of points[b] 1	2	3	4	6
Endometrial implants					
Peritoneal	< 1 cm	1–3 cm	> 3 cm	—	—
Tubal	—	< 1 cm	—	> 1 cm	Tubal occlusion
Peritoneal adhesions	Filmy	Dense with partial cul-de-sac obliteration	Dense with complete cul-de-sac obliteration	—	—
Periovarian adhesions	Filmy	—	—	Dense with partial ovarian enclosure	Dense with complete ovarian enclosure
Peritubal adhesions	Filmy	—	—	Dense with tubal distortion	Dense with tubal enclosure
Endometriomas	—	< 1 cm	—	1–3 cm	> 3 cm or ruptured

[a]----->, no change between stages or subdivisions.

[b]Assigned for the sum of diameters of implants or endometriomas or for the texture and pathologic effect of all adhesions in each half of pelvis. Stage I (mild), 1–5; stage II (moderate), 6–15; stage III (severe), 16–30; stage IV (extensive), 31–54.

upon statistical comparisons between the stages. In an endeavor to ameliorate the clinician's recognition of endometriosis in its various modes, Kistner et al.[39] incorporated a presumed natural history of endometriosis into their classification system. Attention was focused upon both the mobility of the broad ligament in relation to the ovaries and to the fallopian tubes and the patency of the tubal fimbria. Endometriosis was depicted as a serpiginous growth from central structures to more lateral ones.[39] However, neither classification proposal reflected unilateral involvement with gross preservation of single tubo-ovarian anatomy. For this purpose The American Fertility Society (AFS)[40] system assigned points to the number, size, and location on the peritoneum, ovary, or tube of the same basic triad of endometrial implants, endometriomas, and adhesions but added the dimensions of isolating enclosures of tube and ovary. The aggregation of points reflected the pervasiveness of the disease on each side, and the total score indicated the stage of the disease. Table 4 attempts to relate the three staging systems as a guide in normalizing studies based on the different classifications.

Experience with this initial AFS scoring system, as highlighted by Buttram,[41] has revealed its failure to weight points appropriately to adhesions of the tubes and ovaries, to invasive versus superficial endometriosis, to complete enclosure of the fimbriated end of the fallopian tubes, and to complete posterior cul-de-sac obliteration. Consequently, a revised AFS classification, instituting a "minimal" and eliminating an "extensive" category, has been drafted and approved.[42] It is hoped to provide a standard scheme for all gynecologists that will permit more interpretable data collection, more objective evaluation of therapeutics, and more justifiable prognostication for patients with endometriosis. The updated charts can be readily obtained from The AFS for consistent postoperative staging by the surgeon.[42] As we have learned from the retrospective studies of the past decade, interpretation of clinical trials during the phase of transition from the initial[40] to the revised[42] AFS scoring systems would be facilitated by dual classification of each case.

HORMONAL VERSUS SURGICAL TREATMENT

HORMONAL THERAPY

Pseudopregnancy and Progestins

The amelioration of endometriosis that seemed to accompany pregnancy both incited much debate in the 1950s and fostered initial treatment with progestin therapy and oral contraceptives (OCs). Kistner[43] introduced the pseudopregnancy regimens by uninterrupted administration of one of the combination OCs for 6 to 9 months. Pseudopregnancy relieves dysmenorrhea and pelvic pain in > 80% of patients, but frequently transiently. However, reported pregnancy rates of between 20% and 40%[44] do not approach rates achieved with recent treatment with danazol or surgery. It must be appreciated that the OC literature suffers from a paucity of prospective studies to determine both pregnancy rates and recurrence rates.

In a similar manner, progestin therapy was fashioned on the production of decidualization and eventual atrophy of endometrial like tissue. Medroxyprogesterone acetate dosages of 30 mg daily for 90 days administered to women with minimal to moderate endometriosis were associated with subjective and objective improvement. In eight of ten infertile women without male factor problems and in two of ten women with spouses with sperm abnormalities, continuing pregnancies were achieved.[45] Significant breakthrough bleeding and/or depression frequently detracted from medroxyprogesterone acetate regimens, even when the "depo" form was employed. Comparisons of this treatment to either control or placebo-treated groups of women with endometriosis matched according to stage are sorely lacking.

There also remains a dearth of knowledge about the exact recurrence rate of endometriosis after treatment with pseudopregnancy. The larger series of patients are marred by short periods of follow-up, whereas only limited numbers of patients have been followed for longer intervals of observation. During a 1-year period after completion of oral therapy with norethynodrel, Riva and co-workers[46] reported recurrences in 17.8% of patients, as did Kistner[47] in 16.6% of women.

Androgens

The scenario of critical studies remains the same for treatment with androgens before the synthesis of danazol. Furthermore, the daily dose of 5 to 10 mg of methyltestosterone sublingually, although effective in relieving dysmenorrhea and dyspareunia, does not consistently inhibit ovulation. However, higher dosages of methyltestosterone can be flagrantly masculinizing.[1] Hence, treatment with this agent poses the possibility of inadvertent genitourinary teratogenicity or virilization of a female fetus.

Danazol

The isoxazol derivative of 17α-ethinyl testosterone, danazol, has become the mainstay in the hormonal armamentarium effective against endometriosis. Although introduced through the literature by Greenblatt and associates in 1971,[48] it was not until a decade later that the intricate pharmacology of this drug was characterized.[49] Danazol effects a state of "pseudomenopause" by creating an endocrine environment that inhibits the growth of endometrial tissue. As summarized by Barbieri and Ryan,[49] this milieu is established by at least four major actions: (1) gonadotropin-releasing hormone (GnRH) and/or gonadotropin suppression, (2) direct interaction with androgen and P receptors; (3) direct inhibition of ovarian steroidogenesis; and (4) increased metabolic clearance of estradiol and P. The first of these effects of danazol can be further attributed to the prevention of the midcycle surge in the gonadally intact animal without significant depression of the basal levels of luteinizing hormone/follicle-stimulating hormone in gonadally intact women. However, danazol can prevent the compensatory rise in luteinizing hormone/follicle-stimulating hormone in castrated animals.[49]

In an attempt to evaluate the direct effect of danazol on endometriosis, 39 patients diagnosed at laparoscopy were relaparoscoped at the end of 3 to 11 months of this therapy.[50] At second-look laparoscopy, approximately 59% of these women had no evidence of disease, 26% had peritoneal adhesions and hemosiderin deposits without active disease, and 15% had residual, grossly identified endometriosis with inactive glands and stroma only.[50] In a more comprehensive clinical study, the same team of Dmowski and Cohen[51] followed 99 women who were diagnosed at laparoscopy or laparotomy, staged according to a self-defined classification similar to that of Acosta et al.,[38] treated with 800 mg daily of danazol for 3 to 18 months, and reevaluated clinically an average of 37 months later.[51] Symptomatic and clinical improvement was noted in > 85% of these women; and objective decreases in the extent of endometriotic lesions, with reduced congestion of pelvic organs, were visualized in 37 women who underwent repeat laparoscopy on the last day of treatment. Of 84 involuntarily infertile women, 39 conceived (46.4%), with the majority of pregnancies (23 of 39) occurring within the first 6 months of completing treatment and a total of 30 within the first year. The beneficial aspects of danazol were counterbalanced by a disturbing recurrence rate of 20% in the first year and 5% per year thereafter. These statistics of Dmowski and Cohen[51] were remarkably echoed by the prospective study of 100 consecutive cases of endometriosis diagnosed at laparoscopy, staged according to Kistner et al.,[39] treated with 800 mg of danazol daily for a mean of 17.3 weeks, and surgically reevaluated.[52] Symptoms decreased in 89%, lesions regressed in 94%, and pregnancies resulted in 46% (26 of 56) of patients. However, 15 of these 26 patients subsequently underwent conservative surgery, so the role of danazol cannot be fully evaluated. The important finding was that a course of danazol as outlined above resulted in a 40.9% uncorrected fertility rate in 22 patients with stage I endometriosis. Over the 5-year period of follow-up, 33% of the patients suffered recurrences, as judged by physical examination or symptoms.[52]

Tables 5 and 6 present the data relating to the two pivotal issues of pregnancy rate and recurrence rate in women with endometriosis after treatment with danazol. Particular attention has been focused upon inclusion of subsequent surgery in these patients in an effort to prognosticate more realistically the efficacy of danazol alone according to degree of endometriosis. From these studies it appears that danazol as sole therapy has been associated with pregnancy rates ranging from 30.9% to 52.6% in mild endometriosis, from 23.1% to 50% in moderate endometriosis, and from 0% to 100% in severe disease (Table 5).[51-57] The estimation of success rates in the latter category must be considered tenuous because of the small number of women in these groups. Hence, danazol appears better tailored to the woman with a mild to moderate degree of endometriosis. Although dosages of danazol cannot be conclusively compared in the same arena, 800 mg daily accompanies the higher pregnancy rates. Studies relating tubo-ovarian anatomical distortion to the percentages of conception are not available.

One of the most frustrating aspects of treating patients with endometriosis has been the recurrence rate. Danazol has fared tantamount to other regimens in this regard. As seen in Table 6, endometriotic lesions have been detected in 7.1% to 28.6% of women as early as the last day of danazol treatment.[50] Although the highest recurrence rates (51.6% overall)[55] have been reported when symptoms served as the diagnostic parameter, implants have been noted at repeat laparoscopy in 23.1% of patients 6 months after completing therapy.[53] Therefore, this temporizing, rather than curative, effect of danazol[50-54, 57] must be foremost in both rational design of our clinical protocols and appropriate education of our patients.

Dmowski and Cohen[51] observed two second- and third-trimester fetal deaths in women who had conceived within the first 3 months after discontinuing danazol. However, a subsequent series has not confirmed any deleterious effect of danazol on the outcome of proximally conceived pregnancies.[53] In this latter study of 36 pregnancies in 66 women after the end of danazol treatment, 5 normal full-term pregnancies were in women who had conceived without an intervening menstrual period after the end of danazol.[53] Barbieri et al.[52] found that in their series, the five pregnancies associated with danazol therapy that terminated in first-trimester spontaneous abortions were conceived more than 15 months after the completion of danazol.[52] Although 85 of 100 patients complained of significant side effects related to androgenicity and estrogen deprivation, only 1

Table 5. *Summary of Danazol Dose, Stage of Endometriosis, and Conceptions*

Reference	Dosage of danazol	Classification system	Stage of endometriosis	Pregnancy rate after danazol				Pregnancy rate after adjuvant surgery
				Gross		Corrected		
				%	(n)[a]	%	(n)[a]	
Dmowski and Cohen[51]	800 mg daily for 3–18 mos	Self-defined, approximating Acosta et al.[38]	Mild	52.6		83.3		—
			Moderate	45.7		72.7		—
			Severe	27.3		37.5		—
			Overall	46.4	(39/84)	72.2		—
Daniell and Christianson[53]	800 mg daily for 25 days, then 600 mg daily for 4 mos (mild) or 6 mos (moderate)	Acosta et al.[38]	Mild	57.1	(20/35)	70	(20/28)	—
			Moderate	56.0	(14/25)	64	(14/22)	—
			Severe	33.0	(2/6)[b]	—		1/2[b]
			Overall	55.0	(36/66)[b]	—		1/36[b]
Puleo and Hammond[54]	800 mg daily for 6 mos (mild and moderate) or 9 mos (severe)	Acosta et al.[38]	Mild	40.0	(4/10)	80.0	(4/5)	—
			Moderate	23.1	(3/13)	37.5	(3/8)	—
			Severe	33.0	(2/6)	66.7	(2/3)	—
			Overall	33.0	(9/29)	56.3	(9/16)	—
Barbieri et al.[52]	800 mg daily for 4–31 wks, mean of 17.3 wks	Kistner et al.[39]	I	50.0	(11/22)[b]	—		2/11[b]
			II	37.5	(6/16)[b]	—		5/6[b]
			III	45.5	(5/11)[b]	—		4/5[b]
			IV	57.1	(4/7)[b]	—		4/4[b]
			Overall	46.4	(26/56)[a]	—		15/26[b]
Moore et al.[55]	600 mg daily	Acosta et al.[38]	Mild, moderate, or severe	20.0	(2/10)	—		—
	400 mg daily			0	(0/5)	—		—
	200 mg daily			50.0	(4/8)	—		—
	100 mg daily for 6 mos			28.6	(2/7)	—		—
			Overall	26.7	(8/30)	—		—
Butler et al.[56]	800 mg daily	Acosta et al.[38] or AFS[40]	Mild	30.9	(17/55)	—		—
	600 mg daily		I	20.0	(1/5)	—		—
	400 mg daily for 6 mos			20.0	(3/15)	—		—
			Overall	28.0	(21/75)	—		—
Buttram et al.[57]	800 mg daily	Acosta et al.[38]	Mild	50.0	(6/12)	—		9/11
			Moderate	50.0	(1/2)	—		12/16
			Severe	—	(0)	—		9/16
			Overall	50.0	(7/14)	—		30/43
	400 mg daily		Mild	36.0	(9/25)	—		2/2
			Moderate	50.0	(8/16)	—		6/10
			Severe	100	(3/3)	—		10/20
			Overall	45.5	(20/44)	—		18/32

[a]Number of women conceiving/total number of infertile women.

[b]Pregnancy rate after danazol includes surgical therapy because ratio reflects the number of patients treated with danazol and conservative laparotomy/number of patients conceiving.

discontinued therapy because of the side effects.[52] The common and uncommon side effects are listed in Table 7. Considering the pharmacology of danazol in the light of known side effects, the contraindications to this therapy remain few. Obviously, pregnancy and breast-feeding would expose a fetus to the potential induction of urogenital abnormalities[58] or the neonate to virilization.

Although the diminutive effect of danazol on active endometriotic tissue has been well documented and pregnancies have followed treatment, the efficacy of danazol versus OCs is not a well-traversed subject. Noble and Letchworth[59] conducted a small prospective, randomized study that compared 17 patients who received 75 μg mestranol/5 mg norethynodrel with 25 women

Table 6. *Recurrence Rate After Danazol Treatment with Reference to Stage of Disease, Method of Determining Recurrence, and Interval of Observation After Completing Danazol Therapy*

Reference	Method of determining recurrence	Stage or dosage of danazol[a]	Recurrence rate		Interval between completion of danazol therapy and recurrence
			Ratio	%	
Dmowski and Cohen[50]	Repeat laparoscopy	Mild	1/14	7.1	None (performed on last day of danazol therapy)
		Moderate	3/18	16.7	
		Severe	2/7	28.6	
		Overall	6/39	15.4	
Dmowski and Cohen[51]	Patient symptoms	Mild	11/44	25.0	48 mos
		Moderate	20/42	47.6	
		Severe	8/13	61.5	
		Overall	39/99	39.4	
Daniell and Christianson[53]	Repeat laparoscopy	Mild	1/8	12.5	6 mos
		Moderate	2/11	18.2	
		Overall	3/13[b]	23.1	
Puleo and Hammond[54]	Recurrent dysmenorrhea or pelvic pain	Mild	4/12	33.3	3–9 mos
		Moderate	6/16	37.5	
		Severe	5/11	45.5	
		Overall	15/39	38.5	
Moore et al.[55]	Patient symptoms	Minimal	2/11	18.2	1 yr
		Moderate	4/8	50.0	
		Severe	10/19	52.6	
		Overall	16/31[c]	51.6	
		600 mg	7/11	63.6	
		400 mg	2/9	22.2	
		200 mg	4/10	40.0	
		100 mg	3/8	37.5	
		Overall	16/31[c]	51.6	
Barbieri et al.[52]	Physical findings or symptoms	I	9/41	22.0	5 yrs
		II	13/32	40.6	
		III	5/15	33.3	
		IV	6/12	50.0	
		Overall	33/100	33.0	
Buttram et al.[57]	Second-look laparoscopy or laparotomy	800 mg			None
		Mild	38% peritoneal, 58% ovarian[d]		
		Moderate			
		Severe			
		400 mg			
		Mild	45% peritoneal, 56% ovarian[d]		
		Moderate			
		Severe			

[a]Daily dose. Where dosage not specified, patients treated as a group with 800 mg daily or slight variation as described in Table 7.
[b]Denominator reflects 6 of 19 women were lost to follow-up.
[c]Denominator reflects 7 of 38 women were lost to follow-up.
[d]Based upon resolution rates determined by surgeon.

who were treated with danazol in dosages of 400 to 800 mg daily to the point of amenorrhea (Table 8).[59] Although danazol dramatically reduced endometriotic plaques, large masses, dense fibrosis, and scar tissue were not resolved by either treatment. Danazol emerged superior to mestranol/norethynodrel treatment for symptomatic relief of mild to moderate disease. However, a high at-

Table 7. *Side Effects Associated with Danazol Treatment Compiled from Barbieri et al.[52] and Buttram et al.[57]*

	Side effects
Common	Weight gain
	Edema
	Decreased breast size
	Acne, hirsutism, oily skin
	Deepening of voice
Uncommon	Menorrhagia
	Headache
	Vaginitis
	Decreased libido
	Muscle cramps
	Hot flashes
	Mood changes
	Skin rash
	Nausea
	Fatigue
	Sweating

trition rate secondary to side effects of the OCs may have skewed objective results. Of note is the lack of difference in subsequent pregnancy rate and the absence of follow-up for the determination of comparative recurrence rates.[59]

GONADOTROPIN-RELEASING HORMONE

In addition to pseudopregnancy and pseudomenopause, the availability of the GnRH agonist offers the most recent weapon in hormonal therapy. This "medical oophorectomy" allows temporary suppression of ovarian function without the transient stimulation of estrogenic substances or the inconveniences of androgenic ones. A pilot 28-day study of five women with proven endometriosis treated daily with subcutaneous doses of a potent GnRH agonist showed suppression of ovarian estrogens and androgen levels like that in oophorectomized women[60] and popularized the potential use of "medical oophorectomy" for endometriosis. In six women, including four prior danazol failures, a 6-month course of a long-acting GnRH analog ([imB21] DHis^6, Pro^6-NET)-GnRH on a daily subcutaneous injection protocol produced subjective improvement but also resulted in hot flashes after 1 month of therapy.[61] On repeat laparoscopy, five women had histologically inactive peritoneal endometriosis, whereas one had active ovarian disease. Steingold et al.[61] admit that although treatment effects castrate estrogen levels associated with regression of lesions, menopausal symptoms of vaginal thinning and increased calcium excretion are also induced. Long-term consequences and recurrences have not yet been determined. The possible addition of estrogen/progestin replacement to a GnRH eradication therapy for endometriosis may be a viable alternative to women's suffering from hypoestrogenicity.

The crux of the treatment of endometriosis is the efficacy of intervention in early stage disease because the natural progression of endometriosis remains elusive. This dilemma has been approached from two directions. First, the role of expectant management in minimal to mild endometriosis has been explored in comparison to surgical and hormonal therapies. This literature will be perused after addressing the effect of surgical management. Second, in an attempt to reduce variation in patient selection and to establish danazol effectiveness in mild endometriosis, Butler et al.[56] preceded danazol therapy with a postlaparoscopy 3-month interval of coital exposure. In this collaborative study at six medical centers, 75 patients were treated with danazol for 6 months in dosages of 800 mg (73.3% of patients), 600 mg (6.7% of patients), and 400 mg (20.0% of patients). Only 28.0% of patients conceived, and only 20.0% of patients had viable pregnancies. These investigators concluded that the pregnancy rate in infertile patients with mild endometriosis treated with danazol is lower than previously reported and probably similar to spontaneous conception rates. Their failure to report the number of patients conceiving immediately after laparoscopy detracts from the homogeneity of their group of danazol-treated patients. Furthermore, the higher pregnancy rate (30.9%) in patients taking 800 mg/day needs to be compared more systematically with conception rates in women receiving

Table 8. *Comparison of Symptomatic and Laparoscopic Improvement, Requirement for Total Abdominal Hysterectomy and Bilateral Salpingo-oophorectomy (TAHBSO), Severity of Side Effects, and Pregnancy Rates in Women Treated with Danazol or 75 μg Mestranol/5 mg Norethynodrel (Data Summarized from Noble and Letchworth[59])*

	Danazol	Mestranol/ norethynodrel
Total no. of patients with endometriosis	25	17
Symptomatic improvement	18/21 (86%)	3/10 (30%)
Improvement on laparoscopy after treatment	21/25 (84%)	3/17 (18%)
TAHBSO required	1/25 (4%)	3/17 (18%)
Discontinuation secondary to side effects	1/25 (4%)	7/17 (41%)
Pregnancy rate	58% (7/12)	40% (4/10)

600 mg (20%) and 400 mg (20%). No reference was made to the menstrual status of the women during danazol therapy in the sense that only amenorrhea may bespeak an adequate dosage.[56] The question of optimal dosage has been addressed, but not answered, by Moore et al.[55] in a randomized double-blind study of 38 women given 100 to 600 mg/day. Although 71% of women (27 of 38) were found to have improvement at repeat laparoscopy, conceptions occurred in only 28% of those women (8 of 28), with a follow-up ranging from 6 to 14 months. Again, their lower conception rate may reflect insufficient dose or duration of medication, as is consistent with the 51% recurrence rate within 1 year of the discontinuation of danazol. Alternatively, the group studied may not have been homogeneous because 10 of the 38 women had previously undergone conservative surgery.[55]

CONSERVATIVE SURGERY

Although the definition of conservative surgery has remained "the destruction of as much endometriosis as possible with preservation of childbearing function," the technical advances of in vitro fertilization-embryo transfer and embryo donation permit maintenance of a uterus to be the sole prerequisite for implantation and delivery of a viable infant. Therefore, our ideas of surgical removal of endometriosis in the woman interested in bearing a child will evolve dramatically over the next few years. Similarly, the tools of surgery are expanding from the scalpel to include the laser used at both laparoscopy and laparotomy. Critical studies of this latter instrument in treatment of endometriosis are limited. Therefore, a review of more traditional surgical methods will serve as a basis for later comparisons.

Without segregation according to the stage of endometriosis, pregnancy rates after conservative surgery range from 33.3% to 87.5%.[62] On the other hand, intelligent reference to the stage of disease more succinctly describes chances of conception as 66.0% to 75.0% in mild disease, 36.8% to 74.0% in moderate endometriosis, and 0% to 48% in severe endometriosis.[62]

In addition to pregnancy rates, the incidence of subsequent operations after conservative surgery also appears to correlate with the severity of disease at the initial surgery. Of 117 patients followed for 3 years after conservative operations for endometriosis, a second operative procedure for recurrent pain and/or infertility occurred in 14.3% of women with mild endometriosis, 23.5% of patients with moderate disease, and in 40.6% of women with severe endometriosis.[63] Three of 26 of these women whose second operation had been conservative achieved a pregnancy, and another 3 required definitive surgery for relief of recurrent pain. Hence, the chance of pregnancy (approximately 12%) after a second palliative procedure equaled the possibility of castration. It must be realized that only four of the six patients who underwent repeat removal of endometriosis had infertility workups that identified endometriosis as the sole factor in infertility.[63] This shortcoming in defining different groups of patients with endometriosis was reflected in a later review from the same senior author.[64] Of 423 patients treated by conservative operations, 62 required second procedures; but the severity of endometriosis was not predictive of the operative recurrence rate. Furthermore, this larger analysis revealed a more favorable prognosis for conception after second conservative operation in that 10 of 20 patients (50%) desiring pregnancy did conceive. Therefore, these two reports[63, 64] illustrate that the contrasting results of different institutions concerning success rates and recurrences cannot be explained simply by the differing nuances of operative techniques. Not only was the private practice base unchanged, but the time overlap may have signaled incorporation of some of the same patients into both these reports. Hence, the predictive capacity of any retrospective study not using stringent criteria to reevaluate surgically all patients after conservative operations needs to be viewed at face value. In both these studies, pregnancy after the first operative procedure seemed to affect the occurrence of the second procedure by either decreasing the incidence of reoperation from 40.6% in persistently infertile women to 3.7% in women who had conceived[63] or by increasing the interoperative interval from a mean of 37 months to a mean of 47 months.[64] Again, psychologic ramifications of successful attainment of a conception may have obviated the need for follow-up surgical manipulation, which would be guided instead by the patient's tolerance of painful recurrences. The enigmatic spectrum of this disease also must be considered.

Improved pregnancy rates have been reported with atraumatic microsurgical techniques that employ loupes and the microscope for magnification and the intraabdominal laser. The former procedures were used in 176 infertile women whose cumulative pregnancy rates with the use of life-table methods were 28.8% after 1 year, 40.5% after 2 years, and 60% after 4 years.[65] There was no statistically significant difference in the cumulative pregnancy rates between mild, moderate, or severe groups. Therefore, these authors[65] suggest that careful reconstruction of tubo-ovarian interfaces and the surrounding peritoneum, without incidental appendectomy or presacral neurectomy, may equalize the chances of conception among the stages of endometriosis.

Similarly, the carbon dioxide laser has been proposed to be optimal for endometriotic resection. Vaporization of focal implants, excision of endometriotic cysts, and lysis of adhesions were performed in 54 patients with stage II to IV endometriosis. Although 66.7% of the patients were followed for a period of less than 1 year, pregnancies resulted in 14 of 23 women interested in conceiving (60.8%).[66] Of the 14 women who became pregnant, 11 had received 800 mg of danazol daily for 6 to 9 months after the laser operative procedure. Although Chong and Baggish[66] detail both laser equipment and manipulation for vaporization, lysis of adhesions, and ovarian excision, they concede that the merit of this treatment requires prospective randomized scrutiny.

COMBINED THERAPY

The coupling of hormonal suppression with surgical therapy in either the immediately preoperative or postoperative period has remained controversial. In a study before the era of the staging of endometriosis, Andrews and Larsen[67] found that the pregnancy rate of 39 infertile women treated with operation alone (59%) was significantly higher than the pregnancy rates of 7 women given pseudopregnancy alone (43%) or of 24 women treated with combined sequential therapy of operation and pseudopregnancy (21%).[67] Although the failure to randomize treatment prohibits direct comparison of the two modalities, this study does suggest the detrimental postoperative effect of "precious time lost by iatrogenically induced anovulation."[67] Contradictory evidence for postoperative suppression of ovarian function emerges from a pregnancy rate of 79% in 19 women with severe endometriosis treated with extirpative laparotomy immediately followed by danazol therapy versus 30% in 119 women with severe disease treated with comparable laparotomy alone.[68] Six of the 19 patients required 200 mg of danazol twice daily to achieve the prescribed 3 months of amenorrhea, whereas 13 of these women achieved this goal only in response to 600 to 800 mg daily for a period of up to 6 months. Although the two groups of patients are characterized by Wheeler and Malinak,[68] the reason fostering adjuvant danazol is not explored. Furthermore, correction of concomitant infertility factors, present in 47% of the surgery group versus 21% of the combined group, or previous nonperioperative hormonal treatment may have skewed results.[68] In fact, a more recent report[57] of a prospective, nonrandomized evaluation of danazol from the same institution portrays the addition of danazol to surgical treatment as less effective than surgery alone. Only 32% of 24 patients treated with 800-mg or 400-mg regimens of danazol conceived, compared with 56% of an "historical control group." However, preoperative danazol therapy resulted in a higher pregnancy rate (64%) than its use postoperatively or when conservative surgery alone was used.[57] Thus, Buttram et al.[57] suggest that decreased pelvic vasculature and inflammation in patients with endometriosis treated with danazol may reduce the risk of postoperative adhesion formation. They advise a short preoperative course of a reduced dosage of danazol to effect this amelioration.[57]

DANAZOL VERSUS CONSERVATIVE SURGERY IN MILD TO MODERATE DISEASE

Dissolution of thick adhesions, deagglutination of distally occluded fallopian tubes, or correction of a distorted tubo-ovarian juxtaposition have not been accomplished by danazol therapy alone. Therefore, surgical correction must be efficaciously chosen in such cases of severe endometriosis. In contrast, minimal to moderate endometriosis invites a direct comparison. Guzick and Rock[69] retrospectively analyzed the cumulative pregnancy rates of 224 infertile women, without other obvious causes of infertility, diagnosed with mild or moderate endometriosis, comparing 91 women who chose to receive 4 to 12 months of 400 to 800 mg/day danazol with 133 women who underwent conservative surgery as their sole mode of therapy. A shorter follow-up period for the danazol group was offered to explain the higher gross pregnancy rate for the surgery group (57%) than for the danazol group (33%). However, cumulative pregnancy curves for the two groups "virtually coincided." There was no statistically significant difference between the cure rate effected by danazol (68.3%) and that associated with surgery (74.0%). Similarly, spontaneous abortions terminated 10% of pregnancies in each group. Although the expert use of statistical tools critically evaluates the two therapies, the authors acknowledge the element of patient preference guided by physician prejudice in choosing therapy.[69]

EXPECTANT MANAGEMENT IN PATIENTS WITH MINIMAL TO MILD ENDOMETRIOSIS

The final "Pandora's box" to be opened during this review is the role of the passage of undisturbed menstrual cycles, artfully exposed to coital experience, in the woman suffering from minimal to mild endometriosis. Initiation of therapy is clinically warranted when disease is severe and probably when it is moderate. However, the decision to subject an infertile patient to either surgical resection or 6 months of hormonal intervention has rested, as presented, on uncontrolled retrospective results without comparisons to appropriate control populations.

Despite the reams of literature attesting to the efficacy of danazol in effecting pregnancies in women with early stage disease, Seibel et al.[70] conducted a long-awaited, justified prospective study. Stage I endometriosis, as classified according to Kistner et al.,[39] was diagnosed by laparoscopy in 65 women who underwent dilatation and curettage and tubal lavage and who were randomly assigned to receive either no treatment for 6 months or danazol for 6 months followed by no treatment for an additional 6 months.[70] Twenty of 32 "danazol patients" completed the study (only 3 patients failed to continue taking danazol), as did 28 of the 32 "no danazol patients." Pregnancies occurred in 30% of the danazol patients and 50% of those managed expectantly, which is not a statistically significant difference. As suggestd by these authors, a beneficial effect on infertility may be wrought by diagnostic laparoscopy, a dilatation and curettage, or mechanical tubal lavage.[70] Alternatively, their removal of dye at termination of the procedure may have altered the peritoneal macrophages[13] or prostanoid concentration.[17, 18, 20, 21] This prospective study[70] reiterates the data suggested by the cumulative pregnancy rate of 61.2% within 18 months in a small group of 31 patients not treated after laparoscopy.[71]

Table 9. *Therapeutic Recommendations for Women with Endometriosis*

Therapy	Disease factors
Expectant management	Infertility with minimal to mild disease after diagnostic laparoscopy and chromotubation (possibly dilatation and curettage)
Danazol	1. Infertility with mild to moderate disease 2. Future fertility desired with mild or moderate disease 3. One year after conservative surgery without conception
Pseudopregnancy	As for danazol when cost is a factor
Androgens	1. Fertility not desired 2. Few symptoms 3. Surgery not appropriate
Conservative surgery	1. Infertility with moderate to severe disease 2. Future fertility with severe disease 3. Failed hormonal therapy 4. Infertility with age as additional factor
Total abdominal hysterectomy and bilateral salpingo-oophorectomy	1. Future fertility not desired 2. Failed conservative surgery or hormonal therapy

The merit of expectant management was evident in two other studies in which the treated groups had undergone surgical resection. Of 17 patients with minimal endometriosis who received only emotional support after their diagnostic endoscopies, 11 (64.7%) became pregnant.[72] This mirrored the 66.7% conception rate in three patients treated surgically.[72] Similarly, Schenken and Malinak[73] retrospectively studied 45 infertile patients with mild endometriosis diagnosed by endoscopy and followed with dilatation and endometrial biopsy. Twenty-one of 29 patients (72.4%) who had undergone conservative surgery conceived within 1 year, as did 12 of the 16 patients (75%) who had fortuitously decided to postpone surgery. Whether or not those patients had also undergone tubal lavage during the diagnostic endoscopy was not revealed, but tubal patency had been evaluated previously by hysterosalpingogram.[73]

Incorporating the appropriate potency of expectant management in treating women with mild endometriosis, a schema of therapeutic recommendations is proposed in Table 9. The intention of this menu is to reflect the composite of clinical studies surrounding endometriosis and not to limit the practitioner in making cogent decisions about each patient's treatment.

SUMMARY

The enigmatic disease of endometriosis continues to baffle both the scientist and the clinician. An encompassing theory of pathogenesis has failed to emerge from contemporary understanding of the immunologic manifestations, the hormonal aberrations, or the evasive infertility associated with endometriosis. Similarly unsettling is the failure of medical or conservative surgical maneuvers to eradicate endometriosis in a manner commensurate with castration. It is hoped that further insight into these areas of research will resolve both of these dilemmas.

Acknowledgment. I would like to thank Ms. Audrey Bergenty for her diligent assistance in preparation of this manuscript.

REFERENCES

1. Kistner RW: Endometriosis and infertility. Clin Obstet Gynecol 22:101, 1979
2. Sampson JA: Peritoneal endometriosis due to the menstrual dissemination of endometrial tissue into the peritoneal cavity. Am J Obstet Gynecol 14:422, 1927
3. Novak E: The significance of uterine mucosa in the fallopian tubes with a discussion of the origin of aberrant endometrium. Am J Obstet Gynecol 12:484, 1926
4. Halban J: Hysteroadenosis Metastica. Wien Klin Wochenschr 37:1205, 1924
5. Halme J, Hammond MG, Hulka JF, Raj SG, Talbert LM: Retrograde menstruation in healthy women and in patients with endometriosis. Obstet Gynecol 64:151, 1984
6. Simpson JL, Elias S, Malinak LR, Buttram VC Jr: Heritable aspects of endometriosis: I. Genetic studies. Am J Obstet Gynecol 137:327, 1980
7. Muse KN, Wilson EA: How does mild endometriosis cause infertility? Fertil Steril 38:145, 1982
8. Weed JC, Arquembourg PC: Endometriosis: can it produce an autoimmune response resulting in infertility? Clin Obstet Gynecol 23:885, 1980
9. Badawy SZA, Cuenca V, Stitzel A, Jacobs RDB, Tomar RH: Autoimmune phenomena in infertile patients with endometriosis. Obstet Gynecol 63:271, 1984
10. Mathur S, Peress MR, Williamson HO, Youmans CD, Maney SA, Garvin AJ, Rust PF, Fudenberg HH: Autoimmunity to endometrium and ovary in endometriosis. Clin Exp Immunol 50:259, 1982
11. Barbieri RL, Bast RC, Niloff JM, Kistner RW, Knapp RC: Evaluation of a serological test for the diagnosis of endometriosis using a monoclonal antibody OC-125. Presented at the Annual Meeting of the Society for Gynecologic Investigation, March 1985. Abstract 33/P
12. Steele RW, Dmowski WP, Marmar DJ: Immunologic aspects of human endometriosis. Am J Reprod Immunol 6:33, 1984
13. Muscato JJ, Haney AF, Weinberg JB: Sperm phagocytosis by human peritoneal macrophages: a possible cause of infertility in endometriosis. Am J Obstet Gynecol 144:503, 1982
14. Halme J, Becker S, Hammond MG, Raj MHG, Raj S: Increased activation of pelvic macrophages in infertile women with mild endometriosis. Am J Obstet Gynecol 145:333, 1983
15. Haney AF, Misukonis MA, Weinberg JB: Macrophages and infertility: oviductal macrophages as potential mediators of infertility. Fertil Steril 39:310, 1983
16. Gleicher N, Dmowski WP, Siegel I, Liv TL, Friberg J, Radwanska E, Toder V: Lymphocyte subsets in endometriosis. Obstet Gynecol 63:463, 1984
17. Drake TS, O'Brien WF, Ramwell PW, Metz SA: Peritoneal fluid thromboxane B_2 and 6-keto-prostaglandin $F_{1\alpha}$ in endometriosis. Am J Obstet Gynecol 140:401, 1981
18. Badawy SZA, Marshall L, Gabal AA, Nusbaum ML: The concentration of 13,14-dihydro-15-keto prostaglandin $F_{2\alpha}$ and prostaglandin E_2 in peritoneal fluid of infertile patients with and without endometriosis. Fertil Steril 38:166, 1982
19. Rock JA, Dubin NH, Ghodgaonkar RB, Bergquist CA, Erozan YS, Kimball AW Jr: Cul-de-sac fluid in women with endometriosis: fluid volume and prostanoid concentration during the proliferative phase of the cycle—days 8 to 12. Fertil Steril 37:747, 1982
20. Dawood MY, Khan-Dawood FS, Wilson L: Peritoneal fluid prostaglandins and prostanoids in women with endometriosis, chronic pelvic inflammatory disease, and pelvic pain. Am J Obstet Gynecol 148:391, 1984
21. DeLeon FD, Vijayakumar R, Rao CV, Yussman MA: Correlation of peritoneal fluid prostaglandin (PG) to estradiol (E_2) and progesterone (P) levels in women with endometriosis. Presented at the Annual Meeting of the Society for Gynecologic Investigation, March 1984. Abstract 269P
22. Maathuis JB, VanLook PFA, Nichie EA: Changes in volume, total protein and ovarian steroid concentration of peritoneal fluid throughout the human menstrual cycle. J Endocrinol 76:123, 1978
23. Roddick JW Jr, Conkey G, Jacobs EJ: The hormonal response of endometrium in endometriotic implants and its relationship to symptomatology. Am J Obstet Gynecol 79:1173, 1960
24. Prakash SJ, Ulfelder H, Cohen RB: Enzyme-histochemical observations on endometriosis. Am J Obstet Gynecol 91:990, 1965
25. Schweppe KW, Wynn R: Ultrastructural changes in endometriotic implants during the menstrual cycle. Obstet Gynecol 58:465, 1981
26. Gould SF, Shannon JM, Cunha GR: Nuclear estrogen binding sites in human endometriosis. Fertil Steril 39:520, 1983
27. Vierikko P, Kauppila A, Rönnberg L, Vihko R: Steroidal regulation of endometriosis tissue: lack of induction of 17β hydroxysteroid dehydrogenase activity by progesterone, medroxyprogesterone acetate, or danazol. Fertil Steril 43:218, 1985
28. Maslar I, Riddick DH: Prolactin production by human endometrium during the normal menstrual cycle. Am J Obstet Gynecol 135:751, 1979
29. Haney AF, Handwerger S, Weinberg JB: Peritoneal fluid prolactin in infertile women with endometriosis: lack of evidence of secretory activity by endometrial implants. Fertil Steril 42:935, 1984

30. Schmidt CL, Demopoulos RI, Weiss G: Infected endometriotic cysts: clinical characterization and pathogenesis. Fertil Steril 36:27, 1981
31. Schmidt CL: Unpublished data
32. Hirschowitz JS, Soler NG, Wortsman J: The galactorrhea-endometriosis syndrome. Lancet 1:896, 1978
33. Hargrove JT, Abraham GE: Abnormal luteal function in endometriosis. Fertil Steril 34:302, 1980
34. Brosens IA, Koninckx PR, Corvelyn PA: A study of plasma progesterone, oestradiol-17β, prolactin and LH levels, and the luteal phase appearance of the ovaries in patients with endometriosis and infertility. Br J Obstet Gynaecol 85:246, 1978
35. Pittaway DE, Maxson W, Daniell J, Herbert C, Wentz AC: Luteal phase defects in infertility patients with endometriosis. Fertil Steril 39:712, 1983
36. Radwanska E, Henig I, Rana N, Dmowski WP: Nocturnal prolactin (PRL) levels in infertile women with and without endometriosis. Presented at the Annual Meeting of the Society for Gynecologic Investigation, March 1985. Abstract 109P
37. Daly DC, Walters CA, Soto-Albors CE, Riddick DH: Endometrial biopsy during treatment of luteal phase defects is predictive of therapeutic outcome. Fertil Steril 40:305, 1983
38. Acosta AA, Buttram VC Jr, Besch PK, Malinak LR, Franklin RR, Vanderheyden JD: A proposed classification of pelvic endometriosis. Obstet Gynecol 42:19, 1973
39. Kistner RW, Siegler AM, Behrman SJ: Suggested classification for endometriosis: relationship to infertility. Fertil Steril 28:1008, 1977
40. American Fertility Society: Classification of endometriosis. Fertil Steril 32:633, 1979
41. Buttram VC Jr: Evolution of the Revised American Fertility Society Classification of Endometriosis. Fertil Steril 43:347, 1985
42. American Fertility Society: Revised American Fertility Society Classification of Endometriosis: 1985. Fertil Steril 43:351, 1985
43. Kistner RW: The treatment of endometriosis by inducing pseudopregnancy with ovarian hormones: a report of 58 cases. Fertil Steril 10:539, 1959
44. Luciano AA, Pitkin RM: Endometriosis: approaches to diagnosis and treatment. Surg Annu 16:297, 1984
45. Moghissi KS, Boyce CR: Management of endometriosis with oral medroxyprogesterone acetate. Obstet Gynecol 47:265, 1976
46. Riva HL, Wilson JH, Kawasaki DM: Effect of norethynodrel on endometriosis. Am J Obstet Gynecol 82:109, 1961
47. Kistner RW: Infertility with endometriosis: a plan of therapy. Fertil Steril 13:237, 1962
48. Greenblatt RB, Dmowski WP, Mahesh VB, Scholer HFL: Clinical studies with an antigonadotropin—danazol. Fertil Steril 22:102, 1971
49. Barbieri RL, Ryan KJ: Danazol: endocrine pharmacology and therapeutic applications. Am J Obstet Gynecol 141:453, 1981
50. Dmowski WP, Cohen MR: Treatment of endometriosis with an antigonadotropin, danazol: a laparoscopic and histologic evaluation. Obstet Gynecol 46:147, 1975
51. Dmowski WP, Cohen MR: Antigonadotropin (danazol) in the treatment of endometriosis: evaluation of post-treatment fertility and three-year follow-up data. Am J Obstet Gynecol 130:41, 1978
52. Barbieri RL, Evans S, Kistner RW: Danazol in the treatment of endometriosis: analysis of 100 cases with a 4-year follow-up. Fertil Steril 37:737, 1982
53. Daniell JF, Christianson C: Combined laparoscopic surgery and danazol therapy for pelvic endometriosis. Fertil Steril 35:521, 1981
54. Puleo JG, Hammond CB: Conservative treatment of endometriosis externa: the effects of danazol therapy. Fertil Steril 40:164, 1983
55. Moore EE, Harger JH, Rock JA, Archer DF: Management of pelvic endometriosis with low-dose danazol. Fertil Steril 36:15, 1981
56. Butler L, Wilson E, Belisle S, Gibson M, Albrecht B, Schiff I, Stillman R: Collaborative study of pregnancy rates following danazol therapy of stage I endometriosis. Fertil Steril 41:373, 1984
57. Buttram VC Jr, Reiter RC, Ward S: Treatment of endometriosis with danazol: report of a 6-year prospective study. Fertil Steril 43:353, 1985
58. Duck SC, Katayama KP: Danazol may cause female pseudohermaphroditism. Fertil Steril 35:230, 1981
59. Noble AD, Letchworth AT: Medical treatment of endometriosis: a comparative trial. Postgrad Med J (Suppl 5) 55:37, 1979
60. Meldrum DR, Chang RJ, Lu J, Vale W, Rivier J, Judd HL: "Medical Oophorectomy" using a long-acting GnRH agonist—a possible new approach to the treatment of endometriosis. J Clin Endocrinol Metab 54:1081, 1982
61. Steingold KA, Lu JKH, Randle D, Moore JG, Judd HL, Meldrum DR: Treatment of endometriosis with a long acting GnRH analog—a blinded evaluation. Presented at the Annual Meeting of the Society for Gynecologic Investigation, March 1985. Abstract 246
62. Malinak LR: Infertility and endometriosis: operative technique, clinical staging, and prognosis. Clin Obstet Gynecol 23:925, 1980
63. Schenken RS, Malinak LR: Reoperation after initial treatment of endometriosis with conservative surgery. Am J Obstet Gynecol 131:416, 1978
64. Wheeler JM, Malinak LR: Recurrent endometriosis: incidence, management, and prognosis. Am J Obstet Gynecol 146:247, 1983
65. Gordts S, Boeckx W, Brosens I: Microsurgery of endometriosis in infertile patients. Fertil Steril 42:520, 1984
66. Chong AP, Baggish MS: Management of pelvic endometriosis by means of intraabdominal carbon dioxide laser. Fertil Steril 41:14, 1984
67. Andrews WC, Larsen GD: Endometriosis: treatment with hormonal pseudopregnancy and/or operation. Am J Obstet Gynecol 118:643, 1974
68. Wheeler JM, Malinak LR: Postoperative danazol therapy in infertility patients with severe endometriosis. Fertil Steril 36:460, 1981
69. Guzick DS, Rock JA: A comparison of danazol and conservative surgery for the treatment of infertility due to mild or moderate endometriosis. Fertil Steril 40:580, 1983
70. Seibel MM, Berger MJ, Weinstein FG, Taymor ML: The effectiveness of danazol on subsequent fertility in minimal endometriosis. Fertil Steril 38:534, 1982

71. Portuondo JA, Echanojauregui AD, Herran C, Alijarte I: Early conception in patients with untreated mild endometriosis. Fertil Steril 39:22, 1983
72. Garcia C-R, David SS: Pelvic endometriosis: infertility and pelvic pain. Am J Obstet Gynecol 129:740, 1977
73. Schenken RS, Malinak LR: Conservative surgery versus expectant management for the infertile patient with mild endometriosis. Fertil Steril 37:183, 1982

Chapter 22

Peritoneal fluid environment and infertility

Craig H. Syrop, M.D.
Jouko Halme, M.D., Ph.D.

The University of Iowa Hospitals and Clinics, Iowa City, Iowa and University of North Carolina School of Medicine, Chapel Hill, North Carolina

Although the presence of small amounts of fluid in the pelvis has been recognized for over 60 years,[1] the widespread use of laparoscopy has generated further interest in peritoneal fluid. Changes in fluid volume as well as concentration of a variety of cells, hormones, and other compounds have been characterized during normal menstrual cycles and in pathologic conditions.[2] The peritoneal fluid (PF) microenvironment has been recognized as a dynamic zone of gamete interaction, sensitive to the influences of pathologic conditions and possessing constituents capable of having impact on reproductive processes. Further exploration of this compartment that bathes the fallopian tubes and ovaries and provides the stage for sperm-oocyte transport, fertilization, and cleavage may grant insight into the various mechanisms of reproductive failure.

Although ongoing interactions between the cellular and molecular components of PF must be assumed, each will be considered separately in normal conditions, pathologic states, and as potential mediators of infertility.

CELLULAR AND ACELLULAR COMPONENTS OF PERITONEAL FLUID UNDER PHYSIOLOGIC CONDITIONS

Peritoneal Fluid Volume

PF does not arise as a result of tubal secretory activity,[3] but is considered to be an ovarian exudate. Although the total peritoneal fluid volume (PFV) receives a contribution from follicular rupture, follicular contents do not account exclusively for persistently high PFV.[4] Indeed, PFV of women without an ovulation stigma noted does not differ from that in ovulatory women.[3,4] PFV depends on follicular activity, corpus luteum vascularity, and hormonal production[4–6]; it reaches its peak during the third week of the menstrual cycle.[2,5] Women on oral contraceptives have decreased PFV,[2] approaching that of menopausal women.[6]

Cellular Components

In women with patent fallopian tubes, PF receives a portion of menstrual detritus on a cyclic basis. Halme et al.[7] found that significantly fewer perimenstrual samples from women with occluded tubes had red blood cells present compared to women with patent tubes. Approximately 90% of normal women experience retrograde menstruation, with 70% exhibiting grossly bloody PF during menstruation. Endometrial glands, presumably transported via the fallopian tubes, have been noted in PF under normal circumstances[8,9] and following uterine procedures.[8,10] Excluding these few endometrial cells, approximately 82% to 98% of nucleated peritoneal cells are peritoneal macrophages (PMs), lymphocytes constituting the remaining 10%.[11,12] It is generally assumed that peripheral blood monocytes[13] migrate into the peritoneal cavity and differentiate into actively phagocytizing macrophages[11,14] that are also present in the oviducts.[15] In the older literature,[1] the PMs were often described as mesothelial cells; however, it is now recognized that they are, in fact, the same entity. Approximately 6 to 7 million macrophages are normally present in the peritoneal cavity and, although disputed,[16] no proven cyclic changes have occurred in the PM concentration and total count.[5] The main physiologic function of the PMs is considered to be phagocytosis of cellular debris, sperm, and red blood cells. Other potentially physiologic functions include a luteotropic effect on the developing corpus luteum and cumulus-corona complex of the ovulated oocyte, since macrophages are capable of influencing granulosa-luteal cell progesterone production.[17]

Acellular Components of Peritoneal Fluid

Just as PFV exhibits cyclic changes, the concentration and/or content of many of its acellular constituents are influenced by the changing hormonal environment, fluid shifts, or ovulation during the menstrual cycle.

Serum Proteins

Maathuis et al.[2] first noted that the total protein concentration of PF remained fairly constant throughout the menstrual cycle, but was lower during the late proliferative phase. Subsequently, others[4,18] have demonstrated that PF total protein, transcortin, and sex hormone binding globulin increase in the luteal phase while serum levels remain constant. Peritoneal fluid concentrations of albumin, α_1-globulins, β-globulins, α_1-antitrypsin, C_3 and C_4 proteins are all cycle-dependent, but levels of IgA, IgM, and possibly IgG are not.[4] In general, the higher the molecular weight of a given protein, the lower its PF concentration.[4]

Protein Hormones

Koninckx et al.[18] found PF follicle-stimulating hormone (FSH), luteinizing hormone (LH), and prolactin (PRL) levels to be lower than in serum. This contrasts with the work of Bouckaert et al.[19] who, based upon the date of the LH surge (LH day 0), noted a phase dependency of PF to serum ratios for FSH and LH. PF levels correlated with serum levels except during LH days −6, −5, and −4. The presence of FSH and LH could not be explained by simple diffusion or exudation alone because PF levels were equal to or greater than serum throughout the study. The carbohydrate and particularly sialic acid content of these hormones may influence diffusion and probably lead to PF accumulation of FSH especially. The physiologic significance of this remains to be determined.[19]

Steroids

Sex steroid hormones are found in PF and are significantly influenced by ovarian activity.[2,6,20,21] PF estrogen is predominantly estradiol (E_2). Individuals may demonstrate peritoneal fluid E_2 levels lower than, equal to, or greater than plasma E_2 preceding ovulation.[22] While PF E_2 rises gradually throughout the preovulatory period, it exhibits a more discernible elevation with ovulation. This increase in PF E_2 has been reported[6,20,22] to be from 45 to 1840 ng/ml before to 450 to 9000 ng/ml[22] after follicular rupture.

Progesterone (P) accumulates within follicular fluid (FF) during the late follicular period because only small amounts pass through the follicle wall.[22] The mechanical rupture of the follicle and release of the FF into the peritoneal cavity immediately augments PF P, with the highest concentrations noted after ovulation.[6,20] P levels (mean, 254.6 ± 69.5 ng/ml) remain high throughout cycle days 17 to 19,[6] when secretion of the early, less vascular corpus luteum is preferentially directed to the peritoneal cavity.[22] PF P decreases significantly thereafter.[6] Of unknown physiologic importance is the interaction of PF with available granulosa cell components to further enhance P production.[23]

Other Components

The exact role of many substances identified within PF is unclear. Relaxin, rarely identified in follicular phase PF samples, reaches high levels in PF during cycle days 20 to 24 as a result of corpus luteum secretion.[24] While high PF relaxin levels correspond to the period of nidation, the link is speculative. Progestin-dependent endometrial protein (PEP)[25] and PRL[26] have both been detected in PF, yet a defined physiologic role for their presence in PF is unknown. PF content of epidermal growth factor appears to be dependent on menstrual cycle because higher levels have been demonstrated in the secretory phase.[27]

Prostaglandins (PGs) and prostanoids (PN) have recognized effects on smooth muscle within the reproductive tract. Their possible pathophysiologic effects and PF levels in endometriosis will be discussed subsequently. Under physiologic conditions, however, no significant cyclicity variation of PG levels has been found.[27] This finding suggests that the ovarian follicle and corpus luteum do not serve as the primary source of PF PGs.[27]

PERITONEAL FLUID ENVIRONMENT IN PATHOPHYSIOLOGIC STATES

The cellular and acellular constituents of PF are often altered in pathophysiologic conditions associated with infertility, even without gross distortion of pelvic anatomy.

Peritoneal Cells in Endometriosis

As noted previously, red blood cells are frequently present in PF as a result of retrograde menstruation.[7] During the nonmenstrual phase, however, subjects with endometriosis have blood in PF significantly more often than other women.[3,7] Endometrial cells have been found in the PF in endometriosis as often as in women without endometriosis.[10,28] However, patients with endometriosis may have more endometrial cells in the fluid late in the luteal phase and following uterine irrigation than subjects without endometriosis.[10] Other cellular components are also affected by the presence of endometriosis. The number of peritoneal macrophages (PMs) in normal subjects, patients with adhesive disease, and those with unexplained infertility is similar[5] and is not significantly influenced by cycle week.[5] Many studies have confirmed elevated peritoneal or oviductal macrophage numbers in patients with mild endometriosis when compared with fertile controls or other infertile patients.[5,12,29–31] The extent of endometriosis generally does not appear to correlate with PM count, although a tendency toward higher numbers has been observed in women with mild stages of endometriosis.[30]

Investigations into the influence of disease processes on the cytochemical characteristics of PMs have revealed differences in patients with endometriosis compared with fertile or infertile controls.[31] Fewer peritoneal macrophages of patients with endometriosis exhibited positive myeloperoxidase staining, indicating that either fewer fresh macrophages (monocytes) were present among the PMs or that more rapid differentiation occurred.[31] PMs in endometriosis display higher acid phosphatase activity and increased ectoenzyme (leucine aminopeptidase) levels.[11] This finding corresponds to an increase in PM size and activity present over the menstrual cycle in women with endometriosis, but not in fertile subjects.[11]

PMs of patients with endometriosis also appear functionally different.[32,33] While standard measures of phagocytosis of opsonized zymosan were not different in PMs of normal subjects and women with endometriosis,[11] animal models have suggested the ability of macrophages to attack gametes[34,35] via different membrane receptors. Muscato et al.[32] found that PMs of patients with endometriosis phagocytized significantly more normal sperm in vitro than PMs of fertile or other infertile women. This was not dependent upon opsonization; however, the presence of antisperm antibodies enhanced spermiophagy and lysis by PMs of women with tubal adhesive disease. In patients with antisperm antibodies, increased numbers of PMs could promote sperm phagocytosis.[36] Olive et al. suggested that this increase reflects the presence of infertility without a mechanical cause.[30] Of interest is the hypothesis presented by Halme et al.,[37] which suggests that the altered function and maturation of PMs may be responsible for the pathogenesis of endometriosis rather than being secondary to the disease process itself.

ACELLULAR COMPONENTS IN ENDOMETRIOSIS OR UNEXPLAINED INFERTILITY

Peritoneal Fluid Volume

The acellular constituents of PF are also influenced by pathologic processes. As previously reviewed, PFV changes in response to ovarian activity during the normal menstrual cycle. Alterations in PFV resulting from or associated with endometriosis or unexplained infertility have been debated.[5,21,27,30,38–42] In interpreting these reports, one should consider differences in the menstrual cycle and diagnostic grouping because both affect PFV.[5] Rock et al.[38] found no increase in PFV in patients with endometriosis compared with infertile patients without endometriosis during the follicular phase. Olive et al.[30] detected no significant difference in the PF of infertile patients with endometriosis compared with fertile women undergoing sterilization without a reference to the cycle phase. Sgarlata et al.[39] found no difference in PFV during the follicular phase when endometriosis subjects were matched with disease-free women. DeLeon et al.[27] and Badawy et al.[42] include infertile women without endometriosis as controls. This control group would include many women with unexplained infertility. Koninckx et al.[3] did not distinguish fertile from infertile women, yet noted an increased PFV in the follicular phase of women with mild or moderate endometriosis. Severe endometriosis was associated with significantly lower PFV in the luteal phase than in women without endometriosis or disease rated as mild to moderate.[3]

By comparison, Drake et al.[40] believed PFV was increased throughout the cycle in patients with endometriosis and especially in those with advanced disease. Oak et al.[41] found increased PFV in women with unexplained infertility and endometriosis when either was compared with fertile subjects in the early luteal phase. In the most recent study, Syrop and Halme[5] examined the PFV of 426 patients and performed careful statistical evaluation of the data: women with endometriosis had a greater PFV than fertile control women, patients with adhesive disease, or unexplained infertility. The fluid volume in unexplained infertility was also higher than in controls. In summary, it appears that increased PFV is commonly associated not only with endometriosis, but also with longstanding, unexplained infertility.

Prostaglandins and Prostanoids in Endometriosis/Infertility

Considerable controversy exists over prostaglandin (PG) and prostanoid (PN) concentrations or content in the PF of patients with endometriosis or unexplained infertility. Because the PF is in direct contact with gametes, fallopian tubes, and ovaries, abnormal alterations in PG levels leading to infertility via ovulatory or tubal dysfunction poses an attractive consideration.[27,31,38,39,42–49] Rabbits with surgically induced endometriosis demonstrated impaired fertility primarily because of a defect in ovulation.[50] A postovulatory defect could not be excluded as only two of four ovulatory animals achieved pregnancy. Significant increases in prostaglandin F (PGF) but not prostaglandin E (PGE) were found in rabbits with endometriosis when compared with controls. Monkeys autografted with endometrium[51] produced increased concentrations of $PGF_{2\alpha}$ only if they had moderate or severe disease. Levels of $PGF_{2\alpha}$ were not different in monkeys with luteinized unruptured follicles (LUF) and luteal phase defects than in those with ovulatory cycles. Levels of $PGF_{2\alpha}$ and PGE in peritoneal washings were not different in monkeys that aborted or produced term pregnancies.[51] Unfortunately, it is difficult to evaluate the diverse findings of several papers reporting on PG and PN in human PF. Table 1 represents a compilation of these studies[27,31,38,39,42–49] with clarification of control groups and cycle phase. While a definitive conclusion regarding concentrations of PF PGs in infertility is hazardous, 6-keto-$PGF_{1\alpha}$ is the most consistently elevated PN when cycle phase[27,48] is controlled and patients with endometriosis or other disease categories are compared with fertile women.[48]

Peritoneal Fluid Hormones in Infertility/ Luteinized Unruptured Follicles

PF steroid hormones E_2 and P levels are not different in endometriosis when compared with controls either in proliferative or secretory phase.[26,27] These steroid hormone assays have been suggested as being useful in making the diagnosis of luteinized unruptured follicle syndrome (LUF).[52,53] However, an overlap exists between PF steroid hormone levels in women with and without an ovulation stigma. Furthermore, some women without an ovulation stigma may have high steroid concentrations in PF.[52] Lesorgen et al.[53] found 21% of control patients to have a corpus luteum without a stigma and biochemical criteria for LUF were found in 7% of controls and more often in all pathologic groups. In contrast, Dhont et al.[54] noted ovulation stigma in one-half of patients regardless of fertility status, the presence of endometriosis, or the time of the luteal phase. Peritoneal fluid E_2 and P levels did not correlate with the presence or absence of a stigma. No discriminatory PF hormone level could be established that would ascertain the diagnosis of LUF. In contrast to the premise that LUF should occur repeatedly in order to cause infertility, the authors found that 9 of 22 patients without a stigma conceived without therapy; this lack of a relationship with fertility status made it doubtful that the absence of an ovulation stigma on laparoscopic examination could be equated with LUF. Toward a less variable measure of follicular rupture, Padilla et al.[55] examined the PF content of plasminogen in the pre- and postovulatory period of fertile women. Total plasminogen and its PF concentration increased only in the early luteal phase. Since PF plasminogen concentration exhibited less variation than E_2 or progesterone, it was suggested that PF plasminogen may be useful in documenting ovulation or LUF.

OTHER PERITONEAL FLUID CONSTITUENTS IN INFERTILITY

Alterations in the health of the PF environment may lead to changes in its cellular or acellular constituents. Such changes may either directly result from infertility or from alterations associated with disease processes. Several proteins in PF have been examined as indicators of pelvic pathology. PF total protein content was unchanged by the presence of endometriosis,[31] yet acid phosphatase enzyme level has been found to be elevated in women with endometriosis when compared with unex-

Table 1 Prostaglandin (PG)/Prostanoid (PN) Concentration (C) or Content (T) Measured in Study Versus Control Group

	Controls[a]	Study group[a]	Cycle phase[b]	(C)/(T)	$PGF_{2\alpha}$	PGE_2	TxB_2[c]	6 KF[c]	MPG $F_{2\alpha}$[c]	Comment
Drake et al.[43]	FR + ADz	EM	NR	(C)/(T)			↑[e]	↑		
Rock et al.[38]	UEx*	EM	Pr	(C)	→[f]	→	→		→	*Infertile "disease-free" with "normal pelvis"
Badawy et al.[44]	BTL + Dys	EM	Pr/Se†	(C)					NR	†Author states "no difference in (C) PGE_2 + $MPGF_{2\alpha}$" in various parts of the cycle in patients with endometriosis.
	UEx	EM	PR/Se	(C)		→			→	
	BTL + Dys	UEx	Pr/Se			NR[d]			↑	
Halme et al.[31]	FR	EM	Se	(C)	→	→				
	FR	UEx	Se	(C)	→	→				
Drake et al.[45]	FR + BTL	UEx	Pr/Ov/Se	(C)			↑	↑		
Sgarlata et al.[39]	DF	EM	Pr	(C)	Δ	Δ	→	→		Δ, no significant difference in PGE + PGF (C)
Dawood et al.[46]	FR	EM	Pr/Se	(C)	→	→	→	↑		
	FR	EM	Pr/Se	(T)	→	→	→	→		
	FR	ADz	Pr/Se	(C)/(T)	→	→	→	→		
	ADz	EM	Pr/Se	(C)/(T)	→	→	→	→		
Koskimies et al.[47]	FR	EM	Pr/Ov/Se	(C)			↑	↑		
	FR	UEx	Pr/Ov/Se	(C)			↑	↑		
Ylikorkala et al.[48]	FR‡	EM	Pr/Se	(C)			↑	↑		‡FR includes women with male factor infertility
	FR	UEx	Pr/Se	(C)			↑	↑		
	FR	ADz	Pr/Se	(C)			↑	↑		
Badawy et al.[42]	DF§	EM	Cycle days 1–8	(C)	↑	→	→	→		§Author defined controls as infertile without endometriosis
	DF§	EM	Cycle days 9–16 and 17–24	(C)	↑	↑	→	→		
Mudge et al.[49]	UEx, ADz, UEx	EM	Se	(C)/(T)				→		
	FR	EM	Se	(C)/(T)				→		
DeLeon et al.[27]	BTL/UEx	EM	Pr	(C)	→	→	→	→		
	BTL/UEx	EM	Se	(C)	↑	↑	↑	↑		

[a] FR, fertile volunteers; BTL, prior tubal ligation; DF, "disease free"; EM, endometriosis; UEx, unexplained infertility; ADz, pelvic/tubal adhesive disease; Dys, dysmenorrhea.
[b] Pr, proliferative; Se, secretory; Ov, periovulatory.
[c] TxB_2, thromboxane B_2; 6-KF, 6-keto-$PGF_{1\alpha}$; $MPGF_{2\alpha}$, 13,14 dihydro 15-keto $PGF_{2\alpha}$.
[d] NR, not reported.
[e] ↑, significantly increased in the study group.
[f] →, not significantly increased in the study group.

plained infertility or fertile controls.[31,56] Reduced plasminogen activator activity (PAA), at least 50%, was associated with the presence of pelvic adhesions; however, no difference in peritoneal PAA was found in the follicular or luteal phase of patients with or without endometriosis.[57] Similarly, severity of endometriosis did not alter PAA levels. PF lysozyme, a ubiquitous product of macrophages, is no different in endometriosis or infertility when compared with controls.[58] PF epidermal growth factor (EGF) level appears increased in the secretory phase, but no differences were noted in women with or without endometriosis.[27] PF PRL levels failed to be indicative of ectopic endometrial activity, perhaps because all implants were not functionally active in secreting PRL or the stromal component was too scant to cause significant increase.[26] PEP in the PF of women with moderate or severe endometriosis was, however, approximately 10-fold the level noted in mild disease or controls.[24] PEP therefore may correlate to the extent of ectopic endometrium present.

In view of data suggesting qualitative and quantitative changes in PMs in endometriosis and infertility, Syrop and Halme[59] attempted to determine the impact of macrophage numbers and PF volume upon fertility. After initial sampling of PF at laparoscopy, 124 infertile patients were followed for a minimum of 2 years or until pregnant. The outcome in all patients bore no correlation to PFV or macrophage count. However, when patients with endometriosis were examined separately, those who achieved a pregnancy had a significantly lower PFV than those who did not achieve pregnancy. Thus, in endometriosis, PFV had an inverse correlation to the subsequent occurrence of pregnancy. PM count was not a predictor variable for pregnancy. These data indirectly suggest that an alteration in the PF itself may affect the reproductive process and may be associated with relative subfertility at least in mild endometriosis.

POSSIBLE MECHANISMS BY WHICH PERITONEAL FLUID CONSTITUENTS MAY CAUSE INFERTILITY

To influence fertility, PF components must interact in a potentially adverse fashion with either ovulatory function, gamete transport or survival, sperm-ovum interaction, early embryonic development, or implantation.

Ovulatory Function/Corpus Luteum Function

Macrophages are found within developing follicles and PMs stimulate granulosa-luteal cell P production in vitro.[17] Thus, a similar physiologic or pathophysiologic effect of PMs on the cumulus mass or early corpus luteum in this manner must be considered. Preliminary studies have demonstrated that, in some cases of endometriosis, PMs decrease granulosa cell P production.[17] However, a more detailed investigation is warranted. PF PGs, whether derived from macrophages or elsewhere, could potentially affect either the ovulation mechanism or granulosa luteal cell function in an adverse fashion. As pointed out previously, the data on PF PNs is not definitive.

Gamete Transport or Survival

The number of oviductal and peritoneal macrophages is increased in women with endometriosis.[15] PMs in animal[34] and human[32] studies exhibited spermiophagy in the absence and presence of opsonized antibodies. Elevated numbers of macrophages in women with endometriosis and without mechanical infertility might then have an impact on oviductal transport of sperm or their survival within the peritoneal compartment. This concept is strengthened by the observation that Ethiodol (Savage Laboratories, Melville, NY), having been associated with increased fertility after hysterosalpingography (HSG), inhibits spermiophagy of PMs in vitro.[60] Oak et al.[41] incubated normal sperm in the presence of PF and found a significantly reduced proportion of motile sperm in endometriosis or unexplained infertility when compared with controls. While the velocity of sperm increased in fluid of fertile women, it was significantly reduced by the PF obtained from subjects with endometriosis or unexplained infertility. Motility reduction was independent of the velocity reduction. Not all investigators agree that PF affects sperm motility,[61,62] although others have noted toxic effects of PF.[63,64]

Ovum or embryo transport alterations by PF substances were recently demonstrated in elegant work by examination of the oocyte-cumulus complex (mouse)/fimbrial (hamster) interaction.[65] Oocyte capturability was significantly diminished by incubating the fimbria with native or cell-free PF of endometriosis patients. The substance that diminished oocyte capturability was water soluble with a molecular weight of >100,000. Increased levels of PGs can potentially affect tubal transport function, but as previously noted, the data are inconsistent and difficult to interpret.

Sperm/Oocyte Interaction

Secretory products of PMs may adversely affect fertilization. Chacho et al.[16] demonstrated that medium conditioned with macrophages from fertile or infertile women with or without endometriosis had no adverse effect on sperm penetration of hamster ova.

Fertilization in a mouse assay was significantly diminished over that of controls in a dose-dependent fashion by a filterable and heat labile factor within the PF of patients with endometriosis.[66] Heat lability of such a factor would be consistent with previous findings by Halme and Hall[67] using a hamster penetration assay in which heat-treated samples of PF showed no difference in penetration rates between groups of infertile women with and without endometriosis.

Early Embryonic Development/Implantation

Secretory products of PMs, such as interleukin-1 (IL-1),[68] have been demonstrated to have an adverse effect on early embryonic cleavage and development. This preliminary work has implied that such a mechanism is responsible for the subfertility in endometriosis. Heat-tested and filtered PF of patients with endometriosis maintained irreversible toxicity to mouse embryo development and was significantly more toxic than fluid from patients without endometriosis.[63] Rabbit studies[69] demonstrated that the number of corpora lutea and fertilized ova in surgically induced endometriosis was no different than in controls, although rabbits with endometriosis displayed significantly decreased numbers of fetuses and implantation sites. A markedly reduced implantation rate following intraperitoneal injections of endometriosis-associated PF was also noted. Human in vitro fertilization experience in women with endometriosis runs counter to this animal model.[70] Rates of oocyte recovery and fertilization are not affected by endometriosis. Stage I and II disease provide pregnancy rates approximating success rates for tubal disease with IVF. Pregnancy rates for severe endometriosis are reduced in IVF; this reduction is related, in part, to the reduced number of oocytes recovered.

SUMMARY

The PF environment is one that hosts the processes of ovulation, gamete transportation, fertilization, and early embryonic development. The cellular and acellular constituents of this dynamic fluid are in a constant interactive state, being influenced by the physiologic events of the menstrual cycle and pelvic disease processes; these constituents probably influence disease manifestation and reproduction. The importance of understanding this zone of early reproductive life has been now recognized. We hope that future investigations will define the exact role(s) of known components and some yet-to-be defined substances of PF in disease processes that affect reproductive function. With better understanding of normal and abnormal events in this pelvic microenvironment, we can develop rationales for novel treatment modalities.

REFERENCES

1. McGowan L, Bunnag B: Morphology of mesothelial cells in peritoneal fluid from normal women. Acta Cytol (Baltimore) 18:205, 1974
2. Maathuis JB, Van Look PFA, Michie EA: Changes in volume, total protein and ovarian steroid concentrations of peritoneal fluid throughout the human menstrual cycle. J Endocrinol 76:123, 1978
3. Koninckx PR, Ranaer M, Brosens IA: Origin of peritoneal fluid in women: an ovarian exudation product. Br J Obstet Gynaecol 87:177, 1980
4. Bouckaert PXJM, Evers JLH, Doesburg WH, Schellekens LA, Brombacher PH, Rolland R: Patterns of changes in proteins in the peritoneal fluid of women during the periovulatory phase of the menstrual cycle. J Reprod Fertil 77:329, 1986
5. Syrop CH, Halme J: Cyclic changes of peritoneal fluid parameters in normal and infertile patients. Obstet Gynecol 69:3, 1987
6. Donnez J, Langerock S, Thomas K: Peritoneal fluid volume and 17-β-estradiol and progesterone concentrations in ovulatory, anovulatory, and postmenopausal women. Obstet Gynecol 59:687, 1982
7. Halme J, Hammond MG, Hulka JF, Raj SG, Talbert LM: Retrograde menstruation in healthy women and in patients with endometriosis. Obstet Gynecol 64:151, 1984
8. Beyth Y, Yaffe H, Levij I, Sadovsky E: Retrograde seeding of endometrium: a sequela of tubal flushing. Fertil Steril 26:1094, 1975
9. Portuondo JA, Herran C, Echanojauregui AD, Riego AG: Peritoneal flushing and biopsy in laparoscopically diagnosed endometriosis. Fertil Steril 38:538, 1982
10. Bartosik D, Jacobs SL, Kelly LJ: Endometrial tissue in peritoneal fluid. Fertil Steril 46:796, 1986
11. Halme J, Becker S, Wing R: Accentuated cyclic activation of peritoneal macrophages in patients with endometriosis. Am J Obstet Gynecol 148:85, 1984
12. Haney AF, Muscato JJ, Weinberg JB: Peritoneal fluid cell populations in infertility patients. Fertil Steril 35:696, 1981
13. Parwaresch MR, Radzun HJ, Dommes M: The homogeneity and monocytic origin of human peritoneal macrophages evidenced by comparison of esterase polymorphism. Am J Pathol 102:209, 1981
14. Bercovici B, Gallily R: The cytology of the human peritoneal fluid. Acta Cytol (Baltimore) 22:124, 1978
15. Haney AF, Misukonis MA, Weinberg JB: Macrophages and infertility: oviductal macrophages as potential mediators of infertility. Fertil Steril 39:310, 1983
16. Chacho KJ, Chacho MS, Andreson PJ, Scommegna A: Peritoneal fluid in patients with and without endometriosis: prostanoids and macrophages and their effect on the spermatozoa penetration assay. Am J Obstet Gynecol 154:1290, 1986
17. Halme J, Hammond MG, Syrop CH: Peritoneal macrophages modulate human granulosa-luteal cell progesterone production. J Clin Endocrinol Metab 16:912, 1985
18. Koninckx PR, Heyns W, Verhoeven G, Van Baelen H, Lissens WD, DeMoor P, Brosens IA: Biochemical characterization of peritoneal fluid in women during the menstrual cycle. J Clin Endocrinol Metab 51:1239, 1980
19. Bouckaert PXJM, Evers JLH, Doesburg WH, Schellekens LA, Rolland R: Patterns of changes in glycoproteins, polypeptides, and steroids in the peritoneal fluid of women during the periovulatory phase of the menstrual cycle. J Clin Endocrinol Metab 62:293, 1986
20. Loumaye E, Donnez J, Thomas K: Ovulation instantaneously modifies women's peritoneal fluid characteristics: a demonstration from an in vitro fertilization program. Fertil Steril 44:827, 1985
21. Crain JL, Luciano AA: Peritoneal fluid evaluation in infertility. Obstet Gynecol 61:159, 1983
22. Zorn JR, Roger M, Savale M, Grenier J: Steroid hormone levels in peritoneal fluid during the periovulatory period. Fertil Steril 38:162, 1982
23. Dingman C, Syrop CH, Halme J: Peritoneal fluid from fertile and infertile women stimulates granulosa-luteal cell progesterone production in vitro (Abstr 21). Presented at the Forty-Second Annual Meeting of The American Fertility Society, the Eighteenth Annual Meeting of the Canadian Fertility and Andrology Society, Toronto, Ontario, Canada, September 27–October 2, 1986. Birmingham, The American Fertility Society, p 7
24. Loumaye E, Depreester S, Donnez J, Thomas K: Immuno-

reactive relaxin surge in peritoneal fluid of women during the midluteal phase. Fertil Steril 42:856, 1984
25. Joshi SG, Zamah NM, Raikar RS, Buttram VC, Henriques ES, Gordon M: Serum and peritoneal fluid proteins in women with and without endometriosis. Fertil Steril 46:1077, 1986
26. Haney AF, Handwerger S, Weinberg JB: Peritoneal fluid prolactin in infertile women with endometriosis: lack of evidence of secretory activity by endometrial implants. Fertil Steril 42:935, 1984
27. DeLeon FD, Vijayakumar R, Brown M, Rao CV, Yussman MA, Schultz G: Peritoneal fluid volume, estrogen, progesterone, prostaglandin, and epidermal growth factor concentrations in patients with and without endometriosis. Obstet Gynecol 68:189, 1986
28. Koninckx PR, Ide P, Vandenbroucke W, Brosens IA: New aspects of the pathophysiology of endometriosis and associated infertility. J Reprod Med 24:257, 1980
29. Halme J, Becker S, Hammond MG, Raj S: Pelvic macrophages in normal and infertile women: the role of patent tubes. Am J Obstet Gynecol 142:890, 1982
30. Olive DL, Weinberg JB, Haney AF: Peritoneal macrophages and infertility: the association between cell number and pelvic pathology. Fertil Steril 44:772, 1985
31. Halme J, Becker S, Hammond MG, Raj MHG, Raj S: Increased activation of pelvic macrophages in infertile women with mild endometriosis. Am J Obstet Gynecol 145:333, 1983
32. Muscato JJ, Haney AF, Weinberg JB: Sperm phagocytosis by human peritoneal macrophages: a possible cause of infertility in endometriosis. Am J Obstet Gynecol 144:503, 1982
33. Henig I, Zeller JM, Rana N, Radwanska E, Dmowski WP: Chemiluminescence activities of peripheral blood monocytes and peritoneal macrophages in infertile women with endometriosis (Abstr 12). Presented at the Forty-Second Annual Meeting of The American Fertility Society, the Eighteenth Annual Meeting of the Canadian Fertility and Andrology Society, Toronto, Ontario, Canada, September 27–October 2, 1986. Birmingham, The American Fertility Society, p 4
34. Ball RY, Scott N, Mitchinson MJ: Further observations on spermiophagy by murine peritoneal macrophages in vitro. J Reprod Fertil 71:221, 1984
35. Weissmann G, Finkelstein MC, Csernansky J, Quigley JP, Quinn RS, Techner L, Troll W, Dunhan PB: Attack of sea urchin eggs by dogfish phagocytes: model of phagocyte-mediated cellular cytotoxicity. Proc Natl Acad Sci USA 75:1825, 1978
36. London SN, Haney AF, Weinberg JB: Macrophages and infertility: enhancement of human macrophage mediated sperm killing by antisperm antibodies. Fertil Steril 43:274, 1985
37. Halme J, Becker S, Haskill S: Altered maturation and function of peritoneal macrophages: a new hypothesis for pathogenesis of endometriosis. Am J Obstet Gynecol 156:783, 1987
38. Rock JA, Dubin NH, Ghodgaonkar RB, Bergquist CA, Erozan YS, Kimball AW: Cul-de-sac fluid in women with endometriosis: fluid volume and prostanoid concentration during the proliferative phase of the cycle—days 8 to 12. Fertil Steril 37:747, 1982
39. Sgarlata CS, Hertelendy F, Mikhail G: The prostanoid content in peritoneal fluid and plasma of women with endometriosis. Am J Obstet Gynecol 147:563, 1983
40. Drake TS, Metz SA, Grunert GM, O'Brien WF: Peritoneal fluid volume in endometriosis. Fertil Steril 34:280, 1980
41. Oak MK, Chantler EN, Williams CAV, Elstein M: Sperm survival studies in peritoneal fluid from infertile women with endometriosis and unexplained infertility. Clin Reprod Fertil 3:297, 1985
42. Badawy SZA, Marshall L, Cuenca V: Peritoneal fluid prostaglandins in various stages of the menstrual cycle: role in infertile patients with endometriosis. Int J Fertil 30:48, 1985
43. Drake TS, O'Brien WF, Ramwell PW, Metz SA: Peritoneal fluid thromboxane B_2 and 6-keto-prostaglandin $F_{1\alpha}$ in endometriosis. Am J Obstet Gynecol 140:401, 1981
44. Badawy SZA, Marshall L, Gabal AA, Nusbaum ML: The concentration of 13,14-dihydro-15-keto prostaglandin $F_{2\alpha}$ and prostaglandin E_2 in peritoneal fluid of infertile patients with and without endometriosis. Fertil Steril 38:166, 1982
45. Drake TS, O'Brien WF, Ramwell PW: Peritoneal fluid prostanoids in unexplained infertility. Am J Obstet Gynecol 147:63, 1983
46. Dawood MY, Khan-Dawood FS, Wilson L Jr: Peritoneal fluid prostaglandins and prostanoids in women with endometriosis, chronic pelvic inflammatory disease and pelvic pain. Am J Obstet Gynecol 148:391, 1984
47. Koskimies AI, Tenhunen A, Ylikorkala O: Peritoneal fluid 6-keto-prostaglandin $F_{1\alpha}$, thromboxane B2 in endometriosis and unexplained infertility. Acta Obstet Gynecol Scand [Suppl] 123:19, 1984
48. Ylikorkala O, Koskimies A, Laatkainen T, Tenhunen A, Viinikka L: Peritoneal fluid prostaglandins in endometriosis, tubal disorders, and unexplained infertility. Obstet Gynecol 63:616, 1984
49. Mudge TJ, James MJ, Jones WR, Walsh JA: Peritoneal fluid 6-keto-prostaglandin $F_{1\alpha}$ levels in women with endometriosis. Am J Obstet Gynecol 152:901, 1985
50. Schenken RS, Asch RH: Surgical induction of endometriosis in the rabbit: effects on fertility and concentrations of peritoneal fluid prostaglandins. Fertil Steril 34:581, 1980
51. Schenken RS, Asch RH, Williams RF, Hodgen GD: Etiology of infertility in monkeys with endometriosis: measurement of peritoneal fluid prostaglandins. Am J Obstet Gynecol 150:349, 1984
52. Koninckx PR, DeMoor P, Brosens IA: Diagnosis of the luteinized unruptured follicle syndrome by steroid hormone assays on peritoneal fluid. Br J Obstet Gynaecol 87:929, 1980
53. Lesorgen PR, Wu CH, Green PJ, Gocial B, Lerner LJ: Peritoneal fluid and serum steroids in infertility patients. Fertil Steril 42:237, 1984
54. Dhont M, Serreyn R, Duvivier P, Vanluchene E, De Boever J, Vandekerckhove D: Ovulation stigma and concentration of progesterone and estradiol in peritoneal fluid: relation with fertility and endometriosis. Fertil Steril 41:872, 1984
55. Padilla SL, Galle PC, Ellegood JO, Mahesh VB, McDonough PG: Plasminogen in peritoneal fluid: a possible nonsteroidal indicator of ovulation. Fertil Steril 46:1071, 1986
56. Badawy SZA, Cuenca V, Marshall L, Munchback R, Rinas AC, Coble DA: Cellular components in peritoneal fluid in infertile patients with and without endometriosis. Fertil Steril 42:704, 1984
57. Batzofin JH, Holmes SD, Gibbons WE, Buttram VC Jr: Peritoneal fluid plasminogen activator activity in endometriosis and pelvic adhesive disease. Fertil Steril 44:277, 1985
58. Olive DL, Hobbs MM, Misukonis MA, Weinberg JB, Haney

AF: Macrophages and infertility: the association between lysozyme activity and cell number (Abstr 318). Presented at the Forty-Second Annual Meeting of The American Fertility Society, the Eighteenth Annual Meeting of the Canadian Fertility and Andrology Society, Toronto, Ontario, Canada, September 27–October 2, 1986. Birmingham, The American Fertility Society, p 110

59. Syrop CH, Halme J: A comparison of peritoneal fluid parameters of infertile patients and the subsequent occurrence of pregnancy. Fertil Steril 46:631, 1986
60. Boyer P, Territo MC, de Ziegler D, Meldrum DR: Ethiodol inhibits phagocytosis by pelvic peritoneal macrophages. Fertil Steril 46:715, 1986
61. Muse K, Estes S, Vernon M, Zavos P, Wilson E: Effect of endometriosis on sperm motility in peritoneal fluid in vitro (Abstr 286). Presented at the Forty-Second Annual Meeting of The American Fertility Society, the Eighteenth Annual Meeting of the Canadian Fertility and Andrology Society, Toronto, Ontario, Canada, September 27–October 2, 1986. Birmingham, The American Fertility Society, p 99
62. Stone SC, de la Maza LM, Peterson EM: Recovery of microorganisms from the pelvic cavity after intracervical or intrauterine artificial insemination. Fertil Steril 46:61, 1986
63. Morcos RN, Gibbons WE, Findley WE: Effect of peritoneal fluid on in vitro cleavage of 2-cell mouse embryos: possible role in infertility associated with endometriosis. Fertil Steril 44:678, 1985
64. de Ziegler D, Cedars M, Boyer P, Hamilton H, Moreno T, Meldrum D: Peritoneal fluid (PF) of some IVF patients is toxic to sperm (Abstr 62). Presented at the Forty-Second Annual Meeting of The American Fertility Society, the Eighteenth Annual Meeting of the Canadian Fertility and Andrology Society, Toronto, Ontario, Canada, September 27–October 2, 1986. Birmingham, The American Fertility Society, p 22
65. Suginami H, Yano K, Watanabe K, Matsuura S: A factor inhibiting ovum capture by the oviductal fimbriae present in endometriosis peritoneal fluid. Fertil Steril 46:1140, 1986
66. Sueldo CE, Lambert H, Steinleitner AJ, Swanson JA: Effect of peritoneal fluid from endometriosis patients on murine sperm-ova interaction (Abstr 23). Presented at the Forty-Second Annual Meeting of The American Fertility Society, the Eighteenth Annual Meeting of the Canadian Fertility and Andrology Society, Toronto, Ontario, Canada, September 27–October 2, 1986. Birmingham, The American Fertility Society, p 8
67. Halme J, Hall JL: Effect of pelvic fluid from endometriosis patients on human sperm penetration of zona-free hamster ova. Fertil Steril 37:573, 1982
68. Fakih H, Baggett B, Holtz G, Tsang K-Y, Lee JC, Williamson HO: Interleukin-1: a possible role in the infertility associated with endometriosis. Fertil. Steril. 47:213, 1987
69. Hahn DW, Carraher RP, Foldesy RG, McGuire JL: Experimental evidence for failure to implant as a mechanism of infertility associated with endometriosis. Am J Obstet Gynecol 155:1109, 1986
70. Matson PL, Yovich JL: The treatment of infertility associated with endometriosis by in vitro fertilization. Fertil Steril 46:432, 1986

SECTION V

In Vitro Fertilization

In the first volume of *Modern Trends* published in 1979, only a single reference was made to in vitro fertilization (IVF) in the human. That reference described the first reported attempt at IVF by Steptoe and Edwards which resulted in a tubal pregnancy.[1] Three years later, in the second volume of *Modern Trends,* Blandau's contribution pessimistically concluded with a statement urging couples "not to expect that this method of procreation will afford relief of infertility problems to many in the foreseeable future."[2] By the time Volume III was published in 1985, IVF had become firmly established as a standard therapy for certain types of infertility. IVF had progressed from a procedure for which the most clear-cut indication was absence of fallopian tubes to one which encompassed a variety of other conditions resulting in infertility. Indeed, at that time Lopata's chapter on IVF cited tubal disease as the indication in only 54.2% of his patients.[3] Fully 45% of the procedures were already being performed for other indications. Volume III also included a review of the equipment and laboratory instruments required for establishment of an IVF program. By 1985 more than 300 IVF programs were operational throughout the world, yielding 9,641 reported treatment cycles, 24,037 oocytes collected, and 7,722 embryos transferred.

As this fourth volume is beng prepared, over 2,000 babies have already been born throughout the world as a result of IVF. In the United States 800 IVF babies have been born, and 150 facilities are in operation since 1981. These figures accentuate the rapid development of IVF in the short space of a decade from a procedure originally viewed with skepticism as experimental to a well-accepted therapeutic technique now considered to be a key component of infertility programs throughout the world.

As predicted, the growth of this modality has led to challenging issues. Among them have been the following: (1) means for improving success rates; (2) reduction in cost; (3) technological advances to simplify the procedure and enhance its safety; (4) critical questions regarding ethical aspects of IVF and related technologies geared towards improved reproductive performance. Many of these challenges are interrelated. For example, how can reduction in cost and increased availability be considered without the appreciation of the potential impact of IVF on industry, providers, and entrepreneurs? Or, how can we attempt to maximize reproductive performance without provoking society's reaction as to whether physicians and scientists have the right to regulate procreation?

In 1984, Charles B. Hammond, as President of The American Fertility Society, appointed Howard W. Jones, Jr., to chair a Committee on Ethics. The Committee was specifically charged to assume a leadership position in addressing ethical issues in reproduction. Explicit in the charge to the Committee was to consider various ramifications of IVF including surrogacy, gamete donation, cryopreservation, and genetic manipulation. The multidisciplinary committee met formally on eight occasions, and in September, 1986, its report was released as a supplement to *Fertility & Sterility*.[4] The Committee incorporated into its conclusions the concept that the human person should be regarded as "integrally and adequately considered," taking into account that the basis for IVF outweighed foreseeable risks to the potential offspring thereform and to the specific couple as well as to society in general. Recognizing that there is a potential role for certain types of surrogacy (specifically surrogate gestational motherhood), the report expressed serious ethical reservations about surrogacy in general. Appropriate data on risks and benefits of surrogacy are required to enable comprehensive evaluation of this procedure. Gamete donation and the use of donor pre-embryos for clear-cut indications were considered ethically acceptable. Although cryopreservation was a desirable adjunct, the Committee considered that cryopreservation of pre-embryo and egg was still in an experimental stage. At the time of this writing, an instance of a child from a cryopreserved egg has been reported in Letters to the Editor of the *New England Journal of Medicine*. Quality assurance is naturally a major concern and the Ethics Committee recommended ongoing analysis of procedures involved for reproductive enhancement.

This section represents several advances in the field of IVF over the past 3 years and addresses several of the challenges alluded to above. Trounson summarizes the world literature and his own experience regarding cryopreservation of eggs and embryos. In addition to describing technical aspects of cryopreservation as it applies to eggs and embryos, Trounson critically evaluates the applications of this process in human reproductive medicine. The technical considerations include choice of a cryoprotectant (dimethyl sulfoxide [DMSO], glycerol), and the rates of freezing and thawing. The recognition that eggs and pre-embryos differ dramatically in their ability to withstand freezing and thawing and that species differences occur in intracellular and membrane responses to freezing are also important. With the confidence that sufficient scientific expertise ultimately will be developed to enable both egg and pre-embryo cryopreservation, the applications of cryopreservation are manifold. We may then have acceptable solutions to the problem of disposition of excess oocytes and fertilized eggs. The opportunity to cryopreserve for future cycles relieves us of the burden of transferring large numbers of pre-embryos at one time and of the pressure to consider discarding and not transferring or donating them. It also reduces the need for multiple surgical attempts at oocyte recovery. The technique of cryopreservation makes possible an efficient means for synchronization between donors and recipients in egg or embryo donation programs. It also provides a method whereby patients in jeopardy of losing ovarian function through disease, surgery, radiation, or chemotherapy can retain the prospect of childbearing.

Genetic diagnosis of a blastomere of a pre-implantation embryo becomes a possibility in the era in which deoxyribonucleic acid (DNA) probes are widely used to identify genetic defects. Although these possibilities can have a positive effect on the future of human reproductive potential, they nonetheless raise sensitive questions regarding safety, appropriateness, and custodianship of cryopreserved gametes and embryos. In this section, John Robertson, a member of The AFS Ethics Committee and a Professor of Law at the University of Texas, reviews both the ethical and legal issues associated with cryopreservation. Robertson urges that each couple's dispositional instructions be carefully spelled out in detail at the outset, including specifications in the event of parental death, divorce, nonavailability, or failure to pay storage charges. If, as the author states, the major distinguishing feature separating cryopreservation of embryos from other noncoital techniques used to manage infertility is the temporary suspension of further cleavage following conception and prior to intrauterine placement, cryopreservation of the human embryo can be evaluated using criteria similar to those used for IVF and gamete donation. On the other hand, the world may not be ready for the concept that the fused gametes of two individuals may remain in the frozen state awaiting indefinitely the decision of the couple as to their ultimate fate. The interpersonal vicissitudes within the marriage relationship over time enter into the formula. Development of the technical expertise to preserve oocytes effectively can eliminate many, if not all, of the problems associated with preservation of the fertilized egg. Unlike spermatozoa, which are abundantly available without the need for an invasive procedure, oocytes are far less plentiful and require an invasive technique for their recovery. This invasive technique could be a spin-off of a primary procedure, e.g., laparotomy, laparoscopy, oocyte recovery for IVF or gamete intrafallopian transfer (GIFT), or it could actually require a freestanding procedure. In either event, planning for IVF of oocytes identified for donation requires significant cyclic coordination, as is the case with artificial insemination by donor (AID). The ability to cryopreserve eggs would help to resolve the logistics of this problem, at least in part.

The current state-of-the-art using donor eggs is articulated in Zev Rosenwaks' chapter. That oocyte donation is more intricate than sperm donation should be obvious immediately. The vast experience of Dr. Rosenwaks and his group at Norfolk testifies to the need for careful monitoring, the synchrony of natural cycle with in vivo embryonic development, and attention to the differences in embryonic developmental rate in vitro and in vivo. The terms "window of receptivity" and "window of transfer" have been coined to apply to the receptive period of the endometrium for implantation. The spin-offs of basic IVF become readily apparent now that we have a model for investigating interactions among conceptus, endometrium, and circulating steroid levels. When we consider the success of oocyte donation in achieving pregnancy among patients with ovarian failure, the boundaries between what is and what is not possible seem limitless in their extension. These boundaries remain restricted only by technologic capacity and by the extent of man's creativity and determination.

IVF has advanced so remarkably in this decade that ultrasound has become standard for several facets of the procedure. We depend upon sonography not only for monitoring follicle growth, but also for oocyte retrieval. Vaginal probes have increased the scope of sonography. More refined protocols for follicle maturation have evolved, and our understanding of oocyte and embryonic potential is just now being developed. The success of GIFT as an alternative to IVF has also broadened our horizons. All in all, we've learned that what can be derived from a new procedure often significantly exceeds the original expectations for it. Overlying all of these positive aspects of IVF and related technologies is the compelling question which requires resolution, namely whether society has truly had an opportunity to register its response regarding its reproductive aspirations and the methods whereby they should be attained.

Edward E. Wallach, M.D.

REFERENCES

1. Steptoe P, Edwards R: Reimplantation of a human embryo with subsequent tubal pregnancy. *Lancet* 1:880, 1976
2. Blandau RJ: In vitro fertilization and embryo transfer. In Modern Trends in Infertility and Conception Control, Vol. 2, Edited by EE Wallach, RD Kempers. Philadelphia, Harper & Row Publishers, 1982, p 239
3. Lopata A: Concepts in human in vitro fertilization and embryo transfer. In Modern Trends in Infertility and Conception Control, Vol. 3, Edited by EE Wallach, RD Kempers. Chicago, Year Book Medical Publishers, Inc., 1985, p 420
4. Ethics Committee of The American Fertility Society: Ethical Considerations of the New Reproductive Technologies. Fertil Steril 46:(Suppl. 1), 1S-94S, 1986

Chapter 23

Preservation of human eggs and embryos

Alan Trounson, Ph.D.

Centre for Early Human Development, Monash University, Queen Victoria Medical Centre, Melbourne, Australia

The introduction of superovulation techniques[1] into human in vitro fertilization (IVF) raised an immediate dilemma that large numbers of human eggs and embryos would be produced because it has never been possible to control precisely the number of follicles that develop in response to the administration of high doses of ovulation-inducing drugs such as clomiphene citrate and human menopausal gonadotropin. The alternatives have been to restrict the number of eggs recovered or eggs inseminated to that required for replacement in utero; to replace all the embryos that develop; to discard eggs or embryos in excess of the number required for immediate replacement in utero; and to use the excess eggs or embryos for research purposes. It is apparent that most IVF groups have chosen one or more of these alternatives because very few groups have successfully integrated egg or embryo cryopreservation into their clinical IVF programs, thereby avoiding the inherent disadvantages of the other alternatives to the infertile patients. For example, the restricted collection of eggs risks that the viable eggs remain in follicles, that nonviable eggs are inseminated, and that unaspirated follicles persist as ovarian or luteal cysts. If the number of eggs inseminated is restricted and the excess discarded, the number of embryos available for replacement in utero will be reduced and have the direct effect of reducing the IVF pregnancy success rate.[2] The replacement of large numbers of embryos is an exceedingly risky proposition for maternal health and fetal normality. The sequelae of triplet, quadruplet, and larger multiple pregnancies are well known, and the consequences in IVF are already becoming apparent in perinatal statistics.[3]

The discarding of eggs and embryos is undoubtedly a widespread practice in human IVF. However, in my own view, this procedure is the least desirable or ethical alternative. It would be much better to study excess eggs or embryos so that we might improve IVF procedures, reduce embryonic defects, and increase the application of IVF and related technologies. It is unfortunate that most IVF groups are ill-equipped for embryonic research and that ethical approval of this type of research is becoming difficult to obtain. Given these situations and the present attitude of many communities toward embryonic research, egg and embryo cryopreservation offers an attractive alternative to those mentioned earlier. This consideration was the basis for our own arguments[4] for the development of human embryo cryopreservation. Our own hospital's Ethics Committee supported the proposal in 1981, and funding for the work was provided in 1982 by our government's National Health and Medical Research Council.

DEVELOPMENTS IN EMBRYO FREEZING

The first successful reports of mammalian embryo freezing were published in 1972.[5, 6] Live mice were obtained following slow cooling of 8-cell embryos to temperatures of −196°C in a dimethyl sulfoxide (DMSO)-based cryoprotectant. Modification of these methods was used successfully to cryopreserve rabbit,[7] sheep,[8] goat,[9] and cow embryos.[10, 11] These animal experiments showed that slow freezing of embryos to low subzero temperatures (−80°C) requires slow thawing,[5] transfer of embryos to liquid nitrogen at relatively high subzero temperatures (−30° to

−40°C) requires rapid thawing,[12] embryos of many species have stage-specific requirements for successful cryopreservation,[11] and glycerol could also be used successfully as a cryoprotectant for late-stage embryos.[13] These important observations became the basis for which a substantial commercial industry developed in cattle and sheep embryo banking, which is used extensively in these animal breeding industries. Mouse embryo banks have also been extensively developed for the genetic conservation and breeding of rapidly proliferating mouse strains.[14, 15] Analyses of the data generated from embryo banking in the mouse and a wide variety of other species have shown that embryo freezing is a safe and effective method in animal breeding and that there is no evidence to suggest genetic alteration of well-defined, inbred strains of mice, increased birth defects, or any other abnormality, even when embryos are exposed to high levels of ionizing radiation;[14] a consideration in the long-term preservation of embryonic material.

DEVELOPMENT OF HUMAN EMBRYO FREEZING

In 1981 we began to apply the principles developed for mouse and cattle embryo freezing to cryopreservation of the human embryo. Our preliminary studies[16] showed that embryos of all the developmental stages examined (2-cell to blastocysts) survived freezing and thawing in DMSO- and glycerol-based cryoprotectants when frozen to either relatively high or low subzero temperatures. The survival of 4- to 8-cell human embryos is in direct contrast to the failure of embryos of many other species, in particular, domestic animals such as the cow, which survive freezing only at the late morula to expanded blastocyst stages.[17] This observation led us to concentrate on the 4- to 8-cell human embryo because nonfrozen embryos of these stages resulted in pregnancies when replaced in utero in routine IVF practice. These observations were reported at a number of conferences in 1981,[18, 19] and by the end of 1982 we were successful in establishing a pregnancy from a frozen-thawed 8-cell human embryo.[20] The observations of interest at that time included the success of a DMSO-based cryoprotective medium for freezing, the apparent cell-fusagenic properties of glycerol-based cryoprotective medium and the relatively low cell-permeability of glycerol in early cleavage stage embryos,[16] the success of freezing to relatively low subzero temperatures (−80°C), and the viability of embryos despite freezing damage to some of the original blastomeres.[20] We also made detailed observations on the ultrastructure of frozen-thawed human embryos[21-23] and thereby confirmed the fusagenic properties of glycerol, which is lethal for embryonic development, and showed that extensive cell damage can result from intracellular ice formation, that abnormal embryo development can occur if damage to more than half the number of original blastomeres results, and that embryos may survive freezing and thawing with no apparent intracellular or membrane damage.

The clinical results of pregnancies and births obtained in the initial studies on human embryo cryopreservation using DMSO as the cryoprotectant were published in 1985 by Mohr.[24] It was apparent in this report that slow freezing to low subzero temperatures (−80°C) before storage in liquid nitrogen resulted in significantly higher embryo survival rates than slow cooling to higher subzero temperatures (−30° to −40°C). Zeilmaker et al.[25] reported two pregnancies and births from a method of freezing in DMSO to a relatively high subzero temperature (−40°C). However, no further reports have been published by this group, and high rates of success in the use of this method have not been confirmed by others.

Successful freezing and thawing of human blastocysts by use of the freezing methods developed for cryopreservation of cow blastocysts has been reported by Cohen et al.[26] They used a glycerol-based cryoprotective medium normally used to preserve cattle embryos and slow-cooled blastocysts to relatively high subzero temperatures (−40°C) before storage in liquid nitrogen. The cryopreservation of later stage embryos by use of this method appears to be a good alternative to slow-freezing early cleavage stage embryos to low subzero temperatures.[20]

REQUIREMENTS OF HUMAN EMBRYO FREEZING

A number of additions to normal IVF facilities are required for incorporating human embryo freezing clinically into infertility practice. A controlled biologic freezer is necessary for cooling accurately to subzero temperatures at rates of 0.1 to 0.5°C/minute. In our program we use Planar Biological Freezers (Planar Products, Sunbury-

Table 1. *Method for Slow Freezing Early Cleavage Embryos at Monash University*

Process	Medium	Time or freezing rate
Embryo culture	T6 + 10% MHS[a]	40–84 hours
Addition of cryoprotectant	PBI + 10% FCS[b]	10 minutes
	0.25 M DMSO	10 minutes
	0.5 M DMSO	10 minutes
	1.0 M DMSO	10 minutes
	1.5 M DMSO	10 minutes
Packaging in glass ampoule	1.5 M DMSO	2 minutes
Cooling to −6°C	1.5 M DMSO	2°C/minute
Seeding at −6°C	1.5 M DMSO	30 minutes
Cooling to −32°C	1.5 M DMSO	0.3°C/minute
Cooling to −35°C	1.5 M DMSO	0.1°C/minute
Cooling to −80°C	1.5 M DMSO	0.3°C/minute
Cooling to −110°C	1.5 M DMSO	10°C/minute
Storage in liquid nitrogen	1.5 M DMSO	< 5 years[c]

[a]Whittingham's T6 + 10% maternal human serum.

[b]Phosphate-buffered Dulbecco's medium plus 10% fetal calf serum.

[c]Maximum determined by Victoria's Infertility Medical Procedures Bill, 1984.

on-Thames, UK), but a number of other controlled biologic freezers are also suitable. Liquid nitrogen facilities are also needed, including substantial liquid nitrogen storage tanks that must be maintained by automatic liquid nitrogen filling or by close supervision.

It is absolutely essential that the embryologists who do the embryo freezing have substantial experience in the cryopreservation of animal embryos. We would normally expect embryologists to achieve a consistent survival rate of more than 60% of 2-cell mouse embryos frozen, developing the blastocyst stage when cultured in vitro after thawing. If survival rates are reduced after thawing or if embryos fail to develop normally to blastocysts, errors have been made in the cryopreservation technique; and these must be corrected before progressing to human embryo freezing. Some support of the importance of this experience is that all IVF groups that have been successful in developing and introducing embryo freezing into their IVF programs have experienced cryobiologists. There have been a large number of other groups who have had no success to date, and very few of the latter have had embryologists with any experience in cryobiology.

There is also a need for additional clinical responsibilities for counseling patients on the implications of embryo preservation and for the management and tracking of patients for ovulation during the cycle of thawing and embryo transfer.

METHODS OF EMBRYO FREEZING

The methods used for routine embryo freezing and thawing at Monash University are shown in Tables 1 and 2. These methods follow the stepwise evaluation of different cooling and warming rates. The continued cooling from −80°C to −110°C reduces damage to the zona pellucida, and the step of cooling very slowly between −32° and −35°C increases the survival rate of embryos, presumably through achieving greater dehydration of blastomeres.

Other methods that have been investigated include the replacement of 1.5 M DMSO with 10% glycerol,[20, 26] cooling to higher subzero temperatures (−35° to −40°C) before plunging into liquid nitrogen,[20, 25] reduction of the equilibration time at −6°C after seeding,[27] and the use of different base culture medium for mixture with the cryoprotectant.[26, 27] The replacement of DMSO with glycerol reduced early cleavage stage embryo viability,[20] and the transfer of embryos to liquid nitrogen at higher subzero temperatures reduced embryo survival.[24] It is not certain whether the other modifications benefit embryo survival and viability. In addition to these methods, our own group and others in Australia and France are examining variations of the procedure described by Renard and Babinet[28] for the rapid thawing of mouse embryos frozen in propanediol, the cryoprotectant. Preliminary data indicate that high survival rates may be obtained with very early cleavage stages (1-cell pronuclear and 2-cell embryos), a phenomenon that has been difficult to achieve in the past.[16]

Table 2. *Method for Thawing Early Cleavage Stage Embryos at Monash University*

Process	Medium	Time or thawing rate
Thawing between −80° to +4°C	1.5 M DMSO	8°C/minute
Mixing during dissolution of ice	1.5 M DMSO	1 minute
Removal of cryoprotectant	1.5 M DMSO	12–15 minutes
	1.25 M DMSO	10–12 minutes
	1.0 M DMSO	10–12 minutes
	0.75 M DMSO	7.5–10 minutes
	0.5 M DMSO	7.5–10 minutes
	0.25 M DMSO	5–7 minutes
Embryo culture	T6 + 10% FCS	1–4 hours

The freezing of human blastocysts[26, 29] involves the use of glycerol instead of DMSO and slow freezing to about −40°C before plunging into liquid nitrogen. Embryos are always thawed rapidly from −196°C by agitation of the frozen ampule in a water bath at +20° to +30°C, when transferred to liquid nitrogen at high subzero temperatures. The reason for rapid thawing is to prevent the regrowth of minute intracellular ice crystals that may be formed during freezing through incomplete dehydration of the embryos.

There are some critical steps in the embryo freezing and thawing technique, irrespective of the methods used. It is important to mix cryoprotective solutions completely because cryoprotectants such as DMSO, glycerol, and propanediol do not immediately mix when added to culture medium. One must adequately expose the embryos stepwise to increasing (before freezing) or decreasing (after thawing) concentrations of cryoprotectant to ensure that equilibration occurs before moving to the next concentration. This step requires careful pipetting of embryos through the various solutions. During dissolution of ice when thawing, it is important to mix completely the cryoprotective solution to avoid exposing embryos to excessive concentrations of cryoprotectant caused by layering when these solutions thaw. When ice crystallization (seeding) is induced, it is essential not to precool the ampule below −10°C and to induce the formation of ice crystallization at the liquid meniscus rather than inducing the rapid and complete solidification of the medium at the time of seeding, a procedure that risks rapid precooling and rewarming. One should check the ampule to ensure ice formation after seeding and before beginning to cool to lower temperatures.

Embryos may also be frozen successfully in plastic straws. The straws are sealed with a heat sealer, and air spaces are usually used to isolate the embryo from the extremities of the plastic straws. The straws are also seeded at −6°C with precooled forceps, and the straws are touched toward their extremities and not directly over the embryos.

THAWING AND TRANSFER OF FROZEN EMBRYOS

Patients requesting the thawing and transfer of their embryos advise the IVF program at the beginning of their menstrual cycle. The method we use for determining the onset of the luteinizing hormone (LH) surge has been described by Freemann et al.[30] The 95% confidence interval for the LH surge is calculated from past menstrual cycle lengths, and blood samples are obtained twice daily, beginning on the first day of this confidence interval, and assayed for estrogen, progesterone, or LH. Less precision is obtained with urine samples, although a selftest urinary dipstick assay[31] is presently under evaluation for timing of the onset of the LH surge and transfer of frozen embryos. Ovulation is confirmed by assay of plasma progesterone levels on the day before embryo transfer.

Embryos are thawed usually 4 to 8 hours before the calculated time of exact synchrony of postinsemination age and the time after ovulation (40 hours after the onset of the plasma LH surge).

Embryos are thawed slowly (8°C/minute) from −80° to +4°C in a biologic freezer, the cryoprotectant removed (Table 2), and embryos cultured in vitro for 1 to 4 hours before transfer to the patients. Only embryos with 50% or more of their original cell numbers are transferred, and no more than 3 embryos are transferred on any one occasion.

RESULTS OF EMBRYO CRYOPRESERVATION

The value of embryo cryopreservation may be assessed in many different ways. One could argue that the 20 pregnancies achieved in the Monash IVF Program (Table 3) would never have occurred in the absence of cryopreservation; the eggs or embryos would have been discarded or used in other ways. It could be argued that unless cryopreservation achieves success rates approaching that of normal IVF, then it is not worth the effort. It is almost impossible for pregnancy rates after frozen embryo transfer to be equated

Table 3. *Summary of Pregnancies from Frozen-Thawed Embryos at Monash University 1983 to 1985*

No. of pregnancies	20
No. of chemical pregnancies	2
No. of spontaneous abortions	3
No. of therapeutic abortions	1
No. of ongoing pregnancies	4
No. of births	10
Stillborn female[a]	1
Single male	3
Single female	5
Twin females	1

[a]Due to premature membrane rupture and intrauterine infection.[20]

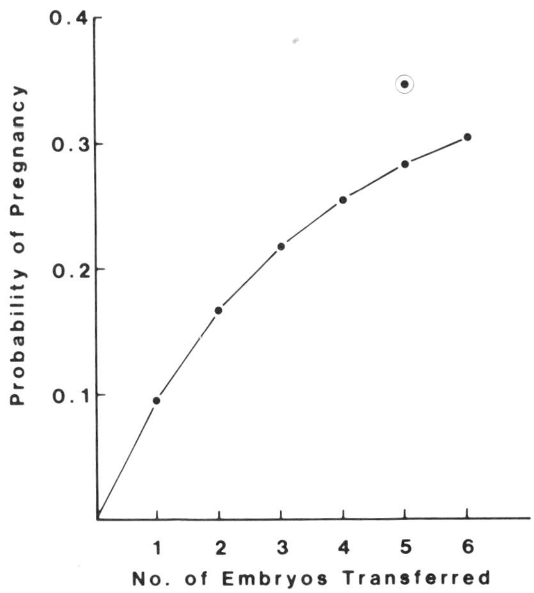

Figure 1
Calculated probability of pregnancy from the Monash University data with increasing numbers of embryos transferred. The *point* above the curve is the probability of pregnancy when five embryos are obtained and three embryos are replaced on the cycle of IVF treatment and the other two embryos frozen and thawed transferred in another ovulatory cycle. (Reproduced with permission of the publisher. From Trounson A, Hoppen H-O, Lutjen PJ, Mohr LR, Rogers PAW, Sathananthan AH: In vitro fertilization: the state of the art. In Gamete Quality and Fertility Regulation, Edited by R Rolland, MJ Heineman, SG Hillier, H Vemer. Amsterdam, Excerpta Medica, 1985, p 325.)

with that obtained after routine IVF, because fewer embryos are replaced on average, and the embryos have been subject to a major manipulation (frozen and thawed). If this view predominated, there would clearly be no progress in new IVF techniques and applications, nor would IVF itself have been developed in the first place.

The pregnancies established in our own IVF program involving cryopreserved embryos are tabulated in Table 3. There have been ten births, including a set of twins and a stillborn baby following premature membrane rupture and development of a septic infection at 26 weeks' gestation.[20] One therapeutic abortion has been carried out because of a severe fetal limb deformity. This defect was not due to chromosomal abnormality and is of concern, although it is highly unlikely for it to have arisen as a result of cryopreservation. The spontaneous pregnancy loss rate is equivalent to that observed for our own IVF program and lower than that recorded for Australian IVF pregnancies.[3]

There is only one publication[30] with sufficient unselected data to make meaningful predictions concerning cryopreservation success rates. Freemann et al.[30] reported the results for 205 patients who had all of their excess 402 embryos frozen. Of these frozen embryos, 396 were thawed and 229 (58%) were transferred to 144 (70%) of the patients, resulting in 16 (11%) pregnancies. All excess embryos were frozen, irrespective of their age after insemination and morphologic quality from the 2-cell to the 12-cell stage of development. The mean number of embryos transferred was 1.6 embryos per patient, and the mean embryo viability was 8% (number of fetuses per number of embryos transferred). The pregnancy rate per patient who had embryos frozen was also 8%. This means in practice that a further 8% may be added to IVF success rates calculated per laparoscopy for patients having four or more embryos available for transfer. When five embryos are available, and only three are transferred and two frozen, then thawed, and replaced during a subsequent ovulatory cycle, there is an advantage for IVF patients as illustrated in Figure 1. There also appears to be a distinct advantage in terms of pregnancy rate in freezing three or more embryos during the cycle of IVF treatment (Table 4). This concept is consistent with the observation that the pregnancy rate increases with the number of embryos produced and transferred in routine IVF.[2]

The calculated success rates in published reports[32] of embryo cryopreservation programs vary from 11% to 28% pregnancies of patients in whom embryos were transferred and 8% to 14% pregnancies of patients who had embryos frozen. In some reports it is difficult to determine the criteria of selection for the data presented. Cohen et al.[26, 29] reported a relatively high success rate of thawing and transfer of blastocysts: 23 blastocysts of 44 thawed were transferred to 18 patients, resulting in eight pregnancies. However,

Table 4. *Relationship of the Number of Embryos Frozen and Pregnancy Rate After Freezing and Thawing (Modified from Freemann et al.[30])*

No. of embryos frozen each IVF cycle	No. of patients with embryos frozen	No. of patients transferred embryos	Pregnancy rate/transfer
			%
1	91	52	10
2	70	51	2
3	23	20	30
4	11	11	27
5+	10	10	10

Table 5. *Success Rate of Embryo Freezing at Specific Cell Stages*[a]

% Pregnancy rate	4-cell	6-cell	7-cell	8-cell
Frozen embryos	5%	4%	2%	15%[b]
Transferred embryos	8%	9%	4%	32%[b]

[a]From Trounson A, Freemann L: The use of embryo cryopreservation in human IVF programs. Clin Obstet Gynaecol 12:825, 1985.
[b]$P < 0.001$.

data were excluded on the results of freezing and thawing when blastocysts were thawed and transferred on days 3 and 5 after ovulation. Data from Bourn Hall[33] indicate that about 40% of fertilized eggs develop to blastocysts in vitro and that about 25% are arrested from the 8-cell stage onward. The freezing of blastocysts selects only those embryos capable of continued development and excludes embryos that are arrested, fragment, or develop abnormally. This phenomenon would account for some of the differences between the results obtained with early cleavage stages and those with blastocysts. However, it is probably necessary to carry out a large-scale trial within one clinic for the determination of whether a significant advantage occurs in the results of freezing with one of the two different stages of embryonic development. The criteria used for selection of embryos for freezing will also have a major influence on the success rates achieved. For example, if only 8-cell embryos had been chosen for freezing (Table 5), the success rate achieved in our own IVF program would have been substantially higher.

FACTORS AFFECTING SUCCESS RATE OF EMBRYO CRYOPRESERVATION

Factors influencing the success rate of cryopreservation have been reviewed recently by Trounson and Freemann.[32] The number of embryos frozen (Table 4) and the developmental cell stage (Table 5) both affect the success rate of embryo cryopreservation. Embryo viability appears to increase with increasing stage of development.[29, 31] Embryo quality as assessed by the degree of regularity or fragmentation also has a significant effect[30, 32] on embryo viability. Completely regular and unfragmented embryos had the highest viability (15% developed to pregnancies), compared with those with a few fragments (12%), those with a number of irregular cells and fragments (5%), and those that were badly fragmented (0%). It has also been noted that survival rates of "irregular blastocysts" were lower than those classified as "regular."[29] The more rapidly dividing embryos were also more likely to result in pregnancies in the data reported by Cohen et al.,[29] but this trend was only apparent at the 8-cell stage in the data reported by Freemann et al.[30]

It has been surprising that damage to the blastomeres of embryos after freezing and thawing does not correlate closely with the viability of embryos, except when more than 50% of the original cell number are damaged.[30, 32] However, it was notable that 47% of undamaged 8-cell embryos contributed to all the pregnancies reported by Freemann et al.[30] and that both pregnancies obtained by Zeilmaker et al.[25] were undamaged embryos. Additional data may be required for adequate demonstration of the significant effects of freezing damage. Cohen et al.[29] reported that disruption to the zona occurs more frequently in early cleavage stage embryos and is lethal. Removal of the zona pellucida per se is probably not responsible for this effect, and damaged zonae may be associated with even more serious damage to cell function.

There is a remarkable association of pregnancy in the cycle of IVF treatment and pregnancy with the same cohort of embryos after freezing and thawing (Table 6). Only 6% of patients who failed to become pregnant on the cycle of IVF treatment became pregnant when transferred frozen-thawed embryos, compared with 41% of patients who became pregnant on the cycle of IVF treatment. It is tempting to speculate that this significant ($p < 0.001$) association is due to the collection of a cohort of viable embryos. It is not possible to exclude a hostile uterine environment in patients who fail to conceive on both the cycle of IVF treatment and the natural ovulatory cycle when frozen-thawed embryos are transferred.

Table 6. *Association of Pregnancy in the Cycle of IVF Treatment and Pregnancy After Freezing and Thawing the Same Cohort of Embryos*[a]

Outcome of transfer of frozen-thawed embryos	Outcome of transfer of fresh embryos on cycle of IVF treatment (no. of patients and pregnancy rate)			
	Not pregnant	Aborted (A)	Delivered (B)	A + B
Not pregnant	113	12	1	13 (19%)
Aborted (C)	2	1	1	2 (50%)
Ongoing/delivered (D)	5	6	1	7 (58%)
C + D	7 (6%)	7 (37%)	2 (67%)	9 (41%)

[a]Cryopreservation data modified from Freemann et al.[30]

Table 7. *Pregnancy Rate and Degree of Synchrony Between Embryo Age and Time After Ovulation for Embryo Transfer*

Factor	Time (hrs.) from calculated exact synchrony					
	+7 to +12	+3 to +6	−2 to +2	−3 to −6	−7 to −12	−12 to −24
No. of patients transferred embryos	3	2	67	27	30	18
No. of patients pregnant	0	0	9	4	3	1
%	—	—	13%	15%	10%	6%

The life-table data reported by Kovacs et al.[34] show that it takes six treatment cycles by IVF before there is a significant decline in IVF success rates. This observation would suggest that a hostile uterine environment is most unlikely to be governing the association observed in Table 6 because such defects at present require repeated failure of embryo transfer to be identified.

Cohen et al.[26, 29] transferred their frozen-thawed 5- to 10-cell embryos on day 2 after ovulation, a day earlier than the postinsemination age of the embryos, and reported that blastocysts only implant when transferred on day 4 but not on day 3 or day 5. Quinn and Kerin[27] also argued that embryos should be replaced a day earlier than the postinsemination age of the embryos. With the method described by Freemann et al.[30] for identifying the onset of the LH surge, the trend to the highest pregnancy rate in our own data is closest to exact synchrony of embryo age after insemination and the time after expected ovulation (Table 7).

The time embryos are stored in liquid nitrogen appears to have no effect on the survival or viability of embryos.[30, 32] Pregnancies have been obtained from embryos stored up to 21 months in liquid nitrogen,[32] and it could be expected that embryos will survive indefinitely in liquid nitrogen, provided they remain fully immersed.

PRESERVATION OF MANIPULATED EMBRYOS

Our own group has an interest in the micromanipulation of embryos, particularly for the identification of genetic and embryonic developmental abnormalities. We have conducted a series of experiments,[35] summarized in Table 8, in which we enzymatically removed the zona pellucida of mouse embryos and then cooled them to −6°C, froze them to −80°C, or froze and stored them in liquid nitrogen using the procedures described in Table 1. The embryos were thawed and then cultured in vitro to the expanded blastocyst stage. The data shown in Table 8 demonstrate a number of interesting principles of cryobiology:

1. The freezing and thawing of embryos to −80°C may have a relatively minor effect on embryo viability.
2. The handling of embryos at temperatures below −80°C can have a major effect on embryo viability, despite the presumption that slow cooling to −80°C should have completed blastomere dehydration and ice formation. It is frequently presumed that damage to embryos occurs at relatively high subzero temperatures. This presumption may be erroneous.
3. The removal of the zona pellucida reduces embryo viability; and the effects are greater, the earlier the cleavage stage. The role of the zona in protecting the embryo against freezing damage is not certain, but the zona may protect the embryos against intracellular ice formation during dehydration. Blastomeres may also lose their intercellular connections during freezing and thawing, and an intact zona pellucida will prevent separation and loss of blastomeres from the embryonic cell mass. It has been reported that in the human embryos disruption of the zona is lethal.[29] Our own observations in women show that the capacity of further embryonic development is severely reduced when the zona is disrupted, although this damage may not be lethal.[21] The effect of

Table 8. *Survival and Development of Mouse Embryos Frozen With or Without a Zona Pellucida*

Cell stage	Presence of the zona	% Development of blastocysts of embryos frozen		
		Cooled to −6°C	Frozen to −80°C	Frozen and stored at −196°C
2-cell	Yes	96	88	31
	No	65	36	12
8-cell	Yes	95	95	42
	No	72	60	20
Morula	Yes	85	76	43
	No	61	43	30

removing the zona may be seen even on cooling embryos to −6°C (Table 8).

4. The viability of early cleavage stage embryos following freezing and thawing is generally lower than that of later cleavage stages. Similar observations have been made with human embryos.[29, 30] This phenomenon may be due to the difference in the size of the component blastomeres, a difference which will affect the degree of dehydration, osmotic damage, and the probability of intracellular ice formation. The intracellular composition of lipid and other temperature-sensitive substances and organelles may vary according to the cell stage, possibly prejudicing the survival of certain cell stages when frozen and thawed.[17] Statistically there is also a greater chance of affecting embryo viability by the damage of a small number of large cells than a small number of small cells. The extreme example of this effect is observed with the oocyte in which, if any part of the cell membrane is damaged, survival cannot occur, whereas loss of up to 50% of cells of an 8-cell embryo will not necessarily mean the loss of embryo viability.[30, 32]

The implication of these observations for micromanipulation is that biopsied embryos[36] should probably be grown to the morula or blastocyst stage before cryopreservation. Studies on the biopsy and preservation of embryos, with a zona partially opened for retrieval of cells, indicate that disruption of the zona has less effect on embryo viability than complete removal.

CRYOPRESERVATION OF HUMAN EGGS

Our group has studied the cryopreservation of human eggs. Our initial studies[37] some years ago showed that immature eggs recovered from ovarian wedge biopsies and matured in culture for 48 hours could be frozen and thawed successfully by the use of the methods of slow freezing employed for mouse eggs[38] or human embryos, but survival rates were only about 20% of those frozen. At the time the possibility of increased aneuploidy resulting from exposure of mature eggs to cryoprotectants and to freezing and thawing was of concern. The ovulating oocyte is arrested at the metaphase of the second meiotic division with chromosomes attached to the temperature-sensitive spindle microtubules.[39] Depolymerization of the microtubules by cryoprotectants or by cooling may prevent the normal separation of sister chromatids at fertilization and thus lead to chromatid nondisjunction and the state of aneuploidy after extrusion of the second polar body. The egg is theoretically more susceptible to aneuploidy because normal separation of sister chromatids requires intact spindle microtubules at the time of sperm penetration for the immediate activation of the egg and resumption of meiosis. Aneuploidy as a result of failure to eject one chromosome would result in trisomy, and the ejection of an additional chromosome would result in monosomy. These chromosomal abnormalities are, for the most part, lethal; but if embryos do survive, infants may be born with major developmental and mental defects, such as Down's syndrome.

Whittingham and his colleagues have undertaken a major study of the chromosome complement of embryos derived from frozen-thawed mouse eggs and compared the results with the rate of defects found in eggs fertilized in vivo and in vitro. The results have been summarized by Wood,[40] who reported reduced fertilization rates and an increased incidence of chromosomal defects in embryos derived from frozen-thawed eggs; these were due primarily to an increase in polyploidy. Transfer of embryos derived from frozen-thawed embryos to recipients resulted in the same proportion of normal fetuses as embryos derived from nonfrozen eggs. Given this information, our own group continued experiments to locate a suitable freezing method for human eggs.

We have examined a number of methods for egg cryopreservation; these methods are summarized in Table 9. Since mature human oocytes were not available for screening embryo freezing methods, we used aged human eggs that had failed to fertilize when inseminated from patients enrolled in the Monash IVF program. These aged eggs (24 to 72 hours after insemination) are not viable[41] and are normally discarded, but serve as an appropriate model for studying the response of frozen-thawed mature human oocytes. Survival of these aged eggs, which have an intact plasma membrane, after thawing was considered a good index for the survival of mature unfertilized eggs. The limitations of mouse eggs and those of other species include the disparity in size and susceptibility to cooling damage because of differences in membrane and intracellular composition.

Slow and rapid cooling of aged human eggs in 1.5 M DMSO yielded results (Table 10) similar to those obtained in the original studies with ovarian wedge oocytes. Increased egg survival rates of

Table 9. *Summary of Freezing Methods Used for the Cryopreservation of Human Eggs*

Procedure	Slow[a]	Rapid	Ultrarapid	Vitrification
Addition of cryoprotectant				
Temperature	20°	20°	20°	4°
Time	10-minute steps	10-minute steps	2–3 minutes	10-minute steps
Cooling rate	0.3°/min to −50°	0.3°/min to + 35°	Plunge to −196°	Plunge to −196°
Thawing	8°/min −80° to +4°	30° Water bath	37° Water bath	0° Water bath
Removal of cryoprotectant				
Temperature	20°	20°	20°	4°
Time	10-minute steps	10-minute steps	10 minutes in sucrose	10 minute steps

[a]In DMSO or propanediol cryoprotectant.

about 50% were obtained with the use of a new ultrarapid freezing method developed in our own laboratory.[42] The use of a modified vitrification technique[43] also gave very encouraging survival rates of 75% of those eggs frozen (Table 10).

A number of mature human oocytes has been donated by IVF patients for studies of egg freezing. A summary of the results of these studies is included in Table 11. Even though small numbers of mature oocytes were involved in these experiments, it has been shown that oocytes may survive freezing and thawing and be fertilized after insemination. At least two different methods give reasonable survival rates. Oocytes vitrified with their cumulus intact, fertilized, and developed to at least the 8-cell stage and oocytes slow-frozen with propanediol as the cryoprotectant, resulted in high survival and fertilization rates (Table 11). It is likely that other methods will also be devised for egg cryopreservation, and recently a pregnancy following egg freezing has been announced publicly.[44]

Despite the development of these methods for egg cryopreservation in mid 1985, our group has been unable to take the next obvious step and transfer developing embryos to patients. This situation has developed in response to the Victorian State's Infertility Medical Procedures Bill, which prevents embryo experimentation. We have indicated to our own hospital's Ethics Committee that a small number of embryos derived from frozen-thawed eggs should be analyzed for their chromosomal and developmental normality before progressing to transfer of such embryos to patients in order to confirm the experiments on mouse eggs.[40] We agreed to a self-imposed moritorium on this work while the state government's Standing Review and Advisory Committee on IVF considered our application to study these embryos. No decision has been made on the matter to date. The hospital's Ethics Committee has also been awaiting this decision before agreeing to the transfer of embryos resulting from egg cryopreservation. The ultimate result is that we cannot progress either to examine the embryos or to transfer them to patients.

APPLICATIONS OF HUMAN EGG AND EMBRYO CRYOPRESERVATION

Egg and embryo cryopreservation has numerous and diverse applications in human medicine. These applications include the following:

1. A solution to the collection of excess oocytes and the development of more embryos than is required for transfer in human IVF.

2. An adjunct for procedures where oocytes are transferred directly to the oviducts (gamete intrafallopian transfer or GIFT procedure)[45] or to the uterus[46] for fertilization and embryo development in vivo. It is usual to transfer a maximum of four eggs in these programs, and excess eggs may be cryopreserved or fertilized in vitro and the embryos cryopreserved for transfer in later ovulatory cycles.

Table 10. *Survival of Aged Human Eggs After Freezing and Thawing by a Variety of Methods*

Freezing method	No. of eggs frozen	No. of eggs surviving after thawing
Slow cooling in 1.5 M DMSO	17	3 (18%)
Rapid cooling in 1.5 M DMSO	8	2 (25%)
Ultrarapid cooling		
in 1.5 M DMSO	62	32 (52%)
in 3.0 M DMSO	33	17 (52%)
Vitrification	12	9 (75%)

Table 11. *Freezing and Thawing Mature Human Eggs*

Freezing method	No. of eggs frozen	Survival on thawing	Survival after culture	Fertilized	Developed to 8 cells or more
Slow cooling					
1.5 M DMSO	3	0	—	—	—
1.5 M propanediol	6	4	4	4	[a]
Ultrarapid cooling	18	9	0	—	—
Vitrification					
Cumulus removed	6	4	4	3	0
Cumulus intact	16	10	10	4	3

[a]Pronuclear eggs not cultured in vitro.

3. A method for overcoming problems of synchronization between donors and recipients in egg or embryo donation programs. In our own donation program we have recently achieved a pregnancy using cryopreserved embryos in a woman who had primary ovarian failure.[47]

4. A method for preserving eggs or embryos for patients who are at risk of losing ovarian function through pelvic disease, surgery, or therapy involving radiotherapy or chemotherapy. Semen banking has been available for men at risk of losing reproductive function, and the availability of egg or embryo banking for young women seems entirely reasonable. The creation of frozen egg banks for donation would provide selection of the alternatives that are available in donor semen banks.

5. Use in new methods being developed for the diagnosis of genetic defects in preimplantation embryos. The rapid proliferation of dioxyribonucleic acid probes for the identification of chromosomal and gene defects will enable the identification of genetic abnormalities in embryonic biopsies. Embryo cryopreservation may be needed to enable sufficient time to amplify the dioxyribonucleic acid of biopsied cells and to enable in situ hybridization or the use of other molecular biologic techniques for identifying genetic abberations.

In the future it may be possible for couples to defer the formation of families by using semen, egg, or embryo banking facilities. At present there is little medical or community support for this proposal. However, this could be viewed as insurance against the development of sterility and the increased incidence of birth defects that occurs with increasing age.

CLINICAL CONSIDERATIONS OF EGG AND EMBRYO CRYOPRESERVATION

In our own IVF program the majority of patients choose to have their embryos cryopreserved in preference to other alternatives presented to them. The other options include inseminating no more than four oocytes, donation of oocytes or embryos to other infertile couples or to research, and disposal of eggs or embryos.[48] This results in about one-third of all IVF patients using cryopreservation facilities. The clinical implications of egg and embryo cryopreservation need to be carefully and fully explained to all couples receiving IVF treatment, particularly those requesting cryopreservation. Counseling on this subject is mandatory in the state of Victoria. The couple advises the IVF program's management in writing of their wishes in the event of disagreement, separation, divorce, or death of one or both partners regarding the destination of any cryopreserved embryos or eggs. More than 75% of couples wish their eggs or embryos to be donated to other couples, 15% wish them to be donated to research, and less than 5% wish them discarded. The importance of these stipulations is exemplified by the controversy surrounding the death of a wealthy American couple in an airplane accident who had two cryopreserved embryos in our own IVF program.[48] In this instance, written advice from the couple on the destination of these embryos was lacking, and the attorney general of the state of Victoria decided that the embryos would be donated to another infertile couple and included this procedure in the Infertility Medical Procedures Bill. Under the Status of Children Act in Victoria, couples agreeing to be recipients of donated eggs, sperm, or embryos are considered the parents in law, so that the donating biologic parents are not responsible for the care or financial support of children arising through donation procedures. Therefore, inheritance from the biologic parents is no longer an issue in the state of Victoria.

There are limitations for the length of time embryos can remain in cryostorage. The Infertility Medical Procedures Bill limits cryostorage to

5 years in Victoria unless there are particular circumstances requiring notification to the government. Under the Australian National Health and Medical Research Council's guidelines for IVF, cryostorage is limited to 10 years. Unlimited cryostorage, particularly across generation intervals, raises concerns in the community, although in Australia the majority view supports embryo cryopreservation in IVF.[49] The cryopreservation of eggs appears to raise few ethical concerns, and at the present time the only regulations relating to eggs are in the area of donation.

REFERENCES

1. Trounson AO, Leeton JR, Wood C, Webb J, Wood J: Successful human pregnancies by in vitro fertilization and embryo transfer in the controlled ovulatory cycle. Science 212:681, 1981
2. Wood C, McMaster R, Rennie G, Trounson A, Leeton J: Factors influencing pregnancy rates following in vitro fertilization and embryo transfer. Fertil Steril 43:245, 1985
3. Lancaster P: In vitro fertilization pregnancies Australia and New Zealand, 1979 to 1984. Report of the National Perinatal Statistics Unit, Sydney, University of Sydney, 1985, p 1
4. Trounson AO, Wood C, Leeton J: Freezing of human embryos: an ethical obligation. Med J Aust 2:332, 1982
5. Whittingham DG, Leibo SP, Mazur P: Survival of mouse embryos frozen to −196°C and 269°C. Science 178:411, 1972
6. Wilmut I: The effect of cooling rate, cryoprotective agent and stage of development on survival of mouse embryos during freezing and thawing. Life Sci 11:1071, 1972
7. Whittingham DG, Adams CE: Low temperature preservation of rabbit embryos. J Reprod Fertil 47:269, 1976
8. Willadsen SM, Polge C, Rowson LEA, Moor RM: Deep freezing of sheep embryos. J Reprod Fertil 46:151, 1976
9. Bilton FJ, Moore NW: In vitro culture, storage and transfer of goat embryos. Aust J Biol Sci 29:125, 1976
10. Willadsen SM, Polge C, Trounson AO, Rowson LEA: Transplantation of sheep and cattle embryos after storage at −196°C. In The Freezing of Mammalian Embryos, Ciba Foundation. Amsterdam, Excerpta Medica, 1977 p 190
11. Trounson AO, Shea BF, Ollis GW, Jacobson ME. Frozen storage and transfer of bovine embryos. J Anim Sci 47: 677, 1978
12. Willadsen SM: Factors affecting the survival of sheep embryos during deep-freezing and thawing. In the Freezing of Mammalian Embryos, Ciba Foundation. Amsterdam, Excerpta Medica, 1977, p 175
13. Bilton RG, Moore NW: Factors affecting the viability of frozen stored cattle embryos. Aust J Biol Sci 32:101, 1979
14. Glenister PH, Lyon MF: Long-term storage of 8-cell mouse embryos at −196°C. J In Vitro Fertil Embryo Trans 3:20, 1986
15. Mobraaten LE: Mouse embryo cryobanking. J In Vitro Fertil Embryo Trans 3:28, 1986
16. Trounson A: In vitro fertilization and embryo preservation. In In Vitro Fertilization and Embryo Transfer, Edited by A Trounson, C Wood. Edinburgh, Churchill Livingstone, 1984, p 111
17. Mohr LR, Trounson AO: Structural changes associated with freezing of bovine embryos. Biol Reprod 25:1009, 1981
18. Trounson AO, Mohr LR, Pugh PA, Leeton JR, Wood C: The deep-freezing of human embryos. (Abstr 111) Presented at the Third World Congress of Human Reproduction, 1981, Berlin, West Germany, p 367
19. Trounson AO, Mohr LR, Pugh PA, Leeton JF, Wood C: Deep-freezing of human embryos. (Abstr.) Presented at the 13th Annual Meeting of the Australian Society of Reproductive Biology, August, 1981, Canberra, Australia, p 82
20. Trounson A, Mohr L: Human pregnancy following cryopreservation, thawing and transfer of an eight-cell embryo. Nature 305:707, 1983
21. Mohr LR, Trounson AO, Leeton JF, Wood C: Evaluation of normal and abnormal human embryo development during procedures in vitro. In Fertilization of the Human Egg In Vitro, Edited HM Beier, HR Lindner. Berlin, Springer-Verlag, 1983, p 211
22. Mohr L, Trounson A: In vitro fertilization and embryo growth. In Clinical In Vitro Fertilization, Edited C Wood, A Trounson. Berlin, Springer-Verlag, 1984, p 99
23. Mohr LR: Assessment of human embryos. In In Vitro Fertilization and Embryo Transfer, Edited by A Trounson, C Wood. Edinburgh, Churchill Livingstone, 1984, p 159
24. Mohr LR, Trounson A, Freemann L: Deep-freezing and transfer of human embryos. J In Vitro Fertil Embryo Trans 2:1, 1985
25. Zeilmaker GH, Alberda AT, van Gent I, Rifkmans CMPM, Drogendijk AC: Two pregnancies following transfer of intact frozen-thawed embryos. Fertil Steril 42:293, 1984
26. Cohen J, Simons RF, Edwards RG, Fehilly CB, Fishel SB: Pregnancies following the frozen storage of expanding human blastocysts. J Vitro Fertil Embryo Trans 2:59, 1985
27. Quinn P, Kerin JPF: Experience with the cryopreservation of human embryos using the mouse as a model to establish successful techniques. J In Vitro Fertil Embryo Trans 3:40, 1986
28. Renard JP, Babinet C: High survival of mouse embryos after rapid freezing and thawing inside plastic straws with 1-2 propanediol as cryoprotectant. J Exp Zool 230: 443, 1984
29. Cohen J, Simons RF, Fehilly CB, Edwards RG: Factors affecting survival and implantation of cryopreserved human embryos. J In Vitro Fertil Embryo Trans 3:46, 1986
30. Freemann L, Trounson A, Kirby C: Cryopreservation of human embryos: progress on the clinical use of the technique in human IVF. J In Vitro Fertil Embryo Trans 3:53, 1986
31. Martinez F, Trounson A, Besanko M: Detection of the LH surge for AID, AIH and embryo transfer using a twice daily dipstick assay. J Clin Reprod Fertil. In press
32. Trounson A, Freemann L: The use of embryo cryopreservation in human IVF programmes. Clin Obstet Gynecol 12:825, 1985

33. Fishel S: Embryo culture and replacement. Presented at Jan Pfalfin Symposium, September 1985, Antwerp, Belgium
34. Kovacs GT, Rogers P, Leeton JF, Trounson AO, Wood C, Baker G: In vitro fertilization and embryo transfer—prospects of pregnancy by life table analysis. Med J Aust. In press
35. Jessup D, Trounson A: Unpublished data
36. Trounson A: Recent progress in human in vitro fertilization and embryo transfer. In Manipulation of Mammalian Development, Edited by R Gwatkin. New York, Plenum Press, 1985, p 149
37. Whittingham DG, Trounson A: Unpublished data
38. Whittingham DG: Fertilization in vitro and development to term of unfertilized mouse oocytes previously stored at −196°C. J Reprod Fertil 49:89, 1977
39. Magistrini M, Szollosi D: Effects of cold and of isopropyl-N-phenyl carbamate on the second meiotic spindle of mouse oocytes. Eur J Cell Biol 22:699, 1980
40. Wood MJ: Recent progress in animal embryo cryopreservation. In Proceedings of the Fourth World Congress on in Vitro Fertilization, Edited by I Johnston. New York, Plenum Press. In press
41. Trounson A, Webb J: Fertilization of human oocytes following reinsemination in vitro. Fertil Steril 41:816, 1984
42. Peura A, Trounson A, Freemann L: Ultra-rapid embryo freezing. (Abstr.) Presented at the Proceedings of the Fourth World Congress on In Vitro Fertilization, Melbourne, Australia, November 1985, p 244
43. Rall WF, Fahy GM: Ice-free cryopreservation of mouse embryos at −196°C by vitrification. Nature 313:573, 1985
44. Chen C: Unpublished data
45. Asche RH: GIFT (gamete intra fallopian transfer), a new treatment of infertility. (Abstr.) Presented at the Proceedings of the Fourth World Congress on In Vitro Fertilization, Melbourne, Australia, November 1985, p 203A
46. Craft IL, Djahanbakheh O, McLeod F, Bernand A, Green S, Twigg H, Smith W, Edmonds DK, Lindsay KS: Human pregnancies following intrauterine transfer of preovulatory oocytes and sperm. Lancet 2:1031, 1982
47. Lutjen P, Trounson A, Leeton J, Findlay J, Wood C, Renou P: The establishment and maintenance of pregnancy using in vitro fertilization and embryo donation in a patient with primary ovarian failure. Nature 307:174, 1984
48. Wood C, Downing B, Trounson A, Rogers P: Clinical implications of developments in in vitro fertilization. Br Med J 289:978, 1984
49. Kovacs GT, Wood C, Morgan G, Brumby M: The attitudes of the Australian community to treatment of infertility by in vitro fertilization and associated procedures. J Vitro Fertil Embryo Trans 2:213, 1985

Chapter 24

Ethical and legal issues in cryopreservation of human embryos

John A. Robertson
Baker & Botts Professor of Law

The University of Texas at Austin, School of Law, Austin, Texas

Some in vitro fertilization (IVF) programs in the United States, Australia, Great Britain, and Europe are offering cryopreservation of human embryos as a component of infertility treatment. Although still experimental, the freeze-thawing of embryos is likely to prove effective and eventually be incorporated into routine IVF practice. This communication reviews legal, ethical, and policy issues that arise for society and for physicians and patients considering human embryo freezing.

ADVANTAGES OF CRYOPRESERVATION

Embryo freezing enhances the ability to initiate pregnancy through IVF. Cryopreservation of embryos allows all eggs to be retrieved and inseminated after superovulation, with the excess of embryos required for IVF transfer stored for later use. By ensuring more embryos for transfer, cryopreservation is expected to increase pregnancies per laparoscopy in IVF treatment by 8% to 12%.[1] Patients will also find the reduced physical, psychological, and financial costs of IVF treatment on subsequent cycles attractive. Many patients undergoing IVF are likely to freeze excess embryos.

Cryostorage of embryos will also facilitate such novel means of family formation as egg and embryo donation and gestational surrogacy. Persons at risk of loss of ovarian function may also select this technique to ensure genetic offspring. Indeed, couples not ready to form a family might bank embryos as insurance against future sterility or age-related birth defects. Embryo freezing may also facilitate embryo biopsy and preimplantation diagnosis and treatment of genetic defects. In the more distant future Grobstein speculates that cryopreservation may play a role in space exploration and migration to distant planets.[2]

REQUIREMENTS FOR EMBRYO CRYOPRESERVATION

Early research suggests that embryo freezing will prove as successful in human beings as in animal breeding, in which a substantial industry now exists. Freezing at both early and late cleavage stages for indefinite periods appears feasible. Successful pregnancies have been reported after freeze-thawing of human embryos in the United States, Australia, and the Netherlands. A growing number of IVF programs are now offering cryopreservation on an experimental basis.

Successful cryopreservation, however, will require special skills and equipment and may place additional burdens on an IVF program.[1] A controlled biologic freezer capable of cooling accurately to subzero temperatures and liquid nitrogen storage system are necessary. Embryologists experienced in cryopreservation of animals are essential for a successful program. Additional counseling of patients about the implications of embryo freezing is needed. Finally, an efficient system for tracking patients, including accurate means of storage and recontact of patients at periodic intervals, is also needed.

Although every IVF program may not wish to take on these burdens, the space and equipment investment is relatively low and can be rapidly amortized in large programs. Given patient demand, many IVF programs are likely to incorporate human embryo freezing into infertility practice. The result is that thousands of embryos will be stored for varying periods across the country in

IVF clinics and embryo banks. In time an entire industry devoted to embryo banking with regionalized storage facilities and transport of embryos may emerge.

Because embryos are genetically unique living human material that can initiate pregnancy, widespread cryopreservation has medical, social, ethical, and legal significance. Numerous questions about decisional authority over stored embryos need resolution if cryopreservation is to be successfully integrated into infertility treatment.

LEGAL STATUS OF HUMAN EMBRYO CRYOPRESERVATION

Although still experimental, cryopreservation of human embryos is legally acceptable in most western countries. A number of uncertainties and unresolved questions exist. The main legal questions concern not the acceptability of freezing but particular questions of dispositional authority, length of storage, posthumous use, inheritance rights, and family relations after embryo donation and surrogacy.

No jurisdiction has yet legislated directly on embryo freezing, although official advisory bodies or commissions have addressed certain aspects of human cryopreservation in some countries. The Warnock Committee, which has conducted the most extensive review of issues in embryo freezing, endorsed cryopreservation when certain conditions were met.[3] Official advisory bodies and commissions in Australia, Ontario, and Israel have also approved cryopreservation in principle and made recommendations for length of storage, disposition of embryos, the need for prior licensing, and the like.[4, 5] Most recently, the Ethics Committee of the American Fertility Society endorsed cryopreservation as an experimental procedure.[6]

In the United States cryopreservation is legally available as an adjunct to infertility practice, although federal research funding for cryopreservation is not currently provided.[7] A few states have broadly worded fetal research laws that may appear to impinge on clinical uses of embryo freezing. But these laws were not passed to regulate embryo freezing and should not be interpreted to ban medically acceptable research or clinical uses of the technique. If they were so interpreted, they would likely be struck down as an unconstitutional interference with procreative liberty.[8]

ETHICAL ISSUES IN CRYOSTORAGE OF HUMAN EMBRYOS

Embryo freezing raises a number of ethical issues, aside from practices such as egg and embryo donation and surrogacy that it might facilitate.

A major issue is whether freeze-thawing of human embryos produces a higher rate of abnormal or defective births and thus will damage resulting offspring. Although freeze-thawing damages some embryos, the work with animals and early human data strongly suggests that a high rate of deformities is unlikely. Only the hardiest and healthiest embryos are likely to survive freeze-thawing, be implanted, and come to term.[1] Embryo freezing will not be attractive if a high rate of handicaps occurs.

A second ethical concern arises for the minority that views the preimplantation embryo itself as a subject of rights. Because freeze-thawing may damage blastomeres and render some embryos nonviable, this minority views freezing as a direct harm or wrong to embryos. Persons who object to cryopreservation on this ground often oppose IVF as well.[9]

The majority view, however, is that embryos, while deserving special respect, do not themselves have the rights or status of persons and therefore cannot be wronged.[6] Because most embryos do not implant, freezing might not damage embryos that would have implanted and come to term. In fact, freeze-thawing seems to increase the overall rate of embryo survival. Embryos that would not have been transferred (or created in the first place) may now be stored and transferred at a later time. Thus cropreservation may reasonably be viewed as showing special respect for embryos.

A third ethical issue is the psychological effect on offspring of suspended development before implantation. While suspending human development at early cleavage stages is a new development for human beings, it is akin to freezing sperm or other tissue and should not itself be psychologically problematic for offspring. For example, freezing at an early cleavage stage would not have the same impact that suspending development of a child or adult already embedded in a set of human relations would.

Yet suspended development could have psychological importance in several situations. If the period of suspension were long, it could lead to rearing by older parents or nonbiologically related persons. Freezing could also lead to novel and problematic relations with genetic parents as a result of embryo donation and gestational surrogacy. Policies about length of storage, decisional authority over stored embryos, and the relations among the participants in embryo donation and surrogacy must address the questions about offspring welfare that arise with these uses of cryopreservation.

A final set of ethical concerns in human embryo freezing is more broadly philosophic or even theologic. Some persons view embryo freezing as an unacceptable intrusion into natural processes of reproduction, or the next step on a slippery slope toward a Brave New World of governmental genetic engineering. Such concerns have arisen since the inception of IVF and are not a sufficient basis for prohibiting the practice. Indeed, such views support leaving decisions about embryo freezing to private sector actors. Moral condemnation alone is an insufficient basis for public prohibition when strongly different moral judgments exist. Individuals who find freezing objectionable need not participate in the practice.

In sum, the emerging moral consensus is that cryopreservation of human embryos is now acceptable as an experimental procedure, and if transferred thawed embryos achieve an acceptable rate of healthy births, cryopreservation would be ethically acceptable as a routine part of infertility treatment. Important ethical and legal questions remain, however, about who may properly exercise decisional authority over stored embryos and the limits of that authority.

DECISION-MAKING AUTHORITY OVER CRYOSTORED EMBRYOS

The couple or persons providing the egg and sperm would have primary decision-making authority over the embryos that were cryostored at their request. Their right to transfer their decision-making authority to others, such as the embryo bank or storage facility, is also almost certain to be recognized.

Although law and ethics have not directly addressed this issue, such a result is strongly suggested by precedents concerning control and disposition of organs, semen, blood, and other body parts.[10] A person's interest in having or avoiding biologic heirs also supports the gamete providers' authority over embryos formed from their gametes. While persons do not have unlimited freedom (property or ownership) in their body parts, the gamete providers, rather than others to whom they have not transferred their authority, have whatever property or quasi-property rights of ownership in embryos is legally available. Some right would also exist to transfer their authority to others, who would step into their shoes in deciding the disposition of stored embryos.

For implementation of their authority it is essential that persons give instructions at the time of storage concerning disposition of embryos if they do not choose to have the embryo thawed for transfer to the egg provider. These instructions could include consulting them at a later time for further instructions about continued storage or disposition (every 5 years according to Warnock).[3] They should also include specifications if they die, divorce, are unavailable for later consultation, or fail to pay storage charges. Advance instructions will avoid the problem that arose in the Rios case, in which a wealthy couple died in a plane crash without instructions about disposition of their cryopreserved embryos.[11]

Consideration of these options will require extensive counseling and discussion with couples. In considering various contingencies, couples will have to clarify the meaning or significance that stored embryos have for them. Only IVF programs able to undertake this counseling should engage in cryostorage.

TRANSFER OF DECISION-MAKING AUTHORITY

Several other questions follow from this initial assignment of property or quasi-property rights in stored embryos. One question is the storing couple's right to transfer decisional authority over cryostored embryos to others. The joint decision-making authority of the gamete providers could be transferred to one of them, to the storage facility, or to others. In general a person who receives authority from the gamete providers (or their transferee) may exercise the same rights of disposition that the gamete providers did concerning continued storage, discard, donation, and research. However, the transferee's right to discard or donate for transfer may be restricted if he or she lacks a reproductive interest in the embryo.

The gamete providers need to specify at the time of storage dispositional alternatives if joint decision-making is not possible. In the case of death, a workable solution would be to have authority pass to the survivor, with instructions specified about disposition in case of the survivor's death. In the case of divorce or separation the parties should specify that the embryo will be discarded, donated to the storage facility, or disposed of as the parties otherwise agree. They might also agree to transfer control to the storage facility in case of disagreement, as Warnock recommends.[3]

An important question concerns their right to designate or transfer decisional authority over the embryo to others if one or both of them dies. Transfer of decisional authority to the survivor of the couple, or to the storage facility if the survivor dies or is unavailable, is a workable solution that will be adopted by many couples and programs. However, some persons may wish to designate another person, for example, to assure that the decedent's wishes concerning remaining embryos are followed. Law, policy, or practice should not prematurely exclude this possibility.

A final question is whether the gamete providers' right to transfer dispositional control of embryos permits them to receive money or other consideration for doing so. While many people object to the symbolic connotations of "selling" embryos, few laws appear to prohibit directly the receipt of consideration at the present time.[8] However, official bodies in Britain and Australia have recommended against payment for gametes, embryos, and surrogacy and thus are likely to legislate against the practice if payments do occur.[3]

The question of payment is most likely to arise when the recipient or transferee of an embryo is asked to pay a fee to cover acquisition and storage costs. Because creation of embryos is expensive ($700 to $1000 per embryo in many American programs) and cryopreservation charges will arise, it is not necessarily unreasonable to ask the recipient of an embryo donation to share production and storage costs. Recoupment of costs can be distinguished from payments that reflect "profit" or other monetary gain from embryo donation.

The parallel with organ donation is instructive. The recipient of an organ transplant, rather than the donor family, pays the costs of maintaining brain-dead cadavers and surgically removing donated organs. Such payments are consistent with a firm policy against the buying and selling of organs.[12] A similar policy with embryo donations might permit the recipient to share the costs of embryo production and storage.

POSTHUMOUS THAWING AND EMBRYO TRANSFER

Cryostorage also raises the possibility of thawing and transfer to a uterus after one or both of the gamete providers has died. Such a disposition may be specified by the gamete providers at the time of storage or in their will or by the survivor of the two, or result from a transferee's donation of the embryo to an infertile couple.

The posthumous birth of children has occurred to a limited extent—fathers have died after conception and mothers in childbirth—but it remains controversial. For example, the postmortem use of stored sperm has been problematic in France and several other countries.[13] With cryopreservation of human embryos, transfer to the uterus, implantation and birth may not occur until long after the gamete source or sources have died. If cryostorage is widely practiced, there will be many more occasions to thaw and transfer embryos posthumously.

Some persons have questioned the desirability of posthumous transfer because of the feared impact on offspring of being raised by single or elderly parents or by parents who are not genetically related (as in the case of posthumous embryo donation). None of these concerns seems adequate to prevent couples storing embryos from providing for posthumous transfer. Reliance on them would be inconsistent with other accepted practices, such as embryo donation itself and elderly men fathering children. Moreover, a policy that prevents existence altogether hardly protects offspring, when rearing by nongenetically related, single, or elderly parents does not alone render a child's life not worth living. Indeed, prohibition on posthumous transfer of stored embryos might violate procreative rights of the gamete providers to reproduce after death.

However, the inheritance rights of children born posthumously from stored embryos must be clarified for this practice to occur. The ability to transfer thawed embryos to a uterus posthumously means that all biologic heirs may not be in utero or be born at the time of death, the usual requirement for a person to be the legal heir of a decedent. Should embryos "en ventre sa frigidaire" be treated like embryos "en ventre sa mere?"[14]

The possibility has enormous implications for estate planning and the orderly administration of probate. If persons born posthumously from frozen embryos are considered heirs, estates could be tied up as long as embryos are cryostored. Delays in settling estates could be enormous.

A workable policy to ensure the efficient administration of estates would be that no embryos not in utero at the time of death would qualify under intestacy statutes (which control when there is no will) or under wills that devise property to "heirs," "children," or other designations that could include posthumous offspring from thawed embryos.

However, a person's stated wish to transfer property to biologic offspring born posthumously has some appeal, particularly when the surviving wife carries the embryo. Thus an exception to the proposed inheritance policy might be considered when the testator specifically devises property to offspring "born from embryos stored at time of death." However, the risk of long delays in settling estates will still exist unless a time limit for thawing and transfer after death is specified.

LENGTH OF STORAGE

Assuming that indefinite storage of embryos is clinically feasible, the length of storage should be determined in the first instance by the gamete providers and embryo banks. Although most couples will thaw embryos to initiate pregnancy within a few months or years, situations leading to storage for 5, 10, or more years can easily be imagined. Embryo banking early in marriage to protect against later sterility or birth defects could also lead to long storage.

Embryo banks may be of two minds concerning indefinite storage. As long as charges are being paid, they might have no objection to and even desire lengthy storage. After all, the business of embryo banking is to bank embryos for paying clients.

However, IVF programs offering cryopreservation as an adjuvant infertility treatment may wish to reduce the administrative burdens of maintaining many embryos and periodically recontacting the storing parties concerning disposition. It may be administratively easier for some programs to set a time limit of 2 to 5 years, at the end of which the storing couple will be contacted and asked to decide about discard or donation to infertile couples or researchers. If the couple is not available, previously given instructions for disposal of remaining embryos will then be followed. Couples seeking longer storage may bank their embryos elsewhere.

With clear instructions concerning disposition at key decisional points, there is no need for law or public policy to specify the maximum length of storage. Indeed, such limits might interfere with the procreative goals of persons who desire longer storage and with the business of banks willing to serve them.

Storage limits recommended by various official bodies therefore need further consideration. Warnock, for example, recommended a maximum of 10 years for storage of embryos, after which time decisional authority would pass to the storage facility.[3] Other bodies have recommended limits such as 5 years or not beyond the reproductive life of the storing woman.[6]

Concerns about clinical efficacy will not support time limits if indefinite storage is compatible with thawing and healthy birth. Nor is a time limit needed to avert complications in the case of the death or divorce of the storing parties as long as clear instructions about these contingencies are given at the time of storage. Storage limits also do not protect offspring born after long storage, because the alternative for them is no life at all.

Indeed, policies limiting the length of storage could unfairly discriminate against women. A time limit based on the woman's reproductive capacity would prevent continued storage and eventual transfer to a surrogate of embryos stored shortly before a woman had to undergo a hysterectomy for medical reasons. Yet she still has an important reproductive interest in the stored embryos despite her inability to gestate, as does her spouse or partner. Similarly, 5- or 10-year limits might impair the reproductive interests of both men and women.

DISCARD OR NONTRANSFER OF FROZEN EMBRYOS

Although cryopreservation avoids the current IVF dilemma of not inseminating or transferring all fertilized eggs, the question of discard or nontransfer of embryos will inevitably arise even with cryopreservation. If the couple no longer wishes embryos thawed for transfer to the egg source, they may wish them to be discarded rather than donated to others.

Although many IVF programs insist on transferring all fertilized eggs to the uterus, this is not a legal requirement. Legally, the gamete providers, their transferees, and the storing facilities may discard embryos that they do not wish transferred to a uterus. Destruction or discard of an embryo is not covered by homicide or feticide laws, because it would not be destruction of a live-born person or fetus.[8]

Although embryo discard is a legal option, some persons have argued that respect for human life requires the embryos either not be created or that they be donated to others if they will not be transferred to the uterus of the woman providing the egg. The minority that views the preimplantation embryo as a person or moral subject in its own right holds that there is a moral obligation to transfer all embryos to a uterus.

Other persons argue for a duty to transfer all embryos on symbolic grounds, rather than as a question of moral duties owed embryos themselves. David Ozar, a philosopher, has articulated this position as follows:[15]

> The value that we as individuals and as a community attach to human life . . . is nurtured in many subtle ways in our habits and mores, and in our institutions. Thus . . . widespread public acceptance of a practice in which human embryos are made when it is efficient and economical to make them and disposed of when it is efficient and economical to dispose of them (might) have an effect on the community's valuing of human life in other contexts, an impact that would put the life of those already born at risk when tradeoffs of efficiency and economics did not favor them. We know far too little to predict that something like this will certainly occur. But we also know far too little to predict that it certainly will not. Certainly enough is at stake that we would be foolish not to acknowledge the risk. Only reasons of economy and efficiency support a policy of disposal.

In response, it may be argued that Ozar overinflates the symbolic effects of embryo discard and undervalues its procreative importance for gamete providers. At a time when more powerful symbols of human life—fetuses—may be killed in utero, the additional devaluation of human life from embryo discard appears to be minimal. After all, early cleavage embryos lack human form, are not sentient, and are not yet clearly individual.

Moreover, this position ignores the reproductive and personal significance of potential biologic offspring for the gamete source.[8] A person's interest in avoiding biologic heirs, even if they do not rear them, is significant and deserves respect. A desire to symbolize respect for human life may not be sufficient to justify laws or public policy overriding this very personal interest.

Nevertheless, the power of the state to take such a position may exist. In the United States a person's constitutional right to avoid conception and pregnancy would not necessarily provide a right to have stored embryos discarded. That right may not encompass a person's wish to avoid biologic heirs when no rearing duties are imposed, as might occur with a law requiring that unwanted embryos be donated to willing recipients.[8]

Although mandatory embryo donation laws may be within state power, the need for them can be questioned. The social importance traditionally assigned to blood relationships argues for allowing gamete providers to discard unwanted embryos. IVF programs, however, are legally free to encourage or require all patients to accept transfer of stored embryos or permit donation for transfer to others.

DONATION OF EMBRYOS FOR TRANSFER

Although embryo donation for transfer to an infertile couple may occur independent of freezing, cryopreservation increases the likelihood of donation, because synchronization of menstrual cycles is facilitated. Although few infertile couples will lack both egg and sperm and thus need an embryo donation, such cases will occasionally occur. Widespread embryo banking with shipment to distant points will increase the choice of prospective recipients, just as sperm banking does. At the present time there appears to be no ethical or legal barrier to such donations.

Embryo donations enable embryos that would otherwise have been discarded to be transferred and possibly brought to term. The separation of genetic from gestational and rearing parents that results is not so harmful to offspring that donation should be prohibited in all cases. But for the donation the offspring would never have existed. Indeed, embryo donation provides a closer link with rearing parents than does postbirth adoption because the rearing mother will also have gestated.

Legally, no states have laws specifically regulating embryo donations and few that apply by analogy. Although sometimes referred to as embryo "adoptions," legal provisions applying to postbirth adoptions of children do not apply to donation of preimplantation embryos. Thus no prior agency or court review of parental fitness is legally required. Embryo donations are so close to sperm and egg donations that they should be treated similarly.

IVF programs and physicians, however, should use due care in arranging embryo donations, as they would in using donor sperm. They should require the donating couple to execute a form relinquishing their rights and interests in the embryo. The recipient should sign a form acknowledging the donation and agreeing to rear any children born as a result. Records of the transactions should be maintained in case the offspring is accorded a legal right to learn of his or her genetic roots.[6]

As a legal transaction, the donating couple transfers their decisional authority over the embryo and rearing rights and duties in resulting offspring to the recipient. The recipient assumes rearing rights and duties in the embryo that she gestates and brings to term. The genetic parents are eliminated as rearing or social parents, with the gestational parent and her consenting partner taking on rearing rights and duties. The offspring becomes the legitimate child of the recipient couple for all purposes unless specified otherwise.[8]

Although legislation specifying this result is probably desirable, it is likely that an embryo donation agreement will be recognized by courts adjudicating disputes about custody, support, visitation, and inheritance even in the absence of legislation. Indeed, Warnock and other advisory groups have recommended a similar result in the case of embryo donations for transfer.[3]

An exception to the donor and recipient's right to settle rearing relationships in resulting offspring might arise from the offspring's interest in knowing his or her genetic roots. Because adopted children and offspring of donor sperm often have strong desires to learn their genetic roots, offspring born of embryo donations might also wish to know their genetic parents. Although most states do not currently give adopted children this right, laws permitting offspring to learn their genetic identities would appear to be a valid ground for overriding promises of anonymity or confidentiality in the donation contract.[8] In the meantime, IVF programs participating in embryo donations should maintain records on donors so that such information is available if the right is later granted to offspring.

SURROGATE GESTATORS

IVF programs cryopreserving embryos may occasionally be asked to thaw the embryo and place it in the uterus of a woman who has agreed to be a surrogate carrier for the woman providing the egg.

The main indication for surrogacy arises when the woman providing the egg lacks uterine function or is unable to complete pregnancy because of hysterectomy, endometriosis, incompetent cervix, or other medical factors. (Surrogacy for career or life-style "convenience" is discouraged at the present time.) Surrogacy is thus an alternative to embryo discard or donation when the woman providing the egg is unable to maintain a pregnancy herself. Cryopreservation greatly facilitates gestational surrogacy because it avoids the need for synchronizing the surrogate's cycle with egg retrieval from the egg source.

Surrogacy is the most controversial of all the new collaborative reproductive techniques because of the intensity and length of the surrogate's contribution and the importance of the gestational bond to mothers, offspring, and society. Such a placement is not illegal and is not necessarily unethical or undesirable if the surrogate has knowingly chosen this role. Although most surrogates to date have also provided the egg (in essence a preconception agreement to be inseminated and relinquish rearing rights and duties at birth to the father and his partner), the use of surrogates to gestate the embryo of another couple has occurred and will increase with cryopreservation.

The legal issues in surrogate gestation are still being clarified and controversy remains. Although the birthing woman has always been considered the legal rearing mother, the separation of female genetic and gestational parentage will cause this presumption to be reevaluated. Indeed, in the one known case of a surrogate gestator in the United States, a court permitted the genetic mother to be listed as the mother on the birth certificate and recognized as the rearing mother.[8]

Surrogate gestation itself is not illegal in most countries, although some American states may penalize money payments to surrogates under state baby-selling laws or refuse to enforce custody or behavior provisions of surrogate contracts.[16] However, such laws may be subject to constitutional challenge, because payment and contract enforcement is usually necessary to enable an infertile couple to reproduce in this way.[8] Other countries may not permit surrogacy at all. Warnock, for example, condemned surrogacy and recommended criminal penalties for persons arranging surrogate transactions.[3]

A major issue with surrogate gestation is whether the surrogate who changes her mind can abort or refuse to relinquish the child at birth. A surrogate who has not provided the egg is less likely to be free legally to breach her agreement. If she aborts contrary to contract, she would probably be liable for damages for destruction of the couple's embryo. Her claim to retain custody at birth is also less compelling, because she never would have received the couple's embryo for gestation unless she had agreed to relinquish the child at birth.[8]

Gestational surrogacy is best viewed, as the Ethics Committee of the American Fertility Society recommended, as a clinical experiment until more data on its effects are available.[6] It is not unethical for a program to offer surrogacy as an option for placement of stored embryos when a valid need arises and the surrogate is adequately informed. In such cases the couple and their brokering agents rather than the IVF program storing embryos will probably recruit the surrogate. The IVF program should ensure that the surrogate is freely consenting and is medically fit to carry a child. A copy of the agreement between the parties should be examined and placed in the medical records of each. The program should also cooperate with research studying the effects of surrogacy on the parties involved. Physicians who object to such arrangements or who have doubts about the validity of the surrogate's consent may choose not to participate in surrogate gestation.

DONATION FOR RESEARCH

Cryopreserved embryos may also be donated for research, if the storing couple no longer wishes them transferred to initiate pregnancy. In most cases embryos donated for research will be discarded after completion of the research. In a few cases, however, transfer to a uterus may occur, in effect making it a donation for research and possible transfer.

The question of embryo research has been controversial in Australia, Great Britain, and, to a lesser extent, the United States. To avoid controversy, many researchers are reluctant to conduct studies on human embryos. However, developments in IVF and other fields will increasingly draw researchers to human embryos as vehicles for research in infertility, contraception, genetics, cancer, and other fields.

Despite the cautious approach taken to embryo research, a consensus recognizing the ethical and legal acceptability of embryo research can be identified. Official and advisory bodies in the United States, Great Britain, Canada, and Australia have considered embryo research and found it acceptable in well-designed studies approved by institutional review boards.[17] Most of these bodies would limit extracorporeal embryo research to 14 days. They would also permit transfer to a uterus when there is reasonable grounds for thinking that the resulting offspring will be healthy. With the exception of Victoria in Australia, they would even permit research on embryos created solely for that purpose.[17]

Thus there is no question that stored embryos created to treat infertility may be donated for research before discard. Such research does not harm embryos and thus does not raise the ethical problems of research with nonviable abortuses and dying persons. If done for valid purposes, it is as consistent with respect for embryos as is research with human subjects generally. A few American states have broadly drawn fetal research laws that might appear to prohibit any embryo research. However, unless narrowly interpreted, such laws are vulnerable to constitutional challenge as an interference with first amendment and procreative rights.[17]

IVF programs that offer cryopreservation should therefore inform couples storing embryos of their right to donate them for research if they do not wish them thawed and transferred to a uterus. This option should be explored at the time of initial storage and when later decisions are made. By analogy to organ donation, request for donation of embryos for research should be considered in all cases in which embryos will not be placed in a uterus.[18]

Such requests will be helpful to researchers who need discarded embryos to conduct studies that will benefit infertile couples and others in the future. Donation of embryos for research may also provide meaning for couples when the embryo cannot be placed in the woman or donated to an infertile couple. It will also lessen the need to create embryos solely for research, although it will not eliminate this controversial issue altogether.

REGULATION OF CRYOPRESERVATION

As an experimental procedure involving human subjects, cryopreservation of human embryos currently should be conducted according to a research protocol that has been reviewed and approved by an institutional review board or similar body. Some countries may require that such review occur on a national rather than local level. In the United States this review is conducted at a local level only. Federal funding (currently unavailable for any research with human embryos) would require some form of national approval.

Once cryopreservation is routinely practiced, no special regulatory oversight seems needed. Such review is not necessary for IVF or for highly risky procedures such as heart transplants. It would be anomalous to single out cryopreservation for special licensing when accepted medical procedures of greater risk do not require this, for cryopreservation does not appear to impose risks that justify special concern. In the United States IVF programs wishing to cryopreserve human embryos are free to do so, as long as they meet institutional requirements for review of human subjects research.

Some countries, however, might opt for a special license requirement for physicians or programs wishing to conduct IVF and variations such as cryopreservation. The Warnock committee recommended such an approach for Great Britain, and several countries including Australia and Israel now take such an approach.[3]

In most countries the main regulatory mechanism will be professional practice standards and competition for patients rather than direct governmental regulation. The experience with human sperm banking, while mixed, suggests that the private sector can ensure high-quality services and avoid major problems that warrant governmental intervention.

IVF programs and embryo banks, for example, have strong incentives to comply with professionally determined standards for freezing equipment, counseling patients, recordkeeping, and the like. Given the legal rights of patients storing embryos, they are likely to respect the decisional authority of the gamete providers. Although some embryo banks may be unwilling to meet all patient demands, alternative banking facilities are likely to be available.

Reliance on the private sector, however, assumes that it will develop reasonable standards of practice and ensure that valid patient and societal interests are considered in providing this service. It would be helpful if the professional groups directly involved with infertility practice and embryo freezing convened special advisory or ethics committees, with interdisciplinary membership, to monitor developing practices. Future developments in the embryo banking industry may also require monitoring.

In litigious societies such as the United States the threat of lawsuits against IVF programs and embryo banks for negligent destruction of embryos or disregard of decisional authority should ensure compliance with professional standards and patient desires. This solution to the regulatory problem, however, requires that there be a legal remedy for negligent destruction of embryos and mistakes in recordkeeping. This remedy should not unduly add to insurance costs or be difficult to pursue by aggrieved patients.

However, the legal right to recover for negligent loss of embryos is not yet clearly established. In the *Del Zio* case in 1979 a New York jury awarded $50,000 to a couple when a physician deliberately destroyed an embryo to prevent an experimental transfer.[19] However, the basis for the award was the intentional infliction of emotional distress, rather than destruction of a property or quasi-property interest in embryos or future offspring.

Whether compensation for negligent destruction or misidentification of cryopreserved embryos will be available is unclear. Because there is no way to show that particular embryos would have implanted and gone to term, negligent loss cannot be equated with wrongful death of a child or fetus. Moreover, the loss is purely psychological and ordinarily will not occur in the presence of the parent, a situation that the tort system does not usually recognize.[20] In addition, given the uncertainty of successful pregnancy with any stored embryo, damages may be too small to support the costs of suit in most cases.

The courts will inevitably be drawn into determining whether negligent destruction of embryos is actionable. Because the storing couple does have an important procreative interest at stake, some remedy for negligent destruction seems justified. Legal concepts of tort and property may have to evolve to take care of this situation. A practical solution would be to have the couple and storage bank set liquidated damages for negligent destruction of embryos in the initial storage contract. A sum based on the cost of creating the embryo might be a reasonable basis for most losses. The apparent valuing of life that occurs here is no more offensive than provisions in accident or life insurance policies.

The private sector, however, may not adequately consider the larger societal ramifications of cryopreservation. Grobstein and others have suggested that an ongoing national commission or other deliberative body should be convened to consider the ethical and social issues that arise with cryopreservation and other novel reproductive techniques.[2] Such bodies can play useful roles in identifying consensus and problems that need to be addressed. It is not clear, however, that a national body is needed to consider further developments with embryo freezing. As discussed previously, cryopreservation poses few unique ethical and social issues, although it does facilitate extensions of IVF that may need further examination. Further developments in this field are likely to occur without such a deliberative body.

CONCLUSION

Technical advances in the safety and efficacy of human embryo cryopreservation may lead to incorporation of cryostorage into routine IVF practice. Many persons undergoing IVF are likely to choose cryopreservation of embryos not transferred during an IVF treatment cycle.[1] Embryo banking on a wide scale in many countries will probably result.

Review of legal and ethical issues shows that cryopreservation as an experimental and eventually as an established procedure is ethically and legally acceptable in most countries now offering IVF. The couple providing the gametes for the embryos exercises primary decisional authority over stored embryos and their disposition when thawed. Their right to store, transfer, discard, and donate to infertile couples or to research has wide legal and ethical acceptance. Indeed, some countries, such as the United States and Canada, may permit placement of a thawed embryo in a surrogate. For effectuation of the couple's decisional authority, it is essential that couples state their dispositional desires at time of storage in case they are not available at later decisional points.

This review has shown that cryopreservation of human embryos is less problematic ethically and legally than has originally been thought. Only the suspension of further cleavage after conception and before placement in a uterus distinguishes embryo freezing from IVF and other noncoital techniques though it does facilitate the use of some controversial techniques that can occur without freezing. Suspension of embryonic development, however, turns out to have few risks for offspring and enables embryos that would have otherwise been discarded to be placed in a uterus and brought to term. Although the possibility of long storage and posthumous transfer requires continued attention, the case for cryopreservation of human embryos to treat infertility is strong.

REFERENCES

1. Trounson A: Preservation of human eggs and embryos. Fertil Steril 46:1, 1986
2. Grobstein G, Flower M, Mendeloff J: Frozen embryos: policy issues. N Engl J Med 312:1584, 1984
3. Report of the Committee of Inquiry Into Human Fertilisation and Embryology. Warnock, M (Chairwoman). London, Her Majesty's Stationary Office, 1984, p 53
4. Victoria Committee to Consider the Social, Ethical and Legal Issues Arising from In Vitro Fertilization. Report on the disposition of embryos produced by IVF, 1984
5. Ontario Law Reform Commission, 1985
6. The Ethics Committee of The American Fertility Society: Ethical considerations of the new reproductive technology. Fertil Steril 46 (Suppl 1) 1986
7. U.S. Department of Health, Education and Welfare (HEW), Ethics Advisory Board. HEW support of research involving human in vitro fertilization and embryo transfer. 44 Fed. Reg. 35, 033, 1979
8. Robertson JA: Embryos, families and procreative liberty: the legal structure of the new reproduction. S California Law Rev 59:501, 1986
9. Hearings Before the Subcommittee on Investigations and Oversight of the House Committee on Science and Technology. (Statement of Reverand Donald McCarthy.) 98th Congress, 2d Session. 1984, p 350
10. Andrews L: My body, my property. Hastings Center Report 16:18, 1986
11. Australia dispute arises on embryos. New York Times, June 11, 1984 (A30, column 4)
12. National Organ Transplant Act of 1984.
13. Dionne, Widow wins Paris case for husband's sperm. New York Times, August 1, 1984 (A96, column 4)
14. Wadlington W: Artificial conception: the challenge of family law. Virginia Law Review 69:488, 1983
15. Ozar D: The case against thawing unused frozen embryos. Hastings Center Report 15:10, 1985
16. Doe v. Kelley, 100 Mich. App. 169, 207 N.W.2d 428, 1981

17. Robertson JA: Embryo research. Western Ontario Law Rev 24:15, 1986
18. U.S. Department of Health and Human Services: Report of the Task Force on Organ Transplantation, Organ Transplantation: Issues and Recommendations, 1986, p 31
19. No. 71-3588 (S.D.N.Y. 1978) (memorandum decision)
20. Dillon v. Legg, 441 P2d 912 (Calif. 1986)

Chapter 25

Donor eggs: their application in modern reproductive technologies

Zev Rosenwaks, M.D.

Jones Institute for Reproductive Medicine, Department of Obstetrics and Gynecology, Eastern Virginia Medical School, Norfolk, Virginia

Recent advances in reproductive medicine and reproductive technology have provided novel avenues for the treatment of infertility and have made the achievement of pregnancy possible in conditions previously thought to be irreversibly sterile.

The development of human in vitro fertilization (IVF) successfully overcame female sterility due to absent, obstructed, or irreparable fallopian tubes and has allowed the extension of this technique to any etiologic infertility factor that cannot be satisfactorily treated with conventional methods, provided the partners involved have normal gametes and the female partner has a normal uterus. Recently, the successful transfer of donor embryos[1-3] and of donor oocytes fertilized in vitro to recipient endometria has extended the use of IVF technology for conditions where the female gametes are absent, are not readily accessible to oocyte harvest,[4-10] or where there is gametic abnormality resulting in IVF failure. Moreover, the availability of donor oocytes has allowed the use of such gametes for testing fertilization potential in couples where repetitive IVF trials have resulted in lack of fertilization of apparently normal oocytes by seemingly normal spermatozoa. Thus, oocyte donation programs can be used in the treatment of human infertility as well as diagnostically to assess sperm oocyte interactions. Although oocyte donation is medically analogous to sperm donation, the relative inaccessibility of female gametes and the relative difficulty of synchronizing the ovulatory process in the donor with endometrial maturation in the recipient make the procedures quite different technically. Because the temporal window of endometrial receptivity and indeed the window of transfer in the human is unknown, the great challenge and possible reward of a donor oocyte program will be the scientific information derived from these clinical experiments.

HISTORICAL ASPECTS AND ANIMAL EXPERIMENTATION

Although the use of embryo transfer technology to alleviate infertility has been relatively recent, this technology has been under investigation for a century. The first successful embryo transfer was performed in rabbits 96 years ago.[11] This transfer was followed by experimentation in many species, with the greatest number of studies performed in the mouse, rabbit, sheep, and cow. Indeed, the first successful bovine embryo transfer was reported in 1951.[12] Since that time, many advancements and refinements have led to a high success rate and the routine use of these techniques in the cattle industry.[13] Briefly, these procedures involve the steps illustrated in Figure 1: superovulation of the donor with gonadotropins, insemination (allowing fertilization to occur in vivo), embryo recovery, isolation of the embryos, and the transfer of embryos to a recipient uterus. An alternative to immediate transfer is cryopreservation of embryos for later transfer into a suitable recipient. Thus, the donor is the genetic mother while the host or recipient is the surrogate who will carry and give birth to the young.

It appears fairly conclusive that, in order to optimize success in the bovine model, the recipient must be at the same stage of the estrous cycle as the donor. Asynchrony between the donor and recipient estrous cycle of 2 days or more in the luteal phase results in poor pregnancy rates.[14] In mice, synchrony between donor and recipient must be within one-quarter of a day for implanta-

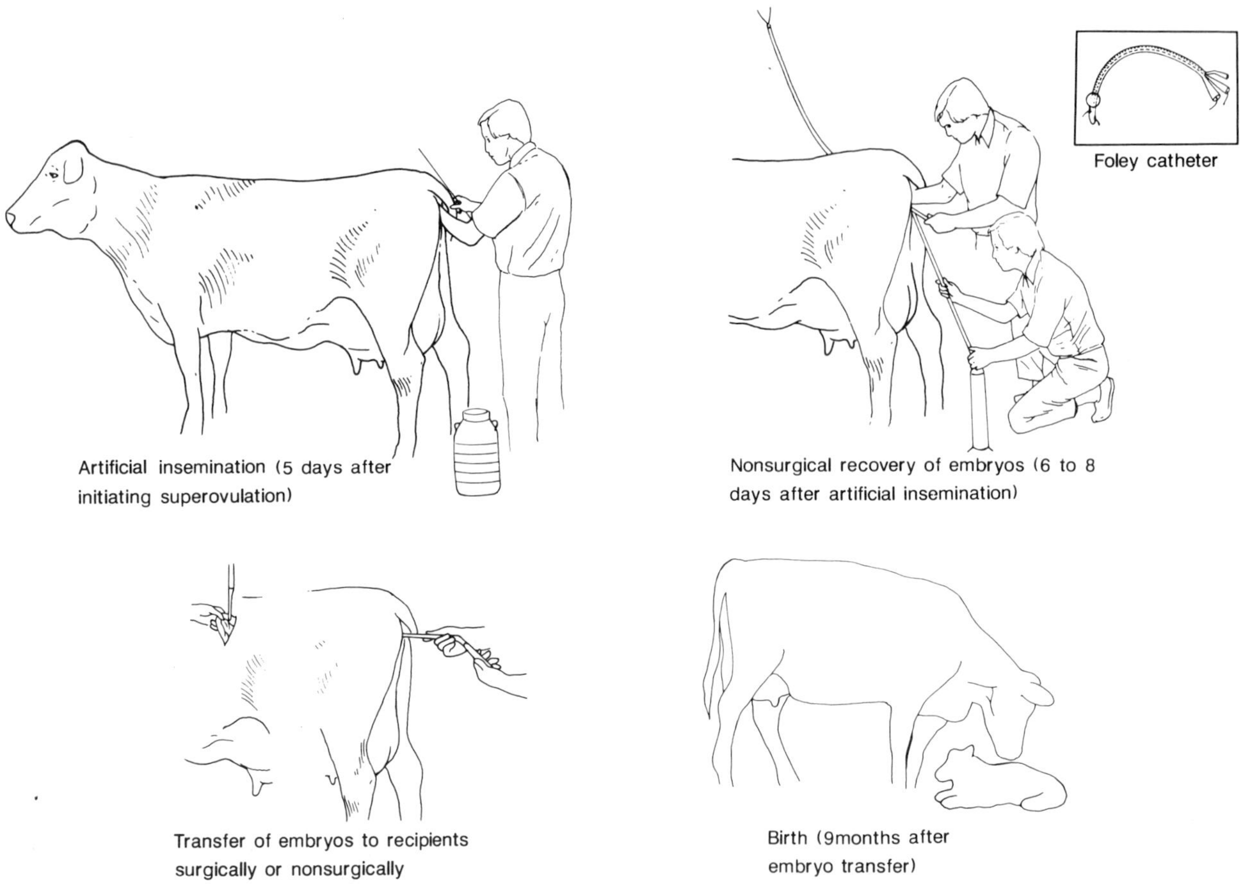

Figure 1
Schema for bovine in vivo fertilization.

tion to take place.[15] In sheep, when synchronization of donor and recipient is exact, 75% of all recipients become pregnant; a relatively high pregnancy rate is also obtained when there is asynchrony of up to 2 days. When there is a difference of 3 or more days, however, only 8% of ewes become pregnant.[16] In cattle, transfer efficiency approaches 70%.[17] Hodgen reported a 36% pregnancy rate (4 of 11 monkeys) in oophorectomized recipient monkeys replaced with subcutaneous estradiol (E_2) and progesterone (P) capsules[18] with a tolerance of 3 days of asynchrony between embryo and endometrium.

TEMPORAL WINDOW OF TRANSFER IN THE HUMAN

Hertig and Rock[19] observed that the early embryo floats freely in the endometrial cavity during the postovulatory stage of the menstrual cycle. Croxatto et al.[20, 21] and Diaz et al.[22] described the sequence of ovum tubal transport and arrival in the endometrial cavity. Their collective findings implied that the ovum arrives in the endometrial cavity most commonly on days 18 or 19 of an idealized menstrual cycle if day 14 is arbitrarily designated as the day of the luteinizing hormone (LH) surge. However, ova also could be recovered from the endometrial cavity 6 days after the LH surge. It has been suggested that in vivo egg transport is programmed in such a way as to allow adequate time for fertilization and development of the embryo to a stage that optimizes its survival and implantability in the synchronously developed endometrial environment.[21] Embryo transfer procedures should ideally mimic nature's optimization by attempting to best duplicate the in vivo sequence of events. Buster et al. relied heavily on this information when developing the temporal lavage window for their nonsurgical ovum transfer procedures.[1-3]

The procedure involved donor and recipient synchronization of ovulation. To achieve synchronization, daily serum LH and E_2 were measured in the periovulatory phase of the menstrual cycle. The objective was to synchronize LH peaks to within ± 2 days. Phenotypically matched female donors were inseminated with the infertile recipient's husband's semen on the day of or 1 day after the LH peak. Fertilization was allowed to occur in the reproductive tract of the donor woman. Nonsurgical recovery of the early conceptus by lavage of the donor uterus was performed transcervically on days 5 to 7 after the donor's LH peak, as first described by Seed and Seed in 1980 (Fig. 2).[23] Success of the nonsurgical recovery and transfer of in vivo fertilized ova must depend on the efficiency of embryo recovery and the consistency of synchronization of donor and recipient. Since Buster et al.[1] used the "natural" cycle, with its limitation of single embryo recovery, their efficiency was not optimal.

The transfer of in vitro fertilized donated oocytes to appropriately synchronized recipients (Fig. 3) has been a different approach with wider clinical applications. This procedure provides the added advantage of multiple oocyte collection in donors who are being stimulated with gonadotropins. Moreover, IVF does not require the in vivo insemination of a donor with its inherent risk of undesired retained tubal or intrauterine pregnancy and the possibility of transmitting semen-born infectious diseases. In vivo fertilization and lavage provide the advantages of retrieval of an embryo that has developed in a natural environment versus the artificial incubator environment. To optimize retrieval, one could stimulate the ovaries before in vivo fertilization and lavage.

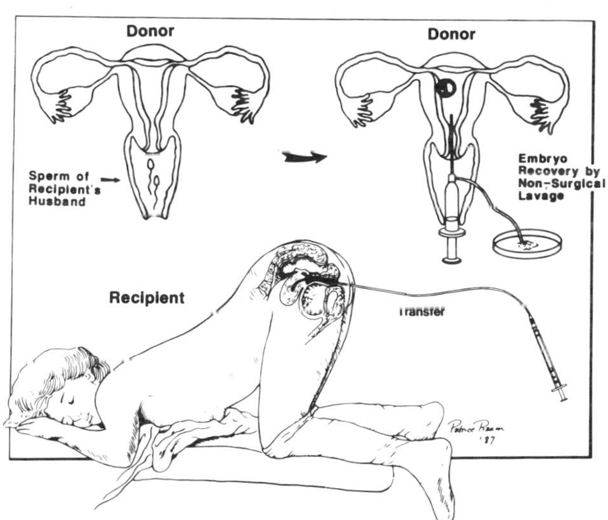

Figure 2
Schema for human in vivo fertilization; lavaged embryos are transferred to synchronized donors.

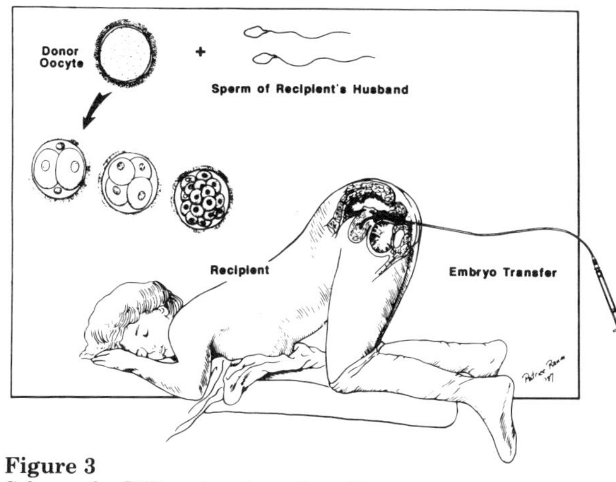

Figure 3
Schema for IVF and embryo donation.

Success of all donor oocyte procedures depends on appropriate embryo-endometrial synchronization. Critical to the achievement of pregnancy is the procurement of a viable embryo that can be transferred into a receptive endometrial milieu. It must be stressed that, in the human, the optimal conceptus stage with the corresponding critical endometrial developmental day necessary for normal implantation is unknown. Indeed, donor oocyte programs can be designed to answer this and other fundamental physiologic questions.

SIGNIFICANCE

Although IVF technology has greatly expanded our ability to treat many factors of infertility, it also has provided evidence that infertility may be due to subtle gamete abnormalities. Not only can the oocyte be the culprit, oocyte interaction with particular spermatozoa also may be at fault. Thus, the availability of both male and female donor gametes allows the study and treatment of "gametic infertility." Obvious extensions to this new technology are the use of donated oocytes for women with ovarian failure, for women with problems related to oocyte harvest, or when there is an abnormality of the oocyte.

INDICATIONS

Candidates for oocyte donation fall into two major categories: those with or without ovarian function. Conditions that may require oocyte donation in the presence of ovarian function include: (1) anatomically inaccessible ovaries; (2) repetitive failure with basic IVF; (3) repetitive lack of fertilization in vitro of apparently normal oocytes and spermatozoa; (4) genetic abnormalities (including significant autosomal dominant or sex-linked disorders or autosomal recessive traits where the couple is reluctant to use donor insemination); (5) medical contraindication to surgical ovum harvest; (6) recurrent, persistent ovarian cysts, precluding the use of ovarian stimulants; and (7) abnormal oocytes. Conditions that are amenable to ovum donation with gonadal failure include: (1) gonadal dysgenesis; (2) insensitive ovary; (3) autoimmune ovarian failure where glucocorticoid treatment has failed; and (4) premature menopause of any etiology (surgically absent ovaries or chemotherapy- and/or radiotherapy-induced ovarian failure).

With the advent of improved ultrasonographic-guided oocyte harvest techniques, fewer patients will require oocyte donation due to ovarian inaccessibility, although this still may be required where massive bowel adhesions or large blood vessels are overlying the ovaries. Multiple failures with basic IVF may result from oocyte abnormalities, lack of adequate follicular development reflected by a poor E_2 response to stimulation, or repetitive lack of fertilization. Whereas it is clear that oocyte donation should be used soon after discovery of oocyte unfertilizability or when there is repeated poor follicular development and poor oocyte harvest, it is less clear when one should resort to oocyte donation if basic IVF fails after securing normal oocyte harvest, fertilization, and transfer. In these circumstances, one can elect to cryopreserve concepti, which will be transferred later into a defined, ideally receptive endometrium. This latter step will ensure that an inadequate endometrium was not responsible for the IVF failure. It has been shown previously that endometrial histology on the day of embryo transfer may be retarded, normal, or advanced in relation to the day of human chorionic gonadotropin (hCG) administration.[24] However, it should be emphasized that, despite this attempt to define the endometrial histology on the day of embryo transfer, failure to achieve a pregnancy with cryopreserved concepti may result from the inefficiency of the cryopreservation technique itself rather than from the endometrial environment.

CANDIDATES FOR OOCYTE DONATION

Oocyte donation may be performed in three clinical situations. The protocol to be followed is dictated by the recipient's particular diagnosis or circumstance. All protocols are aimed at transfer of concepti into a defined endometrial bed, characterized histologically as day 17 to 19 endometrium by the criteria of Noyes et al.[25] This characterization seemed reasonable at the inception of the donor egg program because, in the human, the ovum arrives at the endometrial cavity at that time. It was recognized that, in the in vivo situation, a morula or blastula enters the endometrial cavity; in the in vitro fertilized donor oocyte circumstance, the 2 to 16 blastomeric embryo is transferred. Taking into consideration the presumed embryo growth in vivo, it also would seem reasonable to transfer pre-embryos on days 16 or 17, as they will continue to develop to the morula or blastula stage in the endometrial cavity by days 18 to 20, respectively, thus mimicking nature's synchrony of conceptus and endometrium. This program, with its inherent ability to manipulate the peri-implantation events (namely, conceptus stage and endometrial environment at transfer), can be used to elucidate the width of the embryo transfer window as well as the temporal window of implantation in the human.

DONORS

Donors may be IVF patients who agree to donate excess oocytes. To minimize the occurrence of multiple pregnancies, the Norfolk program policy has been to inseminate no more than five mature oocytes, with the remaining oocytes being made available for either donation or scientific study. With availability of cryopreservation as an option, most patients choose to inseminate all of their own oocytes, transfer five, and freeze any remaining concepti. Consequently, the donor program must depend upon the availability of specific donors. In some instances, a sister has provided oocytes; at other times, patients requesting tubal sterilization will agree to undergo gonadotropin stimulation before their surgical procedures. The program policy discourages payment to donors (as recommended by the Ethics Committee of The American Fertility Society).[26] All donors undergo gonadotropin stimulation. Whereas a particular stimulation protocol may be used for an IVF patient who might donate excess oocytes,[27-29] designated donors have all been stimulated with a combination of pure follicle-stimulating hormone (FSH; Metrodin, Serono Laboratories, Randolph, MA) and human menopausal gonadotropin (hMG;

Pergonal, Serono Laboratories) protocols. Gonadotropin stimulation is begun on days 3 and 4 of the menstrual cycle with the administration of 2 ampules of FSH in the morning, followed by 2 ampules of Pergonal in the afternoon. Beginning on day 5, 2 ampules of Pergonal are administered daily until critical follicular development is achieved, as judged by daily serum E_2, ultrasonograms, and cervical mucus changes as previously described.[30, 31] Typically, hCG is administered in the evening of day 9 of the menstrual cycle, and oocyte harvest is scheduled approximately 34 to 36 hours later.[32] After the harvest, the oocytes are inseminated with the infertile woman's husband's spermatozoa, as described for our basic IVF insemination procedures.[33] Typically, transfer of concepti occurs 44 to 74 hours after insemination, depending upon the recipient's luteal day and the previously defined endometrial histology for the day of transfer, thus allowing for maximal synchronization of endometrium and conceptus. For example, if on the day of the donor's oocyte harvest, the recipient is on day 14 of her cycle, one may consider transferring the pre-embryo on day 17, or 3 days after insemination. Day 17 may be more suitable for transfer than day 16, because it allows for 1 more day of endometrial maturation.

RECIPIENTS WITH NORMAL MENSTRUAL FUNCTION

OOCYTE DONATION DURING A NATURAL MONITORED CYCLE

Given the previous discussion, early attempts at donor recipient synchronization endeavored to provide a donated conceptus for transfer on days 18 or 19 of the natural cycle. Therefore, recipients were monitored for 1 or 2 months preceding the donor oocyte transfer. Serum E_2 and LH assays were performed during the early follicular phase and daily in the periovulatory phase of the menstrual cycle. A single daily LH measurement appeared to be adequate for detecting the LH surge. It is recommended that a basal body temperature (BBT) chart as well as daily P determinations in the early luteal phase be used to confirm the timing of the LH surge and ovulation. During the preparatory monitored cycle, a late luteal phase endometrial biopsy should be performed to assess the endometrial implantation bed and corpus luteum adequacy, especially in the infertile woman. Recent information suggests that synchronization of donor and recipient should be aimed at furnishing a 4- to 6-cell embryo for transfer on days 17 to 19 of the recipient's cycle. The day of the LH surge is arbitrarily defined as day 14, day 15 being designated as the day of ovulation. Figure 4 represents an example of oocyte donation in the natural cycle. Note that the recipient was a 40-year-old woman who had multiple IVF failures; the donor was a 32-year-old IVF patient who agreed to donate all mature oocytes in excess of five. Four donated oocytes were inseminated; three fertilized and were transferred on day 20 of the recipient's cycle, defined herein as day 19 relative to the LH peak, which occurred on day 15. As previously reported, a β-subunit hCG was positive 8 days after transfer and the patient delivered an infant at term.[5] Another successful recent example was of a 39-year-old woman with a 15-year history of infertility who had repeated failed IVF attempts because of an oocyte abnormality. A suitable matched donor was found who agreed to donate excess oocytes. Two 16-cell pre-embryos were transferred on the third day after the LH peak, designated herein as day 17 of the natural cycle. The recipient's LH surge occurred on the day of the donor oocyte harvest. To allow for 1 more day of endometrial maturation, the pre-embryos were placed in the uterus 3 days, rather than the customary 2 days, after in vitro insemination. Thus, 16-cell pre-embryos implanted when placed into histologic day 17 endometrium. The patient delivered a healthy infant at term.

OOCYTE DONATION DURING A FAILED IVF CYCLE

In women who have had repeated failed IVF attempts, one can be prepared to use donor oocytes during an anticipated failed cycle. Repeated IVF failures may be due to abnormalities of the ovaries and/or gametes. In such patients, previous attempts are characterized by deficient E_2 responses to ovarian stimulants in successive cycles, by recurrent poor oocyte harvests and, more infrequently, by the collection of morphologically abnormal oocytes. Oocyte abnormalities include failure of final maturation and repetitive failure of fertilization by seemingly normal spermatozoa. A cytoplasmic refractile body has been associated with lack of fertilization in some women.[34]

To maintain the anonymity of these potential recipients, it is preferable to use predesignated

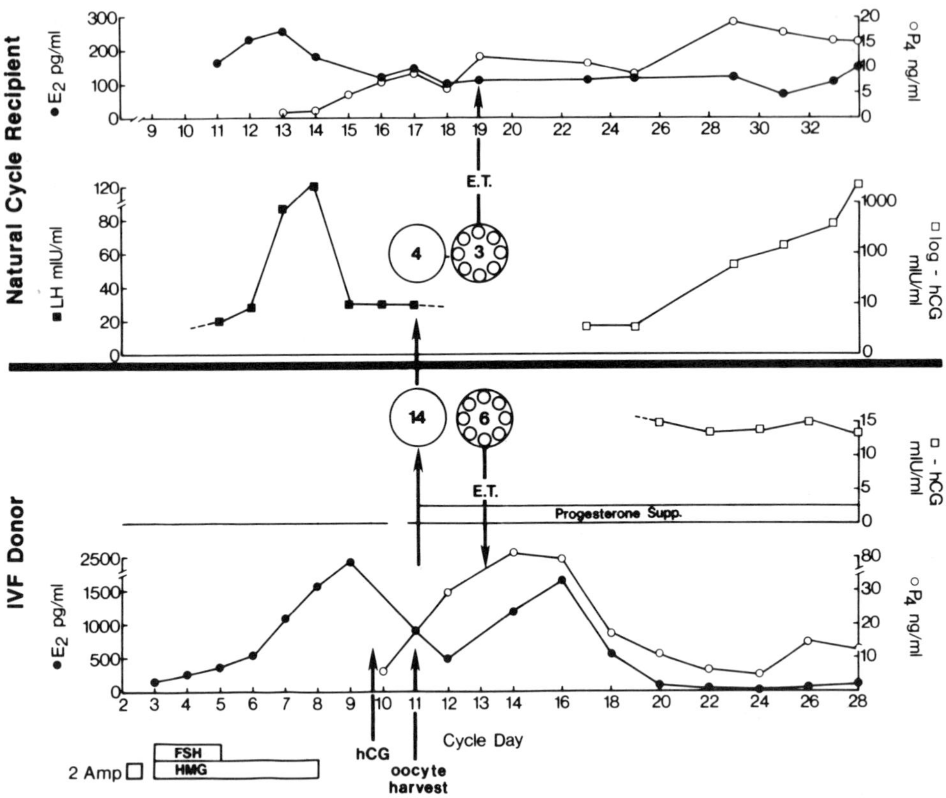

Figure 4
Oocyte donation of excess oocytes to a natural cycle recipient. The day of LH surge is arbitrarily defined as day 14. Four excess oocytes were inseminated with the recipient's husband's spermatozoa. Embryo transfer of three concepti was accomplished on day 19. , an 8-cell conceptus was the most advanced embryo transferred.

donors rather than excess oocytes from women who are co-participants in the IVF program.

Gonadotropin stimulation of donor and recipient must coincide to allow for optimal synchrony of oocyte retrievals and embryo transfers. In the event that no oocytes are obtained from the potential recipient, one can inseminate the donor oocytes with the recipient's husband's spermatozoa, aiming at a transfer day that is within 1 to 2 days of the previously anticipated transfer day. Figure 5 represents an example of oocyte transfer to both a donor and recipient who were undergoing simultaneous gonadotropin stimulation for IVF. No fertilizable oocyte was harvested from the recipient while the donor made available a single extra mature oocyte to the recipient. Both donor and recipient underwent transfer of 4-cell pre-embryos. The donor was transferred on the second day after oocyte retrieval while the recipient, who had oocyte harvest 1 day before the donor, received a 4-cell conceptus on the third day after her own failed retrieval.[9] In this example, although the actual histologic stage of the endometrium is unknown, there was tolerance, in the IVF model, of at least 1 day of asynchrony between the endometrium and conceptus. Both donor and recipient became pregnant and both delivered healthy infants at term.

OOCYTE DONATION IN RECIPIENTS WITHOUT OVARIAN FUNCTION

There have been several recent reports on the establishment and maintenance of pregnancies after transfer of donor oocyte-derived concepti to women with ovarian failure who were replaced with estrogen and P. These successful pregnancies, also accomplished in the oophorectomized nonhuman primate, suggest that pregnancy can be established and maintained, in the absence of ovaries, with replacement of estrogen and P only. While estrogen is necessary for endometrial proliferation and induction of endometrial P receptors in the follicular phase, it is unclear whether luteal phase estrogens are necessary for implantation and pregnancy maintenance in the primate. It has been firmly established, however, that luteal P is necessary to allow implantation and to maintain pregnancy in most species, whereas the estrogen requirements in the luteal phase vary from species to species. For example, estrogen is critical for normal implantation in the

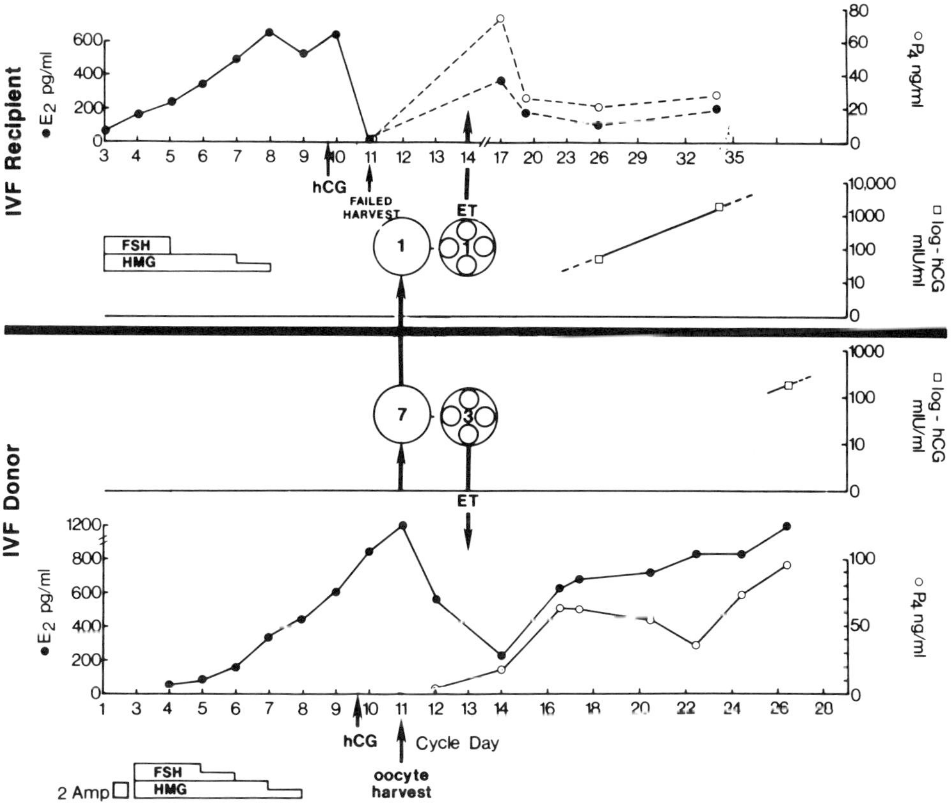

Figure 5
Embryo transfer to both a donor and recipient undergoing IVF. A donated oocyte was inseminated 1 day after the recipient's laparoscopy and a 4-cell conceptus was transferred 2 days later. Both donor and recipient conceived. *Number in circle* represents the oocytes retrieved or transferred.

rodent,[35] while it may be facilitatory in the rhesus monkey.[36] Meyer et al.[37] were able to maintain pregnancy with administration of P alone in rhesus monkeys who were ovariectomized between days 2 and 6 after ovulation. Hodgen[38] was able to allow implantation and maintain pregnancies after transfer of donated embryos in 4 of 11 P-replaced rhesus monkeys who were ovariectomized after ovulation. Supraphysiologic E_2 levels inhibited implantation. P in increasing doses was able to antagonize the deleterious E_2 effects. More importantly, P alone could maintain a pregnancy in the ovariectomized rhesus monkey.[38] Similar data on human E_2 and P requirements are lacking. Csapo et al.[39] suggested that P replacement therapy in women undergoing luteectomy during the first 50 days of gestation could maintain a pregnancy, whereas E_2 alone could not do so. Thus, the role of P in establishing and maintaining a pregnancy in the primate has been confirmed, while the relative importance of E_2 is unclear. Until further information in the human is available, it seems reasonable to simulate the menstrual cycle in ovarian failure patients who are prepared for ovum donation. Although several steroid replacement protocols have been proposed, they all endeavor to mimic the steroidal milieu of the normal menstrual cycle.

REPLACEMENT PROTOCOLS

Lutjen et al.,[4] who reported the first pregnancy in an ovarian failure patient, used oral E_2 valerate (Progynova, Schering, Sydney, Australia) and vaginal P suppositories for steroid replacement. Following embryo transfer and for the maintenance of pregnancy, they used intramuscular P injections. Navot et al.[10] modified the Lutjen protocol by using only intramuscular P for luteal phase replacement. Briefly, 1 mg/day E_2 valerate was administered orally on days 1 to 5. The dosage was increased to 2 mg/day on days 6 to 9 and to 6 mg/day on days 10 to 13. The dosage was reduced to 2 mg/day on days 14 to 17, then increased to 4 mg/day on days 18 to 26, and then reduced to 1 mg/day on days 27 and 28.[10] It should be noted that the reduction of E_2 valerate on days 14 to 17 was used to mimic the drop in E_2 that one observes during the natural cycle after the LH surge. P was administered in a single intramuscular dose, 25 mg on days 15 and 16, increasing to 50 mg on days 17 through 26, then reduced to 25 mg/day on days 27 and 28. Navot's protocol[10] appears to result in satisfactory serum levels of both steroids as well as adequate endometrial development as judged by luteal biopsy.

A number of replacement protocols have been evaluated in Norfolk. E_2 has been delivered by the vaginal route using polysiloxane-impregnated E_2 rings, provided by Paul Stumpf, M.D.[40, 41] (Jersey Shore Medical Center, Neptune, NJ) or by the oral route using micronized E_2 (Estrace, Mead-Johnson, Evansville, IN) following a modification of the Lutjen protocol.[4] P has been administered most frequently by vaginal suppository or by intramuscular injection. Although early studies suggested that 2000 mg intravaginal polysiloxane cylinders (also provided by Paul Stumpf, M.D.) were adequate for achieving appropriate P blood levels, their use was soon abandoned because of vaginal discomfort and/or infection. The surface area necessary for delivery of nanogram levels of P made the cylinder too cumbersome and impractical.

E_2 REPLACEMENT

Two micrograms of micronized E_2 are administered orally on cycle days 1 to 5. The dosage is increased to 4 mg/day (given at 12-hour intervals) on days 6 to 9, and to 6 mg/day (given at 8-hour intervals) on days 10 to 13. The dosage is then decreased to 4 mg/day on days 14 to 28 (Fig. 6). Serum E_2 and estrone levels are measured to ensure adequate absorption and to permit dose modification as necessary. An alternative method for estrogen replacement uses E_2-impregnated vaginal rings. These rings are placed in the vagina, thus allowing a steady release of E_2 into the bloodstream. The replacement schedule is highly individualized to ensure optimum simulation of the menstrual cycle hormonal milieu. It may be necessary to monitor patients for 2 to 3 cycles before adequate hormonal replacement is achieved. A typical replacement protocol is represented in Figure 7. Note that a new ring is replaced on days 1, 9, 11, and 13. Absorption data reveal that, with each insertion of a "new" ring, one observes a "burst" of E_2 before a steady state of absorption is maintained. One can use this phenomenon in order to achieve super high E_2 levels at the simulated midcycle by reintroducing a new ring every other day. It became evident early on, however, that vaginal P suppositories inhibited the absorption of E_2, probably by coating the ring surface. Therefore, it was necessary to add oral E_2 to achieve adequate estrogen levels in the luteal phase.

PROGESTERONE REPLACEMENT PROTOCOLS

Adequate P levels can be achieved by vaginal suppository or by intramuscular administration. We have used 75 mg vaginal-administered P (given every 8 hours in divided doses) on days 15 and 16. The dosage was increased to 150 mg of P (given every 8 hours in divided doses) from days 17 to 26; it then was decreased to 25 mg three times per day on days 27 and 28. Absorption studies confirm the adequacy of replacement as compared with normal control luteal phase levels, as illustrated in Figure 8. P replacement also can be accomplished by intramuscular injection, as demon-

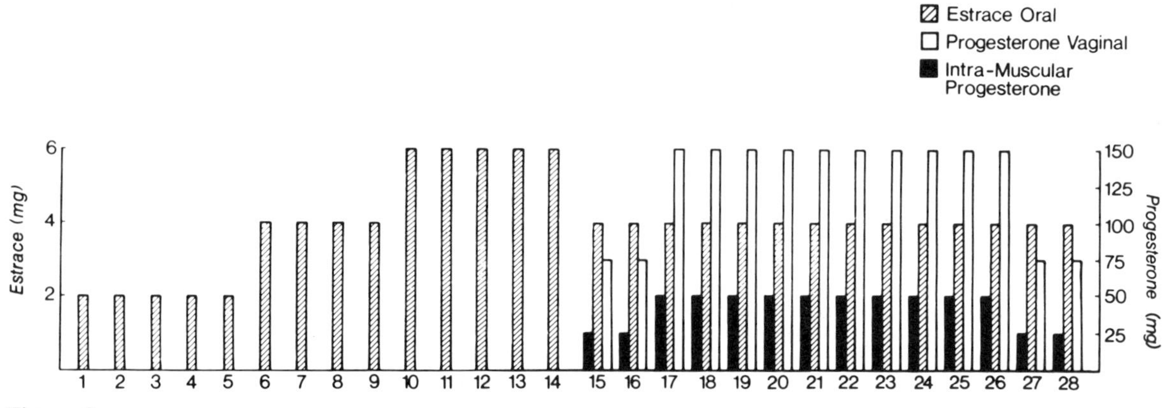

Figure 6
Estrogen and P replacement protocols currently used in Norfolk.

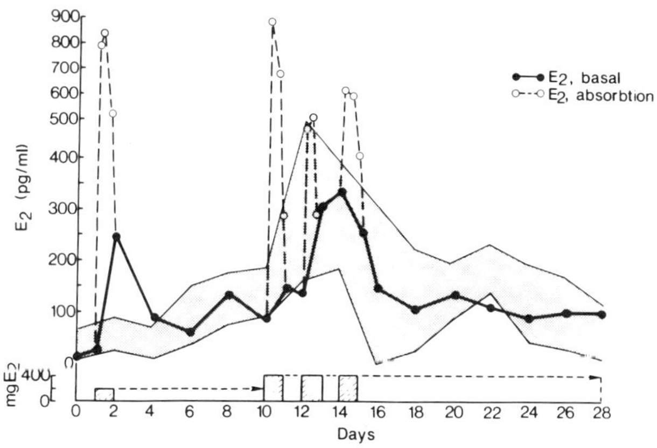

Figure 7
Vaginal E_2 impregnated polysiloxane rings protocol. (●), Baseline morning serum levels. (○), Absorption levels at 1, 2, and 6 hours after ring insertion. *Shaded area* represents the E_2 ranges in normal cycling women.

strated by Navot et al.[10] (Fig. 9). Alternatively, P suppositories can be used during the monitored, simulated preparatory cycles (to assess the adequacy of endometrial maturation), later to be supplemented or changed to the intramuscular route of administration during the cycle of embryo transfer.

Final judgment on the suitability of a given replacement protocol depends on the histologic assessment of the endometrium. Secretory changes, which compare favorably with the expected natural cycle day histology, would be the desired end point.

Endometrial biopsies are performed during two replacement cycles. An early to midluteal biopsy is followed by a late days 26 to 27 biopsy in a second estrogen and P replacement cycle.

We have observed that early biopsies, performed on days 20 to 22, display days 17 to 18 glandular architecture, along with a characteristic days 21 to 23 stroma. A typical early biopsy performed on day 21 is depicted in Figure 10. Note the subnuclear vacuolization and linear arrangement of nuclei characteristic of day 18 architecture, juxtaposed with edematous stroma suggestive of days 21 to 22 endometrium. This asynchrony occurs despite seemingly adequate P absorption. In contrast, biopsies performed on day 26 reveal the characteristic pseudodecidual changes in the stroma of days 25 to 26 endometrium. Thus, early endometrial gland development seems to be lagging behind the stroma, though the endometrium appears to catch up in the late luteal phase. It should be emphasized that the early luteal phase biopsy findings were confirmed on repeated biopsies, suggesting that the lag in glandular maturation was not due to "first cycle" exposure to steroids, but rather this lag may indicate that the glands may require a longer, albeit lower threshold exposure to P in order to achieve prompt and timely secretory changes.

It is possible that, during the natural cycle, the early rise in P on day 14 allows the gradual development of the glandular endometrial compartment, whereas during replacement therapy, the endometrium is exposed to progesterone 1 to 2 days later, thus explaining the disparity between glands and stroma in the day 20 or day 21 biopsies. Conversely, the stroma may mature more rapidly when exposed to a threshold level of P.

That the apparent lag in development of the glands does not appear to interfere with implantation is suggested by a pregnancy resulting from the transfer of two concepti into endometrium on day 18 of a simulated cycle, which had previously shown such dysynchrony between glands and stroma. The patient was a 39-year-old woman with secondary ovarian failure caused by radiation exposure. She was replaced with E_2 vaginal rings and P vaginal suppositories. Transfer of two pre-embryos (of 6 and 4 blastomeres) on day 18 of the cycle resulted in a singleton pregnancy. After

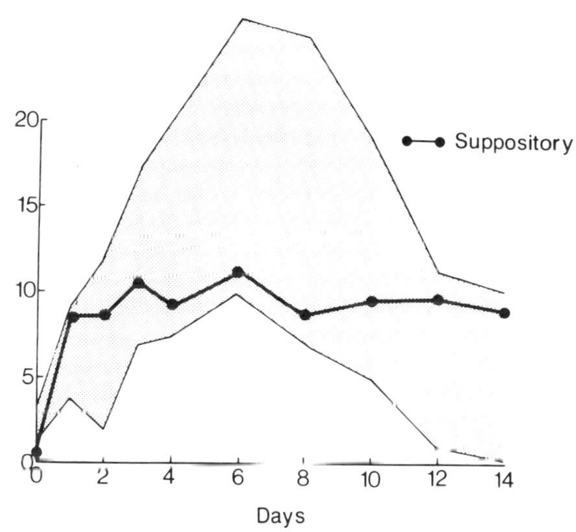

Figure 8
Representative daily P concentrations after treatment with P vaginal suppositories in the simulated luteal phase. *Shaded area* depicts the luteal range of P levels in normal cycling women. P (75 mg) is administered on days 15 and 16 in three divided doses, 150 mg on days 17 to 25 in divided doses, then decreasing to 75-mg on days 27 and 28.

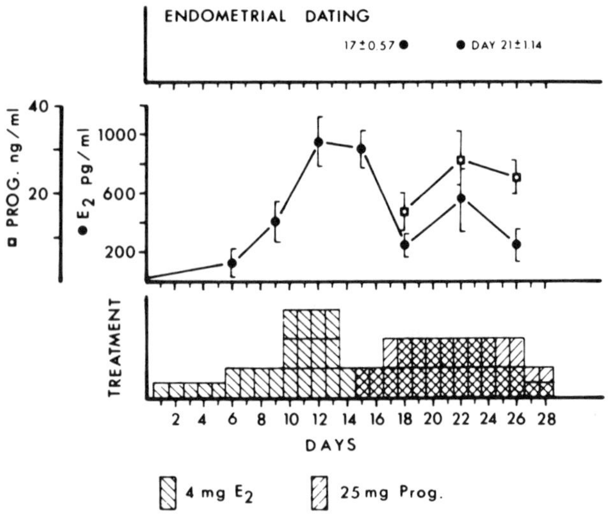

Figure 9
Exogenous hormonal treatment, serum estrogen and P levels in eight patients undergoing estrogen and P replacement. Adapted from Navot et al.[10]

transfer, intramuscular P was administered until midtrimester. Serum P levels were maintained between 20 and 70 ng/ml. An oral E_2 (Estrace) dosage between 3 and 5 mg/day was maintained in the first trimester, then tapered and discontinued by week 13 of pregnancy.

The mere fact that pregnancies have occurred after transfer of concepti on days 18 and 19 of the replaced cycle suggests that the retarded glandular development may not be as critical for implantation as the stromal developmental stage. It should be noted that Navot and co-workers[10] found a greater conformity between the day of biopsy and the expected histologic architecture in women receiving intramuscular P for luteal phase replacement. Similarly, Lutjen et al.[7] reported that endometrial biopsies obtained on luteal day 21 or 22 in patients treated with P vaginal suppositories (50 mg on days 15 and 16, followed by 100 mg on days 17 to 26) were histologically dated as day 20 ± 2.1 days endometrium (mean ± standard deviation; range, 17 to 23) in nine women with ovarian failure.[42] The disparity in endometrial dating between the Norfolk and Melbourne findings, despite Norfolk's higher P dosage, may represent a different interpretation of similar histologic findings. Conversely, the (retarded) delayed glandular development observed in the Norfolk series may be secondary to the somewhat lower serum E_2 concentrations seen in some women who were replaced with oral E_2 (Estrace). It may be that inadequate or suboptimal estrogen replacement could result in diminished follicular proliferation, decreased induction of P receptors in the glands, and consequent delayed glandular maturation.

DONOR OOCYTE PREGNANCIES

There have been few published reports[6, 7, 10] of pregnancies after donation of in vitro fertilized oocytes. The Monash group has widely reported on their experience in ovarian failure patients who were treated with oral E_2 valerate and P vaginal suppositories. Lutjen reported six ongoing pregnancies after 28 embryo transfers.[43] Approximately 60% of transfers were with "fresh" embryos, with the remaining constituting cryopreserved-thawed embryos. Navot and co-workers[10] reported on two successful pregnancies in eight ovarian failure patients who were treated with oral E_2 and intramuscular P. In Norfolk, five pregnancies have resulted from transfer of embryos to E_2- and P-replaced women. Two pregnancies occurred after replacement with E_2 vaginal rings, whereas three occurred after oral E_2 (Estrace). Three of the five pregnancies are ongoing at 37 weeks', 24 weeks', and 13 weeks' gestation, respectively. Three other pregnancies have resulted from the transfer of in vitro fertilized donated oocytes during the natural cycle. The reported world IVF experience with donated oocytes is depicted in Table 1.

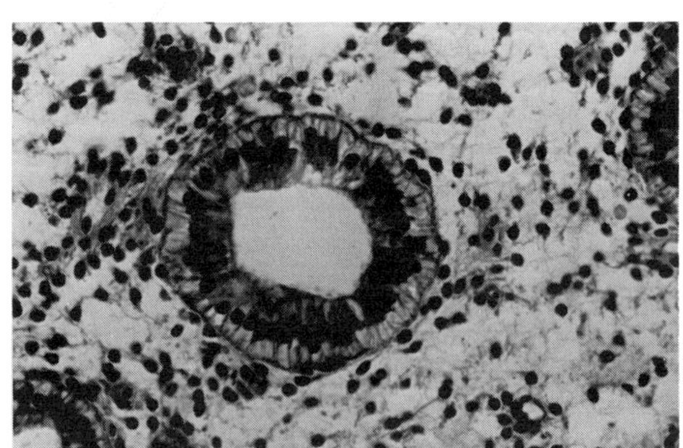

Figure 10
Histology of day 21 endometrial biopsy after estrogen-P replacement of an ovarian failure patient. Note the subnuclear vacuolization and linear arrangement of nuclei characteristic of day 18 glands juxtaposed with edematous stroma characteristic of days 21 to 22 endometrium.

Table 1. *IVF of Donated Oocytes: The World Experience*[a]

Author	No. of embryo transfers	Days of transfer[b]	No. of pregnancies	No. of viable pregnancies
			(%)	(%)
Rosenwaks	21	17–19	8 (38)	6 (28.6)
Rosenwaks	11	20–24	0 (0)	0 (0)
Lutjen et al.[4]	31	16–18	6 (19)	4 (13)
Navot et al.[10]	8	16–21	2 (25)	2 (25)
Levran[45]	27	17	10 (37)	4 (15)
Feichtinger and Kemeter[44]	4	17	1 (25)	1 (25)
Devroey et al.[49]	31	—	3 (9.7)	2 (6.5)

[a]Fresh oocytes only.
[b]First day of P is day 15. Day of spontaneous LH surge is normalized to day 14.

WINDOW OF TRANSFER

Clinically, the goal of a donor oocyte program is the achievement of a pregnancy in an infertile or sterile woman. Scientifically, such a program may serve as a tool to answer critical physiologic questions. By transferring concepti into previously histologically defined endometrial environments, we can determine the width of the window of transfer and implantation in the human. Navot et al.[10] transferred concepti (pre-embryos) into eight women between days 16 and 21 of the estrogen and P replacement cycles. Two women with primary ovarian failure, transferred on days 18 and 19, respectively, became pregnant. Four embryos, two 6-cell and two 4-cell, were transferred on day 19 in one, whereas one 6-cell and three 4-cell embryos were transferred on day 18 of the replaced cycle in the other. The six unsuccessful transfers were performed on days 16, 17, 18 (two), 19, and 21.

The Monash group[7] typically performed embryo transfers on day 17 ± 1 of the replaced cycle. Whereas the Hadassah group[10] used predesignated assigned donors who were stimulated with gonadotropins, with subsequent multiple transfers for all their recipients, the majority of the Monash transfers were of embryos derived from IVF patients who were willing to donate excess oocytes. Thus, they transferred single embryos in most donation cycles. Because it has been shown that the IVF success rate is increased after transfer of increasing numbers of embryos,[46] it is expected that transfers of multiple concepti to recipients would result in an improved success rate. Perhaps more importantly, excess oocytes obtained from IVF patients tend to be the least desirable morphologically because the oocytes with the best morphology are saved for the IVF patient. Thus, clinics using excess oocytes may have a lower pregnancy rate than clinics that use designated fertile donors. For the most part, we have used excess oocytes in Norfolk, although sisters of patients and women undergoing sterilization procedures have been donors as well.

To determine the window of transfer in the human, we have transferred available embryos on different days of the luteal phase. Of 21 transfers performed with multiple concepti derived from mature oocytes, seven patients became pregnant. All 7 (or 7 of 14) were transferred on days 17 to 19 of an idealized menstrual cycle, while none of the remaining 7 patients who were transferred on day 20 or later became pregnant. These preliminary observations taken together with the reported world experience, suggest that placing embryos of four or more blastomeres into an endometrium that is histologically developed to days 17 to 19 is more likely to result in implantation and pregnancies. A pregnancy following gamete interfallopian tube transfer of donated oocytes to E_2- and P-replaced ovarian failure patients has been reported by Asch et al.[47] In this circumstance, P administration is begun as the day of tubal transfer. Thus, the conceptus arrives in the endometrial cavity after in vivo tubal transfer, presumably on days 18 to 19 of the simulated cycle. A recent report by Formigli et al.[48] suggests that a blastula may implant when placed into day 22 endometrium. However, the Formigli report lacked precise delineation of the occurrence of the LH surge and ovulation. More data must accumulate to further define the window of transfer and implantation in the human.

MAINTENANCE OF PREGNANCY IN THE OVARIAN FAILURE PATIENT

Detailed experience on the requirements for pregnancy maintenance has been reported by several investigators. A positive β-hCG titer can be expected approximately on days 26 to 28 or 10 to 12 days after embryo transfer. If the pregnancy test is negative, one tapers the E_2 and P dose to allow endometrial shedding and menstruation to occur. If positive, most investigators have immediately and substantially increased the E_2 dose. Lutjen et al.[7] maintained their patients on 2 mg of E_2 valerate in the luteal phase of the transfer cycle, increasing the dosage to 8 or 9 mg/day as soon as the β-hCG titer became positive. At the same time, they placed the patient on intramuscular P at 50 to 100 mg/day. They suggest that this regimen maintains the plasma steroid levels at concentrations that are within the normal ranges for pregnancy. Their goal is to maintain E_2 concentrations at 100 to 500 pmol/l and P within the 100 to 200 nM/l range. Lutjen et al. discontinued E_2 treatment at 12 weeks of pregnancy, whereas P injections were maintained through the 16th week. Withdrawal of medication was predicated on observing a rise in endogenous steroids from the placenta. From the observations of Csapo and associates[39] in luteectomized women, one would expect adequate placental steroidal production after days 50 to 60 of pregnancy. Navot and co-workers[10] maintained steroid concentrations at supraphysiologic levels. At time of embryo transfer, they increased the intramuscular P dose from 50 to 100 mg/day. They then increased the P dose by 25 mg/week, to a maximum of 200 mg of P/day by the eighth week. The E_2 valerate dose was increased by 4 to 6 mg/week until the seventh week, when the amount of E_2 valerate administered reached 24 mg/day. In contrast to the described Australian[4] and Israeli[10] protocols, the Norfolk pregnancy maintenance protocol is highly individualized. Dosage adjustment is liberal and is highly dependent on the measured serum steroidal concentration. The P dose is maintained at 50 mg/day administered intramuscularly, rarely exceeding 75 mg/day. The E_2 (Estrace) dosage has ranged from 3 to 10 mg/day. One pregnancy, currently at 24 weeks, was maintained on 3 to 6 mg/day of Estrace until week 15 of pregnancy. We have attempted to minimize the dosage of replaced E_2 in view of the observations in the rhesus monkey by Meyer et al.[37] and Hodgen,[38] which suggested that E_2 replacement may not be necessary in the primate. In our first ovarian failure pregnancy, however, we attempted to maintain the pregnancy with P injections only. The E_2 levels remained between 10 and 30 pg/ml during the luteal phase. No attempt was made to appreciably increase the E_2 levels. Although the β-hCG titers were increasing properly for 7 days after pregnancy diagnosis, they soon began to drop in the ensuing week, finally decreasing to 0 by week 6. During a second established pregnancy in the same patient, E_2 rings were used for follicular phase E_2 replacement. Micronized E_2 was administered at 3 mg/day doses in the luteal phase, increasing to 5 mg/day by week 7, then decreasing until week 12 of pregnancy to 1 mg/day, with discontinuation of Estrace by the 13th week. E_2 levels were maintained at 100 to 300 pg/ml and endogenous placental E_2 began to rise on the 8th week of gestation. Maintenance of a fixed steroid dose allowed the assessment of onset of endogenous E_2 and P production by the placenta. Navot et al.[10] observed an E_2 surge during the 11th week, and began stepwise withdrawal of E_2 at that time. P appeared to rise during the 12th week of pregnancy. Lutjen et al.[7] reported earlier increases in steroid production, with withdrawal of steroids being started on days 65 and 38 of pregnancy in two recent patients, respectively. Cessation of replacement was completed on day 80. In comparison, earlier patients required greater dosages for replacement and steroids were withdrawn in the second trimester.[4] It appears that, in the human, E_2 concentration requirements for implantation and early pregnancy maintenance may be less than previously used. Further investigations are needed to specifically determine the ideal E_2/P ratio necessary for implantation and pregnancy maintenance in the human.

USE OF DONOR OOCYTES FOR DIAGNOSIS OF INFERTILITY

It has been suggested that repetitive lack of fertilization in vitro, during clinical attempts with basic IVF, is an indication for a trial of fertilization with donated oocytes. The practice of donor insemination for male factor infertility is widely accepted and is used with increasing frequency in IVF where the semen profile suggests that lack of fertilization is most likely due to a qualitative problem in the male. Similarly, in cases where there appears to be "normal" spermatozoa, with repeated lack of fertilization, one can use donated oocytes to assess spermatozoan fertilizability. Many programs continue to transfer all fertilized embryos, making oocyte-sperm interaction testing only possible in couples who agree to accept the transfer of concepti derived from donated oocytes. This clinical tool then can be used successfully as a test of gametic infertility.

We have used donated oocytes twice for testing sperm-oocyte interaction in couples with failed IVF. In one circumstance, there appeared to be morphologically "normal"-appearing oocytes, whereas harvested oocytes in the other situation did not undergo final oocyte maturation in vivo. In the second instance, fertilization occurred sporadically, after maturation of the patient's oocytes in vitro, but no pregnancy resulted. After IVF and transfer of mature donated oocytes, the patient became pregnant and carried a pregnancy to term. In the first instance, insemination of donated oocytes by the husband's seemingly normal spermatozoa resulted in lack of fertilization, confirming a fertilizing defect by the husband's spermatozoa. The couple was advised to undergo artificial donor insemination, demonstrating that a donor oocyte program can be used effectively as a diagnostic tool for unexplained infertility.

CONCLUSIONS

Oocyte donation has extended our ability to treat women previously thought to be irreversibly sterile. Basic IVF combined with oocyte donation procedures have provided insights into hitherto undefineable causes of infertility. The direct observation of gametic interaction and the ability to substitute the male or female gametes allows the assessment of infertility at the microscopic level. The transfer of embryos into defined endometrial environment continues to provide critical scientific information on the "window of receptivity" of human endometrium. Although the quality of transferred embryos remains enigmatic and confounds the interpretation of the data, our results strongly suggest that the window of transfer in the human for the 4- to 16-cell embryo extends to day 19 (perhaps day 20) of the idealized 28-day cycle, with the proximal width of the window as yet undefined. If one assumes that the 4- to 16-cell conceptus becomes a blastula within 2 to 3 days in vivo, then it can be surmised that the window of implantation in the human does not extend beyond day 22 or 23 of the menstrual cycle.

Estrogen and P replacement in ovarian failure patients allows assessment of the relative roles of these steroids in endometrial proliferation and differentiation. The transfer of defined staged concepti into specific endometrium has enabled the assessment of the window of implantation in the human. Clearly, precise manipulation of endometrial proliferation and differentiation, by varying E_2 and P regimens in ovarian failure patients, will allow the separation of endometrial from ovarian factors. The ability to manipulate the estrogen and P dosages during pregnancy in ovarian failure patients will precisely define the roles of these steroids in the establishment and maintenance of pregnancy.

A donor oocyte program, while being an exciting and gratifying treatment modality for infertility, has provided a unique human model for the study of conceptus, endometrial and steroidal interactions. It may elucidate previously unapproachable questions of human reproduction and infertility.

Acknowledgments. I thank all the members of the Jones Institute for their collaboration and Darlene Caryl for preparing the manuscript.

REFERENCES

1. Buster JE, Bustillo M, Thorneycroft IH, Simon JA, Boyers SP, Marshall JR, Louw JA, Seed RW, Seed RG: Nonsurgical transfer of in vivo fertilized donated ova to five infertile women: report of two pregnancies. Lancet 2:223, 1983
2. Bustillo M, Buster JE, Cohen SW, Thorneycroft IH, Simon JA, Boyers SP, Marshall JR, Seed RW, Louw JA, Seed RG: Nonsurgical ovum transfer as a treatment in infertile women: preliminary experience. JAMA 25:1171, 1984
3. Bustillo M, Buster JE, Cohen SW, Hamilton F, Thorneycroft IH, Simon JA, Rodi IA, Boyers SP, Marshall JR, Louw JA: Delivery of a healthy infant following nonsurgical ovum transfer. JAMA 251:889, 1984
4. Lutjen P, Trounson A, Leeton J, Findlay J, Wood C, Renov P: The establishment and maintenance of pregnancy using in vitro fertilization and embryo donation in a patient with primary ovarian failure. Nature 307:174, 1984
5. Trounson A, Leeton J, Besanka M, Wood C, Conti A. Pregnancy established in an infertile patient after transfer of a donated embryo fertilized in vitro. Br Med J 286:835, 1983
6. Rosenwaks Z, Veeck LL, Liu H-C: Pregnancy following transfer of in vitro fertilized donated oocytes. Fertil Steril 45:417, 1986
7. Lutjen PJ, Leeton JF, Findlay JK: Oocyte and embryo donation in IVF programs. Clin Obstet Gynaecol 12:799, 1985

8. Leeton J, Trounson A, Wood C: The use of donor eggs and embryos in the management of human infertility. Aust NZ Obstet Gynaecol 24:265, 1984
9. Rosenwaks Z: Donor eggs. In In Vitro Fertilization, Norfolk, Edited by HW Jones Jr, GS Jones, GD Hodgen, Z Rosenwaks. Baltimore, Williams & Wilkins, 1986, p 270
10. Navot D, Laufer N, Kopolovic J, Rabinowitz R, Birkenfeld A, Lewin A, Granat M, Margaliot E, Shenker JG: Artificially induced endometrial cycles and establishment of pregnancies in the absence of ovaries. N Engl J Med 314:806, 1986
11. Heape W: Preliminary note on the transplantation and growth of mammalian ova within a uterine foster mother. Proc R Soc Lond 48:457, 1890
12. Wilett EL, Black WG, Casida LE, Stone WH, Buckner PJ: Successful transplantation of a fertilized bovine ovum. Science 113:247, 1951
13. Seidel GEJ Jr: Superovulation and embryo transfer in cattle. Science 211:351, 1981
14. Newcomb R, Rowson LE: Conception rate after uterine transfer of cow eggs in relation to synchronization of oestrus and age of eggs. J Reprod Fertil 43:539, 1975
15. Beatty RA: Transplantation of mouse eggs. Nature 168:2995, 1951
16. Rowson LEA, Moor RM: Embryo transfer in the sheep: the significance of synchronizing oestrus in the donor and recipient animal. J Reprod Fertil 11:201, 1966
17. Rowson LEA, Lawson RAS, Moor RM, Baker AA: Egg transfer in the cow: synchronization requirements. J Reprod Fertil 28:427, 1972
18. Hodgen GD: Surrogate embryo transfer combined with estrogen-progesterone therapy in monkeys, implantation, gestation and delivery without ovaries. JAMA 250:2167, 1983
19. Hertig AT, Rock J: A series of potentially abortive ova recovered from fertile women prior to the first missed menstrual period. Am J Obstet Gynecol 58:968, 1949
20. Croxatto HB, Diaz S, Fuentealba B, Croxatto HD, Carrillo D, Fabres C: Studies on the duration of egg transport in the human oviduct. I. The time interval between ovulation and egg recovery from the uterus in normal women. Fertil Steril 23:447, 1972
21. Croxatto HB, Ortiz ME, Diaz S, Hess R, Balmaceda J, Croxatto HD: Studies on the duration of egg transport by the human oviduct. Am J Obstet Gynecol 132:629, 1978
22. Diaz S, Ortiz M-E, Croxatto HB: Studies on the duration of ovum transport by the human oviduct. III. Time interval between the luteinizing hormone peak and recovery of ova by transcervical flushing of the uterus in normal women. Am J Obstet Gynecol 137:1161, 1980
23. Seed RG, Seed RW: Artificial embryonation—human embryo transplant. Arch Androl 5:90, 1980
24. Garcia JE, Acosta AA, Hsiu J-G, Jones HW Jr: Advanced endometrial maturation after ovulation induction with human menopausal gonadotropin/human chorionic gonadotropin for in vitro fertilization. Fertil Steril 41:31, 1984
25. Noyes RW, Hertig AT, Rock J: Dating the endometrial biopsy. Fertil Steril 1:3, 1950
26. The Ethics Committee of The American Fertility Society: Ethical considerations of the new reproductive technologies. Fertil Steril (Suppl 1) 46:1S, 1986
27. Garcia JE, Jones GS, Acosta AA, Wright G Jr: Human menopausal gonadotropin/human chorionic gonadotropin follicular maturation for oocyte aspiration: phase I, 1981. Fertil Steril 39:167, 1983
28. Garcia JE, Jones GS, Acosta AA, Wright G Jr: Human menopausal gonadotropin/human chorionic gonadotropin follicular maturation for oocyte aspiration: phase II, 1981. Fertil Steril 39:174, 1983
29. Bernardus RE, Jones GS, Acosta AA, Garcia JE, Liu H-C, Jones DL, Rosenwaks Z: The significance of the ratio of follicle-stimulating hormone and luteinizing hormone in induction of multiple follicular growth. Fertil Steril 43:373, 1985
30. Muasher SJ, Garcia JE, Rosenwaks Z: The combination of follicle-stimulating hormone and human menopausal gonadotropin for the induction of multiple follicular maturation for in vitro fertilization. Fertil Steril 44:62, 1985
31. Rosenwaks Z, Muasher SJ, Acosta AA: Use of hMG and/or FSH for multiple follicle development. Clin Obstet Gynecol 29:148, 1986
32. Rosenwaks Z, Muasher SJ: Recruitment of fertilizable eggs. In In Vitro Fertilization, Norfolk, Edited by HW Jones Jr, GS Jones, GD Hodgen, Z Rosenwaks. Baltimore, Williams & Wilkins, 1986, p 30
33. Veeck LL, Maloney M: Insemination and fertilization. In In Vitro Fertilization, Norfolk, Edited by HW Jones Jr, GS Jones, GD Hodgen, Z Rosenwaks. Baltimore, Williams & Wilkins, 1986, p 168
34. Veeck LL: Failure of fertilization in vitro. In Atlas of the Humans Oocyte and Early Conceptus, Edited by LL Veeck. Baltimore, Williams & Wilkins, 1986, p 314
35. Findlay JK: The endocrinology of the pre-implantation period. In The Endocrinology of Pregnancy and Parturition: Current Topics in Experimental Endocrinology, Vol 4, Edited by L Martin, VHT James. New York, Academic Press, 1983, p 35
36. Hearns JP: Primate models for early human pregnancy. In Animal Models in Human Reproduction, Edited by M Serio, L Martini. New York, Raven Press, 1980, p 319
37. Meyer RK, Wolf RC, Arslan M: Implantation and maintenance of pregnancy in progesterone-treated ovariectomized monkeys (*Macaca mulatta*). Presented at the 2nd International Congress of Primatology. Vol 2. Edited by H Hofer. Atlanta, GA, 1968, p 30
38. Hodgen GD: Presented in part at the 4th International Congress of In Vitro Fertilization, Melbourne, Australia, November 19 to 22, 1985
39. Csapo AI, Pulkinnen KO, Wiest WG: Effects of luteectomy and progesterone replacement therapy in early pregnant patients. Am J Obstet Gynecol 115:759, 1973
40. Stumpf PG, Maruca J, Santen RJ, Demers LM: Development of a vaginal ring for achieving physiologic levels of 17 beta-estradiol in hypoestrogenic women. J Clin Endocrinol Metab 54:208, 1982
41. Stumpf PG: Selecting constant serum estradiol levels achieved by vaginal rings. Obstet Gynecol 67:91, 1986
42. Lutjen PJ, Findlay JR, Trounson AO, Leeton JF, Chan LK: Effects on plasma gonadotropins of cyclic steroid replacement in women with premature ovarian failure. J Clin Endocrinol Metab 62:419, 1986
43. Lutjen PJ: Unpublished data
44. Feichtinger W, Kemeter P: Pregnancy after total ovariectomy achieved by ovum donation. Lancet 2:722, 1985

45. Levran D: Unpublished data
46. Jones HW Jr, Acosta AA, Andrews MC, Garcia JE, Jones GS, Mayer J, McDowell JS, Rosenwaks Z, Sandow BA, Veeck LL, Wilkes CA: Three years of in vitro fertilization at Norfolk. Fertil Steril 42:826, 1984
47. Asch R, Balmaceda J, Rochester M: Pregnancy following GIFT (gamete intrafallopian transfer) in premature ovarian failure. Presented at the Conjoint Annual Meeting of The American Fertility Society, the Canadian Fertility and Andrology Society, Toronto, Canada, September 27 to October 2, 1986. Published by The American Fertility Society, in the 1986 abstracts of the scientific paper and poster sessions, p 54
48. Formigli L, Formigli G, Roccio C: Donation of fertilized uterine ova to infertile women. Fertil Steril 47:162, 1987
49. Devroey P, Braeckmans P, Camus M, Khan I, Smitz J, Staessens C, Van Der Abbeel E, Van Waesberghe L, Wisanto A, Van Steirteghen AC: Pregnancies after replacement of fresh and frozen-thawed embryos in a donation program. In Future Aspects of Human In Vitro Fertilization, Edited by W Feichtinger, P Kemeter. Berlin, Springer-Verlag, 1987, p 133

SECTION VI

Male Infertility

The traditional investigation of the infertile couple includes a critical assessment of the husband's reproductive capabilities. Although the exact incidence is unknown, a male factor has been found to be significant in 15% to 30% of infertility couples and may play a contributing role in another 10% to 20% of cases. Because early classic investigation placed undue emphasis on sperm concentration, other determinants of male fertility potential often went unrecognized in the past. Today the physician managing the infertile couple must have a broad understanding of the endocrinology, genetics, immunology, and pathophysiology of the male reproductive system in order to provide appropriate investigation and sound management. An understanding of spermatogenesis and techniques to evaluate sperm quality is imperative. Important factors to be considered in the evaluation include possible autoimmunity to sperm, microbial factors, anatomic alterations such as varicoceles, possible ejaculatory dysfunction, and psychological factors. It is clear that close cooperation between the gynecologist, andrologist, and urologist is critical to successful management of male infertility.

Fertilizing determinants of sperm include their ability to fertilize the ovum itself. In this section Rogers provides a reevaluation of the sperm penetration assay (SPA) and the controversies surrounding the utilization of this test. In 1979 she and her associates recognized the potential of using the zona-free hamster eggs as surrogate eggs to evaluate fertilizing potential of human sperm and reported ranges for fertile and infertile men.[1] When there is well defined male infertility, the range of penetration is very low. The percent penetration should be reported with reference to a donor of known potential. Rogers proposes a standardized methodology for the SPA which includes eight factors such as strict adherence to abstinence time, washing procedure, and time of sperm and egg interaction. The SPA has its most significant correlation with semen analysis in the areas of motility, quality, and morphology. In vitro fertilization (IVF) programs have made available the opportunity to perform simultaneous inseminations using both zona-free hamster eggs and zona-intact human eggs. In her laboratory 86% of the results are concordant. Cryopreservation of semen samples has proved an unacceptable means of preserving the fertilizing potential for this assay. Potential pitfalls which plague the SPA are discussed. Rogers makes the interesting observation that approximately 16% of men with no definite sperm abnormality have 0% SPA and would have been missed by routine semen analysis. Rogers concludes that while SPA does not faithfully reproduce in vivo conditions, this test comes the closest to adequately evaluating the functioning potential a sperm was designed to achieve—egg penetration. While SPA appears to correlate well with male fertility in vivo, the value of SPA in IVF remains controversial. Kuzan and coauthors have reported that pregnancy rates were similar in patients with low and normal SPA scores and found no correlation between SPA and IVF in their study.[2]

The indications for intrauterine insemination (IUI), the direct transfer of sperm to the uterine cavity, are examined by Allen and associates at Vanderbilt University. Wide discrepancies in reported pregnancy rates result from dissimilar methods of sperm preparation, protocols for insemination, and criteria employed for patient selection. Techniques for sperm washing and preparation are reviewed in this report. Appropriate timing and duration of therapy are extremely important. Controversy surrounds the effectiveness of IUI for infertility due to male factor from such conditions as oligospermia and poor SPA. While some reports suggest a 25% pregnancy rate for IUI-treated male infertility, many others report a poor success rate. The results of IUI for patients with infertility associated with cervical factor achieve a pregnancy rate of 50% to 70%. While the criteria for establishing the presence of cervical factor infertility varies widely from study to study, most authors base their diagnosis on abnormal postcoital tests. The use of IUI for the treatment of immunological defects remains controversial. IUI may help when cervical mucus antibodies are the primary obstacle to fertility. However, surface antisperm antibodies produced in the male genital tract are insufficiently separated by the multiple washings and centrifugation techniques. IUI would not be expected to correct infertility problems in these patients and may in fact increase the risk of sperm sensitization in these women.

The timely overview and the recommendations for screening therapeutic insemination donors for sexually transmitted diseases is contributed by Greenblatt and coauthors at the University of Washington in Seattle, Washington. Sexually transmitted pathogens are associated with a wide variety of disease states now including acquired immunodeficiency syndrome (AIDS). Guidelines for minimizing the transmission risk and these consequences are formulated on the basis of estimates of prevalence and associated morbidity. The authors provide a table of 13 pathogens, noting in each case the presence in semen, reported transmission by donor semen, and likelihood of transmission in the few cases in which it has not yet been reported. While the AIDS virus has been reported to be transmitted by donor semen, the hepatitis B virus has not. Interestingly, *Chlamydia trachomatis* transmission by therapeutic donor insemination has not yet been documented.

In recommending donor screening guidelines the authors suggest a two-step procedure. In the first step potential donors are screened by history and serologic screening for cytomegalovirus (CMV). The second step involves the physical examination, urethral cultures, and additional serologic testing to include HTLV-III, the AIDS virus. Surveillance and follow-up include rescreening of donors at least every six months. The use of frozen semen provides a number of advantages but also has some drawbacks. For many physicians the recommended screening process is too cumbersome. Where facilities for cryopreservation are available, semen can be frozen pending the results of cultures and serologic testing. It has been suggested that freezing may reduce the concentration of some viral and bacterial pathogens, but this concept is not yet well documented.

Haas and Beer combined to provide a comprehensive chapter on the immunological influence of sperm gametogenesis and maturation in the male and female genital tracts. They describe the immune protection of sperm during their development, the development of sperm antibodies which react with only a select subpopulation of sperm because sperm in the male genital tract undergo a constant maturation process, and the immunoregulatory factors which have been hypothesized. During passage of spermatozoa through the female genital tract, cervical mucus aids in sperm selection, acting as both a mechanical and immunological filter. Immunoglobulins are produced not only by cervical cells but by endometrial and oviductal cells as well, where immunological clearing of sperm continues. Exposure of sperm to capacitating conditions results in a redistribution of the sperm surface antigens. The sperm membrane is a dynamic surface that is constantly varying its presentation to its environment.

Another chapter on the immunology of semen is contributed by Alexander and Anderson, who review recent basic research concepts and clinical implications of both immunostimulatory and immunosuppressive aspects of semen immunology. Listed in tabular form is the large number of known human sperm antigens of possible immunologic significance, while many more still are being defined by sperm specific monoclonal antibodies. Because antisperm antibodies are associated with infertility, it may be possible to develop contraceptive vaccines based on sperm antigens. Alexander and Anderson observe that antisperm immunity may be naturally controlled by male reproductive immunosuppressive factors and individuals lacking such factors and their spouse may experience immunosuppressive infertility. By regulating immunosuppressive factors produced in male reproductive tissues, it may be possible to treat infertility, to aid in the irradication of pathogenic organisms residing in these tissues, or to develop more effective sperm antigen vaccines in men.

The final chapter in this section written by Zamboni discusses the relevance to infertility of ultrastructural examination of semen. Transmission electron microscopy (TEM) may help to identify a variety of sperm defects and developmental abnormalities not diagnosable by conventional methods of semen analysis. The electron microscope can identify flagellar defects which impair motility through pathology of the flagellar axoneme and the outer dense fibers. It also makes possible evaluation of acrosomal defects such as hypoplasia and agenesis which are important causes of infertility. Similarly, the structural organization of the sperm nucleus and the connecting piece can be readily evaluated by TEM. Defects of the sperm nucleus and separation of the head from the tail are of ominous significance in infertility. Ultrastructural examination is indicated for patients with normal semen analysis, yet long standing unexplained infertility, patients with negative zona-free hamster egg penetration assays, and those with abnormal sperm motility and head configuration. This review will make the reader more aware of the wide constellation of sperm defects and developmental abnormalities, only a few of which can be identified by routine evaluation of human semen.

Roger D. Kempers, M.D.

REFERENCES

1. Rogers BJ, Van Campen H, Ueno M, Lambert H, Bronson R, Hale R. Analysis of human spermatozoal fertilizing ability using zona-free ova. Fertil Steril 32:664, 1979
2. Kuzan FB, Muller CH, Zarutskie PW, Dixon LL, Soules MR: Human sperm penetration assay as an indicator of sperm function in human in vitro fertilization. Fertil Steril 48:282, 1987

Chapter 26

The ultrastructural pathology of the spermatozoon as a cause of infertility: the role of electron microscopy in the evaluation of semen quality

Luciano Zamboni, M.D.

Department of Pathology, Los Angeles County, Harbor-UCLA Medical Center, Torrance, California, and University of California School of Medicine, Los Angeles, California

The classification of male infertility from pretesticular, testicular, and post-testicular causes,[1-5] still widely used in modern textbooks and treatises of pathology[6] and urology and infertility,[7-10] does not include the pathology of the spermatozoon among the causative factors of reproductive failure, and modern reviews of methods of semen analysis[10-12] are still based on old seminal cytologic classification schemes, such as those proposed by MacLeod[13] in the early 1960s. This is in sharp contrast to the significant progress that has been made in the last 25 years in the elucidation of the complex structural organization of the spermatozoon (Fig. 1) and the highly specialized functions of its components.[14-21] This progress, in turn, has been instrumental in the clarification of major aspects of the reproductive process that had been unclear for a long time (such as capacitation and its structural manifestations and the mechanisms that facilitate the progression of the spermatozoon through the egg investments and its conjugation with the female gamete). Since man expresses his fertility potential through the sperm, the insufficient attention and the inadequacy of the methods with which the structural integrity and functional fitness of the cell are studied in the everyday clinical evaluation of male infertility are disturbing and certainly not commensurate with the depth at which the same parameters are researched in reproductive biology. This article is aimed at alerting the reader to the existence of a variety of sperm defects and developmental abnormalities that are causes of infertility and are not identifiable by conventional methods of semen analysis. It is also meant to make the reader aware of the potential and relevance of the ultrastructural examination of the semen for the diagnostic assessment of infertile conditions and for their prognosis and management.

To express its fertility potential and fulfill its reproductive function, the spermatozoon must be viable and must possess the following: (1), an efficient motor apparatus required to cover the relatively large distance separating the vagina from the oviduct and overcome the formidable obstacles encountered along the way (the cervical mucus, the stricture of the uterotubal junction, the anfractuosities of the oviductal wall, the downward direction of the beating of the cilia of the oviductal epithelium, the prevailing direction of the current of the tubal fluid), and to penetrate through the egg investments; (2) an intact acrosome to acquire fertilizing competence through capacitation and realize it through the acrosome reaction; and (3) an intact nucleus for the establishment of the genomic patrimony of the embryo at syngamy. None of these parameters can be evaluated precisely in the course of the conventional semen analysis because of one or more of the following: (1) the crude methods by which the seminal fluid is prepared for microscopic analysis, (2) the extremely small dimensions of most of the sperm organelles and their being beyond the limits of resolution of the optic microscope, (3) the limited applicability of the few staining methods that have been devised either to assess sperm viability or for the selective demonstration of individual cellular components, and (4) the common practice of having the semen analysis performed as a doctor's office procedure by nonspecialized personnel. While the analysis of semen

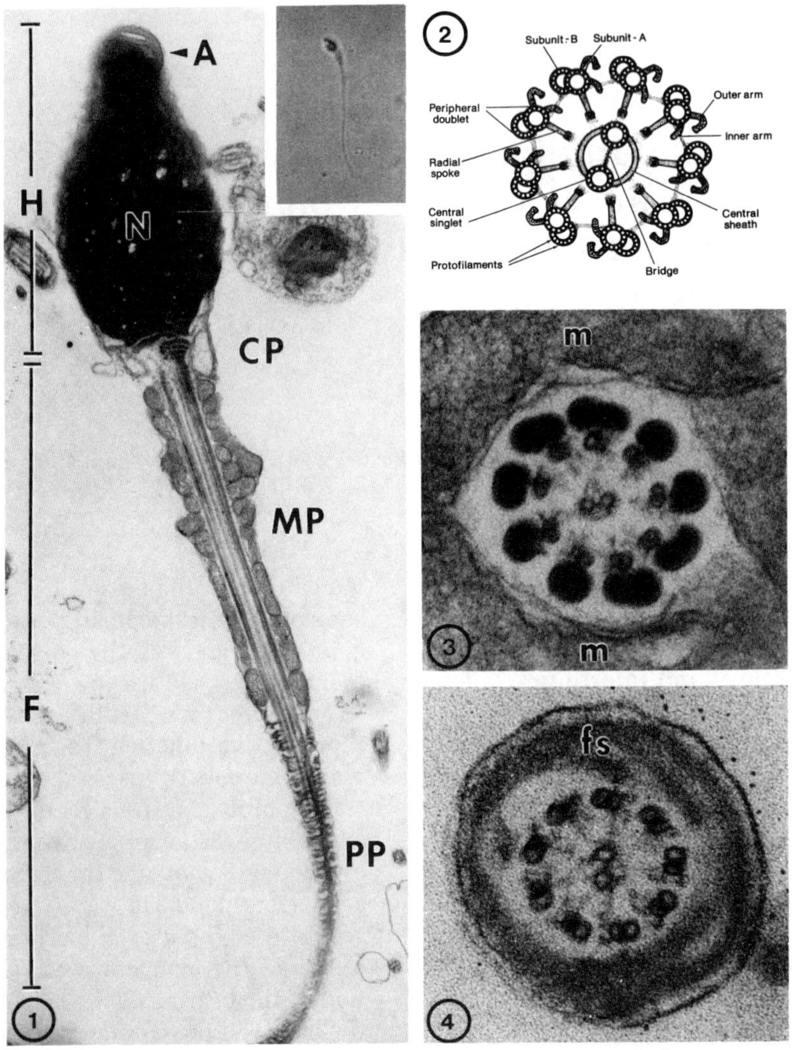

Figure 1 Ultrastructural overview of a morphologically normal spermatozoon (the *insets* in this and other illustrations depict the light-microscopic appearance of sperm analogous to those shown in the electron micrographs). *H,* sperm head comprised of the acrosome (*A*) and the nucleus (*N*); *F,* flagellum consisting of the connecting piece (*CP*), midpiece (*MP*), and principal piece (*PP*) (×19,500). **Figure 2** Diagrammatic representation of the ultrastructural organization of the elements of the flagellar axoneme. (From Fawcett.[31] Reproduced with the permission of the publisher.) **Figures 3 and 4** The axonemal complex as seen in flagella transversely sectioned at the level of the midpiece (Fig. 3) and the principal piece (Fig. 4). In Figure 3, the nine plus two system of axonemal microtubules is surrounded by the nine outer dense fibers, which terminate in the distal segment of the midpiece. *m,* mitochondria; *fs,* fibrous sheath (Fig. 3, ×155,000; Fig. 4, ×150,000).

continues to be the most important tool for the evaluation of the male fertility potential, the assessment of sperm morphology, one of the three most important parameters to be evaluated by the procedure (numbers and motility are the other two), needs to be improved considerably and must be performed as critically as is done customarily in reproductive biologic investigations. The morphologic features of the sperm currently are assessed as if the cells consisted simply of a head and a tail. They are therefore classified and rated exclusively on the basis of the overall appearance of these two components and only "gross" defects are noted, such as obvious aberrations of head shape, presence of multiheaded and multiflagellated spermatozoa, and conspicuous flagellar defects. The finer abnormalities, which frequently subtend the patient's infertility, remain undetected. If the assessment of the functional morphology of the sperm is meant to be an evaluation of the structural integrity of the cell as a prerequisite for its preparedness for the reproductive function, more refined methods of investigation must be used. Because the organization of subcellular elements is an important component of the overall evaluation, it is logical that the study be performed using ultrastructural methods of morphologic analysis.

The ultrastructural pathology of the human spermatozoon as cause of infertility has been fragmentarily documented in the literature in the form of isolated case reports (to be appropriately cited in this article); a few comprehensive reviews were published,[21–25] but most of them appeared outside the mainstream of the specialized North American literature. A systematic classification of the ultrastructural pathology of the human sperm is difficult to compile because of the well-known pleomorphism of the cell,[14,15,21] its organizational complexity[14–21] and thus the large variety of ultrastructural defects and developmental abnormalities that may occur, and the frequent presence in the same cell of associations of defects.[22–26] To avoid assembling a pedantically exhaustive anatomic list of questionable significance, this review (like a previous one by the same author[26]) will be based exclusively on functional perspectives and will be devoted only to the consideration of those structural defects that limit or negate the ability of the sperm to either reach the site of fertilization or acquire and express its fertilizing competence.

FLAGELLAR DEFECTS

Because the flagellum is the effector of sperm motility, any structural anomaly of its various components is of consequence. These anomalies range from "gross" defects that can be detected by light microscopy (such as bending, coiling, knotting) to those that affect subcellular components (such as the mitochondria, the outer dense fibers, and the fibrous sheath) and that cannot be detected by conventional methods of semen analysis because of the extremely small size of these elements. For the sake of conciseness, only the severe impairment of motility that is caused by the pathology of the flagellar axoneme and the outer dense fibers will be considered.

Functional Anatomy of the Flagellar Axoneme

The axoneme or axonemal complex (for reviews, see references 27 to 30) consists of a system of microtubules extending from the connecting piece where they implant on the proximal centriole situated just below the sperm head, to the tip of the flagellum (Fig. 1). Its organization is best appreciated in transverse sections (Figs. 2 to 4). The system consists of nine double microtubules (also referred to as doublets) circularly arranged around two single microtubules situated in the center of the system (referred to also as singlets) and forming with them the "nine plus two" microtubular pattern that is characteristic of the flagellar (and ciliary) organization of all eukaryotic organisms.[30] Each peripheral doublet consists of a subunit A, a complete microtubule, and a subunit B, which is incomplete, C-shaped, and attached with its extremities to the wall of subunit A. The two singlets in the center of the system are complete microtubules. The microtubules are made up of heterodimers of tubulin, a protein that is M_2 10,000. Subunit A of each doublet and the two central singlets contain 13 dimers of tubulin, whereas subunit B of each peripheral doublet only has 10 dimers of the protein. If cross-sectioned flagella are examined at high magnification, other functionally important elements become evident. The two central microtubules are surrounded by a central sheath consisting of a helicoidal system of filamentous projections departing from their wall and are connected at their closest points by 6-nm long bridges organized like the rungs of a ladder. Subunit A of each peripheral doublet is provided with two arms (an outer and an inner) that extend with slightly diverging courses toward subunit B of the next doublet in a clockwise direction. The arms are made up of dynein, a heterogenous protein M_2 500,000 possessing adenosinetriphosphatase (ATPase) activity[27] and contain, for the most part, dynein fraction 1, which accounts for 75% of the total ATPase of the axoneme.* Also departing from each subunit A of the peripheral doublet microtubules are the nexin links that traverse the interdoublet space and connect subunit A of each doublet with the B of the adjacent one[34], and the radial spokes, hammer-shaped structures that extend toward, and attach to, the helical sheath surrounding the singlet microtubules. An identical organization characterizes the axonemal system of the cilia of respiratory, oviductal, and endometrial epithelia, except that, whereas in the spermatozoa the axonemal elements are surrounded by the outer dense fibers, the mitochondria, the fibrous sheath, and, obviously, the

* A dynein fraction 2 also has been isolated; it represents 15% of the axonemal ATPase and appears to be localized in the two central microtubules.[32,33]

cell membrane, the axonemal system of the cilia is surrounded only by the latter.

The role of the various axonemal components in flagellar (and ciliary) motility has been elucidated using as prime experimental models demembranated cilia and flagella, axonemes deprived of their dynein arms by chemical methods, and flagellar mutants (for reviews, see references 30, and 35 to 37). These studies[30,35-37] have confirmed the view, first formulated by Afzelius[38] in 1959, that the undulating motion of beating flagella and the oscillating motion of the cilia are not the result of conformational changes in the molecules of their contractile proteins and consequent shortening of their axonemal microtubules (as previously thought), but are induced by the sliding movements of the microtubules—movements that are comparable to those of the actin and myosin filaments of the skeletal muscle during the contraction-relaxation cycle. The movements of the microtubules are dependent upon the presence of an intact plasma membrane and the availability of ATP synthesized by the mitochondria in the midpiece of the flagellum; in the presence of Mg_2^+, the ATP is hydrolyzed by the dynein arms, and chemical energy is thus converted into mechanical movements. The function of the other axonemal elements is less clear; it is presently understood, however, that the radial spokes regulate the sliding movements of the peripheral microtubules and provide the shear resistance that is necessary to convert sliding movements into bending by becoming alternatively detached from, and reattached to, the central sheath surrounding the singlet microtubules in the center of the axoneme.[39]

Axonemal Defects

Abnormalities of the various components of the flagellar axoneme occasionally may be noted in the spermatozoa of normal individuals,[26,40,41] a finding obviously of scarce diagnostic relevance and of insignificant consequences for fertility, and one that is to be anticipated considering the massive production of flagella during spermiogenesis. It is, however, when the vast majority or the totality of the sperm in a sample display either the same axonemal defect or repeat associations of defects that the finding is of diagnostic and prognostic relevance. The most important axonemal defects for the objectives of this review are the numeric aberrations of the microtubules and the structural defects of their associated elements. These abnormalities, which usually occur in otherwise structurally normal spermatozoa, are the expression of specific alterations of spermiogenesis of congenital origin (see subsequent discussion).

Numerical aberrations can be in excess or in defect, i.e., the number of microtubules may be greater or less than that required for the normal "nine plus two" organization. Both aberrations result in lack of movement coordination and considerable reduction of movement efficiency. The first aberration may be represented by supernumerary doublet (Fig. 5) or singlet microtubules (Fig. 6) at the periphery, or in the center of the axoneme, or both. The much more severely limiting numerical aberrations in defect are represented by the deletion of one or more of the peripheral doublets (Fig. 7) or of one or both of the central singlets (Figs. 8 and 9), the latter being referred to as the "nine plus zero" defect.[32,42] For evident reasons, the different varieties of numeric aberrations often result in derangement of the normal axonemal topography; in extreme cases, a veritable organizational anarchy[26] may occur (Fig. 10), as noted by others.[43,44] The deletion of all axonemal microtubules is rare (Fig. 11). In one case,[45] an infertile man with chronic respiratory tract infections had the defect not only in the sperm flagella but also in the cilia of the tracheal and bronchial epithelium, one of several situations that have contributed to the formulation of the concept that the same gene(s) may be responsible for both flagellar and ciliary axonemal defects; other evidence militates against this hypothesis, however (see subsequent discussion).

The structural defects of the axonemal complex are essentially represented by the absence of the delicate elements that are associated with the microtubules, especially the dynein arms. Despite the general awareness of their existence (awareness that is due to their being part of the pathologic constellation of the so-called immotile or dyskinetic cilia syndrome [see subsequent discussion]) and of their being one of the best documented and frequently occurring sperm abnormalities,[46-51] in this author's experience, these defects are infrequently considered in situations characterized by generalized or universal lack of motility—situations that, for the most part, are indiscriminately diagnosed as necrospermia (see subsequent discussion). The most frequent of these defects is the complete and systemic absence of both outer and inner arms (Fig. 12), followed by the selective absence of either the inner (Fig. 13) or the outer arm; focal absence of the dynein arms only in some doublets also can occur (Fig. 14). The systemic, selective, or focal

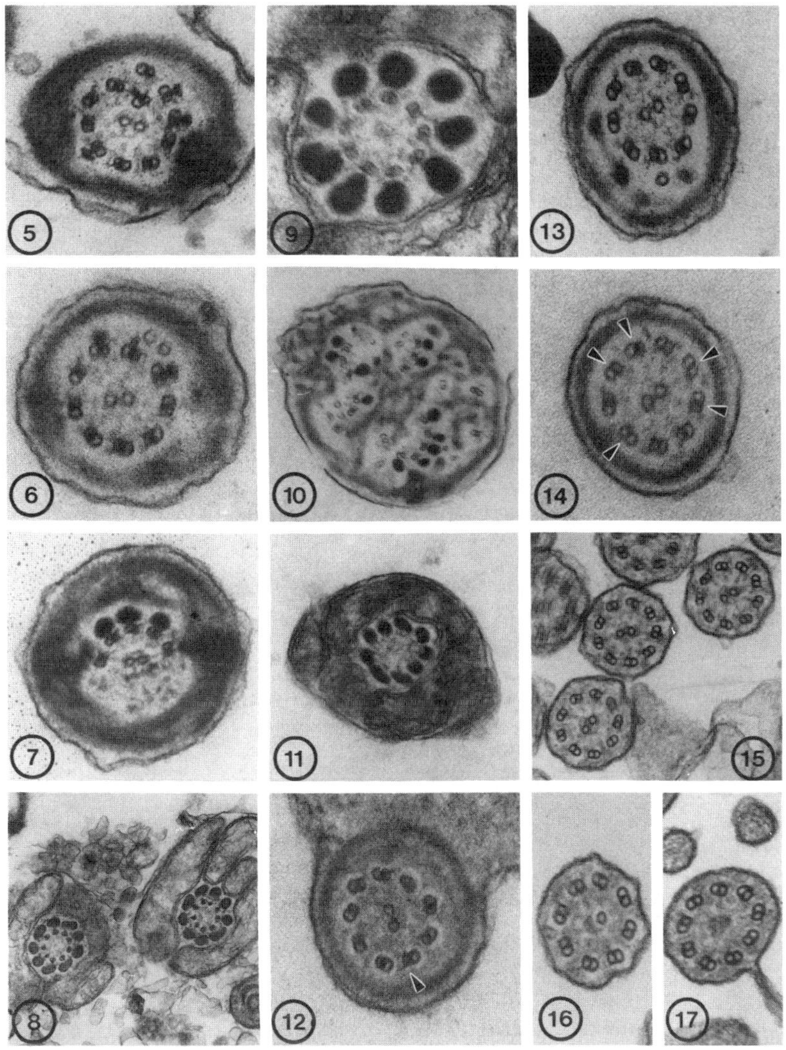

Figures 5 to 9 Numeric aberrations of the axonemal microtubules. The sperm flagellum in Figu 5 contains two supernumerary doublets, that in Figure 6 has two supernumerary singlets in ectopic position, that in Figure 7 shows the deletion of four peripheral doublets, and the flagella in Figures 8 and 9 have the deletion of the two microtubules in the center of the axoneme (the nine plus zero defect) (Fig. 5, ×100,000; Fig. 6, ×105,000; Fig. 7, ×75,000; Fig. 8, ×35,000; Fig. 9, ×50,000). **Figure 10** Organizational anarchy of the axonemal microtubules, outer dense fibers and fibrous sheath (×52,500). **Figure 11** Total deletion of the axonemal microtubules (×55,000). **Figures 12 to 14** Absence of dynein arms. Complete (i.e., involving both arms) and nearly systemic in Figure 12 (the outer arm is present in the doublet at *arrowhead*); selective in Figure 13, where only the inner arms are missing; and focal (i.e., involving only some of the peripheral microtubules; those indicated by *arrowheads*) in Figure 14. Notice the absence of the radial spokes and central sheath in the flagella in Figures 12 and 13, and the supernumerary single microtubule in the flagellum in Figure 13. (Fig. 12, ×100,000; Fig. 13, ×120,000; Fig. 14, ×145,000). **Figures 15 to 17** Complete and systemic absence of dynein arms in the cilia of the respiratory epithelium. In Figure 16, the defect is associated with the deletion of one peripheral doublet and one central singlet (an eight plus one organization); in Figure 17, the defect is associated with the deletion of the two central singlets (the nine plus zero defect) (Fig. 15, ×60,000; Fig. 16, ×60,000; Fig. 17, ×60,000).

absence of the arms is frequently associated with other abnormalities, such as numeric aberrations of the axonemal microtubules (Fig. 13) and absence of the radial spokes and of the central sheath around the microtubules in the center of the axoneme (Figs. 12 and 13). Generally, but not regularly (see subsequent discussion), these defects result in complete sperm immotility. That the infertile condition of these patients mainly results from the incapacity of their sperm to ascend the female reproductive tract and reach the site of fertilization has been confirmed by recent studies[52,53] showing that spermatozoa with this type of axonemal defects can undergo the acrosome reaction and penetrate the zona-free hamster eggs.[54] Thus, it would appear that spermatozoa with structural defects of their axonemes still may be competent to fertilize when placed in close proximity to the female gamete as it is done, for example, in procedures for extracorporeal fertilization. This consideration alone, which incidentally reinforces the validity of in vitro fertilization as a treatment of selective conditions of male infertility,[55,56] justifies electron microscopic examination of the semen in cases of diffuse or generalized immotility.

The numeric and structural defects of the axoneme (the latter especially) are frequently associated in the same patient with analogous abnormalities of the cilia of, among others, the respiratory epithelium (Figs. 15 to 17), and, as such, are a part of the pathologic constellation of the "immotile cilia syndrome"[57–63] characterized by chronic ear and sinopulmonary infections and reduced or absent mucociliary clearance; in about 50% of the patients, these manifestations are associated with bronchiectasis and situs viscerum inversus, thus constituting the Kartagener's syndrome.[64] The prevalence of these defects in Polynesians has been established.[65–67] Recently, the structural bases of the immotile cilia syndrome were enlarged to include abnormalities of the radial spokes,[68] the transposition of one set of doublets from the periphery to the center of the axoneme to substitute for the deletion of the central singlets (a defect that is referred to as the "eight plus two" condition,[69,70] the absence of the central sheath around the central microtubules,[71] and others.[72] The anatomic heterogeneity of the immotile cilia syndrome[61,71–73] has a functional counterpart since these structural abnormalities do not always result in complete ciliary and flagellar immotility; spermatozoa selectively lacking the outer but possessing the inner dynein arms may still retain some degree of motility,[24,51,60,71] and residual motility also may be present in cilia and flagella with the "eight plus two" defect.[69,70] Consequently, the original term, "immotile cilia syndrome," has been replaced by "ciliary dyskinesis" or "dyskinetic cilia syndrome,"[74] of which three major variants are presently recognized: type 1 with defective dynein arms, type 2 with defective radial spokes, and type 3 with microtubule translocation (the "eight plus two" defect). The structural and functional heterogeneity of the clinical conditions resulting from these flagellar and ciliary defects has been emphasized further by reports of infertile individuals with the structural defects of the immotile cilia syndrome only in their sperm flagella,[75] and of patients with Kartagener's syndrome who either possessed normal ciliary organization[76–79] or had normal dynein arms in their sperm flagella[79] and allegedly fathered children.[78,79] This evidence does not reconcile with the concept that the same gene(s) is (are) responsible for both the flagellar and the ciliary defects of the immotile cilia syndrome,[70] and suggests that the production of human dynein may be regulated by different genes.[73,75,80,81] The occurrence of different axonemal patterns in the cilia and the flagella of the same individual[63,82] indicates that the "nine plus two" microtubular organization of the flagella of the spermatozoa and of the cilia of the epithelial cells also is under the control of different genes.

Functional Anatomy and Structural Defects of the Outer Dense Fibers

The axonemal microtubules are surrounded for most of their length by a system of nine outer dense fibers (Fig. 3), a situation that results in the "nine plus nine plus two" flagellar organization typical of the spermatozoon of animals with internal fertilization.* The fibers seem to have keratin-like properties[83]; their amino acid profile differs from that of contractile proteins,[84] and they possess a high cystein content[85] and a high number of S–S bonds.[86–88] Thus, they are considered not to fulfill contractile functions but to be resilient stiffening structures[16,89–91] that probably impart elastic rigidity to the flagellum,[92,93] assist in its motility,[20] and protect its delicate axonemal elements from damage during transit through the female reproductive tract. The structural anomalies of the outer dense fibers are less frequent than those of the axonemal elements. As in the latter case, they are represented by numeric aberrations in excess (Figs. 18 and 19) or in defect (Fig. 20), topographic derangements, and structural malformations, such as shape deformations (Fig. 21) and fusion of two or more fibers together. Spermatozoa with outer dense fiber defects are dyskinetic; they display sliding motility patterns and are incapable of penetrating the cervical mucus.[94] These observations corroborate the concept that, despite their not being contractile el-

* The outer dense fibers are not present in the sperm flagella of aquatic phyla, which shed semen in the water.

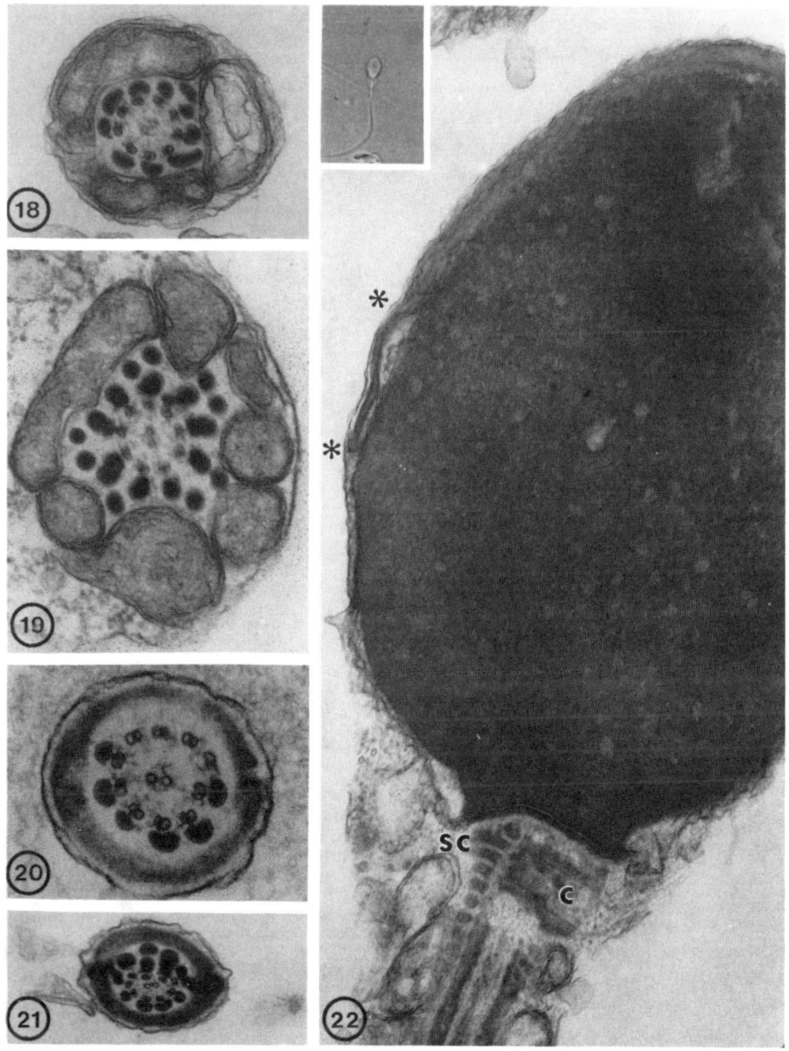

Figures 18 to 21 Outer dense fiber defects: numeric aberrations (in excess, Figs. 18 and 19; in defect, Fig. 20) and shape deformations (Fig. 21) (Fig. 18, ×51,000; Fig. 19, ×52,000; Fig. 20, ×72,000; Fig. 21, ×52,000). **Figure 22** The head and the connecting piece of a morphologically normal spermatozoon at relatively high magnification. Notice the ovoidal shape of the head (see also *inset*), the highly compacted aggregation of the uniformly dense chromatin, and the acrosome covering the rostral two thirds of the nucleus (its thin equatorial segment is demarcated by the *asterisks*). One of the segmented columns (*sc*) and the proximal centriole (*c*) are evident in the connecting piece. Notice the implantation fossa in the posterior aspect of the nucleus just above the connecting piece (for explanation, see text) (×45,000).

ements, the outer dense fibers assist the sperm in its forward progressive motility.

HEAD DEFECTS

Functional Anatomy and Abnormalities of the Acrosome

The acrosome, the nuclear cap of early morphologists, covers the anterior three quarters of the sperm nucleus and is the most rostral element of the sperm (Fig. 22). The organelle is limited by a continuous membrane and consists of a homogeneous matrix of medium electron opacity. In its posterior fifth, it is usually much thinner and tapered; since this occurs where the nucleus is at its widest, this region of the acrosome is referred to as "equatorial segment." The acrosome develops from the Golgi apparatus during early stages of spermatid differentiation, and its definitive shape results from profound remodeling processes that also involve the nucleus and, possibly, cytoplasmic components such as the system of the "manchette" microtubules.[95,96] Because of its Golgi origin and the fact that its matrix and limiting membrane contain hydrolytic enzymes of which hyaluronidase and acrosin are of the greatest functional importance,[20,97–101] the acrosome was originally considered analogous to a primary lysosome[102,103]; however, because of its involvement in an exocytotic process at the time of the acrosome reaction (see subsequent discussion), the organelle presently is viewed as being more akin to a secretory (zymogen) granule.[99,104] Its role in the acquisition and expression of fertilizing competence during and as the result of capacitation,[105,106] respectively, now appears to be established on the basis of evidence (for reviews, see references 98, 101, and 107 to 109) indicating that the latter prepares[110] the sperm to undergo the structural changes of the acrosome reaction that, together with hyperactivated motility,[111] seems to be necessary for its penetration through the egg investments.

Since it was first observed by Austin and Bishop[112] in 1958, the acrosome reaction has been the subject of a large number of investigations on sperm–egg interactions in vivo and in vitro in different mammalian species, including humans.[113] Copious morphologic studies generally have confirmed the original ultrastructural observations by Barros et al.,[114] indicating that the structural expression of the reaction is the multifocal fusion of the outer acrosomal membrane surrounding the region of the acrosome anterior to the equatorial segment, followed by the rapid dismantling of the fused membranes with consequent exocytosis of the organelle and extracellular liberation of the enzymes that are contained in its matrix and the inner aspect of its limiting membrane.* It is fair to state, however, that the true functional role of the acrosome reaction in the fertilization process remains to be elucidated convincingly. For example, whether the reaction is important for the physical penetration of the sperm through the egg envelopes as proposed originally, or for the unmasking of specific sperm surface components that recognize and bind to the zona pellucida,[115] or for both, has not yet been established; and the specific role of the individual enzymes that are released during the exocytosis of the acrosome,[99,101] and even the site where the reaction begins and becomes completed,[100,116–118] are still unclear. Even though our knowledge in this regard is very fluid, it is unquestionable that the acrosome plays (a) pivotal role(s) in the reproductive process.[108,109] As such, it is not surprising that structural defects of the organelle cause infertility very likely due to the impossibility for the affected spermatozoa to become capacitated, a pathogenetic mechanism that appears to be supported by their inability to penetrate the denuded hamster egg.[26,119–121]

Because the acrosome cannot be clearly visualized in live and unstained human spermatozoa due to its relatively small size and translucency, special staining procedures were devised to evaluate its morphology by light microscopy. These procedures include the Papanicolau stain,[122] the eosin-fast green-naphthol yellow staining method proposed by Bryan,[123] the naphthol yellow-S and erythrosin B stain of Bryan and Akruk,[124] the use of chlortetracycline,[125] lectins,[126] and monoclonal antibodies[127] as fluorescent labels, the triple staining method of Talbot and Chacon,[128] and the application of supravital stains coupled with other techniques, such as indirect immunofluorescence labeling[129] or differential interference contrast microscopy.[130] These procedures, however, are of limited diagnostic relevance not only because of their complexity and, therefore, minimal applicability to routine semen analyses, but also and especially because they serve mostly for the visualization of the acrosome reaction and/or to distinguish the true acrosome reaction that occurs as a result of the capacitated condition of the spermatozoon, from the spurious or false acrosome reaction, which is a manifestation of cell degeneration.[103,131] As such, these procedures are of only limited assistance, if any, for the evaluation of the structural integrity of the organelle and the prospective assessment of its functional fitness as a key participant in the reproductive process. Considering how essential the normalcy of the acrosome is for fertilization, the inability of assessing its morphologic features is, in itself, one of the most severe limitations of conventional methods of semen analysis. This parameter can be evaluated easily by electron microscopy.

Of the relatively broad spectrum of acrosomal defects,[132–136] two need to be reviewed in detail since both constitute important causes of infertility: acrosomal hypoplasia and fragility, and acrosomal agenesis.

The first defect is characterized by production of sperm all possessing extremely thin acrosomes

* The equatorial region does not participate in the acrosome reaction; the mechanisms responsible for this exclusion phenomenon and its functional implications are unknown.

(Figs. 23 to 27); the reduction in organelle size often is so pronounced as to efface the differences between its anterior four fifths and its equatorial segment. These hypoplastic acrosomes also display distorted, bizarre shapes (Figs. 24, 26, and 27), are detached from the underlying nucleus (Figs. 26 and 27), have rarefied matrices, (Fig. 24) and/or are undergoing dissolution (Fig. 25). The presence of intact plasma membranes over the defective organelles rules out the possibility that these changes may be induced artefactually. Spermatozoa with these acrosomal defects are otherwise normal; because of this fact and because of the impossibility of visualizing the acrosome with the light microscope, these spermatozoa are classified as normal in routine semen analyses or, if the eye of the analyst is particularly well trained, as having a reduced head size. As already mentioned elsewhere,[26] the hypoplasia of the acrosome is not being paid the attention that its frequency and its devastating impact on fertility would demand. Even in major reviews of seminal pathology,[22,25] the abnormality is superficially treated under the heading of, or together with, "microcephaly." The defect is typical of patients with a long history of infertility and whose spermatozoa fail to penetrate the zona-free hamster eggs, despite the fact that repeated semen analyses had consistently shown "normal sperm numbers, motility and morphology."[26]

The other major acrosomal defect is the agenesis

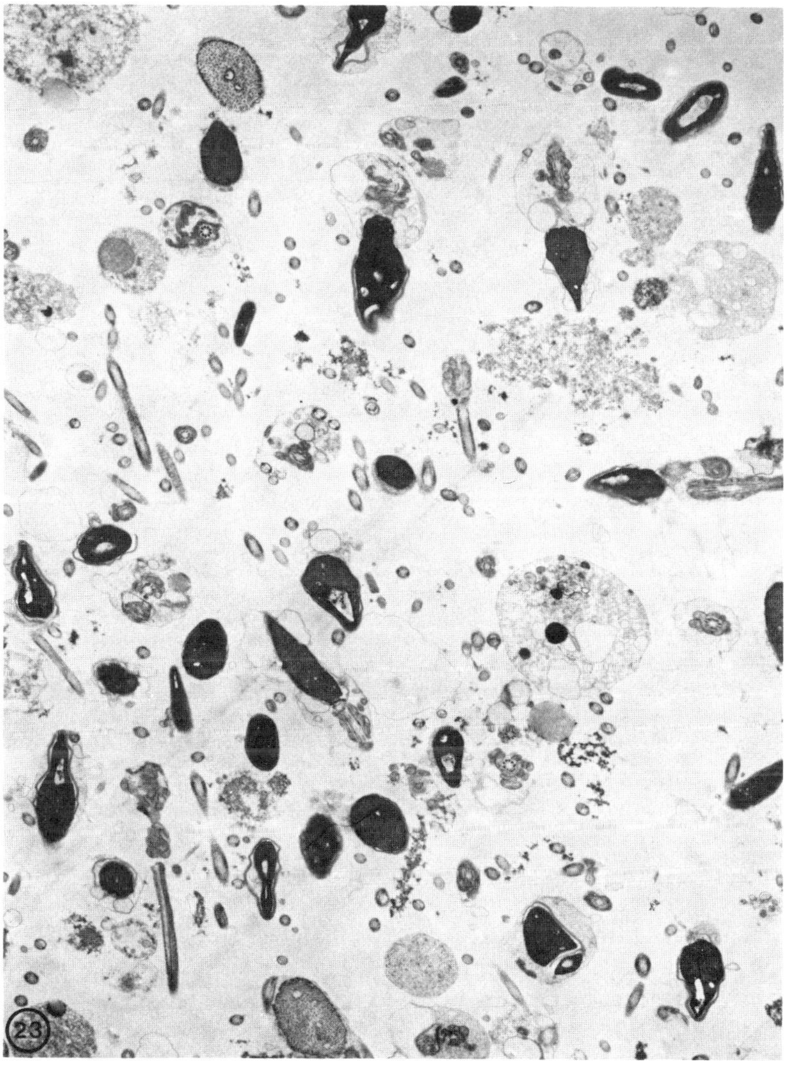

Figure 23 Universal hypoplasia and fragility of the acrosomes in the semen of an infertile patient (×5000).

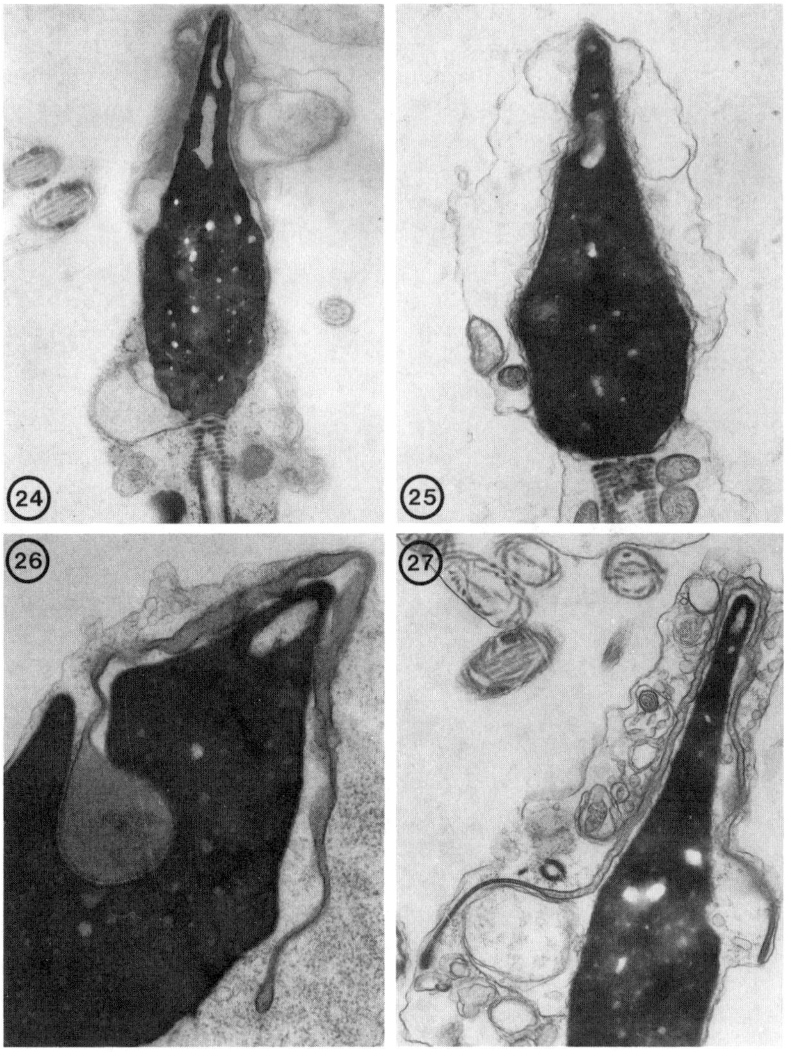

Figures 24 to 27 Acrosomal hypoplasia associated with deformations of the normal shape of the organelle (Figs. 24 and 26) and its separation from the nucleus (Figs. 26 and 27). The defect also is frequently associated with swelling (Fig. 24), rarefaction (Figs. 24 and 27), and dissolution of the matrix (Fig. 25) (Fig. 24, ×20,000; Fig. 25, ×33,000; Fig. 26, ×37,000; Fig. 27, ×33,000).

of the organelle (Figs. 28 to 31): since it is frequently associated with a spherical shape of the sperm nucleus, this abnormality conventionally is misleadingly referred to as "round head defect." The vast majority of spermatozoa with agenesis of the acrosome also have abnormal, immature patterns of chromatin aggregation (Figs. 28, 30 and 31; see subsequent discussion). The triad—agenesis of the acrosome, sphericity of the nucleus, and immaturity of the chromatin—has been documented in all cases so far consigned to the literature[137–142] and has been demonstrated also by studies that have monitored its morphogenesis in testicular biopsies by ultrastructural,[23,133,143–146] histocytochemical,[144,145] and immunohistochemical methods.[147] The defect develops as the result of an abnormal topographic relationship between the Golgi complex and the nucleus of the spermatid prior to acrosome development, defective secretory activity of the Golgi complex, and rudimentality or absence of the cytoplasmic microtubules of the manchette,[144] the participation of which in the remodeling processes leading to the definitive shape of the sperm nucleus and the acrosome has been postulated but never demonstrated.[95,96] The concomitant occurrence of acrosome agenesis, abnormality of

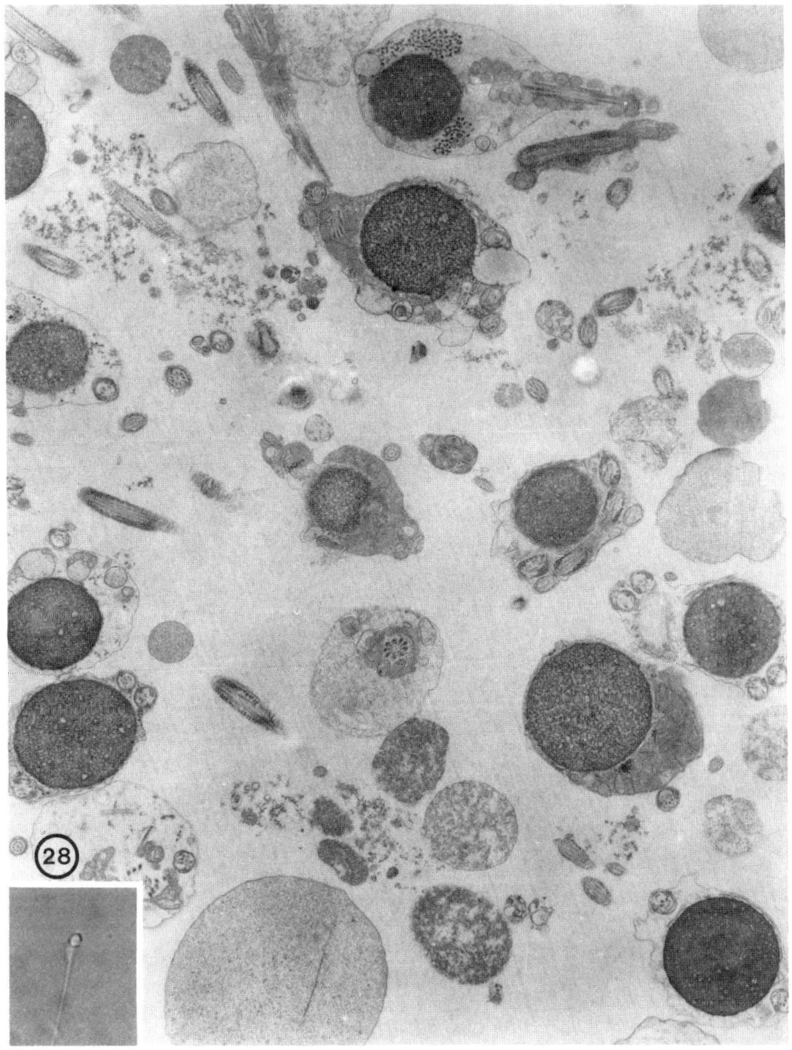

Figure 28 Universal agenesis of the acrosome in the spermatozoa of an infertile patient. Notice the spherical shape of the sperm heads and the immature pattern of aggregation of the chromatin (compare with the nucleus of the spermatozoon in Fig. 22) (×10,000).

nuclear shape, and chromatin immaturity would suggest that the physical-chemical organization of the sperm head as a whole is influenced by either identical or concomitantly operating mechanisms. The agenesis of the acrosome has a familial trait[26,139,141,148] and is congenital; a polygenic rather than a monogenic mode of inheritance has been suggested.[148] In routine semen analyses, the defect should be suspected whenever large numbers of round-headed spermatozoa are visualized; its actual occurrence should be verified by electron microscopy also because the sphericity of the sperm head does not always signify the absence of the organelle. While the defect is probably one of the least ignored in the clinical practice of andrology, it recently has been reported[142] that not everyone recognizes that the spheroidal shape of the sperm head is an ominous sign of irreversible infertility.

Functional Anatomy and Abnormalities of the Nucleus

The conventional methods of assessing the morphology of the sperm at routine semen analysis allow the visualization of the entire head but not that of the nucleus as an individual entity mostly because the nucleus is covered by the acrosome for most of its extension; the structural organization of

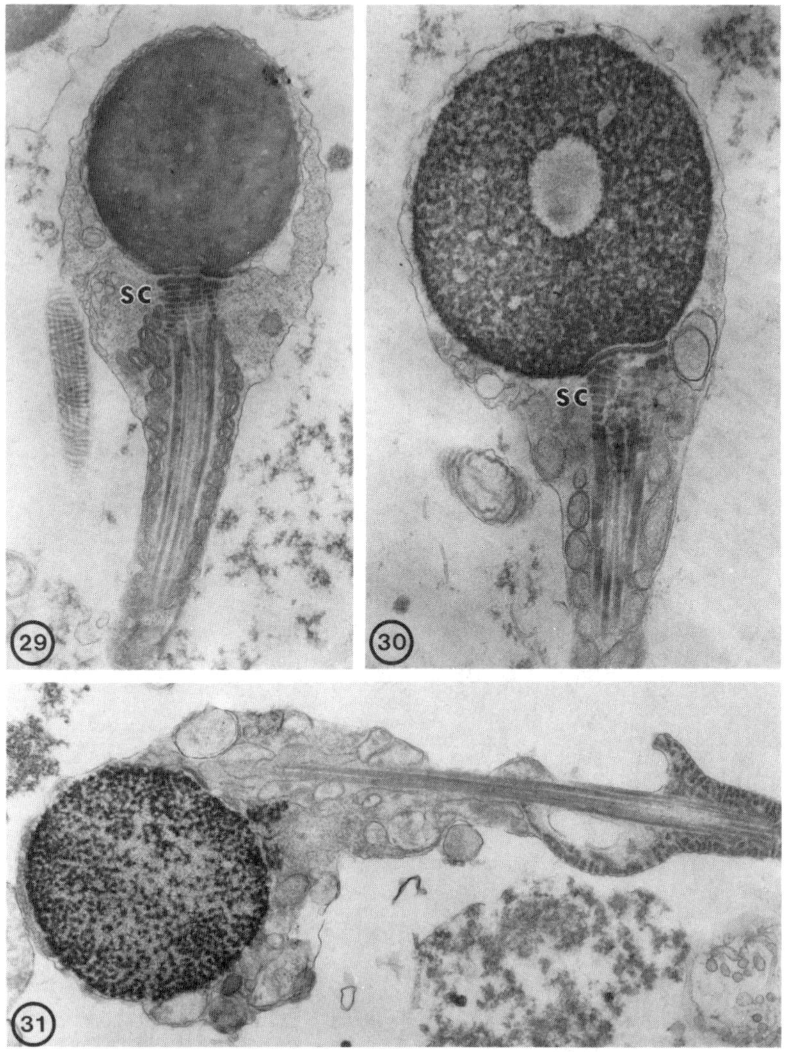

Figures 29 to 31 Other examples of agenesis of the acrosome. The sperm in Figure 29 has a normal pattern of chromatin aggregation, but immature patterns are displayed by those in Figures 30 and 31. All spermatozoa have spheroidal head shapes. *sc,* segmented columns (Fig. 29, ×22,000; Fig. 30, ×28,000; Fig. 31, ×17,500).

the sperm nucleus can, instead, be evaluated in electron-microscopic preparations without any difficulty. The nucleus of the mature human spermatozoon (Figs. 1 and 22) consists of a uniformly compact, keratinoid mass of chromatin made up prevalently of deoxyribonucleic acid (DNA) coupled to basic proteins. This organization is the result of profound physical-chemical transformations that occur in late stages of spermiogenesis and continue during sperm transit through the epididymis; they include the elimination of the ribonucleic acid (RNA),[149] the replacement of somatic histones by protamines,[150] the formation of disulfide bonds that are essential for chromatin stability,[151,152] and the gradual transformation of the finely granular chromatin of the young spermatid nucleus at first into the globular variety of the late spermatid and, ultimately, into the uniformly compact and densely aggregated organization typical of the mature spermatozoon.[96,103] Mature sperm nuclei are highly resistant to disruption; their DNA can be neither unraveled by sonication nor digested by DNAse[31,153] and can be partially decondensed only by strong agents such as detergents,[154,155] acids,[156] and lytic enzymes of bacterial origin[157] (for a review, see reference 20). Such a high degree of unreactivity may well serve to protect the genomic patrimony of the sperm from physical or chemical injuries during transit through the female reproductive tract.[31,158] Often enclosed in the dense mass of its chromatin are one or two small vacuoles appearing as nonmembrane-bound areas of rarefaction containing sparse, granular, or filamentous material; these vacuoles form as the consequence of uneven processes of chromatin condensation.[96,103]

The defects of the sperm nucleus are of ominous significance for fertility. Frequently noted in infertile patients are intranuclear vacuoles and inclusions often so large as to result in conspicuous deformations of the nucleus and overall head shape (Figs. 32 to 35). The vacuoles may be optically empty but, more frequently, contain pleomorphic inclusions such as whorls or parallel stacks of membranes (Figs. 33 and 34), vesicles of different size (Fig. 35), lipid droplets (Fig. 35), and cytoplasmic organelles, especially mitochondria. This nuclear defect often occurs in association with abnormal patterns of chromatin condensation (see subsequent discussion) and is most frequently noted in spermatozoa with hypoplastic acrosomes (Figs. 32 and 33), again indicating the existence of abnormal remodeling patterns during spermiogenesis; its morphogenesis was carefully documented by Hol-

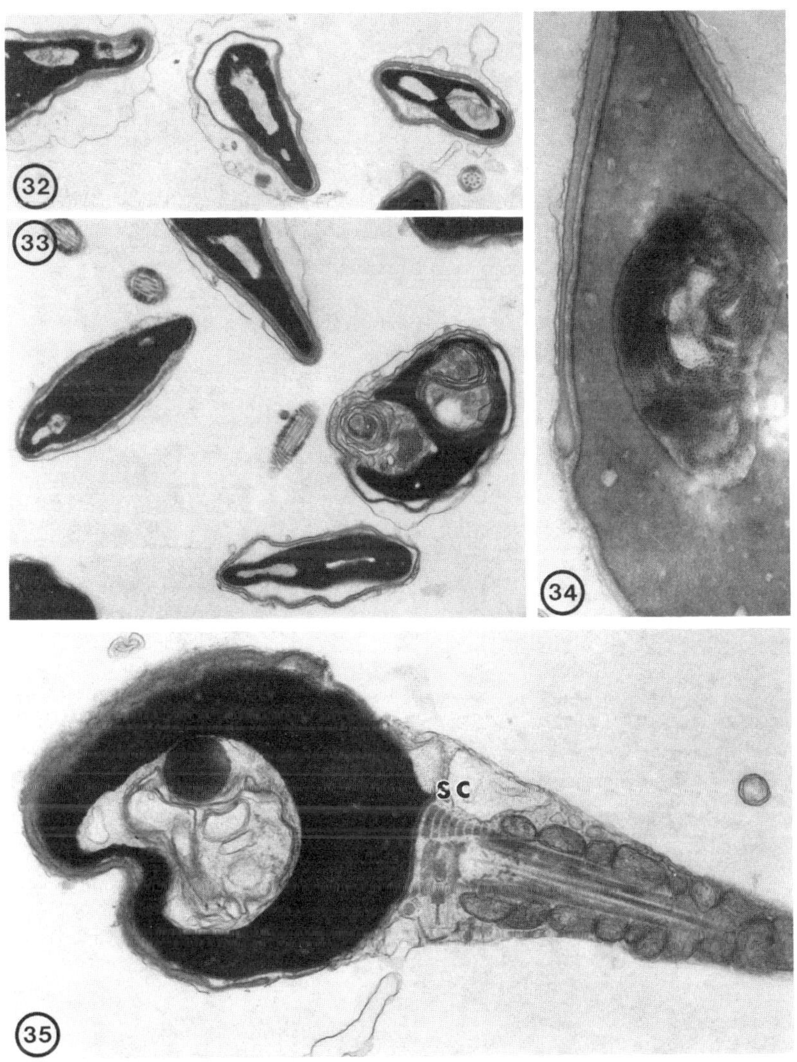

Figures 32 to 35 Intranuclear inclusions. Figures 32 and 33 illustrate the universality of the defect in the semen of two infertile patients whose spermatozoa are also characterized, as often is the case, by hypoplasia and fragility of their acrosomes. Notice the deformation of the nucleus of one of the sperm in Figure 33. Whorls of parallel membranes have been sequestered in the inclusion in Figure 34. The spermatozoon in Figure 35 has an intranuclear inclusion containing, among others, a lipid droplet. *sc*, segmented column (Fig. 32, ×13,500; Fig. 33, ×16,500; Fig. 34, ×52,500; Fig. 35, ×28,000).

stein[23] in testicular biopsies from 128 subfertile or infertile patients with a variety of andrologic disorders characterized by oligo-, terato-, or azoospermia. The defect also is frequent in infertile patients with inflammatory bowel disease[159] where it appears to be a direct consequence of the disease rather than of the medication with sulfa-drugs, as originally postulated when the association of inflammatory bowel disease with infertility, inferior semen quality, and abnormal sperm morphology was first noted.[160–164]

Another fertility-limiting nuclear defect is the immaturity of the chromatin (Figs. 36 to 39), an abnormality that is almost invariably associated with other head defects such as multiple nuclei, acrosome hypoplasia (Figs. 36 and 39), and nuclear inclusions. Spermatozoa with this defect usually have coarsely granular chromatin identical to that characteristic of spermatids at the stage of incipient nuclear elongation,[96,103] hence the term "chromatinic" or "nuclear immaturity."[26] The most extreme cases are characterized by a true nucleomalacic condition (Figs. 38 and 39). While the infertility of the patients with nuclear immaturity may be co-induced by its association with other sperm abnormalities, especially acrosome hypoplasia, we know that the defect is in itself capable of preventing fertility. The DNA of these sperm is prevalently single- rather than double-stranded and, as such, has a markedly decreased resistance

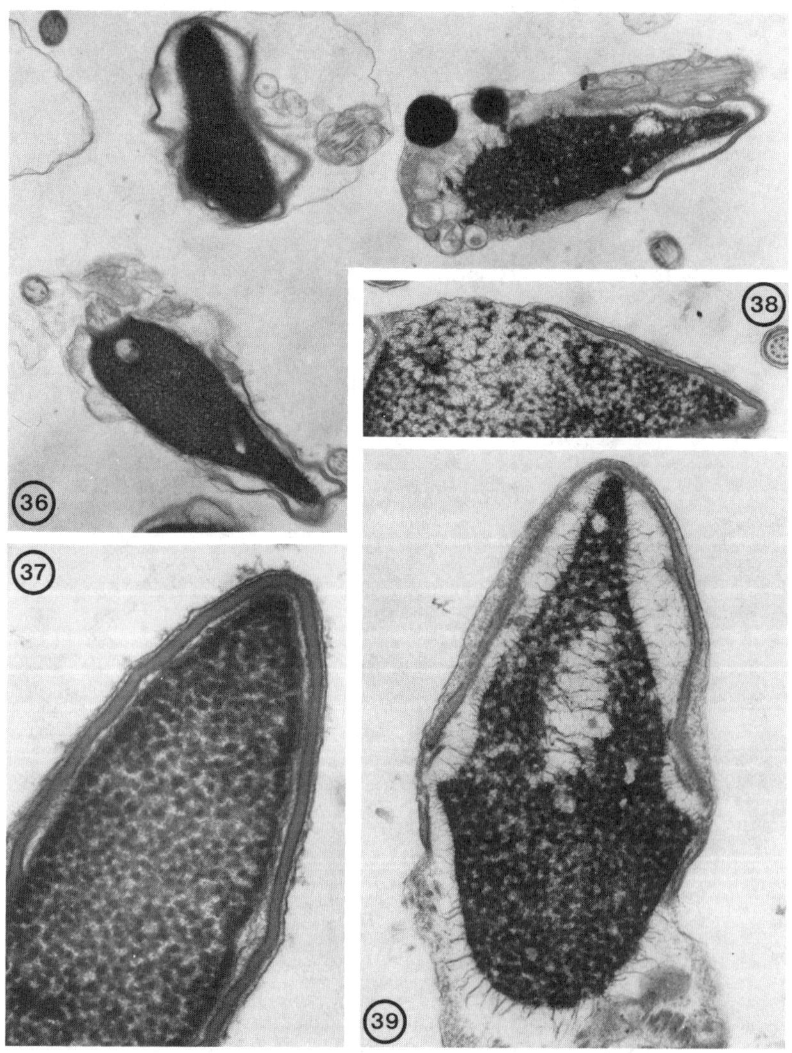

Figures 36 to 39 Chromatin immaturity. Notice the universality of the defect in the spermatozoa in Figure 36 and the truly nucleomalacic condition of the spermatozoa in Figures 38 and 39 (Fig. 36, ×15,500; Fig. 37, ×42,000; Fig. 38, ×22,000; Fig. 39, ×30,000).

to thermal denaturation compared with the DNA of normal spermatozoa.[165] Lower phosphorus concentrations, higher-than-normal zinc content, and persistence of variable amounts of lysin also have been found; the latter observation suggests that somatic histones have not been replaced by basic proteins, which are, instead, rich in arginine and cystein,[144] a hypothesis supported indirectly by the finding that the spermatozoa of infertile men frequently contain histones rather than protamines.[166] The association of low degrees of chromatin aggregation with chromosomal abnormalities has also been well documented.[167–170]

FUNCTIONAL ANATOMY AND DEFECTS OF THE CONNECTING PIECE

As its name indicates, the most important function of the connecting piece, or neck, is to maintain the connection between, and coordinate the movements of, the head and the flagellum; it may also play a role in the generation of motility (see subsequent discussion). The connecting piece constitutes the most cranial segment of the flagellum, situated just behind the nucleus (Figs. 1, 22, 24, 25, 29, 30, 35, and 40). Its most cranial component is the capitulum, a convex structure that articulates

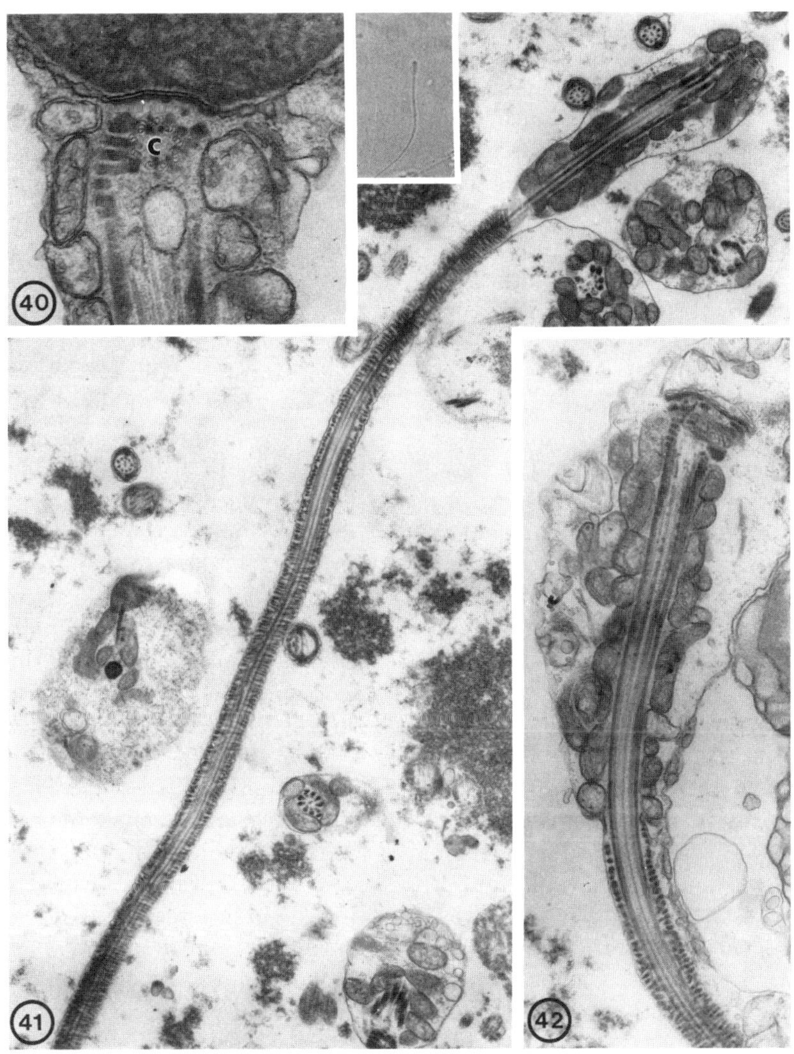

Figure 40 The connecting piece of a morphologically normal spermatozoon. The plane of section is perpendicular to those in Figures 22 and 35; the triplet microtubular organization of the centriole (*c*) is evident (×58,000). **Figures 41 and 42** Decapitated sperm flagella. Because of the cytoplasmic droplet that surrounds their most cranial segments, these headless flagella can, and frequently are, interpreted as microcephalic spermatozoa at conventional semen analysis (see *inset*) (Fig. 41, ×12,000; Fig. 42, ×22,000).

with the basal plate, a concave element lining the implantation fossa on the posterior surface of the nucleus (these structures are visible in Figs. 22, 30, 35, and 40). The capitulum is supported by a circular system of nine segmented columns (Figs. 1, 22, 24, 25, 29, 30, 35, and 40), each made up of a craniocaudal series of alternating dense segments and clear spaces, and fusing with a corresponding outer dense fiber at its caudal extremity. At their apices, the segmented columns surround the proximal centriole (Figs. 22, 35, and 40) consisting, as any other centriole, of a circular array of nine triplet microtubules (Fig. 40) and oriented with its long axis perpendicular to the flagellum. Together with the underlying distal centriole, whose presence in human spermatozoa and in those of few other species was demonstrated by Zamboni and Stefanini,[171] the proximal centriole is responsible for the assembly of the axonemal microtubules during the development of the sperm flagellum.[172] The proximal centriole also has been considered the site of generation of the flagellar movements,[103,171] a hypothesis, however, which is not supported by evidence, showing that there are animals whose spermatozoa lack the proximal centriole[173] and that flagella of bull sperm dissected distal to the neck are still capable of motility.[174]

The most important abnormality of the connecting piece is the separation of the head from the tail; this abnormality, which constitutes the most severe sperm defect irreconcilable with any fertility potential, is generally referred to as decapitation or decapitated sperm defect.[175,176] Patients with this structural defect produce an ejaculate containing exclusively or prevalently headless but vigorously motile flagella, the heads very likely having separated in the epididymis at the time the spermatozoa acquire motility. This defect is congenital and is due to either a faulty head-flagellum connection[177] or an abnormal position of the proximal centriole with respect to the spermatid nucleus at the time of flagellar development during late stages of spermiogenesis.[178,179] Ultrastructural examination of these headless flagella reveals interesting features. First, their ultrastructural organization is normal[26,179]; second, their uppermost segments regularly include a complete connecting piece together with the proximal centriole and are surrounded by a voluminous, elliptic cytoplasmic droplet containing a variety of organelles (Figs. 41 and 42). Because of their shape, these droplets are easily misinterpreted as small-sized heads with the light microscope; thus, the defect either goes unnoticed or is classified as a microcephalic or pin-headed sperm condition.[180] The abnormality may be more common than the sparsity of the cases reported in the literature indicates; in fact, decapitation is a common sperm defect in farm animals, especially bulls, where it constitutes an irreversible cause of sterility.[181–187] It is tempting to speculate that the vigorous motility of these decapitated sperm could be maintained by the persistence of the proximal centriole in the most cranial portion of their flagella.

NECROSPERMIA

The spermatozoa of many infertile patients often display sluggish, ineffective motility (asthenospermia) or total immotility; this could be the expression of either sperm agony or death (necrospermia), or of defects of the motor apparatus. However, it is difficult, if not impossible, to distinguish dead from live spermatozoa on purely morphologic bases by light microscopy and, therefore, to answer the question: are the sperm weakly motile or immotile because they are agonic or dead, or because of structural defects of their flagellar elements? Several staining procedures, mostly based on the use of supravital dyes,[128,129,188–190] have been devised to assess sperm viability or lack thereof. These procedures, however, are neither precise nor entirely reliable. In any case, experience shows that they are used only exceptionally in the course of routine semen analysis. Consequently, the most common method to evaluate sperm viability (unfortunately) remains the estimation of motility. In general, therefore, any condition characterized by sperm immotility is indiscriminately diagnosed as necrospermia because of the lack of awareness regarding the existence of submicroscopic flagellar defects that prevails among those who perform semen analyses. In some cases, the diagnosis may be of disastrous consequences since a true necrospermic condition has etiopathogenetic and prognostic implications different from those of conditions characterized by presence of viable but immotile spermatozoa as the consequence of defects of their motor apparatus. For example, whereas generalized sperm death hardly reconciles with any fertility potential, we have already noted that sperm with flagellar defects may still express residual fertilizing competence under special conditions, such as in vitro fertilization.

The identification of sperm degeneration or death is easily made by electron microscopy and it

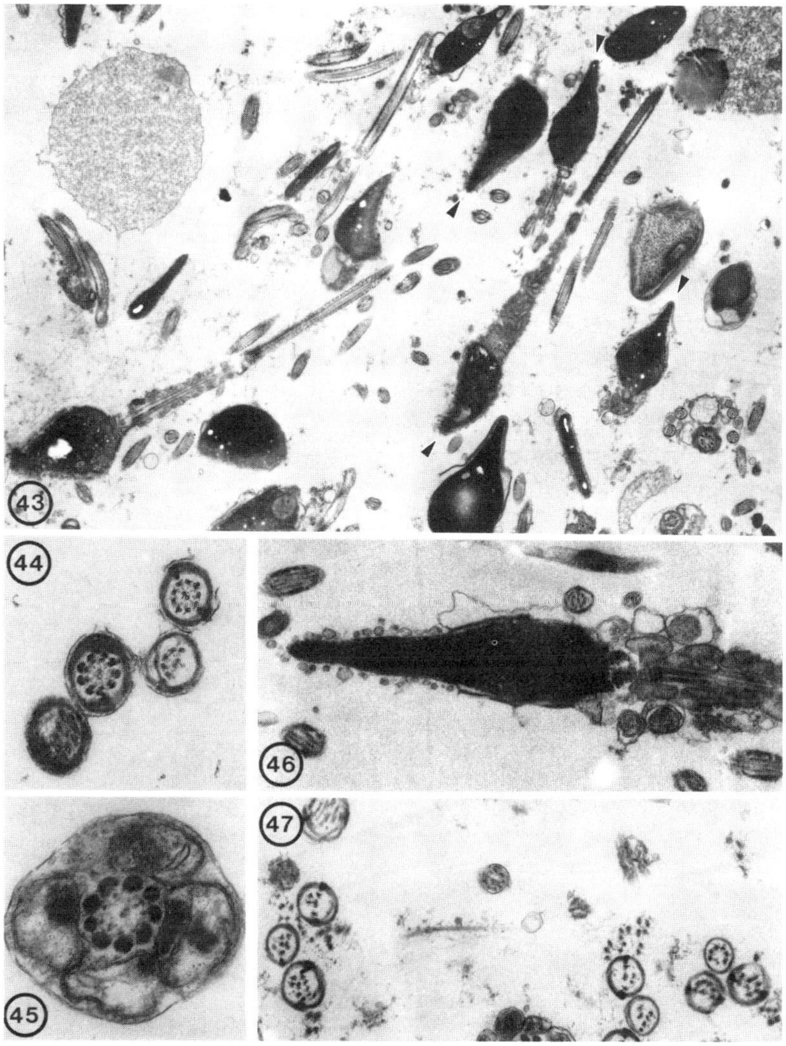

Figure 43 Generalized necrospermia in the semen of an infertile patient. All spermatozoa show evident signs of regression and necrosis, such as fragmentation and loss of the plasma membrane, swelling of the mitochondria with obliteration of their cristae, dissolution of the acrosome (*arrowheads*), and others. Many of these regressive changes are illustrated in greater detail in Figures 44 to 47 (×7500). **Figures 44 to 47** Regressive changes in necrospermia: fragmentation and/or disappearance of the plasma membrane and obfuscation of the normal structural organization of the fibrous sheath in Figures 44 and 47, spurious acrosome reaction (see text) in Figure 45, swelling of the mitochondria, obliteration of the cristae, and presence of dense "toxic" granules in their matrix, together with "filamentous" transformation of the axonemal microtubules in Figure 46 and subversion of the normal axonemal architecture and "filamentous" transformation of the microtubules in Figure 47 (Fig. 44, ×33,000; Fig. 45, ×60,000; Fig. 46, ×13,000; Fig. 47, ×30,000).

is based on the observation of degenerative changes that usually involve all sperm components (Figs. 43 to 47). There is fragmentation or complete disappearance of the plasma membrane (Figs. 43 and 46), extreme rarefaction of the matrix of the acrosome, vesiculation of the periacrosomal membrane and extracellular dissolution of the acrosomal substance (the spurious acrosome reaction; Figs. 43 and 46), karyolysis, swelling of the mitochondria and fragmentation of their cristae (Fig. 45), rarefaction of the striated columns and outer dense fibers, disorganization and breakdown of the rib-like structures of the fibrous sheath (Fig. 44), and filamentous transformation and/or disappearance of the microtubules of the proximal centriole and of the axoneme (Figs. 44, 45, and 47). Generalized necrospermia has different etiologies that include the production of nonviable spermatozoa in the seminiferous tubules, the inability of the epididymis to sustain sperm viability and/or assist in their maturation and in the acquisition of motility, and the effects of physical factors and of toxic substances.

GENERAL CONSIDERATIONS

Under what clinical and laboratory conditions is an ultrastructural examination of the semen required or indicated? It is not simple to answer this question considering the well-known variegation of the clinical and laboratory situations that characterize different subfertile or infertile conditions. In this author's opinion, however, the examination is diagnostically indicated in situations where repeated semen analyses have consistently shown that the patient has normal sperm concentrations, normal and effective motility, and "normal" morphologic features, and yet there is a long history of infertility and/or a negative zona-free hamster egg–sperm penetration assay.* [54] In agreement with the opinion of others,[22,195] the analysis is also indicated in situations characterized by immotility or abnormal motility and "normal" morphologic features to distinguish a true necrospermic condition from impairments of motility because of submicroscopic defects of the flagellum; it is also strongly recommended any time the conventional semen analysis detects generalized deviations of normal head shape and size such as, for example, head sphericity to rule out agenesis of the acrosome, and microcephaly to rule out acrosome hypoplasia or decapitation. Finally, it also is strongly indicated in those situations, and they are very frequent, where the patient has gone for months or years from one semen analysis to the next and from one form of therapy to the other without any significant improvement in the quality of his semen, and/or whenever the couple wishes to precisely assess the causes of the inferior quality of the semen. In these situations, the ultrastructural examination of the semen is likely to bring to an end protracted periods of clinical trials, spare the patient from the necessity of repeated semen analyses and from further investment of time and money, and permit the physician to advise the couple swiftly regarding the availability of alternative methods for the resolution of their infertile condition. We have already seen that one of these methods is extracorporeal fertilization.[55,56] Thus, an elucidation of the ultrastructural basis of "poor semen quality" could also contribute to providing the infertile couple with alternatives that would not be available otherwise.

Preparation of the semen for ultrastructural analysis does not represent a problem provided that there has been previous communication with the pathologist or the personnel in the electron microscopy laboratory where the sample is to be sent. After liquefaction, the sample is fixed in toto (i.e., without separating the cellular fraction from the seminal plasma) in large volumes of any of the primary fixatives for electron microscopy—preferable are those having a high osmolarity, such as that of Ito and Karnovsky,[196] or the picric acid-formaldehyde (PAF) fixative of Stefanini, De Martino, and Zamboni,[197] commonly referred to as Zamboni's fixative, which was devised specifically for the ultrastructural preservation of spermatozoa. These specialized fixatives are highly recommended since the induction of artifactual changes may render the visualization of the sperm ultrastructural organization extremely difficult and may considerably confuse the issue. After appropriate primary fixation (extremely rapid since one deals with a suspension of cells), the specimen is placed in buffer where it can remain indefinitely, and it is in buffer that it is usually sent to the electron microscopy laboratory for further processing and evaluation. It is recommended that the semen be produced at the site where it will be prepared for analysis (either the physician's office or the electron microscope laboratory) since some patients may be tempted to submit semen samples other than their own. It is difficult to resist the temptation to report a situation that occurred recently in this author's laboratory. One of our hospital patients of Polynesian extraction with chronic sinopulmonary infections and reduced mucociliary clearance had a bronchial biopsy that revealed universal absence of the dyn-

* The progressively wider use of this assay,[191] which incidentally is a product of basic research on gamete physiology,[192] despite its cost and the unsatisfactory reproducibility of its results[193] mostly due to methodologic vagaries, has further widened the dichotomy between the practice of clinical andrology and the progress made in the current understanding of sperm morphophysiology. It is difficult, in fact, to reconcile a vision of spermatozoa as cells consisting only of "a head and a tail" with an assay that should evaluate functional parameters (in this case, the competence of the acrosome) based on the structural integrity of subcellular components.[194] Practically, this translates into the difficulty, frequently experienced by the andrologist, to correlate the results of the bioassay with those of the analysis of the semen, especially when the patient with a "normal or just subnormal semen quality," as assessed by conventional laboratory methods, is to be explained the reason why "he failed the hamster test."

ein arms in the cilia of the respiratory epithelium. Considering that the patient had been married 7 years without conceptions, an ultrastructural examination of his semen was thought to be indicated. Since the patient was hospitalized, it was not believed to be necessary to have him come to the pathology department to produce the sample, which he provided from his room. Examined fresh prior to fixation for electron microscopy, the semen showed complete and generalized immotility; however, electron microscopy revealed that the lack of motility was due to universal deletion of the two microtubules in the center of the axonemes (the nine plus zero defect), a condition which did not readily reconcile with the absence of the dynein arms in the cilia. Confronted with the issue, the patient reluctantly admitted to giving us the semen of one of his friends; being another Samoan, this individual also happened to have dyskinetic cilia syndrome.

Since ultrastructural abnormalities may be sporadically found even in spermatozoa of normal and fertile individuals,[26,40,41] the diagnosis of a true pathologic situation depends on the careful examination of a large number of spermatozoa studied on planes of sections favorable to the visualization of the relevant structures. How many sperm constitute a sufficient number? This depends on the structures that are involved, the type of defect that is being researched, and the degree by which the ultrastructural findings correlate with the observations made upon semen analysis. For example, considering that only a minimal percentage of the randomly oriented sperm flagella in any given sample will be sectioned along a perfectly transverse plane, the consistent absence of dynein arms in 20 to 25 cross-sectioned flagella provides nearly absolute mathematical evidence of the existence of a ciliary dyskinetic condition, especially if the finding correlates with generalized immotility. In this case, the number of properly examined structures is low, even though the amount of time required to find 20 to 25 flagella in transverse sections is considerable. The diagnosis of acrosome hypoplasia will have to be based instead on the examination of a much larger number (minimum, 75 to 100) of sperm heads in longitudinal planes of section since it is difficult to assess the volume of the organelle in any other plane because of its nonuniform thickness: in this case, however, the time required for the examination is much shorter because of the ease by which the acrosome can be appropriately visualized as the result of its relatively large size.

CONCLUSIONS

This selective review is intended to render the reader more aware of the fact that, of the wide constellation of sperm defects and developmental anomalies, only a few can be identified by the methods employed for the routine evaluation of the human semen. Because of the superior preservation of the specimen and the high power of resolution of the electron microscope, the ultrastructural analysis considerably increases the quantity and greatly enhances the precision of the information to be derived from the study of the semen. Because of these considerations, it would be difficult to justify not exploiting its diagnostic and prognostic potential for the sake of practicality.[10] A considerable wealth of knowledge has been gained from studying the fine morphologic features of the spermatozoon in various phases of maturation and participation in the reproductive process; ignoring this knowledge in the assessment of the reproductive potential of a patient is no longer excusable.

Acknowledgments. I thank the technical personnel of the Electron Microscopy Laboratory, especially Mr. William Lungo, who patiently and skillfully printed all the micrographs. I also thank Ms. Elizabeth Neal who patiently typed the manuscript many times.

REFERENCES

1. Wong T-W, Straus FH, Warner NE: Testicular biopsy in the study of male infertility. I. Testicular causes of infertility. Arch Pathol 95:151, 1973
2. Wong T-W, Straus FH, Warner NE: Testicular biopsy in the study of male infertility. II. Posttesticular causes of infertility. Arch Pathol 95:160, 1973
3. Wong T-W, Straus FH, Warner NE: Testicular biopsy in the study of male infertility. III. Pretesticular causes of infertility. Arch Pathol 98:1, 1974
4. Wong T-W, Straus FH, Jones TM, Warner NE: Pathological aspects of the infertile testis. Urol Clin North Am 5:503, 1978
5. Wong T-W, Jones TM: Evaluation of testicular biopsy in male infertility studies. In Infertility in the Male, Edited by LI Lipshultz, SS Howards. New York, Churchill Livingstone, 1983, p 217
6. Mostofi KF, Davis CJ Jr: Male reproductive system and prostate. In Anderson's Pathology, Edited by JM Kissane. St. Louis, CV Mosby, 1985, p 791
7. Chan SL, Cunningham GR, Lipshultz LI: Testicular and post-testicular causes of male infertility. In Aspects of Male Infertility, Edited by R deVere White. Baltimore, Williams and Wilkins, 1982, p 116
8. Lipshultz LI, Cunningham GR, Howards SS: Differential diagnosis of male infertility. In Infertility in the Male, Edited by LI Lipshultz, SS Howards. New York, Churchill Livingstone, 1983, p 249
9. Lipshultz LI, Howards SS: Evaluation of the subfertile

male. In Infertility in the Male, Edited by LI Lipshultz, SS Howards. New York, Churchill Livingstone, 1983, p 187

10. Sherins RJ, Howards SS: Male Infertility. In Campbell's Urology, Vol 1, Edited by PC Walsh, RF Gittles, AD Perlmutter, TA Starney. Philadelphia, WB Saunders, 1986, p 640
11. World Health Organization: Laboratory manual for the examination of human semen and semen cervical mucus interaction. In World Health Organization Special Programme of Research, Development and Research Training for Human Reproduction, Edited by MA Belsey, KS Moghissi, CA Paulsen, AJ Gallegos, MRN Pusard. Singapore, Singapore Press Concern, 1980
12. Hargreave TB, Nilsson S: Seminology. In Male Infertility, Edited by TB Hargreave. Berlin, Springer-Verlag, 1983
13. MacLeod J: Human seminal cytology as a sensitive indicator of the germinal epithelium. Int J Fertil 9:281, 1964
14. Zamboni L, Zemjanis R, Stefanini M: The fine structure of monkey and human spermatozoa. Anat Rec 169:129, 1971
15. Bedford JM: Biology of primate spermatozoa. Contrib Primat 3:97, 1974
16. Fawcett DW: The mammalian spermatozoon: a review. Dev Biol 44:394, 1975
17. Phillips DM: Mammalian sperm structure. In Handbook of Physiology, Edited by DW Hamilton, RO Greep. Washington, American Physiology Society, 1975, p 405
18. Pedersen H, Fawcett DW: Functional anatomy of the human spermatozoon. In Human Semen and Fertility Regulation in Men, Edited by ESE Hafez. St. Louis, CV Mosby, 1976, p 65
19. Setchell BP: Spermatogenesis and spermatozoa. In Germ Cells and Fertilization, Edited by CR Austin, RV Short. Cambridge, Cambridge University Press, 1982, p 63
20. Bellvé AR, O'Brien DA: The mammalian spermatozoon: structure and temporal assembly. In Mechanisms and Control of Animal Fertilization, Edited by JF Hartman. New York, Academic Press, 1983, p 56
21. Baccetti B: The human spermatozoon. In Ultrastructure of Reproduction, Edited by J Van Blerkom, P Motta. Boston, Martinus Nijhoff Publishers, 1984, p 110
22. Bisson JP, David G: Anomalies morphologiques du spermatozoide humain: 2. Étude ultrastructurale. J Gynecol Obstet Biol Reprod (Paris) 4(suppl 1):37, 1975
23. Holstein AF: Morphologische Studien an abnormen Spermatiden und Spermatozoen des Menschen. Virchows Arch A 367:93, 1975
24. Escalier D, David G: Pathology of the cytoskeleton of the human sperm flagellum: axonemal and periaxonemal anomalies. Biol Cell 50:37, 1984
25. Nistal M, Paniagua R: Testicular and Epididymal Pathology. New York, Thieme Stratton, 1984
26. Zamboni L: Sperm ultrastructural pathology and infertility. In Pathology of Infertility, Edited by B Gondos, D Riddick. New York, Thieme Medical Publishers, 1987, p 281
27. Gibbons IR: Structure and functions of flagellar microtubules. In International Cell Biology, Edited by BR Brinkley, KR Porter. New York, Rockefeller University Press, 1977, p 348
28. Olson GE, Linck RW: Observations on the structural components of flagellar axonemes and central pair microtubules from rat sperm. J Ultrastruct Res 61:21, 1977
29. Linck RW: Advances in the ultrastructural analysis of the sperm flagellar axoneme. In The Spermatozoon: Maturation, Motility, Surface Properties and Comparative Aspects, Edited by DW Fawcett, JM Bedford. Baltimore, Urban and Schwarzenberg, 1979, p 99
30. Gibbons IR: Cilia and flagella of eukaryotes. J Cell Biol 91:107s, 1981
31. Fawcett DW: The Cell. Philadelphia, WB Saunders, 1981
32. Baccetti B, Burrini AG, Maver A, Pallini V, Renieri T: "9 + 0" immotile spermatozoa in an infertile man. Andrologia 11:437, 1979
33. Baccetti B, Burrini AG, Pallini V, Renieri T: Human dynein and sperm pathology. J Cell Biol 88:102, 1981
34. Baccetti B, Porter KR, Alrich M: High voltage electron microscopy of sperm axoneme. J Submicrosc Cytol 17:171, 1985
35. Gibbons BH: Studies on the mechanisms of flagellar movement. In The Spermatozoon: Maturation, Motility, Surface Properties and Comparative Aspects, Edited by DW Fawcett, JM Bedford. Baltimore, Urban and Schwarzenberg, 1979, p 91
36. Satir P: Basis of flagellar motility in spermatozoa: current status. In The Spermatozoon: Maturation, Motility, Surface Properties and Comparative Aspects, Edited by DW Fawcett, JM Bedford. Baltimore, Urban and Schwarzenberg, 1979, p 81
37. Haimo LT, Rosenbaum JL: Cilia, flagella and microtubules. J Cell Biol 91:125s, 1981
38. Afzelius BA: Electron microscopy of the sperm tail: results obtained with a new fixative. J Biophys Biochem Cytol 5:269, 1959
39. Brokaw CJ, Luck DJL, Huang B: Analysis of the movement of *Chlamidomonas* flagella: the function of the radial-spoke system is revealed by comparison of wild type and mutant flagella. J Cell Biol 92:792, 1982
40. Pryor JP, Collins WP, Landon G, Tyler JPP: The clinical application of electron microscopy and the heterologous ova penetration test to the assessment of spermatozoa from infertile men. Br J Urol 53:660, 1981
41. Hunter DG, Deretzer FL: Abnormal axonemes in sperm of fertile men. Arch Androl 16:1, 1986
42. Nistal M, Paniagua R, Herruzo A: Absence de la paire centrale du complex axonemique dans une tératospermie avec flagelles courts et épais. J Gynecol Obstet Biol Reprod (Paris) 8:47, 1979
43. Pedersen H, Hammen R: Ultrastructure of human spermatozoa with complete subcellular derangement. Arch Androl 9:251, 1982
44. McClure RD, Brawer J, Robaire B: Ultrastructure of immotile spermatozoa in an infertile male: spectrum of structural defects. Fertil Steril 40:395, 1983
45. Baccetti B, Burrini AG, Pallini V: Spermatozoa and cilia lacking axoneme in an infertile man. Andrologia 12:525, 1980
46. Afzelius BA, Eliasson R, Johansen O, Lindholmer C: Lack of dynein arms in immotile human spermatozoa. J Cell Biol 66:225, 1975
47. Baccetti B, Burrini AG, Pallini V, Renieri T, Rosati F, Menchini-Fabris GF: The short-tailed human spermatozoa: ultrastructural alterations and dynein absence. J Submicrosc Cytol 7:349, 1975
48. Pedersen H, Rebbe H: Absence of arms in the axoneme of immotile human spermatozoa. Biol Reprod 12:541, 1975
49. Baccetti B, Burrini AG, Dallai R, Pallini V: The dynein electrophoretic bands in axoneme naturally lacking the inner or the outer arm. J Cell Biol 80:334, 1979

50. Terquem A, Dadoune JP: Les anomalies de structure dans les troubles du la mobilité di spermatozoide humain à propos de 60 cas d'asthenospermie. Bull Assoc Anat (Nancy) 64:567, 1980
51. Jouannet P, Escalier D, Serres C, David G: Motility of human sperm without outer dynein arms. J Submicrosc Cytol 15:67, 1983
52. Aitken RJ, Ross A, Lees MM: Analysis of sperm function in Kartagener's syndrome. Fertil Steril 40:696, 1983
53. Moryan AI, Gray AT, Tulchinsky D: Normal penetration of hamster ova by human spermatozoa with dyskinetic motility. Fertil Steril 45:735, 1986
54. Yanagimachi R, Yanagimachi H, Rogers B: The use of zona-free animal ova as a test system for the assessment of the fertilizing capacity of human spermatozoa. Biol Reprod 15:471, 1976
55. Cohen J, Fehilly CB, Fishel SB, Edwards RG, Hewitt J, Rowland GF, Steptoe PC, Webster J: Male infertility successfully treated by *in vitro* fertilization. Lancet 1:1239, 1984
56. Cohen J, Edwards R, Fehilly C, Fishel S, Hewitt J, Purdy J, Rowland G, Steptoe P, Webster J: In vitro fertilization: a treatment for male infertility. Fertil Steril 43:422, 1985
57. Afzelius BA: A human syndrome caused by immotile cilia. Science 193:317, 1976
58. Eliasson R, Mossberg B, Camner P, Afzelius BA: The immotile cilia syndrome: a congenital ciliary abnormality as an etiologic factor in chronic airway infection and male sterility. N Engl J Med 297:1, 1977
59. Afzelius BA: The immotile-cilia syndrome and other ciliary diseases. Int Rev Exp Pathol 19:1, 1979
60. Camner P, Afzelius BA, Eliasson R, Mossberg B: Relation between abnormalities of human sperm flagella and respiratory tract disease. Int J Androl 2:211, 1979
61. Afzelius BA: Genetic disorders of cilia. In International Cell Biology, Edited by HG Schweiger. Berlin, Springer-Verlag, 1980, p 440
62. Afzelius BA, Mossberg B: Immotile cilia. Thorax 35:401, 1980
63. Walt H: Untersuchungen an Spermieflagellen und Zilien mit pathologischer Motilität and Ultrastruktür. Schweiz Med Wochenschr 114:1442, 1984
64. Kartagener M: Zur Pathogeneses der Bronchiektasien: Bronchietasien bei Situs Viscerum Inversus. Beitr Klin Tuberk 83:489, 1933
65. Waite D, Steele R, Ross I, Wakefield J St J, Mackay J, Wallace J: Cilia and sperm tail abnormalities in polynesian bronchiectatics. Lancet 2:132, 1978
66. Wakefield J St J, Waite DA: Abnormal cilia in Polynesian with bronchiectasis. Am Rev Respir Dis 121:1003, 1980
67. Waite DA, Wakefield J St J, Mackay JB, Ross IT: Mucociliary transport and ultrastructural abnormalities in Polynesian bronchiectasis. Chest 80:896, 1980
68. Sturgess J, Chao J, Wong J, Aspiri N, Turner P: Cilia with defective radial spokes: a cause of human respiratory disease. N Engl J Med 300:53, 1979
69. Sturgess J, Chao J, Turner P: Transposition of ciliary microtubules: another cause of impaired ciliary motility. N Engl J Med 303:318, 1980
70. Sturgess J, Chao J: Ultrastructural features of a human genetic defect of cilia. Progr Clin Biol Res 80:7, 1982
71. Afzelius BA, Eliasson R: Flagellar mutants in man: on the heterogeneity of the immotile-cilia syndrome. J Ultrastruct Res 69:43, 1979
72. Schneeberger EE, McCormack J, Issenberg HJ, Schuster SR, Gerald PS: Heterogeneity of ciliary morphology in the immotile-cilia syndrome in man. J Ultrastruct Res 73:34, 1980
73. Afzelius BA: Genetical and ultrastructural aspects of the immotile cilia syndrome. Am J Hum Genet 33:852, 1981
74. Rossman CM, Forrest JB, Less RMKW, Newhouse AF, Newhouse MT: The dyskinetic cilia syndrome: abnormal ciliary motility in association with abnormal ciliary ultrastructure. Chest 80:860, 1981
75. Walt H, Campana A, Balerna M, Domenighetti G, Hedinger C, Jakob M, Pescia G, Sulmoni A: Mosaicism of dynein in spermatozoa and cilia and fibrous sheath aberrations in an infertile man. Andrologia 15:295, 1983
76. Herzon FS, Murphy S: Normal ciliary ultrastructure in children with Kartagener's syndrome. Ann Otol Rhinol Laryngol 89:81, 1980
77. Schidlow DV, Katz SM: Immotile cilia syndrome. N Engl J Med 308:595, 1983
78. Greenstone M, Rutman A, Pavia D, Lawrence D, Cole PJ: Normal axonemal structure and function in Kartagener's syndrome: an explicable paradox. Thorax 40:956, 1985
79. Johnsson MS, McCormick JR, Gillies CG, Gondos B: Kartagener's syndrome with motile spermatozoa. N Engl J Med 307:1131, 1982
80. Lungarella G, Fonzi L, Burrini AG: Ultrastructural abnormalities in respiratory cilia and sperm tails in a patient with Kartagener's syndrome. J Ultrastruct Res 3:319, 1982
81. Chao J, Turner JAP, Sturgess JM: Genetic heterogeneity of dynein deficiency in cilia from patients with respiratory disease. Am Rev Respir Dis 126:302, 1982
82. Baccetti BA, Burrini AG, Pallini V: Different axonemal patterns in cilia and flagella of the same animal. J Submicrosc Cytol 13:479, 1981
83. Calvin HI, Hwang FH-F, Wohlrab H: Localization of zinc in a dense fiber-connecting piece fraction of rat sperm tail analogous chemically to hair keratin. Biol Reprod 13:228, 1975
84. Olson GE, Sammons DW: Structural chemistry of outer dense fibers of rat sperm. Biol Reprod 22:319, 1980
85. Baccetti B, Pallini V, Burrini AG: The accessory fibers of the sperm tail. I. Structure and chemical composition of the bull "coarse fibers." J Submicrosc Cytol 5:237, 1973
86. Baccetti B, Pallini V, Burrini AG: The accessory fibers of the sperm tail. II. Their role in binding zinc in mammals and cephalopods. J Ultrastruct Res 54:261, 1976
87. Baccetti B, Pallini V, Burrini AG: The accessory fibers of the sperm tail. III. High sulphur and low sulphur components in mammals and cephalopods. J Ultrastruct Res 57:289, 1976
88. Baccetti B: The evolution of the sperm tail. Symp Soc Exp Biol 35:521, 1982
89. Phillips DM: Comparative analysis of mammalian sperm motility. J Cell Biol 53:561, 1972
90. Phillips DM, Olson G: Mammalian sperm motility. In The Functional Anatomy of the Spermatozoon, Edited by BA Afzelius. New York, Pergamon Press, 1975, p 117
91. Fawcett DW: Unsolved problems in morphogenesis of the mammalian spermatozoon. In International Cell Biology, Edited by BR Brinkley, KR Porter. New York, Rockefeller University Press, 1977, p 588
92. Bedford JM, Calvin HI: Changes in S-S linked structure of the sperm tail during epididymal maturation with compar-

ative observations in submammalian species. J Exp Zool 187:181, 1974
93. Swan MA, Linck RW, Ito S, Fawcett DW: Structure and function of the undulating membrane in spermatozoan propulsion in the toad, *Bufo marinus.* J Cell Biol 85:866, 1980
94. Feneux D, Serres C, Jouannet P: Sliding spermatozoa: a dyskinesia responsible for human infertility? Fertil Steril 44:508, 1985
95. Fawcett DW, Anderson WA, Phillips DM: Morphogenetic factors influencing the shape of the sperm head. Dev Biol 26:220, 1971
96. Holstein AF: Ultrastructural observations on the differentiation of spermatids in man. Andrologia 8:157, 1976
97. Bhattacharyya AK, Zaneveld LJD: The sperm head. In Biochemistry of Mammalian Reproduction, Edited by LJD Zaneveld, RT Chatterton. New York, John Wiley & Sons, 1982, p 119
98. Rogers JB, Bentwood BJ: Capacitation, acrosome reaction, and fertilization. In Biochemistry of Mammalian Reproduction, Edited by LJD Zaneveld, RT Chatterton. New York, John Wiley & Sons, 1982, p 203
99. Harrison RAP: The acrosome, its hydrolases, and egg penetration. In The Sperm Cell, Edited by J André. The Hague, Martinus Nijhoff Publisher, 1983, p 259
100. Frazer LR: Mechanisms controlling mammalian fertilization. In Oxford Reviews of Reproductive Biology, Vol 6, Edited by JR Clarke. Oxford, Clarendon Press, 1984, p 144
101. Austin CR: Sperm maturation in the male and female genital tracts. In Biology of Fertilization, Vol 2, Edited by CB Metz, A Monroy. Orlando, Academic Press, 1985, p 121
102. Allison AC, Hartree EF: Lysosomal enzymes in the acrosome and their possible role in fertilization. J Reprod Fertil 21:501, 1970
103. Zamboni L: Fine Morphology of Mammalian Fertilization. New York, Harper and Row, 1971
104. Friend DS: The organization of the sperm membrane. In Immunobiology of Gametes, Edited by M Edidin, MH Johnson. Cambridge, Cambridge University Press, 1977, p 5
105. Austin CR: Observations on the penetration of sperm into the mammalian egg. Aust J Sci Res (Series B) 4:581, 1951
106. Chang MC: Fertilizing capacity of spermatozoa deposited into the fallopian tubes. Nature 168:697, 1951
107. Yanagimachi R: Mechanisms of fertilization in mammals. In Fertilization and Embryonic Development in Vitro, Edited by L Mastroianni, Jr, D Biggers. New York, Plenum Publishing, 1981, p 81
108. Bedford JM: Significance of the need for sperm capacitation before fertilization in eutherian mammals. Biol Reprod 28:108, 1983
109. Moore HDM, Bedford JM: The interaction of mammalian gametes in the female. In Mechanism and Control of Animal Fertilization, Edited by JF Hartman. New York, Academic Press, 1983, p 453
110. Chang MC: The meaning of sperm capacitation: a historical perspective. J Androl 5:45, 1984
111. Yanagimachi R: The movement of golden hamster spermatozoa before and after capacitation. J Reprod Fertil 23:193, 1970
112. Austin CR, Bishop MWH: Role of the rodent acrosome and perforatorium in fertilization. Proc R Soc Lond [Biol] 149:241, 1958
113. Nagae T, Yanagimachi R, Srivastava PN, Yanagimachi H: Acrosome reaction in human spermatozoa. Fertil Steril 45:701, 1986
114. Barros C, Bedford JM, Franklin LE, Austin CR: Membrane vesiculation as a feature of the mammalian acrosome reaction. J Cell Biol 34:C1, 1967
115. Saling PM: Involvement of trypsin-like activity in binding of mouse spermatozoa to zonae pellucidae. Proc Natl Acad Sci USA 78:6231, 1981
116. Florman HM, Storey BT: Mouse gamete interactions: the zona pellucida is the site of the acrosome reaction leading to fertilization *in vitro.* Dev Biol 91:121, 1982
117. Phillips DM: Problems in the analysis of mammalian fertilization. In Ultrastructure of Reproduction, Edited by J Van Blerkom, PM Motta. Boston, Martinus Nijhoff Publishers, 1984, p 166
118. Storey BT, Lee MA, Muller C, Ward CR, Wirtshafter DG: Binding of mouse spermatozoa to the zonae pellucidae of mouse eggs in cumulus: evidence that the acrosome remains substantially intact. Biol Reprod 31:119, 1984
119. Weissenbergh R, Eshkol A, Rudak E, Lunenfeld B: Inability of round acrosomeless human spermatozoa to penetrate zona-free hamster ova. Arch Androl 11:167, 1982
120. Syms AJ, Johnson AR, Lipshultz LI, Smith RG: Studies on human spermatozoa and round head syndrome. Fertil Steril 42:431, 1984
121. Jeyendrau RS, Vanderven HH, Kennedy WP, Heath E, Perez-Pelalz M, Sobrero AJ, Zaneveld LJD: Acrosomeless sperm: a cause of primary male infertility. Andrologia 17:31, 1985
122. Singer R, Sagir M, Barnet M, Alahouf D, Landau B, Segenreich E, Servadio C: Head abnormalities: assessment of sperm in the routine laboratory. Andrologia 13:236, 1981
123. Bryan JHD: An eosin fast green-naphthol yellow mixture for differential staining of cytologic components in mammalian spermatozoa. Stain Technol 45:231, 1970
124. Bryan JHD, Akruk SR: A naphthol yellow-S and erythrosin B staining procedure for use in studies of the acrosome reaction of rabbit spermatozoa. Stain Technol 52:47, 1977
125. Saling PM, Storey BT: Mouse gamete interaction during fertilization *in vitro:* chlortetracycline as a fluorescent probe for the mouse sperm acrosome reaction. J Cell Biol 83:544, 1979
126. Talbot P, Chacon R: A new procedure for rapidly scoring acrosome reaction of human sperm. Gamete Res 3:211, 1980
127. Wolf DP, Boldt J, Byrd W, Bechtol KB: Acrosomal status evaluation in human ejaculated sperm with monoclonal antibodies. Biol Reprod 32:1157, 1985
128. Talbot P, Chacon R: A triple stain technique for evaluating normal acrosome reactions of human sperm. J Exp Zool 215:201, 1981
129. Cross NL, Morales P, Overstreet JW, Hanson FW: Two simple methods for detecting acrosome-reacted human sperm. Gamete Res 15:213, 1986
130. Aalseth EP, Saacke RG: Vital staining and acrosomal evaluation of bovine sperm. Gamete Res 15:73, 1986
131. Saacke RG, Almquist JO: Ultrastructure of bovine spermatozoa. I. The head of normal, ejaculated sperm. Am J Anat 115:143, 1964
132. Bisson JP, David G, Magnin C: Étude ultrastructurale des anomalies de l'acrosome dans les spermatozoïde à tête irrégulière. Bull Assoc Anat (Nancy) 59:345, 1945

133. Holstein AF, Schirren C: Classification of abnormalities in human spermatids based on recent advances in ultrastructure research on spermatid differentiation. In The Spermatozoon: Maturation, Motility, Surface Properties and Comparative Aspects, Edited by DW Fawcett, JM Bedford. Baltimore, Urban and Schwarzenberg, 1977, p 341
134. Brun B, Clavert A: Modifications morphologiques de l'acrosome chez un homme exposé à la chaleur. J Gynecol Obstet Biol Reprod (Paris) 6:907, 1977
135. Camatini M, Chiara F, Franchi E, Bellone L: Acrosomal cap abnormalities of spermatids from infertile men. In Recent Progress in Andrology, Edited by A Fabbrini, E Steinberger. London, Academic Press, 1978, p 403
136. Soderstrom KO: An acrosomal abnormality in spermatids from infertile men. Arch Androl 7:275, 1981
137. Holstein AF, Schirren C, Schirren CG: Human spermatids and spermatozoa lacking acrosomes. J Reprod Fertil 35:489, 1973
138. Pedersen H, Rebbe H: Fine structure of round-headed human spermatozoa. J Reprod Fertil 37:51, 1974
139. Kullander S, Rousing A: On round-headed human spermatozoa. Intern J Fertil 20:33, 1975
140. Anton-Lamprecht I, Kotzur B, Schöpf E: Round-headed human spermatozoa. Fertil Steril 27:685, 1976
141. Nistal M, Herruzo A, Sanchez-Corral F: Teratozoospermia absoluta de presentacion familiar: espermatozoides microcefalos irregulares sin acrosoma. Andrologia 10:234, 1978
142. Tyler JPP, Broadle RA, Stevens SMB: Round-headed spermatozoa: a case report. Pathology 17:67, 1985
143. Schirren CG, Holstein AF, Schirren C: Ueber die Morphogenese Rundkopfiger Spermatozoen des Menschen. Andrologia 3:117, 1971
144. Baccetti B, Renieri T, Rosati F, Selmi MG, Casanova S: Further observations on the morphogenesis of the round headed human spermatozoa. Andrologia 9:255, 1977
145. Castellani L, Chiara F, Cotelli F: Fine structure and cytochemistry of the morphogenesis of round-headed human sperm. Arch Androl 1:219, 1978
146. Nistal M, Paniagua R: Morphogenesis of round-headed human spermatozoa lacking acrosomes in a case of severe teratozoospermia. Andrologia 10:49, 1978
147. Florke-Gerloff S, Krause W, Topfer-Petersen E, Tschesche H, Muller-Esterl N, Engel W: On the teratogenesis of round-headed spermatozoa: investigations with antibodies against acrosin, an intra-acrosomally located acrosin-inhibitor, and the outer acrosomal membrane. Andrologia 17:126, 1985
148. Florke-Gerloff S, Topfer-Petersen E, Muller-Esterl W, Mansouri A, Schatz R, Schirren C, Schill W, Engel W: Biochemical and genetic investigation of round-headed spermatozoa in infertile men including two brothers and their father. Andrologia 16:187, 1984
149. Monesi V: Chromosome activities during meiosis and spermiogenesis. J Reprod Fertil [Suppl] 13:1, 1971
150. Bellvé AR: The molecular biology of mammalian spermatogenesis. In Oxford Reviews of Reproductive Biology, Edited by CA Finn. London, Oxford University Press, 1979, p 159
151. Bedford JM, Calvin HI: The occurrence and possible functional significance of -S-S- crosslinks in sperm head with particular reference to Eutherian mammals. J Exp Zool 188:137, 1974
152. Saovaros W, Panyim S: The formation of disulfide bonds in human protamines during sperm maturation. Experientia 35:191, 1979
153. Meistrich ML, Reid BO, Barcellona WJ: Changes in sperm nuclei during spermiogenesis and epididymal maturation. Exp Cell Res 99:72, 1976
154. Everson DP, Witkin SS, De Harven E, Bendich A: Ultrastructure of partially decondensed human spermatozoal chromatin. J Ultrastruct Res 63:178, 1978
155. Gusse M, Chevailler P: Electron microscopic evidence for the presence of globular structure in different sperm chromatins. J Cell Biol 87:280, 1980
156. Tanphaichitr N, Sobhon P, Chalermisarachai P, Patilantakarnkool M: Acid-extracted nuclear proteins and ultrastructure of human sperm chromatin as revealed by differential extraction with urea, mercaptoethanol and salt. Gamete Res 4:297, 1981
157. Sobhon P, Chutatape C, Chalermisarachai P, Vongpanyabal P, Tanphaichitr N: Transmission and scanning electron microscopic studies of the human sperm chromatin decondensed by micrococcal nuclease and salt. J Exp Zool 221:61, 1982
158. Bustos-Obregon E, Leiva S: Chromatin packing in normal and teratozoospermic human ejaculated spermatozoa. Andrologia 15:468, 1983
159. Hrudka F, Singh A: Sperm nucleomalacia in men with inflammatory bowel disease. Arch Androl 13:37, 1984
160. Levi AJ, Fisher AM, Hughus L, Hendry WF: Male infertility due to sulphasalasine. Lancet 2:276, 1979
161. Toth A: Reversible toxic effect of salicylazosulfapyridine on semen quality. Fertil Steril 31:538, 1979
162. Traub AL, Thompson W, Orville J: Male infertility due to sulphasalazine. Lancet 2:639, 1979
163. Toovey S, Hudson E, Hendry WF, Levi AJ: Sulphasalazine and male infertility: reversibility and possible mechanism. Gut 22:445, 1981
164. Hudson E, Doré C, Sowter C, Toovey S, Levi AJ: Sperm size in patients with inflammatory bowel disease on sulphasalazine therapy. Fertil Steril 38:77, 1982
165. Evenson DP, Darzynkiewicz Z, Melamed MR: Relation of mammalian sperm heterogeneity to fertility. Science 210:1131, 1980
166. Silvestroni L, Frajese G: Abnormal structure of "spermatozoa" in infertile oligospermic men. In Recent Progress in Andrology, Edited by A Fabbrini, E Steinberger. London, Academic Press, 1978, p 415
167. Kjessler B: Karyotype, meiosis and spermatogenesis in a sample of men attending an infertility clinic. Monogr Hum Genet 2:10, 1966
168. Kjessler B: Facteurs génétiques dans la subfertilité male humaine. Fecondité et Sterilité du Male. Acquisitions Récentes Paris, Masson, 1972
169. Kjessler B: Chromosomal constitution and male reproductive failure. In Male Fertility and Sterility, Edited by RE Mancini, L Martini. London, Academic Press, 1974, p 231
170. Abramsson L, Beckman G, Duchek M, Nordenson I: Chromosomal aberrations and male infertility. J Urol 128:52, 1982
171. Zamboni L, Stefanini M: The fine structure of the neck of mammalian spermatozoa. Anat Rec 169:155, 1971
172. Fawcett DW, Phillips DM: The fine structure and development of the neck region of the mammalian spermatozoa. Anat Rec 165:153, 1969

173. Woolley DM, Fawcett DW: The degeneration and disappearance of the centrioles during the development of the rat spermatozoon. Anat Rec 177:289, 1973
174. Lindeman CB, Rikmenspoel R: Sperm flagella: autonomous oscillations of the contractile system. Science 175:337, 1972
175. Lüders G: Ein Defekt der Kopf-Schwanz-Verknüpfung beim menschlichen Spermatozoen. Andrologia 8:365, 1976
176. Perotti ME, Giarola A, Gioria M: Ultrastructural study of the decapitated sperm defect in an infertile man. J Reprod Fertil 63:543, 1981
177. LeLannou D: Teratospermie consistant en l'absence de tête spermatique par defaut de connexion tête-col, chez l'homme. J Gynecol Obstet Biol Reprod (Paris) 8:43, 1979
178. Baccetti B, Selmi MG, Soldani P: Morphogenesis of "decapitated" spermatozoa in a man. J Reprod Fertil 70:395, 1984
179. Chemes HE, Carizza C, Scarinci F, Brugo S, Neuspiller N, Schwarsztein L: Lack of a head in human spermatozoa from sterile patients: a syndrome associated with impaired fertilization. Fertil Steril 47:310, 1987
180. Zaneveld LJD, Polakoski KL: Collection and physical examination of the ejaculate. In Techniques of Human Andrology, Edited by ESE Hafez. Amsterdam, North Holland Biomedical Press, 1977, p 147
181. Hancock JL, Rollinson DHL: A seminal defect associated with sterility of Guernsey bulls. Vet Rec 61:742, 1949
182. Hancock JL: The disintegration of bull spermatozoa. Vet Rec 67:825, 1955
183. Jones WA: Abnormal morphology of the spermatozoa in Guernsey bulls. Br Vet J 118:257, 1962
184. Williams G: An abnormality of the spermatozoa of some Hereford bulls. Vet Rec 77:1204, 1965
185. Van Rensburg SW, Van Rensburg SJ, de Vos WA: The significance of the cytoplasmic droplet in the disintegration of semen in Guernsey bull. Anderstpoort J Vet Res 33:169, 1966
186. Settergren I, Nicander L: Ultrastructure of disintegrated bull sperm. Proceedings of the 6th International Congress on Animal Reproduction and Artificial Insemination, Edited by C Thibault. Paris, Institut National de La Recherche Agronomique, 1968, p 191
187. Blom E, Birch-Andersen A: Ultrastructure of the "decapitated sperm defect" in Guernsey bulls. J Reprod Fertil 23:67, 1970
188. Blom E: A one minute live-dead sperm stain by means of eosin-nigrosin. Fertil Steril 1:176, 1950
189. Williams WW, Pollack OJ: Study of sperm vitality with the aid of eosin-nigrosin stain. Fertil Steril 1:178, 1950
190. Eliasson R, Treichl L: Supravital staining of human spermatozoa. Fertil Steril 22:134, 1971
191. Yanagimachi R: Zona-free hamster eggs: their use in assessing fertilizing capacity and examining chromosomes of human spermatozoa. Gamete Res 10:187, 1984
192. Hanada A, Chang MC: Penetration of zona-free eggs by spermatozoa of different species. Biol Reprod 6:300, 1972
193. Lipshultz LI: Beyond the routine semen analysis. Fertil Steril 38:153, 1982
194. Gould JE, Overstreet JW, Yanagimachi H, Yanagimachi R, Katz DF, Hanson FW: What functions of the sperm cells are measured by in vitro fertilization of zona-free hamster eggs? Fertil Steril 40:344, 1983
195. Pedersen H, Rebbe H, Hammen R: Human sperm fine structure in a case of severe asthenospermia-necrospermia. Fertil Steril 22:156, 1971
196. Ito S, Karnovsky MJ: Formaldehyde-glutaraldehyde fixatives containing trinitro compounds. J Cell Biol 39:168a, 1968
197. Stefanini M, De Martino C, Zamboni L: Fixation of ejaculated spermatozoa for electron microscopy. Nature 216:173, 1967

Chapter 27

The sperm penetration assay: its usefulness reevaluated

B. Jane Rogers, Ph.D.

Division of Infertility/Endocrinology, Department of Obstetrics and Gynecology, Vanderbilt University, Nashville, Tennessee

The sperm penetration assay (SPA) is a potentially valuable new tool in the investigation of infertility. The appearance of over 200 publications in the last 4 years alone attests to the tremendous interest which this technique has evoked. With this mushrooming literature and utilization of the test, of course, has come controversy. Agreement has not even been reached on the name of the test. Besides SPA it is also called the hamster test, the "humster" (human + hamster) test, the heterologous ovum penetration test, and hamster zona-free ovum test. The basic questions could be simplistically phrased as follows: "What does the SPA really tell us?" "How can it be used clinically?" "Is it an asset to an infertility workup?" The purpose of this review is to reevaluate this test objectively. Recent reviews[1-4] have provided comprehensive accounts of various aspects of the SPA. This review is not intended to be an exhaustive compilation of all articles on the subject. This contribution will specifically address some of the controversies surrounding utilization of the test so that the clinician can decide personally whether it would be valuable in his or her own infertility workup.

HISTORY OF SPERM PENETRATION ASSAY

The methodology that is critical for the SPA can be traced back to the preparation of zona-free mouse eggs by Beatrice Mintz in 1962.[5] Zona-free eggs were inseminated by sperm of heterologous species in 1972.[6, 7] In 1976 we showed that zona-free hamster eggs could be penetrated by human sperm.[8] The potential of using this surrogate egg as a means of evaluating fertilizing potential was immediately obvious. Other species were tested and proved not to be as receptive as the hamster. The mouse ovum, in particular, was found to allow no penetration by human sperm. The hamster egg is unique in that in its zona-free state it can be penetrated by every species of sperm tested thus far (guinea pig,[7, 9] mouse,[6, 10] deer mouse,[11] rat,[6, 10, 11] rabbit,[9] boar,[12-18] bull,[17, 19, 20] horse,[20] goat,[21] bat,[22] dolphin,[23] marmoset monkey,[24] rhesus monkey,[25] cynomolgus monkey[26]).

METHODOLOGY AND TECHNIQUES OF TEST PERFORMANCE

The method for performance of the SPA has been described in detail and is depicted in Figure 1.[27, 28] The critical steps in performing the procedure will be discussed, and evidence will be provided to substantiate the choice of a method. Recommendations for a standardized procedure are given in Table 1. The first consideration of any analysis of semen quality is *abstinence time*. The possible effect of a reduced abstinence time on penetration of zona-free eggs was previously demonstrated by us.[28] In four cooperative fertile donors a reduction in abstinence from 48 hours to either 12 or 24 hours produced a substantial reduction in penetrating potential which was not always accompanied by a reduction in count or motility. Longer abstinence, up to 5 days, is acceptable but presumably produces no enhancement of results. False negative results could be obtained with abstinence of less than 48 hours, and thus short periods of abstinence are not recommended.

After the sample is collected, the *time in seminal plasma* becomes critical. This variable has been loosely controlled in some settings, because the detrimental effect has not been appreciated. Many samples have been collected outside the

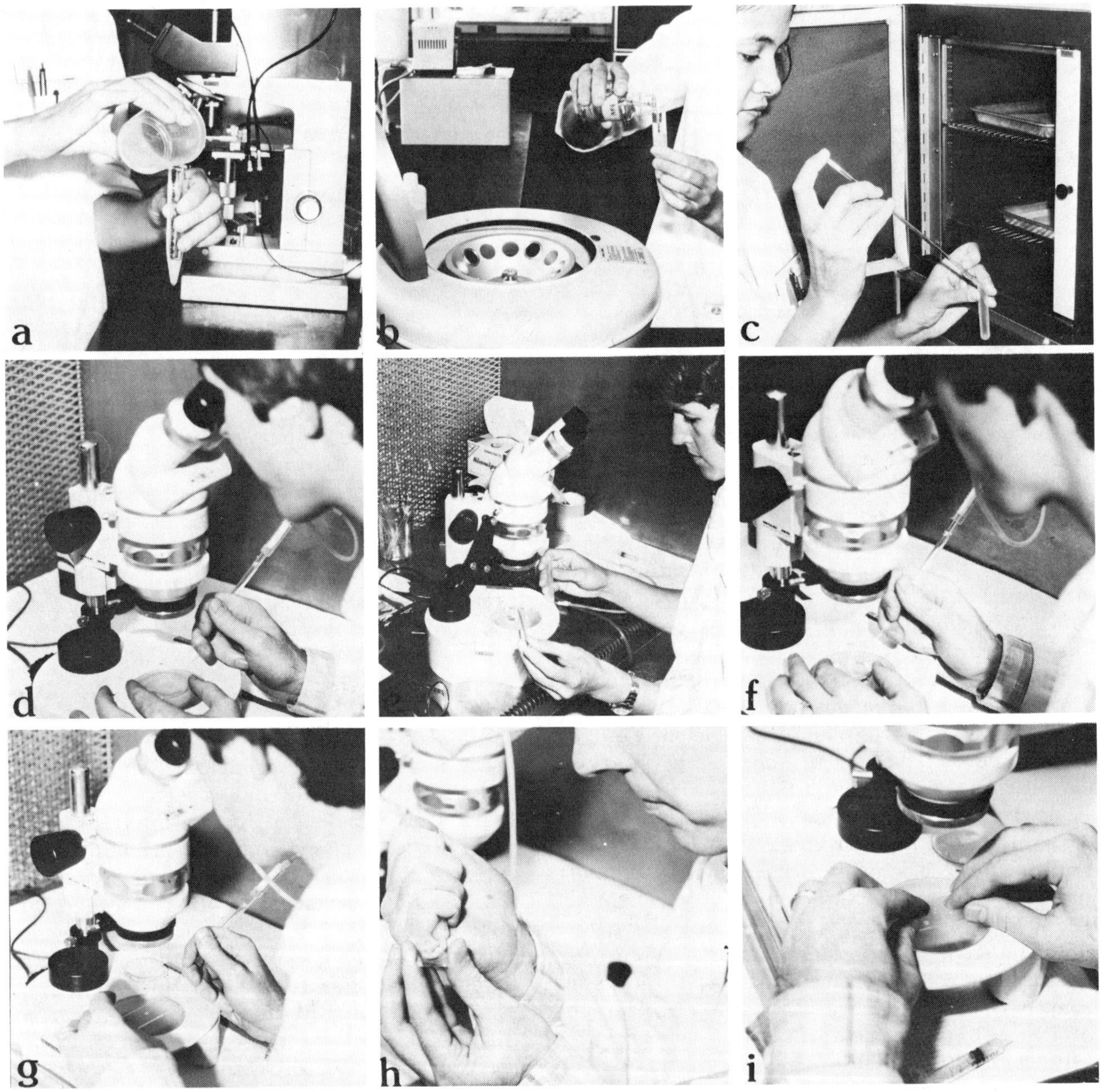

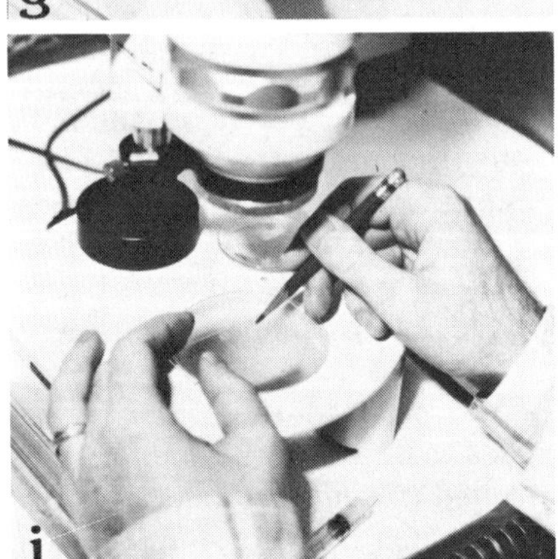

Figure 1
Methodology and techniques of test performance. (**a**), Semen sample poured from a sterile disposable collection container after 30 minutes' liquefaction at room temperature into a 15-ml conical centrifuge tube. (**b**), Addition of Biggers, Whitten and Whittingham (BWW) culture medium up to 10 ml prior to washing in a desk-top centrifuge. (**c**), Transfer of 0.5 ml of washed resuspended sperm at a concentration of 1×10^7 sperm/ml into Falcon tubes prior to incubation horizontally in an air incubator at 37°C for 18 hours. (**d**), Manipulation of eggs in a watch glass during hyaluronidase and trypsin treatment to remove cumulus cells and zona pellucida. Each enzymatic treatment is followed by three washes in watch glasses containing BWW culture medium. (**e**), Transfer of a 0.1-ml aliquot of preincubated sperm to a Falcon Petri dish followed by covering with mineral oil and addition of 20 to 25 zona-free eggs per drop. (**f**), Removal of eggs from the sperm drop after 2 to 3 hours' incubation. (**g**), Placing 12 to 15 eggs on a slide in a small drop (10 to 15 μl) after one wash for removal of excess adherent sperm. (**h**), Application of Vaseline/paraffin mixture contained in a tuberculin syringe to the four corners of the coverslip. (**i**), Pressing down the coverslip carefully over the drop containing eggs. (**j**), Further positioning of the coverslip by pressing at the four corners with a pencil while viewing eggs through a dissecting microscope to monitor the extent of flattening.

Table 1. *Proposed Standardized Methodology for SPA*

Procedure	Range of variation	Recommended procedure
Abstinence time	2 to 5 days	2 days
Time in seminal plasma	30 to 120 minutes	30 minutes, room temperature
Washing procedure	Centrifugation or sperm rise	Centrifugation three times at 600 × g for 5 minutes
Preincubation time of sperm	1 to 24 hours	18 hours
Time of sperm and egg interaction	2 to 8 hours	2 to 3 hours
Sperm concentration	1×10^6–1×10^7/ml (total sperm or motile sperm)	1×10^7 total sperm/ml
Hamster-egg recruitment	Immature or cycling female hamsters	Injections of mature females on days 1 and 3
Medium composition and gas phase	BWW with or without BSA or HSA at 0.3% to 3.5%, 5% CO_2 or air	BWW with HSA at 3.5% air

clinic, and the sperm have been allowed to reside in seminal fluid 1 to 2 hours before the initiation of processing. Figure 2 indicates in five donors tested that extended time in seminal plasma reduced the fertilizing potential to the point of shifting the results of three individuals from the fertile to the infertile range. Therefore, insistence on sample collection in an area of the clinic is preferable.

The preincubation of the sperm is preceded by a *washing procedure*. This is usually done by centrifugation in a simple desk-top centrifuge at 600 × g for 5 minutes. After three washes the sperm are suspended in a final sperm concentration of 1×10^6 to 1×10^7. An alternate procedure recently utilized for sperm processing in the SPA is called "sperm rise." This procedure allows a concentrated sample of sperm to " swim up" into an overlay of buffer, thus providing an actively motile "cleaned-up" sample of sperm. This procedure, which is routinely used in vitro fertilization (IVF) gives an enhanced penetration when compared with an unrisen sample.[29] Of the samples tested in our laboratory, all had an enhanced penetration in the risen samples. Wolf and Sokoloski[30] showed inconsistent results in their report. For two of four donors, sperm penetration increased significantly. One sample showed a decrease with the use of the "swim-up" sperm, and another showed a nonsignificant increase. Cohen et al.[31] reported that the spermatozoa of seven individuals that passed into the upper medium layer fertilized more zona-free hamster eggs than did spermatozoa that failed to migrate into the upper layer. Because the usefulness of SPA lies primarily in differentiating between fertile and infertile samples, an enhanced penetration produced by the rise procedure may in effect reduce the discriminating potential of the assay. This author's recommendation for sperm processing would be to use centrifugation rather than the sperm rise procedure.

The *preincubation time of sperm* is an extremely important variable in the procedure. In our original article,[8] human sperm were preincubated from 2 to 7 hours. Significant percent penetration was observed at 4 hours in air and 5 hours in 5% CO_2 and air. Since that report, preincubation times varying from 1 to 24 hours have been reported. No clear evidence has been provided to indicate the absolute superiority of any given preincubation time. The underlying assumption has been that human sperm would exhibit a capacitation time that would be uniform or consistent from individual to individual. This was shown not to be the case by Perreault and Rogers[32] when they studied various time points for individual donors. We discovered that the optimal penetration rate for a given person may be after 3 hours of preincubation or 10 hours or even 18 hours of preincubation. Because no single time would be optimal for every individual, the rationale for choosing a long preincubation period would be to give every sample tested the possibility of reaching a measurable level of penetration. If a given

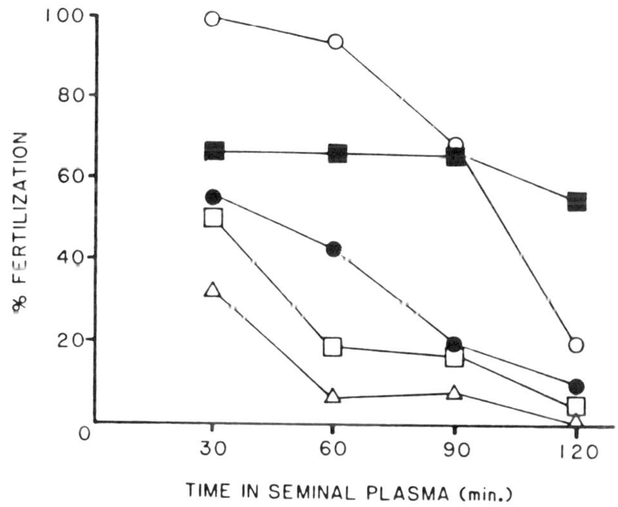

Figure 2
Time in seminal plasma.

individual's sperm penetrates none of the zona-free hamster eggs after an overnight incubation accompanied by a significant motility reduction, this individual should then be retested with a shortened preincubation period (3 to 5 hours). In general, the longer preincubation period has been selected because it allows sufficient time for capacitation and acrosome reaction to take place and is logistically optimal in a clinical setting. Recently, results have been reported[33] that show that a 20-hour preincubation period gives higher levels of penetration than a 7-hour preincubation period. The point was made that of the donors tested 33% had < 10% penetration when preincubated for the short interval, while all of the donors had penetration rates in the fertile range after 20 hours of incubation. A point to be made about preincubation times is that the fertile ranges were established with the use of the long preincubation times; so it would seem invalid to classify an individual as being in the fertile range when the conditions under which the test is performed have been altered. The suggestion would be that when a diagnostic procedue is being performed, the procedure used for the assay should be the same as that used when the ranges for fertile and infertile samples were established.

The *time of sperm and egg interaction* has varied from investigator to investigator. The range of variability for this coincubation time has been 2 to 8 hours. The original procedure used a 2- to 3-hour time interval for the sperm and eggs to interact. Our subsequent work has shown that optimal hamster-egg penetration can occur at 3 hours.[28] Other investigators have suggested that longer sperm/egg interaction times produce higher levels of penetration. The possible flaw in the logic associated with this interpretation could be that because of a shortened preincubation time the sperm/egg interaction time had to be lengthened in order to allow for an optimal capacitation time for the sperm. If, however, the sperm are adequately capacitated in a long preincubation period, an extended sperm/egg interaction time is not required. If an 18-hour preincubation is used, then the recommended sperm/egg interaction time would be 2 to 3 hours. If, however, a shortened preincubation time of 1 to 3 hours is utilized, then the sperm/egg interaction time might be extended from 3 to 6 hours for achievement of higher penetration rates.

The *sperm concentration* in the preincubation medium will affect the level of acrosome reaction that occurs in the sperm population and subsequently the percent penetration of the zona-free hamster eggs. Numerous investigators have looked at sperm concentrations ranging from 5×10^4 to 2×10^7 sperm/ml.[28, 34-37] In addition, the consideration of motile sperm per milliliter compared with total sperm per milliliter has been a source of controversy. Martin and Taylor[36] reported that the optimum concentration for ovum penetration was 10^7 sperm/ml. We found no difference between 0.5 and 1.0×10^7 sperm/ml. In the original establishment of fertile and infertile ranges of penetration,[27] the sperm concentration utilized was 10^7 sperm/ml. This sperm concentration was not adjusted for motile sperm. Adjusting for motile sperm again biases the assay toward enhancement of the results. When the test is being used for discriminating purposes, it seems somewhat illogical to attempt to enhance the results. The recommendation for a standardized methodology in this area would be a concentration of 10^7 sperm/ml incubated in a 0.5 ml volume.

The *hamster-egg recruitment* and processing is a portion of the procedure that has remained reasonably standardized with most investigators. In our original methodology[8] mature cycling hamsters were used. Injections of pregnant mare serum (PMS) and human chorionic gonadotropin (hCG) were given on days 1 and 3 of the hamster's 4-day cycle. A variation on the procedure has been to use immature uncycling hamsters,[37] giving them an injection of PMS on any day and hCG 52 to 57 hours later. No evidence is available to indicate that immature animals provide more eggs or eggs of better quality. The recommendation in this area of methodology is to use mature females at least 6 weeks old, but preferably 8 to 12 weeks old. The injection schedule is PMS on the morning of day 1 when the postestrus discharge is obvious as a stringy material. The hCG injection which is given on day 3 is 15 to 17 hours prior to the time that the eggs are needed.

Medium composition and gas phase constitute another area in which the basic methodology has been maintained to a large degree. The major variables in the medium have been the use of either bovine serum albumin (BSA) or human serum albumin (HSA) and the concentration of the albumin. Some investigators[30] have found that increasing the albumin concentration from 0.3% to 3.5% enhances the percent penetration rate. Others have not observed this enhance-

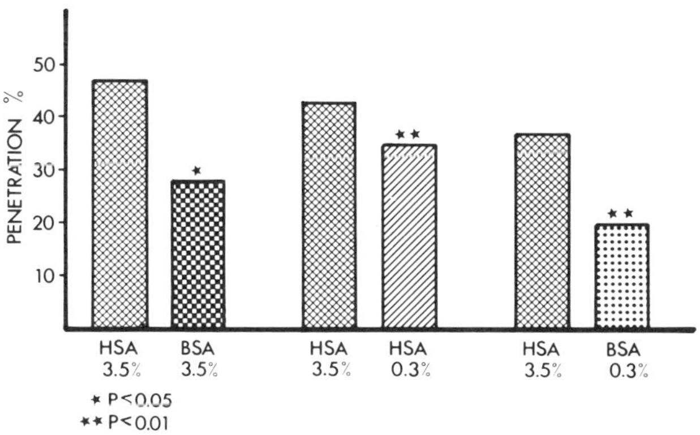

Figure 3
Effect of albumin type and concentration on penetration. (From Margalioth.[39] Reproduced with the permission of the author.)

ment.[38] Figure 3[39] shows a comparison of the two albumin types at different concentrations, and the best result is with 3.5% HSA. The other area of variation with regard to medium is the gas phase that is utilized. Both air and 5% CO_2 and air have been used successfully to allow human sperm to capacitate, undergo the acrosome reaction, and penetrate eggs. In our original work[8] it appeared that capacitation occurred slightly faster in air than in 5% CO_2 and air. The pH in air would be higher than that in CO_2 and would be a factor in the rate of occurrence of the acrosome reaction. The recommendation in this area is using air as the gas phase primarily for simplicity. This will allow adequate capacitation and the acrosome reaction if an extended preincubation period is used.

ESTABLISHMENT OF ASSAY AS DIAGNOSTIC TOOL FOR INFERTILITY EVALUATION

The usefulness of the SPA as a potential diagnostic tool was obvious at the time of the initial publication[8] concerning the penetration of human sperm into zona free hamster eggs in 1976. We published the first report establishing fertile and infertile ranges for humans in 1979.[27] Since that time numerous investigators have reported validating results for the ranges of fertile and infertile individuals. The data of many of these investigators are shown in Table 2.[27, 33, 34, 40-54] This table is restricted to investigators who published ranges of predictability and therefore excludes the original work of Barros et al.[55] This group carried out the early work using zona-free hamster eggs and human patients from an infertility clinic. They considered penetration of one egg as positive, and in their original work[55] no details of egg numbers or methodology were made available.

A key factor in the establishment of the fertile and infertile ranges is the definition that the investigator uses for fertile and infertile. These definitions are listed in Table 2, and it becomes apparent that in most instances the infertile group is *not well defined*. The range for the fertile men is reasonably consistent for each investigator, the lower limit varying between 11% and 25%. Most investigators will agree that spermatozoa from men of proven fertility almost consistently penetrate > 10% of the eggs. Only four investigators in the table have reasonably well defined infertility groups. The best definition of an infertile male would be the partner in an infertile marriage of a woman who has previously been pregnant by another partner. The next best category for an infertile male would be a partner in an infertile couple where the wife has no demonstrated evidence of an infertility factor. There are four studies[27, 34, 43, 45] that have infertile men defined in either of these two categories. When these four studies are examined, the ranges of penetration for the potentially infertile men are 0 to 10, 0 to 8.7, 0 to 11, and 0 to 11, respectively. In all other groups where the infertility definition is limited only to patients attending an infertility clinic or individuals of unexplained infertility, ranges can extend from 0% to 100%. This is actually not an unexpected finding, because a large number of the male subjects who are tested in an infertile couple would, in fact, be fertile.

REPORTING SPERM PENETRATION ASSAY RESULTS (VARIABILITY, SENSITIVITY, AND SPECIFICITY)

The results of the sperm/egg interaction were originally reported as percent penetration or fertilization on fresh or stained preparations. The inseminated eggs are transferred to a slide after a wash step and examined at × 400 magnification with a phase contrast microscope. The swollen heads are readily visible (Fig. 4) if a coverslip resting on a Vaseline/paraffin mixture is pressed down over the eggs almost to the point of rupture. The clear areas of the heads must be attached to or associated with a tail to be counted. Alternatively, staining with 1% acetolacmoid or 0.25% acetocarmine allows visualization as dark spots

Table 2. *Establishment of Penetration Ranges in SPA for Fertile and Infertile Men*

Investigator	Year	No. of subjects in study	Range for fertile men	Range for potential infertile men	Definition of fertile (f) and infertile (i) populations
Rogers et al.[27]	1979	94	14–100	0–10	f—fathered a child i—wife previously pregnant[a]
Overstreet et al.[40]	1980	27	11–100	0–100?	f—fathered a child in past 2 years i—marriage infertile for at least 2 years
Hall[41]	1981	65	20–100	0–100	f—fathered one or more children i—male partner of couple consulting at infertility clinic
Siddiquey[42]	1981	39	56–100	0–90	f—normal donors i—apparently unexplained infertility with many years' duration
Tyler et al.[34]	1981	39	23.5–88.9	0–8.7	f—proven fertility i—infertility of more than 1 year and wife with no cause for fertility[a]
Karp et al.[43]	1981	133	15–96	0–11	f—wife pregnant at time of testing i—wife previously conceived pregnancy with another man[a]
Zausner-Guelman et al.[44]	1981	45	15–100	0–100	f—established a pregnancy in previous 12 months i—infertility patient
Shy et al.[45]	1982	59	15–100	0–11	f—a pregnant spouse at time of SPA i—spouse who had prior pregnancy, current evaluation with no infertility factors and 1 year infertile[a]
Junca et al.[46]	1982	33	8–100	—	f—candidates for IVF i—infertile couple
Cohen et al.[47]	1982	122	11–100	0–100	f—fathered one or more children i—from infertile couples
Martin and Taylor[48]	1982	69	15–60	0–51	f—fathered a pregnancy i—unexplained infertility for 3 years
Aitken et al.[49]	1982	35	14–90	—	f—fathered a child within the previous 3 years
Stenchever et al.[50]	1983	340	11–100	—	f—wives were pregnant i—no conception for 1 year of contraception-free coitus
Comhaire and Vermeulen[51]	1983	—	25–100	—	f—proven fertility
Wickings et al.[52]	1983	80	15–83	8–83	f—proved fertility in last 4 years i—attending infertility clinic
Margalioth et al.[53]	1983	54	20–100	0–100	f—fathered a child within the past year i—infertile couple for 3 to 7 years without a known cause
Albertsen et al.[54]	1983	85	0–100	0–90	f—men who had impregnated their wives within 1.3 ± 1 years i—men presenting for evaluation of infertility
Johnson and Alexander[33]	1984	9	12.0–64.3	—	f—proven fertility

[a]Infertility definition with reasonably careful delineation of fertility status.

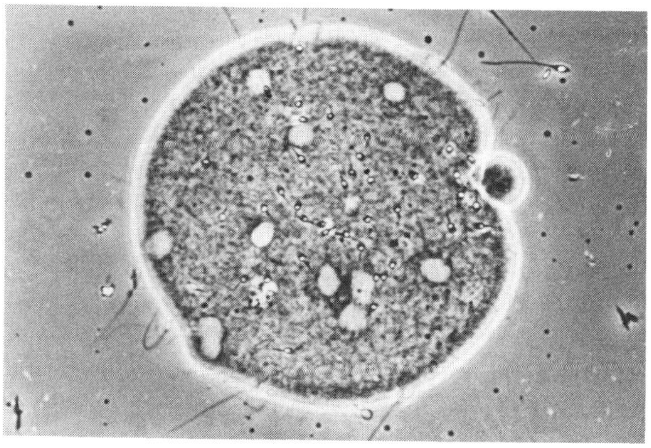

Figure 4
Zona-free hamster egg with polyspermic penetration by human spermatozoa.

instead of clear areas. Usually 40 to 50 eggs are examined per patient, and the percentage penetration is simply the number of eggs with swollen heads divided by the total number of eggs inseminated multiplied by 100. An additional parameter we have used is the fertilization index (FI), which is equal to the total number of swelling heads divided by the number of eggs examined. This number is really a reflection of the extent of acrosome reaction in the sample, because there is no block to polyspermy in zona-free hamster eggs. The FI gives an extended range of comparison, because 100% penetration could have FIs of 1.00, 2.00, or 3.00, etc., depending on the degree of polyspermic penetration exhibited. The reporting of the FI without a percent figure may not be appropriate, however, because most ranges for fertility evaluation have been reported as percentages. A binding score can also be reported, which reflects the number of sperm attached to each egg. The actual importance of such a score has not been quantitated in a clinical sense.

The percent penetration of any individual should be reported with reference to a donor of known penetrability. Tables 3 and 4 present results over an 11-month period for two donors. One would be considered a "high penetrator," and the other a "medium range" penetrator. It is immediately obvious that there is variability in their scores. The higher scorer penetrated < 50% on only 3 occasions and penetrated 100% on 19 occasions but still had a wide range of 9% to 100%. The other donor had a range of 0% to 100% and was less consistent in his score. From these results and our previous experience it is clear that an individual will not have the same percentage of penetration every time tested. However, the test can prove diagnostic, because an individual tends to have a penetration rate consistently in the fertile or the infertile range.

The sensitivity and specificity of the assay need to be evaluated. For this evaluation, data from fertile and infertile groups have been compared. We consider a man fertile (group A) if he claims paternity and infertile (group B) if he is married to a woman who has had a normal current gynecologic evaluation, who has failed to achieve pregnancy after 1 year of appropriate exposure, and who has been previously pregnant by another partner. We defined fertile and infertile ranges empirically. As a result of our early experience, we defined the fertile range for the SPA as 10% or

Table 3. *Donor Variability in SPA for a "High Penetrator"*

Date	Volume (ml)	Sperm/ml $\times 10^6$	% Motile	% Normal	% SPA
3/19/84	5.5	104	78	75	80
4/2/84	2.0	76	70	79	100
4/9/84	4.0	96	77	84	61
4/16/84	4.0	121	66	78	84
4/23/84	4.5	126	73	78	83
4/30/84	4.0	170	77	79	94
5/7/84	5.0	103	77	71	79
5/14/84	4.5	87	82	75	100
5/22/84	4.0	110	74	80	92
6/4/84	5.5	104	81	82	9
6/18/84	4.3	192	72	78	100
6/25/84	5.0	123	77	81	27
7/1/84	5.5	136	81	77	87
7/23/84	3.5	80	75	82	86
7/30/84	4.5	91	75	82	100
8/14/84	6.0	162	73	87	55
8/20/84	5.0	185	70	67	92
8/27/84	5.0	112	73	68	95
9/10/84	5.5	112	74	72	90
9/18/84	5.0	150	75	74	97
9/24/84	5.0	114	72	70	100
10/1/84	5.0	110	70	78	100
10/8/84	5.5	159	79	69	100
10/15/84	5.0	94	72	70	100
10/29/84	5.0	177	72	78	72
10/31/84	5.0	97	76	70	100
11/5/84	5.0	153	77	85	100
11/12/84	5.0	177	78	75	91
11/19/84	3.0	155	76	73	100
11/27/84	5.5	174	76	72	100
12/3/84	4.0	169	73	70	100
12/10/84	5.0	118	76	74	100
12/17/84	4.5	100	79	81	100
12/19/84	4.5	113	78	83	100
1/7/85	5.0	117	67	84	69
1/14/85	4.0	117	79	80	100
1/21/85	4.5	113	73	72	100
1/29/85	5.0	135	80	75	38
2/5/85	4.5	187	73	67	89
2/11/85	5.0	154	72	74	92
2/18/85	5.5	137	83	84	100

Table 4. *Donor Variability in SPA for a "Medium Penetrator"*

Date	Volume (ml)	Sperm/ml × 10^6	% Motile	% Normal	% SPA
3/21/84	3.0	109	56	54	60
3/26/84	3.0	84	55	61	95
4/11/84	3.0	114	61	69	70
4/18/84	3.0	129	49	66	90
5/9/84	2.5	84	70	58	33
5/16/84	2.5	104	59	71	30
5/23/84	3.5	136	64	69	60
5/30/84	2.5	121	58	64	17
5/30/84	2.5	153	56	66	60
6/7/84	3.5	152	55	75	100
6/20/84	3.0	106	52	58	100
6/27/84	3.3	142	60	60	56
7/18/84	3.5	109	40	57	59
7/25/84	3.5	114	57	71	0
8/1/84	3.5	123	49	18	3
8/8/84	3.0	120	52	64	50
8/15/84	2.5	99	50	53	19
8/29/84	2.5	154	50	57	92
9/5/84	2.5	146	63	68	81
9/12/84	3.0	95	55	72	97
9/19/84	2.5	101	48	68	62
9/26/84	3.5	95	57	54	54
10/3/84	3.0	102	48	66	64
10/17/84	3.0	125	65	58	47
11/7/84	3.0	82	60	68	55
11/28/84	3.5	128	55	69	11
12/5/84	3.0	185	63	64	71
12/12/84	3.0	155	51	59	24
1/9/85	3.5	153	57	54	45
1/16/85	3.0	156	55	66	59
1/31/85	4.0	208	55	62	61
2/7/85	2.5	272	60	57	78
2/14/85	3.5	159	58	62	5

more of ova penetrated and the infertile range as < 10%. However, having evaluated over 1500 assays, we now feel that any individual penetrating at any level is potentially fertile, but that correlation with clinical fertility status is superior with our original definition of normality. We looked at the semen analysis (SA) and SPA results of 62 men in group A and 53 men in group B. Table 5 demonstrates no significant discordance of average conventional semen parameters between clinically fertile and clinically infertile men. On the other hand, penetration rates are significantly discriminating ($P < 0.0001$). An analysis of the occurrence of noncorrelation in test results is shown in Table 6. Thirty-two percent of clinically fertile men (group A) showed at least one abnormality on standard SA (false-negative), whereas 30% of clinically infertile men (group B) had a normal SA (false-positive). Analysis of individuals whose SPA result did not correlate with clinical fertility status discloses a false-negative rate (sensitivity) of 18% and a false-positive rate (specificity) of 2%. Thus, the false-positive and false-negative rates for the SPA are much lower than for the SA. Of the 11 patients testing false-negative on SPA, 3 had sperm concentrations $< 2 \times 10^7$/ml, and 3 had increased numbers of white blood cells ($> 10^7$/ml) in the semen sample tested. One patient's sample showed both low sperm concentration and increased white blood cells. Obviously, low sperm concentrations raise questions concerning paternity history, and we have demonstrated previously clear inhibition of sperm penetration rates in samples with large numbers of white blood cells.[56] If we exclude these seven men, the false-negative rate drops to 6.5%. Further, improper sexual abstinence and technical error may contribute to a false-negative result. We conclude that the SPA is clearly superior to conventional SA as a predictor of clinical fertility status. Additionally, we note that clinically fertile men may have negative results in the SPA (false-negative), but that clinically infertile men seldom have positive test results. That is, a positive SPA more probably correlates with fertility potential than a negative assay.

CORRELATION OF SPERM PENETRATION ASSAY WITH CONVENTIONAL SEMEN ANALYSIS PARAMETERS

When we originally reported the fertile and infertile ranges,[27] we also reported no significant correlation between either sperm concentration or percentage motile sperm and the penetration

Table 5. *Semen Parameters (Averages and Ranges) of Clinically Fertile (Group A) and Clinically Infertile (Group B) Men*

	Sperm concentration[a]	% Motile[a]	% Normal forms[a]	% Penetration[b]	Penetration index[b]
	10^6/ml				
Group A (n = 62)	88 (2–282)	64 (29–90)	62 (20–90)	40 (0–100)	0.56 (0–2.36)
Group B (n = 53)	37 (1–404)	48 (2–80)	45 (7–76)	0.8 (0–12)	0.01 (0–0.12)

[a]Normal values: sperm concentration, ≥ 20 × 10^6/ml; progressive motility, ≥ 50%; normal forms, ≥ 45%. No significant discrimination between fertile (A) and infertile (B) groups.

[b]Normal if 10% of eggs were penetrated. Penetration rates discriminate fertile (A) and infertile (B) groups at $P < 0.0001$.

Table 6. *Noncorrelation of SA and SPA with Clinical Fertility Status*

	SA	SPA
False-negative, group A[a]	32% (20/62)	18% (11/62)
False-positive, group B[b]	30% (16/53)	2% (1/53)

[a]Group A consisted of 62 fertile men. "False-negative" indicates an abnormal semen parameter in a fertile man.

[b]Group B consisted of 53 infertile men. "False-positive" indicates a normal semen parameter in an infertile man.

percentages in the zona-free hamster eggs. Numerous investigators have looked at the SPA results, compared with semen parameters since that time. In 1981 three groups[34, 41, 44] reported no correlation between the percentage of penetrated ova and the original sperm density, motility, or morphology. The results of Tyler et al.[34] and Hall[41] were only for the "fertile" men. When applied to patients, Hall[41] found significant correlations for both sperm concentration and percent progressively motile spermatozoa versus SPA results. Aitken et al.[49] looked at correlates of fertilizing capacity in normal fertile men, oligospermic men,[57] and patients with unexplained infertility.[58] In the normal fertile group the differences in sperm function could not be correlated with any of the conventional parameters of semen analysis or any of a large number of sperm movement characteristics. In contrast to these data in normal fertile men, statistically significant associations were observed in oligospermic men between the penetration rate and both percentage of motile sperm (0.414, $P < 0.05$) and percentage of normal forms (0.443, $P < 0.05$). In the cases of unexplained infertility there was a significant relationship between morphology and fertilizing capacity in the hamster egg assay. In the same year three other groups reported conflicting results in sperm correlations.[48, 59, 60] Martin and Taylor[48] reported no correlation between penetration rates and any of the traditional measures of SA. Cohen et al.[59] found low correlations between the SPA and both sperm concentration and motile sperm count. Berger et al.,[60] however, found significant positive correlations between the SPA and sperm count, sperm motility, and morphologically normal sperm. They felt that the most important predictors of the SPA were total numbers of leukocytes per milliliter, sperm count, and sperm motility. The issue of correlation between conventional semen parameters and the egg penetration results seems somewhat unclear.

More recent work in 1983 stresses morphology and motility characteristics as the most correlated parameters. We reported that penetration correlated best with morphology ($r = 0.73$).[61] Aitken et al.[62] and Albertsen et al.[54] report motility parameters as being highly predictable of lowered penetrating capacity. Figure 5, from Albertsen's article, gives an excellent overview of the relative ability of each of the parameters to be diagnostic. The penetration of zona-free eggs is the most successful at predicting infertility, with an identification score of 66%, followed by multiple-exposure photomicrography (a quantitative measure of sperm motility), with a score of 54%, followed by normal sperm morphology, with a score of 27%. In simplistic terms, the SPA does correlate with some of the routine SA parameters. The degree of correlation reported may depend on the selection of the group of samples. The most significant correlations with egg penetration seem to be motility *quality* and morphology.

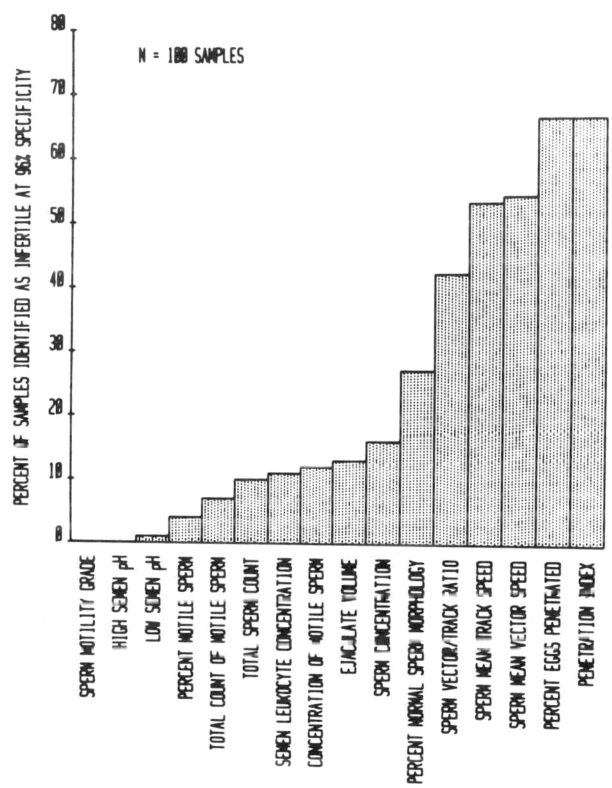

Figure 5
Identification of samples as infertile by different semen parameters. (From Albertsen.[54] Reproduced with the permission of the publisher.)

CORRELATION OF SPERM PENETRATION OF ZONA-FREE HAMSTER EGGS AND HUMAN EGGS

Some people believe the ultimate validation of the SPA is comparison of human and hamster egg penetration. IVF programs have availed us of the opportunity to perform these simultaneous inseminations using a single semen sample with both zona-free hamster eggs and zona-intact human eggs. Prior to the comparison in IVF programs, Overstreet et al.[40] published a report comparing penetration of nonliving zona-intact human eggs and living zona-free hamster eggs. They found positive correlations (both human and hamster eggs were penetrated or neither human nor hamster eggs were penetrated) in 85% of the samples ($n = 27$) tested. Four cases that showed hamster penetration did not penetrate the human eggs.

When Wolf et al.[63] compared the penetration of human eggs and hamster eggs, they tested 24 husbands and found 18 cases with human eggs fertilized. They reported that in 89% of the husbands who fertilized their wives' eggs, a positive fertility assessment was obtained ($\geqslant$ 10% penetration). The two patients with false-negative assessments did have limited penetration (6% and 7.7%). They concluded that fertility assessment with the SPA is highly correlated with the fertilization of human eggs in vitro.

Margalioth et al.[64] presented 20 IVF patients for whom SPAs had been run. They found seven patients with pathologic results in the SPA that penetrated 0% of their human eggs. Of the 13 patients with a normal SPA (20% to 100%), 10 (77%) had fertilization of at least one of their human eggs. They felt that the good correlation between the pathologic results in the SPA and failure of IVF stressed the clinical value of the assay. They suggested the use of the SPA for patient selection.

A more recent report by Foreman et al.[65] takes a more negative view on the usefulness of the SPA as a screening procedure for IVF. They present hamster and human egg penetration results from three distinct groups of patients: (1) spermatozoa failing to fertilize human oocytes; (2) spermatozoa occasionally fertilizing human oocytes; and (3) spermatozoa capable of fertilizing human oocytes. In group 1, 7 of 15 failed to penetrate human eggs but penetrated > 10% of the hamster eggs. In group 2, all seven men penetrated some percentage of the hamster and human eggs. In group 3, all 15 men penetrated both the hamster and the human eggs well. The authors[65] use these results to conclude that "positive results in this assay are an unreliable guide to human in vitro fertilization." Their own data show concordance in human and hamster egg results over 81% of the time. They also suggest that the test gives a high incidence of false-positives, although false-negatives are rare. A potential flaw in their report seems worth considering. Of the seven patients with discordant penetration results, three had only one human egg inseminated. There is no certainty that these individual eggs were of good quality. Another problem with the hamster results is that they are based on relatively small numbers of hamster eggs in most cases. In spite of the fact that they conclude that the hamster test will not predict the success or failure of human IVF, their data are reasonably supportive of a predictive value. Looked at from a positive viewpoint, all the patients they presented who fertilized human eggs either occasionally ($n = 7$) or consistently ($n = 15$) penetrated hamster eggs (with a range of 8% to 93%). In addition, all the patients presented ($n = 6$) who penetrated 0% in the hamster test also penetrated 0% of human eggs. In spite of their negative conclusion, this seems rather compelling support of the hamster assay. A more appropriate conclusion might be that the assay has a high degree of prognostic value but can produce false-positives.

Other investigators have reported positive correlations between hamster egg penetration and human IVF results.[66-68] In our laboratory[69] simultaneous inseminations have been done on 29 IVF patients. The results presented in Table 7 indicate that 86% of the results are concordant. The occurrence of false-positives is not an unexpected result, because the human egg has an additional step of zona penetration that is not measured by the zona-free assay. A false-positive re-

Table 7. *Distribution of Penetration by Human Sperm in Two Types of Eggs (n = 29)*

	Hamster egg penetrated	Hamster egg nonpenetrated
Human egg penetrated	23[a]	2[b]
Human egg nonpenetrated	2[b]	2[a]

[a]Concordance = 86% (25/29).
[b]Discordance = 14% (4/29).

sult could, however, be an indicator of a potential problem in the quality of human eggs.

The absolute value of a screening SPA for potential IVF candidates is controversial. Due to the difficulty of assay performance and limited assay availability, it seems prudent to recommend SPAs only for couples with a potential male factor or unexplained infertility. Positive results would be interpreted as indicative of a high probability of success in IVF, and negative results would be interpreted as predictive of a low probability. The couple would not be eliminated from an IVF attempt because of a negative SPA, but would be apprised of the potential of failed fertilization. In such instances donor backup could be planned if desirable. In all unscreened couples where human egg fertilization is unsuccessful, an SPA would be performed to assess the potential contribution of the sperm to this failure. A high degree of penetration of hamster eggs with no simultaneous human egg penetration *could* be interpreted as an egg quality problem meriting a modification of the stimulation protocol.

CORRELATION OF SPERM PENETRATION ASSAY WITH OTHER MALE FERTILITY TESTS (BIOCHEMICAL AND FUNCTIONAL)

In addition to routine semen parameters and more sophisticated motility evaluations, other measurements of seminal plasma and sperm components as well as mucus penetration tests have been compared with SPA results. In general, these other tests are performed in the hope that they will be simpler, more objective, more diagnostic, and thus capable of replacing the SPA. In general, the results have been relatively discouraging.

A few of the biochemical correlates that have been evaluated are seminal fumarase,[70] adenosine triphosphate (ATP),[71] and protein carboxylmethylase (PCM).[72] Fumarase activity was measured in 69 men attending an infertility clinic and compared with SPA results. There was no significant relationship between fumarase activity and hamster egg fertilizing ability by the spermatozoa. ATP concentrations measured in 20 semen donors and 10 infertile men were found to correlate significantly with the percentage of hamster ova penetrated in both groups.[71] They suggest that ATP is a useful biochemical characteristic of semen, allowing predictability of fertilizing potential. PCM activity was assayed in sperm cytosol preparations from fertile and infertile males with varying degrees of motility.[72] PCM activity had been reported to be reduced in necrospermic patients, and the rationale was that this enzymatic activity might be a biochemical index of both motility and fertility. PCM values ranged from 2.2 to 105 pmol of tritiated *s*-adenosyl methionine/ml protein and related to motility only at the extreme ends of the range. No correlation ($r = 0.032$) was apparent for percentage motile versus PCM activity. Simultaneous SPA values did not significantly correlate ($r = 0.374$) with PCM activity. This lack of correlation of PCM activity suggests that PCM determinations are inadequate for fertility diagnosis.

The functional tests related to sperm fertilizing potential other than egg penetration are those involving mucus penetration. Comparisons have been made between SPA results and postcoital tests (PCT),[73] human cervical mucus (HCM) penetration,[74, 75] and bovine cervical mucus (BCM) penetration.[76] A retrospective study was done on 79 couples attending an infertility clinic who had both a PCT result and an SPA result.[73] The correlation was insignificant ($r = 0.17$) between the PCT and the SPA. However, the partner of a male deemed fertile by the SPA was more likely to have a clinically acceptable PCT result (five or more motile sperm per high power field). When HCM penetration in vivo was evaluated and related to the hamster-egg penetration test a correlation coefficient of 0.623 ($P < 0.01$) was found.[74, 75] We have looked at a large group of patients ($n = 136$), using the SPA and BCM penetration. The correlation coefficient for the egg and mucus penetrations was 0.40 ($P < 0.01$). If samples were divided into three groups based on their ability to penetrate BCM, the other semen parameters were seen to increase with increasing mucus penetration (Fig. 6). Penetration of 0 to 20 mm is considered inadequate, 21 to 30 is the unclear range, and > 30 mm is considered adequate. When known fertile and infertile groups were tested, the mucus test predicted 74% correctly, and the SPA predicted 90% correctly. Although the SPA is more predictive, the inclusion of both tests in a complete infertility evaluation is recommended.

CRYOPRESERVATION OF EITHER EGGS OR SPERM TO FACILITATE UTILIZATION OF SPERM PENETRATION ASSAY

The logistics of the SPA can become somewhat cumbersome, because the hamsters require

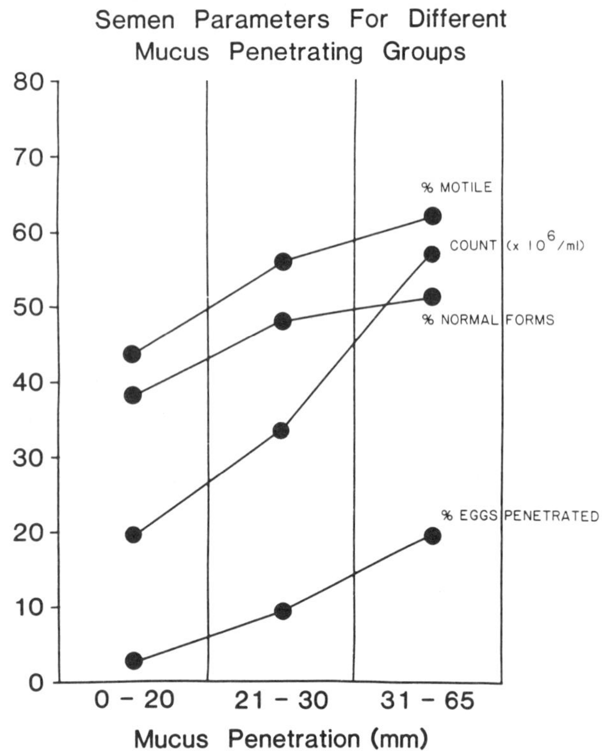

Figure 6
Semen parameters for different mucus-penetrating groups.

scheduled injections prior to egg collection, and the patients need to collect their samples at a certain time fixed by egg availability. It would seem conceptually reasonable to freeze either the eggs or the sperm for more flexibility in the performance of the assay. The value of preserved eggs is even more significant for infertility clinics where animals are not readily available and for countries such as Australia where the hamster is not available. Preserved sperm would allow transportation of these samples to centers where the test is performed routinely.

Cryopreservation of hamster eggs has been accomplished.[77-80] The two original reports of freezing hamster eggs used zona-intact ova. Fleming et al.[79] used only zona-free ova, whereas the Australian workers[80] used both zona-free and zona-intact hamster eggs. The procedure recommended by Quinn et al.[80] is to cool zona-intact ova slowly (~ 0.3°C/minute) in HEPES-buffered Tyrode's medium containing 30 mg BSA/ml and 2.0 M dimethylsulfoxide (DMSO) to −80°C and then transfer them to liquid N_2. They suggest thawing slowly at ~ 8°C/minute and diluting out the DMSO at room temperature by a single addition of 1 ml DMSO medium to 0.2 ml of the freezing medium. They wash the ova twice and after 1 hour's incubation, remove the zona with trypsin. There was no difference in penetration rate of human sperm into frozen or fresh oocytes when handled this way. If, however, a lower albumin concentration was used, then the number of ova penetrated was significantly reduced. They found that between 70% and 80% of the zona-intact ova survived this freezing procedure. They suggest that survival of hamster oocytes stored at −196°C offers a convenient means of supplying and transporting these ova. Fleming et al.[79] had claimed ~ 90% survival with their freeze-thawing procedure with zona-free eggs, whereas Quinn et al.[80] found survival percentages of 16% and 46% using zona-free ova. The sharp contrast in survival rates underscores the fact that attempting to use frozen embryos adds another degree of complexity to an assay that is already difficult. Frozen eggs would not, therefore, be the method of choice. However, if fresh eggs are not available, the freezing of zona-intact eggs with a controlled freezing rate protocol is the next best alternative.

Cryopreservation of human sperm would seem at first glance the easiest approach to simplify the logistical considerations of performing the SPA. Unfortunately, this approach is fraught with problems. Sperm freezing is not the major problem. Cryopreservation of sperm has been routinely performed for use in artificial insemination and other situations requiring sperm banking. The reduced viability of sperm after thawing makes it impossible to perform the SPA by the long preincubation methodology which was employed when the original fertile and infertile penetration ranges were established. Although postthawing viability varies with individuals, most samples of human sperm do not retain reasonable motility longer than 5 hours after thawing. The method used to test the samples must then be modified to accommodate this reduced viability. Penetration rates of thawed sperm samples have been reported as almost the same as those of fresh spermatozoa[81, 82] and as reduced.[31, 83, 84] Urry et al.[82] claim that frozen sperm retained 86% of the fresh sperm penetration values, but to achieve this result they eliminated nine samples from their results which had "an insufficient motile sperm density following freezing." This elimination of over 15% of the study group from analysis makes the suggested result equivocal. It appears obvious that cryopreserved sperm do not retain their fresh

Table 8. *Comparison of Fertilization Rates for Fresh and Frozen Samples*

Donor	Count × 10^6/ml	% Fertilization (fresh sample with long incubation)	% Fertilization (frozen sample with short incubation)
206-A	154	100	0
189-V (7/23)	174	100	0
189-V (7/31)	200	100	24
189-V (8/1)	123	100	4
189-V (8/13)	160	100	17
238-R	147	100	38
182-H	232	99	44
46-N	21	95	0
249-G	101	92	57
235-W	38	61	36
15-F	54	55	0
239-A	19	12	0
240-M	25	8	7
236-W	104	7	0
244-T	19	6	0
248-B	97	6	0

penetration values consistently enough to prove useful in a diagnostic procedure. Using frozen sperm in the SPA would make a positive result diagnostic, but a negative result would be of limited value because of the strong possibility of a false-negative. Cohen et al.[31] concluded that there was, in general, a marked decrease of in vitro fertilizing capacity in frozen and thawed spermatozoa. However, in some cases the in vitro fertilizing capacity of frozen and thawed sperm was comparable to that of fresh sperm. They also make the point that a high prefreezing fertilizing capacity does not guarantee a high postthawing fertilization percentage. Our own data[84] indicate that individual variation is high in postthawing penetration rates (Table 8). The unpredictable nature of the freezing/thawing effect on the penetration rate makes extrapolation to fresh values from frozen values virtually impossible. Testing of frozen samples, although logistically desirable, enhances the complexity of interpretation and thus makes cryopreservation of semen samples an unacceptable means of preserving the fertilizing potential for assay.

TEST-YOLK BUFFER PRESERVATION OF SPERM FERTILITY

Because freezing sperm reduces the assayable fertilizing potential by shortening the viable postthawing period and reducing motility, an alternative preservation procedure is desirable. Such a procedure was reported by Bolanos et al.,[85] involving storing the semen for 48 hours at 2° to 5°C in a TEST-yolk buffer prior to evaluating their fertilizing potential. This provides a mechanism for shipping samples from any location to a central laboratory where the assay is performed routinely. This eliminates the necessity of setting up the hamster test individually in every infertility clinic.

In addition to preserving the fertilizing potential, the TEST-yolk buffer enhances the sperm sample's penetration rate of zona-free hamster eggs. Our recent results comparing fresh and preserved samples are shown in Table 9. Seventy-

Table 9. *Comparison of SPA Results With and Without TEST-Yolk Buffer*

Patient	Fresh semen				Buffer-treated semen			
	Count	% Motile	% Normal	% SPA	Count	% Motile	% Normal	% SPA
	× 10^6/ml				10^6/ml			
J. K.	55	40	55		22	50	55	46
T. R.	109	57	59		92	48	70	68
J. B.	4	31	33		5	22	42	35
T. B.	16	40	62	0	38	41	55	42
S. C.	18	47	40	0	26	43	65	7
G. C.	5	25	37	8	6	31	47	0
P. P.	40	57	71	6	47	63	67	31
D. R.	75	55	60	0	63	45	54	100
C. T.[a]	17	21	46	0	17	21	46	0
P. Y.	74	52	52	0	42	44	54	31
D. H.[a]	12	34	42	0	12	34	42	0
C. S.[a]	34	25	57	4	34	25	57	100
R. S.[a]	77	72	64	11	77	72	64	10

[a]The same sample was processed with and without buffer.

seven percent (10 of 13) showed enhancement of egg penetration due to buffer treatment. Similar results have been reported previously.[85-87] Bolanos et al.[85] tested 10 fertile donors and 19 patients with and without buffer treatment. The enhancement of mean percent penetration was from 64% to 90% (fresh versus stored) in the donor group. The infertile samples were divided into two groups on the basis of the normality of semen parameters. The normal semen group ($n = 11$) showed a mean percent penetration increase from 30% to 67% (fresh versus stored), whereas the abnormal group ($n = 8$) showed an increase from 35% to 53%. The increase differed from man to man, and in some cases it was not significant. However, one key point is that in four patients the test results changed from "negative" to "positive" when fresh versus stored results were compared. Jeyendran et al.[86] showed an increase in penetration from 12.9% for seven semen samples stored in glycerol to 46.7% for samples stored in TEST-yolk buffer. Johnson et al.[87] more recently tested 66 individuals and found that the number of penetrations per egg increased by an average of 2.5 times when capacitated in TEST-yolk buffer for 42 hours, as compared with 18 hours. These authors suggest that the buffer enhancement may eliminate some false-negative results in the SPA. No one has, however, addressed the possibility of creating false-positives with this buffer treatment. Because the original "fertile ranges" were established without buffer treatment, it is certainly possible that these buffer treatment results cannot be evaluated with the use of the same ranges. On the other hand, a sperm sample that does not show enhancement with buffer treatment may very well represent a truly negative result.

The intriguing aspect of buffer enhancement is in the area of treatment of impaired fertility even more than in diagnosis of subfertility. If a sample can be enhanced to penetrate zona-free hamster eggs, could this treatment be used to enhance penetration of human eggs in vivo or in vitro? This merits attention as a potentially fruitful area of investigation. We have recently achieved successful fertilization by buffer enhancement of sperm in a couple who had previously failed in an IVF attempt. Their SPA result was improved from 0% to 31% by buffer enhancement. Whether this buffer treatment can enhance fertilizing potential sufficiently to be an effective treatment remains to be established.

MODIFICATION OF PENETRATING ABILITY BY VARIOUS ADDITIVES

The fertilizing potential which is assayable by penetration of zona-free hamster eggs has been modified by the incorporation of a wide range of substances in the incubation medium. These agents include dibutyryl-3′,5′-cyclic adenosine monophosphate (dbcAMP),[88] caffeine,[89, 90] theophylline,[89] trypsin or chymotrypsin,[91] 17β-estradiol (E_2),[92] and ionophore A23187.[93] Whether these substances will prove beneficial from a therapeutic standpoint is unresolved. The existence of some of these enhancement possibilities will be explored to provide an awareness of possible innovative treatment.

We demonstrated that the phosphodiesterase inhibitors, caffeine and theophylline,[89, 94] could stimulate the penetration rates, compared with those of controls, after 6 hours of preincubation. If caffeine (7 mM) or theophylline (10 mM) were added to washed sperm before insemination either in vivo or in vitro, the potential of fertilization of human eggs might be optimized. Such experiments and clinical procedures have yet to be implemented to resolve such questions. An enhancement of zona-free hamster egg penetration does not necessarily translate to improved human egg penetration. Weeda and Cohen[90] report that they have done pilot experiments which confirm our observations of caffeine shortening the capacitation time, but they do not find improved in vitro fertilizing capacity when caffeine is added to the semen for 1 hour before processing for the SPA. Their average penetration rates, however, are quite low, both with and without caffeine (29%). More recently, Chan et al.[88] demonstrated stimulation of human spermatozoal fertilizing ability by both dbcAMP and theophylline in vitro for groups of patients with suspected fertility and subfertility. They suggested that these compounds might be of clinical value in improving the fertilizing ability of human semen samples with poor penetrating efficiency under artificial insemination conditions.

Other stimulatory additives that have potential clinical application are the proteolytic enzymes chymotrypsin and trypsin.[91] These have been used to decrease the viscosity of highly viscous semen of subfertile patients, but they also increase the in vitro fertilizing ability as measured with zona-free hamster eggs in sperm from both normal and highly viscous semen. The enzymes were added (5 mg/ml) to the semen samples for 1 hour before a 1-hour sperm rise procedure. The upper layer was washed and preincubated 4 to 5 hours before the addition of zona-free hamster ova. This procedure thus has the potential of not only decreasing viscosity but also improving sperm quality.

The penetration efficiency of human sperm has been shown to be stimulated by E_2.[92] The mean penetration rates for fertile men increased from 35.6% to 60.1% when E_2 was added during the 5-hour incubation, whereas the subfertile group mean penetration rate changed from 10.2% to 30.5%. It is suggested that E_2 may be of clinical value in artificial insemination conditions by the use of a preinsemination estrogen treatment to ensure adequate stimulation of spermatozoal penetration efficiency.

More recently, the ionophore A23187 was added to the hamster egg assay for sperm function with interesting and potentially useful results.[93] The ionophore at 50 and 100 μM caused a significant increase in fertilization rates for sperm from fertile controls, whereas the oligospermic patients did not exhibit a significant change in most cases. Using the ionophore would reduce the time to run the assay to 3.5 hours and achieve a greater degree of separation of normal from abnormal semen samples.

None of these additives has been validated in the human egg penetration situation. The fact that enhancement of the zona-free hamster eggs is achieved does suggest that capacitation and acrosomal reaction of the human sperm has been stimulated. To effect enhanced zona penetration of the human egg sufficient motility would have to accompany the acrosome reaction to allow fertilization. Although we have no guarantees that any of these procedures would be effective in the clinical setting, they definitely merit further exploration as possible new therapeutic approaches for reduced sperm fertilizing potential.

PITFALLS IN PROCEDURE AND INTERPRETATION OF RESULTS

The implementation of the SPA is plagued by potential pitfalls. Initial collection of the sample has potential problems with reduced abstinence and extended time in seminal plasma. Inadequate abstinence reduces penetration, as does an extended time in seminal plasma before processing. In a clinical setting this can be a major obstacle for patients who are unwilling to collect their samples at the clinic. Washing the sample can be problematic if the sample is stringy and does not pellet well. Resuspension of the sample and incubation overnight can result in invalid results if the tubes are not capped tightly and the sample loses a large percentage of motility. In treating the eggs with hyaluronidase and trypsin, a serious pitfall can be timing. If the time for the enzymatic treatment steps is prolonged, the eggs tend to be less fertilizable. This is a serious problem for a novice "egg handler" and will be remedied as speed is acquired with practice. The trypsin step has at least two possible problems. One is not leaving the eggs in trypsin long enough for removal of all of the zona, thus preventing sperm penetration. The other is letting the eggs get stuck in the pipette by drawing them up too far. Their enhanced stickiness after zona removal requires keeping them in the lower part of the pipette to prevent sticking. The most serious pitfalls in the entire procedure are associated with the actual evaluation of sperm penetration. The eggs must be pressed down sufficiently so that the swollen heads can be visualized, but not so much that the eggs rupture. The consistency of the Vaseline/paraffin drops that the coverslip rests on is crucial in this step. Most investigators have problems initially with the egg-mounting steps. Done well, the assay provides useful information in a clinical workup; but done incorrectly, it can produce invalid results that could be more detrimental than valuable.

The major pitfall in interpreting the results may come from overinterpreting. The test has never been intended to predict the relative ease with which a man can impregnate his wife. No one claims that a 100% SPA result means a greater ability to achieve pregnancies than a 70% SPA result. A positive SPA result should be interpreted as representing potential fertility. On the other hand, one 0% SPA result should not be used as the basis of a potentially devastating clinical diagnosis. Because false-negatives occur in this assay, an effort to eliminate all extenuating circumstances should be made before a repeat SPA is done. Such things as inadequate abstinence, improper sample collection or handling, and a high number of white cells in the sample should be immediately corrected. Other possible problems could be a concurrent illness or medication taken at the time of the SPA. Potential technical problems should always be considered, because

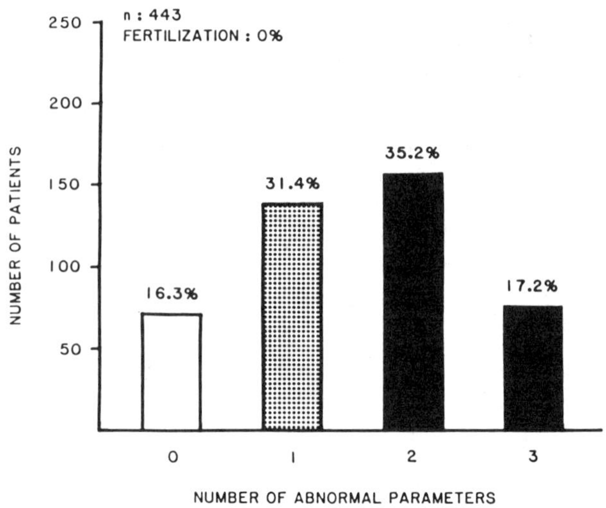

Figure 7
Distribution of abnormal parameters in patients with 0% fertilization potential in SPA.

this is an extremely sensitive bioassay. If all problems are ruled out, a second 0% in the SPA could be taken as indicative of male factor subfertility.

ROLE OF THE SPERM PENETRATION ASSAY IN ASSESSING AND TREATING THE INFERTILE COUPLE

The expensive SPA ($150 to $325) does not replace the standard SA in evaluation of the infertile couple. If repeated routine SAs are neither clearly normal nor abnormal, we perform an SPA, referring the male or female for further evaluation according to the results. If the routine SA is normal, we initiate the evaluation for a female factor. If that evaluation uncovers no abnormality and infertility persists, or if expensive or invasive therapy of the female is planned, the SPA is done. Because of the comparatively low sensitivity of the standard SA, using the SPA, we not infrequently discover a male factor. On the other hand, because of the high concordance between an abnormal standard SA and an infertile-range SPA in the clinically infertile male, we recommend proceeding directly to further evaluation and/or therapy for the male factor in the patient whose standard SA is subnormal. One point to be emphasized is that there is a subset of individuals in the subfertile population that do not have apparent semen abnormalities (Fig. 7). The 16.3% of the 443 men with 0% SPA had no readily detectable semen abnormalities and would have been missed by a routine SA.

Monitoring of treatment of the male factor is possible with the SPA. We have monitored surgical treatment of varicocele, the most commonly diagnosed cause of male infertility, using the SPA.[95] In 194 men presenting with varicocele at an infertility clinic, of whom 59 elected to undergo repair of varicocele, we found that pregnancy ($n = 7$) occurred when the SPA result improved into the fertile range postoperatively ($n = 14$). Of these 14 men showing improvement into the fertile range, 3 are single, 1 is separated, and 1 is married to a woman with endometriosis. Hence, seven men impregnated their partners of the nine who had a reasonable opportunity to do so. Of note are two men who presented with 0% penetration, improved to a normal SPA range postoperatively, and achieved impregnation. In the subset of 45 men who demonstrated no improvement in SPA postoperatively, only 2 achieved an impregnation. In one of these patients the SPA was normal preoperatively, suggesting that the varicocele may not have been contributing to subfertility in his marriage. In the other patient standard SA was abnormal (sperm concentration 50,000/ml, 35% motile, 36% normal forms); the SPA could not be performed because of the low sperm concentration; and the pregnancy was initiated less than 2 months following surgery. For apparent reasons we suspect the patient's claim to paternity may be in question.

Because of the uncommon occurrence of a false-positive SPA (2%), and because these impressive pregnancy data strongly correlated with a positive SPA following varicocele repair, we believe that it may be inappropriate to recommend surgery in those patients with varicocele in an infertile marriage whose SPA result is positive (54 of 194, or 27.8% of our patients). Further, if the SPA improves to normal postoperatively, and if pregnancy is not achieved, we recommend exhaustive evaluation for a female factor causing the infertile union. Finally, we speculate that if the SPA does not improve following varicocele repair, surgery was incomplete, or irreversible damage to spermatogenic cells had already occurred, or the varicocele was not the cause of infertility. Again, in the unimproved group after varicocele repair, the prognosis for eventual pregnancy is extremely poor.

Any treatment regimen can be monitored with the SPA. We have also done a preliminary study to evaluate clomiphene citrate.[96] Antibiotic therapy has been monitored.[56, 97] The potential for testing new and innovative therapies is available. The major drawback is the paucity of treatment regimens for the infertile male. The outlook presently is rather bleak. However, we are currently testing the potential therapeutic value of clomiphene citrate and tamoxifen in males. The real value of the SPA is the ability to monitor male improvement per se without the confounding variable of the woman. If pregnancy does not occur in association with an improved SPA, in our estimation the etiology of the infertility would be presumed to be related to the woman.

It needs to be stressed that the SPA does not faithfully reproduce in vivo conditions. Specifically, sperm concentration is adjusted, sperm migration within the female genital tract is not assessed, and the barriers of cumulus and zona pellucida are removed. It is unlikely, however, that sperm will fertilize an ovum in vivo if the sperm entry test is negative. On the other hand, a positive SPA does not guarantee successful in vivo fertilization. How, then, should our original questions be answered? What does the SPA really tell us? It gives us an evaluation of the man's sperm that is highly correlated with true fertility in vivo. How can it be used clinically? It can be used in determining male factor infertility and in monitoring treatment. Is it an asset to an infertility workup? Yes, but it may not be required as an integral part of an initial workup. It is especially useful in unexplained infertility and varicocele where obvious routine semen parameters are not abnormal. The SPA is certainly not "the test" to answer all male infertility questions. However, it comes closest to adequately evaluating the functional potential a sperm was designed to achieve—egg penetration.

REFERENCES

1. Rogers BJ. Hamster egg: evaluation of human sperm using in vitro fertilization. In In Vitro Fertilization and Embryo Transfer, Edited by PG Crosignani, BL Rubin. London, Academic Press, 1983, p 101
2. Blasco L: Clinical tests of sperm fertilizing ability. Fertil Steril 41:177, 1984
3. Prasad MRN: The in vitro sperm penetration test. Int J Androl 7:5, 1984
4. Yanagimachi R: Zona-free hamster eggs: their use in assessing fertilizing capacity and examining chromosomes of human spermatozoa. Gamete Res 10:187, 1984
5. Mintz B: Experimental study of the developing mammalian egg: removal of the zona pellucida. Science 138:594, 1962
6. Hanada A, Chang MC: Penetration of zona-free eggs by spermatozoa of different species. Biol Reprod 6:300, 1972
7. Yanagimachi R: Penetration of guinea-pig spermatozoa into hamster eggs in vitro. J Reprod Fertil 28:477, 1972
8. Yanagimachi R, Yanagimachi H, Rogers BJ: The use of zona-free animal ova as a test system for the assessment of the fertilizing capacity of human spermatozoa. Biol Reprod 15:471, 1976
9. Hanada A, Chang MC: Penetration of the zona-free or intact eggs by foreign spermatozoa and the fertilization of deer mouse eggs in vitro. J Exp Zool 203:277, 1978
10. Pavlok A: Interspecies interaction of zona-free ova with spermatozoa in mouse, rat and hamster. Anim Reprod Sci 2:395, 1979
11. Hanada A, Chang MC: Penetration of hamster and rabbit zona-free eggs by rat and mouse spermatozoa with special reference to sperm capacitation. J Reprod Fertil 46:239, 1976
12. Imai H, Niwa K, Iritani A: Penetration in vitro of zona-free hamster eggs by ejaculated boar spermatozoa. J Reprod Fertil 51:495, 1977
13. Imai H, Niwa K, Iritani A: Time requirement for capacitation of boar spermatozoa assessed by their ability to penetrate the zona-free hamster egg. J Reprod Fertil 56:489, 1979
14. Imai H, Niwa K, Iritani A: Ultrastructural observations of boar spermatozoa penetrating zona-free hamster eggs. Biol Reprod 23:481, 1980
15. Pavlok A: Penetration of hamster and pig zona-free eggs by boar ejaculated spermatozoa preincubated in vitro. Int J Fertil 26:101, 1981
16. Pavlok A, Trávník P, Kopěcny V, Stastna J: Fusion of hamster and pig zona-free eggs stimulated by boar and guinea pig sperm at fertilization in vitro. Gamete Res 6:189, 1982
17. Hanada A, Nagase H: Effects of sperm preincubation in rabbit uterus and imidazol on the penetration of zona-free hamster eggs by bull and boar spermatozoa in vitro. Jpn J Anim Reprod 27:113, 1981
18. Smith M, Peterson RN, Russell L: Penetration of zona-free hamster eggs by boar sperm treated with ionophore A23187 and inhibition of penetration by antiplasma membrane antibodies. J Exp Zool 225:157, 1983
19. Bousquet D, Brackett BG: Penetration of zona-free hamster ova as a test to assess fertilizing ability of bull sperm after frozen storage. Theriogenology 17:199, 1982
20. Brackett BG, Cofone MA, Boice ML, Bousquet D: Use of zona-free hamster ova to assess fertilizing ability of bull and stallion. Gamete Res 5:217, 1982
21. Kim CI, Niwa K, Imai H, Iritani A: Penetration of zona-free hamster eggs in vitro by goat spermatozoa preincubated in the reproductive tract isolated from a maturing gilt. J Exp Zool 213:181, 1980
22. Lambert H: Temperature dependence of capacitation in bat sperm monitored by zona-free hamster ova. Gamete Res 4:525, 1981
23. Fleming AD, Yanagimachi R, Yanagimachi H: Spermatozoa of the Atlantic bottlenose dolphin, *Tursiops truncatus*. J Reprod Fertil 63:509, 1981

24. Moore HDM: An assessment of the fertilizing ability of spermatozoa in the epididymis of the marmoset monkey (*Callithrix jacchus*). Int J Androl 4:321, 1981
25. Boatman DE, Bavister BD: Stimulation of rhesus monkey sperm capacitation by cyclic nucleotide mediators. J Reprod Fertil 71:357, 1984
26. Hoffman ML, Curtis GL: Prevention of monkey sperm penetration of zona-free hamster ova by sperm antibody obtained from vasectomized cynomolgus monkeys. Fertil Steril 42:108, 1984
27. Rogers BJ, Van Campen H, Ueno M, Lambert H, Bronson R, Hale R: Analysis of human spermatozoal fertilizing ability using zona-free ova. Fertil Steril 32:664, 1979
28. Rogers BJ, Perreault SD, Bentwood BJ, McCarville C, Hale RW, Soderdahl DW: Variability in the human-hamster in vitro assay for fertility evaluation. Fertil Steril 39:204, 1983
29. Rogers BJ: Unpublished data
30. Wolf DP, Sokoloski JE: Characterization of the sperm penetration bioassay. Andrology 3:445, 1982
31. Cohen J, Felten P, Zeilmaker GH: In vitro fertilizing capacity of fresh and cryopreserved human spermatozoa: a comparative study of freezing and thawing procedures. Fertil Steril 36:356, 1981
32. Perreault SD, Rogers BJ: Capacitation pattern of human spermatozoa. Fertil Steril 38:258, 1982
33. Johnson JP, Alexander NJ: Hamster egg penetration: comparison of preincubation periods. Fertil Steril 41:599, 1984
34. Tyler JPP, Pryor JP, Collins WP: Heterologous ovum penetration by human spermatozoa. J Reprod Fertil 63:499, 1981
35. Binor Z, Sokoloski JE, Wolf DP: Sperm interaction with zona-free hamster egg. J Exp Zool 222:187, 1982
36. Martin RH, Taylor PJ: Effect of sperm concentration in the zona-free hamster ova penetration assay. Fertil Steril 39:379, 1983
37. Berger T, Marrs RP, Saito H, Kletzky OA: Factors affecting human sperm penetration of zona-free hamster ova. Am J Obstet Gynecol 145:397, 1983
38. Aitken RJ, Wang YF, Liu J, Best F, Richardson DW: The influence of medium composition, osmolarity and albumin content on the acrosome reaction and fertilizing capacity of human spermatozoa: development of an improved zona-free hamster egg penetration test. Int J Androl 6:180, 1983
39. Margalioth EJ: Unpublished data
40. Overstreet JW, Yanagimachi R, Katz DF, Hayashi K, Hanson FW: Penetration of human spermatozoa into the human zona pellucida and the zona-free hamster egg: a study of fertile donors and infertile patients. Fertil Steril 33:534, 1980
41. Hall JL: Relationship between semen quality and human sperm penetration of zona-free hamster ova. Fertil Steril 35:457, 1981
42. Siddiquey AKS: Human/hamster in-vitro fertilization: a useful test for fertility status in male. INSERM 103:285, 1981
43. Karp LE, Williamson RA, Moore DE, Shy KK, Plymate R, Smith WD: Sperm penetration assay: useful test in evaluation of male fertility. Obstet Gynecol 57:620, 1981
44. Zausner-Guelman B, Blasco L, Wolf DP: Zona-free hamster eggs and human sperm penetration capacity: a comparative study of proven fertile donors and infertility patients. Fertil Steril 36:771, 1981
45. Shy KK, Soules MR, Karp LE: The SPA—a new test of male infertility. Contemp Obstet Gynecol 19:210, 1982
46. Junca A, Mandelbaum J, Plachot M, DeGrouchy J: Evaluation de la fecondance du sperme humain par la fecondation in vitro interspecifique (homme-hamster). Ann Gynecol 25:93, 1982
47. Cohen J, Weber RFA, van der Vijver JCM, Zeilmaker GH: In vitro fertilizing capacity of human spermatozoa with the use of zona-free hamster ova: interassay variation and prognostic value. Fertil Steril 37:565, 1982
48. Martin RH, Taylor PJ: Reliability and accuracy of the zona-free hamster ova assay in assessment of male fertility. Br J Obstet Gynaecol 89:951, 1982
49. Aitken RJ, Best FSM, Richardson DW, Djahanbakhch O, Lees MM: The correlates of fertilizing capacity in normal fertile men. Fertil Steril 38:68, 1982
50. Stenchever MA, Spadoni LR, Smith WD, Karp LE, Shy KK, Moore DE, Berger R: Benefits of the sperm (hamster ova) penetration assay in the evaluation of the infertile couple. Am J Obstet Gynecol 143:91, 1982
51. Comhaire F, Vermeulen L: Effect of high dose oral kallikrein treatment in men with idiopathic subfertility: evaluation by means of in vitro penetration test of zona-free hamster ova. Int J Androl 6:168, 1983
52. Wickings EJ, Freischem CW, Langer K, Nieschlag E: Heterologous ovum penetration test and seminal parameters in fertile and infertile men. J Androl 4:261, 1983
53. Margalioth EJ, Laufer N, Navot D, Voss R, Schenker JG: Reduced fertilization ability of zona-free hamster ova by spermatozoa from male partners of normal infertile couples. Arch Androl 10:67, 1983
54. Albertsen PC, Chang TSK, Vindivich D, Robinson JC, Smyth JW: A critical method of evaluating tests for male infertility. J Urol 130:467, 1983
55. Barros C, Gonzalez J, Herrera E, Bustos-Obregon E: Fertilizing capacity of human spermatozoa evaluated by actual penetration of foreign eggs. Contraception 17:87, 1978
56. Maruyama DK, Hale RW, Rogers BJ: Effects of white blood cells on the in vitro penetration of zona-free hamster eggs by human spermatozoa. J Androl 6:127, 1985
57. Aitken RJ, Best FSM, Richardson DW, Djahanbakhch O, Templeton A, Lees MM: An analysis of semen quality and sperm function in cases of oligozoospermia. Fertil Steril 38:705, 1982
58. Aitken RJ, Warner P, Best FSM, Templeton AA, Djahanbakhch O, Mortimer D, Lees MM: The predictability of subnormal penetrating capacity of sperm in cases of unexplained infertility. Int J Androl 6:212, 1983
59. Cohen J, Mooyaart M, Vreeburg JTM, Zeilmaker GH: Fertilization of hamster ova by human spermatozoa in relation to other semen parameters. Int J Androl 5:210, 1982
60. Berger RE, Karp LE, Williamson RA, Koehler J, Moore DE, Holmes KK: The relationship of pyospermia and seminal fluid bacteriology to sperm function as reflected in the sperm penetration assay. Fertil Steril 37:557, 1982
61. Rogers BJ, Bentwood BJH, Van Campen H, Helmbrecht G, Soderdahl D, Hale RW: Sperm morphology assessment as an indicator of human fertilizing capacity. J Androl 4:119, 1983

62. Aitken RJ, Best FSM, Richardson DW, Djahanbakhch O, Mortimer D, Templeton AA, Lees MM: An analysis of sperm function in cases of unexplained infertility: conventional criteria, movement characteristics, and fertilizing capacity. Fertil Steril 38:212, 1982
63. Wolf DP, Sokoloski JE, Quigley MM: Correlation of human in vitro fertilization with the hamster egg bioassay. Fertil Steril 40:53, 1983
64. Margalioth EJ, Navot D, Laufer N, Yosef SM, Rabinowitz R, Yarkoni S, Schenker JG: Zona-free hamster ovum penetration assay as a screening procedure for in vitro fertilization. Fertil Steril 40:386, 1983
65. Foreman R, Cohen J, Fehilly CV, Fishel SB, Edwards RG: The application of the zona-free hamster egg test for the prognosis of human in vitro fertilization. J In Vitro Fertil Embryo Trans 1:166, 1984
66. Ausmanas M, Tureck RW, Mastroianni L Jr, Kopf G, Ribas J, Blasco L: The zona-free hamster penetration assay as a prognostic indicator in an in vitro fertilization program. Fertil Steril (Abstr) 41:106S, 1984
67. Berger T, Marrs RP, Sato F, Brown J: Comparison of the hamster penetration test and human in vitro fertilization. Fertil Steril (Abstr) 41:106S, 1984
68. Hall JL, Engel D, Berger GS, Dingfelder JR, Marik J: Use of the hamster zona-free ovum test in human in vitro fertilization program. Fertil Steril (Abstr) 41:105S, 1984
69. Rogers BJ, Herbert CM, Wentz AC: Comparison of human egg and hamster zona-free egg penetration. Presented at the III World Congress of In Vitro Fertilization and Embryo Transfer, May 14 to 17, 1984, Helsinki, Finland (Abstr)
70. Aafjes JH, Cohen J, Vreeburg JTM, Wolffensperger-Van Oort HJ: Fumarase activity in human ejaculate relationship to sperm motility or penetration of zona-free hamster eggs. Andrologia 13:578, 1981
71. Comhaire F, Vermeulen L, Ghedira K, Mas J, Irvine S, Callipolitis G: Adenosine triphosphate in human semen: a quantitative estimate of fertilizing potential. Fertil Steril 40:500, 1983
72. Rogers BJ, Nelson J: The relationship of protein carboxylmethylase to motility and fertility of human spermatozoa. J Androl 3:17, 1982
73. Soules MR, Moore DE, Spadoni LR, Stenchever MA: The relationship between the postcoital test and the sperm penetration assay. Fertil Steril 38:384, 1982
74. Aitken RJ, Templeton A, Schats R, Best F, Richardson D, Djahanbakhch O, Lees M: Methods for assessing the functional capacity of human spermatozoa: their role in the selection of patients for in vitro fertilization. In Fertilization of the Human Egg In Vitro, Edited by HM Beier, HR Lindner. New York, Springer-Verlag, 1983, p 147
75. Schats R, Aitken RJ, Templeton AA: The role of cervical mucus-semen interaction in infertility of unknown aetiology. Br J Obstet Gynaecol 91:371, 1984
76. Takemoto F, Rogers BJ, Wiltbank MC, Soderdahl DW, Vaughn WH, Hale RW: Comparison of the penetration ability of human spermatozoa into bovine cervical mucus and zona-free hamster eggs. J Androl 6:162, 1985
77. Tsunoda Y, Parkening TA, Chang MC: In vitro fertilization of mouse and hamster eggs after freezing and thawing. Experientia 32:223, 1976
78. Parkening TA, Chang MC: Effects of cooling rates and maturity of animals on the recovery of fertilization of frozen-thawed rodent eggs. Biol Reprod 17:527, 1977
79. Fleming AD, Yanagimachi R, Yanagimachi H: Fertilizability of cryopreserved zona-free hamster ova. Gamete Res 2:357, 1979
80. Quinn P, Barros C, Whittingham DG: Preservation of hamster oocytes to assay the fertilizing capacity of human spermatozoa. J Reprod Fertil 66:161, 1982
81. Hall JL, Sloan CS, Williams WD: Evaluation of freeze preserved human sperm fertilizing potential using zona-free animal ova. Biol Reprod (Suppl 1) 20:94a, 1979
82. Urry RL, Carrell DT, Hull DB, Middleton RG, Wiltbank MC: Penetration of zona-free hamster ova and bovine cervical mucus by fresh and frozen human spermatozoa. Fertil Steril 39:690, 1983
83. Binor Z, Sokoloski JE, Wolf DP: Penetration of the zona-free hamster egg by human sperm. Fertil Steril 33:321, 1980
84. Fujita JS, Van Campen H, Rogers BJ: The effect of freezing on fertilizing capacity of human spermatozoa using zona-free eggs. J Androl 1:77a, 1980
85. Bolanos JR, Overstreet JW, Katz DF: Human sperm penetration of zona-free hamster eggs after storage of the semen for 48 hours at 2° C to 5° C. Fertil Steril 39:536, 1983
86. Jeyendran RS, van der Ven HH, Kennedy W, Perez-Pelaez M, Zaneveld LJD: Comparison of glycerol and a zwitter ion buffer system as a cryoprotective media for human spermatozoa. J Androl 5:1, 1984
87. Johnson AR, Syms AJ, Lipshultz LI, Smith RG: Conditions influencing human sperm capacitation and penetration of zona-free hamster ova. Fertil Steril 41:603, 1984
88. Chan SYW, Tang LCH, Ma H-K: Stimulation of the human spermatozoal fertilizing ability by dibutyryl 3′5′-cAMP and theophylline in vitro. Arch Androl 11:19, 1983
89. Perreault SD, Rogers BJ: Relationship between fertilizing ability and cAMP in human spermatozoa. J Androl 3:396, 1982
90. Weeda AJ, Cohen J: Effects of purification or split ejaculation of semen and stimulation of spermatozoa by caffeine on their motility and fertilizing ability with the use of zona-free hamster ova. Fertil Steril 37:817, 1982
91. Cohen J, Aafjes JH: Proteolytic enzymes stimulate human spermatozoal motility and in vitro hamster egg penetration. Life Sci 30:899, 1982
92. Chan SYW, Tang LCH, Ma H-K: Stimulation of the zona-free hamster ova penetration efficiency by human spermatozoa after 17β-estradiol treatment. Fertil Steril 39:80, 1983
93. Aitken RJ, Ross A, Hargreave T, Richardson D, Best F: Analysis of human sperm function following exposure to ionophore A23187. J Androl 5:321, 1984
94. Rogers BJ: Factors affecting mammalian in vitro fertilization. In Bioregulators of Reproduction. New York, Academic Press, 1981, p 459
95. Mygatt GG, Soderdahl DW, Rogers BJ: In vitro fertilization rates after varicocele repair. J Urol 127:1103, 1982
96. Rogers BJ, Maruyama D, Linsenmeyer TA, Soderdahl DW: The effect of clomiphene citrate on oligospermic male infertility as monitored by the sperm penetration assay. Presented at the III International Congress of Andrology, April 27 to May 2, 1985, Boston, Massachusetts (Abstr)

97. Berger RE, Smith WD, Critchlow CW, Stenchever MA, Moore DE, Spadoni LR, Holmes KK: Improvement in the sperm penetration (hamster ova) assay (SPA) results after doxycycline treatment of infertile men. J Androl 4:126, 1983

Chapter 28

Immunology of semen

Nancy J. Alexander, Ph.D.
Deborah J. Anderson, Ph.D.

Oregon Regional Primate Research Center, Beaverton, and Oregon Health Sciences University, Portland, Oregon; Fearing Research Laboratory, Harvard Medical School, Boston, Massachusetts

Sperm express unique differentiation antigens that can elicit autoimmune responses in men and alloimmune responses in women. Antisperm immune responses occur as a result of a breakdown or imbalance in normal protective mechanisms, which include the blood-testis barrier system in men, and seminal plasma immunosuppressive factors and active immunoregulatory mechanisms operative in both men and women. Antisperm antibodies are frequently detected in sera and semen of men with a history of reproductive tract trauma (i.e., vasectomy) or infection (i.e., mumps), and are also detectable in sera and cervical mucus of approximately 5% of sexually active women in North America. Antisperm antibodies are clinically significant because of an association with infertility in both men and women. It is therefore important to understand the mechanisms underlying the generation and potential reversal of this type of immune response. Furthermore, it is increasingly recognized that the immunoprotective environment of reproductive tissues harbors viruses and other microorganisms and is an important element in the sexual transmission of disease. In this article, we will review recent basic research concepts and clinical implications of both the immunostimulatory and immunosuppressive aspects of semen immunology.

IMMUNOGENICITY OF SPERM AND SEMINAL PLASMA

BASIC STUDIES

During meiosis, unique differentiation molecules are expressed by germ cells in the testis. Testis-specific autoantigens appear on late pachytene spermatocytes and persist through spermiogenesis in the mouse.[1] Additional antigens appear on the plasma membrane after the midspermatid stage of spermatogenesis[2] and on the sperm surface during epididymal transit.[3] Similar germ cell- and sperm-specific antigens, revealed by mapping studies with monoclonal antibodies, develop during human spermatogenesis.[4] As has been demonstrated many times by immunization studies, various sperm and germ cell antigens can stimulate the production of antisperm antibodies (Fig. 1) and/or experimental allergic orchitis.[5] However, under normal conditions, humoral immune responses to testicular germ cell or sperm antigens are usually not detected.

At puberty, commensurate with the development of these immunologically unique antigens within the male reproductive tract, barriers form that protect reproductive tissue-specific products from recognition and destruction by the immune system. Surrounding the seminiferous tubules, the Sertoli cells abut in the tightest union between cells anywhere in the body, excluding the passage of lymphocytes and high-molecular-weight proteins such as immunoglobulin and complement.[6, 7] One of the functions of the Sertoli cell is to maintain a specialized intraluminal environment, free of serum components and with a distinctive composition of sugars, proteins, and ions.[8, 9] Sertoli cells also form an immunologic barrier by actively phagocytosing and degrading sperm and residual body products which would be a major source of antigenic stimulation if permitted to leak from the seminiferous tubule. Only one-fifth of the total number of sperm produced actually leave the testis; they and numerous residual bodies which also express sperm antigens

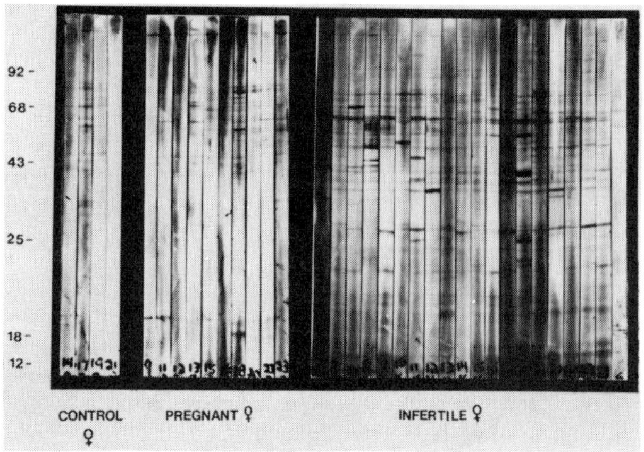

Figure 1
Antisperm antibodies detected by Western blot assay in serum from infertile women. This study reveals the heterogeneity of antisperm immune responses in patient populations.

are resorbed by the germinal epithelium.[10, 11] The physical barrier system of the testis, the blood-testis barrier, provides an immunologically sequestered intratubular environment in which germ cells can undergo meiosis and development. All germinal cell stages with the exception of spermatogonia and preleptotene spermatocytes reside in this protected environment. Additionally, Sertoli cells themselves secrete specific proteins, possibly including immunoregulatory factors. It has been reported that unfractionated proteins of Sertoli cells inhibit lymphocyte blastogenesis and complement-mediated cell lysis.[12]

Tight junctions, although not as extensive as those between Sertoli cells, are found throughout other regions of the male reproductive tract. However, these junctions are weak in the rete testis and efferent ducts, and these locations are sites for entrance of immune mediators into the sperm compartment. Recent studies indicate that initiation of experimental allergic orchitis may occur in the straight tubules of the rete.[13] Furthermore, after vasectomy, sperm antigens escape from the efferent ducts into the surrounding basal lamina (Fig. 2). The anatomic structure of the blood-testis barrier varies among mammalian species, and incidences of antisperm immunity and allergic orchitis differ depending on the experimental animal model under study. As described in detail below, immunosuppressive factors present in male reproductive tract fluids serve as a backup to the structural immunological barriers of the male reproductive tract and modulate humoral and cellular immune responses to sperm in men. These potent immunosuppressive factors are also present in seminal plasma and are speculated to prevent immune reactions to sperm following intercourse in women.

CLINICAL RELEVANCE

Male

Occasionally the mechanisms that prevent generation of adverse reactions to testicular germ cell or sperm antigens fail. The blood-testis barrier in men can break down as a result of chemical or physical trauma or infection.[14, 15] Exposure of the male immune system to sperm antigens frequently results from vasectomy. Spermatozoa continue to be produced after vasectomy, degenerate in the male reproductive tract, and leak soluble products through distended rete testis, epididymis, and efferent ductules into interstitial spaces which are accessible to immunological mediators.[16] The millions of sperm that continue to be produced daily after vasectomy often stimulate high titers of antisperm antibodies that persist for years.[17] However, only 40% to 60% of vasectomized men develop detectable antisperm antibodies; nonresponder individuals could be genetically predisposed to low immunological response to sperm antigens.[18, 19] In support of the possibility of immunogenetic influences on antisperm anti-

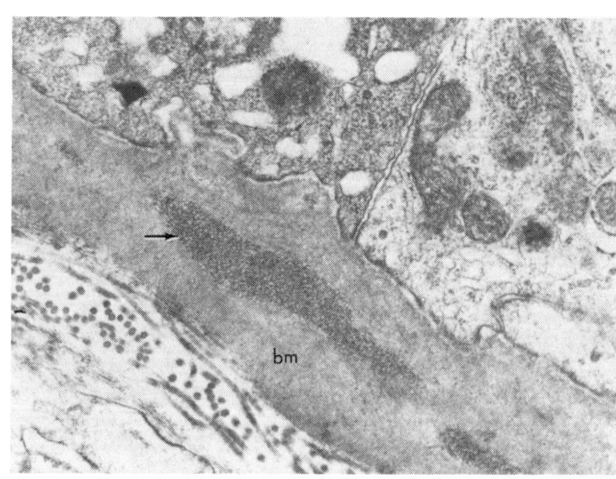

Figure 2
After vasectomy in rhesus monkeys, sperm antigens may escape and combine with circulating antisperm antibodies to form immune complexes (seen as densities by electron microscopy) in the basement membrane surrounding the efferent ducts. Potassium permanganate and lead citrate. (Magnification, × 16,000.)

body responses in men, Law et al.[20] reported an association between antisperm antibodies in vasectomized men and the HLA phenotypes A-28 and B-22. However, the variability could also be due to as yet undefined surgical or other physical factors.

Female

Unlike that of the male, the female reproductive tract is not sequestered behind a physical barrier system. Yet spermatozoa, which are immunologically foreign to women, usually do not stimulate humoral immune responses. A sexually active woman may be exposed to over a trillion sperm in a lifetime. Fertility would be compromised if women were immunized against sperm with each insemination. Deliberate immunization of women with sperm can impair fertility; underlying causes are probably a combination of antisperm antibody effects such as sperm agglutination, reduced motility, impaired cervical mucus penetration, inefficient sperm-egg fusion, enhanced phagocytosis of sperm, and pre- or postimplantation embryo loss. Antibodies to both intrinsic sperm antigens which are produced during germ cell maturation in the testis, and sperm coating antigens, which are added during passage through the epididymis and on exposure to seminal plasma at ejaculation, are associated with unexplained infertility.[21, 22]

Even though antibodies to sperm do not usually develop after intercourse, there is evidence that the female immune system may regularly respond to antigens present in the ejaculate. In mice, there is an increase in the weight of the draining lymph nodes following exposure to sperm.[23] It is possible that this lymph node response represents activation of a suppressive immune response (see below). Several studies[18, 24, 25] indicate that epididymal sperm are more antigenic than ejaculated sperm. There is evidence that seminal plasma enzymes affect sperm surface antigen expression,[26, 27] and that seminal plasma immunosuppressive factors can abrogate antisperm immune responses in vivo.[25]

Human Sperm Antigens

Antigens of human sperm can be mapped; naturally occurring human antisperm antibodies bind to antigens located on the acrosome (Fig. 3), postacrosome, equatorial region, midpiece, principal piece (tail), and tip of tail. Several sperm-

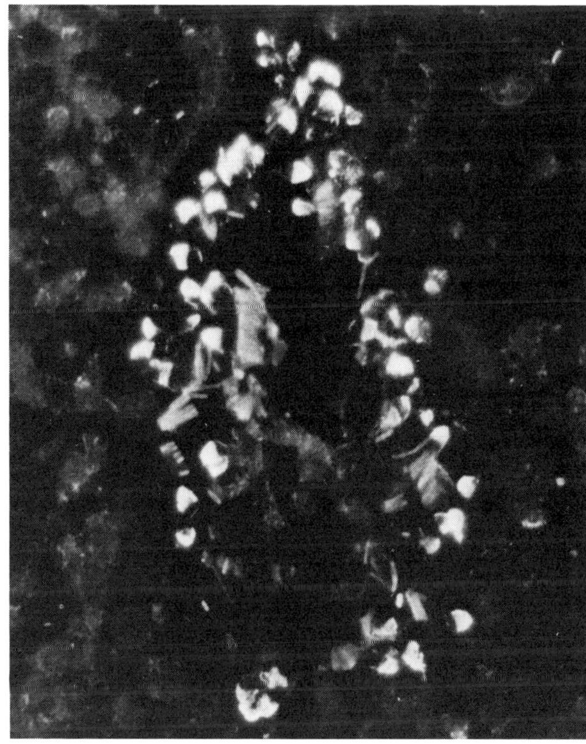

Figure 3
After vasectomy, antibodies to sperm develop to specific regions (in this case, the acrosome). If testicular tissue is exposed, the antibodies react but because of the blood-testis barrier, antigen-antibody complexes are usually not found. Indirect immunofluorescence. (Magnification, × 560.)

specific antigens have been identified (Table 1), and many more are being defined by sperm-specific monoclonal antibodies. Other studies have revealed sperm antigens with limited expression in other tissues including the embryo,[43, 44] placenta,[45, 46] ovary,[4, 44] T-lymphocytes,[47] brain,[43] and a variety of neoplastic tissues.[48] Polymorphic antigens of the major histocompatibility complex which could potentially stimulate vigorous immune reactions in sexually active women are not significantly expressed on sperm.[42, 49] Although ABO blood group antigens are found in the seminal plasma of secretors and are passively adsorbed to the surface of sperm in these individuals,[39, 40] they do not appear to be an important factor in immunologic infertility.

Human sperm antigens are being actively studied through application of monoclonal antibodies (Fig. 4), and their biochemical and functional characterization will provide insight into mechanisms of immunologic infertility as well as contribute to the development of contraceptive vaccines (see below). Monoclonal antibodies have

Table 1. *Human Sperm Antigens of Possible Immunologic Significance*

Antigen name	Description	Reference
LDH-C_4	12 KD testicular isozyme of lactate dehydrogenase; produced abundantly by testicular germ cells, expressed on surface of mature sperm	28-30
Acrosin	Sperm acrosomal enzyme; facilitates penetration of zona pellucida	31, 32
Hyaluronidase	Sperm acrosomal enzyme; facilitates penetration of cumulus mass surrounding egg	33, 34
RSA-1, MA-29, FA-1	Sperm surface antigens identified by heterologous antibodies	35-38
S03, S37, S61, S20	Sperm antigens identified by WHO Monoclonal Antibody Workshop	4
ABO group antigens	Not intrinsic sperm membrane antigens; present in seminal plasma of secretors, can coat the sperm surface	39, 40
HY	Expression on sperm controversial	41
HLA antigens	Not expressed on human sperm	42

also been made against seminal plasma components, and one has recently become an important diagnostic reagent in rape cases.[50] Another clinical application of monoclonal antibodies directed against sperm antigens is in the identification of sperm markers associated with sperm fertilizing capabilities. The WHO Monoclonal Antibody Workshop identified a number of antisperm monoclonal antibodies that recognized functionally significant sperm antigens.[4] For example, one antibody, H316, appears to bind to the human sperm acrosome only after capacitation and may be useful as a probe identifying capacitated sperm.[46] Others caused sperm agglutination, complement-dependent sperm immobilization, and inhibition of cervical mucus and hamster egg penetration. It is envisioned that a panel of such antibodies might be applied clinically to the systematic evaluation of functional defects of infertile semen.[39]

Contraceptive vaccines: The findings that antisperm antibodies are associated with infertility suggest the possibility of development of a contraceptive vaccine based on sperm antigens. The production of monoclonal antibodies directed against sperm provides a powerful tool for definition of new antigens that may be involved in fertilization. To be used for fertility regulation, a vaccine antigen must be expressed on the sperm surface (either an integral membrane protein or epididymal or seminal plasma-derived coating protein) and accessible to immune attack. It must be immunogenic so that either alone or in concert with conjugated proteins or adjuvants, a sustained and effective immunologic contraceptive response can be elicited. Furthermore, the antigen must be sperm specific so that no tissue damage occurs from cross-reactions.[52, 53]

ACCESSIBILITY OF THE MALE REPRODUCTIVE TRACT TO COMPONENTS OF THE IMMUNE SYSTEM

Lymphatics and blood vessels course through the interstitial spaces between the seminiferous tubules of the testis. Furthermore, cells that phenotypically resemble macrophages line the myoid layer surrounding the seminiferous tubules. These cells express abundant HLA-D antigens, molecules which play a role in antigen presentation, which is fundamental to the initiation of immune responses.[54, 55] Thus, mediators of immunologic responses are normally present in the testis. It is widely accepted that cells and high-molecular-weight mediators of immune responses such as immunoglobulin and complement are completely excluded from the sperm compartment in the testis by the Sertoli cell barrier, and therefore the mechanism whereby testicular-an-

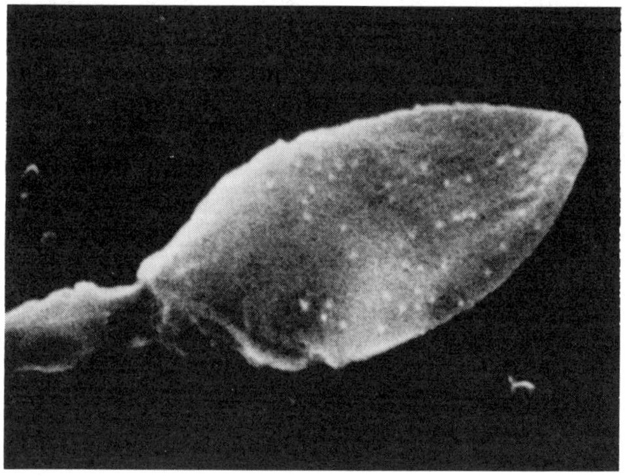

Figure 4
One of our mouse antihuman sperm monoclonal antibodies (MA 19; SO3 in WHO test panel) binds to the acrosome. We used the monoclonal antibody and antimouse immunogold (40 nm) to demonstrate antigen-antibody binding of small gold particles on the acrosome as viewed by scanning microscopy. (Magnification, × 22,000.)

tigen-activated lymphocytes gain access to the sperm compartment in autoimmune orchitis is not understood. The fact that orchitis occurs indicates that testicular antigens may not be completely hidden from the immune system. Evidence that active immunoregulation could normally play a role in suppression of testicular immunologic activity is provided by the studies of Taguchi and Nishizuka,[56] which demonstrated that autoimmune orchitis develops in male mice which have decreased suppressor cell levels due to neonatal thymectomy. Sakaguchi et al.[57] recently demonstrated that the orchitis response in thymectomized mice could be overcome by transfer of Thy-1 positive, Ly-2,3 negative suppressor T cells from normal male mice. This finding suggests that Sertoli cells or local Ia^{+} cells may present testicular antigens to the immune system in a way that induces local tolerance, perhaps by activation of suppressor cells. Local immunoregulation, therefore, may serve as a crucial backup system to insufficient physical barriers in the suppression of testicular autoimmune responses.

Numerous viable lymphocytes and monocytes are present in normal human semen.[58, 59] Because their numbers are greatly reduced after vasectomy, seminal lymphocytes and monocytes appear to principally enter the reproductive tract through the efferent ducts and/or the epididymis (upstream of the vasectomy site).[58, 60] Numerous lymphocytes, primarily of the T8+ (suppressor/cytotoxic) phenotype, are also present in the epithelium of the caput and cauda epididymidis, which also contains many HLA-D positive cells.[54] Until recently, these cells have been considered an unimportant contaminant, and the biologic role of seminal leukocytes has not been defined. However, there is recent evidence that the presence of leukocytes in semen is associated with poor fertilization ability in the hamster egg penetration test,[61] and that factors produced by activated lymphocytes and monocytes affect sperm motility (discussed below). Seminal plasma contains leukocyte chemotactic factors, and large numbers of leukocytes are attracted to the female reproductive tract following insemination.[62] One role of such cells is the phagocytosis and removal of immotile sperm from the insemination site.

Immunoglobulins of the IgG class are detectable in human semen and enter primarily as a transudate through the prostate.[63] IgG has also been detected in low levels in rete testis fluid[64, 65] and epididymal fluid from rabbits[66] and guinea pigs.[67] Antisperm antibodies of the IgA class have been detected in seminal plasma of some infertile men and may be produced locally by plasma cells residing in male reproductive tissues.[68] IgM is usually not detected in human seminal plasma.[69, 70] The complement components C3 and C4 have been found in seminal plasma of infertile men,[71] but are rarely found in semen of normal fertile donors. Other components of the complement cascade have not been measured; whether the full complement system necessary for antibody-mediated lysis is present in seminal plasma is not known. Even if it were, potent complement inhibitors are also present in seminal secretions and suppress the activity of complement (described further below).

Significance of Lymphocytes in Infertility Semen

Numerous viable lymphocytes and macrophages are present in human semen, and recent studies indicate that semen from a significant percentage of infertile men contains dramatically increased numbers and unusual profiles of lymphocytes and activated macrophages[72] (Fig. 5). Furthermore, the effects of products of activated lymphocytes and macrophages on sperm function have recently been investigated, and it was found that leukocyte products affect the hamster egg penetration test[61] and that supernatants from activated lymphocyte cultures and certain purified lymphokines and monokines (products of activated lymphocytes and macrophages, respectively) affect sperm motility and viability.[73] These results indicate that in addition to humoral immunity, cell-mediated immunity could play a significant role in male infertility.

Significance of Antisperm Antibodies in Semen

A majority of men who have had a vasovasostomy and a small percentage of infertile men have antisperm antibodies in their seminal plasma. These antibodies, which are usually of the IgG or IgA subclasses, adhere to sperm and affect fertility. Fertility is suppressed in couples in which the husband has antisperm antibodies. In a study of 254 infertile men, chances of a pregnancy were inversely correlated with antibody titers.[74] In a prospective study of men undergoing vasovasostomy, Fuchs and Alexander[75] also demonstrated poor conception rates in partners of men with elevated antisperm levels as compared to those with low or no measurable levels. The best

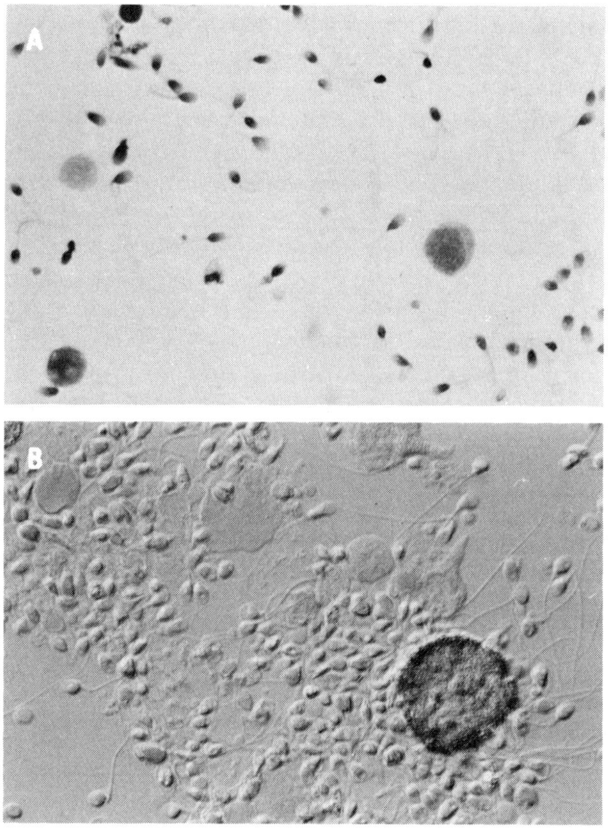

Figure 5
(**A**) Cells of leukocytic morphology in semen sample from normal fertile donor (Hemacolor stain, × 400). (**B**) Cell typed as macrophage (M1 antibody positive) by immunoperoxidase technique in semen sample from subfertile man. (Magnification, × 320.)

method for detection of antisperm antibodies in semen is through the use of immunobeads.[76] This test directly assesses the percentage of spermatozoa coated with antibodies, and the location and class of bound antibodies. Antibody-coated sperm may be impaired in a number of fertility-related functions including motility, cervical mucus penetration, and egg penetration.[77]

Three therapeutic options are available for couples with male factor immunologic infertility: (1) insemination with donor sperm, (2) immunosuppressive therapy, and (3) sperm manipulation. Corticosteroid treatment has been reported to lower antibody levels and improve fertility in some men without altering semen parameters (i.e., sperm count, motility, and percentage of normal forms.)[78, 79] Immunosuppressive therapy, however, is nonspecific and may have severe side effects such as aseptic hip necrosis and exacerbation of incipient duodenal ulcers. Various sperm-processing procedures have been used to remove complexed antibodies from sperm. Sperm washing is usually ineffective because antisperm antibodies have a high affinity for the sperm surface. Dissociation with high-ionic-strength or low pH solutions causes irreversible loss of sperm motility. Bronson et al.[76] have suggested using freeze-thawed sperm from antibody-negative donors as an immunosorbent. Sperm subsequently swim up into overlying buffer layer, but we have found that few sperm are able to migrate into the buffer layer. We have described a method of passing antibody-positive ejaculates through a column of dextran beads that results in an improvement in the hamster egg penetration test.[80] Clinical trials using this technique of antisperm antibody processing are under way. A better understanding of the effects of interactions between antibodies and sperm will promote the development of improved specific treatments for immunologically mediated infertility.

IMMUNOSUPPRESSIVE FACTORS IN SEMEN

BASIC STUDIES

Immunosuppressive Effects of Semen

When added to tests of immune function in vitro, human seminal plasma inhibits activities of most cell types that participate in immune responses and host defense including T cells, B cells, natural killer (NK) cells, macrophages, and polymorphonuclear leukocytes (PMNs). The reported effects of seminal plasma on immune functions are varied and include: (1) inhibition of the ability of T and B lymphocytes to proliferate in response to mitogen or antigen challenge, (2) impairment of the ability of macrophages and PMNs to recognize target antigens by means of surface cytophilic antibodies, (3) impairment of the ability of NK cells and cytotoxic T cells to recognize and destroy tumor and virally infected target cells, and (4) inhibition of phagocytosis by macrophages and PMNs. In addition, human seminal plasma inhibits the action of complement (C1 and C3 components), thereby reducing the lytic effectiveness of antibodies in target cell destruction. In vivo studies of seminal plasma immunosuppression are limited, but on the basis of extensive in vitro studies it can be predicted that seminal plasma immunosuppressive factors would have an overall effect of suppression of the immune mechanisms that could adversely affect spermatozoa (potential immune targets) in men and women. Another consequence of reduced immune activity in reproductive tissues due to the presence of such immunosuppressive factors is compromise of the host mechanisms operative in defense against infection and malignancy.

Cell Viability

Human seminal plasma at high concentrations has been reported to be lymphocytotoxic.[81, 82] The toxic effect of seminal plasma is dramatically enhanced by the presence of fetal calf serum, which contains high levels of polyamine oxidase (PAO), an enzyme which oxidizes spermine and spermidine (present in high levels in semen) to produce complex labile aldehydes which are extremely cytotoxic. Human serum reportedly has little PAO activity. However, many early in vitro immunological tests were performed in the presence of fetal calf serum, and the cytotoxic effects of oxidized polyamines which are artificially induced in this system present a serious artifact. Nonetheless, a number of key studies on immunosuppressive effects of human seminal plasma have taken such cytotoxic effects into consideration and have been performed in systems containing human serum. Furthermore, fractionation of seminal plasma separates immunosuppressive factors from cytotoxic ones; high-molecular-weight seminal plasma fractions which do not contain polyamines are immunosuppressive and not cytotoxic.[81] In addition, mouse male reproductive tract fluids from different anatomic sites have various immunosuppressive effects[25]; seminal vesicle fluid is the only component with a marked cytotoxic effect.[83] These studies indicate that there are numerous factors in seminal secretions that exert a variety of immunosuppressive activities in in vitro systems, not all of which are associated with cytotoxic effects.

Cell Proliferation

Following activation by antigen or mitogen, macrophages and lymphocytes release monokines and lymphokines that stimulate lymphocyte proliferation. Clonal expansion of programmed immunocompetent cells is an important component of host immune defense. A number of studies have documented a potent inhibitory effect of human seminal plasma on lymphocyte proliferation. The mechanisms and factors responsible for this effect have not been adequately defined. Many of the studies on this subject are poorly controlled and are difficult to interpret because (1) seminal plasma components can compete for or alter the structure of mitogens or antigens and prevent their interaction with lymphocyte receptors (i.e., lymphocytes are not activated in the first place), (2) many were performed in the presence of fetal calf serum, which induces the polyamine oxidation artifact, and (3) mycoplasma, a common contaminant of human semen, can dramatically reduce ^{3}H-thymidine uptake in studies of cell proliferation and therefore introduce another potential artifact.[84] Nonetheless, antiproliferative effects of seminal plasma components following lymphocyte activation have been demonstrated.[25] Most studies have closely monitored cell viability and claim no overt cytotoxic effect of seminal plasma at effective doses used in their assays. Several of the components of human seminal plasma, including prostaglandins, polyamines, and pregnancy-associated plasma protein-A, have been demonstrated to suppress lymphocyte proliferation when added in purified form to immunologic assays (Table 2) and may be the factors accountable for this effect. In a recent study we tested human seminal plasma for factors that block Il-2 (T-cell growth factor) activity. Il-2 inhibitors have been found in the decidua during pregnancy and have been ascribed a key immunosuppressive role in the maintenance of the fetal allograft.[101] Our data indicate that human seminal plasma does not inhibit the proliferative effect of purified human Il-2 on human lymphocytes in culture (unpublished). Clearly, the mechanisms and factors involved in the lymphocyte antiproliferative effect of seminal plasma must be further explored.

Cell-Mediated Immunity

Lord et al.[102] reported that human seminal plasma inhibited the generation of cytotoxic T cells in mixed lymphocyte culture but did not affect the lytic activity of cytotoxic T cells in ^{51}Cr-release assays. Other investigators, however, have reported that human seminal plasma does affect the activity of cytotoxic T cells. We have recently found that human seminal plasma inhibits the destruction of cytomegalovirus-infected target cells by activated cytotoxic T cells in vitro.[103] Seminal plasma inhibits the binding of cytotoxic T cells to targets, and the effect is seen when lymphocytes, but not when target cells, are

Table 2. *Components of Human Seminal Plasma with Well-Established or Presumed Immunologic Effects*

Factor	Immunological effect	Reference
Prostaglandins (different forms)	Suppress NK activity	85-87
Polyamines Spermine Spermidine (different forms)	Inhibit lymphocyte proliferation, generation of cytotoxic lymphocytes, cross-link surface peptides in presence of transglutaminase	88, 89, 91
PAPP-A[a]	Inhibits lymphocyte proliferation	90
Transglutaminase	Cross-links receptors	26, 91
Proteases	Alter antigens + receptors	92
Opiates	T rosette inhibition	93
Zn, Zn-peptide complexes	Inhibits lymphocyte proliferation, cytotoxic lymphocyte function	94, 95
Immunoglobulin	Blocking factors (i.e., TLX)	46
Transferrin	Binds to transferrin receptor (NK target)	96
Lactoferrin	Inhibits complement activity	97, 98
α_2-macroglobulin	Antigen masking	99
β_2-microglobulin	Antigen masking	26
Sperm antigens	Induction of suppressor cells, immune tolerance	54
Suppressor T-cell products	Antigen-specific and nonspecific immunosuppression	54
Fc receptor-binding protein	Inhibits binding of cytophilic antibody to Fc receptors on surface of macrophages, PMNs (inhibits recognition of target cells)	100

[a]PAPP-A, Pregnancy-associated plasma protein-A.

preincubated in seminal plasma. This information indicates that seminal plasma may affect the ability of lymphocytes to recognize target cells. Clearly the inhibitory effect of seminal plasma components on the ability of cytotoxic T cells to recognize virally infected targets could be a mechanism promoting the survival of infectious agents in reproductive tissues and the venereal transmission of disease. Also relevant is the observation that human testicular germ cells do not express Class I MHC (HLA-A,B,C) antigens.[49] As these antigenic structures are required in combination with foreign antigen for recognition of target cells by cytotoxic T cells, virally infected germ cells would probably escape recognition and destruction by cytotoxic T cells.

Natural Killer Cells

NK cells operate in the first line of host defense by immediately acting without prior exposure to destroy neoplastic and virally infected cells. Their ability to recognize and destroy target cells has been shown to be dramatically inhibited by seminal plasma[104-106] (Fig. 6). Tarter et al.[85] recently reported that PG-19-OH isolated from human seminal plasma was largely responsible for this effect. The abrogation by seminal plasma of host defense mechanisms could contribute to the development of sexually transmitted organisms and neoplasias.

Anticomplementary Effects

Human seminal plasma has also been shown to inhibit the lytic effect of complement, an important family of enzymes involved in cytolytic mechanisms of humoral immunity. Human seminal plasma inhibits complement-dependent, antibody-mediated killing of bacteria and lysis of

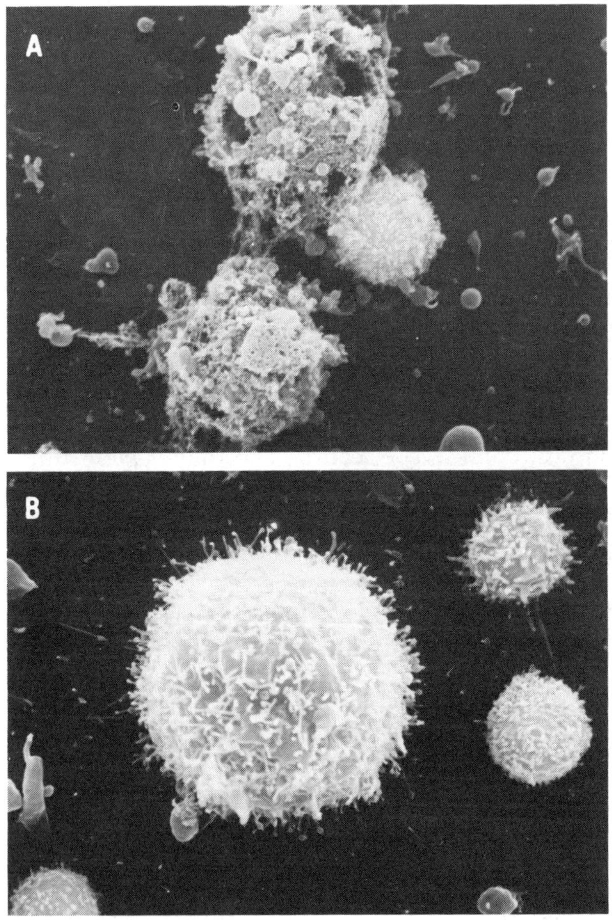

Figure 6
(**A**), Scanning electron micrograph showing lysis of K562 (erythroleukemia) target cell by NK cells isolated from peripheral blood. (**B**), Inhibition of K562 target cell lysis in NK cell assay by human seminal plasma (dilution of 1/100). (Magnification, × 1600).

sheep erythrocytes. The complement-inhibiting factors are concentrated in the prostate of mice and rhesus monkeys[25, 107] but appear to be ubiquitous in the human male reproductive tract.[108] Complement components have been detected in the female reproductive tract (discussed previously), and seminal plasma complement inhibitors could serve to protect spermatozoa from antibody-mediated lysis. The presence of such factors in the male reproductive tract and in the reproductive tracts of sexually active women could inhibit natural humoral immune mechanisms in the elimination of microorganisms. Human seminal plasma at a dilution of 1/1000 inhibited complement-dependent antibody mediated lysis of *Neisseria gonorrhoeae* and a number of gram-negative organisms.[109]

Phagocytic Function

Human seminal plasma has been shown to inhibit the opsonization (immunoglobulin-mediated recognition and phagocytosis) of gram-negative bacteria by leukocytes.[109-111] A possible mechanism accountable for this effect is inhibition by seminal plasma factor(s) of the binding of cytophilic antibodies to Fc receptors on phagocytic cells.[100] Seminal plasma Fc blocking factors also may block the arming of leukocytes and monocytes with cytophilic antibody, which enables them to recognize foreign target cells. Seminal plasma also affects phagocytic activities of both macrophages and PMNs and suppresses the generation of reactive oxygen species, factors involved in the killing of internalized microorganisms.[110-112]

In Vivo Studies

Studies on the in vivo effects of seminal plasma immunosuppressive factors are few. In 1980 Hurtenbach et al.[113] published that intravenous injection of washed epididymal sperm into mice totally paralyzed NK cell and cytotoxic T-cell activities. This finding is intriguing and potentially very important but has not been confirmed. We found in an early study[25] that mouse seminal plasma (a mixture of prostatic, seminal vesicle, and epididymal fluids) decreased the immunogenicity of epididymal sperm when injected in combination with low doses of sperm or at a distant site. Mouse seminal plasma also suppressed the in vivo antibody response to bovine serum albumin. Recent studies have indicated that rectal administration of seminal plasma into rabbits,[114] and prostaglandin E_2 (PGE_2) into male (but not female) rats,[115] inhibits parameters of immune response. Rectal administration of seminal plasma may have dramatic systemic effects due to the absorptive nature of the colon. When human seminal plasma is rectally infused into rhesus monkeys, PGE_2 metabolites peak in blood plasma samples after 2 hours, indicating that immunologically active factors are readily absorbed from the gut.[116]

CLINICAL RELEVANCE OF MALE REPRODUCTIVE TRACT IMMUNOSUPPRESSIVE FACTORS

Antisperm immunity may be naturally controlled by male reproductive tract immunosuppressive factors, and individuals lacking such factors and their spouses could experience immunologic infertility. We have reported that 20% of the human seminal plasma samples tested in one series lacked complement-inhibiting activity.[108] We speculate that some semen samples may lack other components that play a vital role in immune response control.

The sexually transmitted diseases such as gonorrhea, syphilis, and chlamydia are probably promoted by male reproductive tract immunosuppressive factors which inhibit their recognition and destruction by antibodies, cytotoxic T cells, and phagocytes. The same is probably true for the newly recognized sexually transmitted viruses, such as HIV,[59, 117] herpes,[118] CMV, and papilloma virus,[119] which appear to be harbored by male reproductive tissues.[120] NK cell and cytotoxic T-cell mechanisms that are key to host defense against viral infection are dramatically inhibited by human reproductive tract secretions. Herpes virus type 2, cytomegalovirus, and hepatitis B have been shown to reside in male reproductive tissues over prolonged periods of time without evidence of overt disease.[121] The AIDS virus HIV may reside unchallenged by the immune system in $T4^+$ (helper) lymphocytes in the human epididymis.[60] A better understanding of the activities and locations of immunosuppressive factors in the male reproductive tract could provide insight into approaches to inactivate immunosuppressive mechanisms in the reproductive tissues, enabling the destruction of viruses and microorganisms harbored there. Malignancies of the male and female urogenital tracts may also be promoted by seminal immunosuppressive factors which inhibit immunosurveillance mechanisms. In the man, local immunosuppression by prostatic secretions may prevent the host from responding to neoplastic transformation in the prostate. Cervical cancer which is associated with sexual activity and particularly multiple sexual partners is now thought to have a viral etiology and may be promoted as a result of immunosuppressive effects of seminal plasma factors on NK cells, cytotoxic T cells, and macrophages.[106, 122]

CONCLUSIONS AND QUESTIONS

Surprisingly little is known about the role of seminal plasma in fertilization. Animal studies have demonstrated that removal of individual male accessory glands does not affect fertility. Furthermore, other studies have shown that sperm from the caudal epididymis are fertile. These data suggest that the primary role of seminal plasma may be only as a diluent and transport vehicle. However, the complex chemical composition of seminal plasma belies this simplistic interpretation. We propose that the immunosuppressive properties of seminal plasma may be its most significant function. Seminal plasma antigen masking and alteration effects and soluble immunosuppressive factors enable immunologically foreign sperm to repeatedly invade the female tract. It is possible that washed sperm used in intrauterine insemination protocols will stimulate antisperm antibody responses because they may be more antigenic than spermatozoa presented to the female reproductive tract in seminal plasma, and more are inseminated than the number of sperm that normally reach the uterus. Immunosuppressive factors may also protect infectious organisms from immune destruction and provide a transport vehicle for venereal transmission of infectious diseases. They may also facilitate the growth of malignancies in both the male and female reproductive tracts. Prostatic cancer is the second most common cancer in men, and cervical cancer is particularly prevalent in sexually active women with multiple sexual partners.

The immunosuppressive factors of seminal plasma must be chemically and physiologically defined so that their effects are better understood. Many studies in the past have been superficial or flawed. Powerful new immunological reagents and techniques now exist to provide answers to many of the questions in this field. Certainly more in vivo studies must be conducted to determine to what extent seminal plasma is a cofactor in the transmission of venereal viruses such as HIV. The seminal plasma of partners of women with antisperm antibodies should be further studied to determine if certain men lack seminal immunosuppressive factors. It may be possible to regulate, hormonally or otherwise, immunosuppressive factor production in male reproductive tissues as a treatment of infertility, to aid in the eradication of pathogenic organisms residing in male reproductive tissues, or to enhance the efficacy of sperm antigen vaccines in men.

The role of antisperm antibodies in infertility is still not clear. Numerous reports indicate that high antisperm antibody levels are inversely correlated with fertility. Exposure of sperm to antibodies can inhibit sperm motility and egg penetration. Studies involving immunologic mapping of the sperm surface in parallel with immunohistologic and functional inhibition tests should provide important information concerning the role of individual sperm antigens in fertility. A better understanding of local antibody production and cell-mediated immune responses in both the male and female reproductive tracts is also essential to the understanding of immunologic infertility. Studies on how reproductive tract and seminal plasma components protect spermatozoa from immune recognition and destruction will promote better treatment of immunologically mediated infertility. The role of the immunologically privileged status of male reproductive tissues and fluids in the transmission of venereal disease is virtually unexplored and provides an important research problem on a topical subject. Sexually transmitted viruses are epidemic and are perhaps the most significant clinical problem of the 1980s.

REFERENCES

1. Millette CF, Bellvé AR: Temporal expression of membrane antigens during mouse spermatogenesis. J Cell Biol 74:86, 1977
2. Romwell LJ, O'Rand MG: Capping and ultrastructural localization of sperm surface isoantigens during spermatogenesis. Dev Biol 63:76, 1978
3. Feuchter FA, Vernon RB, Eddy EM: Analysis of the sperm surface with monoclonal antibodies: topographically restricted antigens appearing in the epididymis. Biol Reprod 24:1099, 1981
4. Anderson DJ, Johnson PM, Alexander NJ, Jones WR, Griffin PD: Report of WHO-sponsored workshops on monoclonal antibodies to human sperm and trophoblast antigens. J Reprod Immunol. In press

5. Brown PC, Holborow EJ, Glynn LE: The aspermatogenic antigen in experimental allergic orchitis in guinea-pigs. Immunology 9:255, 1965
6. Hamilton DW: Structure and function of the epithelium lining the ductuli efferentes, ductus epididymidis and ductus deferens. In Handbook of Physiology, Vol 5, Edited by RO Greep, EB Astwood. Washington, DC, American Physiological Society, 1975, p 259
7. Gilula NB, Fawcett DW, Aoki A: The Sertoli cell occluding junctions and gap junctions in mature and developing mammalian testis. Dev Biol 50:142, 1976
8. Tuck RR, Setchell BP, Waites GMH, Young JA: The composition of fluid collected by micropuncture and catheterization from the seminiferous tubules and rete testis of rats. Pflugers Arch 318:225, 1970
9. Waites GMH: Fluid secretion. In The Testis, Vol IV, Edited by AD Johnson, WR Gomes. New York, Academic Press, 1977, p 91
10. Johnson L, Petty CS, Neaves WB: Further quantification of human spermatogenesis: germ cell loss during postprophase of meiosis and its relationship to daily sperm production. Biol Reprod 29:207, 1983
11. Johnson L, Zane RS, Petty CS, Neaves WB: Quantification of the human Sertoli cell population: its distribution, relation to germ cell numbers, and age-related decline. Biol Reprod 31:785, 1984
12. Skinner MK, Cosand WL, Griswold MD: Purification and characterization of testicular transferrin secreted by rat Sertoli cells. Biochem J 218:313, 1984
13. Tung KSK, Mahi-Brown CA, Yule T: Testicular immunopathology of experimental autoimmune orchitis induced by adoptive tranfer (sic) and active immuniation (sic) are different (Abstr.). J Reprod Immunol [Suppl] 00:72, 1986
14. Eyquem A, Krieg H: Experimental autosensitization of the testis. Ann NY Acad Sci 124:270, 1965
15. Mancini RE, Andrada JA, Saraceni D, Bachmann AE, Lavieri JC, Nemirovsky M: Immunological and testicular response in man sensitized with human testicular homogenate. J Clin Endocrinol Metab 25:859, 1965
16. Marsh LD, Alexander NJ: Vasectomy: effects on the efferent ducts in *Macaca mulatta*. Am J Pathol 107:310, 1982
17. Alexander NJ, Anderson DJ: Vasectomy: consequences of autoimmunity to sperm antigens. Fertil Steril 32:253, 1979
18. Tarter TH, Alexander NJ: Genetic control of humoral immunity to sperm acrosomal and cell surface antigens. J Reprod Immunol 6:213, 1984
19. Anderson DJ: Immunogenetic considerations in the development of contraceptive vaccines based on testicular or sperm antigens and anti-sperm immune responses. In Male Contraception: Advances and Future Prospects, Edited by GI Zatuchni, A Goldsmith, JM Spieler, JJ Sciarra. Philadelphia, Harper & Row, 1986, p 419
20. Law HY, Bodmer WF, Mathews JD, Skegg DCG: The immune response to vasectomy and its relation to the HLA system. Tissue Antigens 14:115, 1979
21. Isojima S, Li TS, Ashitaka Y: Immunologic analysis of sperm-immobilizing factor found in sera of women with unexplained sterility. Am J Obstet Gynecol 101:677, 1968
22. Shigeta M, Watanabe T, Maruyama S, Koyama K, Isojima S: Sperm-immobilizing monoclonal antibody to human seminal plasma antigens. Clin Exp Immunol 42: 458, 1980
23. Beer AE, Billingham RE: Immunoregulatory aspects of pregnancy. Fed Proc 37:2374, 1978
24. Beer AE, Billingham RE: Immunobiology of mammalian reproduction. Adv Immunol 14:1, 1971
25. Anderson DJ, Tarter TH: Immunosuppressive effects of mouse seminal plasma components *in vivo* and *in vitro*. J Immunol 128:535, 1982
26. Mukherjee DC, Agrawal AK, Manjunath R, Mukherjee AB: Suppression of epididymal sperm antigenicity in the rabbit by uteroglobin and transglutaminase in vitro. Science 219:989, 1983
27. Mazzini MN, Ceraci P, de Cerezo JMS, Cerezo AS: Carbohydrates of the surface of the normal human spermatozoon. Am J Reprod Immunol Microbiol 11:107, 1986
28. Wheat TE, Goldberg E: Immunologically active peptide fragments of the sperm-specific lactate dehydrogenase C_4 isoenzyme. In Peptides: Synthesis—Structure—Function, Edited by DH Rich, E Gross. Pierce Chemical Company, Rockford, IL, 1981, p 557
29. Shelton J, Goldberg E: Serum antibodies to LDH-C_4. J Reprod Immunol 8:321, 1985
30. Beyler SA, Wheat TE, Goldberg E: Binding of antibodies against antigenic domains of murine lactate dehydrogenase-C_4 to human and mouse spermatozoa. Biol Reprod 32:1201, 1985
31. Morton DB: Acrosomal enzymes: immunochemical localization of acrosin and hyaluronidase in ram spermatozoa. J Reprod Fertil 45:375, 1975
32. Wincek TJ, Parrish RF, Polakoski KL: Fertilization: a uterine glycosaminoglycan stimulates the conversion of sperm proacrosin to acrosin. Science 203:553, 1979
33. Talbot P, Franklin LE: The release of hyaluronidase from guinea-pig spermatozoa during the course of the normal acrosome reaction in vitro. J Reprod Fertil 39:429, 1974
34. Triana LR, Babcock DF, Lorton SP, First NL, Lardy HA: Release of acrosomal hyaluronidase follows increased membrane permeability to calcium in the presumptive capacitation sequence for spermatozoa of the bovine and other mammalian species. Biol Reprod 23:47, 1980
35. O'Rand MG, Irons GP, Porter JP: Monoclonal antibodies to rabbit sperm autoantigens. I. Inhibition of in vitro fertilization and localization on the egg. Biol Reprod 30: 721, 1984
36. Saling PM, Irons G, Waibel R: Mouse sperm antigens that participate in fertilization. I. Inhibition of sperm fusion with the egg plasma membrane using monoclonal antibodies. Biol Reprod 33:515, 1985
37. Saling PM, Waibel R: Mouse sperm antigens that participate in fertilization. III. Passive immunization with a single monoclonal antisperm antibody inhibits pregnancy and fertilization in vivo. Biol Reprod 33:537, 1985
38. Naz RK, Alexander NJ, Isahakia M, Hamilton MS: Monoclonal antibody to a human germ cell membrane glycoprotein that inhibits fertilization. Science 225:342, 1984

39. Isojima S, Tsuzuku O: Problem of ABO blood group incompatibility and sterility: the effect of blood group antibody on spermatozoa. Am J Obstet Gynecol 102:304, 1968
40. Kerek G: Distribution of the blood group antigens A and B on human spermatozoa. Int J Fertil 19:181, 1974
41. Wachtel SS: H-Y antigen and the genetics of sex determination. Science 198:797, 1977
42. Anderson DJ, Bach DL, Yunis EJ, DeWolf WC: Major histocompatibility antigens are not expressed on human epididymal sperm. J Immunol 129:452, 1982
43. Solter D, Schachner M: Brain and sperm cell surface antigen (NS-4) on preimplantation mouse embryos. Dev Biol 52:98, 1976
44. Menge AC, Fleming CH: Detection of sperm antigens on mouse ova and early embryos. Dev Biol 63:111, 1978
45. Berkowitz RS, Alexander NJ, Goldstein DP, Anderson DJ: Reactivity of anti-human sperm monoclonal antibodies with normal placenta, hydatidiform mole, and gestational choriocarcinoma. Gynecol Oncol 22:334, 1985
46. Anderson DJ, Johnson PM: The monoclonal antibody 316 which recognizes polymorphic antigens expressed on human trophoblast also reacts with human testicular germ cells and capacitated sperm (Abstr.). J Reprod Immunol [Suppl] 00:31, 1986
47. Mathur S, Goust JM, Williamson HO, Fudenberg HH: Cross-reactivity of sperm and T lymphocyte antigens. Am J Reprod Immunol 1:113, 1981
48. Anderson DJ, Alexander NJ, Fulgham DL, Vandenbark AA, Berger DR: Immunity to tumor-associated antigens in vasectomized men. J Natl Cancer Inst 69:551, 1982
49. Anderson DJ, Narayan P, DeWolf WC: Major histocompatibility antigens are not detectable on post-meiotic human testicular germ cells. J Immunol 133:1962, 1984
50. Herr JC, Summers TA, McGee RS, Sutherland WM, Sigman M, Evans RJ: Characterization of a monoclonal antibody to a conserved epitope on human seminal vesicle specific peptides: a novel probe/marker system for semen identification. Biol Reprod 35:773, 1986
51. Hill JA, Anderson DJ, Johnson PM: Clinical relevance of recent World Health Organization workshops on human sperm and trophoblast antigens (letter). Fertil Steril 46:978, 1986
52. Anderson DJ, Alexander NJ: A new look at antifertility vaccines. Fertil Steril 40:557, 1983
53. Simon LL, Alexander NJ: Sperm antigens as immunocontraceptives. In Perspectives in Immunoreproduction: Conception and Contraception, Edited by S Mathur, CM Fredericks. Washington, DC, Hemisphere Publishing. In press
54. Ritchie AWS, Hargreave TB, James K, Chisholm GD: Intraepithelial lymphocytes in the normal epididymis: a mechanism for tolerance to sperm auto-antigens? Br J Urol 56:79, 1984
55. Taylor-Emery S, Battaile A, Anderson D: An immunohistological study of lymphoid cells in the human male reproductive tract (Abstr.). J Reprod Immunol [Suppl] 00:71, 1986
56. Taguchi O, Nishizuka Y: Experimental autoimmune orchitis after neonatal thymectomy in the mouse. Clin Exp Immunol 46:425, 1981
57. Sakaguchi S, Fukuma K, Kuribayashi K, Masuda T: Organ-specific autoimmune diseases induced in mice by elimination of T cell subset. I. Evidence for the active participation of T cells in natural self-tolerance; deficit of a T cell subset as a possible cause of autoimmune disease. J Exp Med 161:72, 1985
58. Olsen GP, Shields JW: Seminal lymphocytes, plasma and AIDS. Nature 309:116, 1984
59. Zagury D, Bernard J, Leibowitch J, Safai B, Groopman JE, Feldman M, Sarngadharan MG, Gallo RC: HTLV-III in cells cultured from semen of two patients with AIDS. Science 226:449, 1984
60. Anderson DJ, Hill JA: CD4 ($T4^+$) lymphocytes in human male reproductive tissues and semen: implications for the venereal transmission of AIDS. (Submitted for publication)
61. Maruyama DK Jr, Hale RW, Rogers BJ: Effects of white blood cells on the in vitro penetration of zona-free hamster eggs by human spermatozoa. J Androl 6:127, 1985
62. Pandya IJ, Cohen J: The leukocytic reaction of the human uterine cervix to spermatozoa. Fertil Steril 43:417, 1985
63. Rümke P: The origin of immunoglobulins in semen. Clin Exp Immunol 17:287, 1974
64. Johnson MH, Setchell BP: Protein and immunoglobulin content of rete testis fluid of rams. J Reprod Fertil 17: 403, 1968
65. Koskimies AI, Kormano M, Lahti A: A difference in the immunoglobulin content of seminiferous tubule fluid and rete testis fluid of the rat. J Reprod Fertil 27:463, 1971
66. Weininger RB, Fisher S, Rifkin J, Bedford JM: Experimental studies on the passage of specific IgG to the lumen of the rabbit epididymis. J Reprod Fertil 66:251, 1982
67. Tung KSK, Unanue ER, Dixon FJ: Pathogenesis of experimental allergic orchitis. II. The role of antibody. J Immunol 106:1463, 1971
68. Ayvaliotis B, Bronson R, Rosenfeld D, Cooper G: Conception rates in couples where autoimmunity to sperm is detected. Fertil Steril 43:739, 1985
69. Quinlivan WLG: Analysis of the proteins in human seminal plasma. Arch Biochem Biophys 127:680, 1968
70. Boettcher B: Antigens of the male tract. J Reprod Fertil Suppl 18:77, 1973
71. Husted S, Hjort T: Microtechnique for simultaneous determination of immobilizing and cytotoxic sperm antibodies: methodological and clinical studies. Clin Exp Immunol 22:256, 1975
72. Anderson DJ, Hill JA: Cell-mediated immune mechanisms in infertility. In Proceedings of the 3rd International Congress of Reproductive Immunology, Edited by DA Clark. Amsterdam, Elsevier Science Publishers. In press
73. Hill JA, Haimovici F, Politch JA, Anderson DJ: Effects of soluble products of activated lymphocytes and macrophages (lymphokines and monokines) on human sperm motion parameters. Fertil Steril. In press
74. Rümke P, Van Amstel N, Messer EN, Bezemer PD: Prognosis of fertility of men with sperm agglutinins in the serum. Fertil Steril 25:393, 1974

75. Fuchs EF, Alexander NJ: Immunologic considerations before and after vasovasostomy. Fertil Steril 40:497, 1983
76. Bronson R, Cooper G, Rosenfeld D: Sperm antibodies: their role in infertility. Fertil Steril 42:171, 1984
77. Alexander NJ: Antibodies to human spermatozoa impede sperm penetration of cervical mucus or hamster eggs. Fertil Steril 41:433, 1984
78. Hendry WF, Stedronska J, Parslow J, Hughes L: The results of intermittent high dose steroid therapy for infertility due to antisperm antibodies. Fertil Steril 36:351, 1981
79. Alexander NJ, Sampson JH, Fulgham DL: Pregnancy rates in patients treated for antisperm antibodies with prednisone. Int J Fertil 28:63, 1983
80. Kiser GC, Alexander NJ, Fuchs EF, Fulgham DL: In vitro immune absorption of antisperm antibodies by immunobead-rise, immunomagnetic and immunocolumn separation techniques. Fertil Steril. In press
81. Prakash C, Coutinho A, Möller G: Inhibition of in vitro immune responses by a fraction from seminal plasma. Scand J Immunol 5:77, 1976
82. Allen RD, Roberts TK: The relationship between the immunosuppressive and cytotoxic effects of human seminal plasma. Am J Reprod Immunol Microbiol 11:59, 1986
83. Jacobsen AH, Anderson DJ: On the role of bovine serum in seminal plasma-induced immunosuppression. Immunol Today 7:357, 1986
84. Sinigaglia F, Talmadge KW: Inhibition of [^{3}H]thymidine incorporation by *Mycoplasma arginini*-infected cells due to enzymatic cleavage of the nucleoside. Eur J Immunol 15:692, 1985
85. Tarter TH, Cunningham-Rundles S, Koide SS: Suppression of natural killer cell activity by human seminal plasma in vitro: identification of 19-OH-PGE as the suppressor factor. J Immunol 136:2862, 1986
86. Svanborg K, Bygdeman M, Eneroth P, Bendvold E: Quantification of prostaglandins in human seminal fluid. Prostaglandins 24:363, 1982
87. Goto T, Herberman RB, Maluish A, Strong DM: Cyclic AMP as a mediator of prostaglandin E-induced suppression of human natural killer cell activity. J Immunol 130:1350, 1983
88. Byrd WJ, Jacobs DM, Amoss MS: Synthetic polyamines added to cultures containing bovine sera reversibly inhibit *in vitro* parameters of immunity. Nature (London) 267:621, 1977
89. Williams-Ashman HG, Lockwood DH: Role of polyamines in reproductive physiology and sex hormone action. Ann NY Acad Sci 171:882, 1970
90. Bischof P, Martin-Du-Pan R, Lauber K, Girard JP, Herrmann WL, Sizonenko PC: Human seminal plasma contains a protein that shares physicochemical, immunochemical, and immunosuppressive properties with pregnancy-associated plasma protein-A. J Clin Endocrinol Metab 56:359, 1983
91. Schrode J, Folk JE: Transglutaminase-catalyzed crosslinking through diamines and polyamines. J Biol Chem 253:4837, 1978
92. Stites DP, Erickson RP: Suppressive effect of seminal plasma on lymphocyte activation. Nature (London) 253: 727, 1975
93. Fabbri A, Gnessi L, Perricone R, de Sanctis G, Moretti C, de Carolis C, Fontana L, Isidori A, Fraioli F: Human semen inhibits T rosette formation through an opiate mediated mechanism. J Clin Endocrinol Metab 60:807, 1985
94. Pitout MJ, Jordan JH: Partial purification of an antimitogenic factor from human semen. Int J Biochem 7: 149, 1976
95. Chvapil M, Stankova L, Bernhard DS, Zukoski CF, Drach GW: Effect of prostatic fluid and its fraction on some functions of peritoneal macrophages. Invest Urol 15:173, 1977
96. Faulk WP, Galbraith GMP: Trophoblast transferrin and transferrin receptors in the host—parasite relationship of human pregnancy. Proc R Soc Lond [Biol] 204:83, 1979
97. Morgan OS, Bankay J, Quash GA: The effect of lactoferrin, an iron-binding protein, on complement activity. West Indian Med J 24:46, 1975
98. Kijlstra A, Jeurissen SHM: Modulation of classical C3 convertase of complement by tear lactoferrin. Immunology 47:263, 1982
99. James K: Alpha-2 macroglobulin and its possible importance in immune systems. Trends Biochem Sci 5:43, 1980
100. Witkin SS, Richards JM, Bongiovanni AM, Zelikovsky G: An IgG-Fc binding protein in seminal fluid. Am J Reprod Immunol 3:23, 1983
101. Clark DA, Slapsys R, Croy BA, Krcek J, Rossant J: Local active suppression by suppressor cells in the decidua: a review. Am J Reprod Immunol 5:78, 1984
102. Lord EM, Sensabaugh GF, Stites DP: Immunosuppressive activity of human seminal plasma. I. Inhibitor of *in vitro* lymphocyte activation. J Immunol 118:1704, 1977
103. Glater GB, Anderson DJ: Seminal plasma inhibition of lysis of viral-infected target cells by natural killer cells and activated cytotoxic T cells. (Submitted for publication)
104. Glater GB, Anderson DJ: Human seminal plasma inhibits the cytotoxic effect of natural killer (NK) cells (Abstr.). J Androl 6:P-57, 1985
105. James K, Szymaniec S: Human seminal plasma is a potent inhibitor of natural killer cell activity in vitro. J Reprod Immunol 8:61, 1985
106. Rees RC, Vallely P, Clegg A, Potter CW: Suppression of natural and activated human antitumour cytotoxicity by human seminal plasma. Clin Exp Immunol 63:687, 1986
107. Tarter TH, Isahakia M: Inhibition of complement-mediated hemolysis by aqueous extracts of monkey prostate and seminal vesicle (Abstr.). J Androl 3:10, 1982
108. Tarter TH, Alexander NJ: Complement-inhibiting activity of seminal plasma. Am J Reprod Immunol 6:28, 1984
109. Brooks GF, Lammel CJ, Petersen BH, Stites DP: Human seminal plasma inhibition of antibody complement-mediated killing and opsonization of *Neisseria gonorrhoeae* and other gram-negative organisms. J Clin Invest 67: 1523, 1981
110. Stankova L, Drach GW, Hicks T, Zukoski CF, Chvapil M: Regulation of some functions of granulocytes by zinc of the prostate fluid and prostate tissue. J Lab Clin Med 88:640, 1976

111. James K, Harvey J, Bradbury AW, Hargreave TB, Cullen RT, Donaldson K: The effect of seminal plasma on macrophage function—a possible contributory factor in sexually transmitted disease. AIDS Res 1:45, 1983
112. Peterson BH, Lammel CJ, Stites DP, Brooks GF: Human seminal plasma inhibition of complement. J Lab Clin Med 96:582, 1980
113. Hurtenbach U, Shearer GM: Germ cell-induced immune suppression in mice: effect of innoculation of syngeneic spermatozoa on cell-mediated immune responses. J Exp Med 155:1719, 1982
114. Richards JM, Bedford JM, Witkin SS: Rectal insemination modifies immune responses in rabbits. Science 224: 390, 1984
115. Kuno S, Ueno R, Hayaishi O: Prostaglandin E_2 administered *via anus* causes immunosuppression in male but not female rats: a possible pathogenesis of acquired immune deficiency syndrome in homosexual males. Proc Natl Acad Sci USA 83:2682, 1986
116. Alexander NJ, Tarter TH, Ducsay CA, Fulgham DL, Huso N: Rectal absorption of semen (Abstr.). J Reprod Immunol [Suppl] 00:82, 1986
117. Ho DD, Schooley RT, Rota TR, Kaplan JC, Flynn T, Salahuddin SZ, Gonda MA, Hirsch MS: HTLV-III in the semen and blood of a healthy homosexual man. Science 226:451, 1984
118. Centifanto YM, Drylie DM, Deardourff SL, Kaufman HE: Herpesvirus type 2 in the male genitourinary tract. Science 178:318, 1972
119. Zur Hausen H: Human genital cancer: synergism between two virus infections or synergism between a virus infection and initiating events? Lancet 2:1370, 1982
120. Greenblatt RM, Handsfield HH, Sayers MH, Holmes KK: Screening therapeutic insemination donors for sexually transmitted diseases: overview and recommendations. Fertil Steril 46:351, 1986
121. Holmes KK, Mardh PA (Eds): International Perspectives on Neglected Sexually Transmitted Diseases. Washington DC, Hemisphere Publishing, 1984
122. Nahmias AJ, Naib ZM, Josay WE: Epidemiological studies relating genital herpetic infection to cervical carcinoma. Cancer Res 34:1111, 1974

Chapter 29

Immunologic influences on reproductive biology: sperm gametogenesis and maturation in the male and female genital tracts

Gilbert G. Haas, Jr., M.D.
Alan E. Beer, M.D.

University of Oklahoma Health Sciences Center, Oklahoma City, Oklahoma, and University of Michigan Medical Center, Ann Arbor, Michigan

Mammalian reproduction involves a series of events mandating either that the immune system of the host is not alerted to respond or that a response when initiated aids in the processes associated with the production, passage, or union of gametes as well as those postimplantation events attendant to a successful pregnancy. This series of events include the following: (1) the production of germ cells in an immunologically mature host long after self-tolerance is established (the male gamete expresses a variety of tissue- and organ-specific antigens not present during the individual's embryogenesis; as such, these antigens are potential targets of immune responses); (2) the union of genetically dissimilar germ cells within the reproductive tract to produce a zygote that is genetically foreign to the maternal host in that it expresses a variety of developmental, tissue-specific, and histocompatibility antigens; and (3) the eventual colonization of the female by trophoblasts locally and systemically as well as her subsequent exposure to blood cellular elements of the developing fetus. The engraftment with the mother is ended at parturition, and her immunologic system readies itself for another exposure that is also successful in the majority of cases. There are, nonetheless, many men and women in whom these normal reproductive events do not occur, and infertility or reproductive wastage after fertilization that has an immunologic basis is experienced.

PASSAGE OF SPERMATOZOA THROUGH THE MALE GENITAL TRACT

Mature sperm possess a variety of unique organ-specific and tissue-specific antigens not present in the host at the time in fetal life when immune self-recognition takes place. It is believed that during this critical time period lymphocyte clones capable of immune reactivity against "self" antigenic determinants are deleted or suppressed. In addition, there is evidence that suppressor lymphocytes present during embryogenesis play a major role in the development of immunologic tolerance to self-determinants. This process(es) prevents the development of autoimmunity in most individuals. Because spermatogenesis is not initiated until puberty, antigens unique to spermatozoa are not included in this recognition process. As a consequence of this sequence of events, postpubertal spermatogenesis must proceed in a milieu that limits the exposure of the male host's immune system to mature sperm antigens that if stimulated can result in cellular and humoral responses that are capable of destroying or inactivating sperm.

Several lines of evidence support the theory that sperm are antigenically foreign to their host and that the spontaneous formation of antisperm antibodies is a reaction against foreign antigens and does not represent a classical autoimmune phenomenon. Of special importance is the incriminating observation that male animals produce sperm antibodies if systemically inoculated with their own gametes.[1] Tung[2] suggested that both the age-related pattern of occurrence of sperm antibodies (they are found relatively early in life) and the heterogeneity of the antigenic response most closely resemble an immune response to foreign antigens, as opposed to an autoimmune phenomenon.

There are two proposed mechanisms for the prevention of an immune response to sperm in all mammalian species tested.[2] The first theory recognizes that sperm maturation occurs in the seminiferous epithelium that establishes an effective compartment shielded from the immune effectors. The tight junctions between the Sertoli cells that line the seminiferous tubules prevent antigen in effective concentrations from reaching antigen-reactive lymphocytes, at the same time blocking effector lymphocytes and antibodies from reaching the lumen of the seminiferous tubules that contain maturing sperm. The second hypothesis is that the barriers created by the tight junctions allow the passage of minute amounts of soluble sperm antigen into the host. Soluble antigen is known to activate suppressor lymphocytes involved in down-regulating cytotoxic immune responses. Similar processes occur in the thyroid gland, which develops late in ontogeny and is frequently involved in autoimmune responses. Thyroglobulin is found in trace amounts in the circulation in normal individuals. Its presence in low levels stimulates suppressor T-lymphocytes that are involved in the homeostatic mechanisms that dampen autoimmune responses.

Conditions that result in a major disruption of the blood-testis barrier are associated with the formation of sperm antibodies. Although vasectomy is the most common cause of antigen leakage,[3] other injuries, such as vas obstruction,[4] testicular trauma,[5] torsion,[6] biopsy study,[7] malignancy,[8] and genital tract infections[9] all have been associated with an increase in the incidence of sperm antibodies. Once antibodies are present in the systemic circulation, the damaged barriers in the testes or other regions of the male genital tract may allow the antibodies access to sperm. Once complexed with the sperm surface, the antibodies can interfere with sperm function.

IMMUNE PROTECTION OF SPERM DURING THEIR DEVELOPMENT

The easily identified tunica albuginea, which loosely surrounds the testicle, provides no barrier to the transfer of antigens or immunoglobulins into or out of the testicle. Radially positioned septa derived from this capsular material divide the testes into radicles containing several coiled seminiferous tubules. Interspersed between the seminiferous tubules are the testosterone-secreting Leydig cells and the lymphatic, vascular, and neuronal elements of the testes.[2, 10] The muscle-like myoid cells that surround the seminiferous tubules act as a partial barrier to the transudation of large molecules in some species[11]; however, they do not appear to perform this protective function in humans.[2] Although appropriate monoclonal antibodies have not identified lymphocytes in the interstitial space between the tubules,[12] mast cells,[13] monocytes,[13] macrophages,[14] and plasma cells[15] have been noted on light-microscopic examinations. The ratio of Leydig cells to macrophages has been estimated to be 4/1.[16] The absence of helper T cell lymphocytes within the interstitium of the seminiferous tubules has been proposed as one mechanism that lessens the possibility of immune stimulation by sperm,[12] because these cells are necessary for helping other lymphocytes in the elicitation and expression of a cytotoxic immune response.

The process of spermatogenesis can be divided into three stages: (1) mitotic division of the primary spermatogonia; (2) meiotic cell division of these sperm precursors to produce haploid spermatocytes; and (3) spermiogenesis, during which the round spermatocytes are metamorphosed into flagellated spermatozoa. The entire process takes approximately 70 days,[17] and it is not very efficient in that only one of five of the mitotic offspring of the spermatogonia successfully matures to spermatocytes.[18] This redundancy usually would be of small consequence, but excess sperm antigenic material that is potentially foreign to the host must be degraded and cleared in a manner that avoids immune stimulation of the host.

During the various stages of spermatogonial maturation, there are continual additions and deletions of spermatogenic cell surface antigens. It has been estimated that up to 50% of the antigens on mature spermatozoa were not present on spermatogonia.[19] The amount of sperm-specific antigen exponentially increases from approximately 4% to greater than 96% by the late spermatid stage.[19] As a result of this evolution of sperm antigens, even if the spermatogonia present during embryogenesis were recognized during the self-recognition process, because of the changes that occur during the maturation process of spermatozoa, mature spermatozoa would not be recognized as self by the host.

Interspersed between the spermatogonia are the nondividing Sertoli cells. These cells are attached firmly to the basement membrane of each seminiferous tubule and extend radially from this membrane toward the tubal lumen. The luminal border of the Sertoli cells possesses filagreed cytoplasmic processes that surround and nurture the maturing germ cells. The primary barrier to ingress of systemic proteins into the seminiferous tubule and egress of intratubular antigens are the special tight junctions between the abutting Sertoli cells.[20] The 40 to 50 tight junctions that exist between each pair of Sertoli cells provide what has been described as the strongest tissue barrier in the body.[21] The association between Sertoli cells is so dense that the intercellular space in some areas can be totally obliterated. This blood-testes barrier limits the transudation of molecules and cells that are involved in immune processes.[22]

The specialized junctions between Sertoli cells separate the seminiferous tubule into the basal and adluminal compartments. As the maturing gamete travels toward the seminiferous tubule lumen, newly created intercellular processes appear immediately below the migrating spermatocytes before dissolution of the more central junctions. As a result, protective cell-junction "doors" close behind the developing gametes, effectively isolating them from the immune system of the host. It can be envisioned that the developing gametes pass from the basilar compartment into a caricature of an "air lock" bounded on both sides by tight inter-Sertoli junctions. Subsequently, the more lumenally placed cell junction disperses and "releases" the developing sperm into the inner compartment, which is in communication with the tubal lumen. This air lock principle prevents inoculation of the male's immune system during spermatogenesis. At first, alterations in sperm morphologic features may merely allow formation of the distinguishing characteristics of the tailed spermatozoa, but the antigenic remodeling also may be critical to the attachment and/or detachment of the mature sperm from its nurturing Sertoli cells.

The antigens on spermatozoal precursors that can elicit an antisperm antibody response in humans have not been widely studied. In guinea pigs, autoimmune orchitis can occur only after injection into the host of germ cells that have matured beyond primary spermatocytes.[23] Similarly, passive transfer of antispermatozoal antibodies does not interfere with reproductive function until the testes of the host animals display germ cells that have matured past the stage of secondary spermatocytes.[24] In humans, this finding may explain why mumps orchitis is seen only in pubertal boys, not in prepubertal boys.

SPERM MATURATION IN THE EFFERENT DUCTS OF THE MALE GENITAL TRACT

The seminiferous tubules converge into common passageways within the central core of the testicle and eventually empty through the rete testes into the ductuli efferentes. The spermatozoa then pass, in successive order, through the epididymis, the vas deferens, and (after the addition of secretions from the prostate gland) into the urethra at the time of ejaculation. Intravenous injection of sperm antibodies results in their attachment to sperm in the rete testes but not on testicular sperm.[25] This and other data imply that the rete testes is more permeable than the seminiferous tubule to the egress of sperm antigens or ingress of circulating antisperm antibodies. However, Jones[26] noted that the concentration of sperm in the rete is only one-half that found in more distal segments of the male genital tract. This dilution of sperm antigens would lessen the possibility of massive antigen stimulation of the host even if antigen leakage occurred. In addition, the poor vascularization of the rete testis[27] may limit interplay of the intraluminal and intravascular compartments. The ductus efferentes is not totally impermeable to circulating substances of small molecular weight. This may be because the intercellular tight junctions are not numerous and do not completely surround the tubule.[28]

The epididymis is divided into three anatomic regions: the caput, corpus, and cauda. It has been suggested that sperm acquire the ability to fertilize during their 2-day[29] passage through the epididymis because of the attachment or inclusion of certain critical cell wall determinants from the epididymal fluids. Sperm also become motile during their passage through the epididymis, and motility processes appear to precede those events that will mature the sperm to fertilizing capability. Sperm can become motile when there is dissociation of the disulfide bonds that have kept the sperm tail rigid.[30] Overstreet[31] suggested that several interdependent processes render sperm capable of fertilization. These are the removal or modification of sperm components, the insertion of new chemical components onto or into the sperm membrane, and the covering or exposure of critical sperm membrane receptors or molecules through adsorption or removal of surface coats. *De novo* synthesis of surface components during epididymal passage has been detected. A variety of probes such as lectins[32] and monoclonal antibodies[33] have verified these alterations of the sperm surface. Many of the molecules involved in these processes are produced in a very limited segment of the epididymis.

Ejaculated sperm are derived from the vas deferens and cauda epididymis in a 2/3 ratio.[31] A single ejaculate apparently represents the product of 2 days of testicular sperm maturation.[29] Sperm are concentrated in the epididymis through a process of water absorption. In the area of the epididymis that contains mature spermatozoa endowed with both motility and fertilization functionality, suppressor T-lymphocytes are present in the surrounding tissues. The presence of cells that are capable of suppressing an immune response may minimize the chance of autoinoculation.[12] The mechanism by which the male genital tract disposes of sperm that are not ejaculated is of considerable interest, because this cellular material must be degraded in a manner that avoids immune stimulation of the host. Sperm that are not ejaculated may leave the male reproductive tract at the time of urination[34] or may undergo phagocytosis by intraluminal macrophages. Although the latter are not present in large numbers, they, like their counterparts in the uterus, are involved in sperm degradation. There are undoubtedly other mechanisms for the elimination of these sperm.

SPERM ANTIBODIES

Sperm in the male genital tract undergo a constant maturational evolution; therefore, antibodies directed against them may react with only a select subpopulation. For example, if the antigenic conformations of sperm change from A to B to C and an antibody forms against antigens present during the B stage of development, then the length of time the sperm is in the B stage has a direct relationship to the probability that the antibody can affect reproductive function. These conformational alterations may further inhibit a male from mounting an immune attack against his gametes. Contrariwise, the specificity of antibodies to certain stage-specific antigens in sperm development explains why only certain regions of the sperm surface bind to antibodies and why only certain steps in reproductive function can be singularly disturbed by a particular antisperm antibody-containing sera. It is not clear why sperm antibodies that form spontaneously are usually against limited numbers of sperm antigens and an individual inoculated with sperm and adjuvant produces antibodies against virtually all sperm antigens and why these antibodies often interfere with all reproductive processes.

Antibodies also can be elicited against internal sperm antigens. Although these antibodies may be sperm-specific, they have little chance of interfacing with the normal function of sperm, because living sperm maintain the integrity of their plasma membrane until they undergo the acrosome reaction. Immunocytochemical assays, such as immunofluorescence and immunoperoxidase, detect antibodies to internal sperm antigens.[35] The methanol (or acetone) used as a fixative in most of these assay techniques to increase the signal-to-noise ratio exposes subsurface sperm antigens. For this reason, the clinical usefulness of these assays is limited. For example, Tung et al.[36] detected, with the use of indirect immunofluorescence, naturally occurring antisperm antibodies in 90% of the sera of children of both sexes before puberty. It was found that these antibodies cross-reacted with certain bacteria and yeast. These antibodies appear to be directed against subsurface sperm antigens that share molecules in common with certain microorganisms. This finding nonetheless alerts us to certain pitfalls of sperm antibody assays as well as to the major problem of "immunologic background noise" in many of our assay systems. It is unfortunate that many investigators use these assays to "prove" that sperm antibodies or isolated monoclonal antibodies are against the sperm surface, even though a positive assay with these techniques often only implies that any sperm antibodies that are present are probably against internal sperm antigens.[37] Assays that employ disrupted or fixed sperm as an antigen source also may give results that are quite different from those of assays that employ intact sperm as an antigen source.[38]

It is unknown whether haploid sperm can express externally antigens coded for by their internal genome. Recent studies have failed to verify that human sperm express major histocompatibility antigens.[39] The inability of the haploid chromosomal content to express their genetic information may explain why it is difficult to separate certain subpopulations of sperm, such as those bearing a Y chromosome,[40] based upon an external expression of the sperm's karyotype. It seems logical that sperm would have limited expression of antigens that would be unique to the male partner, because that type of antigen probably would elicit an immune response in the female partner.

IMMUNOREGULATORY FACTORS

When sperm antibodies are present in a man, there are no clinical symptoms and the genital tract examination is normal. Such men are not at an increased risk to develop orchitis, and the presence of sperm antibodies in a man's genital tract is not associated with other autoimmune conditions. One possible reason for this lack of clinical symptoms is that seminal plasma is anticomplementary.[41] It has been hypothesized that activation of the alternate complement pathway by immature sperm in the female reproductive tract may aid in the selection of mature sperm that will have an increased opportunity to fertilize ova.[42] If sperm are capable of such complement activation, then the anticomplementary effect of seminal plasma may protect the sperm until they have been deposited within the female reproductive tract. The ability to activate complement decreases with the maturity of the sperm, as assessed by the region of the epididymis from which the sperm were collected.[42] This decrease in ability to bind complement gives an advantage to the most mature sperm, because they would have the greatest chance to avoid in vivo complement-mediated cytotoxicity.

The limited amount of seminal plasma complement components implies that complement-mediated cytotoxicity of antibody-bound sperm would not be possible in the male genital tract. If a paucity of complement components were the rule in the genital tracts of all men, then low sperm counts or motility could not be a sequela of the in vivo attachment of antibodies onto the sperm surface. However, certain of the complement components (C3 and C4) have been detected in men who also have sperm antibodies in their seminal plasma.[43] The presence (or leakage) of complement would allow complement-mediated events to occur in the male reproductive tract. However, no correlation has been found between the presence of sperm-associated immunoglobulins and a distinctive semen abnormality.[44-46]

It appears that circulating IgG and IgA transude into the male reproductive tract, with the seminal plasma/serum ratios being in the order of 1/100.[47] The high molecular weight of the pentameric IgM molecule presumably prevents it from transuding from the circulation.[46] The concentration of IgA varies widely; 60% to 90% of this IgA immunoglobulin is secretory IgA.[48] Rumke[47] was the first to suggest that seminal plasma IgA concentrations varied independently from other transuded proteins, implying that the male reproductive tract may be capable of a "local" immune response. Several investigators have reported that the majority of seminal plasma IgA has a molecular weight associated with the dimeric immunoglobulin molecule produced by mucosal surfaces elsewhere in the body.[49, 50]

The bulk of the first portion of an ejaculate is derived from prostatic secretions, and the subsequent portion is derived from the seminal vesicles. Because the majority of seminal plasma sperm antibodies are found in the first portion of an ejaculate, it is thought that transudation of circulating antisperm antibodies occurs via the prostate[47] or that the prostate gland is capable of mounting a local immune response following antigen stimulation.[51]

It is not known at what site in the male reproductive tract antisperm antibodies attach to the sperm surface. The male genital tract proximal to the vas deferens may be capable of mounting an effective local immune response in some instances. Linnet and Fogh-Anderson[52] noted that the presence of sperm antibodies in fluid collected from the testicular side of the vasectomy site correlates well with the subsequent fertility of these men following vasovasostomy. It has been reported[48] that in vasectomized rhesus monkeys that develop vas fistulas; antibodies can be detected on the sperm from the fistula. This indicates antibody production or transudation of immunoglobulins proximal to the vasectomy site. Although these data suggest that the more proximal regions of the male genital tract may be capable of mounting an immune response against sperm following vasectomy, another possibility is that transudation of circulating antibodies might be increased in these regions following vasectomy. This could occur secondary to surgical trauma or increased intraluminal pressure following ligation of the vas. Despite these suggestions of local immunocompetence of the proximal male reproductive tract, it has been reported[48] that the immunoglobulin concentrations in the seminal plasma of vasectomized men was no different from those in nonvasectomized controls.

Human spermatozoa can be agglutinated with infectious and physiochemical agents[53] as well as when sperm antibodies are present. The percentage of sperm that must be agglutinated to correlate with immunologically mediated events is not known, although typically in even the most severe circumstance, there are nonagglutinated sperm swimming free in the ejaculate. The type of sperm agglutination (head-to-head, etc.) does not correlate with the actual site of antibody attachment to sperm.[54]

Although IgG and IgA both are noted to attach to sperm in a single ejaculate, it appears that the two immunoglobulins attach to two different subpopulations.[55] When sperm-associated antibodies are detected by a direct immunofluorescence assay monitored with a fluorescein-activated cell sorter,[56] only a minority of sperm appear to have antibodies on their surface, even in the most antibody-positive man. This is in disagreement with assays done with the use of immunobeads.[57] Whether antibody-free sperm are the only ones capable of successful reproductive function remains problematic.[58] It could be hypothesized that if only a minority of sperm are capable of successful reproductive function, then antibody-mediated infertility could result from the binding of immunoglobulin to critical antigenic sites on those particular sperm.

The number of immunoglobulin molecules in antibody-positive sperm varies from 1 to 10 ng/1 $\times$ 10^6 sperm.[59] The number of antibody molecules occupying a particular region of the sperm surface is not known, although the combination of a sensitive assay for sperm antibodies and an accurate method of localizing an antibody's attachment site should provide this information. It is known that one IgM anti-red blood cell molecule is sufficient to lyse one red blood cell in the presence of the components of the complement cascade.

PASSAGE OF SPERMATOZOA THROUGH THE FEMALE GENITAL TRACT

VAGINA

Repeated intravaginal insemination of women with millions of spermatozoa usually is not associated with the development of immunity to sperm that leads to impaired fertility. There are several reasons for this. Studies in a variety of experimental animals have yielded data that sperm are naturally immunosuppressive (see later discussion). For this reason, the antigen-sensitizing ability of sperm is damped. In addition, the human vagina is limited in its immune affector capabilities. The human vagina has only a limited number of plasma cells beneath its epithelial surface.[60] Only sperm enter the cervical mucus; the seminal plasma remains in the vagina.[61] Thus, if sperm antibodies have not attached to sperm before they enter the cervical mucus, they will be unable to do so at a later time. IgE-mediated allergic responses to seminal plasma protein have been documented, with symptoms ranging from chronic vulvovaginitis[62] to anaphylaxis.[63] Skin testing has confirmed that this is a seminal plasma allergy, not a sperm-mediated problem[63] The use of condoms,[64] antihistamines,[62] or desensitization[63, 65] has been advocated. Although increases in the total level of circulating IgE has been associated with infertility,[66] IgE-mediated events are not an important cause of infertility. The vagina has no glandular structures (except Skene's and Bartholin glands), thus it may not be capable of mounting a local immune (secretory IgA-mediated) response to antigens placed within it. Although the placement of antigenic material in the vagina apparently has elicited an antibody response in some instances, it is difficult, if not impossible, to differentiate the response of the cervix from that of the vagina in inoculation experiments. Certainly, the seminal plasma allergies summarized above imply immunocompetence at some level in the vagina. Such a reaction results from the concomitant presence of several factors[65, 67]: (1) the ability to recognize an allergen as foreign; (2) a possible history of atopy, particularly if the inoculation occurs after delivery or hysterectomy (events that might be associated with an interval of abstinence), which somehow may increase the ability of the woman to respond to allergens presented at mucosal surfaces; and (3) deficiencies of the immunosuppressive effect of seminal plasma.

Raffi et al.[68] identified human IgG, IgM, and IgA in the vaginal fluid of hysterectomized women. Ingerslev[69] hypothesized that pure vaginal fluid from such women is merely a transudate from serum and that the vagina cannot mount a local immune response. However, physical irritation may provoke immunoglobulin production, because plasma cells capable of producing both IgA and IgG were found in biopsy specimens of prolapsed vaginas.[70] With the use of indirect immunofluorescence, Lippes et al.[60] noted localized areas of secretory piece along the vaginal surface. However, due to its superficial location, this may have been a contaminant from the cervix.

CERVIX

The cervix functions as a haven for sperm from the hostile acidic vaginal environment, a barrier to abnormal sperm, a reservoir for sperm that are slowly released or that escape into the upper regions of the female reproductive tract, a capacitating media, and a filter that allows sperm penetration while maintaining an effective barrier against the infiltration of microorganisms into the uterine cavity. Many of the functions are probably immunologically mediated.

Cervical mucus may aid in the selection of the most fertile sperm in an ejaculate by acting as both a mechanical and an immunologic filter.[58, 71, 72] This process may not be related to genetic or morphologic abnormalities of the sperm, but may simply be dependent on the percentage and vigor of sperm motility.[73] Mortimer[73] suggested that the sperm select themselves as a direct result of their level of motility. Sperm recovered from the rabbit fallopian tube or uterus are more fertile, on a percentage basis, than unselected, freshly ejaculated sperm.[71] This suggests that the female reproductive tract has removed sperm with decreased fertilization potential. Because morphologically abnormal sperm are capable of fertilizing ova,[72, 73] it is interesting that the morphologic features of human sperm within cervical secretions are significantly more normal than those of sperm in the fresh semen.[72] The normality of the sperm increases the higher the region of the female reproductive tract that is sampled. The possibility that there are a select number of sperm within any ejaculate that are capable of fertilization is bolstered by the observation that in vitro ovum penetration requires a redundant number of spermatozoa.[74]

Because the greatest gradient in total sperm number occurs at the level of the cervix,[71] the cervix may be the major site for this sperm selection process. Exactly how the cervix selects those sperm that will ascend to the higher reaches of the female reproductive tract is unclear. In fact, the cervix may not select sperm at all; perhaps sperm with greater propulsion qualities enter mucus with greater efficiency. It is known that an antibody attached to a cell usually provokes phagocytosis by macrophages or the reticuloendothelial system, effectively removing the cell and degrading it. Senescent sperm,[75] or sperm with reduced motility,[73] are eliminated from both the cervix and the uterus[76] by such mechanisms. This may be an adjunctive method for reducing the antigenic load presented to the female genital tract.

An alternative mechanism for removing antibody-laden cells from reproductive function is mediated by complement. When a single IgM molecule or two closely adjacent IgG molecules attach in close proximity on a cell, a site near the hinge region of the immunoglobulin molecule is activated, which allows the attachment of C1, the first complement component to the cell/immunoglobulin complex. Through a series of enzyme activation steps, the nine components in the complement cascade are activated sequentially. This ultimately results in the formation of a membrane attack complex that is capable of creating holes in the cell membrane to which the immunoglobulin molecule(s) is attached. If several of these membrane attack complexes are formed, they can act on the cell and result in its destruction by osmotic forces. This complex series of events is called the "classical complement pathway." The alternate complement pathway can be activated in the absence of cell-bound antibody by certain bacteria, viruses, or virus-infected cells; IgA is the intermediary in this system. There are five components of the alternate complement pathway, which, together with C3 of the classical pathway, can effect cell lysis mediated by the same membrane attack complexes produced by the classical system.[76, 77]

The quantity of complement in cervical mucus is too limited to allow protection by the classical cytolytic process, in most instances.[79] This has been determined with the use of red blood cell hemolysis assays in which antibody-coated red blood cells are exposed to the fluid to be assayed for complement activity (in this case, cervical mucus). Experiments done with the use of this assay system applied to cervical mucus have failed to demonstrate any detectable hemolysis. A more sensitive assay measures the release of ^{51}Cr bound to the surface of red blood cells if the cell is hemolyzed in the presence of complement. In one report[80] it was demonstrated that periovulatory cervical mucus from two donors contained 11.5% of the complement activity of human serum. When sperm were incubated with a 11.5% dilution of serum as a complement source and serum containing high-titered immobilizing sperm antibodies, 50% of the sperm were found to be immobilized after 4 hours. It is unclear whether parallels can be made between high-titered antisperm antibody-containing serum and results that would be expected when cervical mucus was substituted as the antibody source. Only 1% of circulating IgG and virtually no serum IgM transudes into cervical mucus from the circulation. Thus, unless a majority of the IgG in cervical mucus is directed against sperm antigens, there will be far fewer IgG molecules against sperm antigens in cervical mucus, compared with that same woman's serum. For these reasons, the 50% immobilization observed in the presence of serum antibodies may never be reached if cervical mucus is used as the antibody source. Because within a few minutes after deposition in the vagina some sperm may be found within the fallopian tube, the sperm's exposure to complement may be brief. Combined with the minimal amount of immunoglobulin and complement in cervical mucus, the ability of cervical mucus to effect complement-mediated cytolysis is doubtful, unless there are concomitant inflammatory conditions that allow transudation of these components into the mucus.

Several investigators have attempted to employ sperm immobilization as an endpoint for assays of cervical mucus antisperm antibodies.[81, 82] In these experiments, sperm were incubated with cervical mucus in the presence of a complement source and the degree of sperm immobilization or cytotoxicity was then quantitated. There is no proof that the immobilization that might have occurred was indeed complement-dependent.[83] Processes that are not immunoglobulin or complement-dependent, such as altered pH of the cervical mucus or an adverse effect of the complement source on sperm motility, may produce sperm immobilization when sperm antibodies are not present in the mucus. Because of this caveat, great care must be taken when established assays for serum antisperm antibodies, such as sperm immobilization, are used to detect cervical mucus antisperm antibodies.

It is incorrect to conclude that impaired sperm passage into or through cervical mucus is always a result of antibody-mediated events. Such thinking has led to the fallacious hypothesis that an abnormal postcoital test invariably results from the presence of antisperm antibodies. Antisperm antibodies, in most instances, do not produce hostile (scant, thick, leukocyte-containing) mucus, but instead prevent sperm from either penetrating or surviving as progressively motile cells within normal-appearing cervical mucus.

If complement-dependent and macrophage-dependent interactions with antibody-bound sperm do not occur routinely in cervical mucus, it then becomes difficult to explain how the cervix can effectively select normal sperm to reach the upper female reproductive tract. Further, it is not clear how an immunocompetent cervix is prevented from initiating an immune response against sperm. Several investigators have found that many sperm in the female reproductive tract are coated with low levels of antibodies.[2, 75, 84] Sperm that succeed in reaching the fallopian tube are not coated. Natural, or "spontaneous," antibodies have been found in virtually all pubertal women.[36] Whether these antibodies are formed as a response to cross-reacting antigens or microorganisms is unknown.[36] Hancock[85] hypothesized that these low levels of natural antibodies block the immunogenicity of the majority of sperm, similar to the blocking effect of anti-A or anti-B antibodies in ABO-incompatible matings that dampens the effect of concomitant isoimmunization against Rh antigens. This process also bears similarities to antibodies that block the immunogenicity of the trophoblast (discussed later). Harmful antisperm antibodies can be produced if the female reproductive tract is overwhelmed with antigen.[86] Whether intrauterine insemination of large amounts of sperm will also activate harmful antisperm antibodies is unknown. Sperm themselves are immunosuppressive when inseminated but not when systemically inoculated,[87] a finding that may have some bearing on the acquired immunodeficiency syndrome.[88]

The influence of the sex hormone on levels of IgG and IgA as well as on secretory component has been studied in reproductive tract secretions.[79] Estradiol induces a significant decline in the content of IgA, IgG, and secretory component in the reproductive tract secretions. However, decreases in concentrations does not indicate a decrease in transudation or production by the endocervix, because the concentration changes may merely be the result of dilutional influences. Estradiol also lowers levels of IgA and secretory component. By contrast, progesterone stimulates the local appearance of IgA-positive cells and increases tissue and intraepithelial content of IgA in the cervix. Progesterone also increases the production of secretory component, which appears to control the movement of polymeric IgA into lumenal secretions.[89] Immunoglobulins produced by tissue lymphocytes within the reproductive tissues are joined to secretory piece produced by the epithelial cells prior to their transport across the epithelium.[90] These responses are blocked by progesterone when administered with estradiol. The effect of estrogen on the uterine secretion of immunoglobulins is opposite that noted at the level of the cervix and vagina.[91]

Cervical cells in tissue culture can produce IgA and, to a lesser extent, IgG.[92] In most instances, the exposure of an antigen to a mucosal surface produces a local secretory IgA and, occasionally, a serum IgG response.[93] Evidently, the latter immune response is secondary to the absorption of significant amounts of antigen by the endocervical mucosa, which pass the antigenic message to the circulating immune system. Immunization of female rabbits by horseradish peroxidase in the cervix and vagina gives rise to both a local IgA and a serum IgG antibody response, and systemic administration of the same antigen produces only a circulating IgG or IgM response.[94] Unfortunately, the response to different antigens is not straightforward. Local administration of polio virus results in only an antibody response detectable in cervical secretions.[95] Thus the local and systemic immune response following application of antigens to the cervix may depend on the nature and amount of the inoculum as well as the mode of inoculation.

Lippes et al.,[60] with the use of fluorescein-labeled monospecific antisera to monomeric IgA, IgG, IgM, and secretory piece, reported that secretory piece, IgA, and IgG were present in the cervix of all human specimens tested; no staining for IgM was observed. Secretory piece appeared to be localized in the glandular epithelium and in the lumen of many of these cryptic glands. Rebello et al.[96] noted IgA-containing lymphoid cells in all endocervical specimens examined. These were particularly apparent at the squamocolumnar junction and beneath areas of squamous metaplasia. The epithelial basement membrane and intracellular spaces of the columnar epithelium fluoresced when antisera against IgA were used. Similar staining for IgG was observed but to a much lesser degree. There was no epithelial staining for other immunoglobulin classes. These investigators considered that the number of IgA-producing plasma cells in the upper reaches of the female genital tract (i.e., the fallopian tube and the endometrium) was too small to contribute significantly to the immunoglobulin content of the secretions of the lower genital tract (i.e., the cervix). Because the majority of the IgA noted along the epithelial surfaces of the female genital tract was in the dimeric secretory form, this suggested that very little of the IgA was derived from serum transudation.

O'Reilly et al.,[97] studying local and systemic antibody responses to *Neisseria gonorrhea*, noted a rapid rise and rapid fall in gonorrhea-specific IgA antibodies within the endocervix of women infected with the organism. The implication from these studies was that local IgA responses may require sustained antigenic stimulation for their maintenance and that cervical mucus antibodies are not a direct reflection of humoral antibody activity.

UTERUS

Austin[76] reported that the number of leukocytes dramatically increases within the rabbit uterus following a single intercourse. He believed that this leukocytosis could account for the immunologic clearing of sperm within the uterus. Collection of uterine fluid is difficult, because of the possible formation of artifacts from sampling procedures, dilutional factors secondary to the phases of the menstrual cycle, and the possibility of tissue damage due to the collection technique. Within the limits of these considerations, all of the major serum fractions, including IgG, IgM, and IgA, appear to be present in uterine fluid.[78]

The uterus appears to be a secondary reservoir for sperm in many species,[98] although the uterus functions in this capacity to a lesser extent than the cervix. The tubouterine junction appears to be another point where there is a gradient in sperm migration.[98] The complement activity in uterine fluids is low (approximately 3% of the serum level).[78] Although IgG-secreting plasma cells are numerous in the uterus, staining for IgM-secreting cells is weak and inconsistent.[60] Secretory component has been identified in the epithelial cells of the endometrial glands.[60, 96] Ingerslev[69] concluded that the rare occurrence of plasma cells beneath the normal human endometrium indicates a low possibility of immunoreactivity against sperm. He admitted that some reports suggest that a local immune response may occur in the uterus in connection with tissue inflammation and infection, but the transuding of circulating antibodies into the uterine secretions may be the primary immunoreactivity of the uterus.

FALLOPIAN TUBE

Oliphant et al.[99] reported that the ability of the oviduct to react with sperm on their way to fertilization and to preimplantation embryos as they pass toward the uterus is inhibited by complement inactivators. The concentration of immunoglobulins within oviductal fluid is approximately one-tenth the concentration of serum.[100] Although the oviduct is permeable to most serum proteins, the complement activity of fallopian tube fluid appears limited.[79, 99] Oviductal fluid appears to be derived from a combination of selected transudation from the blood as well as active secretion from its hormonally influenced epithelial tissues. Collection of fallopian tube fluid is extremely difficult, because indwelling catheters, particularly when positioned for immunologic studies, may increase the vascular permeability of the fallopian tube due to a local inflammatory response.[69] Despite these problems, Yang et al.[101] found that the complement activity in tubal fluid is $< 10\%$ of the activity of the corresponding serum sample and is virtually absent in some specimens.[96] Yang et al.[101] noted that IgM occasionally could be detected in rhesus monkey oviductal fluid, a finding also reported for human tubal fluid. Similar to cervical mucus immunoglobulins, tubal fluid antibodies are noted to undergo a midcycle periovulatory decrease.[101] This implies that the concentration of tubal immunoglobulins are low during the periovulatory period, when sperm migration and fertilization occur. Oliphant et al.[100] reported that fallopian tube IgG, IgA, and IgM levels were 4%, 24%, and 2% of serum levels. Some investigators[102] found that tubal fluid antibodies against acrosin may prevent proteolytic digestion of the tube by this enzyme. This enzyme normally is released before ovum penetration.

Haney et al.[103] reported that oviductal macrophages can be found in all women; they hypothesized that the source of the macrophages was the peritoneal cavity. It has been noted that sperm death increases the ability of the sperm to opsonize or activate macrophages.[104] This may be a mechanism for clearing senescent sperm from the female reproductive tract while preventing cell-mediated immune attack on living sperm in areas of the female genital tract that contain macrophages (e.g., the fallopian tube).

Immunoglobulin-producing plasma cells have been found beneath the epithelium of the fallopian tube in humans,[60] but the results in the literature are so diverse as not to provide a sufficient basis for resolution of the question of whether the fallopian tube is capable of mounting a local secretion of IgA.[69] Ingerslev[69] concluded from the information available in the present literature that circulating antibodies may be detectable only in small amounts in tubal fluid.

FOLLICULAR FLUID

Follicular fluid appears to be an ultrafiltrate of plasma. The levels of follicular fluid immunoglobulins are virtually identical to serum levels. Follicular fluid also appears to contain all of the components necessary to support the complement cascade.[79] Whether follicular fluid components remain associated with the cumulus mass surrounding the ova is unknown. Similarly, it is unknown whether immunoglobulin and complement components derived from peritoneal fluid are important in mediating events involving the ova. Plasma cells have not been observed in ovarian follicles.[69]

SPERM MATURATION IN THE FEMALE REPRODUCTIVE TRACT

Sperm must be altered before they can penetrate ova; this process is called capacitation. Although human sperm do not demonstrate obvious morphologic differences between capacitated and noncapacitated sperm, it is not known whether the two sperm populations could be separated by antigenic differences. It is highly probable that some form of "receptor" on the sperm surface interacts with the sperm's environment to effect capacitation. It is also possible that if an immunoglobulin molecule attached and covered or altered this "receptor," capacitation might be inhibited. The difficulty in identifying the process of capacitation in human sperm has made study of this physiologic event difficult. The use of monoclonal antibodies against the sperm surface has shown that exposure of sperm to capacitating conditions results in a redistribution of the sperm surface antigens.[105] Other investigators have implied that the antigenic makeup of the sperm surface can be divided into distinct regions, each with its own antigenic specificities. Sperm antigens maintain a certain fluidity over the sperm surface prior to exposure to capacitating conditions, but following capacitation their domain becomes more restricted.[106] What is most evident from multiple studies reported in the literature is that the sperm membrane is a dynamic surface that is constantly varying its presentation to its environment. These changes not only include the gross vesiculation of membranes that occurs with the acrosome reaction immediately prior to fertilization, but also involve more subtle changes that occur prior to this event. How these alterations in the antigenic makeup of the sperm surface affect reproductive function in vivo is unknown.

REFERENCES

1. Freund J, Lipton MM, Thompson GE: Aspermatogenesis in the guinea-pig induced by testicular tissues and adjuvants. J Exp Med 97:711, 1953
2. Tung KSK: Autoimmunity of the testis. In Immunological Aspects of Infertility and Fertility Regulation, Edited by DS Dhindsa, GFB Schumacher. New York, Elsevier-North Holland, 1980, p 33
3. Alexander NJ, Anderson DJ: Vasectomy: consequences of autoimmunity to sperm antigens. Fertil Steril 32:253, 1979
4. Hendry WF, Parslow J, Stedronska J, Wallace DMA: The diagnosis of unilateral testicular obstruction in subfertile males. Br J Urol 54:774, 1982
5. Haensch R: Spermatozoen-autoimmunphaenomehe bei genitaltraumen und verschlubbazoospermie. Andrologia 5:147, 1973
6. Mastrogiacomo I, Zanchetta R, Graziotti P, Betterle C, Scrufari P, Lembo A. Immunological and clinical study in patients after spermatic cord torsion. Andrologia 14:25, 1982
7. Hjort T, Husted S, Linnet-Jepsen P: The effect of testis biopsy on autosensitization against spermatozoal antigens. Clin Exp Immunol 18:201, 1974
8. Guazziero S, Lembo A, Ferro G, Artibani W, Merlo F, Zanchetta R, Pagano F: Sperm antibodies and infertility in patients with testicular cancer. Urology 26:139, 1985
9. Witkin SS, Toth A: Relationship between genital tract infections, sperm antibodies in seminal fluid, and infertility. Fertil Steril 40:805, 1983
10. deKretser DM: Light and electron microscopic anatomy of the normal human testis. In Male Reproductive Function, Edited by RJ Santen, RS Swerdloff. New York, Marcel Dekker, Inc., 1986 p 3
11. Fawcett DW, Leak LV, Heidger PM: Electron microscopic observation on the structural components of the blood-testis barrier. J Reprod Fertil Suppl 10:105, 1970
12. El-Demiry, Hargreave TB, Busuttil A, James K, Ritchie AWS, Chisholm GD: Lymphocyte sub-populations in the male genital tract. Br J Urol 57:569, 1985
13. Hermol L, Lalli M: Monocytes and mast cells in the limiting membrane of human seminiferous tubules. Biol Reprod 19:92, 1978
14. Tung KSK, Han L-PB, Evan AP: Differentiation autoantigen of testicular cells and spermatozoa in the guinea pig. Dev Biol 68:224, 1979
15. Tung KSK, Alexander NJ: Monocytic orchitis and spermatogenesis in normal and vasectomized rhesus macaques (*Macaca mulatta*). Am J Pathol 101:17, 1980
16. Christensen AK: Discussion of the chapter: Robin BS, Nankin HR, Troen P: Immunologic studies of patients with idiopathic oligospermia. In The Testis in Normal and Infertile Men, Edited by P Troen, HR Nankin. New York, Raven Press, 1977, p 444
17. Heller CH, Clermont Y: Kinetics of the germinal epithelium in man. Recent Prog Horm Res 20:545, 1964
18. Huckins C: The morphology and kinetics of spermatogonial degeneration in normal adult rats: an analysis using a simplified classification of the germinal epithelium. Anat Rec 190:905, 1978
19. Romrell LJ, O'Rand MG: Capping and ultrastructural localization of sperm surface isoantigens during spermatogenesis. Dev Biol 63:76, 1978
20. Dym M, Fawcett DW: The blood-testis barrier in the rat and the physiological compartmentation of the seminiferous epithelium. Biol Reprod 3:308, 1970
21. Friend DS, Gilula NB: Variations in tight and gap junctions in mammalian tissues. J Cell Biol 53:758, 1972
22. Howards SS, Jessee SJ, Johnson AL: Micropuncture studies of the blood-seminiferous tubule barrier. Biol Reprod 14:264, 1976
23. Katsh S: Localization and identification of antispermatogenic factor in guinea pig testicles. Int Arch Allergy Appl Immunol 16:241, 1960
24. Bishop DW, Narbaitz R, Lessof M: Induced aspermatogenesis in adult guinea pigs injected with testicular antigen and adjuvant in neonatal stages. Dev Biol 3:444, 1961
25. Tung KSK, Unanue ER, Dixon FJ: Pathogenesis of experimental allergic orchitis II: the roles of antibody. J Immunol 106:1463, 1971
26. Jones RC: The nature of the barrier to autoimmunity in the excurrent ducts of the mammalian testes. In Immunological Influences on Human Fertility, Edited by B Boettcher. New York, Academic Press, 1977, p 67
27. Kormana M, Reijonen K: Microvascular structure of the human epididymis. Am J Anat 145:23, 1976
28. Suzuki F, Nagano T: Regional differentiation of cell junctions in the excurrent duct epithelium of the rat testis as revealed by freeze-fracture. Anat Rec 191:503, 1978
29. Amann RP, Howards SS: Daily spermatozoal production and epididymal spermatozoal reserves of the human male. J Urol 124:211, 1980

30. Bedford JM, Calvin H, Cooper GW: The maturation of spermatozoa in the human epididymis. J Reprod Fertil (Suppl) 18:199, 1973
31. Overstreet JW: Human sperm function: acquisition in the male and expression in the female. In Male Reproductive Function, Edited by RJ Santen, RW Swerdloff. New York, Marcel Dekker, Inc., 1986, p 29
32. Olson GE, Orgebin-Crist M-C: Sperm surface changes during epididymal maturation. Ann NY Acad Sci 383: 372, 1982
33. Eddy EM, Vernon RB, Muller CH, Hahnel AC, Fenderson BA: Immunodissection of sperm surface modifications during epididymal maturation. Am J Anat 174: 225, 1985
34. Prins GS, Zaneveld LJD: Radiographic study of fluid transport in the rabbit vas deferens during sexual rest and after sexual activity. J Reprod Fertil 58:311, 1980
35. Boettcher B, Hjort T, Rumke P: Auto- and iso-antibodies to antigens of the human reproductive system. I. Results of an international comparative study. Clin Exp Immunol 30:173, 1977
36. Tung KSK, Cooke WD, McCarty TA, Robitaille P: Human sperm antigens and antibodies. II. Age related incidence of antisperm antibodies. Clin Exp Immunol 25:73, 1976
37. Jones R, Brown CR, Cran DG, Gaunt SJ: Surface and internal antigens of rat spermatozoa distinguished using monoclonal antibodies. Gamete Res 8:255, 1983
38. Hancock RJT, Faruki S: Detection of anti-sperm activities of monoclonal antibodies to human sperm. J Reprod Immunol 7:215, 1985
39. Haas GG Jr, Nahhas F: Failure to identify HLA ABC and Dr antigens on human sperm. Am J Reprod Immunol Microbiol 10:39, 1986
40. Hoppe PC, Koo GC: Reacting mouse sperm with monoclonal H-Y antibodies does not influence sex ratio of eggs fertilized in vitro. J Reprod Immunol 6:1, 1984
41. Price RJ, Roberts TK, Green D, Boettcher B: Anticomplementary activity in human semen and its possible importance in reproduction. Am J Reprod Immunol 6:92, 1984
42. Witkin SS, Richards JM, Bedford JM: Influence of epididymal maturation on the capacity of hamster and rabbit spermatozoa for complement activation. J Reprod Fertil 69:517, 1983
43. Quinlivan WLG, Sullivan H: Antispermatozoal effects of human seminal plasma—an immunologic phenomenon. Fertil Steril 27:1194, 1976
44. Cerasaro M, Valenti M, Massacesi A, Lenzi A, Dondero F: Correlation between the direct IgG MAR test (mixed antiglobulin reaction test) and seminal analysis in men from infertile couples. Fertil Steril 44:390, 1985
45. Haas GG Jr, Schreiber AD, Blasco L: The incidence of sperm-associated immunoglobulins and C3, the third component of complement, in infertile men. Fertil Steril 39:542, 1983
46. Clarke GN, Elliott PJ, Smaila C: Detection of sperm antibodies in semen using the immunobead test: a survey of 813 consecutive patients. Am J Reprod Immunol Microbiol 7:118, 1985
47. Rumke P: The origin of immunoglobulins, in semen. Clin Exp Immunol 17:287, 1974
48. Reported by Hjort T (workshop chairman): Immunological capacity of the male genital tract. In Immunological Influence on Human Infertility, Edited by B Boettcher. New York, Academic Press, 1977, p 114
49. Uehling DT: Secretory IgA in seminal fluid. Fertil Steril 22:769, 1971
50. Witkin SS, Zelikovsky G, Good RA, Day N: Demonstration of 11s IgA antibody to spermatozoa in human seminal fluid. Clin Exp Immunol 44:368, 1981
51. Ablin RJ, Soanes WA, Gonder MJ: *In vivo* bound immunoglobulin in the human prostate—their identification and possible significance. Immunitaetsforsch 144:233, 1972
52. Linnet L, Fogh-Anderson P: Vasovasostomy: sperm agglutinins in operatively obtained epididymal fluid and in seminal plasma before and after operation. J Clin Lab Immunol 2:245, 1979
53. Hekman A, Rumke P: Seminal antigens and autoimmunity. In Human Semen and Fertility Regulation in Men, Edited by ESE Hafez, St. Louis, CV Mosby Co., 1976, p 245
54. Kay DJ, Boettcher B: Common specificities of auto- and iso-antibodies to human spermatozoa. Am J Reprod Immunol Microbiol 8:10, 1985
55. Haas GG Jr, Nahhas F: Unpublished data
56. Haas GG Jr, Cunningham ME: Identification of antibody-laden sperm by cytofluorometry. Fertil Steril 42:606, 1984
57. Bronson RA, Cooper GW, Rosenfeld D: Autoimmunity to spermatozoa: effect on sperm penetration of cervical mucus as reflected by postcoital testing. Fertil Steril 41:609, 1984
58. Cohen J, Gregson SH: Antibodies and sperm survival in the female genital tract. In Spermatozoa, Antibodies and Infertility, Edited by J Cohen, WF Hendry. Oxford, Blackwell Scientific Publications, 1978, p 17
59. Haas GG Jr, Nahhas FN: Quantitation of antisperm antibodies by an indirect inhibition assay. (Abstr.) J Androl 7:P-15, 1986
60. Lippes J, Ogra S, Tomasi TB Jr, Tourville DR: Immunohistological localization of γ G, γ A, γ M secretory piece and lactoferrin in the human female genital tract. Contraception 1:163, 1970
61. Asch RH, Balmaceda J, Pauerstein CJ: Failure of seminal plasma to enter the uterus and oviducts of the rabbit following artificial insemination. Fertil Steril 28:671, 1977
62. Chang T-W: Familial allergic seminal vulvovaginitis. Am J Obstet Gynecol 126:442, 1976
63. Halpern BN, Ky T, Robert B: Clinical and immunological study of an exceptional case of reaginic type sensitization to human seminal fluid. Immunology 12:247, 1967
64. Reunala T, Koskimies AI, Björksten F, Jänne J, Lassus A: Immunoglobulin E-mediated severe allergy to human seminal plasma. Fertil Steril 28:832, 1977
65. Friedman SA, Bernstein IL, Enrione M, Marcus ZH: Successful long-term immunotherapy for human seminal plasma anaphylaxis. JAMA 251:2684, 1984
66. Mathur S, Williamson HO, Baker ER, Fudenberg HH: Immunoglobulin E levels and antisperm antibody titers in infertile couples. Am J Obstet Gynecol 140:923, 1981
67. Levine BB, Siraganian RP, Schenkein I: Allergy to human seminal plasma. N Engl J Med 288:894, 1973
68. Raffi RO, Moghissi KS, Sacco AG: Proteins of human vaginal fluid. Fertil Steril 28:1345, 1977

69. Ingerslev HJ: Antibodies against spermatozoal surface-membrane antigens in female infertility. Acta Obstet Gynecol Scand (Suppl) 100:6, 1981
70. Lai A Fat RFM, Cormane RH, Van Furth R: An immuno-histopathological study on the synthesis of immunoglobulins and complement in normal and pathological skin and adjacent mucous membranes. Br J Dermatol 90:123, 1974
71. Cohen J, McNaughton DC: Spermatozoa: the probable selection of a small population by the genital tract of the female rabbit. J Reprod Fertil 39:297, 1974
72. Barros C, Vigil P, Herrera E, Arguello B, Walker R: Selection of morphologically abnormal sperm by human cervical mucus. Arch Androl (Suppl) 12:95, 1984
73. Mortimer D: Selectivity of sperm transport in the female genital tract. In Spermatozoa, Antibodies and Infertility, Edited by J Cohen, WF Hendry. Oxford, Blackwell Scientific Publications, 1978, p 37
74. Wolf DP: The block to sperm penetration in zona-free mouse eggs. Dev Biol 64:1, 1978
75. Symons DBA, Herbert J: Incidence of immunoglobulins in fluids of the rabbit genital tracts and the distribution of IgG-globulin in the tissues of the female tract. J Reprod Fertil 24:55, 1971
76. Austin CR: Fate of spermatozoa in the uterus of the mouse and rat. J Endocrinol 14:335, 1957
77. Adams DD: Autoimmune mechanisms. In Autoimmune Endocrine Disease, Edited by TF Davies. New York, John Wiley & Sons, 1983, p 1
78. Lint TF: Complement. In Immunological Aspects of Infertility and Fertility Regulation, Edited by DS Dhindsa, GFB Schumacher. New York, Elsevier-North Holland, 1980, p 13
79. Schumacher GFB: Humoral immune factors in the female reproductive tract and their changes during the cycle. In Immunological Aspects of Infertility and Fertility Regulation, Edited by DS Dhindsa, GFB Schumacher. New York, Elsevier-North Holland, 1980, p 93
80. Price RJ, Boettcher B: The presence of complement in human cervical mucus and its possible relevance to infertility in women with complement-dependent sperm-immobilizing antibodies. Fertil Steril 32:61, 1979
81. Moghissi KS, Sacco AG, Borin K: Immunologic infertility. I. Cervical mucus antibodies and postcoital test. Am J Obstet Gynecol 136:941, 1980
82. Menge AC, Medley NE, Mangione CM, Dietrich JW: The incidence and influence of antisperm antibodies in infertile human couples on sperm-cervical mucus interactions and subsequent fertility. Fertil Steril 38:439, 1982
83. Jager S, Kremer J, De Wilde-Janssen IW: Are sperm immobilizing antibodies in cervical mucus an explanation for a poor postcoital test? Am J Reprod Immunol 5:56, 1984
84. Cohen J, Werrett DJ: Antibodies and sperm survival in the female tract of the mouse and rabbit. J Reprod Fertil 42:301, 1975
85. Hancock RJT: Sperm antigens and sperm immunogenicity. In Spermatozoa, Antibodies and Infertility, Edited by J Cohen, WF Hendry. Oxford, Blackwell Scientific Publications, 1978 p 1
86. Schwimmer WB, Ustay KA, Behrman SJ: Sperm-agglutinating antibodies and increased fertility in prostitutes. Obstet Gynecol 30:192, 1967
87. Hancock RJT, Popham AM, Faruki S, Dresser DW: Increases in the numbers of immunoglobulin-secreting cells in lymph nodes responding to sperm and other stimuli: possible relationship to immunosuppression. Immunology 55:233, 1985
88. Hurtenback U, Shearer GM: Germ cell-induced immune suppression in mice: effect of inoculation of syngeneic spermatozoa on cell-mediated immune responses. J Exp Med 155:1719, 1982
89. Murdoch AJM, Buckley CH, Fox H: Hormonal control of the secretory immune system of the human uterine cervix. J Reprod Immunol 4:23, 1982
90. van Kooij RJ, Kathmann GA, Kramer MF: Secretory piece and plasma protein in human cervical mucus during the cycle. J Reprod Fertil 68:63, 1983
91. Wira CR, Sandoe CP: Hormonal regulation of immunoglobulins: influence of estradiol on immunoglobulins A and G in the rat uterus. Endocrinology 106:1020, 1980
92. Behrman SJ, Liebeman ME: Biosynthesis of immunoglobulins by the human cervix. In The Biology of the Cervix, Edited by RJ Blandau, KS Moghissi. Chicago, University of Chicago Press, 1973, p 235
93. Bell EB, Wolf B: Antibody synthesis in vitro by the rabbit vagina against diptheria toxoid. Nature 214:423, 1967
94. McAnulty PA, Morton DB: The immune response of the genital tract of the female rabbit following systemic and local immunization. J Clin Lab Immunol 1:255, 1978
95. Ogra PL, Ogra SS: Local antibody responses to polio vaccine in the human female genital tract. J Immunol 110:1307, 1973
96. Rebello R, Green FHY, Fox H: A study of the secretory immune system of the female genital tract. Br J Obstet Gynaecol 82:812, 1975
97. O'Reilly RJ, Lee L, Welch BG: Secretory IgA antibody response to *Neisseria gonorrhoeae* in the genital secretions of infected females. J Infect Dis 133:113, 1976
98. Overstreet JW, Cooper GW: Sperm transport in the reproductive tract of the female rabbit: II. The sustained phase of transport. Biol Reprod 19:115, 1978
99. Oliphant G, Cabot C, Ross P, Marta J: Control of the humoral immune system within the rabbit oviduct. Biol Reprod 31:205, 1984
100. Oliphant G, Randall P, Cabot CL: Immunological components of rabbit fallopian tube fluid. Biol Reprod 16: 463, 1977
101. Yang S-L, Schumacher GFB, Broer KA, Holt JA: Specific antibodies and immunoglobulins in the oviductal fluid of the rhesus monkey. Fertil Steril 39:359, 1983
102. Go KJ, Mastroianni L Jr, Stambaugh R: Inhibition of acrosin by oviductal secretory immunoglobulin A. Gamete Res 4:15, 1981
103. Haney AF, Misukonis MA, Weinberg JB: Macrophages and infertility: oviductal macrophages as potential mediators of infertility. Fertil Steril 39:310, 1983
104. Vogelpoel FR, Verhoef J: Activation of polymorphonuclear leukocytes by spermatozoa. Arch Androl 14:123, 1985
105. Myles DG, Primakoff P: Localized surface antigens of guinea pig sperm migrate to new regions prior to fertilization. J Cell Biol 99:1634, 1984
106. O'Rand MG: Modification of the sperm membrane during capacitation. Ann NJ Acad Sci 383:392, 1982

Chapter 30

Screening therapeutic insemination donors for sexually transmitted diseases: overview and recommendations

Ruth M. Greenblatt, M.D.
H. Hunter Handsfield, M.D.
Merlin H. Sayers, M.D., Ph.D.
King K. Holmes, M.D., Ph.D.

University of Washington, Seattle-King County Department of Public Health, and Puget Sound Blood Center, Seattle, Washington

In the past 20 years demand for therapeutic insemination by donor has risen sharply. The trend is temporally related to a fall in the number of infants available for adoption as well as to increased acceptance of the procedure. Recent estimates of yearly United States births of infants conceived by therapeutic insemination by donor range from 6000 to 10,000.[1] Each conception is the result of an average of 6 to 7 inseminations, with a range up to 200.[1] Some institutions mix the semen of multiple donors before administering it.[1] Thus, a donor insemination recipient may be exposed to the semen of many donors before conceiving.

Like blood products, semen has been implicated in transmission of a variety of viral pathogens, including hepatitis B virus,[2] cytomegalovirus (CMV),[3] and the retrovirus associated with the acquired immunodeficiency syndrome (AIDS).[4] The latter has been named lymphadenopathy-associated virus (LAV), human T-cell lymphotropic virus type III (HTLV-III), AIDS-associated retrovirus (ARV), and most recently, human immunodeficiency virus (HIV).[5] In this paper, the terms HIV and "AIDS virus" are used to designate any or all of these isolates. Herpes simplex virus (HSV) and human papilloma virus (HPV) are known to infect the urethra and might be transmitted via semen, although HSV is rarely isolated from semen in the absence of overt herpetic lesions.

Semen can be contaminated not only with viral agents, but also with *Neisseria gonorrhoeae* or *Chlamydia trachomatis*, and transmission of gonorrhea via donor insemination has been reported.[6, 7] Spermatozoa have been considered a possible vehicle for carriage of both of these pathogens into the upper genital tract of women.[8]

Treponema pallidum could theoretically also be transmitted via semen, and bacterial agents of lower or uncertain pathogenicity, such as group B streptococcus, *Ureaplasma urealyticum, Mycoplasma hominis,* and *Gardnerella vaginalis* undoubtedly are common contaminants of semen from donors.[9, 10] *Trichomonas vaginalis*, a sexually transmitted protozoan, also can be found in the urethras of asymptomatic men.

These sexually transmitted pathogens are associated with a wide variety of disease states in women, ranging from mild infection of the vagina to severe invasive bacterial infections of the upper genital tract that may cause tubal scarring, and severe systemic viral infections, now including AIDS. In pregnancy, complications caused by certain of these pathogens include abortion, chorioamnionitis, premature rupture of the fetal membranes, premature delivery, stillbirth, and perinatal death, as well as congenital and perinatal infectons and postpartum endometritis. Complications in surviving newborns include blindness, deafness, developmental anomalies, psychomotor retardation, and more subtle intellectual impairment.

The risk of infection with genital pathogens through donor insemination has not been systematically studied (as it should be). However, the high prevalences of one or more of these sexually transmitted diseases (STDs) in all populations that have been studied suggest that the risk must be substantial. The infrequency of reported disease transmission by this route does not necessarily denote a low risk, because the acute infections commonly are subclinical, the link between the long-term complications and the insemination procedure may not be perceived, and because the specific etiologies of the chronic manifestations usually are not known. Guidelines for minimizing the risk of these consequences can be formulated now only on the basis of estimates of the prevalence of each of these infections in semen donors and the probable morbidity associated with each infection for the semen recipient, the conceptus, and the spouse.

VIRAL INFECTIONS

HEPATITIS B VIRUS

In the United States the prevalence of hepatitis B surface antigen (HBsAg) carriage in serum was estimated in 1975 to be 0.13% in whites, 0.55% in blacks, and 2.3% in Orientals.[11] HBsAg has been found in the semen of 10 of 18 men with HBsAg in serum,[12] and there is clear epidemiologic evidence of heterosexual transmission of hepatitis B virus, especially from male to female.[2, 13-15]

The risks of acute hepatitis B virus infection during early pregnancy as a result of therapeutic insemination by donor include maternal hepatitis B, in utero infection of the fetus, and perinatal infection transmitted to the infant at delivery. There are few data on the morbidity of hepatitis B during early pregnancy. Fulminant hepatitis B has been described in pregnancy,[16, 17] but available data suggest that the risks of this complication or of chronic active or chronic persistent hepatitis, or of the viral carrier state are not increased in pregnancy. In utero infection is less common than transmission to the neonate at birth.[16-19]

The incubation period for hepatitis B is 40 to 180 days[13]; in 92% of nonpregnant hospitalized adults with acute hepatitis B, the duration of HBsAg in serum was less than 16 weeks from the date of hospitalization.[20] Therefore, hepatitis B virus infection acquired at the time of insemination appears relatively unlikely to result in perinatal transmission at delivery, unless the duration of HBsAg carriage is longer in pregnancy than in the nonpregnant state. More data are needed on the natural history of hepatitis B in early pregnancy. Maternal hepatitis B apparently is not associated with an increased risk of congenital malformation, stillbirth, abortion, or low birth weight.[21] However, premature delivery has been related to maternal hepatitis, occurring in 32% and 35% of pregnancies complicated by hepatitis B in two studies[21, 15]; prematurity was thought to be independent of whether or not the infant was infected.

The majority of infants acquiring hepatitis B virus infection remain anicteric and have no clinical signs of hepatitis B, but suffer prolonged HBsAg carriage, which is later associated with chronic active hepatitis,[17] postnecrotic cirrhosis, primary hepatocellular carcinoma,[22] and the potential for future horizontal or vertical transmission.

In summary, hepatitis B virus infection acquired at or before conception probably carries the same morbidity as in nonpregnant women and poses a poorly defined but probably small risk of in utero or perinatal transmission to the newborn. Nonetheless, hepatitis B is a serious, potentially life-threatening infection and may lead to premature delivery. Transmission via donor semen is undoubtedly possible, although not yet described. HBsAg can be detected quickly, accurately, and inexpensively in the serum of potential semen donors by readily available methods.

CYTOMEGALOVIRUS

The prevalence of serum antibody to cytomegalovirus (MV) varies widely, depending on geographic region, socioeconomic status, and sexual behavior.[23] Sexual intercourse is probably the major route of acquisition of primary CMV infection among young heterosexual women, including pregnant women.[3, 24] Among San Francisco men 18 to 29 years of age, the prevalence of antibody to CMV was 36% in unselected blood donors and 47% in heterosexual male patients at an STD clinic.[25] Among urban homosexually active men, 93% to 100% have been seropositive.[25, 26] The majority of seropositive immunocompetent individuals are asymptomatic and probably shed virus only intermittently. Among 28 seropositive men studied,[27] 4 (14%) had positive cultures for CMV in semen; this may be a falsely low figure, since it is necessary to dilute semen to avoid host cell cytotoxicity. In another study, CMV was recovered from two of three single semen samples from heterosexual male partners of women who had positive cultures for CMV.[3] By contrast, of 32 CMV seropositive homosexual men who submitted semen and urine cultures four or more times over 10 to 30 months, 72% were culture-positive at least once.[26]

Primary CMV infection during pregnancy resulted in congenital infection in nearly 50% of pregnancies in women of middle and upper income groups studied by Stagno et al.,[28] who concluded that primary infection during pregnancy is more likely than recurrent infection to result in severe, clinically apparent neonatal disease, a conclusion supported by other studies as well. Although published data are not yet conclusive, primary CMV infection in early pregnancy may carry the greatest risk of severe congenital infection and in fact might well represent the major preventable cause of birth defects in the offspring resulting from therapeutic insemination by donor. Thus, a CMV-seronegative woman who receives semen containing CMV is at high risk for acquiring primary CMV infection and, if she conceives, of transmitting infection to the fetus, with attendant consequences of congenital CMV infection. It is not known whether exposure of a seropositive woman to a heterologous strain of CMV carries a risk of infection of the woman or the conceptus by the heterologous strain. Therefore, it may be safer to employ CMV-seronegative donors for all recipients, regardless of the recipient's serologic status.

Freezing of blood products has been shown to decrease the concentration of CMV in blood and, in studies involving historical controls, to reduce the risk of CMV transmission by transfusion.[29-31] It is not yet known whether freezing semen would have a similar effect, because the concentrations of CMV in infected semen are substantially higher than in blood. Because of the special risk associated with primary CMV infection in gestation, CMV-seronegative women certainly should not receive fresh (unfrozen) semen from donors with serum antibody to CMV. The safety of frozen semen with respect to CMV is unknown and requires further study.

HUMAN IMMUNODEFICIENCY VIRUS

The prevalence of serum antibody to the AIDS virus varies with the population examined, from 77% in some hemophiliacs[32] to 0.01% in female blood donors.[33] The prevalence of Western blot-confirmed antibody to HIV in male blood donors during 1985 was approximately 0.1%.[34] Among urban homosexually active men from geographic areas where AIDS is common, the reported prevalence of seropositivity has been as high as 20% to 80%.[35]

HIV has been recovered from mononuclear cells in the semen of individuals in groups with high prevalences of AIDS, including 4 of 19 men at risk for AIDS,[36] and two of two AIDS patients,[37] and from both semen and blood of an apparently healthy homosexual man.[38] HIV was transmitted to four of eight recipients of therapeutic insemination who received semen from a single asymptomatic bisexual man.[4] Among women given semen from this donor, seroconversion occurred in all four given semen stored frozen for 1 to 4 months and in none of four given semen stored frozen for 16 to 17 months.

Data are inadequate on whether pregnancy may influence the risk of development of AIDS or AIDS-related complex (ARC) in women infected with the AIDS virus. For example, in one study, 12 of 16 seropositive women who gave birth to an infant with AIDS later developed AIDS or ARC themselves.[39] The risk of developing AIDS or ARC in seropositive homosexual men has recently been estimated to be about 25% during follow-up periods of up to 5 years.[40]

Although data are not conclusive, the course of pregnancy itself might be affected by maternal AIDS virus infection; for example, three pregnancies of one infected mother each terminated with premature delivery.[41] Among 26 infants with AIDS for whom gestational age was determined, 10 (38%) were premature (less than 37 weeks' gestation).[42]

Vertical transmission of AIDS virus has been documented, but the overall risk and relative importance of in utero transmission, perinatal transmission at delivery, and postpartum transmission by breast-feeding or other mechanisms are not well defined. AIDS virus infection has been identified in several infants delivered by cesarean section[41, 43] and in an infant nursed by a mother who acquired HIV from a postpartum blood transfusion.[44] Rates of perinatal AIDS virus transmission varied among the three available retrospective studies from 65% in infants of 13 women who had previously given birth to infants with AIDS[39] to none of three infants born to women who seroconverted after therapeutic insemination.[4] Preliminary evidence suggests that infected newborns have a substantially higher incidence than adults of developing overt, ultimately fatal AIDS, with a risk of 50% or more during the first 2 years of life.

Thus, AIDS virus transmission represents a major, if uncommon, hazard of therapeutic insemination by donor. Anecdotal information from donor insemination programs, and from patients attending our own STD clinic, suggests that homosexual men have frequently served as semen donors in the recent past.

Men belonging to groups at high risk for AIDS should be excluded as potential donors of semen, and all other potential donors should be serologically tested for antibody to the AIDS virus; seropositive men should be permanently excluded as semen donors. These recommendations are analogous to the now standard practice for blood donations. Enzyme-linked immunosorbent assays (ELISA) for AIDS virus antibody are inexpensive and widely available.[45] Prolonged storage of frozen semen may further reduce the risk of transmission, but the effect of freezing and storage of semen on survival of HIV requires study.

The time from acquisition of AIDS virus infection until seroconversion is not well defined, but was 4 to 12 weeks in a study of men with presumed acute AIDS virus infection.[46] Therefore, even seronegative men outside the high-risk groups should be excluded as donors if they have changed sexual partners or otherwise had any potential risk of AIDS virus exposure in the preceding 3 months. Current evidence suggests that antibody to the AIDS virus and AIDS virus infection itself persist indefinitely.[47, 48] Among individuals with no risk factors for AIDS, absence of serum antibody to HIV can be expected to have a very high negative predictive value, virtually excluding HIV infection.[49]

HERPES SIMPLEX VIRUS

The prevalence of culture-positive genital HSV infection is high in selected populations[50] but has been less well studied in the general population. Recently, Nahmias et al.[51] studied 2475 adults presenting for routine care to a prepaid health plan. Using a new serologic assay for serum antibody to glycoprotein G2 antigen of HSV type 2 (HSV-2), approximately 20% of men were seropositive; only one quarter of seropositive individuals had a history of symptomatic HSV infection.[51]

Several investigators[52-54] have reported the isolation of HSV-2 from 29% of prostatic fluid specimens, 19% of prostatic biopsy specimens, and 8% of urethral swab specimens from men seen in a urology clinic in Florida. These findings have not been confirmed by others. Among men attending an STD clinic in Seattle, HSV was isolated from the urethras of only 4% of men during recurrent episodes of genital herpes, usually in association with symptoms of urethritis,[55] and from 3% of men who had no symptoms or signs of urethritis or genital herpes.[56] Among 1377 men attending an STD clinic in Sweden, 4.3% had positive HSV cultures from the urethra or lesions.[57] HSV was not isolated in the same study from any site from any of 131 men attending a dermatology clinic. Cultures of semen have been uniformly negative for HSV[54, 55]; it may be difficult to isolate HSV from semen when it is present, because of the cytotoxicity of undiluted semen, as mentioned above. Transmission of HSV through artificial insemination has not been reported.

The risk of acquiring genital herpes at the time of conception theoretically could include morbidity in the woman, abortion, congenital infection, and perinatal transmission to the neonate at delivery. Although fulminant, disseminated HSV infection has been described during pregnancy, fulminant infections have not been seen in small prospective studies of primary genital herpes in pregnant women.[58, 59] Nahmias et al.[58] have reported that among women who experienced genital herpes infections prior to 20 weeks' gestation, spontaneous abortion occurred in 5 (54%) of 9 with primary infection, versus 7 (25%) of 28 with recurrent or undetermined types of genital infection. Of the cases of abortion reported by Nahmias et al.,[58] most showed evidence of intrauterine death, but none showed specific evidence of fetal infection. Brown et al.[59] reported that congenital infection accounted for 3 of 42 neonates with herpes.

Brown et al.[59] also reported that the risk of symptomatic recurrences during pregnancy was lower after first episodes of genital herpes in pregnancy than after symptomatic recurrent episodes of genital herpes during pregnancy; but conversely, the risk of asymptomatic viral shedding from the genital tract was significantly greater after first episodes during pregnancy than after recurrent episodes during pregnancy. The risk of severe neonatal infection appears to be greatest after primary maternal infections occurring near term.[59]

Thus, some evidence suggests that primary genital herpes during the first trimester may carry an increased risk of abortion and may lead to increased risk of asymptomatic shedding later in pregnancy, with the attendant risk of perinatal transmission because of absence of symptoms in the mother. The risk of intrauterine infection during primary herpes early in pregnancy requires further study. The risk of HSV transmission through artificial insemination is difficult to assess. Although HSV has not been isolated from semen, recovery of the virus from semen may be technically difficult. At present, it is probably adequate to recommend that men with a history of recurrent genital herpes be excluded as potential semen donors. In the near future, when improved assays for serum antibody to HSV-2 will probably become available, the presence of HSV-2 antibody could be added as an exclusion criterion.

HUMAN PAPILLOMA VIRUS

The prevalence of genital papilloma virus infection in the male urethra has not been well studied, but the number of men presenting for care of symptomatic genital warts is increasing.[60] HPV is a sexually transmitted pathogen and in men frequently involves the urethra.[61] HPV cannot be cultured, but HPV types 5 and 2 have been identified by Southern blot hybridization in the semen of three men.[62] The significance of this is uncertain, because it is HPV types 6, 11, 16, 18, and 31 (not 5 or 2) which account for the vast majority of genital HPV infections. Two of the men had a history of chronic wart disease.[62] There are no reports of transmission of HPV by artificial insemination. However, the recent implication of HPV, especially types 16 and 18, in female genital cancers[63, 64] warrants efforts to exclude men with HPV infection as semen donors.

Genital warts usually increase markedly in size during pregnancy, with regression in the puerperium.[61] Probable perinatal transmission of HPV has been reported, leading to laryngeal papillomatosis,[65, 66] perianal condylomata,[67] and possibly to latent penile infection.[68] Roman and Fife[68] studied unselected infant foreskin tissue via deoxyribonucleic acid (DNA) hybridization techniques and found evidence of HPV in 4 of 70 infants tested. None of the mothers had a history of genital warts. Currently there is no readily available method for detection of HPV in the urethra or semen. DNA probes may become more widely available for detection of HPV in clinical specimens in the future.

EPSTEIN-BARR VIRUS

Transmission of Epstein-Barr virus (EBV) occurs via exposure to oral secretions. Sexual transmission has not been documented, although the virus has been recovered from unexplained genital lesions in a woman with a mononucleosis-like syndrome and serologic evidence of EBV infection,[69] and the virus can be grown in cervical epithelial cells.[70] EBV has not been recovered from semen.[71-73]

Ninety-seven percent to 99% of women in the United States are seropositive for EBV at the time of pregnancy.[74] Antibody to early antigen, suggestive of reactivation, is found with increased frequency in pregnant women.[75] One study suggested a possible risk to the fetus in women with persistent infection during pregnancy,[76] but another found no association between reactivation or persistence and low birth weight, congenital anomalies, and neonatal jaundice.[75]

Screening of potential artificial insemination donors for EBV is therefore not justified by current information. Furthermore, the high rate of seropositivity among potential donors makes elimination of seropositive donors impractical.

BACTERIAL INFECTIONS

NEISSERIA GONORRHOEAE

Over 800,000 cases of gonorrhea were reported in 1984,[77] and an equal number are thought to have gone unreported. The incidence of gonorrhea in the United States increased in 1985 for the first year in over a decade[77] and the increase continued through the early part of 1986. Asymptomatic urethral carriage in men is not uncommon; for example, 2.2% of sexually active enlisted men undergoing routine medical examination in 1972 yielded *N. gonorrhoeae* on urethral culture.[78]

N. gonorrhoeae has been recovered from fresh and frozen semen.[9, 79, 80] The organism has been found to attach to spermatozoa;[81] in theory, motile sperm could transport gonococci to the female upper genital tract.[8] Transmission of gonorrhea by donor insemination has been documented, resulting in cervicitis, pelvic inflammatory disease (PID), or gonococcal arthritis.[6, 7, 82] *N. gonorrhoeae* can colonize the cervix of parous women and be carried for extended periods of time,[83] and gonococcal infection in pregnancy has been associated with increased risk of spontaneous abortion, stillbirth, chorioamnionitis, premature rupture of the fetal membranes, and intrauterine growth retardation.[83-86] An increased risk of disseminated gonococcal infection (DGI) in pregnancy has been suggested,[87] but recent work fails to confirm this.[88] Consequences for the neonate of maternal gonococcal infection include ophthalmia neonatorum,[89, 90] oropharyngeal infections,[88, 91] proctitis, neonatal sepsis, meningitis, and, very rarely, vaginitis.[92]

Transmission of gonorrhea via therapeutic insemination by donor is easily avoidable, because infection in the male urethra is readily detected.[78] *N. gonorrhoeae* should be excluded in semen donors by examination of the urethra for discharge and culture of the urethra. Culture of first voided urine may be a suitable alternative to urethral culture, but this is debated.[93, 94]

CHLAMYDIA TRACHOMATIS

Asymptomatic urethral carriage of *C. trachomatis* has been documented in 2% of a male student population, 11% of a group of enlisted men,[95] and 7% of heterosexual men attending an STD clinic.[96] In higher socioeconomic groups, *C. trachomatis* is recovered substantially more frequently than is *N. gonorrhoeae*. Chlamydial infection in women causes cervicitis, endometritis, and salpingitis, and antibody to *C. trachomatis* is strongly associated with tubal infertility[97] (including women without histories of overt salpingitis) and with ectopic pregnancy.[98]

C. trachomatis has been recovered from the semen of three of six men with urethritis and epididymitis.[99] Transmission via therapeutic insemination by donor has not been documented, but this has not been systematically studied. Acute PID of unknown cause has been observed after therapeutic insemination by donor.[7] *C. trachomatis* adheres to human spermatozoa, particularly at low pH, such as occurs in the normal vagina,[100] and it has been postulated that sperm may carry *C. trachomatis* into the upper genital tract.[8]

Studies of the consequences of *C. trachomatis* infection in pregnancy have not yet given consistent results. Associations of prenatal chlamydial infection with low infant birthweight, premature rupture of fetal membranes, and preterm delivery have been seen in some studies,[101-103] but not in others.[104] Postpartum endometritis and fever have been documented in women with untreated antepartum chlamydial infection and in the mothers of infants with chlamydial conjunctivitis.[104, 105]

Maternal chlamydial infection can be transmitted to the neonate at the time of birth.[104] Approximately two-thirds of infants exposed at birth acquire infections in the conjunctiva, nasopharynx, rectum, or vagina. *C. trachomatis* is the most common cause of neonatal conjunctivitis in the United States and a major cause of pneumonitis in early infancy.[106]

Because of the potential effects of chlamydial infection on female fertility, on the course of pregnancy, and on the newborn, and the likelihood that *C. trachomatis* can be transmitted by donor insemination, chlamydial infection must be excluded in semen donors. Serologic testing is not practical because seropositivity most often reflects past infection, and the diagnosis of chlamydial infection rests on identification of the organism at an infected site. Urethral culture is probably the most sensitive measure of chlamydial infection in heterosexual men. The sensitivity and specificity of newer rapid diagnostic techniques for immunochemical detection of chlamydial antigens at infected sites approach those of culture in men with symptomatic urethritis,[107] but these tests have not yet been adequately evaluated in comparison with those of culture in asymptomatic men. Adjer et al.[108] reported that analysis of first voided urine specimens for pyuria (> 10 leukocytes per high-power (400 ×) field in resuspended urine sediment) can be used to screen men for urethral chlamydial or gonococcal infection. Although this would be convenient for screening semen donors, the sensitivity of this method requires confirmation. Therefore, urethral culture for *C. trachomatis* currently is the preferred screening technique.

TREPONEMA PALLIDUM

Overall, the incidence of syphilis has fallen in the United States in the last 20 years.[109] The highest incidence and prevalence of syphilis are observed in homosexual men.[109] An early study[110] revealed that the semen of 20% of men with primary or secondary syphilis contained *T.*

pallidum, but semen from men with late syphilis rarely was infectious. These studies have not been repeated in recent years. The transmission of syphilis by therapeutic insemination by donor has not been reported.

Syphilis during pregnancy is a serious medical problem, with effects on the course of pregnancy as well as on the fetus. The morbidity of syphilis in the female apparently is not changed by pregnancy,[111] but the disease frequently alters the course of pregnancy.[112] The effects of syphilis on the fetus usually become apparent only after the 18th week of gestation.[113] Transmission is most likely when pregnancy occurs during the first 2 years after infection of the mother. Congenital infection produces numerous well-known life-threatening, developmental, and late manifestations.[113]

Although the prevalence of early syphilis in semen donors should be very low, individuals with positive serologic tests are at risk for other STDs. Donor insemination is an elective procedure, and the cost of serologic tests for syphilis is low. Therefore, serologic screening with the venereal disease research laboratory test (VDRL) the rapid plasma reagin test (RPR), or other reaginic antibody assay (with appropriate confirmatory tests if positive) is recommended for potential semen donors.

OTHER INFECTIONS

GENITAL MYCOPLASMAS AND GROUP B STREPTOCOCCUS

The genital mycoplasmas, *M. hominis* and *U. urealyticum*, have been associated with several genito-urinary syndromes in women, including bacterial vaginosis and pelvic inflammatory disease.[114] These organisms are frequently recovered from the urethras of asymptomatic men; for example, *U. urealyticum* was isolated from 58% and *M. hominis* from 42% of 62 asymptomatic men attending an STD clinic.[56]

U. urealyticum has been recovered from semen,[115, 116] and identified by electron microscopy adhering to spermatozoa.[116] *U. urealyticum* infection may have been transmitted by donor insemination in one case report.[115] *M. hominis* was isolated from blood of a semen recipient in her seventh month of pregnancy, as well as from the urine of the semen donor.[117]

The relationship between abnormal pregnancy outcome and genital mycoplasma infection is currently under study in many centers. *U. urealyticum* has been associated with spontaneous abortion, stillbirth, low birth weight, and chorioamnionitis.[118] *M. hominis* has been associated with postpartum fever and postpartum bacteremia.[102, 119] *U. urealyticum* has been implicated in neonatal pneumonitis.[120]

Because of the ubiquitous presence of genital mycoplasmas in sexually active adults, conflicting results of several clinical studies, and the fact that these organisms often coexist with other pathogens which have generally not been concurrently studied, it is difficult to ascertain the contribution of the mycoplasmas to morbidity during pregnancy, the puerperium, and the neonatal period. Thus, it would be difficult to obtain consensus on the benefit of screening semen donors for mycoplasmas. Such screening potentially could exclude a large number of otherwise acceptable donors. As further data become available regarding the significance of genital mycoplasma infection in pregnancy, a better informed decision regarding donor screening can be made. Similarly, the potential benefit of screening semen donors for group B *Streptococcus*, another ubiquitous organism which has been implicated in pregnancy and neonatal morbidity,[121-123] is uncertain.

TRICHOMONAS VAGINALIS

The prevalence of *T. vaginalis* in sexually active men has ranged from $< 1\%$ of asymptomatic men attending an STD clinic[56] to as many as 100% of male contacts of women with trichomonal vaginitis.[124] This wide range is due to patient selection (low socioeconomic status, sexual promiscuity, and history of exposure are risk factors for trichomonal infection) and also to the use of different methods to test specimens from different anatomic sites. In our experience, the most sensitive and specific of available methods for diagnosis of vaginal trichomoniasis, is culture, followed by wet mount examination, followed by Papanicolaou (Pap) stain.[125] It is not known whether cultures from the urethra, urine, semen, or prostatic expressate are most sensitive for detection of *T. vaginalis* in men. *T. vaginalis* was identified via Pap staining in 8% of semen from 85 men at an STD clinic.[126] Transmission of trichomoniasis through donor insemination has been reported in two women.[127]

Vaginal trichomoniasis during pregnancy has not been conclusively linked with maternal morbidity. One early study failed to show an association between vaginal trichomonal infection and puerperal morbidity, though another suggested such an association.[128]

Treatment of trichomoniasis in pregnancy is problematic, particularly during the first trimester, when metronidazole is not recommended.[129]

Perinatal transmission can occur. Although *T. vaginalis* has been cultured from tracheal aspirates of two neonates with pneumonitis of unclear etiology[130] and from the vaginal fluid of newborn infants,[131] *T. vaginalis* has not been frequently associated with major neonatal morbidity.

DISCUSSION AND RECOMMENDATIONS

Donor insemination is a commonly performed elective procedure that has the potential to cause severe infectious complications. Available data suggest that the standard of current practice is highly variable. In 1979, Curie-Cohen et al.[1] surveyed 711 United States physicians likely to perform donor insemination and found that most physicians identified and used a select group of donors (often young medical professionals); but beyond this selection, the practitioners surveyed did little to screen donors for infectious diseases. A smaller 1983 survey of Ontario fertility specialists also indicated that testing of donors for infection was limited.[132] Great variability also was documented by Curie-Cohen et al.[1] in the number of donors providing semen for each recipient, the use of frozen semen, record keeping on the outcome of insemination, the outcome of pregnancy, and the subsequent health of the recipient, the offspring, and the donor. Although there are few data available on insemination related infections (the AIDS virus transmission that occurred in Australia is an exception), such infections clearly could easily escape detection or might not be traced to the source. The early clinical manifestations of most such infections in women and newborns are subtle or nonspecific, the serious sequelae can occur months or years after exposure, several sources for infection commonly are possible, and record keeping is inadequate. Thus, the infrequent documentation of insemination-related infection is not evidence that current practices are safe. The survey by Curie-Cohen et al.[1] reflected the practices of physicians with expertise in infertility, who performed inseminations frequently, but not those of lay practitioners or physicians performing the procedure less frequently, who may use even less standardized methods. Guidelines are needed for acceptable and safe insemination practices.[133, 134]

Table 1. *Presence of Pathogens in Semen and Reported Transmission by Semen Donors*

Pathogen	Presence in semen	Reported transmission by donor semen	Likelihood of transmission if not yet reported
Hepatitis B virus	Yes	Not reported	High
HIV (AIDS virus)	Yes	Yes	—
EBV	Uncertain	Not reported	Low
CMV	Yes	Not reported	High
HSV	Uncertain	Not reported	Low
HPV	Uncertain	Not reported	Low
N. gonorrhoeae	Yes	Yes	—
C. trachomatis	Yes	Possible	High
T. pallidum	Probable	Not reported	Uncertain
U. urealyticum	Yes	Yes	—
M. hominis	Yes	Yes	—
Group B *Streptococcus*	Yes	No	High
T. vaginalis	Yes	Yes	—

In establishing recommendations for donor screening for genital infections, we have considered several principles for donor selection. It is not possible to exclude infection in the donor without specific testing, but the negative predictive value of specific tests can be increased and the cost of screening decreased by (1) initially excluding high-risk donors on the basis of medical and sexual history and CMV serologic tests and (2) use of more expensive laboratory screening tests only on the remaining low-risk, CMV-seronegative donors.

Recommendations should be mainly aimed at preventing transmission of those pathogens known to be present in semen which have the potential to produce severe sequelae for the recipient and her offspring. Tables 1 and 2 summarize the published data concerning the presence of individual pathogens in semen, the evidence or likelihood of transmission by donor insemination, and the reported effects on pregnancy, the fetus, and the newborn. Firm guidelines are not offered here for prevention of transmission of organisms which may have low prevalence in semen or uncertain morbidity if transmitted around the time of conception.

SCREENING RECOMMENDATIONS

We suggest a two-step screening procedure. As summarized in Table 3, the first step entails screening potential donors by a medical and sex-

Table 2. *Reported Effects of Sexually Transmitted Pathogens on Pregnancy, Fetus, and Infant*

Pathogen	Reported effects on pregnancy[a,b]	Effect on fetus/infant[b]
Viruses		
Hepatitis B virus	None known	Perinatal transmission, chronic carriage, chronic hepatitis
Cytomegalovirus	? Prematurity ? Spontaneous abortion	Congenital and perinatal infection, malformation
Herpes simplex virus	Prematurity, abortion, asymptomatic shedding	Congenital and perinatal herpes, encephalitis
HIV (AIDS virus)	Prematurity	Congenital and perinatal infection, AIDS, ARC
Human papillomavirus	Giant condylomata	Laryngeal papillomatosis, genital warts, ? latency
Epstein-Barr virus	None (?)	None (?)
Bacteria		
N. gonorrhoeae	Abortion, stillbirth amnionitis, endometritis PROM, IUGR	Neonatal conjunctivitis, sepsis
C. trachomatis	LBW, PROM, endometritis	Neonatal conjunctivitis, pneumonitis
T. pallidum	Abortion, stillbirth, prematurity	Congenital syphilis
U. urealyticum	Prematurity, LBW	? Pneumonitis
M. hominis	Postpartum fever, endometritis	Neonatal sepsis (rare)
Group B streptococcus	Prematurity, PROM, chorioamnionitis, postpartum endometritis	Neonatal sepsis and meningitis
Protozoa		
T. vaginalis	Vaginitis	Vaginitis

[a]Effects on pregnancy per se, in addition to usual effects of acute infection; see text for description. Reports based solely on anecdotal observations are not included.

[b]PROM, premature rupture of membranes; IUGR, intrauterine growth retardation; LBW, low birth weight; ARC, AIDS-related complex.

ual history; those who remain acceptable then undergo serologic screening for antibody to CMV.

The second step, conducted at a second predonation visit, consists of a physical examination, including the genitourinary system, with particular attention paid to the presence of condylomata, urethritis, and genital vesicles or ulcers. Individuals without evident STD then should undergo urethral cultures for *N. gonorrhoeae* and *C. trachomatis* and serologic testing for HIV antibody, syphilis, and HBsAg. Cultures of the urethra or the first 10 to 15 ml of voided uring for *T. vaginalis* and perhaps for organisms implicated by some studies in pregnancy or perinatal morbidity (e.g., *M. hominis, U. urealyticum,* and group B *Streptococcus*) are of uncertain value and are considered optional at present. When a specific serologic test for antibody to HSV-2 becomes readily available, this could be added to the second stage tests. If analysis of first voided urine sediment for pyuria is confirmed to be sensitive for detecting asymptomatic urethral infections by *C. trachomatis* or *N. gonorrhoeae*, then urinalysis could be substituted for urethral cultures for these organisms. The urine sediment could also be examined for motile trichomonads.

ADDITIONAL RECOMMENDATIONS

To further reduce the risk of exposure of the semen recipient to potentially infectious semen, one should minimize the number of donors for each recipient. Semen from multiple donors should not be mixed. Intrauterine insemination should be done only in the case of cervical factor infertility, because this procedure may facilitate access of urethral pathogens or opportunistic organisms to the upper genital tract.

To enhance the success of insemination and to reduce potential confusion regarding STD transmission via insemination, the recipient and spouse (if applicable) should undergo screening examinations for the same infections as the donor. Uniform recordkeeping of health status and identity of recipients and donors should be established so that any infection transmission can be traced and other recipients protected.

Quality assurance review should be performed to maintain practice standards for the insemination procedure and to amend the practice when problems are identified or changes occur in the epidemiology of genital infections that have bearing on the practice of insemination.

USE OF FROZEN SEMEN

Although the recommended screening procedures for semen donors are within the capabilities of most practitioners, they constitute a cumbersome process. Some may find it easier to utilize prescreened donor semen from frozen semen banks. Creation of regional semen banks with expertise in screening potential donors for STDs

Table 3. *Protocol for Screening Sexually Transmissable Infections in Potential Semen Donors*

I. First visit
   A. Excluded by history
      1. Homosexual contact since 1978
      2. Parenteral drug abuse since 1978
      3. Hemophiliac
      4. From country with predominant heterosexual transmission of AIDS
      5. Sexual partner in AIDS risk group since 1978
      6. More than one sexual partner within the preceding 6 months
      7. History of STD and related infections within the preceding 6 months, including gonorrhea, nongonococcal urethritis, chlamydial infection, epidydimitis, prostatis, genital ulcer, syphilis, hepatitis
      8. Any past history of genital herpes, genital warts, chronic hepatitis, or prior exclusion from blood donation for an infective IVF reason
      9. Current sexual partner with STD
   B. If history negative, obtain CMV serology; if history positive, defer donation
II. Second visit (CMV serologic test negative)
   A. Physical examination to exclude
      1. Urethral discharge
      2. Evidence of genital warts
      3. Genital ulcers
   B. If physical examation is negative, perform urethral culture for:
      1. *N. gonorrhoeae*
      2. *C. trachomatis*
      3. Optional
         a. *T. vaginalis*
         b. *U. urealyticum, M. hominis,* Group B *Streptococcus*
   C. Serology
      1. HIV (AIDS virus)
      2. HBsAg
      3 Serologic test for syphilis (e.g., VDRL)
      4. Optional: HSV-2
   Accept donor if all negative
III. Surveillance and follow-up
   A. Exclude donors/discontinue donors: new acquisition of STD (e.g., genital warts, genital ulcers, urethritis)
   B. New sexual partner: break in monogamy, break in abstinence
   C. Rescreen donors at least every 6 months

and for genetic factors relevant to donor insemination is a concept analogous to that reflected in current blood banking procedures. Where facilities for frozen storage of semen are available, the entire screening procedure could be accomplished at one visit. Both serum and semen would be collected if the donor is not excluded by history and the physical examination is normal. A small aliquot of semen could be tested for *N. gonorrhoeae, C. trachomatis*, and perhaps *T. vaginalis*, the genital mycoplasmas, and other bacterial pathogens. Semen would then be frozen pending results of these cultures and serologic tests. Analysis of first voided urine for pyuria could be performed before collection of semen to exclude donors at high risk for infection by *C. trachomatis* or *N. gonorrhoeae*; if this proves sufficiently sensitive, culture of semen for *C. trachomatis* and/or *N. gonorrhoeae* could be eliminated from the protocol. CMV serologic testing could then be performed. Serum specimens from CMV-seropositive men would be discarded later, whereas specimens from CMV-seronegative donors would undergo further testing for HBV, HIV, and syphilis. The process would obviate the need for the passage of urethral swabs before other serologic tests, which would be performed only on CMV-seronegative specimens to minimize costs.

Use of frozen semen might have other advantages. The requirement for donors to be CMV-seronegative may greatly reduce the number of available donors in some geographic areas or populations in which the seroprevalence of CMV infection is high. In these settings, semen from CMV-seronegative donors might be selectively banked, which would increase the availability of semen to recipients in these areas. Freezing of semen may reduce the concentration of some viral or bacterial pathogens, although this is not well documented.

Freezing of semen has a number of drawbacks. It reportedly reduces the number of motile spermatozoa and increases the average number of inseminations required for conception. The semen of some men is very sensitive to freezing, eliminating these men as donors for programs that use freezing. Freezing and frozen storage are cumbersome, making the procedure difficult for physicians with small insemination practices. Finally, the sensitivities of semen cultures or antigen detection tests have not been compared with the results on urethral specimens. Dilution of urethral secretions by seminal fluid and cytotoxicity of semen for tissue culture cells might be expected to reduce the yield compared with urethral culture; this issue should be investigated.

Overall, the use of banked or frozen semen needs consideration, particularly by those who find the recommended screening procedures prohibitively cumbersome or who have difficulty in matching recipients with acceptable donors. Research on development of new freezing techniques to increase efficacy of frozen semen should be encouraged.

Finally, the use of volunteer donors, rather than paid donors, could further reduce the risk of transmission of genital infections.

Acknowledgments. We thank Dr. C. Alvin Paulsen for his encouragement and advice, Dr. M. Deborah Gold for her assistance, and Mr. Skylar Carroll for preparation of the manuscript.

REFERENCES

1. Curie-Cohen M, Luttrell L, Shapiro S: Current practice of artificial insemination by donor in the United States. N Engl J Med 300:585, 1979
2. Schreeder MIT, Thompson SIE, Hadler SWC Berquist KR, Zaidi A, Maynard JE, Ostrow D, Judson FN, Braff EH, Nylund L, Moore JN, Gardner P, Doto LL, Reynolds G: Hepatitis B in homosexual men: prevalence of infection and factors related to transmission. J Infect Dis 146:7, 1982
3. Handsfield HH, Chandler SH, Caine VA, Meyers JD, Corey L, Medeiros E, McDougall JK: Cytomegalovirus infection in sex partners: evidence for sexual transmission. J Infect Dis 151:344, 1985
4. Stewart GJ, Cunningham AL, Driscoll GL, Tyler JPP, Barr JA, Gold J, Lamont BJ: Transmission of human T-cell lymphotropic virus type III (HTLV-III) by artificial insemination by donor. Lancet 2:581, 1985
5. Coffin J, Haase A, Levy JA, Montagnier L, Oroszlan S, Teich N, Temin H, Toyoshima K, Varmus H, Vogt P, Weiss R: What to call the AIDS virus? Nature 321:10, 1986
6. Fiumara NJ: Transmission of gonorrhea by artificial insemination. Br J Vener Dis 48:308, 1972
7. Chong AP, Taymor ML: Sixteen years experience with therapeutic donor insemination. Fertil Steril 26:791, 1975
8. Howard TL: Bacterial hitchhikers. J Urol 106:94, 1971
9. Noguchi PD, Kiss JE, Petricciani JC: Microbial contamination of human semen. Presented at the Symposium on the Integrity of Frozen Semen. Proceedings of a Round-Table Conference at the National Academy of Sciences. National Academy of Sciences, 1978, p 216
10. Rehewy MSE, Hafez ESE, Thomas A, Brown WJ: Aerobic and anaerobic bacterial flora in semen from fertile and infertile groups of men. Arch Androl 2:263, 1979
11. Szmuness W, Hirsch RL, Prince AM, Levine W, Harley EJ, Ikram H: Hepatitis B surface antigen in blood donors: further observations. J Infect Dis 131:111, 1975
12. Heathcote J, Cameron CH, Dane DS: Hepatitis-B antigen in saliva and semen. Lancet 1:17, 1974
13. Hersh T, Melnick JL, Goyal RK, Hollinger FB. Nonparenteral transmission of viral Hepatitis B (Australia antigen-associated serum hepatitis). N Engl J Med 285: 1363, 1971
14. Koff RS, Slavin MM, Connelly LJD, Rosen DR: Contagiousness of acute Hepatitis B: secondary attack rates in household contacts. Gastroenterology 72:297, 1977
15. Szmuness W, Much MI, Prince AM, Hoofnagle JH, Cherubin CE, Harley EJ, Block GH: The role of sexual behavior in the spread of hepatitis B infection. Ann Intern Med 83:489, 1975
16. Schweitzer IL, Dunn AEG, Peters RL, Spears RL: Viral Hepatitis B in neonates and infants. Am J Med 55:762, 1973
17. Lee AKY, Ip HMH, Wong VCW: Mechanisms of maternal-fetal transmission of Hepatitis B virus. J Infect Dis 138:668, 1978
18. Stevens CE, Toy PT, Tong MJ, Taylor PE, Vyas GN, Nair PV, Gudavalli M, Krugman S: Perinatal Hepatitis B virus transmission in the United States prevention by passive-active immunization. JAMA 253:1740, 1985
19. Tong MJ, Thursby M, Rakela J, McPeak C, Edwards VM, Mosley JW: Studies on the maternal-infant transmission of the viruses which cause acute hepatitis. Gastroenterology 80:999, 1981
20. Frosner GG, Franco E: New developments and open questions in the serology of hepatitis A and B. In Viral Hepatitis and Liver Diseases, Edited by GN Vyas, JL Dienstag, JH Hoofnagle. Orlando, Grune & Stratton, 1984, p 487
21. Hieber JP, Dalton D, Shorey J, Combes B: Hepatitis and pregnancy. J Pediatr 91:545, 1977
22. Beasley RP, Hwang L: Hepatocellular carcinoma and hepatitis B virus. Semin Liver Dis 4:1213, 1984
23. Lang DJ, Garruto RM, Gajdusek DC: Early acquisition of cytomegalovirus and Epstein-Barr virus antibody in several isolated melanesian populations. Am J Epidemiol 105:480, 1977
24. Chandler SH, Alexander ER, Holmes KK: Epidemiology of cytomegaloviral infection in a heterogeneous population of pregnant women. J Infect Dis 152:249, 1985
25. Drew WL, Mintz L, Miner RC, Sands M, Ketterer B: Prevalence of cytomegalovirus infection in homosexual men. J Infect Dis 143:188, 1981
26. Collier AC, Corey L, Myers JD, Murphy VL, Robert P, Handsfield HH: The epidemiology of cytomegalovirus infection in homosexual men. Presented at the Sixth International Society for Sexually Transmitted Diseases Research, Brighton, England, August 1, 1985
27. Lang DJ, Kummer JF: Cytomegalovirus in semen: observations in selected populations. J Infect Dis 132:472, 1975
28. Stagno S, Pass RF, Dworsky ME, Henderson RE, Moore EG, Walton PD, Alford CA: Congenital CMV infection: the relative importance of primary and recurrent maternal infection. N Engl J Med 306:945, 1982
29. Tolkoff-Rubin NE, Rubin RH, Keller EE, Baker GP, Stewart JA, Hirsch MS: Cytomegalovirus infection in dialysis patients and personnel. Ann Intern Med 89:625, 1978
30. Brady MT, Milam JD, Anderson DC, Hawkins EP, Speer ME, Seavy D, Bijou H, Yow MD: Use of deglycerolized red blood cells to prevent post transfusion infection with cytomegalovirus in neonates. J Infect Dis 150:334, 1984
31. Adler SP, Lawrence LT, Baggett J, Biro V, Sharp DE: Prevention of transfusion associated cytomegalovirus infection in very low birth weight infants using frozen blood and donors seronegative for cytomegalovirus. Transfusion 24:333, 1984
32. Gjerset GF, McGrady G, Counts RB, Martin PJ, Jason J, Kennedy S, Evatt B, Hansen JA: Lymphadenopathy-associated virus antibodies and T cells in homophiliacs treated with cryoprecipitate or concentrate. Blood 66: 718, 1985
33. Recommendations for assisting in the prevention of perinatal transmission of human T-lymphotropic virus

type III/Lymphadenopathy-associated virus and acquired immunodeficiency syndrome. MMWR 34:48, 1985
34. Ward J, Center for Disease Control: Unpublished data
35. Curran JW: The epidemiology and prevention of the acquired immunodeficiency syndrome. Ann Intern Med 103:657, 1985
36. Levy JA, Kaminsky LS, Morrow WJW, Steimer K, Luciw P, Dina D, Hoxie J, Oshiro L: Infection by the retro virus associated with the acquired immunodeficiency syndrome: clinical, biological and molecular features. Ann Intern Med 103:694, 1985
37. Zagury D, Bernard J, Leibowitch J, Safai B, Groopman J, Feldman M, Sarngadharan M, Gallo R: HTLV-III in cell cultured from semen of two patients with AIDS. Science 226:449, 1984
38. Ho DD, Schooley RT, Rota TR, Kaplan JC, Flynn T, Salahuddin SZ, Gonda MA, Hirsch MS: HTLV-III in the semen and blood of a healthy homosexual man. Science 226:451, 1984
39. Scott GB, Fischl MA, Klimas N, Fletcher MA, Dickinson GM, Levine RS, Parks WP: Mothers of infants with the acquired immunodeficiency syndrome: evidence for both symptomatic and asymptomatic carriers. JAMA 253: 363, 1985
40. Francis DP, Jaffe HW, Fultz PN, Getchell JP, McDougal JS, Feorino PM: The natural history in infection with the lymphadenopathy-associated virus human T-lymphotropic virus type III. Ann Intern Med 103:719, 1985
41. Cowan MJ, Hellmann D, Chudwin D, Wara DW, Chang RS, Ammann AJ: Maternal transmission of acquired immune deficiency syndrome. Pediatrics 73:382, 1984
42. Thomas PA, Jaffe HW, Spira TJ, Reiss R, Guerrero IC, Auerbach D: Unexplained immunodeficiency in children: a surveillance report. JAMA 252:639, 1984
43. LaPointe N, Michaud J, Pekovic D, Chausseau JP, Dupuy JM: Transplacental transmission of HTLV III virus. (Letter) N Engl J Med 312:1325, 1985
44. Ziegler JB, Cooper DA, Johnson RO, Gold J: Postnatal transmission of AIDS-associated retrovirus from mother to infant. Lancet 1:896, 1985
45. Petricciani JC: Licensed tests for antibody to human lymphotropic virus type III: sensitivity and specificity. Ann Int Med 103:726, 1985
46. Ho DD, Sarngadharan MG, Resnick L, Dimarzo-Veronese F, Rota T, Hirsch M: Primary human T-lymphotropic virus type III infection. Ann Intern Med 103:880, 1985
47. Jaffe HW, Feorino PM, Darrow WW, O'Malley PM, Getchell JP, Warfield DT, Jones BM, Echenberg D, Francis DP, Curran JW: Persistent infection with human T-lymphotropic virus type III/lymphadenopathy-associated virus in apparently healthy homosexual men. Ann Intern Med 102:627, 1985
48. Feorino PM, Jaffe HW, Palmer E, Peterman T, Francis DP, Kalyanaraman VS, Weinstein RA, Stoneburner RL, Alexander WJ, Raevsky C, Getchell JP, Warfield D, Haverkos HW, Kilbourne BW, Nicholson JKA, Curran JW: Transfusion-associated acquired immunodeficiency syndrome: evidence for persistent infection in blood donors. N Engl J Med 312:1293, 1985
49. Ward J, Center for Disease Control: Unpublished data
50. Koutsky LA, Stevens CE, Kiviat NC, Holmes KK, Corey L: Prevalence and clinical presentation of genital herpes in women attending an STD Clinic. Abstract 488. Presented at the 25th Interscience Conference on Antimicrobial Agents and Chemotherapy, Minneapolis, Minnesota, September 29 to October 2, 1985
51. Nahmias A, Keyserling H, Bain R, Becker T, Lee F, Coleman M, Dragalin D, Pereira L, Wickliffe C, Wells E, Perry L, Muther J: Prevalence of herpes simplex virus 2 specific antibodies in a USA prepaid group medical practice population. Abstract 43. Presented at ISSTDR, Brighton, 1985
52. Centifanto YM, Drylie DM, Deardourff SL, Kaufman HE: Herpes virus type 2 in the male genitourinary tract. Science 170:318, 1972
53. Deardourff SL, Deture FA, Drylie DM, Centifano YM, Kaufman H: Association between herpes hominis type 2 and the male genitourinary tract. J Urol 112:126, 1974
54. Deture FA, Drylie DM, Kaufman HE, Centifanto YM: Herpes virus type 2: study of semen in male subjects with recurrent infection. Urology 120:449, 1978
55. Corey L, Adams HG, Brown ZA, Holmes KK: Genital herpes simplex virus infections: clinical manifestations, course, and complications. Ann Intern Med 98:958, 1983
56. Holmes KK, Handsfield HH, Wang SP, Wentwobdh BBL Turck M, Anderson JB, Alexander ER: Etiology of nongonococcal urethritis. N Engl J Med 292:1199, 1975
57. Jeansson S, Molin L: On the occurrence of genital herpes simplex virus infection. Acta Derm Venereol (Stockh) 54:479,1 974
58. Nahmaias AJ, Josey WE, Naib ZM, Freeman MG, Fernandez RJ, Wheeler JH: Perinatal risk associated with maternal genital herpes simplex virus infection. Am J Obstet Gynecol 110:825, 1971
59. Brown ZA, Vontvner LA, Benedetti J, Critchlow CW, Hickok DE, Sells CJ, Berry S, Corey L: Genital herpes in pregnancy: risk factors associated with recurrences and asymptomatic viral shedding. Am J Obstet Gynecol 153: 24, 1985
60. Oriel JD: Genital warts. In Sexually Transmitted Diseases, Edited by KK Holmes, PA Mårdh, PF Sparling, PJ Weisner. New York, McGraw-Hill, 1984, p 496
61. Oriel JD: Natural history of genital warts. Br J Vener Dis 47:1, 1971
62. Ostrow RS, Zachow KR, Nilmura M, Okagaki T, Muller S, Bender M, Faras AJ: Detection of papillomavirus DNA in human semen. Science 231:731, 1986
63. Durst M, Gissmann L, Ikenberg H, Hausen H: A papillomavirus DNA from a cervical carcinoma and its prevalence in cancer biopsy samples from different geographic regions. Proc Natl Acad Sci USA 80:3812, 1983
64. Boshart M, Gissman L, Ikenberg H, Kleinheinz G, Schuerlen W, Hausen H: A new type of papilloma virus DNA, its presence in genital cancer biopsies and in cell lines derived from cervical cancer. EMBO J 3:1151, 1984
65. Quick CA, Faras A, Krzysek R: The etiology of laryngeal papillomatosis. Laryngoscope 88:1789, 1978
66. Boyle WF, Riggs JL, Oshiro LS, Lennette EH: Electron microscopic identification of papovavirus in laryngeal papilloma. Laryngoscope 83:1102, 1973
67. Eftaiha MS, Amshel AL, Shonberg IL: Condylomata acuminata in an infant and mother: report of a case. Dis Colon Rectum 21:369, 1978
68. Roman A, Fife KH: Human pappillomavirus DNA associated with foreskins of normal newborns. J Infect Dis 153:855, 1986

69. Portnoy J, Ahronheim GA, Ghibu F, Glecner B, Joncas JH: Recovery of Epstein-Barr virus from genital ulcers. N Engl J Med 311:966, 1984
70. Sixeby JW, Veterinen EH, Nedrud JG, Raab-Traus N, Walton LA, Pagano JS: Replication of Epstein-Barr virus in human epithelial cells in vitro. Nature 3036: 480, 1983
71. Ahronheim G: Unpublished data
72. Huang C: Unpublished data
73. Henle W: Unpublished data
74. Fleisher GR, Bolognese R: Seroepidemiology of Epstein-Barr virus in pregnant women. J Infect Dis 145:537, 1982
75. Fleisher GR, Bolognese R: Persistent Epstein-Barr virus infection and pregnancy. J Infect Dis 147:982, 1983
76. Icart J, Didier J: Infections due to Epstiein-Barr virus during pregnancy. J Infect Dis 143:499, 1981
77. Blount J, Center for Disease Control: Unpublished data
78. Handsfield HH, Lipman TO, Harnisch JP, Tronca E, Holmes KK: Asymptomatic gonorrhea in men. N Engl J Med 290:117, 1974
79. Sherman JK, Rosenfeld J: Importance of frozen-stored human semen in the spread of gonorrhea. Fertil Steril 26:1043, 1975
80. Jennings RT, Dixon RE, Nettles JB: The risks and prevention of *Neisseria gonorrhoeae* transfer in fresh ejaculate donor insemination. Fertil Steril 28:554, 1977
81. James-Holmquest AN, Swanson J, Buchanan TM, Wende RD, Williams RP: Differential attachment by piliated and nonpiliated *Neisseria gonorrhoeae* to human sperm. Infect Immun 9:897, 1974
82. Nielson NC, Hansen KB: Establishment of a central semen bank in Denmark supplying 22 gynecological departments. In Human Artificial Insemination and Semen Preservation, Edited by G David, WS Price. New York, Plenum Press, 1980, p 81
83. Edwards LE, Barrada MI, Hamann AA, Hakanson EY: Gonorrhea in pregnancy. Am J Obstet Gynecol 132:637, 1978
84. Handsfield HH, Hodson WA, Holmes KK: Neonatal gonococcal infection. JAMA 225:697, 1973
85. Amstey MS, Steadman KT: Asymptomatic gonorrhea in pregnancy. J Am Vener Dis 3:14, 1976
86. Sarrel PM, Pruett KA: Symptomatic gonorrhea during pregnancy. Obstet Gynecol 32:670, 1968
87. Holmes KK, Counts GW, Beaty HN: Disseminated gonococcal infection. Ann Intern Med 74:979, 1971
88. Handsfield HH: Gonorrhea and uncomplicated gonococcal infection. In Sexually Transmitted Diseases, Edited by KK Holmes, PA Mårdh, PF Sparling, PJ Wiesner. New York, McGraw-Hill, 1984, p 205
89. Rothenberg R: *Ophthalmia neonatorum* due to *Neisseria gonorrhoeae*: prevention and treatment. Sex Trans Dis 6: 187, 1979
90. Thompson TR, Swanson RE, Wiesner PJ: Gonococcal ophthalmia neonatorum: relationship of time of infection to relevant control measures. JAMA 228:186, 1974
91. Urban M, Hervada AR: Gonococcal gum abscess in a 10 week old infant. Clin Pediatr 16:193, 1977
92. Stark AR, Glode MP: Gonococcal vaginitis in a neonate. J Pediatr 94:298, 1979
93. Feng WC, Medeiros AA, Murrah ES: Diagnosis of gonorrhea in male patients by culture of uncentrifuged first-voided urine. JAMA 237:896, 1977
94. Luciano AA, Grubin L: Gonorrhea screening: comparison of three techniques. JAMA 243:680, 1980
95. Podgore JK, Holmes KK, Alexander ER: Asymptomatic urethral infections due to *Chlamydia trachomatis* in male U.S. military personnel. J Infect Dis 146:828, 1982
96. Stamm WE, Koutsky LA, Benedetti JK, Jourden JL, Brunham RC, Holmes KK: *Chlamydia trachomatis* urethral infections in men. Ann Intern Med 100:47, 1984
97. Moore DE, Spadoni LR: Infertility in women. In Sexually Transmitted Diseases, Edited by KK Holmes, PA Mårdh, PF Sparling, PJ Wiesner. New York, McGraw-Hill, 1984, p 76
98. Gump DW, Gibson M, Ashikaga T: Evidence of prior pelvic inflammatory disease and its relationship to *Chlamydia trachomatis* and antibody and intrauterine contraceptive devices in infertile women. Am J Obstet Gynecol 146:153, 1983
99. Berger RE, Alexander ER, Monda GD, Ansell J, McCormick G, Holmes K: *Chlamydia trachomatis* as a cause of acute "idiopathic" epididymitis. N Engl J Med 298:301, 1978
100. Wolner-Hanssen P, Mårdh PA: In vitro tests of the adherence of *Chlamydia trachomatis* to human spermatozoa. Fertil Steril 42:102, 1984
101. Martin DH, Koutsky L, Eschenbach DA, Daling JR, Alexander ER, Benedetti JK, Holmes KK: Prematurity and perinatal mortality in pregnancies complicated by maternal *Chlamydia trachomatis* infections. JAMA 247: 1585, 1982
102. Harrison WR, Alexander ER, Weinstein L, Lewis M, Nash M, Sim DA: Cervical *Chlamydia trachomatis* and mycoplasmal infections in pregnancy: epidemiology and outcomes. JAMA 250:1721, 1983
103. Gravett MG, Nelson HP, DeRouen T, Critchlow C, Eschenbach DA, Holmes KK: Independent associations of bacterial vaginosis and *Chlamydia trachomatis* infection with adverse pregnancy outcome. JAMA. In press
104. Frommell GT, Rothenberg R, Wang SP, McIntosh K, Wintersgill C, Allaman J, Orr I: Chlamydial infection of mothers and their infants. J Pediatr 95:28, 1979
105. Mordhorst CH, Dawson C: Sequelae of neonatal inclusion conjunctivitis and associated disease in parents. Am J Opthalmol 71:861, 1979
106. Harrison HR, English MG, Lee CK, Alexander ER: *Chlamydia trachomatis* infant pneumonitis: comparison with matched controls and other infant pneumonitis. N Engl J Med 298:702, 1978
107. Stamm WE, Harrison HR, Alexander ER, Cles LD, Spence MR, Quinn TC: Diagnosis of *Chlamydia trachomatis* infections by direct immunofluorescence staining of genital secretions. Ann Intern Med 101:638, 1984
108. Adger H, Sweet RL, Shafer M, Schachter J: Screening for *Chlamydia trachomatis* and *Neisseria gonorrhoeae* in adolescent males: value of first catch urine examination. Lancet 2:944, 1984
109. Aral S, Holmes KK: Epidemiology of sexually transmitted diseases. In Sexually Transmitted Diseases, Edited by KK Holmes, PA Mårdh, PF Sparling, PJ Weisner. New York, McGraw-Hill, 1984, p 127
110. Kemp JE: The infectiousness of semen of patients with late syphilis, an experimental study. Am J Syphilis, Gonorrhea, Vener Dis 22:401, 1938
111. Holder WR, Knox JM: Syphilis in pregnancy. Med Clin North Am 56:1151, 1972

112. Stokes JH, Beerman H, Ingraham NR: Familial and prenatal syphilis ("congenital" or "heredosyphilis"). In Modern Clinical Syphilology: Diagnosis, Treatment, Case Study. Philadelphia, W. B. Saunders, 1944
113. Murphy F, Patamasucon P: Congenital syphilis. In Sexually Transmitted Diseases, Edited by KK Holmes, PA Mårdh, PF Sparling, PJ Wiesner. New York, McGraw-Hill, 1984, p 352
114. McCormack WM, Taylor-Robinson D: The genital mycoplasmas. In Sexually Transmitted Diseases, Edited by KK Holmes, PA Mårdh, PF Sparling, PJ Wiesner. New York, McGraw-Hill, 1984, p 408
115. Barwin BN: Transmission of *Ureaplasma urealyticum* by artificial insemination by donor. Fertil Steril 41:326, 1984
116. Gnarpe H, Friberg J: Mycoplasmas on spermatozoa and infertility. Nature 245:37, 1973
117. Caspi E, Herczeg E, Solomon F, Sompolinsky D: Amnionitis and T strain mycoplasmemia. Am J Obstet Gynecol 111:1102, 1971
118. Taylor Robinson D, McCormack WM: The genital mycoplasmas II. N Engl J Med, 302:1063, 1980
119. Lamey JR, Eschenbach DA, Mitchell SH, Blumhagen JM, Foy HM, Kenny GE: Isolation of mycoplasmas and bacteria from the blood of postpartum women. Am J Obstet Gynecol 143:104, 1982
120. Stagno S, Brasfield DM, Brown MB, Cassell GH, Pifer LL, Whitley RJ, Tiller RE: Infant pneumonitis associated with cytomegalovirus, *Chlamydia, Pneumocystis*, and *Ureaplasma*: a prospective study. Pediatrics 68:322, 1981
121. Beargie R, Lynd P, Tucker E: Perinatal infection and vaginal flora. Am J Obstet Gynecol 122:31, 1975
122. Regan JA, Chao S, James LS: Premature rupture of membranes, preterm delivery, and group B streptococcal colonization of mothers. Am J Obstet Gynecol 141:184, 1981
123. Baker CJ: Group B streptococcal infections. Adv Intern Med 25:475, 1980
124. Catteral RD, Nicol CS: Is trichomonal infestation a venereal disease? Br Med J 1:1177
125. Kreiger G, Holmes KK: Unpublished data
126. Bernfeld WK: A note on *T. vaginalis* and seminal fluid. Br J Vener Dis 48:144, 1972
127. Kleegman SJ: Therapeutic donor insemination. Conn Med 31:705, 1967
128. Trussell RE, Wilson ME, Longwell FH, Laughlin KA: Vaginal trichomoniasis: complement fixation, puerperal morbidity, and early infection of newborn infants. Am J Obstet Gynecol 44:292, 1942
129. Brunham R, Holmes KK, Eschenbach DE: Sexually transmitted diseases in pregnancy. In Sexually Transmitted Diseases, Edited by KK Holmes, PA Mårdh, PF Sparling, PJ Wiesner. New York, McGraw-Hill, 1984, p 782
130. McLaren LC, Davis LE, Healy GR, James CG: Isolation of *T. vaginalis* from the respiratory tract of infants with respiratory disease. Pediatr 71:888, 1983
131. Al-Salihi FL, Curran JP, Wang JS: Neonatal *T. vaginalis*: report of three cases and review of the literature. Pediatr 53:196, 1974
132. Jarrell J, Milner R: Artificial insemination by donor in Ontario. Ann Coll Phys Surg Can 19:115, 1986
133. Nielsen JO: AIDS—Status 1985: Implications for sperm banks. Int J Androl 8:97, 1985
134. Schiff I, Correia B, Ravnikar V, Schur P: HTLV-III antibody testing in sperm donors. N Engl J Med 312:1637, 1985

Chapter 31

Intrauterine insemination: a critical review

Nancy C. Allen, M.D.
Carl M. Herbert III, M.D.
Wayne S. Maxson, M.D.
B. Jane Rogers, Ph.D.
Michael P. Diamond, M.D.
Anne Colston Wentz, M.D.

Center for Fertility and Reproductive Research (C-FARR), Division of Reproductive Endocrinology, Department of Obstetrics and Gynecology, Vanderbilt University Medical Center, Nashville, Tennessee

Artificial insemination has long served an important role in the treatment of infertile couples. Indications for artificial insemination include physiologic and psychologic dysfunction, such as severe hypospadias, vaginismus, retrograde ejaculation, and neurologic, psychogenic, or drug-related impotence that prevents adequate intercourse. Other indications are abnormal sperm, cervical mucus, or immunologic parameters. Artificial insemination also has been used as a nonspecific therapy for unexplained infertility. Insemination may be with husband's (AIH) or donor's (AID) semen; the latter therapy is reserved for couples in whom a severe male factor exists that is refractory to other forms of therapy or for couples with genetic abnormalities.

AIH has been performed by various techniques. Intrauterine insemination (IUI), the subject of this review, refers to direct transfer of sperm to the intrauterine cavity. Although intracervical insemination is occasionally referred to as a separate type of AIH, often it is not clearly defined or differentiated from IUI. With intravaginal insemination, sperm are placed high in the vagina with a syringe or, alternatively, introduced into a plastic cup that has been placed over the cervix. The use of the cervical cup has allowed couples to perform AIH in their homes, often with excellent results. Diamond et al.[1] reported an overall pregnancy rate of 53% in 61 couples treated by this method for repeatedly poor postcoital tests (PCTs) and/or subnormal semen analyses. The overall pregnancy rate with combined methods of AIH had previously been reported to be 18% and 22% for oligospermia ($< 20 \times 10^6$/ml) and poor PCT, respectively.[2] Reasons proposed to explain the better results with the cervical cup included minimum semen loss, protection of sperm from vaginal environment, and the ability of the couple to control the timing and the procedure of insemination in their own home, independent of office hours, waiting times, third parties, and the associated stresses. The theoretic advantage of IUI over intravaginal techniques is that IUI may increase the number of sperm arriving at the fertilization site when decreased sperm count, poor sperm motility, impenetrable or absent cervical mucus, or antisperm antibodies are present. However, the efficacy of IUI in each of these circumstances has not been clearly established.

REVIEW OF THE INTRAUTERINE INSEMINATION LITERATURE

IUI has been used for a variety of indications, with greatly varying pregnancy rates. It is rarely used as first-line therapy in the treatment of infertility because of its questionable efficacy and other disadvantages, which include expense (both monetary and psychologic), necessity of multiple properly timed office visits, and potential for infection or severe cramps. A conception rate of

3.4% reported in 1957 by Mastroianni et al.[3] led those authors to conclude that "unless techniques be somehow improved, intrauterine inseminations should be abandoned." Nevertheless, IUI has continued to be used with technical modifications; reports have appeared sporadically in the literature. In a 1979 review of AIH, Nachtigall et al.[2] reported 39 pregnancies in 120 patients treated with IUI because of poor PCT results. Although their review included heterogeneous patient populations and protocols, the overall success rate (30%) was encouraging. The authors[2] warned, however, that because of potential side effects, IUI should be reserved for patients who fail alternative therapy.

The reports contained in the literature to date may create a confusing picture for the clinician who considers IUI as an alternative for patient therapy. This review will examine results from studies published during the last several years and will attempt to clarify the place of IUI in clinical practice.

The results of 18 series since 1957 in which IUI was used are presented in Table 1.[3-20] All couples had either primary or secondary infertility. The duration of infertility was not always specified, but in most studies, the mean was at least 3 years. Infertility of at least 1 year but less than 3 years' duration is associated with a higher pregnancy rate,[21, 22] and this unknown factor may account for some variation in results. In the 18 series, a total of 714 patients were inseminated, with an overall conception rate of 28% (range, 0% to 62%).

LIMITATIONS OF THIS REVIEW

A direct comparison of reported results is frequently invalidated by the variability of indications and techniques or by failure to report or define such parameters adequately. For example, indications for including patients in an IUI treatment group are not always specified; similarly, diagnoses such as cervical factor or male factor may be ascribed without diagnostic criteria being provided. Some studies[4, 5, 7, 10, 12, 13, 15, 16, 18, 20] include patients with a variety of diagnoses, whereas other studies[3, 6, 8, 9, 11, 13, 17, 19] deal solely with a specific patient population. It is important in the diagnosis and treatment of the infertile couple that care is taken to identify all factors contributing to the infertility (i.e., cervical, uterine, tubal, ovulatory, peritoneal, immunologic, and male factors). In fact, at least 40% of women with negative infertility workups before laparoscopy will have a diagnosis identified at surgery.[23] Unfortunately, few studies clearly describe that a complete workup was accomplished. The procedure of sperm preparation is another important variable to consider. Furthermore, the insemination technique may vary as to type of catheter and depth of insertion (from internal os to high fundal) and is not always clearly defined or distinguished from intracervical insemination. The number of inseminations per cycle as well as the number of cycles treated per couple varies from study to study. Perhaps the most important variable is the timing of the insemination. Several methods for predicting ovulation and scheduling insemination have been reported (Table 1), but only one group of authors[3] retrospectively evaluated their series for the number of inseminations that were properly timed, with the success rate accordingly reported. For evaluation of the wide discrepancy in pregnancy rates among studies, it is necessary to consider the methods of sperm preparation, protocols for insemination, and criteria employed for patient selection.

TECHNIQUES USED IN INTRAUTERINE INSEMINATION

PREPARATION OF THE SEMEN SPECIMEN

Several methods of sperm preparation before IUI have been used in attempt to improve the chance of conception and to minimize complications of the procedure. One goal is optimization of the concentration of motile sperm in the specimen, especially in cases of oligospermia. Another is reduction of the content of seminal plasma, which contains factors that may inhibit normal fertilization.[24] Seminal plasma also contains prostaglandins that can cause uterine cramping and may contain immunocompetent cells and antisperm antibodies in patients with genital tract infections.[25] Regardless of the method used for preparation of the specimen, small amounts (0.1 to 1.0 ml) are used to avoid cramping and infection. In some series,[3, 4, 10, 13] antibiotics were added to the specimen before insemination.

Often the sperm are simply separated from seminal plasma and concentrated by centrifugation and then washed with a buffered saline solution suitable for sperm.[5, 12, 15, 20] Urine may be treated in the same manner in retrieval of sper-

Table 1. *Results of IUI Clinical Trials*

Author	No. of patients	Mean no. of treatment cycles	No. of inseminations per cycle	Sperm preparation	Method of timing	Pregnancies No.	Pregnancies %
Barwin (1973)[4]	50	NS[a]	NS	Washed/frozen	BBT, intravenous Premarin (20%)	31	62
Davajan et al. (1983)[5]	120	1–8	NS	Washed	BBT, ultrasound (25%)	53	44
Dmowski et al. (1979)[6]	27	4.7	1–3	Albumin filtration	BBT, mucus, vaginal cytologic examination	4	15
Farris and Murphy (1960)[7]	100	NS	NS	Unwashed, split ejaculate	NS	13	13
Glass and Ericsson (1978)[8]	19	3.5	1–2	Albumin filtration	BBT	0	0
Glezerman et al. (1984)[9]	25	6	4–7	Unwashed, split ejaculate	NS	13	52
Goldfarb et al. (1984)[10]	21	1.4	NS	Washed, capacitated	Serum E_2 ultrasound	1	5
Harris et al. (1981)[11]	20	6	2	Sperm rise	Cycle day, mucus	3	15
Kaskarelis and Comninos (1959)[12]	46	7 minimum	1–3	Washed (34)/unwashed whole (12)	BBT	8	18
Kerin et al. (1984)[13]	35	1–2	1	Sperm rise	Serum LH	8	23
Kremer (1979)[14]	60	7	1–2	Unwashed, split ejaculate	BBT, mucus	17	28
Marrs et al. (1983)[15]	11	2 minimum	1	Washed	Ultrasound	2	18
Mastroianni et al. (1957)[3]	29	NS	NS	Unwashed, concentrated	BBT	1	3.4
Sher et al. (1984)[16]	65	NS	1	Washed, capacitated	hMG/hCG serum E_2	24	37
Shulman et al. (1978)[17]	7	2 minimum	2–4	Washed	BBT	1	14
Ulstein (1973)[18]	35	NS	1	Unwashed/whole	BBT, mucus	10	29
White and Glass (1976)[19]	9	4.4	1–9	Unwashed/whole	BBT, CC	5	56
Wiltbank et al. (1984)[20]	35	2.7	1–2	Washed	NS	6	17
Total	714					200	28

[a]NS, not specified.

matozoa in patients with retrograde ejaculation.[4, 26, 27] In 1959, Kaskarelis and Comninos,[12] who used either washed and concentrated or unwashed semen, reported 46 cases of IUI but failed to demonstrate a difference between the two methods. Pregnancy rates were 17% (n = 12) and 18% (n = 34), respectively, and complications were not reported for either group. Other factors in the protocol (e.g., improper timing of insemination) may have accounted for the poor pregnancy rates and obscured any effects of sperm washing.

Several authors[7, 9, 14, 28, 29] have used the first portion of a split ejaculate. The first portion contains a higher density of sperm in most patients[7] and has lower levels of prostaglandins.[14] Farris and Murphy[7] examined whole and partitioned ejaculates in 98 patients for number of motile sperm. In all cases, one portion of the split ejaculate contained a higher number of motile sperm than in the whole specimen. In 89 men, the first part contained most of the motile sperm in a ratio of 7.4 to 1, and in the remaining 9 men the second part was higher (ratio, 4.5 to 1). These results point out the necessity of examining both parts of the specimen in order to use the one with the highest concentration of sperm when this technique is used.

Methods that significantly increase the percentage of progressively motile sperm include filtration through human serum albumin (HSA) columns and sperm migration, or "sperm rise" techniques. The former was derived from the method of Ericsson et al.,[30] who layered semen on columns containing HSA to isolate sperm fractions with an increased number of Y sperm. Glass and Ericsson[8] used this method to prepare IUI specimens for patients with a decreased sperm count and/or motility. They added washed sperm suspension to columns containing either 10% HSA (one-layer column) or 7.5% HSA layered over 17.5% HSA (two-layer column). After 60 to 90 minutes, the sperm from the distal fraction were washed and resuspended in Tyrode's solution before insemination. The average percentage of motile sperm increased from 36% to 66% in the one-layer technique; however, the motile sperm concentration represented only 28% of the original concentration. The two-layer technique improved motility from 41% to 85% but resulted in recovery of only 13% of the motile sperm. However, when 19 women were inseminated for 67 cycles with an average of 7×10^6 motile sperm obtained by the two-layer techniques, there were no pregnancies. Dmowski et al.[6] used the one- and two-layer techniques for treatment of oligospermic men and recovered an average of 31×10^6 and 5×10^6 motile sperm, respectively. No conception occurred in 21 couples when the two-layer method was used, whereas 4 of 12 couples who used the one-layer method became pregnant. The prepared specimens used in the conception cycles contained sperm with 64% to 85% motility.

In the sperm rise technique, a diluent is layered over a sperm concentrate previously prepared by washing and centrifugation of semen. The motile sperm are allowed to migrate into the diluent from which they are subsequently recovered. Kerin et al.[13] found that this method produced an increase in motility of 1.75 to 3.2 times the original, but the total number of motile sperm recovered was only 2% to 11% of the whole ejaculate. Harris et al.[11] used open-ended tubes that contained diluent and layered 0.05 ml of semen at the bottom of each tube so that a large interface was provided. Fifty-eight percent of the motile sperm were recovered, with a mean motility of 95%. Only 3 of 20 wives of men with asthenospermia became pregnant after a mean of six cycles treated with this method, which again suggests that improvement in motility alone does not increase the chance of conception.

Goldfarb et al.[10] and Sher et al.[16] used preincubation of washed sperm (in vitro capacitation) in a method similar to that used for in vitro fertilization. Pregnancy rates of 5% and 37%, respectively, were achieved, which indicated that other factors in their patients or methods affected the outcome of treatment. Barwin[4] used sperm that had been frozen at $-150°C$ with only a 5% to 10% decrease in motility. He[4] performed daily inseminations with these specimens in the periovulatory period, with an overall pregnancy rate of 62%.

INTRAUTERINE TRANSFER OF SPERM

In IUI, sperm are introduced directly into the uterine cavity through a catheter that has been passed through the cervical canal. Various types of catheters have been used, which include pediatric feeding catheters, an 18-gauge needle inserted into fine vinyl tubing molded with a guidewire, Teflon intravenous catheters, and a device that is being manufactured specifically for IUI (Sefi-Medical Instruments, Haifa, Israel).[31] The devices used must be able to traverse the cervical canal and reach the uterus without causing trauma to the cervical crypts, epithelium, or uterine wall. The prepared sperm, in a volume of 0.1 to 1.0 ml, are introduced through the catheter from a syringe fitted onto the end of the catheter.

Technical difficulties are frequently encountered in intrauterine transfer, especially in the patient with cervical stenosis or a severely retroflexed/anteflexed uterus. These circumstances require individualization of the techniques and devices used as well as patience and the ability to improvise on the part of the clinician. It may be helpful to record position, angle of insertion, and type of catheter used for repeat inseminations. Some authors[4, 28] recommended removing the cervical mucus from the canal before insemination, especially when hostile mucus or antisperm antibodies are suspected. In spite of these suggestions, there are no data to indicate that these manipulations improve pregnancy rates.

TIMING OF INSEMINATION

To schedule insemination, a variety of methods have been used to predict the time of ovulation (Table 1). Methods such as basal body temperature (BBT) records,[3-6, 8, 12, 14, 17-19, 28] evaluation of cervical mucus for spinnbarkeit, ferning, and cellularity,[6, 9, 11, 32] serum luteinizing hormone (LH)[13] or estradiol (E_2) levels (preovulatory peak),[10, 16] and vaginal cytologic examination[6] have been used to monitor the hormonal status of the preovulatory phase. Ultrasonography has been used by some to monitor follicular development radiographically.[5, 10] Hormonal manipulation with human menopausal gonadotropin

Table 2. *Treatment Period Required for Conception*

Author	Pregnancies		Mean no. of treatment cycles per conception
	No.	%	
Barwin[4]	31	62	3
Dmowski et al.[6]	4	15	1.8
Glezerman et al.[9]	13	52	5.7
Harris et al.[11]	3	15	3.3
Kerin et al.[13]	8	23	1.1
Marrs et al.[15]	2	18	2
Mastroianni et al.[3]	1	3.4	2
Shulman et al.[17]	1	14	2
White and Glass[19]	5	56	5
Wiltbank et al.[20]	6	17	2.7
Total	74		3.3

(hMG)[16] or clomiphene citrate (CC)[15] and human chorionic gonadotropin (hCG) have been used, especially in women with irregular cycle length. All methods have been employed separately or in combination in attempt to perform the insemination around the time of ovulation. With the use of the BBT chart, Mastroianni et al.[3] retrospectively analyzed 104 IUIs and found that only 68 were carried out in the periovulatory time period. BBT records had been used in all but a few cases in the prospective timing of IUI. It is reasonable to assume that the rate of properly timed inseminations may be higher in the modern-day practice when other predictive parameters, such as urine LH monitoring by newly developed enzyme-linked immunosorbent assay techniques are included; however, the BBT is still the most frequent means of scheduling inseminations.

Difficulty predicting the time of ovulation may partially be overcome by more frequent inseminations, begun 2 to 3 days before the expected BBT rise or begun with the E_2 surge and continued until evidence of ovulation has occurred (e.g., sustained temperature rise). Timing may be especially important if most of the sperm are rapidly transported from the point of insemination to the peritoneal cavity, with fewer of the sperm being stored in the cervical crypts.[9] Daily inseminations might then increase the exposure of the ovum to sperm. Barwin[4] and Glezerman et al.[9] used daily insemination with favorable results (62% and 52%, respectively).

DURATION OF THERAPY

The mean number of treatment cycles required to achieve pregnancy has been reported by several groups (Table 2). A mean of 3.3 insemination cycles were required for each woman who became pregnant; again, there is substantial variation among studies. This is similar to the mean treatment period reported for successful AIH, for which 3.5 cycles were required (range, 3 to 5.1).[2] It was also noted that few patients conceived after 5 unsuccessful months of treatment. Wiltbank et al.[20] noted that their success rate of 17% increased to 33% when only patients with three or more attempts were considered; therefore, they concluded that this should be a minimum before discontinuing IUI efforts.

OTHER METHODS OF INSEMINATION

In six studies,[4, 6, 7, 17-19] some other form of insemination was used in association with IUI. In most cases, the part of the specimen not injected into the uterus was placed high in the vagina or in the endocervix. Ulstein[18] routinely performed AIH with a cervical cup concurrently with IUI. Similarly, Dmowski et al.[6] provided patients with a cervical cup to be used for home insemination when ovulation occurred on a weekend. This method had been employed in two of their four conception cycles. Although there is no way to distinguish which insemination led to fertilization, IUI was the primary treatment used. These cases may not be significantly different from those that did not have other types of insemination specified, because some of the sample may drain to the cervix and vagina after IUI. Moreover, none of the studies took into account the incidence of natural intercourse and its contribution to pregnancy rates (i.e., treatment-independent pregnancy).

INDICATIONS FOR INTRAUTERINE INSEMINATION

MALE FACTOR INFERTILITY

The most frequently reported indication for treatment with IUI was infertility due to a male factor, which included oligospermia, asthenospermia, poor penetration (< 10%) in the zona-free hamster egg sperm penetration assay (SPA),[20] or semen analysis parameters that were regarded as substandard (Table 3). The criteria used for poor semen quality vary widely. These criteria are specified in Table 3 so that this variation may be taken into consideration when results are analyzed. Only those patients for whom the authors made a clinical diagnosis of male factor infertility

Table 3. *IUI-Treated Male Factor Infertility*[a]

Author	Patient characteristics	Semen analysis of fertile men	Pregnancies No.	Pregnancies %
Barwin[4]	< 20 × 10^6/ml, at least 50% motile	Not specified	8/12	66
	< 10 × 10^6/ml, at least 50% motile	Not specified	3/8	38
Dmowski et al.[6]	Total count 119 × 10^6 (n = 12) 203 × 10^6 (n = 21) Motility 41% and 45%, normal forms 48% and 46%	Total count 6–33 × 10^6, motility 64%–85%, normal forms 22%–73%	1/5	20
Harris et al.[11]	< 50% motile	47 × 10^6/ml, 32% motility; 66 × 10^6/ml, 28% motility	3/20	15
Kerin et al.[13]	< 40 × 10^6/ml, < 45% motile, < 40% normal forms, or total count < 60 × 10^6 (× 3)	Mean 24 × 10^6/ml, 25% motile, 17 × 10^6 total motile sperm	8/35	23
Kremer[14]	< 20 × 10^6/ml and/or < 40% motile	4 × 10^6/ml, excellent motility	1/6	17
Sher et al.[16]	< 20 × 10^6/ml, < 20% motile, and penetration < 20 mm in bovine cervical mucus	< 20 mm penetration, < 5 × 10^6/ml, 10% motile	1/4	25
Wiltbank et al.[20]	< 20 × 10^6/ml and/or < 10% penetration in zona-free hamster egg SPA	51 × 10^6/ml, 0% in SPA	1/14	7
Total			26/104	25

[a]No female pathologic findings.

in the absence of female pathologic findings are included, whether or not all diagnostic parameters were clearly delineated. The definition of oligospermia, in particular, varies from study to study, but is usually defined as sperm density < 20 × 10^6 sperm/ml of semen. This value is consistent with the minimum density determined to be in the fertile range by MacLeod and Gold[33] in 1951, although 5% of fertile men in their study had counts below this value. In 1977, Zukerman et al.[34] reported the frequency distributions of sperm counts in 4122 prevasectomy patients, compared with those in 1000 infertile men. There were significant differences between fertile and infertile groups when counts ≷ 10 × 10^6/ml were compared ($P < 0.001$) and when those with 10 to 20 × 10^6/ml were compared with those > 20 × 10^6/ml ($P < 0.01$). In the group of allegedly fertile men, however, 23% had sperm densities < 20 × 10^6/ml and 12% had densities < 10 × 10^6/ml. Nevertheless, in the couples noted in Table 3, the male factor was the only diagnosis to which the authors attributed the infertility.

Although the overall pregnancy rate for couples with IUI-treated male factor infertility is 25%, several authors had less-favorable results. Individual pregnancy rates in most studies are comparable to the rate of pregnancies reported to occur spontaneously in this population.[32] Only Barwin[4] reported pregnancy rates > 25% for this group; however, only samples with > 50% motility were used. Also, Barwin[4] used semen specimens that had been frozen in multiple aliquots, which allowed daily insemination and pooling of samples when the count was severely decreased (< 5 × 10^6/ml). If the patients in this unique study are excluded, the overall pregnancy rate for male factor infertility treated with IUI drops to 18%.

Other authors have noted a poor success rate with male factor infertility. Davajan et al.[5] found a decreased rate of conception that was related to the degree of oligospermia. One study[20] employed the zona-free hamster egg SPA as one index of male fertility. This assay tests the ability of in vitro-capacitated human sperm to penetrate a hamster ovum after enzymatic removal of the zona pellucida. Results of the SPA have been shown to correlate with fertility to a more significant degree than either sperm count or motility and may identify fertile and infertile men not identified by routine testing.[35] Wiltbank et al.[20] found results of the SPA in combination with postcoital test (PCT) results to be a predictor of IUI success. For couples with poor PCTs, the pregnancy rates were 50% and 8% for those with SPA penetration values > 10% and < 10%, respectively. Thus, the SPA might provide a more

Table 4. *IUI-Treated Cervical Factor Infertility*[a]

Author	Patient characteristics	Semen analysis of fertile men	Pregnancies	
			No.	%
Barwin[4]	Immotile sperm on PCT × 2, negative cervical mucus penetration test × 2	Normal × 2	13/18	70
Glezerman et al.[9]	Low cervical score and negative mucus penetration on high-dose estrogen (n = 9)	Normal	13/25	52
Sher et al.[16]	Cervical score < 8/12 and poor PCT	Normal	2/3	67
White and Glass[19]	Immotile or absent sperm on PCT, normal mucus pH	Normal	5/9	56
Wiltbank et al.[20]	Poor PCT	SPA > 10%, > 20 × 10^6/ml	2/3	67
Total			35/58	60

[a]No male pathologic findings.

reliable means for determination of a subpopulation of infertile men who may benefit from IUI treatment. Kaskarelis and Comninos[12] reported that all men whose wives conceived had at least 40 × 10^6 sperm/ml, 50% motility, and 70% normal forms, whereas Farris and Murphy[7] found that the first part of the partitioned ejaculate of men who achieved pregnancy contained 9 × 10^6 to 58 × 10^6 *motile* sperm/ml. It appears that a decreased number of motile sperm is consistently associated with a decreased pregnancy rate, although some conceptions do occur. Sperm preparation procedures that significantly decreased the number of sperm, as in the two-layer albumin filtration technique, have been associated with very few pregnancies (0%[8] and 15%[6]) in spite of increasing the percentage of motile sperm.

Speichinger and Mattox[36] reported pregnancy in a patient who was treated with IUI because her husband's semen was hypovolemic. The total number of sperm and the volume were not specified; however, sperm density was normal (80 × 10^6/ml and 120 × 10^6/ml) in two specimens.

IUI has been successfully used to treat retrograde ejaculation, as in case reports by Colpi and associates[26] and Scammell et al.,[27] but conceptions required eight to ten cycles of treatment. In contrast, Barwin[4] used IUI for one patient with retrograde ejaculation, and the patient was unable to achieve a pregnancy.

CERVICAL FACTOR INFERTILITY

Patients treated with IUI for infertility associated with a cervical factor have achieved a higher pregnancy rate (Table 4). Guttmacher[37] remarked in 1960 that poor mucus production secondary to radical cervical cauterization was "one of the two situations in which [he thinks] intrauterine insemination was justified. The other is the woman with a pinpoint external os in whom during ovulation watery cervical mucus does not exude from the cervical opening." Cervical abnormalities include cervical stenosis, especially after cervical conization with destruction of mucus glands and crypts, and abnormal cervical mucus that is inadequate in quantity or is persistently thick, cellular, and unsuitable for sperm transport despite the attempt to stimulate production with estrogen therapy. The primary test employed to identify or rule out cervical factor is the PCT. IUI has been used when the abnormal PCT is the only finding, but failure to document diagnostic criteria makes this indication difficult to evaluate. The validity of the PCT has been questioned by some authors. Jette and Glass[38] found similar pregnancy rates in patients with 0 to 20 sperm per high power field and concluded it is difficult to determine what is abnormal in the PCT. In 1962, Cohen[39] reported two pregnancies associated with IUI in patients with poor cervical mucus unresponsive to estrogen therapy. As seen in Table 4, 60% of patients who had only a cervical factor diagnosed, which accounted for infertility, became pregnant from IUI. Note that the criteria for cervical factor as well as the extent of evaluation vary widely from study to study and that only couples in which the man had at least one normal semen analysis are included. Davajan et al.[5] also noted a higher pregnancy rate for patients with a cervical factor. This agrees with what one might logically expect: IUI

Table 5. *IUI-Treated Immunologic Infertility*

Author	Patient characteristics	Semen analysis of fertile men	Pregnancies	
			No.	%
Glass and Ericsson[8]	Male serum sperm agglutinating antibodies		0/1	0
Kremer[14]	Poor PCT, mucus penetration test, strongly + SCMCT,[a] antisperm IgG and IgA in seminal plasma or cervical mucus	Not specified	4/20	20
Shulman et al.[17]	Males with + Franklin-Dukes sperm agglutination titers	Sperm density 99–249 × 10^6/ml, 60% to 80% motile	1/7	14
Ulstein[18]	Male serum sperm agglutinating antibodies	< 60 × 10^6/ml, < 70% motile	2/4	50
Wiltbank et al.[20]	Serum agglutinating or immobilizing antibodies	Total sperm count 51–117 × 10^6	2/8	25
Total			9/40	22

[a]Sperm-cervical mucus contact test.

bypasses the hostile cervical canal so that otherwise normal individuals would be likely to conceive with this method.

IMMUNOLOGIC INFERTILITY

IUI for the treatment of immunologic infertility remains controversial (Table 5). Boettcher et al.[40] reported pregnancy after one cycle of IUI with the use of washed sperm in a patient whose husband had serum and seminal plasma antibodies detected by the gelatin agglutination technique. In this case, an immune factor was the only diagnosis to account for infertility of 6 years' duration. Kremer et al.[14, 28] and Shulman et al.[17] have reported limited success with IUI for patients with antibodies. Kremer et al.[28] treated 20 infertile couples with a strongly positive "shaking" phenomenon in the sperm cervical mucus contact test, all of whom had a moderate to high sperm-agglutination titer in the serum of the male or female partner or in the cervical mucus or seminal plasma. Three couples in whom the man had serum and seminal plasma antibodies and one in whom the woman had serum and cervical mucus antibodies (the latter in very high titer, 1 to 2048) were able to conceive with IUI. Shulman and colleagues[17] treated seven men who had serum antisperm antibodies (determined by either the Kibrick or Franklin-Dukes technique) with sperm washing followed by at least two cycles of IUI. One pregnancy occurred in this group. The results of Kremer et al.[14, 28] and Shulman et al.[17] are somewhat difficult to assess without additional clinical information regarding the presence or absence of other factors in the couple's infertility. Wiltbank et al.[20] reported pregnancies in two of eight couples with antisperm antibodies present in either the husband or wife, but three of these eight couples had other diagnoses as well. Ulstein[18] reported pregnancies for two of four couples in whom the man had serum agglutinating antibodies. Both conceptions were associated with low titers of antibodies, and the two couples in whom the man had very high titers failed to conceive.

IUI may be of help when cervical mucus antisperm antibodies are the primary obstacle to fertility, by impairing sperm migration through the cervical canal. However, surface antisperm antibodies produced in the male genital tract may interfere with the ability of the sperm to attach to the zona pellucida[41] and have been shown to block or reduce penetration of zona-free hamster eggs.[42] In these patients, merely bypassing the cervical mucus with IUI would be insufficient to correct completely the effect of the antibodies on a couple's fertility. Unfortunately, because of the high affinity of antisperm antibodies for the sperm surface antigens, multiple washings and centrifugations fail to separate the bonds between them. Techniques required to remove the antibodies include washing with buffers of high ionic strength and lead to loss of sperm function.[43] For treating antibodies that bind to sperm after ejaculation, immediate placement of the sperm into large diluting volumes or into solutions containing membrane fragments of freeze-thawed sperm as an immunosorbent may reduce the percentage of sperm that are antibody bound.[44] Specimens prepared in this fashion could be used for IUI, but the intrauterine technique would doubtfully be

Table 6. *Spontaneous Abortion in IUI-Associated Pregnancies*

Author	Total pregnancies	Spontaneous abortions	
		No.	%
Barwin[4]	31	7	23
Cohen[39]	3	1	33
Dmowski et al.[6]	4	0	
Glezerman et al.[9]	13	4	33
Harris et al.[11]	3	1	33
Kremer[14]	4	1	25
Mastroianni et al.[3]	1	0	
Sher et al.[16]	24	5	21
Ulstein[18]	10	6	60
White and Glass[19]	5	0	
Total	98	25	26

advantageous over intravaginal or cervical cup techniques in this case. Similarly, if women with high serum titers of antisperm antibodies have significant antibody levels present within the reproductive tract, especially at the site of fertilization, IUI would not be a logical approach.

OTHER INDICATIONS FOR INTRAUTERINE INSEMINATION

In many infertility cases, multiple factors are found during diagnostic workup of the couple. IUI has been used when treatment of these factors has failed to result in pregnancy, usually preceded by another form of AIH. IUI has been used to treat couples with unexplained infertility when all clinically detectable parameters appear normal, and some pregnancies have been reported.[14, 16] These pregnancies may or may not have resulted from IUI, but spontaneous remission of an unknown factor cannot be excluded.

An interesting but rare indication of IUI is reported by Shapiro et al.,[45] who described a pregnancy after IUI with washed sperm in a woman with seminal plasma allergy. This patient was unable to have intercouse without the use of a condom because of severe symptoms of hypersensitivity, whereas IUI with washed sperm resulted in a pregnancy without complications.

COMPLICATIONS

EARLY SPONTANEOUS ABORTION

The rate of early spontaneous abortion was 26% (range, 0% to 60%) in 98 patients (Table 6). Again, this rate is comparable to the rate of miscarriages in AIH as reviewed by Nachtigall et al.[2]: 25% of these pregnancies ended in spontaneous abortion (range, 0% to 45%). This increase in the observed rate of abortion in artificially inseminated patients (normal population, ~ 10% to 15%) may be related to factors reponsible for the infertility (abnormal sperm, luteal phase defects, genetic defects, etc.). Furthermore, early detection of pregnancy in the subfertile population may lead to increased frequency of detection and reporting of early miscarriages.

SIDE EFFECTS

The incidence of serious complications related to IUI is uniformly low, regardless of whether the sperm are washed or unwashed or whether a split or whole ejaculate is used. Severe cramps were reported by Barwin (6%),[4] Glass and Ericsson (5%),[8] and Mastroianni et al. (17%).[3] The higher rate of cramps in the latter study could be related to the use of unwashed sperm, although the specimen was concentrated by centrifugation and should have contained smaller amounts of seminal plasma components.

The theoretic risk of infection because of introducing a nonsterile material into the uterine cavity has been of concern to all who have used this form of therapy. Surprisingly, no serious infections were reported in the series here, and only one patient had a rise in temperature after IUI which returned to normal with antibiotic therapy.[12] Some authors have used antibiotics for the insemination period in either the wife[9, 19, 20] or in the specimen inseminated[3, 4, 10, 13]; however, with the low incidence of infection in untreated women, prophylactic antibodies may not be necessary.

Another consequence of IUI treatment was reported by Kremer,[14] who found IUI led to a significant increase in sperm agglutination titers among women who previously had been shown to have moderate or high titers of these same serum antibodies.[11] Pregnancy was achieved in one woman despite an increase in serum sperm agglutination titer from 1 in 64 to 1 in 512, however, and women with low or negative titers did not form antibodies. Introduction of intact mouse sperm into the peritoneal cavities of mice has been found to lead to production of antibodies against these sperm.[46] Because with normal intercourse only tens of hundreds of sperm reach the peritoneal cavity, perhaps the introduction of large numbers of sperm with IUI leads to an increased risk of sensitization.[43]

DISCUSSION

The difficulty in evaluating uncontrolled studies is a significant drawback to the assessment of any treatment modality. Only one study in this review included a control patient group, wherein each couple engaged in natural or LH-timed intercourse in cycles alternating with IUI treatment in other cycles.[13] The incidence of treatment-independent pregnancy is frequently ignored in attributing conception to a given treatment, although it has been well elucidated by some authors.[32, 47-51] For example, in a series of 16 cases of infertility secondary to a male factor, Glass and Ericsson[32] reported a spontaneous pregnancy rate of 25% during the study period, whereas no patients became pregnant as a result of artificial insemination. The male partners in three of these cases were found to have wide variations in both count and motility of sperm. Occasional normal semen specimens may have accounted for the pregnancies. In the review by Nachtigall et al.,[2] the spontaneous pregnancy rate for six series was 14% in couples who had discontinued AIH. In two of those series, the spontaneous pregnancy rate exceeded that associated with treatment. Collins et al.[47] reported rates of treatment-independent pregnancies in 1145 infertile couples over a 2- to 7-year follow-up period. Thirty-five percent of untreated couples achieved pregnancy, varying from 14% to 44% depending on the cause (excluding patients with bilateral tubal disease or azoospermia, none of whom became pregnant without treatment). An additional 7% of the couples studied achieved pregnancies long after the cessation of therapy.

These examples of treatment-independent pregnancy rates are important considerations in assessing the results of any infertility treatment. An assumption that all pregnancies that occurred within a given treatment cycle can be attributed to IUI will likely lead to an overestimation of its efficacy. On the other hand, the reported pregnancy rates are for a relatively short treatment period (usually less than 8 months), and 1- or 2-year cumulative pregnancy rates would be expected to be in higher. Although pregnancy "expectancy" may be calculated by computer analysis (i.e., cumulative pregnancy rate for an indefinite period of time), pregnancy "rate" is confined to and varies with the length of follow-up.[52]

Despite mixed and often discouraging results, IUI continues to be widely employed for a number of infertility problems. Although it has been successfully used to treat the logical indication of cervical factor infertility, IUI has provided little improvement in the rate of pregnancy in couples with a severe male factor. Its use for other indications has not been well elucidated, and IUI success in patients with multiple infertility diagnoses is variable. Careful patient selection is a crucial factor in the chance for conception with this method.

Other steps that may be important prognostically include sperm preparation, which should be directed to maximize the quality of semen for patients with suboptimal semen parameters and minimize the seminal plasma contaminants. Secondly, proper timing of insemination during the periovulatory period must be assured. Various methods to regulate and monitor cycles have been developed, especially through the establishment of successful in vitro fertilization programs,[16] and can be applied toward the IUI treatment protocol. Frequent inseminations can further increase the chance of ovum fertilization with the use of this method.

There are several advantages to IUI when it is carefully managed and when patients are well chosen. It may be used to bypass the cervix when mucus is insufficient or unsuitable for sperm survival and transport, and it is an alternative method for patients who have failed AIH by other means. It may be used before attempting the more costly and complex in vitro fertilization and embryo transfer procedure and/or for couples who are reluctant to resort to AID or adoption. In addition, it may be useful when cervical mucus antibodies are present, but further studies are needed to demonstrate possible benefits.

Disadvantages of IUI include risks of mild to severe cramping, bleeding, possible increase in titers of antisperm antibodies in the woman, and the theoretic risks of pelvic infection or chemical salpingitis. An increased incidence of spontaneous abortion may be associated with bypassing natural sperm selection processes in the cervix.[9] Furthermore, IUI is relatively expensive and can be technically difficult to perform. Finally, the psychologic costs of artificial insemination and disruption of normal coital patterns could lead to emotional or marital stress and could potentially decrease the rate of spontaneous pregnancy. The dropout rate associated with AIH has been reported to be 17% to 72% by the sixth insemination cycle[2] and may in part be because of these psychologic factors.

CONCLUSIONS

IUI is a treatment that should be reserved for couples with relatively clear indications (e.g., cervical factor infertility) and who are highly motivated to carry out an expensive and stressful program. Although IUI has not been shown to be effective in significantly increasing the overall conception rate for men with oligospermia, there have been some reports of pregnancy with IUI when sperm counts are severely decreased. Further studies are needed for assessment of the use of IUI in immunologic infertility, but preliminary results fail to support this indication and introduce the possibility that IUI may increase the risk of sperm sensitization in women. Sperm preparation should be directed to optimize count and motility and minimize content of seminal plasma, and the timing methods should be assessed carefully for accuracy of predicting ovulation. The treatment period should contain at least three cycles before therapy is abandoned. Patients should be thoroughly counseled about the risks, relative pregnancy rates, and emotional considerations before the initiation of treatment.

Acknowledgment. We would like to acknowledge Ms. Brenda Gibson for her valuable assistance in the preparation of this manuscript.

REFERENCES

1. Diamond MP, Christianson C, Daniell JF, Wentz AC: Pregnancy following use of the cervical cup for home artificial insemination utilizing homologous semen. Fertil Steril 39:480, 1983
2. Nachtigall RD, Faure N, Glass RH: Artificial insemination of husband's sperm. Fertil Steril 32:141, 1979
3. Mastroianni L Jr, Laberge JL, Rock J: Appraisal of the efficacy of artificial insemination with husband's sperm and evaluation of insemination technics. Fertil Steril 8:260, 1957
4. Barwin BN: Intrauterine insemination of husband's semen. J Reprod Fertil 36:101, 1974
5. Davajan V, Vargyas JM, Kletzky OA, March CM, Bernstein GS, Mishell DR Jr, Marrs RP: Intrauterine insemination with washed sperm to treat infertility. Fertil Steril (Abstr) 40:419, 1983
6. Dmowski WP, Gaynor L, Lawrence M, Rao R, Scommegna A: Artificial insemination homologous with oligospermic semen separated on albumin columns. Fertil Steril 31:58, 1979
7. Farris EJ, Murphy DP: The characteristics of the two parts of the partitioned ejaculation and the advantages of its use for intrauterine insemination. Fertil Steril 11:465, 1960
8. Glass RH, Ericsson RJ: Intrauterine insemination of isolated motile sperm. Fertil Steril 29:535, 1978
9. Glezerman M, Bernstein D, Insler V: The cervical factor of infertility and intrauterine insemination. Int J Fertil 29:16, 1984
10. Goldfarb JM, Sheean LA, Utian WH: Intrauterine insemination—reappraisal with a new method. Fertil Steril (Abstr) 41:108S, 1984
11. Harris SJ, Milligan MP, Masson GM, Dennis KJ: Improved separation of motile sperm in asthenospermia and its application to artificial insemination homologous (AIH). Fertil Steril 36:219, 1981
12. Kaskarelis E, Comninos A: A critical evaluation of homologous artificial insemination. Int J Fertil 4:38, 1959
13. Kerin JFP, Peek J, Warnes GM, Kirby C, Jeffrey R, Matthews CD, Cox LW: Improved conception rate after intrauterine insemination of washed spermatozoa from men with poor quality semen. Lancet 1:553, 1984
14. Kremer J: A new technique for intrauterine insemination. Int J Fertil 24:53, 1979
15. Marrs RP, Vargyas JM, Saito H, Gibbon WE, Berger T, Mishell DR Jr: Clinical applications of techniques used in human in vitro fertilization research. Am J Obstet Gynecol 146:477, 1983
16. Sher G, Knutzen VK, Stratton CJ, Montakhab MM, Allenson SG: In vitro sperm capacitation and transcervical intrauterine insemination for the treatment of refractory infertility: Phase I. Fertil Steril 41:260, 1984
17. Shulman S, Harlin B, Davis P, Reyniak JV: Immune infertility and new approaches to treatment. Fertil Steril 29:309, 1978
18. Ulstein M: Fertility of husbands at homologous insemination. Acta Obstet Gynecol Scand 52:5, 1973
19. White RM, Glass RH: Intrauterine insemination with husband's semen. Obstet Gynecol 47:119, 1976
20. Wiltbank MC, Kosasa TS, Rogers BJ: Treatment of infertile patients by intrauterine insemination of washed spermatozoa. Andrologia 17:22, 1985
21. Collins JA, So Y, Wilson EH, Wrixon W, Casper RF: Clinical factors affecting pregnancy rates among infertile couples. Can Med Assoc J 130:269, 1984
22. Dor J, Homburg R, Rabau E: An evaluation of etiologic factors and therapy in 665 infertile couples. Fertil Steril 28:718, 1977
23. Musich JR, Behrman SJ: Infertility laparoscopy in perspective: review of five hundred cases. Am J Obstet Gynecol 143:293, 1982
24. Kanwar KC, Yanagimachi R, Lopata A: Effects of human seminal plasma on fertilizing capacity of human spermatozoa. Fertil Steril 31:321, 1979
25. Witkin SS, Toth A: Relationship between genital tract infections, sperm antibodies in seminal fluid, and infertility. Fertil Steril 40:805, 1983
26. Colpi GM, Sommadossi L, Zanollo A: Infertility caused by retrograde ejaculation: a successfully treated case. Andrologia 15:592, 1983
27. Scammell GE, Stedronska J, Dempsey A: Successful pregnancies using human serum albumin following retrograde ejaculation: a case report. Fertil Steril 37:277, 1982
28. Kremer J, Jager S, Kuiken J: Treatment of infertility caused by antisperm antibodies. Int J Fertil 23:270, 1978

29. Perez-Pelaez M, Cohen MR: The split ejaculate in homologous insemination. Int J Fertil 10:25, 1965
30. Ericsson RJ, Langevin CN, Nishino M: Isolation of fractions rich in human Y sperm. Nature 246:421, 1973
31. Makler A, DeCherney A, Naftolin F: A device for injecting and retaining a small volume of concentrated spermatozoa in the uterine cavity and cervical canal. Fertil Steril 42:306, 1984
32. Glass RH, Ericsson RJ: Spontaneous cure of male infertility. Fertil Steril 31:305, 1979
33. MacLeod J, Gold RZ: The male factor in fertility and infertility. II. Spermatozoan counts in 1000 cases of known fertility and in 1000 cases of infertile marriages. J Urol 66:436, 1951
34. Zukerman Z, Rodriguez-Rigau LJ, Smith KD, Steinberger E: Frequency distribution of sperm counts in fertile and infertile males. Fertil Steril 28:1310, 1977
35. Rogers BJ: Hamster egg evaluation of human sperm using in vitro fertilization. In In Vitro Fertilization and Embryo Transfer, Edited by PG Crosignani, BL Rubin. London, Academic Press, 1983, p 101
36. Speichinger JP, Mattox JH: Homologous artificial insemination and oligospermia. Fertil Steril 27:135, 1976
37. Guttmacher AF: The role of artificial insemination in the treatment of sterility. Obstet Gynecol Surv 15:767, 1960
38. Jette NT, Glass RH: Prognostic value of the postcoital test. Fertil Steril 23:29, 1972
39. Cohen MR: Intrauterine insemination. Int J Fertil 7:235, 1962
40. Boettcher B, Kay DJ, Fitchett SB: Successful treatment of male infertility caused by antispermatozoal antibodies. Med J Aust 2:471, 1982
41. Bronson RA, Cooper GW, Rosenfeld DL: Sperm-specific isoantibodies and autoantibodies inhibit the binding of human sperm to the zona pellucida. Fertil Steril 38:724, 1982
42. Alexander NJ: Antibodies to human spermatozoa impede sperm penetration of cervical mucus or hamster eggs. Fertil Steril 41:433, 1984
43. Bronson R, Cooper G, Rosenfeld D: Sperm antibodies: their role in infertility. Fertil Steril 42:171, 1984
44. Bronson RA, Cooper GW, Rosenfeld D: Use of freeze-thawed sonicated human sperm as an in vitro immunoabsorbent. Am J Reprod Immunol 2:162, 1982
45. Shapiro SS, Kooistra JB, Schwartz D, Yunginger JW, Haning RV Jr: Induction of pregnancy in a woman with seminal plasma allergy. Fertil Steril 36:405, 1981
46. Edwards RG: Immunological control of fertility in female mice. Nature 201:582, 1964
47. Collins JA, Wrixon W, Janes LB, Wilson EH: Treatment-independent pregnancy among infertile couples. N Engl J Med 309:1201, 1983
48. Dixon RE, Buttram VC Jr, Schum CW: Artificial insemination using homologous semen: a review of 158 cases. Fertil Steril 27:647, 1976
49. Drake TS, Tredway DR: Spontaneous pregnancy during the infertility evaluation. Fertil Steril 30:36, 1978
50. Harrison RF: Insemination of husband's semen with and without the addition of caffeine. Fertil Steril 29:532, 1978
51. Uehling DT: Low-dose cortisone for male infertility. Fertil Steril 29:220, 1978
52. Katayama KP, Ju KS, Manuel M, Jones GS, Jones HW Jr: Computer analysis of etiology and pregnancy rate in 636 cases of primary infertility. Am J Obstet Gynecol 135:207, 1979

SECTION VII

Contraception and Sterilization

Public health measures to minimize the uncontrolled population growth in most areas of the world remain an enormous challenge. The global population explosion is causing serious food shortages, inadequate medical care, housing and sanitation, as well as frequent political instability. While efforts are ongoing to develop safe, effective, and economical contraception, the emphasis must remain on finding means of making these widely available and implementing and monitoring their use. Under continuing investigation today are a number of promising new methods of contraception. These include long-acting injectable progestin preparations, antihuman chorionic gonadotropin vaccines, luteolytic agents, inhibitory luteinizing hormone-releasing hormone agonists, prostaglandin synthesis inhibitors, antiprogestational agents, and suppression of spermatogenesis with gossypol. Reports on the clinical applicability of these investigations are anxiously awaited. One such recent report is that of a large clinical study by Chinese investigators on the use of gossypol.[1] Although hypokalemia remains a problem with long term use of this preparation, this method was shown to be a highly effective male antifertility drug. None of the wives of the volunteers became pregnant and the continuation rate for its use after one year was over 61%.

The communication by Kessel, Zipper, and Mumford in this section reports on use of transcervical quinacrine pellets as an acceptable nonsurgical female sterilization method. The authors reassessed the safety and efficacy of this method and indicate that it is 95% effective. It is reported that after brief training nonphysicians can perform this procedure on an outpatient basis, and thus it appears to have advantages for both developing and developed countries. To date in over 1,000 insertions of quinacrine pellets there is a lower ectopic pregnancy rate than that with surgical sterilization and a virtual absence of serious complications. The quinacrine tablets produce inflammation and fibrosis confined primarily to the intramural portion of the fallopian tubes. Whether a second or third insertion contributes to the efficacy of this method remains to be determined.

The comprehensive analysis of pregnancy termination techniques and their risks and complications prepared by Castadot of the Fertility Control Center at the Johns Hopkins Hospital distinguishes three subdivisions by weeks of gestation. While the overall mortality for legal abortion in the United States in 1981 was 0.5/100,000, on the average this rate increases 30% with each passing week of gestation. Before 8 weeks' gestation, suction dilatation and curettage (D & C) is currently the preferred method. The complication rate before 7 weeks is higher than during the 8- to 10-week period. A medical approach, possibly self-administered, during this gestation span awaits only an improvement in side effects. Agents such as RU-486 which block progesterone receptors in the endometrium holds promise. This would greatly reduce the need for suction procedures.

From 8 to 15 weeks the methods used include D & C and dilation and evacuation (D & E). While laminaria tents improve the facility and safety of this procedure and are frequently used, prostaglandin analogs (PG) are also feasible for ripening the cervix. The ideal method for termination between 16 to 20 weeks' gestation remains controversial. While D & E is associated with fewer complications, cost effectiveness has dictated the use of other methods such as hypertonic saline and urea augmented with PG. After 20 weeks the urea-PG method is safer. The author stresses that because of the rapid increase in complications with passing weeks, any delay in providing abortion services should be avoided.

The third chapter in this section is a comprehensive review on the past decade of intrauterine contraception. Specific indications for its use continue to be a means of contraception for women who do not desire permanent sterilization and who are poor candidates for oral contraception. Tatum and Connell provide a detailed tabulation for 17 intrauterine devices (IUDs) regarding such factors as rates of pregnancy, bleeding/pain, expulsion, and continuation. Copper-bearing devices are most effective and can provide a pregnancy prevention level of 0.5 pregnancies/100 women years for a period of 4 years. While bleeding and spotting are the most frequent complications, progestin-bearing IUDs have the least blood loss both due to the small size of the device and the direct effect of progesterone on the endometrial cells. Copper medicated devices appear to exert localized activity in the uterine cavity significantly mobilizing leukocytes from the vascular system. The authors examining the question of possible association of pelvic inflammatory disease with the use of IUDs and the micro-organisms most frequently involved. Whether there is a causal relationship between IUD usage and ectopic pregnancy is not established, but it is clear that the copper medicated devices are associated with a lower ectopic rate than the progesterone bearing devices.

Against the background of improved technology and information we are now faced with the virtual demise of the IUDs in the United States. The authors provide a review of the historical events which culminated in the discontinuation of the availability of all these devices except Progestasert (Alza Corp). The discontinuation of the manufacture of IUDs for use in the United States has jeopardized their use in other countries since the implication is that there is something wrong with the devices. This method of fertility control has been widely used throughout the world and most notably in China where it is the major form of contraception. It is hoped that the ongoing effort to reverse the situation in the United States will be successful, and that improved devices can be made available to American women.

Huggins and Zucker provide an update on the concerns and controversy over a possible association between oral contraceptive (OC) use and the development of human neoplasia. The principle investigative methods in human beings are various epidemiologic approaches. Since the number of long term users of OCs continues to grow, investigative studies are much better able to define critical and confounding data items than in the past. Studies of breast disease have shown that high dose (over 1 mg) progestin in combined OCs have a protective effect on the development of benign breast disease. This protective effect has not been shown for the new lower dose progestin pills. However, OCs protect only against those lesions which are not premalignant. No consistent adverse or beneficial effect has been shown between their use and the development of breast carcinoma in women. Benign liver neoplasia has been associated with long term OC use, but this condition is very rare (1 to 5 per 1 million women). Recent reports suggest an association between OC use and hepatocellular carcinoma, but this lesion is also extremely infrequent.

A significant protective effect against the development of adenocarcinoma of the endometrium appears to be conveyed by long term use of OCs. It is estimated that 2,000 cases of this malignancy are prevented through oral contraception each year in the United States. Low dose OCs do not appear to increase the risk of stimulating growth of leiomyomas. There appears to be an increased risk of cervical neoplasia which is directly proportional to the length of its use. The mechanism for this adverse effect is unclear. Epidemiologic studies capturing other major risk factors such as age at first intercourse and the number of sexual partners are necessary to adequately evaluate this problem. Ovarian functional cysts can be prevented with OCs. In similar fashion OCs can afford protection from malignant ovarian neoplasia. It is believed that annually more than 1,700 cases of ovarian cancer are prevented by OC use in the United States. While it is disturbing to read of the growing evidence to suggest adverse effects of oral contraceptive use on cervical neoplasia, the protective effects provided against endometrial and ovarian carcinoma are heartening. This is important information which should be provided to the patient and carefully considered in weighing the risks and benefits to be derived from OC use.

Roger D. Kempers, M.D.

REFERENCE

1. Liu G, Lyle KC, Cao J: Clinical trial of gossypol as a male contraceptive drug. Part I. Efficacy study. Fertil Steril 48:459, 1987

Chapter 32

A decade of intrauterine contraception: 1976 to 1986

Howard J. Tatum, M.D., Ph.D.
Elizabeth B. Connell, M.D.

Department of Gynecology and Obstetrics, Emory University School of Medicine, Atlanta, Georgia

Pressures stemming from rapidly escalating numbers of human beings are resulting in corresponding reductions in standards of living in many areas of the world. Foremost among the problems that this is causing are serious food shortages leading to mass malnutrition and starvation, depletion of natural resources, under- and unemployment, inadequate housing and sanitation, minimal educational facilities, and widespread political instability. In addition, rapid population growth has led to grossly inadequate public health measures including preventive medical services, and, in many areas of the world, absence of the bare essentials for definitive medical and surgical therapy.

One of the generic requisites of minimizing this uncontrolled population growth is to improve the safety and effectiveness of contraceptive methods. Second, ways must be found to make them available upon request throughout the world.

A paper was published in 1977[1] by one of us (H. J. T.) dealing with intrauterine devices (IUDs) used during the years 1966 to 1976. It is the purpose of this present paper not to repeat material from the earlier work, but to highlight the observations and achievements made during the succeeding decade.

During these years, much has been learned about IUDs and the roles that they can and do play in fertility regulation, both in the United States and in many other countries. Significant breakthroughs have been made in understanding their modes of action and in developing long-acting medicated devices. We have learned to bring into clearer focus those criteria which delineate the indications and the contraindications for safe and effective use of IUDs. Finally, we have identified potentially serious complications and discovered how to prevent or at least to minimize them.

It is proposed in this presentation to discuss the salient features relevant to the IUD which continue to make it an important tool in our contraceptive armamentarium. There is no intent to provide a comprehensive review of the world literature, but merely to emphasize those gains in technology and basic information which have been made during the past 10 years and to bring into perspective the lessons which have been learned.

CONTRACEPTIVE CHOICE

It is of the utmost importance that the clinician explain carefully to the patient seeking contraception the risks and the benefits of each method being considered. The final choice must be made jointly by the contraceptor and her health care provider and must take into account the woman's objectives and the medical judgment of the clinician. The decision by the patient as to how to control her fertility is one of the most vital of her human rights, and we, as her medical advisors, must advise her in a sensitive and scientifically sound manner. Our personal prejudices and religious and/or moral judgments should in no way be allowed to influence the woman's choice of a contraceptive method. A selection should be made only after the patient has been informed of all of the options open to her and the appropriateness of one or several of these for her.

GENERAL INDICATIONS FOR IUD USE

The following general indications must be met prior to considering specific indications and contraindications for a particular IUD.[2] Initially, the woman must have an anatomically normal cervix, uterus, and vagina. The size and shape of the uterus must be within normal limits, and it must have no obvious developmental abnormalities such as uterus didelphus. She must be within the active childbearing age group, generally considered today to be somewhere between 14 and 50 years of age. She must be sexually active or expecting to become sexually active and at risk of becoming pregnant.

Over the past several years it has become increasingly apparent that the risk of acquiring pelvic inflammatory disease (PID) while wearing an IUD is significantly greater if the woman has multiple sexual partners. For this reason, it is highly desirable that both the woman and her sex partner be monogamous. In addition, while the risk of PID and subsequent infertility is increased for nulligravid women, it is not for multiparous patients using copper IUDs. Finally, the selection of an IUD meets the general criteria of a contraceptive which is not temporally related to coitus and requires a minimum of follow-up care.

SPECIFIC INDICATIONS FOR IUD USE

There are a number of clinical situations in which the IUD is probably the method of choice.[2] For example, an IUD provides an excellent reversible substitute for sterilization. If the decision has not yet been reached by the contraceptor or by her sexual partner that permanent contraception is desired, then the IUD offers an important temporary solution. It is a viable option for women who have completed their childbearing or who think that they have probably achieved their desired family size.

The IUD is a good choice for the woman who is over the age of 35 and smokes 15 or more cigarettes per day or one who is over the age of 40. These individuals are poor candidates for an oral contraceptive (OC). There may also be other medical contraindications to the use of OCs, including hypertension, the presence or history of thromboembolic disease, stroke or transient ischemia attack, myocardial infarction, genital or breast malignancies and a variety of other factors that place certain women at high risk. Frequent and severe migraine headaches are also considered to be a relative contraindication to oral contraceptives and thus become one of the group of specific indications for an IUD.

While the presence of hypermenorrhea of a functional nature would generally be a contraindication for the use of a nonmedicated or a copper-bearing IUD, it might be considered an indication for one of the progestin-bearing devices. Women with this condition may be candidates, because these latter IUDs effect a generalized suppression of the endometrium with a corresponding reduction in uterine bleeding.

Endometrial adhesions, or synechiae (Asherman's syndrome), have long been a specific indication for intrauterine contraceptive devices. Experience in the past has shown that the use of a nonmedicated IUD such as the Lippes Loop (Ortho Pharmaceutical Corp., Raritan, NJ) or the Saf-T-Coil (Schmid Products Co., Little Falls, NJ) is of benefit because of its larger size and space-filling characteristics.[3] The use of medicated IUDs for this purpose has not yet been assessed.

ABSOLUTE CONTRAINDICATIONS FOR IUD USE

There are several clinical conditions currently considered to represent absolute contraindications for the insertion of an IUD.[4] One of these is an intrauterine pregnancy, because an insertion will usually be followed by a miscarriage. If pregnancy is suspected, whether intrauterine or ectopic, an IUD should not be inserted until the possibility of a pregnancy has been excluded.

The presence of a gynecologic malignancy must be ruled out prior to the insertion of an IUD. Any abnormal unexplained vaginal bleeding contraindicates the use of an IUD until the cause of the bleeding has been ascertained and appropriately treated. Acute vaginal, cervical, or upper genital tract infections must be accurately diagnosed and effectively treated prior to insertion.

RELATIVE CONTRAINDICATIONS FOR IUD USE

There are a number of relative contraindications for the use of IUDs.[4] Each of these must be considered individually with respect to the general health status of the contraceptor and her particular risk/benefit ratio relevant to the use of an IUD. The following clinical entities should be considered but are not necessarily listed in the order of their importance.

A prior ectopic pregnancy suggests a strong possibility or probability that a second one may occur. It must be assumed that any tubal abnormality that contributed to the initial ectopic gestation may still be present in the same tube (unless a salpingectomy was performed) as well as in the contralateral tube. The development of improved microsurgical techniques has increased the successful reestablishment of tubal continuity. Even with modern technology, however, there is no guarantee that patency of the tube(s) will reestablish normal function and that pregnancy will be attained.

A history of acute PID is considered by many to be an absolute contraindication for the use of an IUD. In certain rare instances, if acceptable alternatives are not available for a particular individual, an IUD may be considered. There should, however, be no clinical evidence of persistent disease at the time of insertion. If the patient has had a recent delivery associated with postpartum endometritis or has had an infected abortion or miscarriage within the preceding 3 or 4 months, an IUD is not a good contraceptive choice for her.

Individuals who have had chronic PID, characterized by recurrent flare-ups during the preceding months or years, are rarely to be considered as acceptable candidates for an IUD. The insertion may contribute to reactivation of a smoldering type of infection or may set the stage for a reinfection. It is important to stress that an IUD *cannot* be inserted transvaginally without introducing microorganisms from the vagina into the endometrial cavity. Preexisting acute or chronic PID may damage the tubal and/or parovarian tissues such that there is lowered resistance to pathogens transmitted by intrauterine contamination.

A history of sexually transmitted disease(s) suggests a life style that may be associated with frequent inoculation with new species or strains of microorganisms, introduced into the vagina by multiple sexual partners. Such a history, particularly if there are repeated episodes, is a relatively strong contraindication for the use of an intrauterine device. If, however, a new and monogamous life style of the contraceptor and of her partner has been assured, an IUD may be considered in a women who has no other contraindications for IUD use.

A woman who has severe dysmenorrhea is not a good candidate for an IUD. The history of excessive menstrual pain should indicate to the clinician that the problem might be exaggerated by the presence of an IUD, because the uterus will try to expel the foreign body. The newer, smaller, medicated IUDs have a much reduced tendency to cause severe menstrual and/or intermenstrual pain, compared with the earlier, larger, nonmedicated varieties.

A history of chronic menorrhagia suggests that bleeding might become more severe if an IUD were to be inserted. If an IUD is still being considered, then a small progestin-bearing IUD may be preferable to a copper-bearing or a larger, nonmedicated IUD because of its local action on the endometrium.

As noted above, untreated acute cervicitis and chronic cervicitis are absolute contraindications for the use of an IUD. Chronic cervicitis is one of the most common lesions of the female genital tract, occurring most frequently in multiparous women. However, once the cervicitis has been accurately diagnosed and effectively treated, an IUD may be inserted.

In the past, iron deficiency anemia was considered to be a relative contraindication, because the nonmedicated IUDs consistently increased the amount of blood lost in each menstrual cycle. Bleeding is also increased with the new copper-bearing IUDs but less so than with the nonmedicated devices. The progestin-bearing devices actually reduce the blood loss below that of control cycles and hence may be a possible indication for IUD use in anemic patients (Fig. 1; Progestasert, Alza Corporation, Palo Alto, CA).

Chronic anemia is defined differently in various parts of the world. It is endemic in many developing countries because of the frequency of nutritional deficiencies and parasitic infestations. On the other hand, reduced hemoglobin levels may be considered "normal" for certain population groups. This type of chronic anemia does not necessarily contraindicate the use of the small, medicated IUDs, because acclimatization to chronically reduced levels of hemoglobin has developed over relatively long periods of time. As in all other instances, the risks and benefits for the use of IUDs, as for any other contraceptive method, must be carefully weighed for each individual. However, in such areas, use of IUDs that may increase the amount of total blood loss should be avoided.

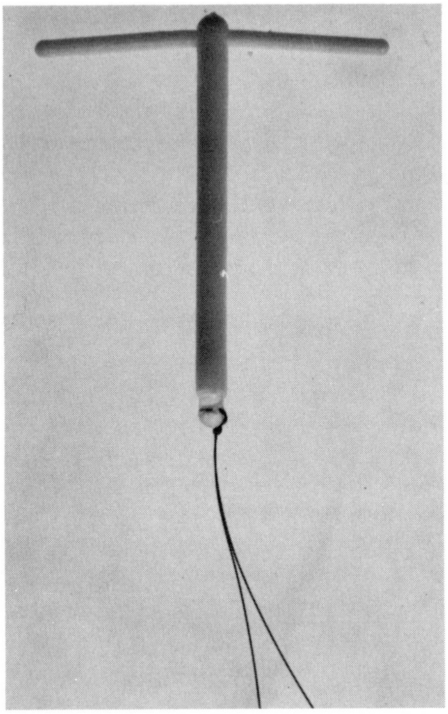

Figure 1
Progestasert.

Congenital anomalies of the external genitalia, vagina, cervix, and uterus can interfere structurally with the insertion of an IUD. These anomalies must be carefully evaluated, because certain of them may lend themselves to surgical correction. If they can be eliminated, use of a contraceptive device may then be considered. However, it must be kept in mind that after reconstructive surgery, the tissues may have an increased susceptibility to pathogenic organisms, and another contraceptive method may be preferred.

Uterine leiomyomas may preclude the use of an IUD if they are of sufficient size as to impinge upon or distort the uterine cavity so that a device cannot readily be accommodated. If the myomats are submucous and are causing irregular uterine bleeding, then an IUD could be expected to increase the amount of bleeding and probably is not the method of choice.

The most important relative contraindication concerns the use of IUDs in nulligravid and/or nulliparous women.[5] As a group, these individuals are known to have a statistically greater risk for the development of ascending pelvic infection than do women who are multiparous. However, it has been clearly demonstrated that the increased risk of infection in these individuals is related far more directly to their nonmonogamous sexual life styles than to their IUDs.[6] There are no scientifically convincing clinical data to indicate that either age or gravidity alone significantly increases the patient's risk of the development of PID in the absence of multiple sexual partners.

The most important serious complication of PID, from whatever cause, is the development of tubal adhesions, which may result in a reduction in fertility. Potential infertility is much more of a problem for women who have not had children or who have not completed their desired family size than it is for women who have had all the children they want. Clinical studies have established that intrauterine contraception can be used safely and effectively by the nulligravid or nulliparous woman *if* the couple is totally monagamous. In this instance, meticulous selection and follow-up is essential if an IUD is to be used successfully as their method of fertility regulation.[2, 6-12]

Sickle cell disease has, in the past, generally contraindicated the use of an IUD because of embolic phenomena and the increased potential risk of infection. However, improved and more effective therapy for sickle cell disease may modify this condition to that of a relative contraindication.[2]

Heart disease of an acquired type is considered by some clinicians to be incompatible with IUD use. It is essential, however, to weigh its risks and benefits as compared to other methods of contraception before deciding that heart disease per se contraindicates the use of an IUD.[2]

Diabetes mellitus was reported by Steel and Duncan[13] to be associated with an unexpectedly high pregnancy rate when using IUDs (five Cu-7s [G.D. Searle & Company, Chicago, IL], five Saf-T-Coils, and one Dalkon Shield [A. H. Robins Company, Richmond, VA]). He suggeted that this high failure rate was due to a metabolic interaction between the diabetic endometrium and the IUD.

These results were not confirmed by Lawless and Vessey,[14] who reported that 13 diabetic women in the Oxford Family Planning Association contraceptive study had used an IUD as their contraceptive method with only one pregnancy during 50 woman-years of observation. The IUDs used in this instance were two Saf-T-Coils, nine Lippes Loops, one Cu-7, and one T Cu 200 (G. D. Searle); the one unplanned pregnancy occurred in the subject wearing the Cu-7. His data were similar to those of Wiese,[15] who reported on the use of the Antigon IUD (Copenhagen, Denmark) in 118 insulin-treated diabetic patients. He reported four pregnancies in the first, but none in the second, year of the study. These results were not significantly different from the data obtained on the use of these same IUDs in nondiabetic women.

Skouby et al.[16] reported on a comparative study of 103 insulin-dependent copper IUD-wearing women and 119 nondiabetic controls. His results indicated that there were no significant differences between the two groups with respect to continuation rates, incidence of PID, or accidental pregnancy. Craig and Newton[17] and the International Planned Parenthood Medical Advisory Panel reviewed the use of IUDs in diabetic women and concluded that diabetes was not a contraindication for the use of an IUD.

The patient who has had one or more expulsions of an IUD is probably not a good candidate for another IUD. If the previous expulsion(s) occurred with a larger, nonmedicated device, insertion of one of the smaller copper-bearing IUDs may be effective in resisting future expulsions.

COMPLICATIONS OF IUD USE

BLEEDING AND SPOTTING

The most frequent complication, or side effect, of all IUDs is bleeding and/or spotting.[2] Both experimental and clinical data have shown that these symptoms are probably related to compression of the delicate endometrial lining of the uterus. With the copper-bearing devices, they may be due as well to the action of the copper itself. As previously noted, the magnitude of the blood loss in women wearing the copper devices is less than that experienced by women wearing the larger, nonmedicated IUDs. However, this reduction in the total amount of bleeding is probably related to their smaller size, which more than compensates for the slight increased bleeding affected by the copper per se. In addition, the IUDs with copper are T- or 7-shaped, to conform to the contours of the uterine cavity at its maximum degree of contraction, whereas IUDs such as the Lippes Loop and Saf-T-Coil force the uterine cavity to conform to the shape of the IUD. This latter distortion results in increased distention of the myometrium and compression of the endometrium.

The early subhuman primate studies conducted in the United States by the Population Council, New York, NY, on the long-term effects of intrauterine copper demonstrated an increased number of days of spotting throughout the duration of use. However, the monkeys did not show any reduction in the body hemoglobin and red blood cell levels during the entire 7-year evaluation.

There have been conflicting clinical studies on women using copper-bearing IUDs. The most recent report, published by Kivijarvi et al.,[18] from Finland showed that about 20% of the women wearing copper IUDs showed some signs of iron deficiency, as measured by ferritin levels, and that 10% of them had clinical anemia at the end of 12 months of use. In contrast, none of the non-copper-bearing IUD controls showed these effects. The authors[18] recommended that iron replacement be instituted when evidence of clinical anemia appeared or that the copper IUD be removed.

A comparative study of the Cu-7 and the Multiload 250 (Multilan S.A., Fribourg, Switzerland) intrauterine devices by Pedron et al.[19] in 1982 indicated that the blood loss was similar for both devices and that there was either no or a slight increase during the 12 months of IUD use. When the IUDs were removed, the menstrual blood loss in both groups returned to the preinsertion levels.

Antihemorrhagic medications, used in the treatment of the increased spotting and bleeding patterns occasionally seen in women wearing copper-bearing IUDs, have generally met with disappointing results. Various combinations of hormonal treatments and vitamin E have produced a moderate degree of success in effecting a return to normal pre IUD menstrual bleeding patterns.[20, 21] However, at the present time, there is no preparation available that results in a significant and consistent reversal of the increased spotting and bleeding patterns associated with the copper-bearing or the nonmedicated IUDs. General discussions of the etiology and management of bleeding problems associated with IUD use are presented in the literature.[1, 4, 22, 23]

The progestin-bearing IUDs have the least blood loss, due both to the small size of the vehicle as well as to the direct local action of the progestin on the endometrial cells. Although there are often increased numbers of days of spotting per cycle, the total quantity of blood lost is generally less than that observed during a preinsertion control cycle.

CRAMPING

Another beneficial effect of the conformation of IUDs to the shape and size of the uterine cavity is a reduction in frequency and severity of cramping and pain. It was shown in early clinical studies that the plain T (used without copper) does decrease the incidence of pain, cramps, and bleeding; but it has an unacceptably high accidental pregnancy rate of 18%. Therefore, adding copper and/or a progestin to a small platform or vehicle designed to approximate the small contracted endometrial cavity not only diminishes the blood loss but also greatly reduces the intensity of uterine cramps while, at the same time, increasing their contraceptive efficacy.[2]

EXPULSION

Explusions are, to a great extent, related to the use of large IUDs, which tend to increase uterine contractions in an attempt to expel the device.[2] With the advent of the diminutive vehicles carrying an active contraceptive agent (the medicated IUDs), the incidence of expulsions has been reduced significantly. In general, the IUDs that have great resistance to expulsion, e.g., the Dalkon Shield, have been shown to be associated with increased bleeding, cramps, and uterine perforations.[2]

Expulsions occur most frequently during the first 3 months after insertion. Thereafter, the uterus adapts to the presence of the IUD, the tendency to expel the IUD is significantly reduced, and expulsions are uncommon after the first year of use. Initial placement of the IUD as high as possible in the endometrial cavity tends to minimize the tendency to expel the device. The rate of success in proper placement has repeatedly been found to be directly related to the experience of the clinician doing the insertion.

Expulsions are generally classified as partial or complete and unnoticed or noticed. Partial expulsions are often associated with increased bleeding, spotting, and uterine cramps. In addition, the incidence of accidental pregnancies is increased since the high fundal position is partially lost, thus diminishing the contraceptive effectiveness. Although complete expulsions are usually noticed, they may not be, and thus are apt to be discovered because of an unintended pregnancy.

Modifications of IUDs developed in order to increase their retention properties will be discussed in the "Time of Insertion" section of this review.

PERFORATION

There are two fundamental types of perforations, those through the fundal wall and those through the cervix.[2] These may be either symptomatic or asymptomatic. Transfundal perforations usually occur at the time of the insertion of an IUD. A change in the linear relationship between the fundal cavity and the cervical canal, such as occurs with acute anteflexion or retroflexion, may increase the risk. Many times, the patient will be aware of a sudden sharp pain in her lower abdomen as the IUD is being inserted. This type of perforation seldom requires emergency surgery, because it is rarely associated with damage to a major blood vessel.

The question has frequently been posed as to whether or not an IUD which is properly placed within the endometrial cavity can gradually erode through the uterine wall as the result of uterine contractions and cause a silent type of perforation. A more likely sequence of events is that a partial perforation occurs at the time of the initial insertion. Then contractions of the uterus force the IUD to continue its passage through the uterine wall, gradually extruding out into the abdominal cavity by a process of pressure necrosis. However, it is virtually impossible to disprove the former possibility, that a normally placed IUD may gradually erode through the endometrium and myometrium without an initial partial perforation of the uterine wall.

When a complete uterine perforation has occurred, the concensus of medical opinion is that the device should be removed as soon as is feasible after the diagnosis has been confirmed.[2] The urgency of the situation and the technique employed vary considerably by the type of IUD that is involved. The nonmedicated IUDs, such as the Lippes Loop and the Saf-T-Coil, do not produce a rapid inflammatory response within the peritoneal cavity; hence removal can, in most instances, be accomplished by laparoscopy.

The copper-bearing IUDs, on the other hand, elicit a rapid inflammatory response and frequently lead to adhesions to adjacent visceral structures and often to engulfment by the omentum. Therefore, the removal of the copper devices should be carried out as soon as possible. If the time span has been less than 2 or 3 days from the time of perforation, they can usually be removed by laparoscopy. On the other hand, if a device has been in the peritoneal cavity for more than 3 days, adhesions will already have been formed, making removal by laparoscopy much more difficult if not totally impossible. In these latter instances, the situation can be assessed initially by laparoscopy, but preparations should be made in advance to proceed to remove the device by laparotomy if necessary.

There are, as yet, inadequate data to indicate how much tissue reactivity occurs with an intraperitoneal progestin-bearing IUD. In areas where the practice of medicine is strongly influenced by the medico-legal climate, however, it is probably advisable to remove a translocated IUD of any type whenever the diagnosis is made.

IUD insertions by the push-out technique such as is used for the Lippes Loop, Saf-T-Coil, and Multiload IUDs result in somewhat greater risk of transfundal perforation than does the withdrawal technique.[2] This latter method, used for the Cu-7 and T Cu devices, consists of the placement of the IUD within an inserter tube, which is then introduced high into the fundal cavity. At that point, the inserter tube is withdrawn over the plunger, which allows the arms of the IUD to be expelled or opened up into the endometrial cavity. There is thus a reduced likelihood of significant upward positioning of the IUD and hence a lessened risk of fundal wall perforation.

A cervical perforation of the dependent portion of an IUD resulting from downward displacement is almost always asymptomatic. The diagnosis is frequently made either by routine pelvic examination, at which time the perforating portion of the IUD can be visualized coming through the cervical tissue into the vagina, or by signs and symptoms of pregnancy. If, in this latter instance, the IUD can be easily and atraumatically removed through the cervical os, it may be possible to allow the pregnancy to continue, if so desired. If the removal procedure proves to be traumatic, there is an increased likelihood that a miscarriage may result from the manipulation.

A double-blind randomized multicentric comparison was made between the T Cu 300 IUDs, half of which had enlarged, ball-like dependent tips. The purpose of this study, carried out at the suggestion of the Food and Drug Authority (Data submitted to the Food and Drug Administration [FDA] in the Population Council's application for a New Drug Authorization), was to evaluate the advantages and disadvantages, if any, with respect to cervical perforations and expulsions. There were no perforations in either group, and there were two early expulsions in the group using the balled dependent tip. The Population Council, with the concurrence of the FDA, agreed to modify the T Cu 200 to bear an enlarged balled tip even though the clinical data did not support this revision.[1]

PELVIC INFLAMMATORY DISEASE

PID is one of the major problems which has been associated with the use of the intrauterine device.[2] The etiology of these infections is varied and not fully understood. However, it has been well established that the insertion procedure is invariably associated with the introduction of microorganisms from the vagina, through the cervical canal, and up into the endometrial cavity. The possible association between ascending pelvic infection and the presence of an intrauterine contraceptive device has been a matter of concern and debate from the time of Graefenberg in the early 1920s. Graefenberg taught that no IUD should have a transcervical appendage because it could theoretically increase the likelihood of microorganisms ascending from the vagina along the string or tail up into the endometrial cavity. More recently, with the advent of the Lippes Loop and Saf-T-Coil, both of which had tails, there were small comparative studies that suggested, but did not establish, a causal relationship between the IUD and PID. However, the earlier studies did not attempt to assess the sexual practices and numbers of sexual partners of the contraceptors. Taking into consideration these additional factors, the concensus at the present time is that the tailed IUD may be associated with a small increase in the relative risk of developing PID, most notably when the wearer has multiple sexual partners.

Mishell showed two decades ago that microorganisms identical to those found in the cervical canal could be cultured from the endometrial cavity for a few days after the insertion of the nonmedicated Lippes Loop.[1, 24] Subsequent cultures obtained from extirpated uteri under sterile sampling conditions showed that fewer and fewer organisms were found, and that by day 30 after the insertion of the IUD the uterus had completely sterilized itself.

Conflicting data were presented in 1976 by Sparks et al.[25] in England. Using what they described as "more sophisticated bacteriologic techniques," they demonstrated the presence of small numbers of bacteria within the endometrial cavity in most of the uteri containing a variety of different IUDs with transcervical tails. When the tails were removed from similar IUDs prior to the insertion, no live microorganisms could be found in the endometrial cavity. Although the time frame relevant to time in utero of the devices is not clear from the paper, the investigation concluded that the presence of the transcervical appendage can and does serve as a "ladder" on which vaginal and exocervical microorganisms can ascend into the endometrial cavity.

There have been several studies comparing the incidence of PID in randomized groups of women in whom identical devices, either with or without a tail, were inserted.[26, 27] In these, with the use of predominantly nonmedicated IUDs, the incidence of pelvic infection was not significantly different.

Batar et al.[28] in 1985 reported a 2-year comparative study of two copper-bearing IUDs in which 581 of the devices inserted were tailless and 602 had conventional monofilament tails. At the end of 2 years of use there were 300 women remaining in the tailless and 304 in the tailed control group. The gross cumulative termination rates were statistically similar for both groups for pregnancy, expulsions, bleeding/pain, other medical reasons, and removals for planning pregnancy. Discontinuation rates for infection, however, were 0.2 for the tailless group and 2.4 for the tailed group. This difference was statistically significant ($P < 0.05$). A total of 12 IUDs were removed specifically for pelvic infection during the 2-year period. Of these, 11 were from the control tailed IUDs, and only 1 was from the tailless group. The infection rate was approximately 13 times greater in the tailed than in the tailless group. The authors[28] concluded that their study supported the concept that the transcervical appendage on an IUD plays an important role in the development of an ascending PID in IUD wearers. They also stressed the need for further research encompassing larger numbers of cases and longer intervals of follow-up to corroborate or refute their conclusions.

It has been found, as in the case of non-IUD wearers, that the incidence of PID is significantly increased when the wearer is polygamous and that even greater differences are detected when the partner(s) of the IUD wearer also has multiple sexual partners.[2] It is believed that the normal vaginal flora established early in the life of the female child exists, for the most part, in a symbiotic relationship with their host. This symbiotic relationship implies that a certain degree of immunity or resistance is developed which may be modified by the addition of different species or strains of microorganisms, as invariably occurs in association with coitus. In this instance, the inherent resistance of the endometrium, parametrium, and tubes and ovaries may be exceeded. The severity of the resulting ascending infection depends entirely upon the relationship between the naturally acquired resistance and the dosage and virulence of the new microorganisms that have entered the vagina.

Another theoretic source of ascending infection has been proposed by Toth et al.[29] They suggest that bacteria in the vagina could ascend through the cervical canal and into the endometrial cavity, attached to sperm. This "piggyback" theory, that sperm serve as vectors for pathogenic organisms and the subsequent development of PID, lacks scientific confirmation. Perhaps the strongest argument against the "piggyback" etiology for the development of PID is that the frequency and incidence of sexual intercourse far exceeds the incidence of PID. If, indeed, the sperm were important as a vector for pathogenic bacteria moving from the vagina into the uterine cavity, most sexually active women would have PID and there would be a universally high incidence of primary tubal infertility. Clearly, the incidence and frequency of sexual intercourse exceeds by far the incidence of both PID *and* primary tubal infertility.

The microorganisms that are frequently associated with PID include *Neisseria gonorrhoeae, Chlamydia, Gardnerella, Escherichia coli*, and, less frequently, anaerobic streptococci and other anaerobic species. It is doubtful that *Trichomonas vaginalis* alone actually causes PID. However, whether or not this organism contributes to the development of PID as a vector remains to be established. Chlamydial and gonorrheal infections are probably the most frequent entities, whereas infections due to tuberculosis and actinomycosis are the least common varieties.

In most instances, PID begins with a cervical infection that extends up through the uterine cavity or out through the parametrial lymphatics into the fallopian tubes and then into the ovaries, parovarian tissues, and beyond. The most severe types of pelvic inflammatory disease result in tuboovarian abscesses. In general, the bacteriologic flora in these abscesses is almost always polymicrobial and is usually predominantly anaerobic in nature. Rupture of a tuboovarian abscess is a very serious, life-threatening complication, demanding systemic antibiotic therapy and, usually, definitive surgical removal of the affected structures. The question of the significance of unilateral versus bilateral tuboovarian abscesses in relation to IUD use has often been raised. The consensus of clinical data indicates that these infections are almost always bilateral. Furthermore, the presence of a clinically apparent unilateral abscess in no way indicates or is diagnostic of an IUD-related infection.

It is not the intention of this presentation to discuss in any detail the signs and symptoms and the general medical management of PID. There is nothing characteristic about the clinical course of PID unique to the use of an IUD. The most important factors that suggest that an IUD is a significant contributing factor are the sexual (polygamous) history of the patient as well as the temporal sequence of clinical events that terminates in a definitive diagnosis of PID.

There continues to be debate as to whether or not the IUD should be removed as soon as the diagnosis of PID is made.[4] Most clinicians agree that the removal will enhance antibiotic effectiveness and should be done at some point in the treatment. A middle-of-the-road approach suggests institution of massive doses of broad-spectrum antibiotics by the intravenous route, coupled with general supportive measures, followed in several hours by removal of the IUD.[2] The degree of severity of the clinical infection should serve as a guide as to whether or not a few hours of antibiotic therapy can be tolerated by the patient prior to removal. There is some increased risk of stirring up the infection in the endometrial cavity by manipulation of the IUD during the removal. In most instances, however, this flare up can be controlled effectively by preliminary intravenous or systemic administration of broad-spectrum antibiotics.

During the past decade much attention has been given to the potential role that *Actinomyces* might play in pelvic infections related to IUDs. Patients with PID in whom actinomycetes are found to be the predominant organisms in surgically removed tissues and/or abscesses are apt to have had *Actinomyces*-like organisms on their Papanicolaou (Pap) smears. When the surgically extirpated structures are found to contain these organisms, they are usually associated with an IUD or with some type of intravaginal, intracervical, or intrauterine pessary.

There are conflicting data as to the presence or absence of *Actinomyces*-like organisms in the vaginal flora of non-IUD wearers.[30, 31] The presence of these organisms on a Pap smear cannot be interpreted as indicative that the patient has or will have pelvic actinomycosis. Therefore, a conservative approach should be followed when the organisms are found on a smear taken from an *asymptomatic* patient. The smears should be repeated at 1- or 2-month intervals. Prophylactic antibiotics are *not* indicated at this time for asymptomatic IUD wearers. If Pap smears remain positive for one, or preferably two, additional menstrual cycles, the IUD should then be removed. Direct scrapings should be obtained from beneath the encrustations on the device and studied for histologic evidence of *Actinomyces*.[32] Antibiotic treatment should be withheld until repeat Pap smears have been obtained for 1 or 2 months after removal of the IUD. If *Actinomyces*-like organisms are no longer present, no antibiotics or other definitive treatment is necessary.

This regimen of conservative management of the asymptomatic patient is usually sufficient. If, on the other hand, the Pap smear continues to remain positive after the removal of the IUD, a 14-day course of penicillin or tetracycline is recommended. Should the Pap smear remain positive after the first course of antibiotics, the same antibiotic regimen should be continued for a second 14-day course. In most instances, subsequent Pap smears will then be negative for the offending organisms. Whether or not an IUD should again be recommended under these specific circumstances has not yet been ascertained, there still being two schools of thought on this matter.

When there is clinical evidence of PID and *Actinomyces*-like organisms predominate in the vagina and beneath encrustations on the IUD, a presumptive diagnosis of pelvic actinomycosis should be made. This disease can only be confirmed by histologic evidence of colonies of actinomycetes (often described as sulfur granules) in abscesses and other diseased pelvic structures removed during surgical exploration. Actinomycetes are strict anaerobes, and culturing is often very difficult. False-negative results are the rule, rather than the exception, probably because of extensive overgrowth by less fastidious and more rapidly growing anaerobes, and because of preoperative systemically administered antibiotics. In general, the histologic evidence of *Actinomyces*-like organisms from affected tissues is considered to be more reliable than cultures.

The recommended definitive surgical procedure consists of removing as much of the diseased tissue as possible. This extensive surgery should be followed by prolonged intensive systemic antibiotic therapy including tetracyclines and broad-spectrum drugs directed toward a mixed group of microorganisms that are predominantly anaerobes. In addition to the actinomycetes, the flora of the abscesses often includes *Bacteroides* species and *Peptostreptococcus* and facultative anaerobic *E. coli*. Because of the severe chronic nature of true pelvic actinomycosis, antibiotic therapy should be continued for at least 4 to 6 weeks after surgery. Prophylactic systemic antifungal treatment must be instituted coincident with the long-term use of antibiotics to protect against severe systemic infections from *Monilia* or other fungi. The mortality associated with pelvic actinomycosis is now between 5% and 10%, whereas prior to the availability of appropriate antibiotics and use of extensive definitive surgery, mortality often reached 70% to 80%.

ACCIDENTAL PREGNANCIES ASSOCIATED WITH WEARING OF AN IUD

Intrauterine Pregnancy

Accidental pregnancies may be either intrauterine or ectopic in location. The initial recommendations for the management of intrauterine pregnancies in women wearing copper-bearing IUDs have been repeatedly confirmed in the United States and throughout the world.[33] If the patient wishes to continue the pregnancy, the intrauterine device should be removed immediately, preferably during the first trimester, provided that this can be accomplished with a minimum of trauma. In order to do this, the tail of the IUD must be within the vagina. If the IUD is removed, the chances of a spontaneous abortion will be diminished from 50% to approximately 25%. If, however, the tail is not visible in the vagina, then no attempt should be made to search for it in women who wish to continue their pregnancies. This procedure itself will, in most instances, initiate an abortion. These recommendations pertain only to those IUDs which have single or double monofilament tails, and clearly exclude the Dalkon Shield with its multifilamented and potentially very dangerous sheathed tail.[4]

If the patient accepts the conditions that she may have a 50% chance of a spontaneous abortion and, in some instances, could develop an intrauterine infection during the remaining portion of her pregnancy with the IUD in place, then careful observation and close follow-up should be advised. It is logical to assume, but has not yet been established, that a tailless IUD can be allowed to remain in a pregnant uterus with a minimum degree of potential danger of intrauterine infection.

If the patient wishes to terminate her pregnancy, since her objective in using the IUD was to prevent conception, then elective termination should be accomplished. However, the IUD should be removed at the time that the diagnosis of pregnancy is made, inasmuch as patients have been known to change their minds and not return for follow-up medical care.

Ectopic Pregnancy

The signs and symptoms suggestive of an extrauterine pregnancy in an IUD wearer are similar to those in non-IUD wearers, and may be confused with PID, appendicitis, ovarian cysts, urinary tract disease, gastroenteritis, or an early intrauterine pregnancy. It has been estimated that an initial correct diagnosis of an ectopic pregnancy is made in no more than 60% to 70% of the cases.[34]

If the pregnancy is accompanied by a clinical picture suggesting that it is ectopic, appropriate measures must be taken promptly to confirm or refute this diagnosis. Ultrasound evaluation, human chorionic gonadotropin (hCG) determinations, laparoscopy, and/or culdocentesis are excellent methods of differentiating between an intrauterine and an extrauterine pregnancy. Obviously, with the presence of free, nonclotting blood in the cul-de-sac, surgical exploration is mandatory. If the quantity of blood found by laparoscopy or culdocentesis is minimal and could conceivably be related to follicular rupture, then laparoscopy will usually assist in the differential diagnosis. When there is evidence of acute blood loss, surgical exploration becomes a life-saving mandate. Every effort should be made to manage a tubal pregnancy as conservatively as possible, the objective being to enhance subsequent microsurgical restoration of the damaged fallopian tube, if that becomes necessary. At the time of surgery, both tubes should be thoroughly inspected for evidence of chronic inflammatory processes.

Whether or not there is a specific causal relationship between the use of an IUD and the incidence of ectopic pregnancy has not yet been established. Tatum and Schmidt, in 1977, indicated that there were data in the United States that suggested such a causal relationship.[35] Sivin, in 1979,[36] reported that ectopic rates in the United States were similar in women who used both copper-bearing and nonmedicated IUDs to those in women who were using barrier contraception and those using no contraceptive method at all. He indicated that the rate of increase in the number of ectopic pregnancies in the United States exceeded by far the increased use of IUDs as a form of contraception.

Ory, in 1981,[37] published a large United States case-control study of the relationship between the IUD and the occurrence of ectopic pregnancy. He concluded that the current use of an IUD was actually protective against ectopics if one compared the rates among users of IUDs with the rates among women who had never used IUDs and women who were using no contraceptive.

In 1985, Sivin[38] reported that the rates for ectopic pregnancies in women wearing copper IUDs were in the range of 0.1 to 0.15/100 woman-years. Dorfman et al.,[39] in 1984, reported that the two IUDs that had the largest surface area of copper (the Multiload 375 and the T Cu 380A) had the lowest risk of an ectopic pregnancy (Fig. 2).

On the other hand, the progesterone-bearing IUD (Progestasert) has been shown in several studies, both in the United States and Europe, to be associated with ectopic pregnancy rates between 0.5 and 1.0/100 woman-years.[39] This represents a five to seven times greater risk than that with copper-bearing IUDs. It has been suggested that this may be related to interference with the normal tubal transport of the fertilized ovum.

Clinicians should always think "ectopic" when a pregnancy is suspected in an IUD wearer. However, with the use of any contraceptive method except the progesterone-bearing IUD and the "mini-pill," both of which have an increased risk, the chances of having an ectopic pregnancy are significantly reduced. There are conflicting data relevant to the influence of long-term use of the IUD on the risk of the development of an ectopic pregnancy. Larger numbers of patients and appropriate controls may resolve this unanswered question.

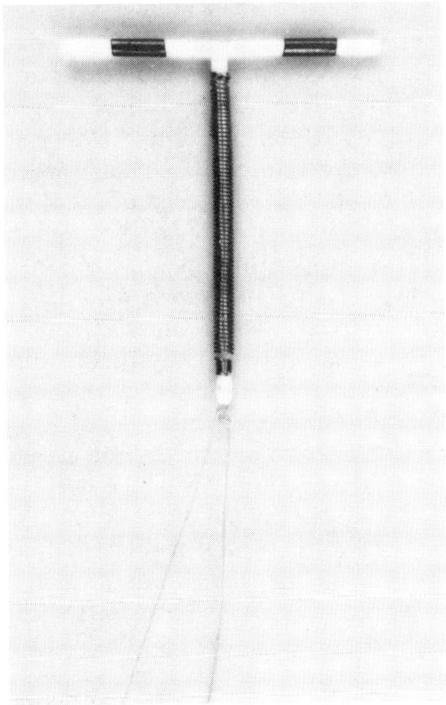

Figure 2
Copper T model T Cu 380A.

INFERTILITY

Tatum et al.[33] reviewed the *incidence of fertility* following discontinuation of the Cu-T for the express purpose of having another pregnancy. Their data as well as the earlier studies dealt with nonmedicated IUDs. Dorfman et al.[39] and Tietze and Lewit[40] indicated that there seemed to be no reduction in fertility in those women who had used IUDs for as long as 3 years and then had them removed for the express purpose of beginning a new pregnancy. It is essential to realize, however, that these data excluded all contraceptors who discontinued the use of their IUD for any other reason.

Those women who have a history of upper genital tract infection(s) may have tubal inflammatory residua, which, in turn, may cause a reduction in fertility. Two recent studies, the first by Daling et al.[41] and the second by Cramer et al.,[42] in 1985, have, for the first time, assessed in separate populations the incidence of tubal infertility, both primary and secondary, in relation to previous IUD use. Daling et al.[41] reported that the risk of infertility in women who had at any time used any IUD was 2.6 times that in women who had never used one. They further reported that the relative risk associated with ever-use of the Dalkon Shield was 6.8 and was 11.3 in those women who had used only a Dalkon Shield. The increased risk associated with use of either the Lippes Loop or the Saf-T-Coil was 3.2. They reported also that the smallest elevation in risk over that of a non-user was found among those who had ever used copper-bearing IUDs, the relative risk in this group being 1.9. The relative risk for women who had used only a copper-containing IUD was 1.3. They concluded that the use of the Dalkon Shield and possibly the nonmedicated Lippes Loop and Saf-T-Coil could lead to infertility in nulligravid women.

Cramer et al.[42] reported a similar study, which, in contrast to the Daling study,[41] compared nulligravid women with primary tubal infertility and women diagnosed as having secondary tubal infertility with women admitted for delivery over the same calendar time span. He found that the relative risk of primary tubal infertility associated with an IUD before a first live birth was 2.0 in relation to non-users. The subjects using the Dalkon Shield had an adjusted risk of 3.3, and users of the Lippes Loop or Saf-T-Coil had an adjusted risk of 2.9. They observed that users of copper IUDs had the lowest relative risk, which was 1.6. Women who reported having only one sexual partner had no increased risk of primary tubal infertility associated with the use of a copper-bearing IUD.

Further, Cramer et al.[42] observed that the adjusted risk was 1.5 for secondary tubal infertility subsequent to the use of a copper IUD, inserted after the first live birth. This risk was not significantly different from that found in non-IUD wearers. A similar comparison was made of the relative risk of secondary infertility following the first live birth between wearers of nonmedicated IUDs and wearers of copper-bearing IUDs. In this instance he determined that the relative risk of the copper IUD was 1.5, whereas that following the use of non-copper devices was 2.8, which is significantly higher. They concluded that secondary and primary infertility are associated with all IUDs, but that this risk is less in association with copper-bearing IUDs.

Several studies over the past decade have assessed the relative risk of the development of severe pelvic actinomycosis in an IUD wearer. Although this is an exceedingly rare type of pelvic inflammatory disease—not more than 100 to 150 cases having been reported in the world literature—an analysis of the data published in review articles strongly suggests that it occurs more frequently in Dalkon Shield wearers than in wearers of nonmedicated IUDs.[2] Moreover, the data reported by Daling et al.[41] and Cramer et al.[42] suggest that copper on an IUD might have some antimicrobial effect.

OPTIONAL TIMES FOR IUD INSERTION

IUDs may be inserted in any phase of the menstrual cycle and following the termination of a pregnancy, whether a delivery, a spontaneous miscarriage, or an early elective therapeutic abortion. Each time has its own advantages and disadvantages. According to White et al.,[43] there is no single time that is preferable in all instances. When IUDs were inserted sometime after the 18th day of the menstrual cycle, the rates for removal because of partial expulsion or infection were lower than when the insertion was performed around the time of the menses. However, at this same time the rates of removal for bleeding or pain or pregnancy were higher. Rates for other medical removals during the first 2 months following delivery were lowest when insertions were performed from the 11th to the 17th day of the postpartum cycle.

Insertion during the bleeding phase of the cycles has a number of advantages:[4] (1) The chance of unrecognized pregnancy is minimal; (2) the cervical canal is relatively patent; (3) discomfort is minimal; and (4) associated spotting is less noticeable.

It also has disadvantages: (1) there is a number of limited days available for insertion; (2) insertion may be psychologically unacceptable because the patient objects to pelvic examination and manipulation at that time; and (3) if insertion is not elected at this time, there is the potential for an unwanted pregnancy to occur prior to a later planned insertion.

For a more complete coverage of optional times for insertion, please refer to a review by Tatum and Connell.[2]

In order to minimize the delay in instituting contraception after termination of a pregnancy, early postpartum insertions of IUDs have been studied. The optimal time is immediately following delivery of the placenta (immediate postplacental insertion). A number of studies using several different IUDs were carried out utilizing the postpartum period for insertions, most of them between the first and fifth days of the puerperium. The expulsion rates were found to be unacceptably high, at the end of 3 months, being almost 21%. The highest rate was 26.5% for the IUDs inserted within 24 hours after delivery.[2]

Laufe et al.[44] affixed three ties of biodegradable chromic suture (Ethicon No. 2) to the upper cross-arm of the Lippes Loop D (Delta Loop). These IUDs were then manually placed high in the fundal cavity immediately after delivery of the placenta. A total of 341 insertions were performed in four separate clinical studies. At the end of 6 months the net expulsion rate as determined by the life-table method was 5.3/100 women. A larger series of 100 women employing the same technique reported a net expulsion rate of 1.2/100 women at 3 months.[45] These studies suggested that an initial "fixation" accomplished by the chromic suture ties imported temporary retention characteristics to the IUD during the period when a nonsutured IUD is most apt to be expelled.

A subsequent multicentric comparative study confirmed the efficacy of chromic ties in enhancing retention of the Delta Loop.[46] At the end of 6 months, the expulsion rate of the Delta Loop was 15.7% in a comparative series consisting of 648 Lippes Loops and 518 Delta Loops. This improvement, based upon gross life-table calculations of expulsion rates per 100 women, is statistically significant ($P < 0.05$). However, these encouraging results were not confirmed by two subsequent studies.[47, 48] Thus, the usefulness of the addition of chromic suture to the IUDs to improve their resistance to early expulsion remains unresolved.

IUD insertions immediately after completion of a miscarriage or following voluntary interruption of an early pregnancy have been reported.[2, 49] These studies indicated that IUDs can be inserted in both of these situations without increasing the complication rates as measured by temperature elevation and by the number of days in a hospital.

Although IUD insertion following termination of an early pregnancy is not an FDA-approved indication, clinical experience throughout the world has established its general safety and efficacy. These insertions are associated with a low rate of expulsion; and, clearly, many patients are highly motivated at that time to accept an effective contraceptive method.[50-55]

POSTCOITAL INSERTION (MORNING-AFTER METHOD)

The first study of the effectiveness of copper IUDs inserted within 7 days after unprotected coitus was reported by Lippes and colleagues[56] in 1979. In 299 subjects there were no pregnancies. There were no annoying side effects such as nausea and vomiting, which are often associated with the postcoital use of hormones. This application of an IUD offers the advantage of providing an effective and continuing method of contraception, if desired, provided there are no medical contraindications for use of an IUD.[57, 58] Although there are ample clinical data establishing the safety and effectiveness of this technique, the FDA has not indicated its approval of the procedure.

MECHANISM(S) OF CONTRACEPTIVE ACTION

There are two general groups of contraceptive mechanisms of action, those generic to all classes of IUDs, and those that are related to specific types of medicated devices.[2, 4]

The mechanisms that represent the known antifertility effects of both the nonmedicated and medicated IUDs originate and act within the endometrial cavity. Their antifertility action(s) are initiated promptly upon insertion, and their contraceptive effect(s) are, in most instances, rapidly reversed when the IUD is removed. These localized changes are not influenced significantly by endocrine control of the menstrual cycle; in other words, except for the progestin-bearing IUDs, the estrogen/progesterone balance within the endometrial cavity is not disturbed. A detailed discussion of these generic mechanisms of contraceptive action was presented in the earlier paper, and will not be repeated here.[1]

In general, the bioantifertility actions which are generic to both nonmedicated and medicated IUDs are elicited by the size, shape, flexibility, and surface area of the device. To a certain extent, the side effects, such as pain, cramps, bleeding, spotting, and partial or complete expulsions, and the magnitude of the mobilization of white blood cells from the vascular system into the endometrial and intratubal cavities reflect the physical characteristics of the IUD itself. It is for this reason that the term "inert" is totally inappropriate in describing any type of IUD.

The era of medicated IUDs began when Zipper et al.[59] noted that copper had an active localized antifertility action in rabbits. Combined with the plastic T-shaped carrier designed by Tatum,[59] this became the first of the medicated IUDs to be evaluated in women. Most, if not all, of the antifertility mechanisms of the nonmedicated IUDs are also involved in the actions of copper in the uterine cavity. However, the magnitude of the leukocytic mobilization is significantly greater with copper than that evoked by the nonmedicated devices. Some of the more recent basic implications of the leukocytic infiltration in relationship to antifertility action were reported by Parr in 1970[60] and Cuadros and Hirsch[61] in 1972. The reader is referred to the earlier paper for details on the information on the mechanism of action gathered prior to 1976.[1]

As long as IUDs have been used for contraceptive purposes, there have been allegations that they act primarily as abortifacients. This concept has been publicized widely by certain religious groups who have therefore proscribed the IUD as an acceptable means of controlling fertility. However, accurate definitions of the terms "pregnancy" and "abortion" and recent scientific data should help to dispel the misconceptions and misinformation which have, in the past, clouded the entire issue of the contraceptive mechanism(s) of action of the IUD.

The American College of Obstetrics and Gynecology (ACOG) in 1972 published its book *Obstetric-Gynecologic Terminology*.[62] In this text, "conception" is defined as "the implantation of the blastocyst." It is *not* synonymous with fertilization. "Pregnancy" is defined as "the state of a female after conception and until termination of the gestation."

The same issues were addressed in September 1985 at a meeting of the International Federation of Gynecology and Obstetrics (FIGO) in West Berlin.[63] At that time, the Committee on Medical Aspects of Human Reproduction, chaired by M. F. Fathalla, M.D., of Egypt, was charged by the FIGO Board, in response to a request from the World Health Organization (WHO), to develop an accurate definition of pregnancy. The Committee agreed on the following: "Pregnancy is only established with the implantation of the fertilized ovum."[63] Based upon the above definitions of "conception" and "pregnancy," an abortifacient acts to interrupt a pregnancy only following implantation.[64]

On the scientific side, a recent publication by Segal et al.[65] reported on sequential serum levels of human chorionic gonadotropin in IUD wearers. He and his co-workers reported: "The study demonstrates that IUD users *do not* retain their natural fertility, and that IUDs do not exert their antifertility effect as abortifacient agents." They conclude: "If a confirmed pregnancy is detected in an IUD user, it may be assumed to represent an isolated case of contraceptive failure."

It is to be hoped that these official definitions and the new scientific data will provide a realistic and scientific foundation for a clearer understanding of the mechanism(s) of action IUDs among the lay public, theologians, politicians, and health care providers in general.

EFFECTIVENESS

The contraceptive effectiveness of an IUD is determined by the summation of the antifertility properties of the shape, size, flexibility, and surface area of the device and the contraceptive action(s) of the added antifertility agent if the IUD is "medicated." The IUDs available until recently in the United States were the nonmedicated Lippes Loop and Saf-T-Coil, the medicated Cu-7 and T Cu 200 (Tatum T) and the progesterone-bearing Progestasert. There have been several other copper-bearing IUDs developed in the United States and in other countries, including Canada, Holland, and Finland. The most effective of these, the T Cu 380A, the T Cu 220C, and the Multiload 375 have not been made commercially available in the United States. Of these latter devices, only the T Cu 380A has been approved for use in the United States by the FDA.

A randomized selection of several studies,[66-70] based upon comparison of reasons for discontinuing use of various IUDs, are shown in Table 1. The pregnancy rate for the most widely used nonmedicated IUD in this selection, the Lippes Loop, was 1.2. For all of the copper-bearing devices, the annual pregnancy rates ranged between 0.5 and 3.1, with an average of 1.2. Of the progestin-bearing devices, the norgestrel-bearing Nova T (Leiras Pharmaceutical, Turku, Finland) had the low-

Table 1. *Annual Discontinuation Rates of IUDs—100 Women/Year*

IUD	Years	Pregnancy	Bleeding/pain	Expulsion	Continuation	No. of women
T Cu 200[70]	2	1.9	6.8	3.3	62.1	5669
T Cu 200[70]	2	0.8	9.9	4.4	59.7	2200
T Cu 220C	10	0.8	2.2	0.9	37.5	906
Cu 7-200[70]	2	3.1	6.7	8.7	54.1	2330
Nova T 200AG[70]	2	0.7	7.8	2.9	65	916
Nova T 200AG	3	0.5	6.0	2.2	39.6	NA[a]
Nova T 200AG	4	0.5	6.0	2.3	48.8	916
Multiload 250[70]	2	1.4	4.5	1.3	90.5	1330
Multiload 375	2	1.1	6.1	1.8	NA[a]	275
T Cu 380A[66]	2	0.6	9.1	4.1	56.9	1051
T Cu 380A	4	0.5	6.3	2.5	35.1	1051
Lippes Loop[70]	2	1.2	6.3	4.9	62.6	3052
T Cu 200[67]	1	2	12	4	76	186
Nova T 200	2	1.7	3.6	3.1	71.9	157
Progestasert[68]	1	2	11	3	76	196
Levo-Norg A[67]	2	0.3	3.8	0.3	66.6	164
Levo-Norg B[67]	2	0.0	3.8	1.6	60.7	163

[a]NA, not applicable.

est rate (0.15). The discontinuation rates presented in Table 1 are from a variety of sources and different populations and hence should be considered as relative values only.

With those data currently available, the contraceptive effectiveness of the copper-bearing device model 380A (Ortho-Canada, Toronto, Canada) has an established pregnancy prevention level of approximately 0.5 pregnancies/100 women/year for a period of 4 years.[66] During those 4 years, no significant reduction in contraceptive efficacy was observed. These data are derived from studies in various parts of the world and show a remarkable degree of similarity. The multisleeved T Cu 220C has only a slightly higher accidental pregnancy rate, approximately 1/100 women/year, but has shown this high rate of protection over a period of at least 10 years.[69]

It is clear from the table that each of these IUDs provides highly effective contraception over a time span ranging from 1 to 10 years. There is no limit placed on the use of the nonmedicated Lippes Loop or Saf-T-Coil. The FDA has placed a time limit approval of 3 years for the Cu-7 and 4 years for the Tatum-T Cu 200 and the T Cu 380A. However, G. D. Searle & Co. has not to date requested a change in their labeling from 3 to 4 years for the Tatum-T.

CURRENT STATUS OF INTRAUTERINE DEVICES

During the past decade, three major milestones have occurred in the field of intrauterine contraception, two of a very positive nature and one extremely negative. First, continued research has resulted in significant improvements in the safety, effectiveness, and utilization of intrauterine devices. Among the more important of these is a new tailless IUD which can be readily detected without expensive equipment or radiologic or invasive procedures. Another innovation is the use of silver-core copper wire, as recommended by Finnish investigators.[2] This has reduced the incidence of segmental loss of wire and hence has increased the contraceptive life of the copper-bearing devices. IUDs that possess an exceptionally high incidence of retention when inserted during the immediate postplacental period are now in clinical trials (Fig. 3, postpartum IUD).

Other innovations, aimed at reducing the incidence of bleeding/spotting and expulsions following interval insertions, are also now in advanced stages of development. In one of these, indomethacin has been incorporated into Silastic IUDs in order to enhance their resistance to expulsion.[71] When tested in experimental animals, a significant increase in retention was effected by this technique, but a similar evaluation has not yet been attempted in the human.

The second major advance has been in the area of study design, data collection, and evaluation. The risks and benefits of the use of the various types of IUDs by specific groups of women have been far better elucidated by studies carried out during the past 10 years.[41, 42, 72] While there has been an unfortunate tendency in the past to consider all intrauterine devices as a single entity, particularly by the media, these papers have pointed out clearly that they are not the same.

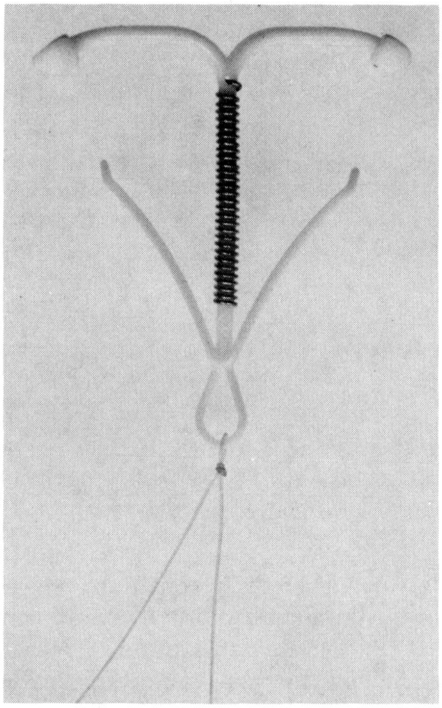

Figure 3
Nova postpartum T Cu 200.

It is essential to realize that the level of risk of developing a pelvic infection while wearing one of the single or double filamented tailed IUDs (Lippes Loop, Saf-T-Coil, Cu-7 or Cu T) may be slightly increased. The risk is significantly increased in wearers of the Dalkon Shield, with its multifilament sheathed tail. With this latter IUD, live bacteria have been cultured from within the sheath between the filaments. Under these circumstances, the cervical mucus barrier cannot protect against the ascent of bacteria from the vagina into the endometrial cavity, as it does when single or double filament tails are used. Furthermore, the nylon sheath of the Dalkon Shield is known to disintegrate while it is in the uterine cavity, thus increasing the risk of bacteria entering the endometrial cavity from the tail.[1, 2] As noted above, the clinical studies carried out to date substantiate this increased risk of PID in wearers of the Dalkon Shield.[41, 42, 72] It is most important that the public be made aware of these significant differences in risk.

In a recent editorial in the *New England Journal of Medicine*, Mishell[73] summarized the two epidemiologic articles[41, 42] published in the same issue. He stressed the importance of and the rational for placing the identifiable risks and benefits of the IUD into proper perspective, as in the case of any contraceptive method or any therapeutic drug. He indicated that it is essential for women to select the IUD as a method of protection against unwanted pregnancy only if they are fully aware of the potential increased risk of subsequent tubal infertility. It is particularly important that they have a monogamous life style and that their sexual partners also be monogamous. Finally, they should have decided that they do not want to have a subsequent pregnancy. The editorial concluded by stating that the IUD continues to be an effective and useful method of contraception for parous women. It emphasized the special usefulness of this method for women over the age of 30, for whom a reversible type of "sterilization" is desired. In this age group, medical problems may make the use of conventional OCs more risky. In addition, the contraceptive effectiveness of the IUD is considerably enhanced in older women as their level of fertility is declining.

It is particularly ironic that against this background of improved technology and information, we are now faced with the third major event, the virtual demise of the IUD in the United States.

The nonmedicated devices were the first to disappear. The Saf-T-Coil was discontinued by Schmid Laboratories in 1984, because it was not economically profitable to manufacture the device because it had a relatively small share of the IUD market. Three events related to the other nonmedicated device, the Lippes Loop, manufactured by Ortho Pharmaceutical Corporation, occurred in 1985. The first of these was a change in the labeling,[74] indicating an increased risk of PID, based upon the papers by Daling et al.[41] and Cramer et al.[42] The second was the decision by the FDA to require additional information on the older medical devices. It requested Lippes Loop data on four safety issues: pelvic actinomycosis, tubal infertility, duration of IUD use, and the safety of leaving the device in postmenopausal women. This request was made in order to apply the requirements of the Medical Device Amendments, enacted on May 28, 1976, to IUDs marketed before that date. The third was the announcement by Ortho Pharmaceutical Corporation that it was no longer going to manufacture the Lippes Loop because of the declining market for nonmedicated devices.[75] A Planned Parenthood memorandum[76] issued following this decision stated that the Lippes Loop was and had "always been categorized as a safe and effective IUD" and its absence would be a "great loss."[76] This discontinuation has had an international impact as well, because the United States Agency for International Development had been supplying Loops as part of their commodity donations.[77] However, the agency was moving to the provision of copper IUDs and was hoping to shift to the T 380A which it believed to be superior to both the Lippes Loop and the T Cu 200.

After the loss of the nonmedicated devices, until January 31, 1986, there were only three IUDs being manufactured in the United States, the Cu-7 and the Tatum-T Cu 200, made by G. D. Searle & Co., and the Progestasert, a product of Alza Corporation. However, during 1984 and 1985, there was an escalating number of lawsuits filed against the Cu-7. In the course of these litigations two major allegations were made. The first was that the design of the insertion system was defective because of the position of the tail in reference to the inserter tube, which was purported to pose certain subsequent health hazards. The second allegation was related to the presumed adverse effects of chronic copper toxicity. It is important to note that neither of these criticisms has ever been substantiated by scientific data.

These events culminated in the announcement on January 31, 1986, by Searle of a product discontinuation, effective immediately, for both the Cu-7 and the Tatum-T.[78] Searle stated that this decision related only to distribution and sales within the United States. It emphasized that their decision was based solely upon the high costs of defending scientifically unwarranted lawsuits and on the fact that further product liability insurance was virtually unobtainable. The company said that it regretted the necessity of taking this stand and acknowledged the hardship that this decision could cause women in the United States. It reaffirmed its position that both devices were safe and effective and pointed out that their approval by the FDA remained in effect. A spokesman for the FDA confirmed that Searle had complied fully with its safety and effectiveness guidelines and that the agency had no intention of discontinuing its approval of these two IUDs. As a result of these multiple corporate actions, the progesterone-bearing Progestasert is now the only IUD being manufactured and sold in the United States.

The extent of the impact which these discontinuations will have on the women in the United States cannot be fully ascertained immediately. Many health care providers have expressed dismay, wondering how to handle patients now for whom the IUD was clearly the contraceptive method of choice. The loss will be particularly felt by older women who have completed their families and who have contraindications for the use of OCs.[79]

There are two additional facets to this new situation. First, because of the current medicolegal climate, none of the research on new and improved IUDs can be carried out in the United States. Second, all of the advances in IUD technology, including the best device developed to date, the T Cu 380A, will probably not become available in the United States because of the untenable liability and malpractice environment.

It is already apparent, based upon comments made by international colleagues, that the impact of these decisions will also jeopardize the use of IUDs throughout the world in a very significant way. Most other countries do not have the same problems of escalating malpractice suits and product liability insurance. Hence, they will infer that if IUDs are not now available for use by women in the United States, then there must be something wrong with the devices. Furthermore, it would be logical for them to come to the conclusion, as they have on similar occasions in the past, that a double standard for safety and effectiveness exists for the United States and the rest of the world.

In November 1985, following the discontinuation of the nonmedicated devices, Planned Parenthood Federation of America, Inc. decided to convene an expert panel on the "Future of the IUD" on February 7, 1986.[80] The removal of the copper devices, shortly before the meeting, made these deliberations even more urgent. It was the expressed opinion of the expert panel that "the IUD is one of the most effective forms of reversible contraception that has yet been approved by the U.S. Food and Drug Administration." It reaffirmed that the IUDs presently approved by the FDA, which include the Cu 7, Tatum-T and Progestasert, continue to be a safe method of contraception for many women. The panel further stated that the loss of the IUDs was "a tragedy for the approximately 2.3 million American women who depend on them for reversible contraception" since "many of these women cannot use the other highly effective reversible method of birth control, the Pill."

Data were presented at the meeting on the demographic impact of the IUD withdrawal, using statistics from the 1982 National Survey of Family Growth. It was noted that 83% of IUD users had previously used OCs, but that 36% had stopped using OCs for medical reasons. When questioned about the desire for future pregnancies, 45% of IUD users indicated that they wanted another baby and 55% did not. On the basis of the previous contraceptive choices made by women discontinuing the use of an IUD, it was estimated that 160,000 more unintended pregnancies might be expected if IUDs were unavailable; 72,000 of the women might continue their pregnancies, and 88,000 might elect termination, given their previously stated desired for future pregnancies.

The panel further recommended that an educational campaign be developed for health care professionals and the public, to put these recent events into proper perspective. It decried "the current litigious climate in the United States and the unavailability of liability insurance to cover product liability" and the fact that the removal of the IUDs "has not only curtailed contraceptive choices for women, but has limited the ability of physicians to provide optimum health care for their patients." Finally, the panel confirmed the fact that the risk of malpractice litigation by the product discontinuations is essentially unchanged as far as providers are concerned. It stated that women may continue to use their present IUDs in accordance with the good medical practice and that current supplies of IUDs can be utilized, if so desired.

Thus, this decade ends on a somewhat mixed note. Significant advances have been made in the field of intrauterine contraception. This method of fertility control is used widely throughout the world, and in some countries, most notably China, is the major form of contraception.[70] Three-quarters of the world's IUD users, 40 million of them, live in China. More than half of the Chinese women who have had one child, the current allowable number, are wearing some type of IUD.

It is ironic that women living in the country which provided much of the expertise and financial support for IUD development will be deprived of their use at the time of maximum achievement. In the words of the panel, it is "a tragedy for American women that they have been disenfranchised in the United States from the use of an effective method of contraception, the copper-bearing IUD, and that to secure a copper IUD they will need to obtain it internationally or on the 'black market,' once existing supplies of Cu-7s and Tatum Ts are exhausted in the United States."

There has been one bright spot in the current bleak litigation scene. This was the March 19, 1986, judgment by a United States District Court judge for the District Court of Maryland. He had presided over a case which consolidated the claims of 17 plaintiffs who were alleged to have been injured by the use of the Cu-7 IUD. After 3 weeks of trial, the jury could not agree on a verdict, and the court declared a mistrial. The judge then evaluated the testimonies of the expert witnesses for the defendant and the plaintiffs. Regarding the latter, he commented on "the scattershot approach of plaintiffs who simply presented a series of alternative unsubstantiated theories." He then concluded that they had "dealt with mere possibilities rather than probabilities." He further stated that "the possibilities may be endless." Yet the probability that any of these events can occur has yet to be proven in this Court. With this type of theoretic proof, the jury was forced into an exercise in speculation, rather than reasoning. In conclusion, the plaintiffs failed to present sufficient evidence of causation and a verdict was rendered in favor of defendant.[81] This decision has clear implications for all subsequent litigation involving the Cu-7.

Reluctantly, it must be concluded that in the United States the IUD, with the important exception of the Progestasert, is dead, at least for the present time. The implications of this fact are especially serious for those women for whom the IUD is truly method of choice. The loss of the IUD as a contraceptive option, either as a new method or as a replacement, is particularly unfortunate for those women we now know are at no increased risk of complications resulting from the use of a copper-bearing IUD. It is very much to be hoped that ongoing efforts to reverse this situation will be successful and that improved devices such as the T Cu 380A will become available to American women during the next decade.

REFERENCES

1. Tatum HJ: Clinical aspects of intrauterine contraception: circumspection 1976. Fertil Steril 28:3, 1977

2. Tatum HJ, Connell EB: Managing Patients with Intrauterine Devices. 1st edition. Durant, Creative Infomatics, Inc., 1985
3. Schenker JG, Margolioth EJ: Intrauterine adhesions: an updated appraisal. Fertil Steril 37:593, 1982
4. Connell EB, Tatum HJ: Reproductive Health Care Manual. 1st edition. Durante, Creative Infomatics, Inc., 1985, p 80
5. Booth M, Beral V: Effect of age on pelvic inflammatory disease in nulliparous women using a copper 7 intrauterine contraceptive device. Br Med J 113:801, 1980
6. Osser S, Gullberg B, Liedho P, Sjobert N: Contraception: is development of pelvic inflammatory disease in women using intrauterine device equal regardless of parity? A one year follow-up study. Popul Rep 17:563, 1978
7. Thiery M: Clinical experience in Belgium and The Netherlands. Br J Obstet Gynaecol (Suppl) 4:51, 1982
8. Graham S, Simcock BW: A review of the use of intrauterine devices in nulliparous women. Contraception 26: 323, 1982
9. Booth M, Beral VA, Guillebaud J: Effect of age on pelvic inflammatory disease in nulliparous women using a copper 7 intrauterine contraceptive device. Br Mod J 281: 114, 1980
10. Tyrer LB: Update on intrauterine devices. Curr Prob Obstet Gynecol 2:1, 1979
11. Eschenback DA, Harnisch JP, Holmes KK: Pathogenesis of acute pelvic inflammatory disease: role of contraception and other risk factors. Am J Obstet Gynecol 128:838, 1977
12. Nahmanovici C, Gelas M: Sterilet et nulliparite (IUD) and nulliparae (FRE). Contraception 8:19, 1980
13. Steel JM, Duncan LJP: Contraception for the insulin-dependent diabetic women: the view from one clinic. Diabetes Care 3:557, 1980
14. Lawless M, Vessey M: Intrauterine device use by diabetic women. Br J Fam Plann 7:110, 1982
15. Wiese J: Intrauterine contraception in diabetic women. Fertil Steril 28:422, 1977
16. Skouby SO, Molested-Pedersen L, Kosonen A: Consequences of intrauterine contraception in diabetic women. Fertil Steril 42:568, 1984
17. Craig G, Newton J: contraception in diabetics. (Letter) Br J Fam Plann 7:121, 1982
18. Kivijarvi A, Timonen H, Rajamaki A, Gronroos M: Iron deficiency in women using copper intrauterine devices. Obstet Gynecol 67:95, 1986
19. Pedron N, Gallegos AJ, Lozano M, Aznar R: Menstrual blood loss estimates in women using copper 7 and multiload-250 intrauterine devices. Contraception 26:475, 1982
20. Batar I: IUD induced bleeding and the way of therapy. Int J Gynaecol Obstet 22:203, 1984
21. Dasgupta PR, Dutta S, Banerjee P: Vitamin E (alpha tocopherol) in the management of menorrhagia associated with the use of intrauterine contraceptive devices (IUCD). Int J Fertil 28:55, 1983
22. Hefnawi F, Yacout MM, Hosni M, El-Sheikha Z, Hassanein M: Medicated intrauterine devices to improve bleeding events. Int J Gynaecol Obstet 15:79, 1977
23. Guillebaud J, Bonnar J, Morehead J, Mathews A: Menstrual blood-loss with intrauterine devices. Lancet 1:387, 1976
24. Tatum HM, Schmidt FH, Phillip D, McCarty, O'Leary M: The Dalkon Shield controversy: structural and bacteriological studies of IUD tails. JAMA 231:711, 1975
25. Sparks RA, Purrier BGA, Watt PJ, Elstein M: Bacteriological colonization of uterine cavity: role of tailed intrauterine contraceptive device. In The Uterine Cervix in Reproduction, Edited by V Insler, G Bettendorf. Stuttgart, George Thieme, 1977, p 271
26. Lehfeldt H: Comparative study of two intra-uterine contraceptive devices. (Abstr) In Intra-Uterine Contraception, Edited by SJ Segal, AL Southam, KD Shafer. Amsterdam, Excerpta Medica (International Congress Series No. 86) 1965, p 237
27. Buchman MJ: A study of the intrauterine contraceptive device with and without an extracervical appendage or tail. Fertil Steril 21:348, 1977
28. Batar I, Lampe LG, Allonen H: IUD and PID: a two-year comparative study of copper-silver devices inserted without the tail. Presented at the Twin Symposia on Contraceptive Delivery Systems, Genetic Disorders and Reproductive Failure, September 22 to 25, 1985, Nairobi, Kenya
29. Toth A, O'Leary WM, Ledger W: Evidence for microbial transfer by spermatozoa. Obstet Gynecol 59:556, 1982
30. Pine L, Malcolm GM, Curtis EM, Brown JM: Demonstration of actinomyces and arachnia species in cervicovaginal smears by direct staining with species-specific fluorescent-antibody conjugate. J Clin Microbiol 13:15, 1981
31. Jones JB, Kaplan W, Brown JM, White W: Studies of cervicovaginal smears for the presence of actinomycetes. Mycopathologia 83:53, 1983
32. Schmidt WA, Bedrossian CWM, Ali V, Webb JA, Bastian FO: *Actinomyces* and intrauterine contraceptive devices: the clinicopathologic entity. Diagn Gynecol Obstet 2:165, 1980
33. Tatum HJ, Schmidt FH, Jain A: Management and outcome of pregnancies associated with the Copper T intrauterine device. Am J Obstet Gynecol 126:869, 1976
34. Kallenberger DA, Ronk DA, Jimerson GK: Ectopic pregnancy: a 15-year review of 160 cases. South Med J 71:758, 1968
35. Tatum HJ, Schmidt FH: Contraceptive and sterilization practices and extrauterine pregnancy: a realistic perspective. Fertil Steril 28:407, 1977
36. Sivin I: Copper T IUD use and ectopic pregnancy rates in the United States. Contraception 19:151, 1979
37. Ory HW: The women's health study: ectopic pregnancy and intrauterine contraceptive devices: new perspectives. Obstet Gynecol 57:137, 1981
38. Sivin I: IUD associated ectopic pregnancies 1974 to 1984. In Intrauterine Contraception: Advances and Future Prospects, Vol 45, Edited by G Zatuchni, A Goldsmith, JJ Sciarra. New York, Harper & Row, 1985, p 340
39. Dorfman SF, Grimes DA, Cates W, Binkin NJ, Kafrisson ME, O'Reilly KR: Ectopic pregnancy mortality, United States 1979 to 1980: clinical aspects. Obstet Gynecol 64:386, 1984
40. Tietze C, Lewit S: Evaluation of intrauterine devices: ninth progress report of the cooperative program. Stud Fam Plann 55:1, 1970
41. Daling JR, Weiss NS, Metch BJ, Chow WH, Soderstrom RM, Moore DE, Spadoni LR, Stadel BV: Primary tubal infertility in relation to the use of an intratuerine device. N Engl J Med 312:937, 1985

42. Cramer DW, Schiff I, Schoenbaum SC, Gibson M, Belisle S, Albrecht B, Stillman RJ, Berger MJ, Wilson M, Stadel BV, Seibel M: Tubal infertility and the intrauterine device. N Engl J Med 312:941, 1985
43. White MK, Rook JB, Strauss L, Rochat RW, Tyler CW Jr, Senanayke P: Current practice concerning time of IUD insertion. IPPF Med 11:1, 1977
44. Laufe LE, Wheeler RG, Friel PG: Methods and devices: modification of intrauterine devices for postpartum insertion. Lancet 1:853, 1979
45. Ezzat KR, Zake ES, Shaaban H, Kessel E: Immediate postpartum insertion of a sutured Lippes Loop. Int J Gynaecol Obstet 18:26, 1980
46. Cole LP, Edelman DA, Potts DM, Wheeler RG, Laufe LE: Postpartum insertion of modified intrauterine devices. J Reprod Med 29:677, 1984
47. Thiery M, Zatuchni GI, Goldsmith A, Sciarra JJ: Timing of IUD insertion. In Intrauterine Contraception: Advances and Future Prospects, Edited by G Zatuchni, A Goldsmith, JJ Sciarra. Philadelphia, Harper & Row, 1984, p 365
48. Thiery M, Laufe LP, Van Der Pas H, Van Kets H, Derom R, Defoort P: Contraception 28:229, 1983
49. Connell EB: Intrauterine devices. In Principles and Practice of Clinical Gynecology, Edited by NG Kase, AB Weingold. New York, John Wiley & Sons, 1983, p 1033
50. Andolsek L: Post-abortion IUD insertion. In Medicated Intrauterine Devices: Physiological and Clinical Aspects, Edited by ESE Hafez, WAA Os Van. The Hague, Martinus Nijhoff, 1980, p 137
51. Bonnar J: Progestagen-only contraception and tubal pregnancies. (Letter) Br Med J 1:287, 1974
52. Goldman JA, Dekel A, Reichman J: Immediate postabortion intrauterine contraception in nulliparous adolescents. Isr J Med Sci 15:522, 1979
53. Nan Lith DAF, Du Plessis-Albas M, Querido L, Van Schie KJ, Beekhuizen W: Post-abortion insertion of Multiload IUD. Leiden, Center for Human Reproduction, 1980, p 28
54. World Health Organization Special Programme of Research, Development and Research Training in Human Reproduction. Ninth Annual Report. Geneva, 1980, p 162
55. Zhang P: Five years experience with the Copper T 200 in Shanghai: 856 cases. Contraception 22:561, 1980
56. Lippes J, Tatum HJ, Maulik D, Sielezny M: Postcoital copper IUDs. Adv Planned Parenthood 14:87, 1979
57. Rowland S, Guillebaud J: Postcoital contraception. Br J Fam Plann 7:3, 1981
58. Tyrer LB: The Cu-7 and postcoital contraception. Adv Planned Parenthood 15:111, 1981
59. Zipper JA, Tatum HJ, Pastene L, Medel M, Rivera M: Metallic copper as an intrauterine contraceptive adjunct to the "T" device. Am J Obstet Gynecol 105:1274, 1969
60. Parr EL: Leucocytes and infertility. J Reprod Fertil 10:153, 1970
61. Cuadros A, Hirsch JG: Copper on intrauterine devices stimulates leukocyte exudation. Am Assoc Adv Sci 175: 175, 1972
62. American College of Obstetrics and Gynecology: Obstetric Gynecologic Terminology. Philadelphia, F. A. Davis, 1972
63. International Federation of Gynecology and Obstetrics, Committee on Medical Aspects of Human Reproduction, M. F. Fathalla, Chairman. World Health Organization, Geneva, Switzerland
64. Tyrer LB: Memorandum to all Planned Parenthood Affiliates, 1985
65. Segal SJ, Alvarez-Sanchez F, Adejuwon CA, Brache de Mejia V, Leon P, Faundes A: Absence of chorionic gonadotropin in sera of women who use intrauterine devices. Fertil Steril 44:214, 1985
66. Sivin I, Tatum HJ: Four years of experience with the TCu 380A intrauterine contraceptive device. Fertil Steril 36: 159, 1981
67. Nilsson CG, Allonen H, Diaz J, Luukkainen T: Two years' experience with two levonorgestrel-releasing intrauterine devices and one copper releasing intrauterine device: a randomized comparative performance study. Fertil Steril 39:187, 1983
68. Larsen S, Hansen MK, Jacobsen JC, Ladehoff P, Sorensen, Westergaard JG: Clinical trials: Comparison between two IUDs: Progestasert and Cu T 200. Contraception Delivery System 2:281, 1981
69. Thiery M, Van der Pas H, Van Kets H: A decade of experience with the CTCu 220 C. Adv Contracep 1:313, 1985
70. Population Information Program: IUDs: on appropriate contraceptive for many women. Popul Rep [B], 1982
71. Dadelszen PV, Hurst PR, Peplow PV: Contraception: effect of indomethacin incorporation on the retention of Silastic intrauterine devices in the rat. Contraception 26:159, 1982
72. Lee NC, Rubin GL, Ory HW, Burkman RT: Type of intrauterine device and the risk of pelvic inflammatory disease. Am J Obstet Gynecol 62:1, 1983
73. Mishell DR: Current status of intrauterine devices. N Engl J Med 312:984, 1983
74. Ortho Pharmaceutical Corporation: Letter, April 1, 1985
75. Casey MD: Ortho Pharmaceutical Corporation to all practicing physicians, September 25, 1985
76. Tyrer LB: Letter from L. B. Tyrer to all Planned Parenthood Federation Affiliates of the United States
77. Assistance for International Development, Population: IUD Procurement Strategy, November 1985
78. Searle letter of February 1, 1986 to the medical professionals in the United States announcing the product discontinuation of the Cu-7 and Tatum-T
79. Connell EB: Contraception for the premenopausal women. The Menopausal Update Series (In press)
80. Minutes of Planned Parenthood Federation of America's Convened Expert Panel on the Future of the IUD. New York, February 14, 1986
81. Memorandum: Joseph H. Young, United States District Judge of Maryland, District Court for the District of Maryland, March 19, 1986. Sue Ellen Marder, lead plaintiff vs G. D. Searle Company, Inc., Chicago, Illinois

Chapter 33

Oral contraceptives and neoplasia: 1987 update

George R. Huggins, M.D.
Peter K. Zucker, M.D.

The Johns Hopkins University School of Medicine, Baltimore, Maryland

Combined estrogen-progestogen oral contraceptives (OCs) have been available in the United States since 1960. The first compound approved contained 10 mg norethynodrel and 150 μg mestranol. Current worldwide use is approximated at 55 million[1] women and United States use at 8 to 10 million women.[2] Clearly, for justification of such wide use of potent drugs, the risk-benefit ratio must weigh substantially in favor of the drug benefits. In the past 26 years more than 40 brands of combined OCs have been sold in the United States. Today, they contain one of five synthetic progestogens (all derived from 19-nortestosterone and one of two estrogens). Most women are now using combined OCs with 0.3 to 1 mg progestogen and 20 to 50 μg estrogen.

Since 1970 all of the newly introduced compounds have used ethinyl estradiol (EE_2) as the estrogen fraction. The progestogens present in the low-dose and triphasic pills are ethynodiol diacetate, norethindrone, norethindrone acetate, and norgestrel.[1] Outside the United States some of the 17α-hydroxyprogesterone derivatives are in use.[1] However, these derivatives were withdrawn from the United States market in response to concerns regarding the occurrence of neoplastic lesions in dogs.

Few issues evoke as much concern and controversy as does the suspected association between OC use and the development of cancer. Isolated case reports and preliminary findings may give rise to overwhelming pressure to discontinue use of the drug with little attempt to weigh its possible risk-benefit ratios. This response is not confined to human evidence. Suspicion of carcinogenicity in any animal species has raised similar concerns and evoked the same demand for drug withdrawal.[3]

Other serious side effects such as cardiovascular problems with use of OCs and severe pelvic infections with use of intrauterine devices (IUDs) have extensive documentation. Morbidity and mortality rates have been estimated.[2, 4, 5] By and large the response of the public and the medical profession has been to evaluate the risk-benefit ratio of contraceptive therapy as related to unplanned pregnancy or induced abortion and to accept the much lower risk of these very effective methods of contraception.

We will survey some of the available data and attempt to evaluate possible associations between OCs and human neoplasia in light of pregnancy risk or benefit for oral contraception. Our first review of this subject was published in 1979.[6] The current discussion will serve as an update to that original presentation. In the past 6 years numerous new data have been published regarding the relationship between OCs and neoplasia that has helped clarify relationships. The most salutary findings have been the protective effect of OCs on endometrial and ovarian cancer. The most disturbing has been the growing consensus regarding an adverse effect on cervical neoplasia.

The more recent epidemiologic studies have been much better able to assess confounding variables and as such appear to have more validity than the older studies.

PROBLEMS OF INVESTIGATION

This investigation is confounded by several problems: (1) there is no suitable animal model in most cases; (2) there is generally a long lag-time, approximately 15 years after exposure to a carcinogen, until the development of overt malignancy[7]; (3) there is a low incidence of malignant disease in the young female population; and (4) there are multiple etiologic influences such as genetic, cultural, geographic, and environmental exposure to many possible carcinogens.

Each steroid formulation used for contraception undergoes extensive testing in several animal species before human investigative use. These animal studies provide only presumptive evidence of carcinogenic potential within a single species and sometimes within a single strain of that species. Extrapolation of conclusions from one species to another has dubious validity. Neither positive nor negative results with animal exposure to suspected carcinogens can be used with any degree of certainty in relation to the human being.[3] The reader is referred to the George Washington University Center Population Reports,[8] which provide an extensive review of animal studies with sex steroids and their relationship to benign or malignant neoplasia. Animal studies are not discussed in detail in this section.

The relationship of OCs to benign neoplasms is germane because some benign neoplastic lesions may predispose or progress to frank invasive cancer. This is especially true with dysplasia of the cervix, hyperplasia of the endometrium, and, to some extent, benign dysplastic breast disease.

INVESTIGATIVE METHODS

The principal investigative methods in human beings include various epidemiologic approaches[9] (Table 1). The methodologies most frequently used are (1) case reports (tumor registries), (2) disease rates and trends, (3) case-control studies, and (4) cohort studies. Each of these approaches provides a specific piece of a very complex puzzle. None of these methods taken by itself will provide a definitive answer as to causal relationships between exposure to an environmental carcinogen and the occurrence of disease. Needless to say, one would be unrealistic to ignore increasing and consistent evidence that is confirmed by these multiple approaches.

CASE REPORTS

The case report (registry) method has served well to alert us to the appearance of new and hitherto unsuspected disease entities. In 1971 Herbst et al.[10] first reported the occurrence of vaginal adenosis and adenocarcinoma in daughters born to women who had taken diethylstilbestrol during early gestation. More recently, Baum et al.[11] reported the occurrence of benign liver tumors in OC users. These initial reports provided the impetus for retrospective case-con-

Table 1. *Four Epidemiologic Methods Used in Studying OCs and Neoplasms*[a]

Method	Description	Functions	Limitations
Case reports	Describe patients, their illnesses, and exposures to environmental factors; discuss suspected interrelationships	Often the source of first suspicions about disease causes; encourage more rigorous study	Few conclusions are made on the basis of case reports alone
Disease rate trends	Examine the incidence or mortality of a disease in a large population	Can be compared with trends in exposure to environmental factors; help assess impact of disease on public health	For detectable changes in rates, exposure to environmental factor must be widespread in the population and must alter the chances of development of the disease
Case-comparison	Compare exposure to environmental factor in groups with a disease with that in similar groups without the disease	Determine relative difference in exposure between those with and those without a disease; appropriate when the disease is rare or quick results are desired	Do not determine the incidence rate in participants, which may be faulty
Cohort studies	Compare disease incidence in groups exposed to an environmental factor with that in groups not exposed	Appropriate when fullest information, least subject to unavoidable possibilities of methodologic bias, is required or when information on more than one disease is sought	Often require study of large groups over long periods of time, especially with rare diseases

[a]Modified from Population Reports: Oral contraceptives: update on usage, safety, and side effects.[9]

trol and prospective cohort studies. As a result of these efforts, the association of maternal diethylstilbestrol ingestion, adenosis, and adenocarcinoma of the vagina in offspring is well established. No conclusions regarding either the incidence of disease or risk of development of the disease can be determined by using only case reports or surveys.

DISEASE RATES AND TRENDS

Disease rates for specific malignancies are available for a number of differing populations.[12] Their incidence varies widely according to geographic location and other subgroups (Table 2). Care must be taken not to extrapolate data to other (dissimilar) populations. This particular approach has been of limited usefulness in evaluating the influence of any single etiologic factor on the development or progression of cancer. It will, however, monitor dramatic changes such as those that have taken place with regard to the increasing incidence of carcinoma of the lung in women.[13]

CASE-CONTROL STUDIES

The main source of useful retrospective information regarding the association between contraceptive steroid exposure and the risk of neoplasia is found in the analysis of case-control studies.[14-20] The approach in case-control or case-comparison studies is to identify patients with the disease to be studied and to match them carefully with patients who are disease free. Factors such as age, parity, race, social class, sexual activity, drug use, concurrent disease, and elimination of exposure to other possible carcinogens are most important in ensuring that the populations studied are as similar as possible. The use of OCs is then compared for both cases and controls. Failure to match for one or more variables can lead to major invalid hypotheses.

The conclusions are usually expressed as relative risk or risk ratio. This is based on the ratio between the incidence of OC use among the cases and the incidence among the controls. With this methodology a relative risk value of 1 would imply neither a positive nor a negative effect of exposure. A relative risk of < 1 implies a negative association, and > 1 a positive association with exposure to OCs. In this type of study highly positive relative risk figures may give rise to unwarranted alarm because the incidence of the disease in the general population is not defined. Five times relative risk for a disease with an incidence of 5/1000 has more important implications than five times relative risk in a disease with a baseline incidence of 5/1,000,000. Unfortunately, case-comparison studies when reported in both the lay and scientific press may not clearly delineate the baseline risk. The potential exists for overestimating the absolute risk to the patient.

Case-comparison studies are relatively inexpensive, can be done quickly, and can be carried out at single institutions that are able to obtain necessary numbers of patients with rare or low-incidence disease.

COHORT STUDIES

The prospective cohort study compares the incidence of disease in patients who are exposed to the suspected environmental factor with other patients who are not so exposed. Cancer has a low incidence among women of reproductive age. The study of possible carcinogenic effects of OCs requires large numbers of patients followed over a long period of time in order to gather enough information for adequate statistical analysis[20] (Table 3).

The cohort study can define the baseline incidence of the disease and compare incidence among users and nonusers in a single population. The cost and logistical problems involved in ade-

Table 2. *Reported Annual Incidence of Cancers of Selected Sites/100,000 Women in Selected Countries, 1960s and 1970s*[a]

Site of cancer	Country				
	Nigeria	United States	Israel	India	Japan
Breast	5.8	89.9	57.6	11.3	14.1
Uterine cervix	7.0	11.4	4.6	14.3	15.2
Uterine corpus	0.5	22.4	11.2	0.7	1.3
Ovary[b]	3.0	15.5	13.4	2.7	3.0

[a]Modified from Waterhouse et al.[12]
[b]Includes tube.

Table 3. *Minimal Samples Required to Detect Differences in Disease Rates Between OC Users and Controls in Prospective Study*[a]

Site of cancer	No. of years after onset of study	Annual incidence rate in controls/10,000	Persons required in each group: incidence 2 times in OC users
Breast	1	2.2	85,000
Corpus uteri	1	0.3	600,000
Cervix	1	3.1	60,000
Breast	10	7.5	25,000
Corpus uteri	10	1.3	140,000
Cervix	10	5.6	35,000

[a]Modified from Seigel and Corfman.[20]

quately conducting a contraceptive cohort study have limited their number. At present there are only two large contraceptive cohort studies in progress—both in the United Kingdom. The Royal College of General Practitioners (RCGP) enrolled 23,611 current OC users and 22,766 nonusers during 1968 to 1969,[21] and Vessey et al.[22] enrolled 9653 OC users and 7379 nonusers during 1968 to 1974 in the Oxford Family Planning Association (OFPA) study.

Care must be taken not to extrapolate data to other (dissimilar) populations. For instance, subjects in the population of the OFPA study[22] were white, married, economically middle class, and 25 to 39 years of age at time of enrollment in the study. Conclusions regarding carcinoma of the breast in this population may have little significance for women in India or Japan.

OCs AND BREAST DISEASE

RISK FACTORS IN CARCINOMA OF THE BREAST

Several major risk factors for carcinoma of the breast have been identified[23, 24] (Table 4). The marked predisposition for this disease in the woman is attributed largely to the endocrine influence of estrogen on breast tissue. Breast cancer has occasionally been reported in men treated with long-term exogenous estrogen for carcinoma of the prostate[25] or in male-to-female transsexuals receiving supplemental estrogen.[26] Studies of postmenopausal estrogen use have yielded conflicting conclusions. Several studies have shown an increased risk of breast cancer associated with estrogen use,[27-29] whereas others have shown none.[30-33] The genetic predisposition is stronger in families with several relatives involved, especially if the disease has been premenopausal and bilateral.[34] The strongly positive relationship with benign breast disease or precancerous mastopathy is most important because of the high incidence of benign breast disease in the general population and the considerable difficulty in defining which type of benign breast neoplasia is "precancerous."[35] Nulliparous women or women who postpone the birth of a first child until after age 34 also show increased risk.[24]

Table 4. *Major Risk Factors in Breast Cancer*[a]

Risk factor	Comparison		Ratio
Sex	Female	Male	99/1
Age	> 40	< 40	85%/15%
Genetic predisposition; family history of breast cancer	Yes	No	3/1
Mother and sister; bilateral and premenopausal	Yes	No	9/1
Previous benign breast disease	Yes	No	3/1
Precancerous mastopathy	Yes	No	5/1
Previous cancer of one breast	Yes	No	5/1
Parity (reflects early first parity)	Nulliparous	Parous	3/1
Age at first birth	Late (> 34)	Early (18)	4/1
Lactation	Yes	No	1/1

[a]Modified from Leis.[24]

BREAST CANCER, PRECLINICAL PHASE

The duration of preclinical or predetected breast cancer may extend over many years. Gullino[36] has estimated this "latent" time on the basis of an assumed 100 days' doubling time for breast cancer cells (Fig. 1). In this model, the major conclusion to be drawn from this estimate is that the clinical phase of breast cancer is by far the shortest phase in the natural history of the disease. Among the problems associated with this model are the realities that the tumor cells do not grow at a constant exponential rate and that a significant portion of the tumor is composed of stroma rather than epithelial cells. However, this assumption has support from the studies of Spratt and Spratt,[37] Collins et al.,[38] and Silvestrimi et al.[39] This long latent, or predetection, phase raises our concerns over the effects of exogenous steroids on the predetected lesion. If the growth of these tumors is stimulated by OC steroids, one possible effect would be the appearance of the

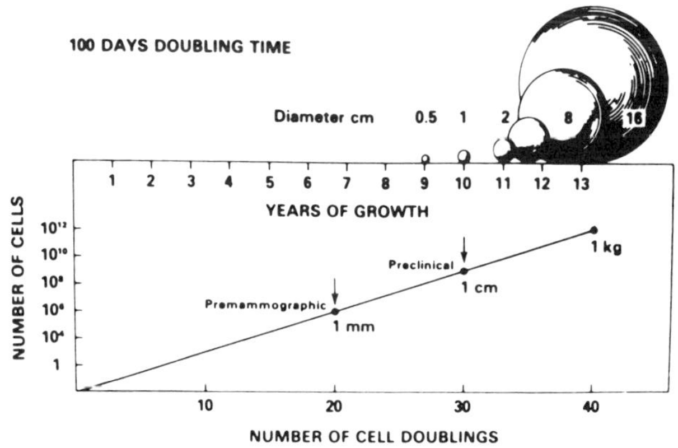

Figure 1
Estimation of duration of preclinical or predetected breast cancer. Reproduced from Gullino[36] with permission.

lesions in younger women, and progression of the lesions, once clearly detected, would be enhanced. There are no firm epidemiologic data at present to support these concerns.

BREAST CANCER AND CHRONIC MASTITIS

Benign breast disease is not a single well-defined process. The histologic descriptive terminology is sometimes confusing and inconsistent. Fibrosis, fibrocystic disease, cystic mastitis, adenosis, fibroadenoma, hypermetaplastic disease, and intraductal papillomas are terms used in discussions of benign breast disease.[40] This inconsistency makes it difficult to compare accurately conclusions from various reports.

McDivitt et al.[41] have shown a much higher risk of cancer associated with lesions having more marked degrees of atypia. Black and Chabon[42] in 1969 proposed a grading system of progressive and atypical proliferative changes in a mammary duct system. These duct changes in sequence were given numerical ranking as follows: (1) control, (2) hyperplasia, (3) and (4) atypia, and (5) carcinoma in situ. An increased relative risk (five times) for development of cancer was shown in atypia grades 3 and 4 as compared with grades 1 and 2.

Kodlin et al.[40] studied 2931 women with at least one benign breast biopsy obtained at the Kaiser-Permanente Medical Center in Oakland, CA, between 1948 and 1973. These patients were followed for an average period of 6.7 years. The incidence of breast cancer in these patients varied between 2.5 and 21.1/1000 person-year rate. According to the Black-Chabon atypia scoring system, the risk increased steadily from 2.5 for lesions classified as types 1 and 2 to 21.1 for type 5.

Kodlin et al.[40] thought that "in general, it appears that looking at the relative risks with respect to population expectations, histology can identify groups of somewhat higher risk than epidemiology. . . ." Cole[43] suggested that when using the Black-Chabon grading scale we have the concept of two types of breast disease, one of which is premalignant and one of which is not.

Few epidemiologic studies before 1975 that investigated risk of breast cancer and benign breast lesions categorized lesions on the basis of pathologic examination of benign breast tissue.

A consensus conference jointly sponsored by the College of American Pathologists and the American Cancer Society convened in 1985 to determine the risk relationship between benign lesions and breast cancer. Risks were determined and categorized by pathologic examination[44] (Table 5).

The most common symptomatic benign breast conditions are lobular hyperplasia, cystic duct dilation, fibroadenoma, and sclerosing adenosis. These are associated with no increased risk of breast cancer. Only those patients with significant hyperplasia show increased risk of breast cancer (1.5 to 5 times). This classification may help to define more clearly subgroups of patients with benign breast disease. Future epidemiologic studies will need to define better patients with "benign breast disease."

Table 5. *Relative Risk for Invasive Breast Carcinoma on the Basis of Pathologic Examination of Benign Breast Tissue*[a]

No increased risk[b]		
Adenosis, sclerosing or florid	Fibroadenoma	Mastitis (inflammation)
Apocrine metaplasia	Fibrosis	Periductal mastitis
Cysts, macro and/or micro	Hyperplasia, mild (> 2 but < 4 epithelial cells in depth)	Squamous metaplasia
Duct ectasis		

Slightly increased risk (1.5 to 2 times)[b]
Hyperplasia, moderate or florid, solid or papillary
Papilloma with fibrovascular core

Moderately increased risk (5 times)[b]
Atypical hyperplasia (borderline lesion)
Ductal
Lobular

[a]Modified from the College of American Pathologists.[44]
[b]For invasive breast carcinoma among women with lesions specified relative to comparable women who have had no breast biopsy.

OCs AND BENIGN BREAST DISEASE

Before 1979 the relationship of combined OCs to benign breast disease was consistently favorable. Most studies[21, 22, 35, 43-48] have shown OC use to be associated with significantly decreased risk of benign breast neoplasia.

In spite of the nearly unanimous agreement that OCs exert a protective effect with relation to benign breast disease, a number of questions and problems persist: (1) Does response differ with respect to duration of use? (2) Does response differ according to histologic cell type? (3) Does response differ for various types and dosages of contraceptive steroids?

DURATION OF USE

Most studies[21, 22, 45-48] have documented with increasing length of OC use a decrease risk that begins to appear after 2 years and persists for more than 4 years of use. There is no suggestion in these studies that the risk increases with longer use. There is some disagreement as to persistence of this protective effect after use of OCs is stopped. Although Ory et al.[45] and Fasal and Paffenbarger[47] have shown some persistence of a protective effect, this finding is not confirmed by most other studies.

RESPONSE BY HISTOLOGIC CELL TYPE

Most studies showing diminished risks for development of benign breast neoplasia during OC use have not analyzed lesions by histologic type. The studies that have examined fibrocystic disease and fibroadenoma separately have reported somewhat inconsistent results. Ory et al.[45] reported decreased risks for both fibrocystic disease and fibroadenoma with combined pills. Sartwell et al.[48] found the decreased risk to hold true only for fibrocystic disease with combined pills.

Brinton et al.[49] analyzed the experience in the OFPA Contraceptive study through 1979. This particular study separated the types of benign breast disease into four separate categories: fibroadenoma, chronic cystic disease, nonbiopsied breast lumps, and other benign breast disease. The protective effect was consistent for all categories. Furthermore each category showed significant trends of decreasing risks with increasing years of use (Table 6). The reductions in risk for current users were 84% for fibroadenoma, 53% for chronic cystic disease, 48% for nonbiopsied breast lumps, and 40% for other breast disease. Women who had discontinued pill use 1 or more years before diagnosis demonstrated no reduction in risk.

Livosli et al.,[50] using a case-control study, investigated the risk of development of fibrocystic disease in OC users by applying the Black-Chabon scoring system. The main purpose of this study was to determine whether the association between OC use and fibrocystic disease varied according to the extent of the breast epithelial atypia. Two hundred five premenopausal women aged 20 to 44 years with a diagnosis of fibrocystic disease, admitted to two hospitals in New Haven, CT, constituted the case population. These patients were matched individually with surgical patients for age, marital status, race, and education. All biopsies were separately classified according to the pathologic criteria of Black-Chabon.[42]

The odds ratio for fibrocystic disease among women who ever used OCs was determined according to the average ductal-atypia score. These

Table 6. *Relative Risks of Benign Breast Disease by Use of OCs; OFPA Contraceptive Study, United Kingdom, 1968–1979*[a]

Measure of exposure	Fibroadenoma (n = 74)	Chronic cystic disease (n = 211)	Nonbiopsied breast lumps (n = 331)	Other breast disease (n = 70)
Ever-use				
No	1.00	1.00	1.00	1.00
Yes	0.35	0.66	0.58	0.63
95% confidence interval	(0.2–0.7)	(0.4–0.9)	(0.4–0.8)	(0.3–1.2)
Years of use				
Never used	1.00	1.00	1.00	1.00
< 2	0.43	1.28	0.84	0.44
2–3	0.46	0.89	0.67	0.51
4–5	0.33	0.49	0.56	0.49
6–7	0.46	0.56	0.44	1.34
8+	0.00	0.35	0.49	0.38
×1 for linear trend	−3.41	−3.41	−3.94	−0.68

[a]Modified from Brinton et al.[49]

determinations were carried out for "ever-users" and for "4-year duration users" compared with patients who had never used OCs. The odds ratio for mild degrees of ductal atypia was less than 1 for both "ever-users" and "4-year users." The odds ratio was 3 for "ever-users" and 3.2 for "4-year users" in patients who had severe ductal atypia. Thus the decreased frequency of fibrocystic disease applied only to those forms of the disease in which epithelial atypia was minimal or absent. Women with marked atypia showed no difference in frequency among long-term users as compared with "never users." Livosli et al.[50] believe that long-term use of OCs protects only against the forms of fibrocystic disease that are not firmly associated with an increased risk of cancer but not against the premalignant forms of breast atypia. There was no suggestion that the use of OCs was associated with a higher incidence of the more advanced grades of atypia.

PROGESTOGEN EFFECT

The women subjects in both the RCGP[21] and the Brinton[49] studies were taking compounds that all contained 50 mg EE_2. The progestogen dosages varied from 1 to 4 mg. The protective effect was significantly greater in the high-progestogen pills (relative risk, 0.27). There was virtually no protective effect (relative risk, 0.8) among the 1-mg progestogen pills.

Berkowitz et al. in 1984[51] provided additional support for the lack of protective effect among women taking low-progestogen-dose pills. This case-control study examined 633 women with biopsy-proved fibrocystic breast disease and 1062 controls from five Connecticut hospitals. For premenopausal women there was no evidence that long-term use of OCs was associated with a decreased risk of fibrocystic breast disease among either current or past users. In an analysis of compounds most frequently used in the United States, estrogen (20 to 50 μg) and progestogens (1 to 2.5 mg) showed relative risks of 0.95 to 1.77, respectively, which are not indicative of a protective effect. Additional studies are needed to clarify these findings further.

Ory et al.[2] estimated that the protective effect of OCs on benign breast disease among the 8,000,000 United States women using OCs results each year in 23,490 fewer breast biopsies. These figures were calculated from estimates of the protective effect of pre-1979 studies.

Should the conclusions of Berkowitz et al.[51] and Brinton et al.[49] be confirmed, the public health benefit of OCs on benign breast neoplasia may be much less than current estimates.

OCs AND BREAST CANCER

Benign breast disease represents a significant risk factor for the ultimate development of carcinoma of the breast. The early studies that show a consistently protective effect on benign disease do not show the same protective effect for breast cancer (Table 7).[21, 22, 45, 47, 52-55]

Most of the derived risk ratios are close to unity. This figure can be interpreted to indicate no evidence of either positive or negative association between breast cancer and up to 4 years' use of OCs.

In a recent review Clavel et al.[56] surveyed 22 major epidemiologic studies that investigated the relationship between OC use and breast cancer. Three cohort studies were analyzed: RCGP study, the OFPA Contraceptive study, and the Walnut Creek Contraceptive Drug study. The only subgroup whose risk reached statistical significance was among young women in the RCGP study (Table 8). Among the 18 case-control studies the overall adjusted relative risk among OC users as compared with nonusers was significantly > 1 in only one study (Clavel et al.[57]). However, there are suggestions that certain subgroups of women may be at increased risk for breast cancer from OC use.[47, 58]

The 1975 case-control study by Fasal and Paffenbarger[47] in which past and current OC usage in 452 premenopausal women with breast cancer was analyzed shows a paradoxical risk pattern. A significantly higher relative risk was found among the cancer patients who had used OCs for 2 to 4 years. However, the risk was not increased

Table 7. *OCs and Breast Cancer: Literature Review*

Report	Type of study	Rate ratio
Arthes et al.[52]	Case-control	0.7
Boston Collaborative Drug Surveillance program[53]	Case-control	0.6
Fasal and Paffenbarger[47]	Case-control	1.1
Kelsey et al.[54]	Case-control	1.35
Vessey et al.[55]	Case-control	0.8
Ory et al.[45]	Cohort	0.7
Royal College of General Practitioners[21]	Cohort	1.1
Vessey et al.[22]	Cohort	0.4

Table 8. *Age-Standardized Risk Ratios of Breast Cancer Among OC Users and Nonusers*[a]

	RCGP		OFPA		Walnut Creek study
	All women	Women aged 15–34	All women	Women aged 25–34	
Never-users	1.00 (39)	1.00[c] (8)	1.00 (52)	1.00 (28)	1.00 (114)
Current users	1.26 (50)	2.81[c,d] (24)	1.04[e] (54)	0.64[e] (18)	1.2 (131)
Ex-users	1.14 (45)		0.87[e] (45)	0.54[e] (15)	

[a]Modified from Clavel et al.[56]
[b]Incidence rates × 10^5 in parentheses.
[c]Also standardized for parity at diagnosis, smoking habit, and social class.
[d]$P < 5\%$.
[e]Ratio of incidence rates of OC users versus nonusers.

for those patients who had taken pills for < 2 years of for 4 to 8 years. The authors proposed two possible conclusions: (1) "that the findings were due simply to chance" or (2) "that oral contraceptives accelerate the growth rate of pre-existing subclinical malignant lesions, with these lesions reaching the level of clinical recognition only after 2 years of drug usage and all being diagnosed within 2 additional years." A second group with increased risk were those patients who had a history of prior breast biopsy and OC usage for 6 or more years. There was no reported analysis of these prior biopsy specimens for degree of atypia or specific cell types.

Pike et al.[58] conducted a case-control study in Los Angeles in 1983. There were 314 women with breast cancer and 314 individually matched controls. He concluded that women < 37 years of age who had used high-progestin OCs before age 25 were at increased risk for breast cancer. He found a steadily increasing risk according to duration of use for all OCs. The relative risk for those women who used high-progestin OCs was further increased (Table 9).

Two studies[58, 59] showed a significance in risk among women who began OC use before age 25. Pike et al.[58] performed the only study that showed a significant linear trend with longer duration of use before age 25.

None of the studies that examined risks by years since initial use or by years since last use found a significant increase in any group. Four studies found some increased risk with OC use before first full-term pregnancy.[60-63] However there was no significant association among nulliparous women. The type and dosage of hormone have not been correlated with risk except for the study of Pike et al.,[58] in which the high-progestogen potency pills were found to carry greater risk. Pike's classification of progestogen potency has been widely questioned.

Paul et al.[64] in 1986 conducted a national population-based case-control study of 433 New Zealand women aged 25 to 54 with newly diagnosed breast cancer compared with 897 control women. Analysis of risk by duration of use, age at first use, and time since first use showed no increased risk. Moreover, even women starting pill use before age 20, who had taken pills more than 15 years previously and had continued to use them for more than 10 years, were not at an increased risk. The authors felt that the statistical power of their study was high because of exceptionally high pill use by New Zealand women. In 1975 the prevalence of pill use was reported to be higher in New Zealand than any other country except Holland.[8]

The largest ongoing United States study designed to evaluate the risks of steroid use and multiple female cancers is the Cancer and Steroid Hormone study of the Centers for Disease Control and the National Institute of Child Health and Human Development.[65] Because of the repeated references to portions of this study, the methods of this investigation will be described in detail. The Cancer and Steroid Hormone study—a multicenter population-based, case-control study—is coordinated by the Division of Reproductive Health, Center for Health Promotion and Education, the Centers for Disease Control, with support from the Center for Population Research of the National Institute of Child Health and Hu-

Table 9. *Relative Breast Cancer Risk*[a]

Months of OC use	Any use	High progestin
0	1.0	1.0
1–14	1.3	1.4
25–48	1.7	2.4
49–72	2.0	4.1
> 73	4.9	∞

[a]Modified from Pike et al.[58]

man Development and the National Cancer Institute (NCI). Enrollment of subjects was begun in December 1980 through the Surveillance, Epidemiology, and End Results (SEER) Centers for the NCI in eight areas (the metropolitan areas of Atlanta, Detroit, San Francisco, and Seattle; the states of Connecticut, Iowa, and New Mexico; and the four urban counties of Utah).

CASES

The case study subjects were women 20 to 54 years of age with histologically confirmed primary breast cancer newly diagnosed between December 1, 1980, and December 31, 1982, who resided in one of the eight SEER reporting areas. A case group of 4711 women was available for analysis.

CONTROLS

Controls were women selected according to Waksberg's method of random-digit dialing[66] in the geographic areas of the cases. Each month, an appropriate proportion of potential controls in each 5-year age group was selected to match the age distribution of women with breast cancer. A control group of 4676 women was available for analysis.

INTERVIEW

Each study participant was interviewed in person according to a pretested standardized questionnaire. The questionnaire focused on reproductive, contraceptive, and family histories of cancer; use of medical services; and personal characteristics and habits.

To asist in recall of the use of OCs and other noncontraceptive hormone therapy, two memory aids were used: a book of photographs of all OC preparations marketed in the United States since 1960, and a calendar on which to record major life events around which contraceptive use might be better remembered.

ANALYSIS

Odds ratios as estimates of the relative risk were calculated according to the method of Mantel and Haenszel,[67] and 95% confidence intervals according to Miettinen's test-bases method.[68] Logistic regression[69] was used to control simultaneously for several variables considered a priority to be potential confounders of the results; variables included in the model were age, menopausal status, age at first term pregnancy, family history of breast cancer, area of residence, and history of benign breast disease before first use of OCs. The results of this logistic regression analysis agreed closely with results from the Mantel-Haenszel procedure[67] to adjust for each of 25 potentially confounding variables individually.

Cases were 4711 women 20 to 54 years of age with newly diagnosed breast cancer selected from eight population-based cancer registries. Controls were 4676 women selected by random-digit dialing in the same population area.

The relative risk of breast cancer among women who had ever used OCs compared with women who had never used them was 1.0. There was no increased risk among long-term users (15 or more years of use) and no increased risk with increase in time since last use. The risk of breast cancer was not significantly different among users of different types of OCs. Analysis was done on women who used either sequential, progestin only, two or more compound, or an unidentified type of OC. Use before first term pregnancy, menopausal status or family history of breast cancer, and history of surgery for benign breast disease did not show increased risk. Those using only mestranol or only EE_2 as the estrogen component showed no increased risk, and there was no significant increased risk by use of any specific progestin contained in combination OC.

No consistent pattern of association between OC use and breast cancer is apparent from the many studies conducted in the past 10 years. Unlike the studies involving ovarian, endometrial, and cervical neoplasia, refinement in study design has not produced consistent findings. These inconsistent findings argue strongly against a significant association between OC use and the risk of breast cancer. Some recent studies continue to raise concern over certain subgroups of women (i.e., nulliparous women and women who began pill use younger than 25). Further studies on these specific populations are necessary.

CERVICAL NEOPLASIA

The epidemiologic factors responsible for the development of cervical dysplasia and subsequent progression to carcinoma in some patients are complex and poorly understood. One of the major epidemiologic factors in carcinoma of the cervix seems to be young age at first intercourse. Others, such as human papilloma virus, multiparity, high frequency of intercourse, multiple partners, and low socioeconomic status, may also relate to early age at the time of first intercourse.[70-72]

Conclusions derived from a number of epidemiologic studies of cervical neoplasia vary considerably. A number of factors contribute to this variability: (1) The histologic interpretation of degrees of dysplasia and carcinoma in situ may vary from one pathologist to another. (2) The most important risk factors (age at first intercourse, frequency of intercourse, and number of sexual partners) are difficult to determine accurately. In spite of the large numbers of both case-control and cohort studies, only one study before 1975 specifically analyzed the issues of age at first intercourse and contraceptive choice.[72] (3) There is a tendency for women using steroidal contraception to avail themselves of medical care more frequently than noncontraceptive users. As a result, certain disease processes may be underreported in populations not using contraceptives. (4) Results are inconsistent in quantitating relative risks. Some reports conclude that there are "remarkable similarities between the test and control group in each age bracket"[73] or "no significant differences in occurrences or duration of use."[74] (5) Some reports concern "prevalence rates," which may include patients with disease at the time they enter the study.[75] (6) There is a confounding influence of sexually transmitted carcinogens.

The carcinogenic effects of human papilloma virus and herpes type II are most important risk factors for this disease.[76, 77] Epidemiologic studies must be designed to detect the incidence of these diseases in their cases and controls. Analysis must also control adequately for these factors. Unfortunately, the authors of the most recent sophisticated case-control studies of OC use and risk of cervical cancer have not been able to accomplish these ends. There are major problems in obtaining an accurate history of specific sexually transmitted diseases. Many patients cannot or will not relate a history of a specific sexually transmitted disease.

Condom and diaphragm use may exert some barrier protective effect against these agents. Comparisons between incidence rates of infection and cervical neoplasia in diaphragm users versus OC users may show a protective effect of diaphragm use rather than an increased rate with OC use.

The 1969 study by Melamed et al.[75] illustrates well some methodologic problems with epidemiologic studies conducted during the 1960s and early 1970s. They surveyed the incidence of cervical carcinoma in situ and a "matched" population of Planned Parenthood patients in New York City.

Five factors were considered in the study design for collection of clinical data: age, ethnic origin, age at first pregnancy, number of children born alive, and net weekly family income. No attempt was made to determine age at first coitus, frequency of coitus, or number of different sexual partners and marital status.

Analysis of the "matched populations" of OC choosers and those who selected the diaphragm revealed significant differences in race, income, and age at first pregnancy. The diaphragm users were predominantly white, of upper-income socioeconomic status, and more likely to have had their first pregnancy after age 20. The OC choosers were predominantly black or Puerto Rican, of lower-income socioeconomic status, and more likely to have had their first pregnancy before the age of 20. Prevalence rates were determined for patients choosing OCs (27,508) and patients selecting the diaphragm (6809). The prevalence rate for carcinoma in situ for OC choosers was 6.6/1000 and 3.8/1000 for diaphragm users. This difference was small but statistically significant.

Assuming that this was not a low-probability statistical variation, three possible explanations were offered: (1) a protective effect of the diaphragm acting as a barrier, (2) a causal effect of steroids acting on the cervicovaginal epithelium, and (3) some unknown factor(s) in the makeup, behavior, or habits of a woman that would alter her probability of development of cervical carcinoma and at the same time impel her to choose a particular contraceptive.

It is important to appreciate that the study by Melamed et al.[75] demonstrated only a tendency of patients with carcinoma in situ to choose OCs more frequently than the diaphragm. No conclusions could be drawn regarding the development of carcinoma in situ in patients using OCs.

Ory et al. in 1977[78] determined the prevalence rates for cervical dysplasia and carcinoma in situ for 15,477 OC users and 6663 IUD users at the Grady Hospital Family Planning Clinic in Atlanta. This study was designed in part to answer the question raised by the study by Melamed et al.,[75] namely, does the prevalence rate of cervical premalignant changes vary according to which contraceptive method is initially accepted by women entering a family-planning program? The IUD and OC acceptors showed similar characteristics: all were black, aged 15 to 44 years, and had lower middle-class incomes. Marital status, age at first pregnancy, and number of pregnancies were similar. For 5164 women with two or more Papanicolaou (Pap) smears choosing the IUD, the crude dysplasia rate was 1.3/100 women. Among 9431 similar OC choosers the dysplasia rate was 2.3/100 women. The calculated risk ratio of 1.5 in this series was considered statistically significant. OC acceptors with Pap smears before initial choice of contraceptive method had a 1.4-fold higher prevalence rate of cervical dysplasia than IUD acceptors. For the same groups of women with two smears the crude prevalence rate of carcinoma in situ was 1.31/100 women for IUD choosers and 0.34/100 women for OC choosers. These differences were not significant.

The group of women studied by Ory et al.[78] was dissimilar to the group of women studied by Melamed et al.[75] The patients in the series of Melamed et al. were older and of higher parity, and fewer were black. Another crucial difference was that Melamed et al.[75] compared only OC and diaphragm users, whereas Ory et al.[78] compared OC and IUD users. Subsequently, Ory[79] conducted a case-control study of 584 women with cervical dysplasia and 148 women with cervical carcinoma in situ, comparing OC versus IUD use. These patients were taken from the same population at Grady Hospital. None of the women with dysplasia and carcinoma in situ had prior abnormal smears, and all had at least two normal smears before entry into the study. Lesions developed over a 2-year period of observation. Diagnoses of abnormal smears were confirmed by cervical biopsies. Controls included 8553 black women matched for age, educational status, marital status, age at first birth, and parity. The control patients had no prior abnormal smears and continued to have normal smears for the 2-year period of the study. Analysis showed a "weak" association between OC use and dysplasia. The relative risk of carcinoma in situ for OC users as compared to nonusers rose linearly from 1.3 (1 to 12 months' use) to 4.7 (> 36 months' use). This trend was statistically significant.

Stern et al.[80] reported a prospective study of 300 women with cervical dysplasia matched with 300 women with normal cervical smears. These patients were obtained from among 6000 women enrolled in a family-planning clinic in Los Angeles. The combined OC chosen for the study contained 100 μg mestranol and 1 mg ethynodiol diacetate. More than 90% of the non-pill users chose an IUD.

The patients with dysplasia and their controls were followed with a Pap smear every 6 months. Total study period for observation was 7 years. In the sample of women with normal smears there was no evidence of a differential effect of the pill. The patients with dysplasia taking OCs showed a significantly increased conversion of dysplasia to carcinoma in situ with extended use (more than 6 years). Analysis was conducted with the life-table method and involved only 32 patients with more than 6 years' use. There was no suggestion of conversion from dysplasia to carcinoma in situ for use less than 6 years.

Other case-control studies before 1977 by Worth and Boyes,[81] Thomas,[82] and Boyce et al.[83] indicated no increased risk of cervical neoplasia associated with OC use.

The early analysis from the cohort studies was reassuring. In their 1976 report Vessey et al.[22] found no cases of cervical dysplasia among 4217 diaphragm users. The incidence of dysplasia among 3162 IUD users and 9653 OC users was similar (0.28 and 0.31/1000 woman-years, respectively). There were but 12 cases recorded, and no valid statistical analysis was possible with so few cases.

The RCGP reported on only "malignant neoplasm of cervix uteri" in 1974.[21] Two cases were observed in OC takers, two cases among "ex-takers," and four cases among the non-OC takers. These numbers were too small for statistical analysis. They have yet to update this report.

The Walnut Creek study[46] involving 17,942 women observed for 37,373 woman-years initially reported a statistically significant association between carcinoma in situ and duration of OC use. This analysis involved only 34 cases of carcinoma in situ and did not include analysis of age at first birth or sexual activity and number of sexual partners. A later analysis of their data in 1977[84] confirmed the significance of these preliminary findings.

In a 1983 update Vessey et al.[85] reported on the incidence of biopsy-proved cervical neoplasia among 6838 parous women taking OCs who had been followed for 10 years in the OFPA study. The control group consisted of 3145 parous women who entered the study while using an IUD.

"Cervical neoplasia" in this study includes biopsy-proved dysplasia, carcinoma in situ, and invasive cancer. All 13 cases of invasive cervical cancer occurred in the OC group ($P < 0.05$). Both carcinoma in situ and dysplasia also had higher overall incidences in the OC group than the IUD groups, although neither difference reached statistical significance.

The aggregated ata for all forms of cervical neoplasia showed a significant association with duration of OC use. The risk for OC users rose from 0.8/1000 woman-years to 2.2/1000 woman-years, whereas the risk among IUD users remained relatively constant at approximately 1/1000 woman-years (Fig. 2).

This study has been criticized in part for the lack of data on age at first intercourse and number of sexual partners. The authors sampled 100 women in the study and obtained detailed sexual histories. The number of women with age at first sexual intercourse of 17 years or less and those having more than one sexual partner were similar among the OC users and IUD wearers. The strengths of this study are its prospective nature, large size, and very low rate of loss to follow-up among its patients. These patients will remain under surveillance, and additional cases should add power to future analysis.

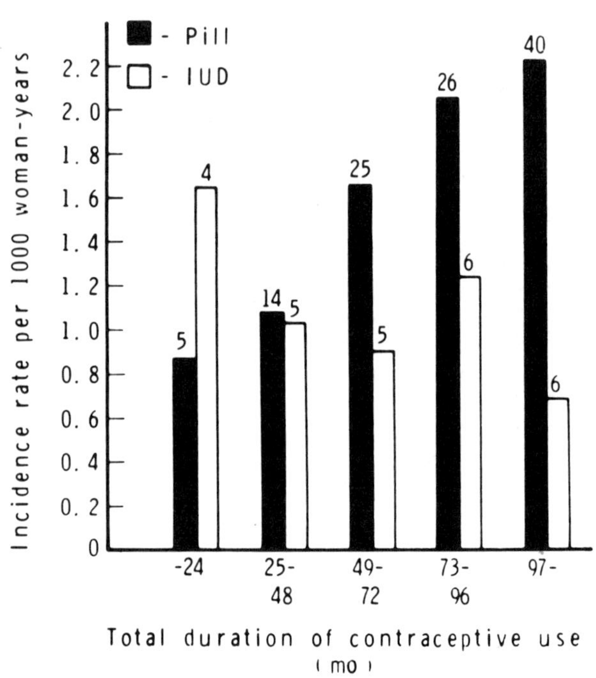

Figure 2
Risk of development of cervical neoplasia among IUD and OC users with respect to total duration of contraceptive use.[85]

Several large studies reported after 1979 have attempted to determine age at first intercourse, age at first birth, number of sexual partners, incidence of sexually transmitted disease, and other factors thought to be important in evaluating the relationship between risk of cervical cancer and OC use.

Harris et al.[86] conducted one of the first case-control studies on the risks of cervical dysplasia and carcinoma in situ in which there was ascertainment of age at first intercourse and number of sexual partners.

Cases were 237 women with abnormal cervical smears matched to 422 controls. Cervical biopsy specimens were taken on each case and were classified as follows: 65 carcinoma in situ, 81 severe dysplasia, 44 mild dysplasia, and 47 normal histology. Significant risk factors were age at first intercourse, multiple sexual partners, and use of OCs.

Statistically significant ($P < 0.05$) linear relationships were seen for length of use of OCs and risk of severe dysplasia and carcinoma in situ. These associations remained significant after adjustment for number of sexual partners.

The NCI undertook a large case-control study in five metropolitan areas in the United States.[87] Incident cases of invasive cervical cancer occurring among women aged 20 to 74 years were accrued over the period 1982 to 1984. Controls for the study were ascertained through random-digit dialing techniques that matched to cases on age, race, and telephone exchange. A total of 479 cases and 789 controls were identified. Interviews elicited detailed information on contraceptive usage as well as demographics, pregnancy history, menstrual history and hygiene practices, sexual behavior, medical events, smoking, diet, and marital and family history.

Analysis found that a number of risk factors were significantly correlated with the probability of exposure to OCs. The most significant confounding variable was interval since last Pap smear. This variable exerted substantial negative confounding, because those with a limited screening history were at extremely low risk for never having used OCs and extremely high risk for invasive cervical cancer (five- to sixfold excess risk for those never having a cervical smear in the 10 years preceding diagnosis). The number of sexual partners, age at first intercourse, and history of a nonspecific genital infection, or sore acted as positive confounders.

After adjustment for pertinent confounding variables, the risk associated with ever-use of OCs was 1.49 (95% confidence interval, 1.1 to 2.1). In addition there was a significant linear increase in risk ($P = 0.003$) with increasing duration of pill use (Table 10).

There was some suggestion that long-term high-potency pill use was associated with a higher risk. There was no evidence that pill associations varied according to number of sexual partners, age at first intercourse, or years of smoking.

Another large multicenter case-control study of cervical cancer and combined OCs is being carried out under the auspices of the World Health Organization (WHO).[88] This study is being carried out by collaborating centers in Australia, Chile, China, Columbia, the German Democratic Republic, Israel, Kenya, Mexico, Nigeria, the Philippines, and Thailand.

Cases were 726 women admitted to a hospital with a histologically-proved diagnosis of invasive carcinoma of the cervix. Controls were 5246 women who were admitted for treatment of nonobstetric or nongynecologic conditions. Matching was done on the basis of age and residence.

Table 10. *Relative Risks[a] of Invasive Cervical Cancer Associated with Varying Parameters of OC Usage[b]*

	Cases	Controls	Relative risk	95% CI[c]
Ever-use				
No	269	386	1.00	—
Yes	210	403	1.49	1.1–2.1
Years of use				
< 5	114	260	1.27	0.9–1.9
5–9	58	83	1.98	1.2–3.2
10+	38	60	1.82	1.1–3.1
Age at first use				
< 20	67	122	1.28	0.8–2.1
20–24	82	167	1.71	1.1–2.7
25–29	36	56	1.92	1.1–3.2
30+	25	58	1.14	0.7–2.0
Years since first use				
< 10	40	86	1.57	0.9–2.8
10–14	75	151	1.41	0.9–2.2
15–19	68	126	1.62	1.1–2.5
20+	27	40	1.35	0.8–2.4
Years since last use				
< 1	47	78	2.00	1.2–3.4
> 1	163	325	1.44	1.0–2.0

[a]Relative risks are adjusted for age, race, number of sexual partners, age at first intercourse, education, interval since last Pap smear, and history of a nonspecific genital infection or sore.

[b]Modified from Brinton et al.[87]

[c]Confidence interval.

To address some of the deficiencies of prior studies the data collection and analysis considered 23 variables of sexual behavior or access to medical care that might have been confounding variables. Included were data on gynecologic and obstetric history, sexual relationships, age at first intercourse, contraceptive history, and prior Pap smears.

The variables most strongly related to risk of cervical cancer or use of OCs were total number of pregnancies, age at first sexual relationship, number of sexual partners, and history of treatment for a vaginal discharge. Vaginal discharge was used as an index of infection by sexually transmitted disease. Among women who had ever used OCs the relationship to invasive cervical cancer showed a relative risk of 1.19 (95% confidence interval, 0.99 to 1.44). When data were analyzed by duration of use the relative risk rose in a linear trend and became significant for those patients who had no history of cervical smears and women analyzed by age and center with more than 60 months' use. The relative risk however, did not reach significance when all six variables were considered (Table 11).

When duration of use was categorized in the same manner as that of Vessey et al.,[85] a similar trend was evident, and a relative risk of 1.63 (95% confidence interval, 1.03 to 2.59) was observed in women who had used OCs for more than 8 years. The patients in this study were taken from populations quite different from that of the British OFPA study[85] or the NCI study[87] in the United States.

The Oxford prospective study[85] analyzed white, married British women. The NCI study[88] analyzed hospitalized women at both rural and urban settings in the United States. The WHO study[88] examined women from diverse geographic, racial, and socioeconomic backgrounds. Because these women came primarily from developing countries, they were drawn from populations with relatively low levels of cervical screening. This approach tends to decrease the risk of selection bias sometimes seen in populations with high levels of cervical screening. These recent reports, like all other epidemiologic studies, suffer from methodologic problems. However, the consistency of their results adds weight to the concern that long-term OC use is associated with an increased risk of cervical neoplasia. Although these results support a direct relationship between extended pill use and an increased risk of cervical dysplasia

Table 11. *Relative Risks of Invasive Cervical Cancer in Users of OCs in Relation to Duration of Use, Adjusted for Various Confounding Variables*

Months of OC use	Age and center	Relative risks (95% confidence[88] intervals)[a]	
		Six variables	No history of smears
None	1.00	1.00	1.00
1–12	1.24	1.00	1.03
13–24	1.08	0.87	1.21
25–60	1.46[a]	1.17	1.24
⩾ 60	1.71[a]	1.37	1.53[a]

[a]Adjusted for age, center, number of pregnancies, age at first sexual relationship, number of sexual partners, and history of vaginal discharge.

and cervical cancer, the mechanisms by which OCs might exert adverse effects on cervical epithelium are unclear.

There is some evidence that cervical tissue has hormone receptor sites[89] and that administration of OCs can result in histologic alterations.[90] There has been some suggestion that OCs may alter progression rates of preinvasive lesions.[91] They may also act as promoters for other risk factors, including herpesvirus or papilloma virus infections.[92] Further studies are necessary to test the biologic possibility of relationships observed in these studies.

BENIGN OVARIAN NEOPLASMS

Several studies have reported a lower incidence of functional ovarian cysts in OC users as opposed to nonusers.[93-95] Ory et al.[2] estimated that the rate of hospitalizations prevented was 35/100,000 pill users. This estimate results in approximately 3000 hospitalizations for treatment of benign ovarian neoplasms prevented in the United States per year.[96]

OVARIAN CANCER

Since 1977 more than nine studies[97-105] have evaluated the risk of ovarian cancer and OC use. All have shown a protective effect of OCs. However, in several of these studies[97-101] the results did not reach statistical significance. As with other studies that first describe new epidemiologic phenomena, the number of subjects was small, and certain confounding factors were not included in the study designs. The smaller studies did not adequately investigate or control for infertility, nulliparity, and small family size, all of which are associated with an increased risk of ovarian cancer.

The Cancer and Steroid Hormone study[105] investigated OC use and the risk of ovarian cancer. Cases were 179 women found to have newly diagnosed ovarian cancer. These were matched for age and residence with 1642 women with intact ovaries.

The study design captured detailed information on contraceptive practices, and 92 other potentially confounding variables. After controlling for age, which was the strongest confounding variable, none of the others appreciably altered the risk estimates.

The age-adjusted relative risk of ovarian cancer among OC users was 0.6 when compared to women who had never used OCs. This protective effect became evident within the first year of use, persisted, and increased through 5 or more years of use (Table 12). This protective effect persists after pill use is stopped, and the magnitude of this effect is virtually unchanged for 10 years after OC use has ceased.

The public health implications of this protective effect are significant. It is estimated that in the United States there were 18,000 new cases and 11,400 attributable deaths from ovarian cancer in 1983. The authors of this study estimate that more than 1700 cases of ovarian cancer are averted each year by past and current OC use among women in the United States.[105]

UTERINE MYOMAS

Estrogens seem to have an association with myomas. Myomas rarely occur before menarche,

Table 12. *Risk of Ovarian Cancer*[a]

Duration of OC use	Relative risk	95% confidence interval
None	1.0	(referent)
Ever	0.6	0.4–0.9
< 3 mo	1.0	0.5–1.9
3–11 mo	0.7	0.4–1.4
1–2 yrs	0.8	0.5–1.4
3–4 yrs	0.5	0.2–1.0
⩾ 5 yrs	0.4	0.2–0.6
Time since last OC use	**Relative risk**	**95% confidence interval**
Never	1.0	(referent)
Ever	0.6	0.4–0.8
> 10 yrs	0.5	0.3–0.9

[a]Modified from the Centers for Disease Control Cancer and Steroid Hormone study.[105]

tend to regress after menopause and may enlarge rapidly during pregnancy or during exogenous estrogen administration.[106] During the early years of OC usage, it was feared that myomas might grow under the stimulation of estrogen contained in the OCs. The presence of myomas has been considered by some to be a relative contraindication for OC use,[1] and many physicians are reluctant to use OCs in patients who have a myoma of any type or size.

At present, there is little objective evidence in the literature to support this concern. The RCGP cohort study[21] found a slightly decreased risk of development of uterine myomas in users as opposed to nonusers. Vessey et al.[22] in their original report found no significant difference in occurrence rates among OC, diaphragm, or IUD users. None of the patients in either of these studies was taking medication containing > 50 μg estrogen.

Ross et al. in 1986[107] updated the analysis of risk factors for uterine fibroids with data from the OFPA study. As of July 1985, 538 women in this cohort study had had pathologically confirmed fibroids. Women with pathologically confirmed fibroids before entrance into the study were excluded. Five hundred thirty-five controls were selected and matched for age, date of entrance into the study, and place of residence. The study found a significant decrease in risk of myomas with increasing number of pregnancies (relative risk, 1.00 with first pregnancy, 0.47 with second pregnancy, and 0.24 with fifth pregnancy). The risk decreased significantly with increasing duration of OC use (relative risk, 0.80 at 2 years and 0.54 at 145 months). The risk of development of myomas was decreased by 31% in women who had used OCs for 10 years. Data from this series were obtained from women who were using pills containing 50 μg EE_2, but with varying amounts of progestogen. There was some suggestion that the higher the dose of progestogen, the more protective the OC. Should these data be confirmed by other studies, the presence of myomas should not be considered a relative contraindication to OC use.

GESTATIONAL TROPHOBLASTIC DISEASE

The potential for persistent trophoblastic proliferation after the initial evacuation of a hydatidiform mole is well documented.[108-110] The successful evaluation and treatment of gestational trophoblastic disease depends on meticulous serial measurement of serum human chorionic gonadotropin (hCG) titers.[111, 112] The failure to note a progressive decline in serum hCG after molar evacuation is generally indicative of trophoblastic malignancy. It may take as long as 100 days for the disappearance of an elevated serum hCG level after the termination of the molar gestation.[113] Pregnancy should be avoided for at least 6 months after negative hCG levels are obtained.[114] A gestation during this follow-up will produce hCG and confound attempts to detect proliferative disease. It is therefore imperative that contraception be used throughout this interval.

The role of OCs as an important method to prevent pregnancy following molar evacuation has been recently reevaluated. Stone et al.[115] investigated the effects of OCs on proliferative trophoblastic sequelae in 611 patients after hydatidiform mole evacuation. After molar evacuation, in 16 of 65 patients (24.6%) who had begun using OCs before normal hCG levels were obtained trophoblastic disease developed requiring cytotoxic chemotherapy. In comparison, among those not using OCs during postmolar follow-up, only 43 of 464 (9.3%) required chemotherapy. This study implied that the administration of OCs to patients before the decline in postmolar hCG levels to normal resulted in a twofold risk of trophoblastic disease requiring chemotherapy. In addition OCs were also found to inhibit the decline in hCG levels even in those not needing chemotherapy. Berkowitz et al.[116] analyzed two groups of patients after molar pregnancy to determine the effects of OCs commenced immediately after molar evacuation on the incidence of trophoblastic disease. Patients were comparable in age, gravidity, tumor histology, pretreatment hCG titers, and exposure to prophylactic chemotherapy. Eleven of 58 (18.9%) using OCs and 6 of 42 (14.3%) using barrier methods developed postmolar trophoblastic disease. These differences were not significantly different, and the authors concluded that OCs do not increase the risk of postmolar trophoblastic disease. They recommended their use during the entire interval of gonadotropin monitoring. They further reported no significant difference in the mean hCG regression time regardless of whether a hormonal or nonhormonal contraceptive was used.

The conflicting conclusions of these two studies prompted further investigation. Yuen and Burch[117] prospectively studied 194 patients with pathologically confirmed molar pregnancies. One hundred seventy-seven patients had β-hCG titers that spontaneously returned to normal. There were no significant differences in the β-hCG-positive interval among those women who used barrier methods, IUDs, or combined OCs. Ninety-three of 97 OC users took compounds with 50 μg or less estrogen. In 17 of the 194 patients invasive complications developed and required therapy. Although the numbers are small there was a significantly greater proportion of women with persistent disease who had used OCs that contained > 50 μg estrogen. However, in determining high versus low estrogen dosage the authors assumed that EE_2 and mestranol were of equivalent potency. There were 21 patients taking OCs containing 50 μg EE_2. Some authors believe that EE_2 may be more potent than mestranol.[118] Had those patients using 50 μg EE_2 been included in the high-estrogen-dose group the results may have been modified to show no added risk for high-estrogen-dose pills.

Morrow et al.[119] studied 149 cases of molar pregnancy from 1977 through 1983. Eighty-four patients seen from 1977 through 1980 received estrogen-progestogen OCs after evacuation. Fifty-five patients seen after 1980 used nonhormonal contraceptives. The groups were similar with respect to age, parity, maternal blood type, and race. Gestational age was significantly shorter and the frequency of cases with a preevacuation β-hCG titer of > 250,000 mIU/ml was significantly higher in the nonhormonal contraception group. There was no significant difference in time of regression for the β-hCG titers between the two groups.

On the basis of the few available studies, use of combination OCs that contain 50 μg or less of EE_2 after evacuation of a hydatidiform mole appears to be safe and effective. Further studies are necessary to elucidate the relationship between high estrogen dose and persistent trophoblastic disease.

OCs AND PITUITARY TUMORS

Recognition of the complex relationship between serum estrogen concentration and potential augmentation of serum prolactin (PRL) release through effects on hypothalamic-pituitary sensors has led to scrutiny of the role that combination OCs might have in altering these neuroendocrine interactions. Estrogen-specific receptors on the lactrotrope with modulation of messenger ribonucleic acid by estradiol in PRL-secreting cells have been studied in vitro.[120] During pregnancy, estrogen is believed to directly stimulate lactotrope PRL production and release. Progressively rising serum PRL levels throughout pregnancy appear to result from lactotrope stimulation by the concomitant gradual elevation of serum estrogen concentrations.[121, 122] Additionally, PRL-secreting pituitary tumors have estrogen receptors, and pregnancy may result in growth of these lesions.[123] It has been speculated that OC-mediated stimulation of pituitary lactotropes by estrogen may cause excessive PRL secretion.[8] Continued uncontrolled estrogenic influence might then lead to hypertrophy and hyperplasia of the lactotrope with possible formation of a pituitary PRL-secreting adenoma.[124]

An awareness of these relationships coupled with a reported rise in the incidence of pituitary adenomas among women of childbearing age has resulted in study of the relationship between the use of combination OCs and pituitary adenomas among various age- and sex-adjusted populations in Olmsted County, Minnesota, during 1935 to 1977. A dramatic increase in the mean annual incidence of these lesions was found in women aged 15 through 44 when data after 1969 were compared with that of prior years. This observation led the authors to conduct a case-control study to determine if OCs were associated with this increased incidence of pituitary adenomas. A decreased relative risk (0.5) was found for pituitary tumors in OC users.[126] The authors concluded that the apparent rise in the incidence of pituitary tumors among women was due to improved diagnostic capabilities, including advances in radiologic technique and endocrinologic assays. This study involved only nine cases. Coulam[126] noted that although several studies had reported a high prevalence of prior OC use by patients with pituitary adenomas (70% to 84%), the frequency of OC use in the general population was frequently unknown.

Sherman et al.[127] carried out a study on the pathogenesis of PRL-secreting pituitary adenomas. Forty-two women with amenorrhea/prolactinemia had histologically verified pituitary adenomas. The authors hypothesized that the estrogen content of OCs presented a greater estrogenic stimulus than the normal menstrual cycle or pregnancy. This relative hyperestrogenic state might stimulate the growth of occult pituitary tumors. Seventy-four percent became symptomatic in the immediate postpartum period, during OC use, or shortly after discontinuation of OCs. Sherman believed that these data suggested that estrogens may facilitate expression of a preexisting lesion. Teperman et al.[128] conducted a case-control study with 20 hyperprolactinemic patients with pituitary adenomas as cases. Controls were 20 patients hospitalized for appendectomy. The incidence of OC use in the 20 cases was 65% (12 patients) and 20% (4 patients among the controls (relative risk, 4.0; $P < 0.025$).

This suggested association between the use of OCs and pituitary adenomas was noted by other small studies before 1980.[129-132] Because of the paucity of data on this important issue, the pituitary adenoma study group was established. They undertook a large multicenter case-control investigation to further analyze the relationship between OCs and PRL-secreting pituitary adenomas.[133] Three case groups consisting of 212 women with adenomas, 119 hyperprolactinemic patients with amenorrhea and/or amenorrhea with normal or equivocal tomograms, and 205 normoprolactinemic women with amenorrhea and/or galactorrhea were matched to neighborhood control subjects. No association was found between OC use and the development of pituitary adenomas within any of the three study groups. The relative risks were 1.33, 1.35, and 0.67, respectively. Further study was recommended to establish whether OCs may promote the growth of a preexisting lesion.

Maheux et al.[134] conducted a case-control study in which 70 patients with histologically proved prolactinomas were matched with three separate control groups: normoprolactinemic women with secondary amenorrhea, infertile women with normal ovulatory cycles, and hospitalized patients without medical or gynecologic problems.[19] The difference in the proportion of OC usage among the four study groups was not statistically significant. The relative risks were 1.1, 1.18, and 1.15, respectively.

Shy et al.[135] conducted a case-control study of 72 women with pituitary prolactinemia matched to 303 neighborhood controls selected by random-digit dialing. A major confounding variable was menstrual pattern. When those patients who were using OCs only for contraception were compared to never-users there was no increased risk of pituitary adenoma (relative risk, 1.3). When patients who were using OCs for menstrual irregularity were compared to never-users, there was a significant increased risk of pituitary adenoma (relative risk, 7.7; confidence interval, 3.7 to 17.0). The data suggest that those patients taking OCs to correct a menstrual disturbance may have had a preexisting, undiagnosed prolactinoma.

On the basis of current available data there appears to be no increased risk of development of a pituitary adenoma in normal patients taking OCs. The question of whether women with menstrual irregularity taking OCs represent a high-risk group for these lesions remains unresolved.

OCs AND ENDOMETRIAL NEOPLASIA

EFFECTS OF ESTROGEN AND PROGESTERONE ON THE ENDOMETRIUM

The endometrium is a hormonally responsive tissue layer whose histologic appearance is directly dependent on intrinsic steroid receptor mediated activity.[136] The interaction of estrogen and progesterone (P) with their individual cytoplasmic protein receptors results in significant endometrial growth effects. Estrogenic influence results in cellular proliferation and further increase in the content of estrogen and P receptors.[137, 138] As estrogen exerts its biologic effects by means of receptors, an increase in the latter facilitates the establishment of an estrogenic responsive mileu. P administration operates in reverse by decreasing levels of estrogen receptors, which results in diminished uterine estrogen response.[138, 139]

Estrogen and P receptors with the same physicochemical characteristics as those found in normal endometrium have been found in endometrial hyperplasia and carcinoma.[140] Some endometrial hyperplasias have been found to have an elevated estrogen and P receptor content.[140, 141] Furthermore, 60% to 90% of hyperplastic tissues contain high P receptor levels.[140, 141] Unopposed estrogenic stimulation is believed responsible for these increased endometrial receptor levels and for the production of hyperplasia.[136] Conversely, P administration in patients with endometrial hyperplasia has been found to decrease hormonal receptor content, with the more pronounced effect on P receptors.[142]

There is convincing evidence that unopposed estrogenic exposure leads to a spectrum of endometrial hyperplastic alterations that can progress to carcinoma.[143] The risk for carcinoma has been found to correlate well with the severity of the endometrial change. Failure to modify these lesions can result in endometrial carcinoma in a significant proportion of patients.[143, 144]

The exposure of the normal estrogen-primed endometrium to P converts the tissue to the typical secretory type seen during luteal phase of the menstrual cycle. This cyclic effect of P prevents the progression of normal proliferative endometrium to hyperplasia.[144, 145] P has also been used therapeutically to convert a spectrum of hyperplastic lesions to normal histology.[144, 145] It is apparent that the delicate balance between circulating estrogen and P levels and their interaction with endometrial cell receptor systems can have profound effects on endometrial growth.

ESTROGEN THERAPY DURING THE MENOPAUSE

Several clinical studies have shown that unopposed estrogen administration increases the risk of endometrial carcinoma in postmenopausal patients.[146-151] Consistent and significantly increased relative risks have been observed (Table 13). Ziel and Finkle[149] in a case-control study reported that conjugated estrogens appear to have an etiologic role in endometrial carcinoma. The risk-ratio estimate increased proportionately with time, reaching 13.9 for 7 or more years' use. The corresponding point estimate of risk ratio was 7.6. McDonald et al.[150] also found that the estimated relative risk of endometrial carcinoma was increased with exposure to conjugated estrogen. The magnitude of the risk was dependent on estrogen dosage as well as duration of use, with the relative risk being increased to 7.9 at 3 years' use and beyond.

Certain objections and criticisms have been raised with respect to these studies: (1) diagnostic surveillance for women taking estrogens may have been increased, so that early lesions would be diagnosed more quickly than lesions in patients not taking estrogens; (2) endometrial hyperplasia may have been misclassified as early endometrial carcinoma, and more advanced stages of endometrial neoplasia have not been studied in adequate numbers; (3) early cases of endometrial carcinoma have inadvertently been treated with estrogens; (4) the history of drug exposure may have been inadequate; and (5) details of estrogen use may not have been sufficient.

Table 13. *Association of Estrogen Use and Adenocarcinoma of the Endometrium: Case-Control Studies*

Author	Year	Relative risk
Smith et al.[148]	1975	7.5
Ziel and Finkle[149]	1975	7.6
Mack et al.[147]	1976	8.0
McDonald et al.[150]	1977	7.9
Antunes et al.[151]	1979	6

In 1978 Antunes et al.[151] conducted a large case-control study of the relationship between estrogen use and endometrial cancer. The study was designed to address the aforementioned criticisms of previous work. Four hundred fifty-one patients with endometrial carcinoma were identified (7% stage 0, 70% stage I, and 23% stages II, III, and IV). These patients were matched with 450 controls.

Pathologic slides were independently reviewed. Information about drug use by type and duration was obtained. There was no difference in time to physician consultation for postmenopausal bleeding between estrogen users and nonusers. No patient in this study with endometrial carcinoma had inadvertently been treated with estrogens.

The overall risk of endometrial carcinoma was sixfold for estrogen users as compared with nonusers. Long-term use of more than 5 years carried with it a 15-fold risk. Despite the failure of case-control, epidemiologic studies to prove a causal relationship, the current evidence seems to suggest that postmenopausal use of estrogens in women with an intact uterus is associated with an increased risk of endometrial carcinoma.

The addition of a progestogen to estrogen replacement regimens has proved helpful in the prevention of most endometrial cancers.[146, 152, 153] Gambrell[146] observed the incidence of endometrial cancer among several groups of postmenopausal women treated with different hormonal replacement schemes from 1975 to 1981: (1) no hormonal replacement, (2) estrogen-only replacement, and (3) estrogen-progestogen replacement. Twenty-eight endometrial cancers were discovered among 5563 women during 20,560 patient-years of observation (Table 14).

Patients using unopposed estrogen had the highest incidence of endometrial adenocarcinoma with a rate of 410/100,000 women per year. Nine women not taking hormones were diagnosed with endometrial carcinoma resulting in a calculated incidence of this disease of 258/100,000 women per year. Estrogen-P users were found to have an annual incidence of 68/100,000 women per year, which was significantly lower than both the unopposed estrogen users as well as the untreated

Table 14. *Incidence of Endometrial Cancer at Wilford Hall USAF Medical Center: 1975–1981*[a]

Therapy group	Patient-years of observation	No. of patients with cancer	Incidence (per 100,000)
Estrogen-progestogen users	11,753	8	68.1
Estrogen users	2434	10	410.8
Estrogen vaginal cream users	1976	1	50.6
Progestogen or androgen users	913	0	—
Untreated women	3484	9	258.3
Total	20,560	28	136.2

[a]Modified from Gambrell.[146]

women. Users of estrogen vaginal cream had a significantly lower rate of endometrial malignancy than did oral estrogen users, but the differences with the other subsets was not of statistical significance. Although these data suggest that progestogen administration in this clinical setting is effective in preventing endometrial cancer, it is unclear whether the subsets were comparable in regard to the various known risk factors for endometrial carcinoma (e.g., obesity, hypertension, early menarche, late menopause, diabetes, and nulliparity).

SEQUENTIAL OCs

Sequential OCs were first marketed in the United States in 1963. Their use was prompted in part by an effort to simulate more closely the natural sequence of estrogen-only followed by estrogen-P found during the normal menstrual cycle. The scheme of administration involved estrogen (80 to 100 μg) along for 14 to 16 days followed by an estrogen-P combination for 5 or 6 days. The progestogen content varied from 2 to 25 μg (1).

Silverberg and Makowski[154] and Lyon[155] in 1975 first reported the occurrence of endometrial carcinoma in young women taking sequential OCs. These reports were quickly followed by others.[156, 157] A "registry" for endometrial carcinoma in young women taking OC agents was established in Denver in 1973. By June 1976 the registry had recorded 30 cases of verified invasive carcinoma of the endometrium occurring in women < 40 years of age who had a documented history of OC use. Twenty patients had documented use of sequential-type preparations; 9 had taken combined formulations, and the type of pill used by 1 patient was unknown. Nineteen of the 20 patients using sequentials had been taking one preparation containing 100 μg of EE_2 as the estrogen and 25 μg of dimethisterone as the progestogen.[158]

Because of the lack of a population-based registry, the previously mentioned authors were unable to establish whether endometrial carcinoma was more common in women using sequential agents than in the general population, or whether the incidence was merely decreased in users of combined agents. Further epidemiologic analysis of this problem in the United States by case-control or cohort studies was not possible. In 1976, the sequential OCs were voluntarily removed from the market by the manufacturers.[159]

COMBINATION OCs

Curently used combination OCs differ from their "sequential" predecessors in administration, composition, and dosage. The addition of a progestogen of higher potency to every pill taken per cycle sufficiently opposes the stimulatory effect of estrogen and prevents hyperplastic growth patterns. Several recent case-control studies found that users of combination OCs have approximately half the risk of development of endometrial carcinoma as compared with women who had never used these preparations.[160-163] This protective effect is evident after 1 year of continuous use.[163] It is unclear whether this protection increases after prolonged use.

Kaufman et al.[161] found the magnitude of protection to be directly proportional to the duration of use of combination OCs with a peak of protection at 3 years and beyond. Similarly, Hulka et al.[162] found that the risk of endometrial carcinoma was reduced further with 5 or more years of combination OC use. However, Weiss and Sayvetz[160] found no relation between duration of use and increased protective effect.

The Center for Disease Control analyzed data from its Cancer and Steroid Hormone study to assess the relationship between use of combination OCs and the risk of endometrial cancer.[163] The study consisted of 187 patients with endometrial cancer obtained through eight population-based cancer registries and 1320 controls randomly selected from the same eight locations. Ever-users of combination OCs had a relative risk of 0.5 of development of endometrial cancer compared with never-users (Table 15). Twelve months of combination OC use was necessary to

Table 15. *Risk of Endometrial Cancer*[a]

Duration of OC use	Relative risk
Never	1.0
< 1 yr	1.1
1–5 yrs	0.4
> 5 yrs	0.6
Time since last OC use	**Relative risk**
Never	1.0
Ever	0.7
≥ 10 yrs	0.8

[a]Modified from Oral Contraceptive Use and the Risk of Endometrial Cancer.[163]

obtain this beneficial effect. The protective effect did not increase after 5 years' continued use. It did persist for 10 or more years after discontinuation of OCs. They estimated that approximately 2000 cases of endometrial cancer are averted each year by past and current use of OCs in the United States. The protective effect of OCs against endometrial cancer has significant public health implications. There remains some disagreement regarding the duration and magnitude of the protective effect after discontinuation of OCs. Several studies have observed a persistent effect for 5 to 10 years,[161-163] whereas others have noted a loss of this protective effect within 3 years.[160, 162]

OCs AND LIVER TUMORS

In 1972 Horvath et al.[164] first suggested a possible association between OCs and ultrastructural findings in the well-differentiated hepatoma. The following year Baum et al.[165] described seven women, all OC users, in whom benign hepatic tumors developed. These lesions were reported as benign hepatic adenomas.

Subsequently, a number of reports indicating an association between OC usage and occurrence of liver tumors have appeared.[166-169] The histopathologic diagnosis has been variously reported as focal nodular hyperplasia, adenoma, hamartoma, benign hepatoma, solitary hyperplastic nodule, and focal cirrhosis.

Reports of these tumors occurring in young women taking OCs immediately engendered grave concern, because before 1970 benign liver tumors in young women were encountered only rarely. Keifer and Scott[168] reviewed the literature and were able to find fewer than 80 cases before 1970.

The Hepatic Branch, Armed Forces Institute of Pathology, and the Family Planning Evaluation Division, Bureau of Epidemiology, Center for Disease Control, in 1977 showed an increasing risk with increased duration of usage[170] (Table 16). Each of 79 living women who had a hepatic adenoma was matched with three neighborhood controls in a case-control study. These groups were similar with regard to age, race, education, marital status, and religion. In addition to duration of use, the study suggests that women 27 years and older who have used high-hormone pills for 7 years are at greatest risk for development of hepatocellular adenoma.

A liver tumor registry was established at the University of California School of Medicine at Irvine in June 1975. Nissen et al.[167] reviewed the literature and the data from the 71 cases at the Irvine Registry in 1977. This report confirmed earlier experience regarding patterns of usage in that 64.2% of these patients had taken mestranol-containing compounds for 71% of the time, and only 17% had taken EE_2-containing compounds for 9.6% of the time. Approximately 85% of the patients had used an OC for more than 4 continuous years. Nissen et al.[167] pointed out that this preponderance of mestranol-containing compounds may have been more apparent than real because the mestranol-containing brands were produced and marketed before the availability of EE_2-containing compounds. Nissen et al.[167] felt that a statistical analysis was not possible and awaited further analysis of larger numbers of patients. Spontaneous rupture of the liver occurred in 18 of these patients, resulting in eight deaths.

In 1977 Keifer and Scott[168] surveyed the available literature and reported 138 cases in United States literature and added their own cases. This report confirmed the predominant usage of mestranol-containing compounds. In discussing the histopathologic diagnosis of these lesions, Keifer and Scott[168] thought that the specific histologic type of tumor might have associated significance.

Table 16. *Increased Risk of Hepatocellular Adenoma in Women with Use of OCs*[a]

Duration of use	Risk ratio
yr	
0–1	1
1–4	9
4–7	120
8	500

[a]Modified from Armed Forces Institute of Pathology, Hepatic Branch and Center for Disease Control, Bureau of Epidemiology, Family Planning Evaluation Division.[170]

They observed that rupture of the liver did not occur in women in whom the pathologic diagnosis was focal nodular hyperplasia. They also noted that most of the patients with ruptured liver had adenomas. Patients taking OCs and having adenomas were at increased risk for rupture as opposed to nonusers: 30 of 69 users as compared with only 6 of 27 nonusers. Nine women with a history of OC use had carcinoma of the liver. There were 11 deaths from hemorrhage. Of these women who died, three had malignancies and eight had benign lesions.

In an attempt to determine more carefully the extent of the problem, the National Cancer Advisory Board requested the American College of Surgeons' Commission on Cancer to conduct a national survey of the extent of primary benign and malignant liver tumors. Four hundred seventy-seven hospitals in the United States searched their tumor registries and reported on all primary benign and malignant liver tumors in male and female patients aged 15 to 45 years from 1970 to 1975.

A total of 543 cases was uncovered, 378 in female and 165 in male patients. These cases were analyzed as to histologic type, age distribution, and contraceptive usage. Analysis of malignant tumors revealed that the frequency increased with age. This finding mirrors the reported distribution in the general population. However, the frequency of the benign lesions showed a large peak in the 26- to 30-year age group. This peak corresponds to increased use of OCs in this age group. This large increase for benign lesions in the 26- to 30-year age group is true only for OC users and only for benign lesions. Vana et al.[171] confirmed the previous reports of the excess occurrence in patients using mestranol-containing compounds (three to one versus those using EE_2-containing compounds). However, Vana et al.[171] found no dose-response relationship and no association with duration of usage. Forty percent of tumors were diagnosed in women exposed for 5 years or less. Hemorrhage was most frequently associated with adenomas and almost exclusively confined to the OC users.

ESTIMATED INCIDENCE OF LIVER TUMORS

Vana et al.[171] estimated the incidence of benign tumors at 4.9/1,000,000. This figure agrees with the estimate of 1/500,000 to 1/1,000,000 by Baum et al.[165] Garcia et al.[172] suggested an incidence at 0.04/1,000,000 women.

These low estimates of occurrence rates were confirmed by Vessey et al.[173] They searched the records of patients enrolled in the RCGP Oral Contraception study (116,000 woman-years' exposure in pill takers) and the OFPA follow-up study of women using different methods of contraception (more than 83,000 woman-years' exposure), and no case of benign or malignant liver tumor was found. In addition, the records of the Oxford Linkage study were searched. This study covers the hospital admissions and deaths in a population of more than 1,000,000. No benign liver tumors were found in women of childbearing age from 1970 through 1975.

One case of benign liver tumor was found in a 23-year-old woman taking OCs for 2 years in a search of the Scottish National Diagnostic Index for the years 1968 through 1974. The system covers hospital admissions and deaths for a population of approximately 5,000,000 people.

CLINICAL ASPECTS

Although benign, these tumors may be life threatening because of their tendency to spontaneous hemorrhage with resultant death. The patient at highest risk for spontaneous hemorrhage seems to be an OC user who has a large mass of the hepatic cell adenoma histologic type and who has taken a high-dose combined pill for more than 4 years.

The lesion can first present itself as an asymptomatic mass, but the majority of patients initially complain of epigastric or right upper-quadrant abdominal pain. Unfortunately, a significant number of these patients also present with signs of intraperitoneal hemorrhage and shock. Timing may be significant in that some of these lesions seem most prone to rupture at or about the time of menstruation.[165, 167-169]

The standard blood liver function tests are of little value in diagnosing these lesions because no consistent abnormalities are found. Computerized tomography, ultrasonography, and liver scan offer the most accurate diagnostic approaches. The need for confirming tissue diagnosis must be weighed against the risk of hemorrhage caused by needle or open biopsy. These lesions are very vascular, and biopsy alone is attendant with significant risk. A number of the reported deaths have occurred secondary to attempts at resection.

There is evidence that these tumors will spontaneously regress after OC use is stopped.[165, 174-176] Pregnancy, with the resultant high levels of sex steroids, may have a particularly stimulating effect and increase the propensity for these lesions to hemorrhage.[177]

For asymptomatic lesions the best and safest course of management would be to discontinue the OCs, urge the patient to avoid pregnancy, and await spontaneous resolution of the lesion.

COMBINATION OCs AND MALIGNANT LIVER TUMORS

Investigation of the possible relationship between OCs and liver cancer has provoked considerable controversy. Synthetic sex steroids are believed to potentiate cholestasis, hypervascularity, microsomal enzyme induction, thrombogenesis, and blood vessel wall thickening, thereby facilitating tumor development.[178] Additionally, steroids can induce hepatic neoplasia in mice[179-181] and in patients receiving anabolic steroids for anaplastic anemia or infertility.[182-185]

The C-17-substituted anabolic steroids, oxymetholone and methyltestosterone, have been specifically implicated in the induction of hepatocellular carcinoma. These compounds closely resemble the C-17-substituted 19-norsteroids used in OCs. Although a direct oncogenic effect remains unproven, these C-17 alkylated steroids are known to promote proliferation of smooth endoplasmic reticulum and production of microsomal hydroxylating enzymes.[186]

Helling et al.[187] reported two cases of hepatocellular carcinoma and reviewed the evidence regarding the association of OCs. They noted the following factors that suggested relationship: (1) women in whom hepatocellular cancer develops tend to be of childbearing age, (2) OCs have been implicated in the induction of benign hepatic tumors, and (3) steroids similar to oxymetholone and methyltestosterone are known to produce malignant liver tumors in men.

In a 1983 review of the literature Gala and Griffin[188] found the average patient age of the 25 cases of hepatocellular carcinoma to be 31 years with a range from 19 to 44. They noted with concern this young age peak and suggest that it may be indicative of a predisposing extrinsic etiologic agent, such as OCs.

Henderson et al.[189] subsequently reported 11 additional cases of malignant liver tumors in young women and found a statistically significant association with OC use. These patients were identified by searching the Los Angeles County Population Based Cancer Registry for all new cases of liver cancer in U.S.-born women aged 18 to 39 years from 1975 to 1980. Two neighborhood controls were selected for each case. Ten of the 11 patients had taken OCs for varying periods of 6 to 168 months. One patient had been given "hormone" shots of undetermined type for menstrual regulation for 9 months before diagnosis. Six of the 11 patients were taking "hormones" at the time of diagnosis. The 11 cases had an average duration of use of 64.7 months versus 27.1 in the control group. This difference was of statistical significance ($P < 0.005$[190]). The authors interpret their data to suggest strongly that long-term OC use may cause malignant liver tumors.

In 1986 Neuberger et al.[191] reviewed a series of 26 women younger than 50 years of age diagnosed with hepatocellular carcinoma in a noncirrhotic liver to determine if OCs had an etiologic role. Eighteen of the 26 patients had used OCs for a median of 8 years. The control group consisted of 1300 women whose history of OC usage was known. The investigators found that although short-term pill usage was not associated with an increased risk of tumor development, there was a 4.4-fold increased risk ($P < 0.01$) for 8 or more years' use. It was concluded that although the overall risk for development of a hepatocellular cancer appeared to be very low, the association should be recognized, particularly in long-term users of OCs. Similarly, Forman et al.[192] carried out a case-control study to investigate this issue. They looked specifically at women aged 20 to 44 who had died of liver cancer between 1979 and 1982. Age-matched controls consisted of women who had died of other causes, unrelated to OC use during the same time period. General practitioners' notes were the source of information regarding use of OCs by both cases and controls. Information was available for 30 patients with histologically verified liver cancer (19 hepatocellular carcinomas and 11 cholangiocarcinomas) and for 147 controls. Analysis of the data showed that ever-use of OCs was associated with a relative risk of 3.8 for hepatocellular carcinoma. The relative risk rose to 20.1 (95% confidence interval, 2.3 to 175.7) after 8 or more years' use. OC use did not appear to significantly increase the risk of cholangiocarcinomas. The authors recognized various methodologic problems with their study. However, they suggest that although liver cancer in young women is an extremely rare disease in most areas of the world, their findings imply that a substantial proportion of the few cases occurring within noncirrhotic livers is related to OC use. The validity of these conclusions has been challenged by some who have underlined problems with interpretation of the data, the limited numbers of patients, study design, and data collection between 1978 and 1983.[193]

Limited data available at present suggest an association between OC use and hepatocellular cancer. The incidence of these tumors is extremely rare. Although there have been anecdotal reports of benign adenomas progressing to malignancy,[194-197] a cause-effect relationship has not been established. Further studies are necessary to clarify the risk that OC use may pose for the development of hepatocellular malignancy.

SUMMARY

Combined OCs have been used by millions of women in the United States for more than 25 years. During this time, the steroid content of these pills has been markedly reduced from the high initial levels. All of the new formulations introduced in the past 15 years contain 50 μg or less of EE_2. The progestogen components are 1 mg or less of norethindrone, 1 mg ethynodiol diacetate, and 0.075 mg or less of levonorgestrel. Investigations in the past 6 years have contributed significant new knowledge to our understanding of the relationships between OCs and neoplasia.

The pool of ever-users of OCs continues to grow substantially. The lag-time from first use is now well into and beyond the range accepted as necessary to promote carcinogenesis. The numbers of long-term users of OCs continue to grow. The investigative studies are much better able to define critical and confounding data items. The analyses of these data have become much more sophisticated and refined. In the United States, because of the suspected association with neoplasia in animals, the 17-hydroxyprogesterones are not in use. Reports of an association between sequential OCs and endometrial carcinoma have contributed to withdrawal of the sequential formulations from the United States market.

The problems in investigating neoplasia and OCs include the following: (1) absence of a suitable animal model, (2) long lag-time from exposure to development of disease, (3) low incidence of specific neoplastic diseases, and (4) multiple etiologic factors in the study population.

The principal investigative methods in the human being are various epidemiologic approaches. The methodologies most frequently used are (1) case reports (tumor registries), (2) disease rates and trends, (3) case-comparison (retrospective) studies, and (4) cohort (prospective) studies. These methods cannot prove a causal relationship between exposure to a possible carcinogen and the occurrence of disease. Care must be taken not to extrapolate epidemiologic conclusions to dissimilar populations. Consistent evidence (positive or negative) confirmed by multiple epidemiologic approaches, can be used to guide physicians and regulatory agencies in formulating policy for the clinical use of OCs.

BREAST DISEASE

The high-dose (> 1 mg) progestogen combined OCs have been shown to have a protective effect on the development of benign breast disease. This protective effect does not appear until 2 years' use and is directly related to the dose of progestogen. The new < 1 mg progestogen pills have not been shown to convey this protective effect.

There may be at least two types of benign breast disease, one of which is premalignant and the other not. The OCs appear to protect only against those benign lesions that are not premalignant.

Current epidemiologic data show no consistent association (either adverse or beneficial) between OC use and the development of carcinoma of the breast in women.

Concerns regarding certain subpopulations (i.e., < age 25 and nulliparous women) persist. Further studies are needed on these specific groups of women.

LIVER TUMORS

Long-term combined OC use appears to be related to the development of benign liver neoplasia. The risk increases with the dose of the steroid and the age of the user. These lesions are quite rare (1 to 5/1,000,000 women). They may be life threatening because of potential spontaneous rupture and hemorrhage. The potential for rupture appears to be related to the histologic type of adenoma rather than focal nodular hyperplasia.

Standard blood liver function tests are of little value for screening diagnostic purposes. Physical examination, ultrasound, computerized tomography, and liver scan are the most useful techniques for diagnosis. Biopsy and resection are attendant with significant risk of hemorrhage. There is some evidence that these lesions will spontaneously regress after discontinuation of the OC. Pregnancy and resumption of use may exacerbate these lesions.

Current data regarding the relationship between OC use and hepatocellular carcinoma are sparse. Several recent reports have shown an increased risk for this very rare tumor and long-term OC use. Additional studies are needed before any valid conclusion can be drawn regarding this relationship.

ENDOMETRIAL HYPERPLASIA

Long-term postmenopausal use of unopposed estrogen significantly increases the risk of development of endometrial hyperplasia and adenocarcinoma of the endometrium. Sequential OCs (14 to 16 days of high-dose, unopposed estrogen followed by estrogen-progestogen for 5 to 6 days) were withdrawn from use in the United States in 1976. This action was in response to a few case reports of endometrial hyperplasia and adenocarcinoma occurring in young women taking these formulations. Recent studies report a significant protective effect on the development of adenocarcinoma of the endometrium by the use of combined OCs. This protective effect becomes evident after 1 year of OC use, and its magnitude reaches 50%. Approximately 2000 cases of endometrial carcinoma are prevented each year among United States women by long-term OC use. This protective effect seems to persist for some years after pill use has been stopped.

LEIOMYOMAS

Estrogens appear to be related to the growth of preexisting uterine leiomyomas. Data on effects of low-dose OCs are sparse. The available studies suggest that there appears to be no increased risk of stimulating the growth of leiomyomas. The most recent study suggests a protective effect. If these data are confirmed, leiomyomata should not be considered a contraindication to use of low-dose OCs.

CERVIX

The most important risk factor for cervical neoplasia appears to be infection with the human papilloma virus. To date there are no large epidemiologic studies that have been able to accurately determine the incidence of this specific disease entity in either case or control populations.

Several large studies conducted since 1979 have captured information on the other major risk factors (age at first intercourse and number of sexual partners). The results of most recent studies appear to be in substantial agreement. They report an increased risk of cervical neoplasia that is directly proportional to the length of OC use. These studies, like all other epidemiologic studies, suffer from some methodologic problems. However, the consistency of their results adds weight to the concern that long-term OC use is associated with an increased risk of cervical neoplasia. Although these results are supportive of a direct relationship between extended pill use and an increased risk of cervical cancer, the mechanisms by which OCs might exert adverse effects on cervical epithelium are unclear.

Further studies are necessary to test the biologic plausibility of the relationships observed in these studies.

GESTATIONAL TROPHOBLASTIC DISEASE

The low-dose (< 50 μg) estrogen combined OCs are appropriate for contraception in the immediate post-molar evacuation period. They do not prolong the time required for the hCG titers to return to normal nor do they increase the rate of conversion to malignant trophoblastic disease.

OVARY

OC use prevents the development of functional ovarian cysts. Approximately 3000 hospitalizations for treatment of benign ovarian neoplasms are prevented in the United States each year. There is a similar protective effect of OCs on the development of malignant ovarian neoplasms. More than 1700 cases of ovarian cancer are averted each year by past and current OC use among women in the United States.

Acknowledgments. We wish to extend our gratitude to Pat Stasuk, Angela Mikles, Victoria Wisniewski, and Janice Scott for their preparation of the manuscript.

REFERENCES

1. Hatcher RA, Guest F, Stewart F, Stewart GK, Trussell J, Cerel S, Cates W: Contraceptive Technology. New York, Irvington Publishers, 1986, p 139
2. Ory HW, Forrest J, Lincoln R: Making Choices Evaluating the Health Risks and Benefits of Birth Control Methods. New York, Alan Guttmacher Institute, 1983, p 11
3. Finkel MJ, Berliner VR: The extrapolation of experimental findings (animal to man): the dilemma of the systemically administered contraceptives. Bull Soc Pharmacol Environ Pathol 4:13, 1973
4. Tietze C, Bongaarts J, Schearen B: Mortality associated with the control of fertility. Fam Plann Perspect 8:6, 1976
5. Population Reports: U.S. morbidity and mortality trends relative to oral contraceptive use 1955-1975. Washington DC, George Washington University Medical Center. Series A4 (Suppl), 1977, p A1
6. Huggins GR, Giuntoli RL: Oral contraceptives and neoplasia. Fertil Steril 32:1, 1979
7. Hueper WC: Environmental cancer. In The Physiopathology of Cancer. Second edition. Edited by F Homburger. New York, 1959, p 919
8. Population Reports: Debate on oral contraceptives and neoplasia continues; answers remain elusive. Washington D.C., George Washington University Medical Center, Series A4, 1977, p 78
9. Population Reports: Oral contraceptives: update on usage, safety, and side effects. Baltimore, Population Information Program, Johns Hopkins University, 1979, p 133
10. Herbst AL, Ulfelder H, Poskanzer DC: Adenocarcinoma of the vagina: association of maternal stilbestrol therapy with tumor appearance in young women. N Engl J Med 284:878, 1971
11. Baum JK, Holtz F, Bookstein JJ, Klein EW: Possible association between benign hepatomas and oral contraceptives. Lancet 2:926, 1973
12. Waterhouse J, Muir C, Correa P, Powell J (editors): Cancer Incidence in Five Continents, Vol 3. Lyon, France, International Agency for Research on Cancer (IARC Scientific Publication No. 15), 1976, p 586
13. Seidman H, Sibberberg E, Holley A: Cancer statistics 1976; a comparison of white and black populations. CA 26:9, 1976
14. Doll R, Vessey MP: Evaluation of rare adverse effects of systemic contraceptives. Br Med Bull 26:33, 1970
15. Dorn HF: Some problems arising in prospective and retrospective studies of the etiology of disease. N Engl J Med 261:571, 1959
16. Hardy RJ, White C: Matching in retrospective studies. Am J Epidemiol 93.75, 1971
17. MacMahon B, Pugh TF: Epidemiology: Principles and Methods. Boston, Little, Brown & Co., 1970, p 376
18. Sartwell PE: Retrospective studies: a review for the clinician. Ann Intern Med 81:381, 1974
19. Schlesselman JJ: Sample size requirements in cohort and case-control studies of disease. Am J Epidemiol 99:381, 1974
20. Seigel D, Corfman P: Epidemiological problems associated with studies of the safety of oral contraceptives. JAMA 203:148, 1968
21. Royal College of General Practitioners: Oral Contraceptives and Health. New York, Pitman Publishing, 1974
22. Vessey MP, Doll R, Peto R, Johnson B, Wiggins P: A long-term follow-up study of women using different methods of contraception: an interim report. J Biosoc Sci 8:375, 1976
23. World Health Organization Technical Report Series: Steroid Contraception and the Risk of Neoplasia. No. 619, 1978
24. Leis HP: Epidemiology of breast cancer: identification of the high-risk woman. In The Breast, Edited by HS Gallagher, HP Leis, RK Snyderman, JA Urban. St. Louis, CV Mosby, 1978, p 38
25. Holleb AL, Freeman HP, Farrow JH: Cancer of the male breast. NY State J Med 68:544, 1968
26. Symmers WE, St. C: Carcinoma of breast in trans-sexual individuals after surgical and hormonal interference with the primary and secondary sex characteristics. Br J Med 2:83, 1968
27. Ross RK, Paganini-Hill A, Gerkins VR, Mack TM: A case-control study of menopausal estrogen therapy and breast cancer. JAMA 243:1635, 1980
28. Brinton LA, Hoover RN, Fraumeni JF: Menopausal estrogen use and risk of breast cancer. Cancer 47:2517, 1981
29. Hoover R, Glass A, Finkle WD: Conjugated estrogens and breast cancer risk in women. JNCI 67:815, 1981
30. Kelsey JL, Fischer DB, Holford TR, LiVolsi VA, Mostow ED, Goldenberg IS, White C: Exogenous estrogens and other factors in the epidemiology of breast cancer. JNCI 67:321, 1981
31. Hulka BS, Chambless LE, Deubner DC, Wilkinson WE: Breast cancer and estrogen replacement therapy. Am J Obstet Gynecol 143:638, 1982
32. Hiatt A, Bawol R, Friedman GD, Hoover R: Exogenous estrogen and breast cancer after bilateral oophorectomy. Cancer 54:139, 1984
33. Kaufman DW, Miller DR, Rosenberg L, Helmrich SP: Noncontraceptive estrogen use and the risk of breast cancer. JAMA 252:63, 1984
34. Petrakis NL: Genetic factors in the etiology of breast cancer. Cancer 39:2709, 1977
35. Stadel BY, Schlesselman JJ: Oral contraceptive use and the risk of breast cancer in women with a "prior" history of benign breast disease. Am J Epidemiol 123:373, 1986
36. Gullino PM: Natural history of breast cancer progression from hyperplasia to neoplasia as predicted by angiogenesis. Cancer 39:2697, 1977
37. Spratt JS Jr, Spratt TL: Rates of growth of pulmonary metastases and host survival. Ann Surg 159:161, 1964
38. Collins VP, Loeffler RK, Tivey H: Observations on growth rates of human tumors. Am J Roentgenol Radium Ther Nucl Med 76:988, 1956
39. Silvestrimi R, Sanfilippo O, Tedesco G: Kinetics of human mammary carcinomas and their correlation with the cancer and the host characteristics. Cancer 34:1252, 1974
40. Kodlin D, Winger EE, Morgenstern NL, Chen V: Chronic mastopathy and breast cancer. Cancer 39:2603, 1977
41. McDivitt RW, Hutter RV, Foote FW, Steward FW: In situ lobular carcinoma, a prospective follow-up study indicating cumulative patient risks. JAMA 201:96, 1967

42. Black MM, Chabon AB: In situ carcinoma of the breast. Pathol Annu 4:185, 1969
43. Cole PT: Oral contraceptives and breast neoplasia. Cancer 39:1906, 1977
44. Consensus Conference: Is fibrocystic disease of the breast precancerous? Arch Pathol Lab Med 110:171, 1986
45. Ory H, Cole P, MacMahon B, Hoover R: Oral contraceptives and reduced risk of benign breast disease. J Engl J Med 294:419, 1976
46. Ramcharan S: The Walnut Creek Contraceptive Drug Study, A Prospective Study of the Side-Effects of Oral Contraceptives, Vol 1, DHEW Publication No (NIH). Washington DC, United States Government Printing Office, 1974
47. Fasal E, Paffenbarger RS Jr: Oral contraceptives as related to cancer and benign lesions of the breast. JNCI 55:767, 1975
48. Sartwell PE, Arthes FG, Tonascia JA: Epidemiology of benign breast lesions: lack of association with oral contraceptive use. N Engl J Med 288:551, 1973
49. Brinton LA, Vessey MP, Flavel R, Yeates D: Risk factors for benign breast disease. Am J Epidemiol 113:203, 1981
50. Livosli VA, Stadel BV, Kelsey JL, Holford TR, White C: Fibrocystic breast disease in oral contraceptive users: a histopathological evaluation of epithelial atypia. N Engl J Med 299:381, 1978
51. Berkowitz GS, Kelsey JL, Livosli VA: Oral contraceptive use and fibrocystic breast disease among pre- and post menopausal women. Am J Epidemiol 120:87, 1984
52. Arthes FG, Sartwell PE, Lewison EF: The pill, estrogens and the breast: epidemiologic aspects. Cancer 28:1391, 1971
53. Boston Collaborative Drug Surveillance Program: Oral contraceptives and venous thromboembolic disease, surgically confirmed gallbladder and breast tumors. Lancet 1:1400, 1973
54. Kelsey JL, Holford TR, White C, Mayer ES, Kitty SE, Acheson RM: Oral contraceptives and breast disease: an epidemiological study. Am J Epidemiol 107:236, 1978
55. Vessey MP, Doll R, Sutton PM: Oral contraceptives and breast neoplasia: a retrospective study. Br Med J 3:719, 1972
56. Clavel F, Benhamou XX, Sitruk-Ware R: Breast cancer and oral contraceptives: a review. Contraception 32:553, 1985
57. Clavel F, Le M, Laplonche A: Étude de la liaison entre le cancer du sein et la puise de medicaments hypotenseurs et: Contraceptifs oraux: resultats d'une etude costemoins. Bull Cancer 68:449, 1981
58. Pike MC, Henderson BE, Krailo MD, Duke A, Roy S: Breast cancer in young women and use of oral contraceptives: possible modifying effect of formulation and age at use. Lancet 2:926, 1983
59. Janerich DT, Polednak AP, Glebatis DM, Lawrence CE: Breast cancer and oral contraceptive use: a case control study. J Chron Dis 36:639, 1983
60. Paffenbarger RS, Kampert JB, Chang H: Characteristics that predict risk of breast cancer before and after menopause. Am J Epidemiol 112:258, 1980
61. Harris NV, Weiss AN, Francis AM, Polissor L: Breast cancer in relation to patterns of oral contraceptive use. Am J Epidemiol 116:643, 1982
62. Pike MC, Henderson BE, Casagronde JT, Rosario I, Gray GE: Oral contraceptive use and early abortion at risk factors for breast cancer in young women. Br J Cancer 43:72, 1981
63. McPherson K, Neila XX, Vessey MP, Doll R: Oral contraceptives and breast cancer. Lancet 2:1414, 1983
64. Paul C, Skagg DCG, Spears GFS, Kaldor JM: Oral contraceptives and breast cancer: a national study. Br Med J 293:723, 1986
65. The Cancer and Steroid Hormone Study of the Centers for Disease Control and the National Institute of Child Health and Human Development: Oral-contraceptive use and the risk of breast cancer. N Engl J Med 315:405, 1986
66. Waksberg J: Sampling methods for random digit dialing. J Am Stat Assoc 73:40, 1978
67. Mantel N, Haenszel W: Statistical aspects of the analysis of data from retrospective studies of disease. JNCI 22:719, 1959
68. Miettinen OS: Estimability and estimation in case-referent studies. Am J Epidemiol 103:226, 1976
69. Schlesselman JJ: Case-Control Studies: Design, Conduct, Analysis. New York, Oxford University Press, 1982, p 227
70. Martin CE: Marital and coital factors in cervical cancer. Am J Public Health 57:803, 1967
71. Rotkin ID: A comparison review of key epidemiological studies in cervical cancer related to current searches for transmissible agents. Cancer Res 33:1353, 1973
72. Merritt CG, Rosenberg SH, Edington E, Losciuto LA: Age at first coitus and choice of contraceptive method: preliminary report on a study of factors related to cervical neoplasia. Soc Biol 22:255, 1975
73. Miller DF: The impact of hormonal contraceptive therapy on a community and effects on cytopathology of the cervix. Am J Obstet Gynecol 115:978, 1973
74. Worth AJ, Boyes DA: A case control study into the possible effects of birth control pills on pre-clinical carcinoma of the cervix. J Obstet Gynaecol Br Commonw 79:673, 1972
75. Melamed MR, Koss LG, Flehinger BJ, Kelisky RP, Dubrow H: Prevalence rates of uterine cervical carcinoma in situ for women using the diaphragm or contraceptive oral steroids. Br Med J 3:195, 1969
76. Meek ES: Herpes virus hominis and cervical carcinoma. In Gynecology and Obstetrics, Edited by JJ Sciarra, HS Buchbaum. Philadelphia, Harper & Row, 1985, p 1
77. Smotkin D, Berek JS, YAOS, Hacker NF: Human papilloma virus deoxyribonucleic acid in adenocarcinoma and adenosquamous carcinoma of the cervix. Obstet Gynecol 68:241, 1986
78. Ory H, Naib Z, Conger SB, Hatcher RA, Tyler CW: Contraceptive choice and prevalence of cervical dysplasia and carcinoma in situ. Am J Obstet Gynecol 124:573, 1976
79. Ory HW, Conger SB, Naib Z, Tyler CW, Hatcher RA: Preliminary analysis of oral contraceptive use and risk of developing premalignant lesions of the uterine cervix. In Pharmacology of Steroid Drugs, Edited by S Garrantini, HW Berendes. New York, Raven Press, 1977, p 211
80. Stern E, Forsythe AB, Coffelt CF: Steroid contraceptive use and cervical dysplasia: increased risk of progression. Science 196:1460, 1977

81. Worth AJ, Boyes DA: A case control study into the possible effects of birth control pills on pre-clinical carcinoma of the cervix. J Obstet Gynaecol Br Commonw 79:673, 1972
82. Thomas DB: Relationship of oral contraceptives to cervical carcinogenesis. Obstet Gynecol 40:508, 1972
83. Boyce JG, Lu T, Nelson JH, Fruchter RG: Oral contraceptives and cervical carcinoma. Am J Obstet Gynecol 128:761, 1977
84. Peritz E, Ramcharan S, Frank S, Brown WL, Huang S, Ray R: The incidence of cervical cancer and duration of oral contraceptive use. Am J Epidemiol 106:462, 1977
85. Vessey MP, Lawless M, McPherson K, Yeates D: Neoplasia of the cervix uteri and contraception: a possible adverse effect of the pill. Lancet 2:930, 1983
86. Harris RWL, Brinton LA, Cowdell DC, Skegg CG: Characteristics of women with dysplasia or carcinoma in situ of the cervix uteri. Br J Cancer 42:359, 1980
87. Brinton LA, Huggins GR, Lehman HF, Mallin K, Savitz D: Long term use of oral contraceptives and risk of invasive cervical cancer. Int J Cancer 38:339, 1986
88. WHO Collaborative Study of Neoplasia and Steroid Contraceptives: Invasive cervical cancer and combined oral contraceptives. Br Med J 290:961, 1985
89. Ford LC, Berek JS, Lagasse LD, Hacker NF, Heins YL, DeLane RJ: Estrogen progesterone receptor sites in malignancies of the uterine cervix, vagina, and vulva. Gynecol Oncol 15:27, 1983
90. Gall SA, Bourgeois CH, Maguire R: The morphologic effects of oral contraceptive agents on the cervix. JAMA 207:2243, 1969
91. Stern E, Forsythe AB, Youkeles L, Coffeit CG: Steroid contraceptive use and cervical dysplasia: increased risk of progression. Science 196:1460, 1977
92. Zur Hausen H: Human genital cancer: synergism between two virus infections or synergism between a virus infection and initiating events? Lancet 2:1370, 1982
93. Ory H: Functional ovarian cysts and oral contraceptives: negative association confirmed surgically: a cooperative study. JAMA 228:68, 1974
94. Ylukorkaia O: Ovarian cysts and hormonal contraception. Lancet 2:1101, 1977
95. Lingeman CH: Etiology of cancer of the human ovary: a review. JNCI 53:1603, 1974
96. Ory HW: The non contraceptive health benefits from oral contraceptive use. Fam Plann Perspect 14:182, 1982
97. Newhouse ML, Pearson RM, Fullerton JM: A case control study of carcinoma in the ovary. Br J Prev Soc Med 31:148, 1977
98. Cassagrande JT, Pike MC, Ross RK: Incessant ovulation and ovarian cancer. Lancet 2:170, 1979
99. McGowan L, Parent L, Lednar W: The woman at risk for developing ovarian cancer. Gynecol Oncol 17:325, 1970
100. Annegers JF, Strom H, Decker DG: Ovarian cancer: incidence and case control study. Cancer 43:723, 1979
101. Hildreth NG, Kelsey JF, LiVolsi VA: An epidemiologic study of epithelial carcinoma of the ovary. Am J Epidemiol 114:398, 1981
102. Weiss NS, Lyon JL, Liff JM: Incidence of ovarian cancer in relation to the use of oral contraceptives. Int J Cancer 28:669, 1981
103. Rosenberg L, Shapiro S, Slone D: Epithelial ovarian cancer and combination oral contraceptives. JAMA 247: 3210, 1982
104. Willett WC, Bain C, Heneckens CH: Oral contraceptives and risk of ovarian cancer. Cancer 48:1684, 1981
105. The Centers for Disease Control Cancer and Steroid Hormone Study: Oral contraceptive use and the risk of ovarian cancer. JAMA 249:1596, 1983
106. Jones HW, Jones GS (editors): Myoma of the uterus. In Novak's Textbook of Gynecology. Tenth edition. Baltimore, Williams & Wilkins, 1981, p 427
107. Ross RK, Pike MC, Vessey MP, Bull D: Risk factors for uterine fibroids, reduced risk associated with oral contraceptives. Br Med J 293:359, 1983
108. Delfs E: Quantitative chorionic gonadotropin: prognostic value in hydatidiform mole and chorioepithelioma. Obstet Gynecol 9:1, 1957
109. Brewer JI, Rinehart JJ, Dunbar R: Choriocarcinoma. Am J Obstet Gynecol 81:574, 1961
110. Hertz R, Lewis J Jr, Lipsett MB: Five years' experience with chemotherapy of metastatic choriocarcinoma and related trophoblastic tumors in women. Am J Obstet Gynecol 82:631, 1961
111. Braunstein GD, Grodin JM, Vaitukaitis JL: Secretory rates of human chorionic gonadotropin by normal trophoblast. AM J Obstet Gynecol 115:447, 1973
112. Bagshawe KD: Trophoblastic disease. In Advances in Obstetrics and Gynecology, Vol 3, Edited by RM Caplan, WJ Sweeney. Baltimore, Williams & Wilkins, 1978, p 225
113. Franke HR, Risse EKJ, Kenemans P, Houx PCW, Stolk JG, Vooijs GP: Plasma human chorionic gonadotropin disappearance in hydatidiform mole: a central registry report from The Netherlands. Obstet Gynecol 62:467, 1983
114. Goldstein DP, Berkowitz RS: Gestational trophoblastic neoplasms. Vol 14. Major Problems in Obstetrics and Gynecology. Philadelphia, WB Saunders, 1982, p 170
115. Stone M, Dent J, Kardana A, Bagshawe KD: Relationship of oral contraception to development of trophoblastic tumour after evacuation of a hydatidiform mole. Br J Obstet Gynaecol 83:913, 1976
116. Berkowitz RS, Goldstein DP, Marean AR, Bernstein M: Oral contraceptives and postmolar trophoblastic disease. Obstet Gynecol 58:474, 1981
117. Yuen BHO, Burch P: Relationship of oral contraceptives and the intrauterine contraceptive devices to the regression of concentrations of the beta subunit of human chorionic gonadotropin and invasive complications after molar pregnancy. Am J Obstet Gynecol 145:214, 1983
118. Mishell DR: Oral steroids. In Reproductive Endocrinology, Infertility and Contraception, Edited by DR Mishell, V Davajan. Philadelphia, FA Davis, 1979, p 487
119. Morrow P, Nakamura R, Schlaerth J, Gaddis O Jr, Eddy G: The influence of oral contraceptives on the postmolar human chorionic gonadotropin regression curve. Am J Obstet Gynecol 151:906, 1985
120. Maurer RA: Estradiol regulates the transcription of the prolactin gene. J Biol Chem 157:2133, 1982
121. Zacur HA, Foster GV, Tyson JE: Multifactorial regulation of prolactin secretion. Lancet 1:410, 1976

122. Archer DF: Current concepts of prolactin physiology in normal and abnormal conditions. Fertil Steril 28:125, 1977
123. Gemzell C, Wang CF: Outcome of pregnancy in women with pituitary adenoma. Fertil Steril 31:363, 1979
124. Tyson JE, Andreasson B, Huth J, Smith B, Zacur H: Neuroendocrine dysfunction with psychogenic implications in postpill galactorrhea-amenorrhea. Obstet Gynecol 46:1, 1975
125. Annegers JF, Coulam CB, Abboud CF, Laws ER Jr, Kurland LT: Pituitary adenoma in Olmsted County, Minnesota, 1935-1977. Mayo Clin Proc 53:641, 1978
126. Coulam CB, Annegers JF, Abboud CF, Laws ER Jr, Kurland LT: Pituitary adenoma and oral contraceptives: a case-control study. Fertil Steril 31:25, 1979
127. Sherman BM, Harris CE, Schlechte J, Duello TM, Halmi NS, VanGilder J, Chapler FK, Granner DK: Pathogenesis of prolactin-secreting pituitary adenomas. Lancet 2:1019, 1978
128. Teperman L, Futterweit W, Zappulla R, Malis LI: Contraceptive history as a risk indicator in patients with pituitary tumors with hyperprolactinemia: a case comparison study of twenty patients. Neurosurgery 7:571, 1980
129. Davajan V, Kletzky O, March CM, Roy S, Mishell DR Jr: The significance of galactorrhea in patients with normal menses, oligomenorrhea, and secondary amenorrhea. Am J Obstet Gynecol 130:894, 1977
130. Chang RJ, Keye WR Jr, Young JR, Wilson CB, Jaffe RB: Detection, evaluation and treatment of pituitary microadenomas in patients with galactorrhea and amenorrhea. Am J Obstet Gynecol 128:356, 1977
131. Shearman RP, Fraser IS: Impact of new diagnostic methods on the differential diagnosis and treatment of secondary amenorrhea. Lancet 1:1195, 1977
132. Hardy J, Beauregard H, Robert F: Prolactin-secreting pituitary adenomas transsphenoidal microsurgical treatment. In Progress in Prolactin Physiology and Pathology, Edited by C Robyn, M Harter. Amsterdam, Elsevier-North Holland, 1978, p 361
133. Pituitary Adenoma Study Group: Pituitary adenomas and oral contraceptives: a multicenter case-control study. Fertil Steril 39:753, 1983
134. Maheux R, Jenicek M, Cleroux R, Beauregard H, De-Muylder X, Gratton NM, VanCampenhout J: Oral contraceptives and prolactinomas: a case-control study. Am J Obstet Gynecol 143:134, 1982
135. Shy KK, McTierman AM, Daling JR, Weiss NS: Oral contraceptive use and the occurrence of pituitary prolactinoma. JAMA 249:2204, 1983
136. O'Malley BW: Mechanisms of action of steroid hormones. N Engl J Med 284:370, 1971
137. Freifeld ML, Feil PD, Bardin CW: The in vitro regulation of the progesterone "receptor" in guinea pigs uterus: dependence on estrogen and progesterone. Steroids 28: 93, 1974
138. Hsueh AJW, Peck EJ Jr, Clark JH: Progesterone antagonism of the estrogen receptor and estrogen-induced growth. Nature 254:337, 1975
139. Hsueh AJW, Peck EJ Jr, Clark JH: Control of uterine estrogen receptor levels by progesterone. Endocrinology 98:438, 1976
140. Pollow K, Schmidt-Gollwitzer M, Pollow G: Progesterone and estradiol binding proteins from normal human endometrium and endometrial carcinoma: a comparative study. In Steroid Receptors and Hormone Dependent Neoplasia, Edited by JL Witliff, O Dapunt. New York, Masson Publishing, 1980, p 88
141. MacLaughlin DT, Richardson GS: Progesterone binding by normal and abnormal human endometrium. J Clin Endocrinol Metab 52:667, 1976
142. Janne O, Kauppila K, Kontula K: Female sex steroid receptors in human endometrial hyperplasia and carcinoma. In Steroid Receptors and Hormone Dependent Neoplasia, Edited by JL Witliff, O Dapunt. New York, Masson Publishing, 1980, p 37
143. Gusberg SB: Hormone dependence of endometrial carcinoma. Obstet Gynecol 30:287, 1967
144. Wentz WB: Progestin therapy in endometrial hyperplasia. Gynecol Oncol 2:362, 1974
145. Kistner RW: The effects of progestational agents on hyperplasia and carcinoma in situ of the endometrium: a 10 year follow-up. Int J Gynaecol Obstet 8:561, 1970
146. Gambrell RD Jr: Hormones in the etiology and prevention of breast and endometrial cancer. South Med J 177:1509, 1984
147. Mack TM, Pike MC, Henderson BE: Estrogens and endometrial cancer in a retirement community. N Engl J Med 294:1261, 1976
148. Smith DC, Prentice R, Thompson DJ: Association of exogenous estrogen and endometrial carcinoma. N Engl J Med 293:1164, 1975
149. Ziel HK, Finkle WD: Increased risk of endometrial carcinoma among users of conjugated estrogens. N Engl J Med 293:1167, 1975
150. McDonald TW, Annegers JF, O'Fallon WM, Dockerty MB, Malkasian GD Jr, Kurland LT: Exogenous estrogen and endometrial carcinoma: case-control and incidence study. Am J Obstet Gynecol 127:572, 1977
151. Antunes CMF, Stolley PD, Rosenshein NB, Davies JL: Endometrial cancer and estrogen use: report of a large case-control study. N Engl J Med 300:9, 1979
152. Nachtigall LE, Nachtigall RH, Nachtigall RB: Estrogen replacement. II. A prospective study in the relationship to carcinoma and cardiovascular and metabolic problems. Obstet Gynecol 54:74, 1979
153. Whitehead MI, Townsend PT, Pryse-Davies J: Effects of estrogens and progestins on the biochemistry and morphology of the postmenopausal endometrium. N Engl J Med 305:1599, 1981
154. Silverberg SG, Makowski EL: Endometrial carcinoma in young women taking oral contraceptives. Obstet Gynecol 46:503, 1975
155. Lyon FA: The development of the endometrium in young women receiving long-term sequential oral contraception: report of four cases. Am J Obstet Gynecol 123:299, 1975
156. Kelley HW, Miles PA, Buster JE, Scragg WH: Adenocarcinoma of the endometrium in women taking sequential oral contraceptives. Obstet Gynecol 47:200, 1976
157. Kreutner A Jr, Johnson D, Williamson HO: Histology of the endometrium in long-term use of a sequential oral contraceptive. Fertil Steril 27:905, 1976

158. Silverberg SG, Makowski EL, Roche WD: Endometrial carcinoma in women under 40 years of age: comparison of cases in oral contraceptive users and non-users. Cancer 29:591, 1977
159. Anonymous: Sequential oral contraceptives removed from the market. FDA Drug Bull 6:26, 1976
160. Weiss NS, Sayvetz TA: Incidence of endometrial cancer in relation to the use of oral contraceptives. N Engl J Med 302:551, 1980
161. Kaufman DW, Shapiro S, Slone D: Decreased risk of endometrial cancer among oral contraceptive users. N Engl J Med 303:1045, 1980
162. Hulka BS, Chambless LE, Kaufman DG: Protection against endometrial carcinoma by combination-product oral contraceptives. JAMA 247:475, 1982
163. The Centers for Disease Control Cancer and Steroid Hormone Study: Oral contraceptive use and the risk of endometrial cancer. JAMA 249:1600, 1900
164. Horvath E, Kovacs K, Ross RC: Ultrastructural findings in a well differentiated hepatoma. Digestion 7:74, 1972
165. Baum JK, Holtz F, Bookstein JJ, Klein EW: Possible association between benign hepatomas and oral contraceptives. Lancet 2:926, 1973
166. Christopherson WM, Mays ET: Liver tumors and contraceptive steroids: experience with the first one hundred registry patients. JNCI 58:167, 1977
167. Nissen ED, Kent DR, Nissen SE: Etiology factors in the pathogenesis of liver tumors associated with oral contraceptives. Am J Obstet Gynecol 127:61, 1977
168. Keifer WS, Scott JC: Liver neoplasms and the oral contraceptives. Am J Obstet Gynecol 128:448, 1977
169. Edmondson HA, Henderson B, Benton B: Liver-cell adenomas associated with use of oral contraceptives. N Engl J Med 294:470, 1976
170. Armed Forces Institute of Pathology, Hepatic Branch and Center for Disease Control, Bureau of Epidemiology, Family Planning Evaluation Division: Increased risk of hepatocellular adenoma in women with long-term use of oral contraceptives. Morbid Mortal Weekly Rep 26:293, 1977
171. Vana J, Murphy GP, Aronoff BL, Baker HW: Study of association between liver tumors and oral contraceptive use. Unpublished data, 1977
172. Garcia CR, Gordon J, Drill VA: Contraceptive steroids and liver lesions. J Toxicol Environ Health 3:197, 1977
173. Vessey MP, Kay CR, Baldwin JA, Clarke JA, MacLeod IB: Oral contraceptives and benign liver tumors. Br Med J 1:1064, 1977
174. Edmondson HA, Reynolds TB, Henderson B, Benton B: Regression of liver cell adenomas associated with oral contraceptives. Ann Intern Med 86:180, 1977
175. Ramseur WL, Cooper MR: Asymptomatic liver cell adenomas: another case of resolution after discontinuation of oral contraceptive use. JAMA 239:1647, 1978
176. Anderson PH, Packer JT: Hepatic adenoma observations after estrogen withdrawal. Arch Surg 111:898, 1976
177. Kent DR, Nissen ED, Nissen SE, Ziehm DJ: Effect of pregnancy on liver tumor associated with oral contraceptives. Obstet Gynecol 51:148, 1978
178. Nissen ED, Kent DR, Nissen SE: Role of oral contraceptive agents in the pathogenesis of liver tumors. J Toxicol Environ Health 5:231, 1979
179. International Agency for Research on Cancer: Evaluation of carcinogenic risk of chemicals to man. Int Agency Res Cancer 6:87, 1974
180. Yager JD, Yager R: Oral contraceptive steroids as promoters of hepatocarcinogenesis in female Sprague-Dawley rats. Cancer Res 40:3680, 1980
181. Wanless IR, Medline A: Role of estrogens as promoters of hepatic neoplasia. Invest 46:313, 1982
182. Bernstein MS, Hunter RL, Yachnin S: Hepatoma and peliosis hepatis developing in a patient with Fanconi's anemia. N Engl J Med 284:1135, 1971
183. Farrell GC, Uren RF, Perkins KW: Androgen-induced hepatoma. Lancet 1:430, 1975
184. Johnson FL, Lerner KG, Siegel M: Association of androgenic-anabolic steroid therapy with development of hepatocellular carcinoma. Lancet 1:1273, 1972
185. Boyd PR, Mark GJ: Multiple hepatic adenomas and hepatocellular carcinoma in a man on oral methyltestosterone for eleven years. Cancer 40:1765, 1977
186. Lengeman CH: Liver-cell neoplasm and oral contraceptives. Lancet 1:64, 1974
187. Helling TS, Wood WG: Oral contraceptives and cancer of the liver: a review with two additional cases. Am J Gastroenterol 77:504, 1982
188. Gala KV, Griffin TW: Hepatomas in young women on oral contraceptives: report of two cases and review of the literature. J Surg Oncol 22:11, 1983
189. Henderson BE, Preston-Martin S, Edmondson HA, Peters RL, Pike MC: Hepatocellular carcinoma and oral contraceptives. Br J Cancer 48:437, 1983
190. Breslow NE, Day NE: Statistical methods in cancer research. Vol 1, The Analysis of Case-Control Studies. International Agency for Research on Cancer, 1980, p 251
191. Neuberger J, Forman D, Doll R, Williams R: Oral contraceptives and hepatocellular carcinoma. Br Med J 292: 1355, 1986
192. Forman D, Vincent TJ, Doll R: Cancer of the liver and the use of oral contraceptives. Br Med J 292:1357, 1986
193. Planned Parenthood Federation of America, Inc, News Release: U.S. Data Fails to Uphold Claims Made in British Medical Journal Showing a Link between Long Term Oral Contraceptive Use and Liver Cancer, 1986, p 1
194. Klatskin G: Hepatic tumors: possible relationship to use of oral contraceptives. Gastroenterology 73:386, 1977
195. Tesluk H, Lawrie J: Hepatocellular adenoma: its transformation to carcinoma in a user of oral contraceptives. Arch Pathol Lab Med 105:296, 1981
196. Goldfarb S: Sex hormones and hepatic neoplasia. Cancer Res 36:2584, 1976
197. Neuberger J, Portmann B, Nunnerlly HB: Oral contraceptive-associated liver tumors: occurrence of malignancy and difficulties in diagnosis. Lancet 1:2734, 1980

Chapter 34

Pregnancy termination: techniques, risks, and complications and their management

Robert G. Castadot, M.D., M.P.H.

Department of Gynecology and Obstetrics, The Johns Hopkins Medical Institutions, Baltimore, Maryland

Over the past 12 years, since the Supreme Court ruling of January 22, 1973, the availability and demand for pregnancy termination in the United States have shown a major expansion (580,000 in 1972 to 1,300,000 in 1981). The techniques and safety of abortion have made major progress: the mortality rate for legal abortion in the United States declined from 8.2/100,000 abortions in 1971 to 1972[2] to 0.5/100,000 in 1981.[2] This progress has been accomplished not by any single major breakthrough, outside of the legalization process itself, but by constant efforts and debates among clinicians, epidemiologists, pharmacologists, public health personnel, and women's groups to improve the solution to an unwanted pregnancy.

Current modalities of pregnancy termination do not fit the traditional subdivision of pregnancy in trimesters. Hence for this review I propose to distinguish three phases: the first phase is up to 49 days past the last menstrual period, the second extends from 8 to 15 weeks, and the third extends from 16 to 24 weeks. Although this subdivision is somewhat arbitrary, in my experience it is useful in terms of therapeutic approach.

EARLY PREGNANCY TERMINATION (UP TO 49 DAYS)

Before 8 weeks of pregnancy, suction dilatation and curettage (D and C) and, to a much lesser extent, sharp curettage are by far the most frequently used techniques for pregnancy termination. There has been, however, some dissatisfaction with these techniques. First, some of the most extensive studies of abortion seem to indicate that the complication rate before 7 weeks is higher than during the 8- to 10-week period.[1, 3] Second, some women have expressed preference for a nonsurgical method that could be self-administered at home. The most common reasons for such preference were "the anonymity of the therapy, the possibility for the husband to participate, and the more 'natural' procedure as compared with vacuum aspiration."[4] Consequently, a number of other surgical and nonsurgical methods were developed, but they did not attain clinical usefulness.

Menstrual regulation, a surgical method developed in the early 1970s,[5, 6] was originally seen as a model for safety, cost-effectiveness, and potential availability as well as a way to avoid psychologic or religious worries for the patient and possible legal implications for both the patient and practitioner where abortion laws were restrictive. Originally defined as a procedure to be done up to the 42nd day after the last menstrual period, the procedure was frequently performed up to 49 days and later. However, broader experience with the method showed several shortcomings.[7] Because the procedure was performed before a pregnancy test became positive, between 27% and 59% of menstrual regulations were done on patients who were not pregnant.[7, 8] Failure rates because of continuing pregnancy or incomplete evacuation were found to be as high as 11% to 12%.[7, 8] This led to a rather elaborate follow-up program that included histologic examination of tissues, a repeat pregnancy test, a repeat pelvic examination, and the requirement of a positive pregnancy test before the procedure.[5, 7-9] Finally, that the complication rates for menstrual regulation were similar to those for early vacuum aspirations (7 to 8 weeks) removed the remaining advantage for the method in the United States.[7] Menstrual regulation, if in disfavor in the United States, appears to have been adopted in countries where fewer resources are available for reproductive health.[10] However, one may question the use of a method with a high failure rate and complication rates around 10% in areas where follow-up services are inadequate.[11]

It has been known for longer than 10 years that prostaglandins (PGs) are effective abortifacients in early pregnancy termination,[12] but naturally occurring PGs ($PGF_{2\alpha}$ or PGE_2) given intravenously or in vaginal suppositories are associated with too high a frequency of gastrointestinal and other side effects at the high doses necessary to terminate a pregnancy.[12, 13] $PGF_{2\alpha}$ and PGE_2, at doses of 5 mg and 1.5 mg, respectively, are effective in inducing abortion with an acceptable level of side effects only if injected in the uterus and require adequate premedication (meperidine, atropine, and diazepam).[14, 15]

PG analogs, such as methyl esters of 15-methyl PGE_2, 15-methyl $PGF_{2\alpha}$, and 16, 16-dimethyl-trans-Δ^2-PGE_1 methyl ester, were also effective administered via the intrauterine route and required less premedication.[4] But the intrauterine route has been largely abandoned because of its invasive nature and because it appears "more painful than vaginal prostaglandin administration or vacuum aspiration."[16] The F analogs are highly effective (from 61% to > 90% complete evacuation[17-19]) and are associated with low complication rates.[4] However, these compounds are associated with a high frequency of gastrointestinal side effects, which limits their general use, when they are administered by a noninvasive route (vaginal, intramuscular).[4] The E analogs produce less gastrointestinal side effects but until recently lacked stability. More stable E analogs, such as 16-phenoxy-ω-17, 18, 19, 20-tetranor-PGE_2 methyl sulfonylamide, 16, 16-di-methyl-trans-Δ^2-PGE_1 methyl ester, and 9-deoxo-16, 16-dimethyl-9-methylene-PGE_2, used in intramuscular injection, vaginal suppositories, or cervical pessaries, have been shown to be very effective (92% to 98% complete evacuation) with side effects (vomiting and/or nausea) found in 40% to 50% of patients.[4, 20, 21] However, the amount of bleeding (mean blood loss by episode, 61.7 ml), the duration of bleeding (1 to 2 weeks), the requirement for analgesia while the patient is in the hospital (32% to 55%), and fever (7% among 9-methylene-PGE_2 users) constitute limitations to the method.[4, 13] But for some patients, a self-administered, medical method may be preferable for reasons of anonymity, "naturalness," and nonhospital atmosphere.[16, 22]

PGs appear so far to be the only abortifacients that can induce uterine contractions leading to separation of the placenta in early pregnancy. This by itself produces a release of endogenous PGs, which increase uterine contractions until evacuation of the uterus is achieved. Hence it appears that endogenous PGs, which are known to regulate uterine contractions in labor and pregnancy,[23] play a role in any abortion induced by such diverse methods as saline or other hypertonic injections, rivanol, and PG analogs.[24] Other drugs that can induce uterine contractions, such as oxytocin, sparteine sulfate, ergot derivatives, and quinine, produce only "erratic results,"[25, 26] and some can create life-threatening situations.[27]

The postcoital use of diethylstilbestrol, oral contraceptives, or intrauterine devices (IUDs) will not be considered, because from a medical point of view these mechanisms act before implantation of the blastocyst and therefore should not be considered abortifacients.[28] Much research has been done on antiprogestational compounds.[25, 29] The disruption of luteal function could be accomplished by inhibition of the early luteotrophic activity of the ovary or of the blastocyst, such as by immunization against human chorionic gonadotropin (hCG) or one of its subunits or by an antihormone effect.[25, 29, 30] Another antiprogestational approach is the blockage of the progesterone receptors in the endometrium.[29, 31] Such an agent, RU-486, appears to be effective as an abortifacient (61% complete abortion) and as a once-a-month contraceptive pill. It has few side effects, but there was occasional heavy bleeding requiring curettage and transfusion in 2 of 37 patients.[31, 32] RU-486 has been termed a "contragestive" by its manufacturer.[31] Testing of compounds that could directly affect the endometrium is still in its infancy.[33]

ANIMAL STUDIES

Segal and Atkinson,[25] in the early 1970s, coined the term "contragestational agents" in their review of possible mechanisms to terminate pregnancy. They included drugs that cause uterine contractions, antiprogestational compounds, uterine luteolysin, immunization against specific placental components, and blastotoxic or embryotoxic agents. Plants, as potential sources of antifertility agents, have generated a great deal of interest,[34] and abortifacient effects have been obtained from several species.[35] Extracts of an African root appear to have consistent abortifacient effects in mice by inducing uterine contractions.[36]

Among the luteolytic agents, compounds that interfere with the cytochrome oxidase system (aminoglutethimide), amine oxidase inhibitors, some ergot derivatives (ergocornine), immunization against hCG or other proteinic substances specific to pregnancy, and drugs that interfere with progesterone receptors have been studied.[25, 29, 30, 37] Antimetabolites and antivitamins have been found to be blastotoxic or embryotoxic but have been largely abandoned because of the double jeopardy represented by their potential teratogenicity and general cell toxicity.[25, 38] Superficial endometrial damage was obtained with several compounds (ethanol, formaldehyde, silver nitrate, iodine, rivanol, cyclizine, urea, methotrexate, and a derivative of 19-nortestosterone) but had limited applicability.[39] The mechanism of action remains to be elucidated for some plant extracts and some polypeptide hormones.[40-42]

PREGNANCY TERMINATION FROM 8 TO 15 WEEKS

There is a broad consensus on the most appropriate technique to be used for pregnancy termination between 8 and 15 weeks.

TECHNIQUE

From 8 to 15 weeks' pregnancy, the suction D and C, and its variant dilatation and evacuation (D and E), has imposed itself as the unchallenged technique for pregnancy termination. Up to 12 weeks of gestation, virtually all pregnancy terminations in the United States are done by suction curettage.[2] Between 13 and 15 weeks and between 16 and 20 weeks, the D and E is the most frequently used technique.[2]

The technique is well-known and needs only to be summarized.[43-45] The procedure is preferably performed on an outpatient basis. The patient reports to the unit early in the morning, having fasted since midnight. After a review of her history and a physical examination, a decision is made to insert one or more laminaria tents or to proceed directly with a vacuum curettage. The use of laminaria tents provides adequate dilatation or facilitates further mechanical dilatation of the cervix, if needed, and makes the suction D and C faster and less painful for the patient, in particular for the nulliparous patient.[46] The number of tents used depends on the size of the cervical canal (i.e., as many tents as the cervix will tolerate are inserted). The laminaria tents are left in place at least 2 hours, during which the patient is encouraged to stay in bed or supine. The use of laminaria tents reduces the risk of cervical laceration or trauma mostly in the nulliparous patient.[46-48] The impact on long-term injury (cervical incompetence, premature delivery, low birth-weight) remains to be ascertained. Osmotic dilators have been shown similarly to reduce the force needed to dilate the cervical canal at the time of first-trimester or midtrimester abortion[49, 50] and can be used to deliver PGs to the uterus.[50]

After the laminaria tents have been removed and the vagina is prepared, the cervix is grasped with a Jacob's tenaculum (American Medical Instrument Company, Flushing, NY) and the direction of the canal is ascertained with a uterine sound. If additional dilatation is required, it is obtained by gentle introduction of Pratt dilators (Sklar Manufacturing Company, Long Island City, NY) whose tapered ends require less force than Hegar dilators (Sklar Manufacturing Company).[51] Suction curettage with a transparent vacurette is performed and followed by a brief sharp curettage to verify the completion of the procedure.

Unless medical reasons or lack of patient cooperation indicate otherwise, the procedure is carried out under cervical block with 10 ml of 0.5% hydrochloride or 2% chloroprocaine hydrochloride or 0.25% bupivacaine hydrochloride and slow intravenous injection of diazepam, 5 mg, and meperidine, 50 mg.

If the patient has requested one and it is not contraindicated, an IUD can be inserted.[52, 53] It is most important for the operator to check the tissue obtained and ascertain the presence of decidua, placenta, and fetal parts. If fetal parts are obtained, it should be verified that all parts have been evacuated and the foot length should be measured. If no fetal parts are seen but placental tissue (villi) is identified, the uterine cavity should be reexplored unless the pregnancy is less than 9 weeks, in which case the fetus is not seen in one half the cases. If no villi are seen, the diagnoses of very early pregnancy, ectopic pregnancy, no pregnancy, failure to complete the abortion, and perforation should be considered.[45] A final diagnosis should be reached as soon as possible. Essential steps in management are a repeat pelvic examination with careful attention given to the adnexae, a repeat procedure, sending of the specimen to the pathology laboratory as a "rush" with results to be communicated by telephone, a repeat pregnancy test before discharge, and 1 week later, the giving of thorough information to the patient about the alternatives and instruction to call in 24 hours for pathologic results.

The transition from suction D and C to D and E is strictly empirical. Further dilatation is required to accommodate larger vacurettes (12- to 14-mm). When vacurettes fail to obtain parts, sponge sticks and, if needed, heavier crushing forceps are used to empty the uterine cavity. Oxytocin is rarely needed and should not be used until after the dilatation has been completed and instruments have easily entered the uterus. The main indications for oxytocin are excessive blood loss and difficulty in delineating a soft uterus.

Ripening of the cervix before vacuum curettage with PG analogs is feasible but not very practical as a routine,[54] but it might be worth undertaking in the young nulliparous patient with a small cervix. There is a physiologic basis to support this concept.[55, 56] Finally, prevention of Rh immunization in Rh-negative women with immunoglobulin should never be omitted.[57]

RISKS AND MANAGEMENT OF EARLY COMPLICATIONS

Like any surgical procedure, vacuum D and C and D and E present a number of risks of complications; these should be both kept in mind and shared with the patient to give substance to her informed consent. These complications have classically been divided into early (i.e., within 1 month of the abortion) and late, or sequelae (i.e., occurring after 1 month). The early complications may be further divided into "immediate" (occurring at the time of the abortion), such as uterine perforation, laceration of the cervix, hemorrhage, and anesthesia-related accidents, and "delayed" (occurring in the following days but within 1 month), such as retention of gestational tissues, infection, venous thrombosis and pulmonary emboli, or depression.[58]

A distinction should be made between complications due to the procedure and those related to preexisting conditions or concurrent surgery, such as a sterilization procedure. Preexisting complications have been well defined by Tietze and Lewit,[1] and often, in my experience, require special management, including specialized anesthesia care. To the list of preexisting complications described by Tietze and Lewit should be added extreme obesity, because of the challenges it offers to both the anesthetist and the gynecologist. The rate of preexisting complications averages 4.2% for all abortions in the original Joint Program for the Study of Abortion (JPSA) study and increases with age, parity, marital status, and gestational age.[1]

Mortality varies much with gestational age, as do complication rates. The mortality rate in the United States between 1972 and 1980 varied between 0.4/100,000 at 8 weeks or less and 14/100,000 after 21 weeks.[58] On an average, the mortality rate increases 30% with each passing week of gestation.[58] Approximately, the mortality rate per 100,000 cases is slightly above 1 at 9 to 10 weeks and around 4 at 13 to 15 weeks.[58] The major causes of death related to abortion recorded in the United States are infection (23%), embolism (23%), hemorrhage (20%), and complication of anesthesia (16%).[58]

Pelvic infection with at least 3 days of fever at 38°C, bleeding requiring transfusion, and unintended surgery (laparotomy, hysterotomy, and hysterectomy) represent 88% of all major complications.[58] Major complications accompanied $<$ 1% of all abortions, varying from a low of 0.25% at 7 to 8 weeks to a high of 2.1% at 15 to 16 weeks in the original JPSA study from 1970 to 1971 by Tietze and Lewit.[1] By 1975 to 1978, the estimated rate of major early complications had decreased to between a minimum of 0.5% and a maximum of 0.67%.[58]

Among immediate complications, hemorrhage, laceration of the cervix, and perforation are rare events, with a total of 1.2% at 8 weeks to 3.6% at 15 weeks and longer.[1] Blood loss increases when the procedure is done with general anesthesia, particularly when agents that produce uterine relaxation, such as halothane, are used. Similarly, perforation and cervical laceration occur more frequently with general anesthesia than with local anesthesia.[58] The risk of death from anesthesia-related and other causes is two to four times greater with general anesthesia than with local anesthesia.[58] Inversely, the risk of convulsion is greater with local anesthesia. Uterine perforation and cervical laceration are best prevented by adequate training of the operator, avoidance of excessive force, and recognition of the direction of the cervical canal by prior sounding. The management of uterine perforation depends on the state of vacuity of the uterine cavity, when it occurs; the type of instrument that causes it; and the chances of perforation of other viscera. If the uterine cavity must be emptied further, it is better done under laparoscopic control. Laparoscopy is also very helpful in assessing the perforation, the bleeding involved, and other possible lesions, such as bladder perforation (blood in the urine is a good sign), but it cannot rule out bowel perforation. Most frequently, perforation requires no other treatment than overnight observation, but occasionally persistent bleeding, extensive perforation, or lesions to other organs require a laparotomy and, exceptionally, a hysterectomy. Cervical lacerations should be sutured even if bleeding is minimal.

Delayed complications are slightly more frequent, ranging from 2.4% at 8 weeks to 5% at 15 weeks.[1] They include postabortion bleeding, tissue retention, anemia, infection, and fever of unknown origin. Venous thrombophlebitis, pulmonary emboli, depression, psychosis, and suicide are so rare as to be very difficult to quantify. Retained placental products, postabortion bleeding, fever, and pelvic infection are all managed by reexploring and emptying the uterine cavity. Oxytocin or methylergonovine may be helpful in decreasing the bleeding and evacuating retained products. If the fever reaches 38°C, antibiotics should be used. Ampicillin by mouth or intravenous or parenteral penicillin plus an aminoglycoside are effective against vaginal flora. Some researchers have advocated the use of tetracyclines, preferably doxycycline prophylactically, as a cost-effective and efficacious preventer of endometritis and pelvic infection.[59]

Failure to interrupt the pregnancy occurs in < 0.5% of suction curettage patients, but the possibility should be kept in mind. It is most likely to occur in abortion performed before 6 weeks' gestation.[58] Unrecognized ectopic pregnancy and continuing pregnancy are prevented with adequate examination of the tissue obtained by curettage, histologic examination, and a repeat pregnancy test when in doubt.

Early termination of pregnancy constitutes the best prevention of all complications except those related to anesthesia. Long-term sequelae will be considered with pregnancy termination after 16 weeks, because the long-term effects cannot be differentiated by gestational age.

PREGNANCY TERMINATION FROM 16 TO 24 WEEKS

There is a considerable amount of controversy on which method of pregnancy termination between the 16th and 24th week of gestation is safest, produces the least number of complications, produces the least acceptable type of complication, produces the least amount of stress for the patient and provider, and is most cost-effective.[60] The key debate concerns the choice between the urea-PG instillation technique and D and E and focuses on the 16- to 20-week period.

TECHNIQUES

The techniques are presented here in their historic order of appearance. The use of hypertonic sodium chloride, PG, or urea-PG injections and of D and E was reviewed recently by Burkman and King[61] and requires only a brief description. All the instillation techniques have similar requirements before the injection of the specific agent. A complete history, physical examination, and laboratory tests allow for the detection of systemic diseases that could increase the expected morbidity or require special management. If there is discrepancy between dates and size of the uterus, abnormality of shape of the uterus, or too close a vicinity to some of the cutoff dates, ultrasonography is helpful.[62] Placement of multiple laminaria tents for at least 4 hours seems to decrease the risk of cervical laceration and may shorten the injection-abortion interval. The technique of the amniocentesis and injection has been described at length.[61] For management and comparison purposes, arbitrary time limits are used to decide when the placenta should be removed with "sponge stick D and C" (2 hours after expulsion of the fetus or when blood loss is excessive) or when the procedure is considered a failure (36 or 48 hours after injection).

There are a number of variations in the techniques used for induction of pregnancy termination with hypertonic saline solutions.[63, 64] Usually, 200 ml of a 20% NaCl solution is slowly injected into the intraamniotic cavity transabdominally after 100 to 200 ml of amniotic fluid has been removed. Frequently, an oxytocic perfusion is added either after the saline injection or at a later time to augment labor. The dosage varies from 40 to 332 mU/minute.[61] Kerenyi[64] indicated that the injection-abortion time ranges between 22 and 38 hours and that a retained placenta is encountered in 13% to 32% of patients.

Several variations of techniques and several PGs are available. The most frequent approach in the United States is the intraamniotic injection of a single dose of 40 or 50 mg of $PGF_{2\alpha}$ or the injection of 25 mg of $PGF_{2\alpha}$ repeated 6 hours later.[61] The use of 15 methyl $PGF_{2\alpha}$ and analogs of the PGE_2 have been successfully used in Scandinavia via the intramuscular route,[65] a controlled-release vaginal delivery system,[66] or vaginal suppositories,[67] or as an intracervical or extraamniotic gel.[68] In many different forms, PGs appear not only to produce uterine contractions, but also to dilate the cervix specifically. They appear to be an effective abortifacient. Suppositories are useful in cases of ruptured membranes. When $PGF_{2\alpha}$ is injected into the amniotic cavity, there is no need to remove amniotic fluid. Oxytocin perfusion may be carefully added if labor fails to ensue or if the placenta is not eliminated within 2 hours of expulsion of the fetus. The average injection-abortion interval ranges between 19 and 22 hours, and the placenta is retained in more than one third of patients.[61] Because of the high frequency of side effects, mostly gastrointestinal, the $F_{2\alpha}$ PGs and analogs are best used in intraamniotic injection. The E analogs are associated with fewer gastrointestinal symptoms but are frequently associated with hyperpyrexia.

Hyperosmolar urea has several advantages over hypertonic sodium chloride or $PGF_{2\alpha}$ injections.[69] The technique includes the removal of 200 ml of amniotic fluid and the subsequent injection of 80 gm of urea in 135 ml of 5% dextrose in water (i.e., a 60% solution of urea). This is augmented by injecting 5 mg of $PGF_{2\alpha}$ after the urea. Earlier attempts to use oxytocin perfusion to augment intraamniotic urea were efficacious but were associated with a longer injection-abortion interval and more problems with water and electrolyte balance.[70] This technique is still used in patients with asthma or other contraindications to PGs. The injection-abortion interval with urea-$PGF_{2\alpha}$ is shorter (16 to 17 hours), but the percentage of retained placenta is high (35% to 46%).[61] Because it is fetotoxic, hyperosmolar urea does not create a problem of live fetal expulsion. Gastrointestinal side effects are less frequent than when PGF_2 alone is used.

During the past 10 years, there has been increasing evidence that suction dilatation modified for extraction of larger volumes through the cervix is feasible and safe even after 16 weeks of gestation.[71, 72] D and E was found to be more cost-effective than saline injection and relatively safe.[73] D and E appears to have less complications than hyperosmolar urea injection when all second-trimester abortions are considered,[74] but this advantage is mainly because D and E allows a large number of second-trimester abortions to be done earlier (i.e., between 13 and 16 weeks). When the complications are measured for the 16- to 20-week period, the complication rates of D and E and urea-PG are similar.[74]

The technique requires placement of multiple laminaria tents with serial replacement if the procedure is performed after 20 weeks' gestation.[75] The dilatation of the cervix is important in view of the need to extract large fetal parts, such as the calvarium.[61, 75] A Bierer-type forceps or a sponge stick is used to grab the anterior lip of the forceps, and generally a Sopher forceps is used to extract fetal parts and the placenta.[61, 76] The suction equipment may be adapted to use vacurettes from size 12 to 16. For late D and E, the suction is still helpful in emptying the amniotic fluid and in bringing parts to the lower uterine segment, where they are more accessible to various forceps. The procedure can be done after cervical block with or without intravenous analgesia.

RISKS AND MANAGEMENT OF COMPLICATIONS

The risks associated with late abortions are much higher than those associated with abortion performed in early pregnancy. Tyler[77] calculated that between 16 and 20 weeks' gestation, the risk of death is 25 times greater than before 8 weeks' gestation. Similarly, morbidity increases markedly during the second trimester, an average of 20% per week for major complications.[58] Also, because this type of management is relatively rare (instillation techniques represent only 4% of all abortions done in the United States), it is probably handled better in a specialized unit, where repeated experience produces specially trained staff. For instillation techniques, complications appear to increase with a prolongation of the injection-abortion interval, age, and parity.[78]

IMMEDIATE COMPLICATIONS

For instillation methods, it is usual to use 48 hours as a cut-off point to acknowledge failure to abort. With hypertonic sodium chloride injection, 1% to 3% of patients fail to abort by 48 hours and will need reinjection. PG intraamniotic injections fail in 14% to 18% of patients.[61] Urea-PG injection is almost always successful (< 1% failure).[61] Failure to abort with D and E is extremely rare. When a patient fails to abort after 48 hours, I recommend proceeding with vaginal evacuation of the uterus, a much easier procedure than a D and E because of the maceration of the fetal parts, dilatation of the cervix, and effects of labor on the lower uterine segment.[79]

Burkman and King[61] showed the following percentage of retained placenta for the three main instillation methods: saline, 13% to 32%; $PGF_{2\alpha}$, 33% to 41%; and urea-$PGF_{2\alpha}$, 35% to 46%. D and E has < 1% retained placental tissue.[71] In patients with the placenta retained for more than 2 hours, temperature elevation, or bleeding, I recommend proceeding with a sponge stick D and C.

Bleeding was associated with 16% of saline injections studied by Tietze and Lewit.[78] The risk of bleeding increases until 20 weeks' gestation, then appears to decline.[80] The frequency of the loss of 500 ml of blood was found by Burkman and collaborators[69] to be around 10% among urea-$PGF_{2\alpha}$ injections. Usually injection of PG is associated with the highest rate of bleeding.

Bleeding at the time of abortion can be caused by retained placenta, atony, or coagulopathy.[61] Retained placenta is easily managed by sponge stick D and C or at the time of D and E by reexploration of the uterine cavity. Atony is treated by intravenous oxytocin or methylergonovine and occasionally by massage of the uterus. Coagulopathy appears to be associated with every form of pregnancy termination,[81] but its frequency has been estimated to be 8/100,000 for suction D and C, 191/100,000 for D and E, and 658/100,000 for saline injection.[81] Coagulopathy with some degree of disseminated intravascular coagulation (DIC) has also been found among urea-PG abortions, but its frequency and severity appear much less than with saline injection.[70] The risk of death from hemorrhage increases with age, gestational age up to 20 weeks, incomplete abortion, and uterine perforation or rupture.[80] Grimes et al.[80] reported that women who sustained a uterine perforation or rupture had a chance of dying from hemorrhage more than 1000 times greater than that of women without that accident.

Uterine perforation is a major but rare (3/1000) complication of D and E.[71] Such perforations are usually more severe than in the first trimester and are sometimes associated with excessive blood loss. The management that I described during the 8- to 15-week period applies, but laparoscopy may be more difficult and laparotomy more likely. Perforations are extremely rare with instillation procedures.

Cervical lacerations are a relatively frequent (3%) complication of PG and urea-PG intraamniotic injections.[69] The use of laminaria tents has reduced the frequency of this complication to < 1%.[61] Because these lacerations rarely bleed, they are often unrecognized unless the cervix is inspected before the patient is discharged. When discovered, they should be repaired after debridement. Burkman and King[61] noted that breakdown is not uncommon and the subsequent obstetric impact of this complication remains to be ascertained. Lacerations of the cervical canal are rare (1%) but potentially more dangerous at the time of D and E or several days later because of occasional severe hemorrhage, which may require vaginal or abdominal sutures and, at times, uterine vessel or hypogastric artery ligation.[61] Sometimes a hysterectomy is the only alternative. Uterine perforation or rupture was frequently present (71%) among patients who died of hemorrhage.[80]

DELAYED COMPLICATIONS

Different definitions used in various studies make infection rates difficult to compare. For saline injection, Tietze and Lewit,[78] in 1973, reported the following rates: infection, 2.5%; hemorrhage and infection, 3.9%; and fever, 3.4%. King et al.[70] found a similar rate of infection in patients with urea-PG injection. The risk of infection increases with the prolongation of the injection-abortion interval. For D and E, the risk of fever is around 1%, and for endometritis it is < 10%.[71] If the interval between injection and abortion extends beyond 24 hours, I give the patient prophylactic antibiotic (cephalothin).[82] Should chorioamnionitis become evident, I routinely use a broad-spectrum antibiotic, such as ampicillin, with or without an aminoglycoside.[61] Burkman and associates[79] reported a patient with chorioamnionitis with *Clostridia perfringens* who required a hysterectomy in addition to high-dose antibiotics.

Burkman et al.[83] reported that 4 of 150 patients had to be readmitted to a hospital after urea-PG abortions, 2 for bleeding, and 2 for infection. In that series, an additional six patients required treatment for infection on an outpatient basis and an additional five patients required treatment for bleeding.[83] From these data the infection rate would approximate 6%, and the bleeding rate would be close to 4.5%. Larger series from my institution yield an infection rate closer to 10% and a bleeding rate around 9%.[69] In Tietze and Lewit's series[78] of almost 14,000 patients who had saline injection abortions, the complication rate for infection appeared to be larger, around 10% and the rate of bleeding was also higher. However, definitions were different. D and E appears to be associated with a lower infection rate, including urinary tract infection, and less bleeding.[71]

METHOD-SPECIFIC COMPLICATIONS

Hypertonic sodium chloride injection is associated with specific accidents and has a distinctly higher frequency of common complications. Sudden death from hypernatremia and necrosis of the uterine wall at the site of injection belong to the first category. DIC and water intoxication are part of the second group of complications. Hypernatremia is probably due to intravascular injection of hypertonic saline. This may lead to immediate cardiovascular collapse or to cerebral edema followed by convulsion, hypoxia, and failure of one of the vital organs.[63] However, this accident is infrequent (1 in 14,000).[78] The extended use of intravenous oxytocin has also led to water intoxication (hyponatremia) and necessitates a careful assessment of intake and output and electrolytes every 12 hours. Clearly, this technique, although efficacious, has potential for major life-threatening complications. One possible remaining indication is previous cesarean section or any other scar on the uterus.[84]

PGs alone have several deficiencies. They are associated with a high rate of gastrointestinal side effects (emesis, 70%; diarrhea, 5% to 10%). The failure rate and the frequency of retained placenta are high. Expulsion of a live fetus is not exceptional. In the case of inadvertent intravascular injection, the patient may present with severe headache, flushing, dizziness, or emesis. The accident is usually contained in time and does not appear to leave sequelae,[61] but cases of sudden death have been reported.[76]

Urea-PG has a shorter injection-abortion interval[83] and is more fetotoxic. Gastrointestinal side effects are less frequent than with PG alone.[61] The risks of intravascular injection and coagulopathy appear much less severe,[61] but the percentage of incomplete abortion is high (35% to 46%) and requires the presence of well-trained staff. The overall risk of major complication is less with urea-PG than with hypertonic saline injection.[85]

D and E offers the possibility of terminating pregnancy between 13 and 16 weeks with the relative safety of that gestational age. After 16 weeks and until 20 weeks, it does not appear safer than urea-PG.[74] After 20 weeks, urea-PG is probably safer. D and E is less expensive and emotionally and physically easier to handle for the patient; however, the emotional trauma is transferred to the clinician and operating room staff.

ABORTION SEQUELAE

Complications of abortion occurring after 1 month are classified as late complications. Among the sequelae, various possibilities of jeopardizing future term delivery have been mentioned: postabortion infertility, cervical incompetence followed by low birth-weight and premature delivery, and Rh isoimmunization.[86] Psychologic sequelae have also been the subject of much debate.

Two recent studies addressed the problem of postabortion infertility.[87, 88] One study, in the United States,[87] showed no increased risk of tubal infertility among women who had one or more induced legal abortions. The second study, by a World Health Organization Task Force,[88] compared one population in Hungary and one in South Korea; no evidence of reduced ability to conceive after an abortion was found, but the study pointed to a number of ectopic pregnancies as a potential subject of further study. Tietze[58] described three clear-cut but very rare complications of abortion that would compromise future reproductive health: hysterectomy, pelvic inflammatory disease, and Rh isoimmunization. Hogue and associates,[89] reviewing available epidemiologic studies, concluded that the distribution of results indicates that it is unlikely that there is an association between first-trimester vacuum aspiration abortion and future reproductive failure and that, if there are increased risks of reproductive failure after such abortion, the risks must be very small. However, the protective effect conferred by a woman's first birth on subsequent pregnancies is not provided by an induced abortion of that first pregnancy.[90] The impact of multiple abortions remains to be ascertained. Tietze[58] stated that long-term effects on fertility of midtrimester abortion have not been adequately studied.

Although it is clear that an abortion can precipitate a psychotic or neurotic crisis, it also appears that relief is the most frequent reaction.[91] A World Health Organization study group stated that there is frequent psychologic benefit and a low incidence of adverse reaction after pregnancy termination.[86]

EPIDEMIOLOGIC OVERVIEW

According to the Centers for Disease Control (CDC), Division of Reproductive Health, there were 1,300,760 abortions in the United States in 1981, the last year for which "abortion surveillance" data have been published.[2] For the same year, the Alan Guttmacher Institute reported 1,577,340 abortions, and for 1982, 1,573,920.[92] The 21% underreporting by CDC is attributed to differences in data collection, because CDC abortion surveillance is more likely to miss abortions done in physicians' offices.[2] After rising each year from 1973 to 1980, the number of abortions performed in the United States reached a plateau in 1980 and remained stable for the following 2 years.[92] The 1973 to 1980 yearly increase appears to be due to increased availability of services and, among other factors, a shift from oral contraception and IUD to less-effective methods.[92]

Almost each year since 1973, abortions have been obtained earlier in pregnancy. According to the CDC abortion surveillance program in 1981, 90% of all abortions had been obtained at 12 weeks, compared with only 83% in 1973.[2] Only 4.7% of abortions were performed after 15 weeks in 1981, compared with 9.7% in 1973.[92] This trend may have played a major role in the decrease in mortality associated with abortions in the United States over the past 12 years.

The average American woman who obtains an abortion is unmarried (81%), white (70%), young (64% are younger than 25 years of age), and nulliparous (58%) and has had no prior abortion (65%).[93] This abortion is probably obtained at or before 12 weeks' gestation (91%) and is performed by mechanical evacuation of the uterus (96% are suction D and C, D and C, or D and E).[93]

The abortion rate in 1982 was 29 abortions/1000 women 15 to 44 years of age (i.e., 3% of women of reproductive age obtained an abortion that year); the 1982 abortion ratio was 299 abortions/1000 live births.[92] Both the abortion rate and the abortion ratio were highest on the East and West Coasts.[92] The highest abortion ratios were found at both extremes of reproductive age: for women younger than 15 years of age the abortion ratio is 1393/1000 live births and for those older than 40 years of age it is 798.[2] The abortion ration among nonwhite women is 56/100 births; among white women it is 24/100 births.[2] Among unmarried women, the abortion ratio is 145 abortions/100 live births.[2] That 92% of abortions are obtained by patients in their state of residence suggests that abortions are available in all states, even if there remain gaps in the availability of services in nonmetropolitan areas.[92]

D and E has become the most frequently used technique for both the 13- to 15-week and 16- to 20-week periods.[2] This trend is attributed to the method's lower cost, greater safety, and relative convenience.[2]

It is remarkable that in 1982, 82% of abortions took place in nonhospital facilities. Even among abortions taking place in hospitals, there was a shift from inpatient to outpatient facilities. Inpatient abortions represented 45% of all hospital abortions in 1980; in 1982, this percentage decreased to 33%.[92]

CONCLUSIONS

Pregnancies of different gestational ages require different termination techniques. Before 8 weeks' gestation, suction D and C is currently the preferred method. A medical approach, possibly self-administered, is feasible, however, and requires only an improvement in side effects. This could dramatically decrease the percentage of suction D and C needed to complete these procedures.

From 8 to 15 weeks' gestation, the suction D and C and D and E methods cannot be challenged. The use of laminaria tents improves both the facility and safety of the procedures in the nulliparous patients and possibly in multiparous patients. The idea of priming the cervix before operation with PG is attractive in selected cases, such as in young primigravida women in late first trimester or early second trimester. It could further decrease the difficulty and risks of the procedure. The use of a hydrogel compound, with its abilities to swell and consequently dilate the cervix and to release PGs, is especially worth consideration.

There is controversy about which method should be used between 16 and 20 weeks' gestation. D and E appears to have fewer complications and be more cost-effective than hypertonic saline injection. Urea-PG appears to have fewer and less-severe complications than saline injection and seems to be more cost-effective than saline injection in terms of duration of hospitalization. The high frequency of failure and side effects combined with the possibility of expulsion of a live fetus make PG-only injection less desirable. A comparison of D and E and urea-PG injection between 16 and 20 weeks' gestation shows similar rates of complication. The decision to choose one over the other may be based more on convenience for either the patient or the providers.

After 20 weeks' gestation, urea-PG injection is probably the safer method. The reasons for very late abortion are, according to the CDC surveillance program, a mixture of delaying factors, such as youth, delayed recognition of pregnancy, geographic and institutional barriers, and financial constraints, or medical indication, such as genetic abnormality.[92] In view of the rapid increase of complications with passing weeks, one of the most important conclusions for clinic managers is to avoid any delay in providing abortion services.

Second-trimester pregnancy terminations are associated with increased mortality and morbidity, particularly after 18 weeks' gestation. Because such procedures represent a very small percentage of all abortions done in the United States, they may be better performed in specialized centers, such as the Fertility Control Center at Johns Hopkins Hospital. In such centers a few providers are exposed to a very large experience and may be better equipped to manage the complications and side effects of the techniques in use.

REFERENCES

1. Tietze C, Lewit S: Joint Program for the Study of Abortion (JPSA): early medical complications of legal abortion. Stud Fam Plann 3:97, 1972
2. Binkin NJ, Lang PRH, Rhodenhiser EP, Hogue CJ, Mackay HT, Berman SM, Buchler JW, Smith JC: Abortion surveillance, 1981. MMWR CDC Surveill Summ 33:1ss, 1985
3. Grimes DA, Schulz KF: Unpublished data. In Induced Abortion, A World Review, 1983, Edited by C Tietze. New York, The Population Council, 1983, p 86
4. Bygdeman M, Christensen NJ, Green K, Zheng S, Lundstrom V: Termination of early pregnancy. Future development. Acta Obstet Gynecol Scand (Suppl) 113:125, 1983
5. Goldsmith S, Margolis AJ: Aspiration abortion without cervical dilatation. Am J Obstet Gynecol 110:580, 1971
6. Karman H, Potts M: Very early abortion using a syringe as a vacuum source. Lancet 1:1051, 1972
7. Hodgson JE: A reassessment of menstrual regulation. Stud Fam Plann 8:263, 1977
8. Atienza MF, Burkman RT, King TM, Burnett LS, Lau HL, Parmley TH, Woodruff JD: Menstrual extraction. Am J Obstet Gynecol 121:490, 1975
9. Irani KR, Henriques ES, Friedlander RL, Berlin LE, Swartz DP: Menstrual induction: its place in clinical practice. Obstet Gynecol 46:596, 1975
10. Laufe LE: Menstrual regulation—international perspectives. In Pregnancy Termination, Procedures, Safety and New Developments, Edited by GI Zatuchni, JJ Sciarra, JJ Speidel. Hagerstown, Harper & Row, 1979, p 78
11. Butler JC: Discussion summary. In Pregnancy Termination, Procedures, Safety and New Developments, Edited by GI Zatuchni, JJ Sciarra, JJ Speidel. Hagerstown, Harper & Row, 1979, p 82
12. Karim SMM, Amy JJ: Interruption of pregnancy with prostaglandins. In Prostaglandins and Reproduction, Edited by SMM Karim. Lancaster, MTP Press Ltd., 1975, p 78
13. Embrey M: Menstrual induction (postconceptional termination). In Postcoital Contraception: Methods, Services and Prospects, Edited by H Grahame. London, Pregnancy Advisory Service, 1983, p 58
14. Mocsary P, Csapo AI: Menstrual induction with $PGF_{2\alpha}$ and PGE_2. Prostaglandins 10:545, 1975
15. Ragab J, Edelman D: Early termination of pregnancy. A comparative study of intrauterine prostaglandin $F_{2\alpha}$ and vacuum aspiration. Prostaglandins 11:275, 1976
16. Bygdeman M, Green KK: Menstrual regulation. Medical techniques. In Pregnancy Termination, Procedures, Safety and New Developments, Edited by GI Zatuchni, JJ Sciarra, JJ Speidel. Hagerstown, Harper & Row, 1979, p 69
17. Brenner PF, Marrs RP, Roy S, Mishell DR Jr: Methods to determine success of attempts to terminate early gestation pregnancies with prostaglandin vaginal suppositories. Contraception 28:111, 1983
18. Bygdeman M, Martin JN, Leader A, Lundstrom V, Ramadan M, Eneroth P, Green K: Early pregnancy interruption by (15S)-15-methyl-prostaglandin $F_{2\alpha}$ methyl ester. Obstet Gynecol 48:221, 1976
19. Wan LS, Stiber AJ, Turkel J: Termination of very early pregnancy by vaginal suppositories: (15S)-15-methyl-prostaglandin $F_{2\alpha}$ methyl ester. Contraception 24:603, 1981
20. Chen JK, Elder MG: Preoperative cervical dilatation by vaginal pessaries containing prostaglandin E1 analogue. Obstet Gynecol 62:339, 1983

21. Ho PC, Liang ST, Tang GW, Ma HK: Pre-operative cervical dilatation in termination of first trimester pregnancies using 16, 16-dimethyl-trans-Δ^2 PGE1 methyl ester vaginal pessaries. Contraception 27:339, 1983
22. Rosen AS, Von Knorring K, Bygdeman M, Christensen NJ: Randomized comparison of prostaglandin treatment in hospital or at home with vacuum aspiration for termination of early pregnancy. Contraception 29:423, 1984
23. Novy MJ, Liggins GC: Role of prostaglandins, prostacyclin and thromboxanes in the physiologic control of the uterus and in parturition. In Prostaglandins in the Perinatal Period. Their Physiologic and Clinical Importance, Edited by MA Heymann. New York, Grune & Stratton, Inc., 1980, p 45
24. Christensen NJ, Green K: Endogenous prostaglandin synthesis and abortion. A mini-review. Acta Obstet Gynecol Scand 113:109, 1983
25. Segal SJ, Atkinson LE: Systemic contragestational agents. In The Abortion Experience: Psychological and Medical Impact, Edited by HJ Osofsky, JD Osofsky. Hagerstown, Harper & Row, 1973, p 400
26. Kumar D, Russell JJ: Controlled oxytocin infusion as a method of therapeutic abortion in early pregnancy. Bull Johns Hopkins Hosp 109:141, 1961
27. Dannenberg AL, Dorfman SF, Johnson J: Use of quinine for self-induced abortion. South Med J 76:846, 1983
28. Brahams D: The postcoital pill and intrauterine device: contraceptive or abortifacient? Lancet 1:1039, 1983
29. Aitken RJ, Harper MJ: New methods for the regulation of implantation. Contraception 16:227, 1977
30. Anonymous: Report of a joint National Institutes of Health/Agency for International Development/Program for Applied Research in Fertility Regulation workshop on research and development of immunological methods of fertility regulation. Contraception 31:11, 1985
31. Anonymous: An all-in-one birth control pill, abortifacient, Cushings's treatment? Medical World News 25:51, 1984
32. Kovacs L, Sas M, Resch BA, Ugocsai G, Swahn ML, Bygdeman M, Rowe PJ: Termination of very early pregnancy by RU 486—an antiprogestational compound. Contraception 29:399, 1984
33. Dubin NH, Burkman RT, King TM, Parmley TH, Blake DA, Cox RT: Research on new approaches to pregnancy termination: ethanol abortifacient activity—animal and human data. A preliminary report. In Pregnancy Termination, Procedures, Safety and New Developments, Edited by GI Zatuchni, JJ Sciarra, JJ Speidel. Hagerstown, Harper & Row, 1979, p 8
34. Farnsworth NR, Bingel AS, Cordell GA, Crane FA, Fong HH: Potential values of plants as sources of new antifertility agents. J Pharm Sci 64:535, 1975
35. Pakrashi A, Basak B, Mookerji N: Search for antifertility agents from indigenous medicinal plants. Indian J Med Res 63:378, 1975
36. Aguwa CN, Mittal GC: Abortifacient effects of the roots of *Momordica angustisepala*. Ethnopharmacol 7:169, 1983
37. Aref I, Hafez ESE: Postcoital contraception: physiological and clinical parameters. Obstet Gynecol Surv 32:417, 1977
38. Morris JM: Postcoital antifertility agents and their teratogenic effect. Contraception 2:185, 1970
39. Conner EA, Blake DA, Parmley TH, Burnett LS, King TM: Efficacy of various locally applied chemicals as contragestational agents in rats. Contraception 13:571, 1976
40. Garg SK: Effect of curcuma longa (Rhizomes) on fertility in experimental animals. Planta Med 26:225, 1974
41. Steinetz BG, Butler MC, Sawyer WK, O'Byrne EM: Effects of relaxin on early pregnancy in rats. Proc Soc Exp Biol Med 152:419, 1976
42. Vaughan MK, Reiter RJ, Vaughan GM: Fertility patterns in female mice following treatment with arginine vasotocin or melatonin. Int J Fertil 21:65, 1976
43. Wentz AC, Burnett LS, King TM: Techniques of pregnancy termination. Part I. Obstet Gynecol Surv 28:3, 1973
44. Burnett LS, King TM, Burkman RT, Atienza MF: An evaluation of abortion: techniques and protocols. Hosp Pract 10:97, 1975
45. Burnhill MS: Reducing complications of first-trimester abortion. Contemp Obstet Gynecol 13:145, 1979
46. Atienza MF, Burkman RT, King TM: Forces associated with cervical dilatation at suction abortion: qualitative and quantitative data in studies completed with a force-sensing instrument. In Dilatation of the Uterine Cervix, Edited by F Naftolin, PG Stubblefield. New York, Raven Press, 1980, p 343
47. Newton BW: Laminaria tent: relic of the past or modern medical device? Am J Obstet Gynecol 113:442, 1972
48. Hale RW, Pion RJ: Laminaria: an underutilized clinical adjunct. Clin Obstet Gynecol 15:829, 1972
49. Nicolaides KH, Welch CC, MacPherson MBA, Johnson LA: Lamicel: a new technique for cervical dilatation before first-trimester abortion. Br J Obstet Gynaecol 90:475, 1983
50. Brundin J, Christensen NJ, Fuchs T, Larsson M: The A-rod—a new possibility for cervical dilation and/or induction of uterine contractions for abortion or delivery by combined pharmacological and mechanical action. Acta Obstet Gynecol Scand (Suppl) 113:159, 1983
51. Hulka JF, Lefler HT, Anglone A, Lachenbruch PA: A new electronic force monitor to measure factors influencing cervical dilation for vacuum curettage. Am J Obstet Gynecol 120:166, 1974
52. Andolsek L: Experience with immediate post-abortal insertions of the IUD. In Proceedings of the Family Planning Research Conference, Edited by A Goldsmith, R Snowden. Amsterdam, Excerpta Medica Foundation, 1972, p 55
53. Burkman RT, Tonascia JA, Atienza MF, King TM: The relationship of immediate post-abortal intrauterine device insertion to subsequent endometritis: a case-control study. Contraception 15:435, 1977
54. Fehrmann H, Practorius B: The cervix-ripening effect of the prostaglandin E analogue sulprostone, before vacuum aspiration in first-trimester pregnancy. Acta Obstet Gynecol Scand (Suppl) 113:141, 1983
55. Uldbjererg N, Ekman G, Herltoft P, Malmstrom A, Ulmsten U, Wingerup L: Human cervical connective tissue and its reaction to prostaglandin E_2. Acta Obstet Gynecol Scand (Suppl) 113:163, 1983
56. Norstrom A, Wilhemsson L, Hamberger L: Experimental studies on the influence of prostaglandins on the connective tissue of the human cervix uteri. Acta Obstet Gynecol Scand (Suppl) 113:167, 1983
57. Keith LG, Method MW, Berger GS: Prevention of Rh immunization after spontaneous and induced abortion. In

Spontaneous Abortion, Edited by ESE Hafez. Lancaster, England, MTP Press, 1984, p 353

58. Tietze C: Induced Abortion, A World Review, 1983. New York, The Population Council, 1983, p 83
59. Grimes DA, Schulz KF, Cates W Jr: Prophylactic antibiotics for curettage abortion. Am J Obstet Gynecol 150:689, 1984
60. Grimes DA, Tyler CW Jr: Controversies concerning midtrimester dilatation and evacuation abortion. In Reid's Controversies in Obstetrics and Gynecology, Vol 3, Edited by FP Zuspan, CD Christian. Philadelphia, W. B. Saunders, 1983, p 386
61. Burkman RT, King TM: Second trimester termination of pregnancy. In Clinical and Diagnostic Procedures in Obstetrics and Gynecology. Part B: Gynecology, Edited by EM Symonds, FP Zuspan. New York, Marcel Dekker, Inc., 1984, p 241
62. Atienza MF, Burkman RT, Wight DJ, King TM: Ultrasonography in the management of the induced abortion. In Ultrasonography in Obstetrics and Gynecology, Edited by R Sanders. Norwalk, Appleton-Century-Crofts, 1977, p 123
63. Burnett LS, Wentz AC, King TM: Techniques of pregnancy termination. Part II. Obstet Gynecol Surv 29:6, 1974
64. Kerenyi TD: Hypertonic saline instillations in second trimester abortion: a global view. In Second Trimester Abortion: Perspectives after a Decade of Experience, Edited by GS Berger, WE Brenner, LG Keith. Littleton, Massachusetts, John Wright/PSG, 1981, p 79
65. Bygdeman M, Christensen NJ: Termination of second-trimester pregnancy by laminaria and intramuscular injections of 15-methyl PGF2 alpha or 16-phenoxy-omega-17, 18, 19, 20-tetranor PGE2 methyl sulfonylamide: a randomized study. Acta Obstet Gynecol Scand 62:535, 1983
66. Bygdeman M, Christensen N, Green K, Vesterqvist O, Roseman TJ, Tuttle ME, Spilman CH: Menses induction and second-trimester pregnancy termination using a polymeric controlled release vaginal delivery system containing (15S)15-methyl PGF2 alpha methyl ester. Contraception 27:141, 1983
67. World Health Organization Task Force on the Use of Prostaglandin for the Regulation of Fertility: Repeated vaginal administration of 15-methyl $PGF_{2\alpha}$ methyl ester for termination of pregnancy in the 13th-20th week of gestation. Contraception 16:175, 1977
68. Kajanoja P: Induction of abortion by prostaglandins in the second trimester of pregnancy. Acta Obstet Gynecol Scand (Suppl) 113:145, 1983
69. Burkman RT, Dubin NH, King TM: The use of hyperosmolar urea for elective abortion of midtrimester pregnancy. In Pregnancy Termination, Procedures, Safety and New Developments, Edited by GI Zatuchni, JJ Sciarra, JJ Speidel. Hagerstown, Harper & Row, 1979, p 261
70. King TM, Burkman RT, Atienza MF: Hyperosmolar urea as a midtrimester abortifacient. In Risks, Benefits and Controversies in Fertility Control, Edited by J Sciarra, GI Zatuchni, JJ Speidel. Hagerstown, Harper & Row, 1977, p 322
71. Grimes DA, Schulz KF, Cates W Jr, Tyler CW Jr: Midtrimester abortion by dilatation and evacuation. N Engl J Med 296:1141, 1977
72. Cates W Jr: D & E after 12 weeks: safe or hazardous? Contempt Obstet Gynecol 13:23, 1979
73. Crist T, Williams P, Lee SH, Hulka JF: Midtrimester pregnancy termination: a study of the cost effectiveness of dilation and evacuation in a free-standing facility. NC Med J 44:549, 1983
74. Kafrissen ME, Schulz KF, Grimes DA, Cates W Jr: Midtrimester abortion. Intra-amniotic instillation of hyperosmolar urea and prostaglandin $F_{2\alpha}$ versus dilatation and evacuation. JAMA 251:916, 1984
75. Hern WM: Serial multiple laminaria and adjunctive urea in late outpatient dilatation and evacuation abortion. Obstet Gynecol 63:543, 1984
76. Speroff L, Cates W Jr, Anderson G, Barr M: Is there a best way to do midtrimester abortions? Contemp Obstet Gynecol 13:106, 1979
77. Tyler CW Jr: Epidemiology of abortion. J Reprod Med 26:459, 1981
78. Tietze C, Lewit S: Early medical complications of abortion by saline: Joint Program for the Study of Abortion (JPSA). Stud Fam Plann 4:133, 1973
79. Burkman RT, Atienza MF, King TM, Burnett LS: The management of midtrimester abortion failures by vaginal evacuation. Obstet Gynecol 49:233, 1977
80. Grimes DA, Kafrissen ME, O'Reilly KR, Binkin NJ: Fatal hemorrhage from legal abortion in the United States. Surg Gynecol Obstet 157:461, 1983
81. Kafrissen ME, Barke MW, Workman P, Schulz KF, Grimes DA: Coagulopathy and induced abortion methods: rates and relative risks. Am J Obstet Gynecol 147:344, 1983
82. Spence MR, King TM, Burkman RT, Atienza MF: Cephalothin prophylaxis for midtrimester abortion. Obstet Gynecol 60:502, 1982
83. Burkman RT, Atienza MF, King TM, Burnett LS: Intra-amniotic urea and prostaglandin $F_{2\alpha}$ for midtrimester abortion: a modified regimen. Am J Obstet Gynecol 126:328, 1976
84. Garbaciak JA Jr, Benzie RJ: Hypertonic saline as an abortifacient in a select group of patients. Obstet Gynecol 61:37, 1983
85. Binkin NJ, Schulz KF, Grimes DA, Cates W Jr: Urea-prostaglandin versus hypertonic saline for instillation abortion. Am J Obstet Gynecol 146:947, 1983
86. World Health Organization: Induced abortion. Geneva, WHO Tech Rep Ser 623, 1978
87. Daling JR, Weiss NS, Voigt L, Spadoni LR, Soderstrom R, Moore DE, Stadel BV: Tubal infertility in relation to prior induced abortion. Fertil Steril 43:389, 1985
88. World Health Organization, Task Force on Sequelae of Abortion, Special Programme of Research, Development and Research Training in Human Reproduction: Secondary infertility following induced abortion. Stud Fam Plann 15:291, 1984
89. Hogue CJ, Cates W Jr, Tietze C: The effect of induced abortion on subsequent reproduction. Epidemiol Rev 4:66, 1982
90. Hogue CJ, Cates W Jr, Tietze C: Impact of vacuum aspiration abortion on future childbearing: a review. Fam Plann Perspect 15:119, 1983
91. Greer HS, Lal S, Lewis SC: Psychosocial consequences of therapeutic abortion. King's termination study III. Br J Psychiatry 128:74, 1976

92. Henshaw SK, Forrest JD, Blaine E: Abortion services in the United States, 1981 and 1982. Fam Plann Perspect 16:119, 1984

93. Henshaw SK, Binkin NJ, Blaine E, Smith JC: A portrait of American women who obtain abortions. Fam Plann Perspect 17:90, 1985

Chapter 35

Quinacrine nonsurgical female sterilization: a reassessment of safety and efficacy

Elton Kessel, M.D., M.P.H.
Jaime Zipper, M.D.
Stephen D. Mumford, Dr.P.H., M.P.H.

International Federation for Family Health, Chapel Hill, North Carolina, Hospital Sotero del Rio, Puente Alto, Chile, and Center for Research on Population and Security, Research Triangle Park, North Carolina

Sterilization is currently the most prevalent contraceptive method in the world; the demand for female sterilization, especially in developing countries, is likely to sharply rise in the remainder of this decade.[1] The need for a safe, inexpensive, and effective method of female sterilization to meet this need is a high priority for fertility research. The acceptable nonsurgical female sterilization method has been described as one that is safe, 95% effective, that can be performed by nonphysicians on an outpatient basis after a brief training period, and that requires only a single visit by the woman.[2]

The transcervical quinacrine pellet method developed by Zipper and co-workers,[3] which utilizes an intrauterine device inserter to deposit 250 mg of quinacrine hydrochloride as pellets in the uterine cavity, has potential for meeting this description. Prehysterectomy studies of the quinacrine pellet method in women showed that quinacrine produces inflammation and fibrosis that is confined primarily to the intramural portion of the fallopian tube.[4]

This method can be performed by nonphysicians on an outpatient basis after a brief training period or by any personnel capable of performing an intrauterine device insertion. In the studies of the quinacrine pellet method for female sterilization reported to date,[5-7] the method appears to be quite safe. No complications or side effects, other than temporary pain and oligomenorrhea, have been reported. However, greater experience is needed to ensure that there will not be a rare, serious complication.

The method does appear to be 95% effective after 3 years[6]; this is with three insertions of quinacrine pellets, each 1 month apart. However, a survey of the literature reveals that three insertions of the pellets has never been clinically shown to be superior to a single insertion.

Both the safety and effectiveness of the quinacrine pellet method must be judged in comparison to surgical methods. In this article, we reexamine reported complications and pregnancy failures of surgical methods and the quinacrine method of female sterilization in order to evaluate each method's relative safety; we also examine the presently assumed need for multiple insertions of quinacrine pellets for the achievement of acceptable efficacy.

RELATIVE SAFETY OF THE QUINACRINE PELLET METHOD

We studied three parameters in order to examine the relative safety of the quinacrine pellet female sterilization method. These were toxicology, complications, and mortality.

TOXICOLOGY

Toxicology studies were previously performed and approved by the United States Food and Drug Administration for premarketing requirements of quinacrine used orally as a malaria suppressant drug during World War II by millions of soldiers in the dose of 100 mg daily. In this extensive experience, there were a few cases of dermatitis and rare cases of convulsions or transient toxic psychosis reported; the only common side effect was discoloration of skin after chronic use.[8]

Toxicology studies of the quinacrine sterilization method in cynomolgus monkeys were encouraging with twice the comparative human dose in the form of a solution for both intravascular and intrauterine administration.[9, 10] Quinacrine was localized in nuclei of epithelial and stromal cells of the endometrium and in epithelial cells of the intramural section of the tube after intrauterine administration, which is consistent with reports that quinacrine intercalates with deoxyribonucleic acid.[11] This however does not appear to be the basis of tissue damage, because quinacrine was detected by histofluorescence in nuclei of these tissues after intravascular quinacrine administration with no histologic damage to any reproductive tissue observed at 24 hours. Within 1 month all tissue levels of quinacrine were at or near the limit of detection.

Intraperitoneal placement of 250 mg of quinacrine pellets in cynomolgus monkeys (approximately 15 times the human dose by body weight) has caused death in two of three monkeys.[12] Blood levels in these monkeys were even higher than those for intravascular administration of quinacrine. No deaths occurred among three monkeys that received 125 mg of quinacrine pellets intraperitoneally. These findings are relevant to possible accidental perforation of the uterus in clinical use of the quinacrine pellet method.

COMPLICATIONS

No serious complications or side effects have been reported to date in over 1000 insertions of quinacrine pellets.[5-7] Earlier studies with a liquid slurry of 1500 mg of quinacrine did produce a 2% rate of transient toxic psychosis shortly after quinacrine instillation, but this has not appeared with the 250-mg quinacrine pellet method.[3] An additional aspect of safety is the complications related to pregnancy failures. Of greatest concern in pregnancy failures is the risk of ectopic pregnancy.

Unlike failures of surgical methods, there is no increase in expected rate of ectopic pregnancy among failures of the quinacrine method. In published reports of pregnancy failures after transcervical application of quinacrine as a slurry or as pellets involving 1723 women, there were 125 pregnancies, of which only 1 (0.8%) was an ectopic pregnancy.[5-7, 13-15] This rate is not significantly different from the expected rate of 1 in 200 to 300 pregnancies in a noncontracepting population.

The ectopic pregnancy rate reported by Chi and co-workers[16] was 7.7% among 194 failures of surgical sterilization methods followed up for 6 months or more in 23,600 women enrolled in clinical studies at the International Fertility Research Program. This rate is probably conservative in view of other reports of higher rates.[17, 18]

The pattern of failures for the quinacrine pellet and the surgical methods are quite different. In the case of surgical methods, the intrauterine pregnancy failure rate declines with time since sterilization, whereas the ectopic pregnancy rate remains constant over time.[16] However, in marked contrast, in the case of the quinacrine pellet method, the intrauterine pregnancy failure rate is constant with time since sterilization,[6] whereas ectopic pregnancies are rare.

Both this difference in pattern of failures resulting in intrauterine pregnancy and the absence of increased risk of ectopic pregnancy for the quinacrine method point to a different biologic process involved in at least some failures of the surgical and quinacrine methods of sterilization.

A possible explanation for these differences in ectopic rates is that surgical sterilization method failures that are ectopic involve fistulae formation secondary to endometriosis in the tubal stump.[19] Extensive damage to the tubal muscularis is likely required for this process, because there is a greater probability of ectopic pregnancy among electrocoagulation-method failures.[18, 20]

It is likely that fistulae formation is more important in ectopic pregnancy failures than in intrauterine pregnancy failures after surgical methods of sterilization. Fistulae require time to develop, and there is an increase in the number of fistulae found in the medial tubal stump with time. There is also a delay in the appearance of ectopic pregnancies compared with intrauterine pregnancy failures after surgical sterilization.[16] Sperm are more likely to traverse the fistula and fertilize the egg in the distal segment of the tube than the egg is to traverse the fistula, which is necessary for intrauterine pregnancy. Indeed, ectopic pregnancies after surgical sterilization are generally found in the distal tubal segment.[21]

Apparently, if there is recovery from the insult of quinacrine to the fallopian tubes, it is relatively complete or in some women there is a way that the tubes are protected from the insult of exposure to quinacrine. The fact that the intramural fibrosis of the quinacrine method in no way interrupts the continuity of the tubal muscularis and leaves no tubal stump to receive an endometrial implant to start a process of endometriosis may explain the absence of increased risk of ectopic pregnancy in failures of the quinacrine method.

In comparing risks of ectopic pregnancy after surgical versus quinacrine pellet methods of sterilization, the following estimates can serve as a guide. At the end of the first year, surgical methods have an ectopic pregnancy rate of approximately 0.75/1000 procedures, which rises to approximately 2.15/1000 procedures at the end of the second year.[16] For the quinacrine pellet method, which has a uterine pregnancy rate of 31/1000 at 1 year[3] and 43/1000 at the end of the second year,[6] the ectopic pregnancy rate is approximately 1/125 pregnancies, or 0.24/1000 sterilizations, at the end of the first year and 0.34/1000 at the end of the second year. These rates are one third and one sixth those of surgical procedures.

In an analysis of 14,910 surgical sterilization procedures, a complication rate of 15/1000 has been reported.[22] However, in this large series none of the complications were nearly as serious as ectopic pregnancy. The surgical sterilization morbidity of 2.15 ectopic pregnancies/1000 procedures should have been added to the 15/1000 other lesser early complications of surgical sterilization. The lower ectopic pregnancy rate of the quinacrine pellet method and the virtual absence of reported serious complications of the method to date would make the quinacrine pellet method favorable except that experience with the method is, as yet, too limited.

MORTALITY

The mortality attributable to sterilization depends upon mortality of the sterilization procedure, maternal mortality related to procedure failure ending in abortion or delivery, and the case fatality of ectopic pregnancies among failures of the procedure. There are marked differences in these risks both for surgical sterilization versus nonsurgical quinacrine sterilization and for developing versus developed countries.

Table 1 illustrates the contrasts in estimated mortality associated with surgical female sterilization and quinacrine nonsurgical female sterilization procedures for Bangladesh and the United States. The surgical procedure mortality estimates are taken from Peterson and co-workers.[23]* We have already estimated the incidence of ectopic pregnancies for the surgical and nonsurgical procedures. The case/fatality rate for ectopic pregnancy in the United States is estimated at 0.08%.[24] Reliable estimates of ectopic pregnancy case/fatality rates do not exist for developing countries. We have applied a rate of 5% for Bangladesh, which is in the same ratio as the reported maternal mortality rates for Bangladesh (570 deaths/100,000 live births)[25] and the United States (7.9 deaths/100,000 live births).[26] This estimate is further supported by the report of Begum,[30] who found a mortality rate of 5.1% among all ectopic pregnancy cases admitted to Dhaka Medical College Hospital in Dhaka, Bangladesh in 1984. The delivery/abortion mortality is calculated by applying the maternal mortality rates to the failures for surgical sterilization, estimated at 0.5%,[22] and for quinacrine nonsurgical sterilization, estimated at 5%.[6]

Table 1. *Estimated Deaths Attributed to Surgical Female Sterilization and Nonsurgical Quinacrine Female Sterilization in Bangladesh and the United States (Per 100,000 Procedures)*

	Surgical sterilization		Nonsurgical sterilization	
	Bangladesh	U.S.	Bangladesh	U.S.
Procedure mortality	19.0	4.0	0.0[a]	0.0[a]
Ectopic pregnancy mortality	10.7	0.2	1.7	< 0.1
Delivery/abortion mortality	2.9	< 0.1	28.5	0.4
Attributable mortality	32.6	4.2	30.2	0.4

[a]Based on limited published reports (see text).

The contrasts by both method and country are dramatic. One third of attributable surgical sterilization mortality is due to ectopic pregnancy in Bangladesh, whereas this accounts for < 5% of

*The estimated rate of surgical sterilization mortality of 0.19/1000 procedures is probably conservative for the Indian subcontinent. Other reports have estimated the rate as five times greater in this region.[27, 28] A lower rate of 0.06/1000 procedures was reported to the International Project of the Association for Voluntary Sterilization in a survey of their funded projects worldwide that had performed 225,812 female sterilizations.[29] This lower rate probably involves both greater underreporting of deaths from service programs without an active surveillance system and actual lower rates in developing countries with better staffing and facilities.

attributable mortality in the United States. The lower ectopic pregnancy and procedure mortality of the quinacrine method in Bangladesh is offset by the method's higher failure rate and the country's high maternal mortality for abortion and delivery. This offset could, however, be moderated by the provision of safe menstrual regulation services for failures of this method. For the United States, a tenfold reduction in attributable sterilization mortality would be expected with the use of the quinacrine pellet method. These estimates are, of course, based on limited experience to date with the quinacrine pellet method.

The main advantage for a country like Bangladesh in using the quinacrine pellet method, besides its lower cost, is its potential for extension of present sterilization services. If two pregnancies are prevented by each sterilization procedure, then over 1000 maternal mortalities (roughly twice the maternal mortality rate) would be prevented for each 100,000 quinacrine pellet sterilizations performed as compared to the method's attributable mortality of 30.2/100,000 procedures. For countries with intermediate maternal mortality and ectopic case mortality between that of Bangladesh and the United States, the quinacrine pellet method has an advantage in terms of reproductive mortality even without consideration of its lower cost or potential for expansion of sterilization services. Again, these projections are based on the limited experience we have with the quinacrine pellet method. But it is also clear from this analysis that the method would have to have a very high procedure mortality in future experience in order to overcome its present apparent favorable risk/benefit ratio in either developing or developed countries.

MULTIPLE QUINACRINE PELLET INSERTIONS

The need for multiple applications of quinacrine for the achievement of a reasonable level of efficacy was demonstrated for the quinacrine liquid slurry formulation.[15] Rates of tubal obstruction, as evidenced by CO_2 insufflation tests, were 54.9% after one instillation and 57.1% after a second instillation 1 month later among those women with tubal patency after one instillation, resulting in a cumulative nonpatency rate of 87.7%.[15] Further evidence for the need of multiple instillations of the quinacrine slurry are the pregnancies occurring between instillations in a three-instillation study.[3] Among 240 women who received a first instillation, 18 became pregnant before the second instillation. An additional 23 women became pregnant before the third instillation. Even after the third instillation, the life-table pregnancy rate was 9.1/100 women at 1 year.[3]

Experience with transcervical insertions of quinacrine pellets is remarkably different. In Zipper and co-workers' first report of 139 women, there was only one pregnancy between the first and second insertion and none between the second and third insertion of quinacrine pellets.[3] The pregnancy rate at 1 year after the third insertion was 3.1.[3] Additional experience confirms both the low pregnancy rate after 1 year and the marked reduction in pregnancies between quinacrine pellet insertions compared with that of quinacrine slurry instillations.[5-7] The combined experience of Zipper and Guzman-Serani and their co-workers[5, 6] shows that among 454 women entering their quinacrine pellet studies of three monthly insertions, 5 women became pregnant between insertions and 1-year pregnancy rates after the third insertion ranged from 0.7/100 women to 4.3/100 women. It appears that pregnancy failures between quinacrine pellet insertions would only marginally affect efficacy of the method. The question remains as to what contribution the second and third quinacrine pellet insertions make to efficacy of this method. This question has not been studied. Only a prospective study of one insertion of quinacrine pellets can provide the answer.

The increased efficacy of quinacrine pellets over the quinacrine slurry is probably related to a more prolonged high concentration of quinacrine in the uterine cavity for the pellets. The pellets used in the referenced studies have a 10-minute release time. Prolongation of this release time may be accompanied by a decline in concentration of quinacrine if quinacrine absorption through the endometrium is greater than the release rate. Studies in cynomolgus monkeys of 800-minute and 7-day quinacrine release preparations showed no damage to the fallopian tubes,[31] whereas a quinacrine slurry or 10-minute pellets did damage the tubes of the cynomolgus monkey.[9, 32] It is likely that the most efficacious release rate for quinacrine pellets lies somewhere between 10 and 800 minutes, but it could also be somewhat less than 10 minutes. Prospective studies in female volunteers are needed to determine the optimal release rate of quinacrine.

The reexamination of the assumption that three monthly insertions of quinacrine pellets are necessary for acceptable efficacy points to an urgent need for a prospective study of one insertion of quinacrine pellets.

CONCLUSIONS

The relative safety and efficacy of surgical methods and nonsurgical quinacrine pellet methods of female sterilization have been reassessed. Although experience with the quinacrine pellet method is limited, it appears to have advantages for both developing and developed countries. Its failure rate at 3 years after three transcervical insertions of 250 mg of quinacrine in pellets is approximately 5%, compared with 0.5% for surgical sterilization. But the method can be delivered in any clinical setting capable of performing an intrauterine device insertion. The absence of increased risk of ectopic pregnancy among quinacrine pellet method failures has been noted. It is estimated that ectopic pregnancy accounts for one third of surgical sterilization mortality in a country like Bangladesh, whereas it accounts for < 5% of sterilization mortality in the United States.

The need for multiple insertions of quinacrine pellets for the achievement of acceptable efficacy has not been demonstrated clinically. A single insertion trial is a high priority for fertility research.

REFERENCES

1. Kessel E, Mumford SD: Potential demand for voluntary female sterilization in the 1980s: the compelling need for a nonsurgical method. Fertil Steril 37:725, 1982
2. Klitsch M: Sterilization without surgery. Int Fam Plann Perspect 8:101, 1982
3. Zipper J, Cole LP, Goldsmith A, Wheeler R, Rivera M: Quinacrine hydrochloride pellets: preliminary data on a nonsurgical method of female sterilization. Int J Gynaecol Obstet 18:275, 1980
4. Bhatt RV, Aparicio A, Laufe LE, Parmley T, King TM: Quinacrine-induced pathologic changes in the fallopian tube. Fertil Steril 33:666, 1980
5. Zipper J, Edelman D, Cole LP, Rivera M: Overview of clinical trials with quinacrine. In Female Transcervical Sterilization: Proceedings of an International Workshop on Nonsurgical Methods of Female Tubal Occlusion, Chicago, Illinois, June 24, 1982, Edited by GI Zatuchni, JD Shelton, A Goldsmith, JJ Sciarra. Hagerstown, Harper & Row, 1983, p 94
6. Guzman-Serani R, Bernales A, Cole LP: Quinacrine hydrochloride pellets: three-year follow-up on a nonsurgical method of female sterilization. Contracept Deliv Syst 5:131, 1983
7. Raj A, Chakravarty S: Permanent female sterilization by chemical method of transcervical insertion of quinacrine. In Proceedings of the Third International Seminar on Maternal and Perinatal Mortality, Pregnancy Termination and Sterilization, Edited by V Hingorani, RD Pandit, VL Bhargava. New Delhi, New Roxy Press, 1980, p 476
8. Steck EA: Chemotherapy of Protozoan Disease, Vol III. Washington, D.C., Walter Reed Army Institute of Research, U.S. Government Printing Office, 1972, p 23
9. Dubin NH, Strandberg JD, Craft CF, Parmley TH, Blake DA, King TM: Effect of intrauterine and intravascular quinacrine administration on histopathology, blood chemistry, and hematology in cynomolgus monkeys. Fertil Steril 38:741, 1982
10. Dubin NH, Blake DA, DiBlasi MC, Parmley TH, King TM: Pharmacokinetic studies on quinacrine following intrauterine administration to cynomolgus monkeys. Fertil Steril 38:735, 1982
11. Wershlem B, deHaseth PL: Quinacrine, a chromosome stain specific for deoxyadenylate-deoxythymidylate-rich regions in DNA. Proc Natl Acad Sci USA 69:629, 1972
12. Dubin NH, Parmley TH, DiBlasi MC, Ghodgaonkar RB, Jiffry MTM, Blake DA, King TM: Pharmacology of quinacrine hydrochloride with emphasis on its use as a tubal occluding agent. In Female Transcervical Sterilization: Proceedings of an International Workshop on Nonsurgical Methods of Female Tubal Occlusion, Chicago, Illinois, June 24, 1982, Edited by GI Zatuchni, JD Shelton, A Goldsmith, JJ Sciarra. Hagerstown, Harper & Row, 1983, p 60
13. Israngkun D, Phaosavadi S, Neuwirth RS, Richart RM: Clinical evaluation of quinacrine hydrochloride for sterilization of the human female. Contraception 14:75, 1976
14. Mehtaji S, Jadwani K, Goyal V: Chemical sterilization with quinacrine. In Fourth Transaction of Scientific Papers, Edited by S Pachauri. Bombay, India Fertility Research Programme, 1977, p 167
15. Zipper J, Stacchetti E, Medel M: Transvaginal chemical sterilization: clinical use of quinacrine plus potentiating adjuvants. Contraception 12:11, 1975
16. Chi I-c, Laufe LE, Atwood RJ: Ectopic pregnancies following female sterilization procedures. Adv Plann Parent 16:52, 1981
17. Cheng MCE, Wong YM, Rochat RW, Ratnam SS: Sterilization failures in Singapore: an examination of ligation techniques and failure rates. Stud Fam Plann 8:109, 1977
18. Phillips JM, Hulka J, Hulka B, Keith L: American Association of Gynecologic Laparoscopists, 1976 membership survey. J Reprod Med 21:3, 1978
19. Rock JA, Parmley TH, King TM, Laufe LE, Su BC: Endometriosis and the development of tuboperitoneal fistulas after tubal ligation. Fertil Steril 35:16, 1981
20. McCausland A: High rate of ectopic pregnancy following laparoscopic tubal coagulation failures. Am J Obstet Gynecol 138:97, 1980
21. Qvigstad E, Jerve F: Ectopic pregnancy following tubal sterilization. Int J Gynaecol Obstet 20:279, 1982
22. Mumford SD, Bhiwandiwala PP, Chi I-c: Laparoscopic and minilaparotomy female sterilization compared in 15,167 cases. Lancet 2:1066, 1980

23. Peterson HB, Lubell I, DeStefano F, Ory HW: The safety and efficacy of tubal sterilization: an international overview. Int J Gynaecol Obstet 21:139, 1983
24. Dorfman SF: Deaths from ectopic pregnancy, United States, 1979 to 1980. Obstet Gynecol 62:334, 1983
25. Chen LC, Gesche MC, Ahmed S, Chowdury AI, Mosley WH: Maternal mortality in rural Bangladesh. Stud Fam Plann 5:334, 1974
26. Advance Report on Final Mortality Statistics, 1982. Monthly Vital Statistics Report 33(9):38, 1984
27. Rosenberg MJ, Rochat RW, Akbar J, Gould P, Khan AR, Measham A, Jabeen S: Sterilization in Bangladesh: mortality, morbidity, and risk factors. Int J Gynaecol Obstet 20:283, 1982
28. Bhatt RV, Pachauri S, Pathak ND, Chauhan L: Female sterilization in small camp settings in rural India. Stud Fam Plann 9:39, 1978
29. Aubert JM, Lubell I, Schima M: Mortality risk associated with female sterilization. Int J Gynaecol Obstet 18:406, 1980
30. Begum SF: Unpublished data
31. Zaneveld LJD, Goldsmith A: Lack of tubal occlusion by intrauterine quinacrine and tetracycline in the primate. Contraception 30:164, 1984
32. Dubin NH, Parmley TH, Ghodgaonkar RB, Strandberg JD, Rosenshein NB, King TM: Effect of intrauterine administration of tetracycline on cynomolgus monkeys. Contraception 29:561, 1984

Chapter 36

Reversibility of female sterilization

Alvin M. Siegler, M.D., D.Sc.
Jaroslav Hulka, M.D.
Alik Peretz, M.D.

State University of New York, Downstate Medical Center, Brooklyn, New York, The University of North Carolina, Chapel Hill, North Carolina, and Rambam Medical Center, Haifa, Bat-Galim, Israel

Sterilization has been incorporated into fertility management techniques in a major way in the past decade. Over 6 million women have been sterilized in the United States, and sterilization is the most common contraceptive method for women over the age of 30.[1] The safety and efficacy of sterilization is unsurpassed by any other contraceptive method, which accounts for its popularity. Half of the sterilizations each year are performed on women under the age of 30,[2] and these are the ones most likely to return later with a request for reversal, usually because of divorce and remarriage.[3 7]

It has been estimated that about 1% of all sterilized women subsequently seek reversal, or about 5000 annually.[8] Because of the widespread acceptance of sterilization and the accompanying problem of requests for reversal, in this section we will review the current status of reversibility of sterilization in the United States and describe both clinical and experimental efforts for developing techniques designed for reversibility.

REGRET AFTER STERILIZATION

Regret is the first stage of reversal. It is clear that a request for sterilization reversal (SR) does not always mean regret for a decision made at the time. Quite often it is a wish to restore fertility because life circumstances have changed after a sterilization that was appropriate at the time it was done.[9]

Schwyhart and Kutner[10] reviewed 22 studies published between 1949 and 1969 in which they found that the percentage of patients regretting the procedure ranged from 1.3% to 15%. The highest dissatisfaction occurred in women who had less than four children and those in whom sterilization was performed with abortion. Marital instability, recent loss of a child, inability to accept the loss, psychologic factors, religious concerns, and misconceptions about the sterilization were considered significant contributing factors. Lack of womanhood, purposeless sexual relations, and increasing guilt over the inability to conceive were other causes for the unhappiness about the sterilization.

Requests for reversal are still quite low in most countries, but if sterilization becomes a more popular method for contraception throughout the world, requests will also increase. The reasons cited are similar from country to country, most frequently being remarriage after divorce or death of the husband, death of one or more children, an improved economic situation, and a psychologic desire to overcome supposed ill effects of tubal sterilization.[3-7, 11, 12]

REVERSAL POTENTIAL OF CURRENT STERILIZATION TECHNIQUES

The ideal operation considered as a reversible method of sterilization should include an easy, reliable outpatient method of tubal occlusion with minimal risk or patient discomfort that subsequently could be reversed without the need for a major surgical intervention. Endoscopic methods have advanced toward the first objective. Although the success of reversing some of these procedures in selected instances is high, the second operation designed to restore normal tubal patency is not easy. The impact of microsurgery in gynecology has involved repair of previously sterilized tubes; and under ideal circumstances, ~ 60% of patients operated upon subsequently achieve a term pregnancy. However, one of the dangers of such success can leave the impression with patients or physicians that sterilization is not to be considered permanent. Success cannot be guaranteed, and extrauterine pregnancies occur with increased frequency in repaired tubes.

A true reversibility rate of a particular sterilization technique can only be ascertained by including all women who consulted a gynecologist primarily for that purpose. Some are dissuaded in continuing the pursuit after learning of the need for major surgery, infertility studies, laparoscopy, and the general preoperative workup. Antoine et al.,[13] in a retrospective study, analyzed 377 requests for reversal and noted that 40% were turned down because of too much tubal destruction. Winston[7] also drew attention to the discrepancy between reversal requests and reversals performed. Although he noted that 7 of 15 of his patients conceived after tubal cornual anastomosis (after unipolar coagulation), he screened 40 women to find the 15 in whom there was sufficient tube to make an attempt at reversal worthwhile, for a reversal rate among those seeking reversal of 18%.

Reversibility also needs to be viewed in the context of current sterilization practices in the United States. About half of the annual sterilizations (250,000) are performed as postpartum procedures, usually by the Pomeroy method. The most mobile portion of the tube (usually at or distal to the isthmic ampullary junction) is removed. Specimens consist of 1 to 2 cm of the excised and contracted segment. About 3 cm of tube is destroyed because of tissue resorption around the ligated stumps. Both operative and pathology reports are essential before reversal is attempted because of the wide variation in the "standard" Pomeroy technique.

The American Association of Gynecologic Laparoscopists conducted surveys of their members; the results showed that bipolar coagulation has replaced the unipolar method within the past 3 years as the most common laparoscopic sterilization technique.[14] At least two contiguous areas of tube are coagulated in the most mobile portion, each resulting in destruction of ~ 1 cm. As the tube contracts during the coagulation, additional destruction occurs, so that > 2 cm is eventually damaged. Subsequent repairs usually require an isthmic-ampullary anastomosis, although some reversals involve tubal implantation because of the extension of the thermal injury into the uterus.

Although bipolar coagulation has replaced the unipolar method for the most part, many women now seeking reversal had undergone sterilization when the unipolar technique was the more common.[15] The mobile tubal segment was grasped and coagulated, with unpredictable results because of the wide variety of generators and forceps. In addition, some physicians advocated tubal division and additional coagulation of the stump. Consequently, operative reports of sterilization with coagulation cannot be used to predict the feasibility of reversal.[16] Preoperative laparoscopy is essential.

The Silastic band type is the most frequently performed noncoagulation method of laparoscopic sterilization. The tubal segment, ~ 3 cm from its uterine origin, is drawn to a depth of 1.4 cm into the hollow metal cylinder. About 3 cm of tube is destroyed above the band, which is released below the drawn loop. Although the amount of tube destroyed is fairly consistent, operative reports are essential because occasionally multiple banding is required, and even coagulation to control bleeding has been reported.

The spring clip is applied across the isthmus ~ 1 to 2 cm from its uterine origin. The clip is 4 mm wide, and, if one allows for resorption of crushed tissue adjacent to the clip, ~ 1 cm of tube is destroyed. Some patients have more than one clip applied to each tube, thus extending the damage. It is advisable to read the operative report of the sterilization to confirm the clip technique. As with other noncoagulation methods, a preoperative laparoscopy is not necessary.

SELECTION OF PATIENTS

It is occasionally difficult to decide whether to accept the challenge to reverse a tubal sterilization previously meant to be permanent. While the chances for success may be acceptable to the patient, the surgeon's enthusiasm should be tempered by experience with the procedure,[17] the patient's general health, and the couple's potential for fertility.

The only criterion for a successful reversal is a term pregnancy. The results are influenced by the amount of remaining tube,[5, 18] the location of the anastomosis,[5, 19, 20] and the experience of the surgeon.[17] The more tubal segment destroyed, the less the chance for a successful reconstruction.

The influence of the age of the patient is difficult to evaluate. Increasing age is associated with longer intervals since sterilization, ovulatory disturbances, and older partners. In the absence of such cofactors, counseling as to medical and social implications of parenthood at or beyond age 40 is appropriate.

Electron-microscopic studies have shown relative atrophy of the tubal epithelium in the proximal stumps of women sterilized more than 5 years prior to reversal.[21] The secretory and ciliary action of the cells are important in sperm and ovum transport, and chronic unrelieved intratubal pressure in these closed stumps may result in dcreased fertility. Although most all women seeking reversal have experienced pregnancy and are therefore documented to have ovulated, normal ovulation cannot be assumed to be present. Some forms of sterilization may alter luteal function, although this possibility is controversial.[22-25] Nevertheless, it is appropriate to document the presence of normal ovulation or easily inducible ovulation.

Although many requests for reversal come from couples in which the male has fathered children, intercurrent illness could affect sperm production. A normal semen analysis and postcoital test are recommended before attempting SR. If a significant male factor is present, donor insemination should be acceptable to the couple before SR. Whether or not to perform a laparoscopy as part of the screening workup appears to be controversial.[26] Most authors did not perform this endoscopic procedure except when sterilization was by coagulation or when the operative and pathology reports were unavailable or ambiguous.[4, 18, 19, 27-29] Mechanical methods (Pomeroy, band, clip) produce fairly consistent injuries, ranging from 1 to 3 cm of tube destroyed. More importantly, proximal isthmic stumps are almost always present, allowing for some form of anastomosis. If the operative report from the sterilization procedure is obtained and an uncomplicated mechanical method is documented, laparoscopic preoperative evaluation may be omitted because the findings are usually favorable for reversal. Both unipolar and bipolar methods inflict unpredictable tubal damage, from surprisingly minimal damage with unipolar to extensive destruction with bipolar methods. Because of this variability, a laparoscopic preoperative evaluation is advised. At laparoscopy, lengths of all four stumps should be estimated so that one can ascertain prognosis or success. Taylor and Leader[30] noted that 27% of patients whose operative pathology reports were quite precise following Pomeroy procedures were found at laparoscopy to have tubes < 4 cm in length or destroyed fimbria. In addition, Cooper et al.[31] suggested that hysteroscopy also be included in the preoperative workup because among women who came for hysteroscopic tubal sterilization, these authors noted a 13% frequency of intrauterine abnormalities.

CURRENT REVERSAL TECHNIQUES

The first operations to correct occluded tubes were described as either a type of salpingostomy or tubal implantation.[32] These were done to overcome inflammatory causes of obstruction. In 1908, Pearl and Surface[33] reported the first experimental end-to-end anastomosis following removal of 10 cm of a hen's oviduct. They approximated the cut ends with silk sutures inserted through all tubal layers. Subsequently the bird laid eggs. Christian and Sanderson,[34] in 1913, reported "successful" isthmic-isthmic anastomoses in three women, and they used "20-day" catgut as a temporary splint.

It is not the purpose of this article to review details of SR procedures other than to state that contemporary methods include some use of magnification, electrosurgery, atraumatic technique, and irrigation of the operative site, accurate approximation of tubal segments and placement of sutures, and the use of fine-gauge needles with nonreactive sutures.

Although it is logical to assume that after most tubal ligations the intramural segment remains normal and anastomosis is possible, both segments should be evaluated and tested intraoperatively prior to reconstruction. Rock et al.[28] found pathologic changes, including endometriosis and hydrosalpinx. Salpingitis isthmica nodosa, fibrosis, and chronic salpingitis also have been detected.[19]

Donnez and colleagues[35] reported histologic findings in 133 previously ligated tubes of women who subsequently had total abdominal hysterectomy and bilateral salpingo-oophorectomy. Dilatation of the proximal tubal lumen, flattening of folds, polyps, and increased mitotic activity of the epithelium were noted regardless of the type of sterilization. Focal endometriosis was found only after tubal ligation with coagulation. Epithelial inclusions were discovered as fragments of tubal epithelium translocated into the tubal wall during the procedure. This finding was increased after coagulation, ligation, and rings but decreased after clips. Endometriosis suggested implantation of expelled menstrual products through the open lumen into the healed ligated area. In 50%, mucosal modifications were represented by deciliation, loss of mucosal folds, and polyposis.

Vasquez et al.[21] did scanning electron microscopy studies on 26 specimens and generally noted increased abnormalities with increasing intervals between sterilization and SR. These included flattening of longitudinal folds, deciliation, and polyposis. Disorders in the tubal isthmus occurred with chronic occlusion. The operating microscope helped to define the extent of polyposis.

Restoration of tubal patency after surgical sterilization in which the luminal continuity has been interrupted requires either implantation of the patent distal segment or resection of the occluded ends and anastomosis of the patent adjacent segments. Anastomoses are classified as intramural-isthmic, intramural-ampullary, isthmic-isthmic, isthmic-ampullary, and ampullary-ampullary.

The techniques described for anastomosis include identification of the proximal obstructed end by instillation of colored solutions into the uterine cavity either by transfundal injection or through a previously placed intrauterine catheter. The distal obstruction is located by retrograde fimbrial perfusion with 1 to 2 ml of solution or gentle passage of a metal probe. The obstructed ends are resected with a small scalpel blade, microscissors, or microsurgical electrodes while selected hemostasis is obtained with electrocoagulation. Splints or nylon threads have been used to bridge the gap or facilitate the repair, and they can be removed postoperatively within a few days.[36] Sutures are inserted in two layers, sometimes without magnification, with the aid of loupes under magnification as high as 20 ×. Some investigators have included the endosalpinx with the repair, and others have excluded it. Patency of the anastomosis is tested by perfusion with a colored solution prior to the abdominal closure.

Prophylactic antibiotics, adjuvants to prevent postoperative adhesions, splints to maintain tubal patency or facilitate the anastomosis, and hydropertubation are of unproven value.

Besides anastomosis, isthmic and ampullary implantation have been used as methods of SR in patients whose intramural segments were occluded.[37] Ampullary salpingoneostomy is required to reverse a previous fimbriectomy.[38] Novy[39] suggested that such women should have at least 8 cm or more of tube, a positive rugal pattern on hysterosalpingogram, minimal peritubal adhesions, and an ampullary width of > 1 cm. Laparoscopy is essential in these patients prior to attempting SR.

RESULTS

There are an estimated 500,000 sterilizations done annually; possibly 5 million have been performed in the past decade. With all the interest in SR and the contributions on that subject to the literature, a recent search uncovered few series[4, 5, 20, 27, 28, 40, 41] of more than 50 cases (Table 1). The 767 operations were analyzed with regard to pregnancy outcome. The percent of live births varied from 47.0% to 78.8%, and the occurrence of tubal pregnancies ranged from 1.7% to 6.5%. A patient with SR has a slightly better than 50% chance of producing a term pregnancy, and the pregnancy will develop in the tube in ~ 4%. These results are significantly better than the 24% reported in a collected series of 201 cases reviewed by Siegler and Perez[42] in 1975. Only five other series of 25 or more cases of SR were found (Table 2).[18, 43-46] Following these 183 operations, intrauterine pregnancies were noted in

Table 1. *Reports of 50 or More Reversals of Sterilization*

Author	Year	No. of patients	Outcome							
			Pregnancy		Live births		Abortions		Tubal	
			No.	%	No.	%	No.	%	No.	%
McCormick et al.[27]	1979	53	33	62.0	25	47.0	—	—	8	15.0
Winston[20]	1980	126	76	60.4	—	73.0	—	58.0	3	2.4
Gomel[41]	1980	118	97	82.5	93	78.8	3	2.6	2	1.7
Rock et al.[28]	1982	125	81	65.0	62	50.0	14	11.0	5	4.0
DeCherney et al.[40]	1983	124	92	74.2	72	58.0	12	9.7	8	6.5
Schlösser et al.[5]	1983	119	72	60.5	44	37.0	11	9.2	3	2.5
Henderson[4]	1984	102	69	68.0	53	52.0	11	11.0	5	5.0
Total		767	520	67.7	349	54.4	51	8.6	34	4.4

about 45%, and almost 6% were tubal gestations. These results are not significantly different from the larger series reported in Table 1. Since there are estimates of about 5000 procedures performed annually and less than 1000 reported, it is obvious that most SR is done by the "silent majority" of gynecologists.

All of the confounding variables in patient selection and small numbers of reported procedures preclude any conclusion concerning the different techniques or the number of operations that give a surgeon a level of expertise. McCormick and co-workers[27] repaired only the better tube while reversing 50 of 53 previous Pomeroy operations. They used 4-0 chromic sutures in a 15-minute procedure.

Few authors[4, 5, 28, 46-49] classify their results of SR according to the original sterilization procedure (Table 3). The most commonly performed sterilization (Pomeroy) was the most frequently reported to have undergone a reversal attempt, with a 50% success rate based on term or intrauterine pregnancies. Electrocoagulation was the next most frequent technique for reversal, with a success rate of 41%. The less destructive mechanical techniques, clip and band, had a reversal rate of 84% and 72%, respectively. In interpreting these results, the disparity between patients requesting procedures and those undergoing procedures,[7, 13] especially after coagulation techniques, needs to be kept in mind.

These results can be summarized by a theoretic flow chart, presented in Figure 1. For every 1000 sterilizations performed, 3% of the patients regret the operation. A sequence of assumptions is presented revealing that consultation, infertility workup, laparoscopy, and ultimate sterilization reversal might yield six intrauterine pregnancies and one tubal pregnancy, and three women would not conceive.

Future reports should also include the number of women who seek reversal, who enter into a true screening procedure, and who actually are operated upon. The results should include all SR patients, even those lost to follow-up or followed for only 3 months (some women, ~ 10%, become pregnant within the first 3 postoperative months). It is important to report the number of patients who had live births and tubal pregnancies. Results should be expressed not only in absolute numbers but also with life-table analyses. With the information gathered today, there is insufficient evidence to state that the interval from sterilization to SR, the site of anastomosis, or the length of the

Table 2. *Reports of 25 to 49 Cases of Reversal of Sterilization*

Author	Year	No. of patients	Outcome					
			Pregnancy		Intrauterine		Tubal	
			No.	%	No.	%	No.	%
Silber and Cohen[18]	1980	25	15	60.0	14	56.0	1	4.0
Grunert et al.[45]	1981	40	24	59.0	23	57.0	1	2.5
Diamond et al.[43]	1982	46	25	54.0	23	50.0	2	4.0
Gantt et al.[44]	1982	40	16	40.0	10	25.0	6	15.0
Wittich[46]	1983	32	13	39.7	12	37.5	1	3.2
Total		183	93	50.8	82	44.8	11	6.0

Table 3. *Term or Intrauterine Pregnancies After Reversal of Different Sterilization Techniques*

Author	Year	No. of patients and intrauterine pregnancies (IUP)							
		Pomeroy		Coagulation		Ring		Clip	
		Done	IUP	Done	IUP	Done	IUP	Done	IUP
Pill et al.[48a]	1981	11	3	8	5	—	—	3	3
Henderson[4]	1984	47	27	33	14	6	5	—	—
Hulka et al.[47b]	1982	—	—	—	—	—	—	85	74
Rock et al.[28a]	1982	31	17	48	17	22	17	1	1
Wittich[46]	1983	14	7	12	4	3	1	—	—
Seiler[49]	1983	40	25	22	15	6	3	—	—
Schlösser et al.[5a]	1983	58	22	52	18	—	—	6	3
Total		201	101	175	73	37	26	91	77
Percentage		50%		41%		72%		84%	

[a]Term pregnancies only listed here.
[b]Gantt et al.[44] are included here.

reconstructed tube (if 4 cm or longer) can influence the outcome.

Although most patients achieve a successful pregnancy following SR, a significant number of failures occur. These can be caused by reocclusion, short tubes (< 3 cm), tubal disease in the newly joined segments, other infertility factors, poor surgical techniques, and inexperience.

The risks of SR, aside from the increased incidence of extrauterine pregnancy, are minimal. Most extrauterine pregnancies seem to occur 1 year or more after SR. Tubal pregnancy is not a partial success; indeed, it is a severe complication. Postoperative infectious morbidity is uncommon, and most fevers are caused by urinary tract or wound infections. No deaths have been reported in the literature. Delayed risks include tubal pregnancy and uterine rupture following tubal implantation. Peterson et al.,[37] in reporting on 8 full-term pregnancies after 16 implantations, stated that the major complication of the procedure was silent dehiscence of the uterine scar, noted at two sections. With this fact in mind, Shortle and Jewelewicz[50] recommended that all patients be clearly informed that the type of tuboplasty might justify a need for cesarean delivery. A clinician who manages the patient after a tuboplasty should consider the obstetric implications of a previous implantation. The authors[50] recommended the avoidance of oxytoxic compounds during labor and performance of elective cesarean section at 38 weeks or at the onset of labor. A more favorable outcome might be anticipated if the placental implantation site was along the anterior or posterior walls or low-lying, rather than in the cornual area, the probable site of the previous tubal implantation.

EXPERIMENTAL APPROACHES TO REVERSAL OF CURRENT TECHNIQUES OF STERILIZATION

Several investigators have been interested in ascertaining the effect of occlusive devices on fallopian tubes and in developing techniques for anastomosis. Boeckx and co-workers[51] applied Falope rings to rabbit oviducts and noted that 10% to 15% of the tube was lost in the ring. After

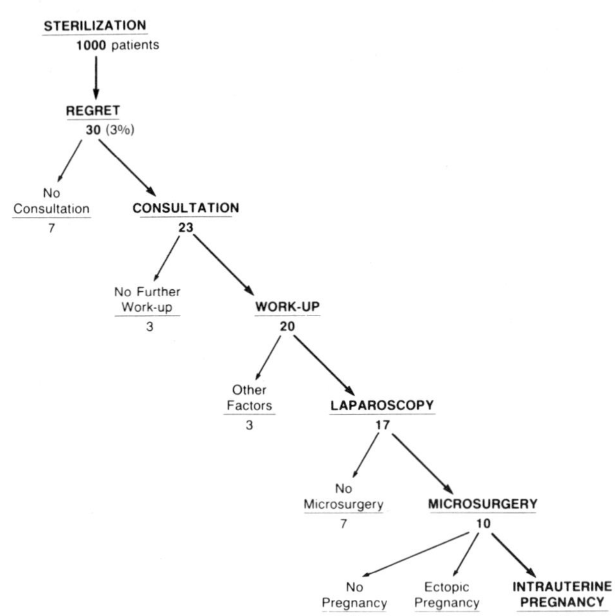

Figure 1
Theoretic flow chart for reversibility prognosis. This flow chart summarizes literature estimates concerning the stages of patient interest in reversing sterilization. Of 1000 patients undergoing sterilization, 1% (10 patients) would be suitable candidates for microsurgical reversal. This would result in six intrauterine pregnancies and slightly fewer live births.

their removal and anastomosis, 86% of the animals had intrauterine pregnancies. Scheidel and colleagues[52] performed end-to-end anastomosis on rabbit oviducts using fibrin glue (biologic tissue allogenic fibrinogen) after removal of 1 to 2 cm of isthmus. The substance is a cryoprecipitate of thrombin, factor XIII, and a proteinase inhibitor. Postoperatively, 12 (60%) of 20 rabbits became pregnant. Histologic examination of the sites of anastomosis showed mild to moderate tissue reaction comparable to results with microsutures. Spernol et al.[53] studied a similar group of animals 3 months postoperatively with light and electron microscopy. Morphologic changes showed minimal tissue reaction and absence of fibrin clots, mild inflammatory reaction, and decreased ciliated cells.

McComb and Gomel[54] designed studies to measure the effect of tubal length on fertility in the rabbit. The animals were subjected to microsurgical resection of different lengths of fallopian tube involving the isthmus in each case. Fertility rates were significantly lower following anastomosis of remaining segments only after 40% of the tubes had been removed. In a follow-up study,[55] these investigators attempted to ascertain the influence of ampullary length on infertility. Based on the results of the new studies, these authors suggested that the length of the distal tubal remnant (ampulla) may influence fertility more than the length of the proximal tubal segment.

Hulka and Ulberg[56] applied clips to female pigs, which were then mated for 3 months; none became pregnant. The animals were reexplored, the clips were removed, and end-to-end anastomoses were performed with only three sutures of 4-0 Dexon from the serosa through the lumen. Six of eight animals became pregnant within 2 months after mating. Zipper and co-workers[57] described the use of chemical agents for transvaginal sterilization and noted that quinacrine caused tubal obstruction by inducing epithelial proliferation. Reversal could be obtained through the administration of exogenous ovarian hormones.

Fayez et al.[58] compared the use of a laser and a microelectrode needle for tubal transection and anastomosis. With the use of a laser beam with a focal spot of 1.8 mm, a 400-mm lens, 20 to 25 W power density, 900 W (cm^2) of continuous power, the tubes were cut and the segments were welded together. Compared with conventional techniques with or without microelectrodes, the results in terms of postoperative pregnancy indicated that the laser beam had no place in tubal reconstruction and resection. Eddy[59] reviewed some of the results of planned iatrogenically traumatized rabbit oviducts to evaluate the physiologic role of various tubal segments in fertility. From his analyses it would appear that fertility can be restored in the absence of fimbria or the uterotubal or isthmic-ampullary junctions. It appears that the isthmus is not a prerequisite for fertility, because ampullary cornual anastomosis and ampullary implantation have enabled pregnancy to occur. A critical length of tube is necessary; but more importantly, it is the ampullary segment that must be present. When sufficient lengths of each tube are present in the sterilized patient seeking reversal, a possible option may be the construction of a single functional tube obtained by surgically combining the left and right tubal remnants.[60, 61]

STERILIZATION PROCEDURES DEVISED FOR REVERSIBILITY

IN HUMANS

Temporary methods of sterilization have been described for almost a century, but in few instances were attempts made to reverse the operation. For the most part, the authors expressed optimism that their procedure would give the patient who changed her mind about the sterilization the opportunity to become fertile again. Initial sterilization required a laparotomy, some had unacceptable failure rates, and a second laparotomy was needed.

The first of these operations was described in 1897 by Beuttner,[62] who performed an infundibulectomy with a serosal covering. Heineberg,[63] in 1916, reviewed causes of failed sterilization and referred to several methods of temporary sterilization as described previously by Rissmann,[64] DeTarnowsky,[65] and Holzapfel.[66] In essence, these involved transection of the tubal isthmus and anchoring of the tubal stumps to the posterior uterine wall. Careful tubal transection with a view to a possible later reversal was reported also by Oberli and Rieben[67] and Chang.[68] Although authors described sterilization by means of fimbrial fixation into a new location, few specifically designed the operation as a method of temporary sterilization. Burying of fimbriae often failed as a method of sterilization; fimbriae tended to become adherent to the broad ligament, and the technique for reversal required a major abdominal operation. Peritoneal exclusion procedures of either the ovary or the tube were described by many investigators.

Hysteroscopy has been used as a visual control for the insertion of various plugs and devices into the uterotubal ostium. Brueschke[69] believed that with a steerable hysteroscope the ostium could be plugged and subsequently the devices could be removed. He never attempted the procedure clinically. Sugimoto[70] described a special intratubal contraceptive device made of silicone rubber (1.2 mm in diameter, 10 mm in length) with three notches 1.5 mm apart to prevent slippage. Under hysteroscopic control, these were pushed into the uterotubal orifices of 32 women scheduled for hysterectomy. In three instances the devices were expelled. No clinical trials for efficacy were described. A recent technique of silicone plugs formed in place has been described by many investigators.[31, 71-75] Over 1000 of these operations have been performed and none of the investigators reported voluntary removal of the plugs followed by pregnancy. Houck et al.,[75] in 1983, reported on 415 patients. They stated that plugs were removed from eight women who desired pregnancy. These women did not conceive, and a post-plug-removal hysterosalpingogram in some of them showed proximal tubal obstruction.[76]

Taylor and Hamou[77] recently described a nylon rigid device with opened loops at each end to prevent migration and connected by a flexible midpiece. Traction on the proximal loop would afford easy retrieval. A multicenter trial is under way. Hysteroscopic sterilization remains experimental, and no proof exists at present that removal of plugs or devices placed in the uterotubal orifices will result in tubal patency and enable subsequent normal intrauterine pregnancy.[78] Hosseinian and Morales[79] inserted either performed silicone or polyethylene blocking devices into the uterotubal junctions of 21 baboons, and none of them became pregnant after breeding. Subsequently they removed these plugs from 15 animals, and 8 became pregnant. Short-term clinical trials were then carried out in 33 women scheduled for hysterectomy. Although tubal patency was shown in 20 women after plug removal, 5 of 11 women became pregnant with the devices in situ.

Wood and Leeton[80] used the term "ovariotexy" to describe the procedure of placing the ovary in a plastic sheet and into the posterior leaf of the broad ligament. Six women had the operation, but none requested reversal. Kady and colleagues[81] created tubal hoods from disposable medical gloves and after appropriate preparation applied them around the oviducts of 35 women. Two unplanned pregnancies occurred, but none of the remaining women requested reversal. These authors believed in its high potential for reversibility and attractiveness to persons with a strong bias against sterilization. A less complicated approach was described by Mahgoub,[82] who passed the ovary through a window in the broad ligament. There were no pregnancies among 30 women followed 4 years and one successful reversal. Steptoe[83] inserted plastic rods (1 mm in diameter, 4.6 cm in length) during laparoscopy into the fimbriated ends of the tube of 50 women. These rods had protuberances, and they were held in place by tantalum clips. Two unplanned pregnancies occurred, one ectopic, but none of the women apparently requested removal of the rods to regain fertility. These procedures are summarized in Table 4.

IN ANIMALS

Hefnawi and co-workers[98] inserted silicone elastomeres into 64 rabbit tubes, but 20% of the animals became pregnant with the plugs in situ. In eight rabbits the plugs were removed and pregnancy resulted. Laufe and colleagues[99] applied silicone rubber fimbrial caps to 20 monkeys, and 5 retained the devices for 14 months and then had them removed. These animals became pregnant. However, in 14 instances unilateral or bilateral hood displacement occurred, resulting in seven unplanned pregnancies. Heesch and Hodgson[100] introduced plastic spheres 1.2 to 1.3 mm in diameter into the ampullae of rabbit oviducts. Some of these beads were impregnated with steroids and chemicals to cause alterations in ovum development and transport. Although the beads remained in the 28 rabbits, 21 of them became pregnant. Meeker[101] sutured Teflon plugs into the fimbrial ostia of rabbits and baboons. These devices completely protected 42 monkeys from pregnancy, and 3 of the 9 rabbits conceived following removal of plugs, which had been in place for 12 weeks.

If reversible sterilization is developed, it must be viewed as temporary contraception. The importance of reversibility and the acceptance of sterilization have not been definitely ascertained.

Table 4. *Sterilization Procedures Devised for Reversibility in Women*

Year	Author	Technique
1897	Beuttner[62]	Infundibulectomy with serosal covering
1905	Rissmann[64]	Cornual wedge resection, tube left intact
1911	Pana[84]	Peritoneal exclusion of ovary
1913	Selheim[85]	Extraperitonealization of fimbria into broad ligament
1913	DeTarnowsky[65]	Distal stumps anchored into subserosal canal on posterior wall
1913	Holzapfel[66]	Tubal transection 2 cm from the uterus and distal ends placed into broad ligament
1915	Stoeckel[86]	Three-fourths of tube placed into rectus fascia and abdominal muscle
1917	Nürnberger[87]	Tube placed in inguinal canal between abdominal muscles and fascia
1919	Turenne[88]	Fimbriated end placed into posterior leaf of broad ligament
1921	Hellendall[89]	Subcutaneous extraperitonealization of tubes
1921	Wessel[90]	Extraperitonealization of ovaries into inguinal canal
1923	Freund[91]	Submucosal extraperitonealization of tubes into anterior vaginal wall
1934	Aldridge[92]	Extraperitonealization of distal ends of tubes into broad ligament
1967	Skouvaklis[93]	Resection of small intramural-isthmic segment
1969	Wood and Leeton[80]	Ovariotexy with ovaries placed into Silastic bags and then into broad ligament
1971	Oberli and Rieben[67]	Resection of small intramural isthmic tubal segment
1976	Brueschke[69]	Hysteroscopic placement of reversible occlusive devices
1976	Camelo et al.[94]	Ovariotexy
1976	Koschnick and Magnus[95]	Vaginal application of plastic clips
1976	Brun and Ducarme[96]	Ovariotexy
1978	Mahgoub[82]	Extraperitoneal anterior transposition of ovaries below round ligaments
1978	Sugimoto[70]	Intratubal contraceptive
1981	Steptoe[83]	Intratubal devices placed by laparoscope
1981	Chang[68]	Transection of tubes, cauterization of transected ends
1982	Tierzi and Zanno[97]	Salpingodeviation, fimbriated ends placed into broad ligament
1983	Taylor and Hamou[77]	Hysteroscopic placement of occlusive device
1983	Reed and Erb[74]	Hysteroscopic occlusive blocking device

The concept of reversibility might enhance the popularity and acceptability of sterilization, helping to eliminate some religious and cultural objections.[26] Nevertheless, the thrust and wisdom of developing reversible methods of sterilization are questionable for several reasons[102]: (1) a large disparity exists between the number of sterilizations performed and requests for reversal; (2) in developing countries the current demand for permanent sterilization exceeds the capacity to deliver these services; (3) the enrollment of women into an experimental program designed to test the efficacy of a reversible method is ethically unfeasible.

Despite these problems, the interest in reversibility remains strong.[103] In 1979 results of a survey of 147 patients of reproductive age suggested that the number of women intending to be sterilized at some future time would more than double if reversal could be 95% effective and comparable in cost to current sterilization procedures.[104] While the goal of a 95% reversible sterilization is not realistic for the near future, the survey showed that reversibility might affect demands for female sterilization.

COMMENTS

Since SR is available and often successful, what should the patient be told before sterilization? This dilemma is best resolved by advising her that sterilization is permanent if no further tubal surgery is performed. Reversal is possible, but it involves a major operation and it is expensive. The decision to undergo sterilization should be made on the basis of acceptance of the procedure as permanent after the above information is understood. SR remains a delicate, expensive procedure with an uncertain outcome that is performed on relatively few sterilized women. It offers an option for patients who have had an unanticipated event in their lives and desire to become a candidate for motherhood again.

Although the demand for reversal remains low, probably $< 1\%$, effective handling of the few requests is important. Large family planning programs providing sterilization should have the backup of skilled surgeons capable of reversing the procedure. The cost of providing such a service would be more than offset by the savings through preventing unwanted pregnancies. These centers should have trained medical personnel, specialized equipment, infertility workup capacity, appropriate surgical volume (experience), a microsurgical laboratory, and relevant research facilities.

REFERENCES

1. Ory HW, Forrest OJ, Lincoln R: Making choices: evaluating the health risks and benefits of birth control methods. New York, The Alan Guttmacher Institute, 1983
2. Center for Disease Control: Surgical Sterilization Surveillance, Tubal Sterilization Summary 1970-1975. Atlanta, Georgia, July, 1979
3. Gomel V: Profile of women requesting reversal of sterilization. Fertil Steril 30:39, 1978
4. Henderson SR: The reversibility of female sterilization with the use of microsurgery: a report of 102 patients with more than one year follow-up. Am J Obstet Gynecol 149:57, 1984
5. Schlösser HW, Frantzen C, Mansour N, Verhoeven HC: Sterilisation Refertilisierung. Erfahrungen und Ergebnisse bei 119 mikrochirurgisch refertilisierten Frauen. Geburtshilfe Frauenheilkd 43:213, 1983
6. Thompson P, Templeton A: Characteristics of patients requesting reversal of sterilization. Br J Obstet Gynaecol 85:161, 1978
7. Winston RML: Why 103 women asked for reversal of sterilization. Br Med J 2:305, 1977
8. Phillips JM, Hulka JF, Hulka B, Keith L, Keith D: American Association of Gynecologic Laparoscopists 1976 membership survey. J Reprod Med 21:3, 1978
9. Divers WA Jr: Characteristics of women requesting reversal of sterilization. Fertil Steril 41:233, 1984
10. Schwyhart WR, Kutner SJ: A reanalysis of female reaction to contraceptive sterilization. J Nerv Ment Dis 156:354, 1973
11. Lambers KJ, Trimbos-Kemper T, van Hall EV: Regret after sterilization. In New Trends in Female Sterilization, Edited by DAF Lith. Chicago, Yearbook Medical Publishers, 1983, p 179
12. Leader A, Galan N, George R, Taylor PJ: A comparison of definable traits in women requesting reversal of sterilization and women satisfied with sterilization. Am J Obstet Gynecol 145:198, 1983
13. Antoine JM, Tournaire M, Lerat H: Les demandes de déstèrilization tubaire. Enquetê du collége national des gynécologiques et obstetriciens français. J Gynecol Obstet Biol Reprod (Paris) 12:583, 1983
14. Phillips JM, Hulka JF, Peterson HB: American Association of Gynecologic Laparoscopists 1982 membership survey. J Reprod Med 29:592, 1984
15. Phillips JM, Hulka JF, Hulka B, Corson SL: 1979 American Association of Gynecologic Laparoscopists membership survey. J Reprod Med 26:529, 1981
16. Cantor B, Riggall FC: The choice of sterilizing procedure according to its potential reversibility with microsurgery. Fertil Steril 31:9, 1979
17. Berger GS: Reversal of female sterilization: an evaluation of results. In Microsurgery in Gynecology, Edited by JM Phillips. Downey, American Association of Gynecologic Laparoscopists, 1977, p 238
18. Silber SJ, Cohen R: Microsurgical reversal of female sterilization: the role of tubal length. Fertil Steril 33:598, 1980
19. Gomel V: Microsurgery In Female Infertility. Boston, Little, Brown & Co., 1983, p 240
20. Winston RML: Microsurgery of the fallopian tube: from fantasy to reality. Fertil Steril 34:521, 1980
21. Vasquez G, Winston RML, Boeckx W, Brosens I: Tubal lesions subsequent to sterilization and their relation to fertility after attempts at reversal. Am J Obstet Gynecol 138:86, 1980
22. Castracane VD, Moore GT, Shaikh AA: Ovarian function in hysterectomized *Macaca fascicularis*. Biol Reprod 20:462, 1979
23. Corson SL, Levinson CJ, Batzer FR, Otis C: Hormonal levels following sterilization and hysterectomy. J Reprod Med 26:363, 1981
24. Donnez J, Wauters M, Thomas K: Luteal function after tubal sterilization. Obstet Gynecol 57:65, 1981
25. Radwanska E, Berger GS, Hammond J: Luteal deficiency among women with normal menstrual cycles, requesting reversal of tubal sterilization. Obstet Gynecol 54:182, 1979
26. Henry A, Rinehart W, Piotrow PT: Reversing female sterilization. Popul Rep [C] 8(5):98, 1980
27. McCormick WG, Torres J, McCanne LR: Tubal reanastomosis: an update. Fertil Steril 31:689, 1979
28. Rock JA, Bergquist CA, Zacur HA, Parmley TH, Guzick DS, Jones HW Jr: Tubal anastomosis following unipolar cautery. Fertil Steril 37:613, 1982
29. Siegler AM: Replacement, repair, and removal of fallopian tubes. Fertil Steril 37:611, 1982
30. Taylor PJ, Leader A: Reversal of female sterilization. How reliable is the previous operative report? J Reprod Med 27:246, 1982
31. Cooper JM, Houck RM, Rigberg HS: The incidence of intrauterine abnormalities found on hysteroscopy in patients undergoing elective hysteroscopic sterilization. J Reprod Med 28:659, 1983
32. Siegler AM: Tubal plastic surgery; the past, the present and the future. Obstet Gynecol Surv 15:680, 1960
33. Pearl R, Surface FM: Resection and end-to-end anastomosis of the oviduct in the hen without loss of function. Am J Physiol 22:357, 1908
34. Christian SL, Sanderson EL: A new method of anastomosing the ovarian tube or vas deferens. JAMA 61:2157, 1913
35. Donnez J, Casanas-Roux F, Ferin J, Thomas K: Tubal polyps, epithelial inclusions, and endometriosis after tubal sterilization. Fertil Steril 41:564, 1984
36. Williams EA: Results of reversal of female sterilization. In Reversibility of Female Sterilization, Edited by I Brosens, RML Winston. London, Academic Press, 1978, p 89
37. Peterson EP, Musich JR, Behrman SJ: Uterotubal implantation and obstetric outcome after previous sterilization. Am J Obstet Gynecol 128:662, 1977
38. Betz G, Engel T, Penney LL: Tuboplasty—comparison of the methodology. Fertil Steril 34:534, 1980
39. Novy MJ: Reversal of Kroener fimbriectomy sterilization. Am J Obstet Gynecol 137:198, 1980
40. DeCherney AH, Mezer HC, Naftolin F: Analysis of failure of microsurgical anastomosis after midsegment, noncoagulation tubal ligation. Fertil Steril 39:618, 1983
41. Gomel V: Microsurgical reversal of female sterilization: a reappraisal. Fertil Steril 33:587, 1980
42. Siegler AM, Perez RJ: Reconstruction of fallopian tubes in previously sterilized patients. Fertil Steril 26:383, 1975
43. Diamond MP, Christianson CD, Daniell JF: Microsurgical reanastomosis of the fallopian tube: increasingly suc-

cessful outcome for reversal of previous sterilization procedures. South Med J 75:443, 1982
44. Gantt PA, Hill JA, McDonough PG: Reversal of female sterilization. South Med J 75:161, 1982
45. Grunert GM, Drake TS, Takaki NK: Microsurgical reanastomosis of the fallopian tubes for reversal of sterilization. Obstet Gynecol 58:148, 1981
46. Wittich AC: Microsurgical tubal reanastomosis in a community hospital: report of a three-year study. J Am Osteopath Assoc 82:695, 1983
47. Hulka JF, Noble AD, Letchworth AT, Lieberman B, Owen E, Gomel V, Taft RC, Haney AF, Wheeless CR, Imrie AH, Winston RML, Loeffler FE: Reversibility of clip sterilization. Lancet 2:927, 1982
48. Pill CF, Noble AD, Letchworth AT: Reversal of female sterilization. Br J Obstet Gynaecol 88:314, 1981
49. Seiler JC: Factors influencing the outcome of microsurgical tubal ligation reversals. Am J Obstet Gynecol 146:292, 1983
50. Shortle B, Jewelewicz R: Uterine rupture following tubal implantation: review of the literature and report of 3 additional cases. Obstet Gynecol Surv 38:407, 1984
51. Boeckx WD, Vasquez G, Brosens IA: Reversibility of tubal ring sterilization. Contraception 15:505, 1977
52. Scheidel PH, Wallwiener D, Wiedemann RA, Hepp HK: Experimental anastomosis of the rabbit fallopian tube using fibrin glue. Fertil Steril 38:471, 1982
53. Spernol R, Riss P, Schindler K, Beck A, Breitenecker G: Morphology of rabbit oviduct after reanastomosis with fibrin glue. Int J Gynaecol Obstet 22:295, 1984
54. McComb P, Gomel V: The influence of fallopian tube length on fertility in the rabbit. Fertil Steril 31:673, 1979
55. McComb P, Gomel V: The influence of fallopian tube ampullary length on the fertility of the rabbit. Int J Fertil 26:30, 1981
56. Hulka JF, Ulberg LC: Reversibility of clip sterilization. Fertil Steril 26:1132, 1975
57. Zipper J, Medel M, Stachetti E, Pastene L, Rivera M, Prager R: Chemical agents for transvaginal sterilization. In Human Sterilization, Edited by RM Richart, DJ Prager. Springfield, Charles C. Thomas, 1972, p 339
58. Fayez JA, McComb JS, Harper MA: Comparison of tubal surgery with the CO_2 laser and the unipolar microelectrode. Fertil Steril 40:476, 1983
59. Eddy CA: Tubal physiology and microsurgery. Aust NZ J Obstet Gynaecol 21:129, 1981
60. Haney AF: Utilization of contralateral fallopian tube segments in tubal reanastomosis. Fertil Steril 37:701, 1982
61. Shapiro SS, Haning RV Jr: Tubal anastomosis of a fimbrial segment pedicle graft. Fertil Steril 32:478, 1979
62. Beuttner O: Sterilisation mittels Tubendurchschneidung nach Laparotomie. Zentralbl Gynakol 21:1227, 1897
63. Heineberg A: Tubal sterilization: pregnancy following bilateral salpingectomy: a report of two cases and a complete review of the literature. NY Med J 104:107, 1916
64. Rissmann P: Die Methoden zur Herbeiführung der weiblichen Sterilität. Zentralbl Gynakol 19:116, 1905
65. DeTarnowsky G: Tubal reimplantation: a new conservative operation for sterilization in women. JAMA 60: 1221, 1913
66. Holzapfel O: Zur Technik der tubaren Sterilisierung. Geburtshilfe Gynakol 74:189, 1913
67. Oberli H, Rieben G: Tubensterilisation, Versagerquote und Moglichkeit der operativen Refertilisierung. Schweiz Med Wochenschr 101:1699, 1971
68. Chang MCE: Abdominal sterilization. In Abortion and Sterilization, Edited by JE Hodgson. New York, Academic Press, 1981, p 398
69. Brueschke EE: Reversible occlusive devices. J Reprod Med 17:103, 1976
70. Sugimoto O: Diagnostic and Therapeutic Hysteroscopy. Igaku-Shoin, Tokyo, 1978, p 208
71. Houck RM, Cooper JM: Hysteroscopic tubal occlusion with formed-in-place silicone plugs. Obstet Gynecol 60: 641, 1982
72. Loffer FD: Hysteroscopic sterilization with the use of formed-in-place silicone plugs. Am J Obstet Gynecol 149:261, 1984
73. Reed TP III: Formed-in-place silicone plugs: improvements and limitations. In Transcervical Sterilization, Edited by GI Zatuchni, JD Shelton, A Goldsmith, JJ Sciarra. Hagerstown, Harper & Row, 1982, p 220
74. Reed TP III, Erb R: Hysteroscopic tubal occlusion with silicone rubber. Obstet Gynecol 61:388, 1983
75. Houck RM, Cooper JM, Rigberg HS: Hysteroscopic tubal occlusion with formed-in-place silicone plugs: a clinical review. Obstet Gynecol 62:587, 1983
76. Cooper J: Personal communication, 1984
77. Taylor PJ, Hamou JE: Hysteroscopy. J Reprod Med 28: 389, 1983
78. Craft I: Intra-uterine sterilization. In Reversibility of Female Sterilization, Edited by I Brosens, R Winston. London, Academic Press, 1978, p 153
79. Hosseinian AH, Morales WA: Clinical application of hysteroscopic sterilization using uterotubal junction blocking devices. In Proceedings of the International Workshop on Nonsurgical Methods for Tubal Occlusion, Edited by GI Zatuchni, JB Shelton, A Goldsmith. Hagerstown, Harper & Row, 1982, p 234
80. Wood EC, Leeton J: Sterilization by ovariotexy: a reversible technique. Lancet 2:1213, 1969
81. Kady AA, Sami G, Laurence KA: The tubal hood: a potentially reversible sterilization technique. In Reversal of Sterilization, Edited by JJ Sciarra, GI Zatuchni, JJ Speidel. Hagerstown, Harper & Row, 1978, p 232
82. Mahgoub S: Mahgoub's operation: a reversible method of sterilization. Fertil Steril 29:466, 1978
83. Steptoe PC: Endoscopic sterilization. In Abortion and Sterilization: Medical and Social Aspects, Edited by JE Hodgson. New York, Academic Press, 1981, p 439
84. Pana M: Contributo anatomo-patologico alla studio dell'esclusione ovarica della cavita abdominale. Ann di Ostet 33:341, 1911
85. Selheim O: Schwangershafts Unterbrechung und Sterilisation in einer Sitzung auf abdominalem Wege. Monatsschr Geburtshilfe Gynakol 38:166, 1913
86. Stoeckel W: Die extraperitoneale Tubenverlagerung als Methode der Sterilisierung. Zentralbl Gynakol 39:161, 1915
87. Nürnberger L: Die sterilisierenden Opertionen an den Tuben und ihre Fehlschläge. Leipzig, J. A. Barth, 1917
88. Turenne A: Temporary sterilization of the female. Surg Gynecol Obstet 29:577, 1919
89. Hellendall H: Eine neue Methode zur temporären Sterilisierung. Zentralbl Gynakol 45:822, 1921

90. Wessel O: Eine neue Methode der zeitweiligen Sterilisation der Frau auf operativem Wege. Zentralbl Gynakol 42:75, 1921
91. Freund H: Die temporäre Sterilisation. Geburtshilfe Gynakol 47:277, 1923
92. Aldridge A: Temporary sterilization with subsequent pregnancy. Am J Obstet Gynecol 27:741, 1934
93. Skouvaklis M: Sterilisation tubaire interstitielle selon Skouvaklis. Bull Fed Gynécol Obstet Franç 19:5, 1967
94. Camelo AA, Garcia J, Neto A: A practical method for reversible sterilization in women. Excerpta Medica 370: 229, 1976
95. Koschnick KF, Magnus J: Zur ambulaten vaginalen Tubensterilisation mit dem Kunstoffclip unter besonderer Berücksichtigung der Reversibilität. Zentralbl Gynakol 98:1518, 1976
96. Brun G, Ducarme AM: L'ovaire après ovariotexie. J Gynecol Obstet Biol Reprod (Paris) 5:957, 1976
97. Tierzi I, Zanno C: Un metodo originale di sterilizzazione chirurica reversible feminile: la salpingodeviazione. Minerva Ginecol 34:797, 1982
98. Hefnawi FF, Fuchs AR, Lawrence KA: Control of fertility by temporary occlusion of the oviduct. Am J Obstet Gynecol 99:421, 1967
99. Laufe LE, Hassler C, Lower BR: A laboratory prototype for reversible female sterilization. In Female Sterilization, Prognosis for Simplified Outpatient Procedures, Edited by GW Duncan, RD Falb, JJ Speidel. New York, Academic Press, 1972, p 65
100. Heesch CM, Hodgson BJ: Medicated intratubal Silastic spheres do not prevent pregnancy in rabbits. Contraception 13:497, 1976
101. Meeker CI: A tubal occlusive device in monkeys. In Reversal of Sterilization, Edited by JJ Sciarra, GI Zatuchni, JJ Speidel. Hagerstown, Harper & Row, 1978, p 226
102. Freedman B, Taylor PJ: Government funding for surgical reversal of voluntary female sterilization: ethical points of reference. J Reprod Med 27:339, 1982
103. Sciarra JJ Jr: Sterilization in women: a review of new and potentially reversible techniques. In Advances in Voluntary Sterilization, Edited by ME Schima, I Lubell, JE Davis, E Connell. New York, American Elsevier Publishing Co., Inc., 1974, p 62
104. Shain RN: Acceptability of reversible versus permanent tubal sterilization: an analysis of preliminary data. Fertil Steril 31:13, 1979

Index

B

C

I

Q

R

S

T